369 0166675

Medical Management of the Surgical Patient

This comprehensive textbook, now fully revised, rewritten and updated in its fourth edition, provides an authoritative account of all aspects of perioperative care for surgical patients. All areas of medical disease are discussed with clear recommendations for work up and management in the perioperative period. Basic discussion of surgical procedures are included to help non-surgeons understand the procedures and their implications for patient care. This definitive account includes numerous contributions from leading experts at national centers of medical excellence. It will serve as a significant work of reference for internists, anesthesiologists and surgeons.

Medical Management of the Surgical Patient

A Textbook of Perioperative Medicine

Fourth Edition

Edited by

Michael F. Lubin

Editor-in-Chief

Robert B. Smith III

Thomas F. Dodson

Nathan O. Spell

H. Kenneth Walke

Associate Editors

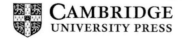

CAMBRIDGE
UNIVERSITY PRESS

CAMBRIDGE UNIVERSITY PRESS
Cambridge, New York, Melbourne, Madrid, Cape Town, Singapore,
São Paulo, Delhi, Dubai, Tokyo

Cambridge University Press
The Edinburgh Building, Cambridge CB2 8RU, UK

Published in the United States of America by Cambridge University Press, New York

www.cambridge.org
Information on this title: www.cambridge.org/9780521180115

First published by Butterworth 1982
Second edition 1988
Third edition published by Lippincott 1995
Fourth edition published by Cambridge University Press 2006
Reprinted 2007
First Paperback Edition 2010

Printed in the United Kingdom at the University Press, Cambridge

A catalog record for this publication is available from the British Library

ISBN-978-0-521-82800-0 Hardback
ISBN-978-0-521-18011-5 Paperback

Cambridge University Press has no responsibility for the persistence or accuracy of URLs for external or third-party internet websites referred to in this book, and does not guarantee that any content on such websites is, or will remain, accurate or appropriate.

Every effort has been made in preparing this publication to provide accurate and up-to-date information which is in accord with accepted standards and practice at the time of publication. Although case histories are drawn from actual cases, every effort has been made to disguise the identities of the individuals involved. Nevertheless, the authors, editors and publishers can make no warranties that the information contained herein is totally free from error, not least because clinical standards are constantly changing through research and regulation. The authors, editors and publishers therefore disclaim all liability for direct or consequential damages resulting from the use of material contained in this book. Readers are strongly advised to pay careful attention to information provided by the manufacturer of any drugs or equipment that they plan to use.

Contents

Editor biographies

Michael F. Lubin

Michael Lubin is the Professor of Medicine at the Emory University School of Medicine, Atlanta, USA. He is a fellow of the American College of Physicians. He is also a Fellow and on the Board of Directors at Phi Beta Kappa Society. He has been the co-editor of three volumes of the *Medical Clinics of North America, on Perioperative Care.*

Henry Kenneth Walker

H. Kenneth Walker is Professor of Medicine at the Emory University School of Medicine. He is on the Board of the National Library of Medicine, USA. In 2000, he was awarded the Best Internal Medicine Professor, Emory University School of Medicine.

Robert B. Smith III

Currently holds the position of John E. Skandalakis, Professor of Surgery Emeritus and Associate Chairman of the Department of Surgery, Emory University School of Medicine, Atlanta, USA. His bibliography includes 219 scientific articles and book chapters and he has coedited five textbooks. His clinical interests have been primarily focused in portal hypertension, and more recently in the surgical treatment of disorders of the carotid artery and the abdominal aorta.

Thomas F. Dodson

Thomas F. Dodson is currently Professor of Surgery and Vice Chairman for Education, Department of Surgery, alongside being the Director of General Surgery Residency at Emory University School of Medicine, Atlanta, USA. He joined the faculty of the Department of Surgery at Emory in the Division of Vascular Surgery in 1988.

Nathan O. Spell III

Nathan O. Spell is currently Emory Clinic Physician as well as being an Assistant Professor of General Internal Medicine at Emory University School of Medicine. He is a member of the American College of Physicians and the Society of General Internal Medicine.

List of contributors

Thomas M. Aaberg Sr., M.D.
F. Phinizy Calhoun Sr.
Professor of Ophthalmology and Chairman
Department of Ophthalmology
Emory University School of Medicine
Atlanta, GA

The Emory Clinic
Room B4404
1365 Clifton Road NE
Atlanta, GA

John Affronti, M.D.
Associate Professor
Department of Digestive Diseases
Emory Clinic – Building A
Atlanta, GA

Joseph D. Ansley, M.D. (retired)
Associate Professor of Surgery
Emory University School of Medicine
Atlanta, GA

Ahsan M. Arozullah, M.D., M.P.H.
Research & Development (151 WS),
Room 6200
Jesse Brown VA Medical Center
820 S. Damen Avenue
Chicago, IL 60612

Daniel L. Barrow, M.D.
MBNA Bowman Professor of Neurosurgery and Chairman
Department of Neurosurgery
Emory University School of Medicine
Atlanta, GA

Jack Basil, M.D.
Assistant Professor of Gynecology and Obstetrics
Emory University School of Medicine
Atlanta, GA

The Emory Clinic
1365 Clifton Road NE
Atlanta, GA 30322

Brian W. Behm, M.D.
University of Virginia HSC
Fellow, Division of Gastroenterology
P.O. Box 800708
Charlottesville, VA 22908

Rafael Bouet Blasini, M.D.
Resident in Urology
Emory University School of Medicine
Atlanta, GA

The Emory Clinic, Building B
1365 Clifton Road NE
Atlanta, GA 30322

Maxwell Boakye, M.D.
Spine Fellow and Instructor
Department of Neurosurgery
Emory University School of Medicine
Atlanta, GA

Atlanta Brain and Spine
2001 Peachtree Road, NE, Suite 645
Atlanta, GA 30309

Duncan Borland, D.O.
0305 SW Montgomery Street
F304
Portland, OR 97201

Jason M. Budde, M.D.
Resident in Cardiothoracic Surgery
Emory University School of Medicine
Atlanta, GA

The Emory Clinic, Building A
1365 Clifton Road NE
Atlanta, GA 30322

Lisa K. Cannada, M.D.
Assistant Professor Orthopedic Surgery
Emory University School of Medicine
Atlanta, GA

Department of Orthopedic Surgery
49 Jesse Hill Jr. Drive SE, Room 301
Atlanta, GA 30303

C. Michael Cawley, M.D.
Assistant Professor of Neurosurgery
Emory University School of Medicine
Atlanta, GA

The Emory Clinic, Building B
1365 Clifton Road NE, Room 6510
Atlanta, GA 30322

Elliot L. Chaikof, M.D., Ph.D.
John E. Skandalakis Professor of Surgery and
Chief Division of Vascular Surgery
Emory University School of Medicine
Atlanta, GA

Woodruff Memorial Building
101 Woodruff Circle, Room 5105
Atlanta, GA 30322

Amy Y. Chen, M.D., M.P.H.
Assistant Professor of Otolaryngology
Emory University School of Medicine
Atlanta, GA

The Emory Clinic, Building A
1365 Clifton Road NE, Room 2315
Atlanta, GA 30322

Stuart H. Cohen
Professor of Medicine
University of California, Davis
4150 V Street
Sacramento, CA 95817

Michelle V. Conde, M.D.
Audie Murphy Division
South Texas Veterans Health Care System
7400 Merton Minter Blvd 11C6
San Antonio, TX 78229-5700

Doyt L. Conn, M.D.
Professor of Medicine
Director, Rheumatology Division
Emory University School of Medicine
49 Jesse Hill Jr. Drive
Atlanta, GA 30303

William A. Cooper, M.D.
Assistant Professor of Cardiothoracic Surgery
Emory University School of Medicine
Atlanta, GA

Medical Office Tower
Emory Crawford Long Hospital
550 Peachtree Street, NE
Atlanta, GA 30308

Anastasios P. Costarides, M.D., Ph.D.
Assistant Professor of Ophthalmology
Emory University School of Medicine
Atlanta, GA

The Emory Clinic, Eye Center
1365 Clifton Road NE, 3rd floor
Atlanta, GA 30322

William A. Cooper, M.D.
Assistant Professor of Cardiothoracic Surgery
Emory University School of Medicine
Atlanta, GA

Medical Office Tower
Emory Crawford Long Hospital
550 Peachtree Street, NE
Atlanta, GA 30308

John M. DelGaudio, M.D.
Assistant Professor of Otolaryngology
Emory University School of Medicine
The Emory Clinic, Building A
1365 Clifton Road NE, Room 1213
Atlanta, GA 30322

Thomas F. Dodson, M.D.
Professor of Surgery
Emory University School of Medicine
Program Director
General Surgery Residency
Atlanta, GA

The Emory Clinic, Building A
1365 Clifton Road NE, Room 3316
Atlanta, GA 30322

Burl R. Don, M.D.
Division of Nephrology
University of California Davis Medical Center
4150 V Street, Suite 3500
Sacramento, CA 95817

James R. Eckman, M.D.
Professor Hematology/Oncology and Internal Medicine
Winship Cancer Institute
Department of Hematology and Oncology
Emory University School of Medicine
49 Jesse Hill Jr. Drive
Atlanta, GA 30303

David V. Feliciano, M.D.
Professor of Surgery
Emory University School of Medicine
Chief of Surgery
Grady Memorial Hospital
Atlanta, GA

Grady Memorial Hospital
Glenn Building
69 Jesse Hill Jr. Drive SE
Atlanta, GA 30303

Lamar L. Fleming, M.D.
Professor of Orthopedic Surgery
Emory University School of Medicine
Atlanta, GA 30329

Michael L. Frankel, M.D.
Professor Neurology
Emory University School of Medicine
Chief of Neurology
Grady Memorial Hospital
Box 036 – 11th floor, C-wing
80 Jesse Hill Jr. Drive
Atlanta, GA 30303

Niall T. M. Galloway, M.D.
Associate Professor of Urology
Emory University School of Medicine
Medical Director
The Emory Continence Center
Atlanta, GA

The Emory Clinic, Building A
1365 Clifton Road NE, Room 3219
Atlanta, GA 30322

Enrique Garcia-Valenzuela, M.D., Ph.D.
Assistant Professor of Ophthalmology
Emory University School of Medicine
Chief of the Retina Service, VAMC
Atlanta, GA

The Emory Clinic, Building B
1365 Clifton Road NE
Atlanta, GA 30322

Ashley D. Gordon, M.D.
Resident in Plastic Surgery
Emory University School of Medicine
Atlanta, GA

Paces Plastic Surgery
3200 Downwood Circle
The Palisades, Suite 640
Atlanta, GA 30327

Joshua A. Greenwald, M.D.
Resident in Plastic Surgery
Emory University School of Medicine
Atlanta, GA

Paces Plastic Surgery
3200 Downwood Circle
The Palisades, Suite 640
Atlanta, GA 30327

William J. Grist, M.D.
Associate Professor of Otolaryngology
Emory University School of Medicine
Atlanta, GA

The Emory Clinic, Building A
1365 Clifton Road NE, Room 2317
Atlanta, GA 30322

Robert E. Gross, M.D.
Assistant Professor of Neurosurgery
Emory University School of Medicine
Atlanta, GA

The Emory Clinic, Building B
1365 Clifton Road NE, Room 6508
Atlanta, GA 30322

Regis W. Haid Jr., M.D.
Atlanta Brain and Spine Care
2001 Peachtree Road, NE, Suite 645
Atlanta, GA 30309

Mark Hanna, M.D.
Resident in Orthopedic Surgery
Emory University School of Medicine
Atlanta, GA

Emory Orthopedic Center
59 Executive Park South
Atlanta, GA 30329

Robert M. Harris, M.D.
Assistant Professor of Orthopedic Surgery
Emory University School of Medicine
2928 Habersham Road
Atlanta, GA 30305

Tommie Haywood, M.D.
Division of Digestive Diseases
Emory Clinic A
Atlanta, GA 30322

John G. Heller, M.D.
Professor of Orthopedic Surgery
Emory University School of Medicine
Emory Orthopedic Center
59 Executive Park South
Atlanta, GA 30329

T. Roderick Hester, M.D.
Assistant Professor of Surgery and Chief
Division of Plastic and Reconstructive Surgery
Emory University School of Medicine
Atlanta, GA

Paces Plastic Surgery
3200 Downwood Circle
The Palisades, Suite 640
Atlanta, GA 30327

Christopher D. Hillyer, M.D.
Professor of Pathology
Emory University Transfusion Medicine
1364 Clifton Road, NE, Room D-655
Atlanta, GA 30322

Krista L. Hillyer, M.D.
Chief Medical Officer
American Red Cross Blood Services
Southern Region
1925 Monroe Drive NE
Atlanta, GA 30324

Assistant Professor
Department Pathology and Laboratory Medicine
Emory University School of Medicine
1364 Clifton Road NE
Atlanta, GA 30322

Eric G. Honig, M.D.
Professor of Medicine
Division of Pulmonary Medicine,
Critical Care & Allergy

Emory University School of Medicine
49 Jesse Hill Jr. Drive
Atlanta, GA 30303

Ira R. Horowitz, M.D.
Willafor Ransom Leach
Professor of Gynecology and Obstetrics
Emory University School of Medicine
Vice Chairman, Dept of Gynecology and Obstetrics
Director, Division of Gynecology and Oncology
The Emory Clinic, 1365 Clifton Road NE
Atlanta, GA 30322

William C. Horton, M.D.
Associate Professor of Orthopedic Surgery
Emory University School of Medicine
Emory Orthopedic Center
59 Executive Park South
Atlanta, GA 30329

G. Baker Hubbard III, M.D.
Assistant Professor of Ophthalmology
Emory University School of Medicine
Director of Retain Fellowship
The Emory Clinic, Building B
1365 Clifton Road NE, Room 3403
Atlanta, GA 30322

Carl C. Hug Jr., M.D., Ph.D.
Professor of Anesthesiology, Emeritus
1873 Kanawha Drive
Stone Mountain, GA 30087-2126

Amy K. Hutchinson, M.D.
Associate Professor of Ophthalmology
Emory University School of Medicine
Atlanta, GA

The Emory Clinic, Building B
1365 Clifton Road NE, Room 4514
Atlanta, GA

Muta M. Issa, M.D.
Associate Professor of Urology
Emory University School of Medicine
Chief of Urology, VAMC
1670 Clairmont Road
Decatur, GA 30033

Michele M. Johnson, M.D.
Resident in Neurosurgery
Emory University School of Medicine
The Emory Clinic, Room B6501
1365 Clifton Road NE
Atlanta, GA 30322

Cassandra D. Josephson, M.D.
Assistant Director
CHOA Blood Banks and Transfusion Services
Assistant Professor
Pathology and Pediatrics
Emory University School of Medicine
1364 Clifton Road NE
Atlanta, GA 30322

Jorge Juncos, M.D.
Associate Professor
Wesley Woods Health Center
Atlanta, GA

Karthikeshwar Kasirajan, M.D.
Assistant Professor of Surgery
Emory University School of Medicine
Emory University Hospital
Room H122
1364 Clifton Road NE
Atlanta, GA 30322

Craig R. Keenan, M.D.
Assistant Professor
University of California, Davis Med. Center
4150 V Street, PSSB Suite 2400
Sacramento, CA 95817

Joe T. Kelley, III, M.D.
943 Beneva Road, Suite 302
Sarasota, FL 34232

Jaffar Khan, M.D.
Assistant Professor of Neurology
Emory University School of Medicine
292 Riverford Way
Lawrenceville, GA 30043

Kathleen Kinlaw, M.Div.
Associate Director
Emory University
Center for Ethics – Dental Bldg., 302
1462 Clifton Road, Suite 302
Atlanta, GA 30322

John G. Kral, M.D., Ph.D.
Professor of Surgery and Medicine
SUNY Downstate Medical Center
Department of Surgery, Box 40
450 Clarkson Avenue
Brooklyn, NY 11203-2098

Sameh A. Labib, M.D.
Assistant Professor of Orthopedic Surgery
Emory University School of Medicine
Atlanta, GA

Emory Orthopedic Center
59 Executive Park South
Atlanta, GA 30329

James J. Lah, M.D., Ph.D.
Assistant Professor, Neurology
Director, Emory Cognitive Neurology Program
Chief of Neurology, Wesley Woods Center
Whitehead Biomedical Research Building
615 Michael St., Suite 505
Atlanta, GA 30322

Omar M. Lattouf, M.D.
Assistant Professor of Cardiothoracic Surgery
Emory University School of Medicine
Medical Office Tower
Emory Crawford Long Hospital
559 Peachtree Street, NE
Atlanta, GA 30308

Valerie V. Lawrence, M.D., M.Sc.
Professor, Department of Medicine
UTHSC at San Antonio – General Medicine
VERDICT 11C-6
ALMD/STVHCS
7400 Merton Minter Boulevard
San Antonio, TX 78229-3900

Jeffrey L. Lennox, M.D.
Professor of Medicine
Grady Memorial/Ponce Center
341 Ponce de Leon Ave., NE
Atlanta, GA 30308-2012

Allan I. Levey, M.D., Ph.D.
Professor and Chairman
Department of Neurology
Emory University School of Medicine
Woodruff Memorial Research/bldg.
1639 Pierce Drive, Suite 6000
Atlanta, GA 30322

Bruce D. Levy, M.D.
Assistant Professor of Medicine
Pulmonary and Critical Care Medicine
Brigham & Women's Hospital
75 Francis Street
Boston, MA 02115

Franklin J. Lin, M.D.
Resident in Neurosurgery
Emory University School of Medicine
Atlanta, GA

The Emory Clinic, Room B6501
1365 Clifton Road NE
Atlanta, GA 30322

Michael F. Lubin, M.D.
Professor of Medicine
Emory University School of Medicine
49 Butler Street
Atlanta, GA 30303

Kamal A. Mansour, M.D.
Professor of Cardiothoracic Surgery
Emory University School of Medicine
The Emory Clinic, Building A
1365 Clifton Road NE, Room 2232
Atlanta, GA 309322

Fray F. Marshall, M.D.
Professor of Urology and Chairman
Department of Urology
Emory University School of Medicine
Atlanta, GA

The Emory Clinic, Building B
1365 Clifton Road NE
Atlanta, GA 30322

Enrique J. Martinez, M.D., F.A.C.P.
Associate Professor of Medicine
Associate Medical Director of Adult
Liver Transplant
UM-JMH Liver Program
1500 NW 12th Ave., Suite 1101
Miami, FL 33136

Douglas E. Mattox, M.D.
Professor of Otolaryngology and Chairman
Department of Otolaryngology
Emory University School of Medicine
The Emory Clinic, Building A
1365 Clifton Road NE, Room 2328
Atlanta, GA 30322

Juliet K. Mavromatis, M.D.
Assistant Professor General Medicine
Emory University School of Medicine
1525 Clifton Road
Atlanta, GA 30322

Gary R. McGillivary, M.D.
Assistant Professor of Orthopedic Surgery
Emory University School of Medicine
Emory Orthopedic Center
59 Executive Park South
Atlanta, GA 30329

Geno J. Merli, M.D.
Sr. Associate Dean for Medical
Education
Jefferson Medical College
Philadelphia, PA

Joseph I. Miller Jr., M.D.
Professor of Cardiothoracic Surgery
Emory University School of Medicine
Medical Office Tower
Emory Crawford Long Hospital
550 Peachtree St NE
Atlanta, GA 30308

Charles E. Moore, M.D.
Assistant Professor of Otolaryngology
Emory University School of Medicine
Chief of Otolaryngology Service
Grady Memorial Hospital
80 Jesse Hill Jr. Drive SE
Atlanta, GA 30303

Praveen V. Mummameni, M.D.
Assistant Professor of Neurosurgery
Emory University School of Medicine
Medical Office Tower
Emory Crawford Long Hospital
559 Peachtree ST. NE, 8th floor
Atlanta, GA 30308

Valli P. Mummameni, M.D.
Emory University School of Medicine
Emory Crawford Long Hospital
559 Peachtree St NE
Atlanta, GA 30308

Peter T. Nieh, M.D.
Associate Professor of Urology
Emory University School of Medicine
The Emory Clinic, Building B
1365 Clifton Road NE
Atlanta, GA 30322

Hien H. Nguyen, M.D.
Fellow, I.D. Division
4150 V Street, Suite G500
Sacramento, CA 95918

Edward R. Norris, M.D.
Vice Chair, Education and Research
Department of Psychiatry
Lehigh Valley Hospital & Health Network
1251 S. Cedar Crest Blvd., Suite 202A
Allentown, PA 18103

Jeffrey J. Olson, M.D.
Professor of Neurosurgery
Emory University School of Medicine
The Emory Clinic, Building B
1365 Clifton Road NE, Room 6470
Atlanta, GA 30322

Nelson M. Oyesiku, M.D., Ph.D.
Associate Professor of Neurosurgery
Emory University School of Medicine
The Emory Clinic, Building B
1365 Clifton Road NE, Room 6512
Atlanta, GA 30322

Alfredo A. Paredes Jr., M.D.
Resident in Plastic and Reconstructive Surgery
Emory University School of Medicine
Paces Plastic Surgery
3200 Downwood Circle
The Palisades, Suite 640
Atlanta, GA 30327

Andrew E. Park, M.D.
Fellow in Spine Surgery
Emory University School of Medicine
Emory Orthopaedic Center
59 Executive Park South
Atlanta, GA 30329

Ted Parran Jr., M.D., F.A.C.P.
Associate Clinical Professor of Medicine
Case Western Reserve Univ. SOM,
Room W-175
10900 Euclid Avenue
Cleveland, OH 44106-4922

L. Reuven Pasternak, M.D., M.P.H., M.B.A.
Vice-Dean for Bayview Campus
The Johns Hopkins University School of Medicine
Pavilion 01-1-22
4940 Eastern Avenue
Baltimore, MD 21224-2780

John G. Pattaras, M.D.
Assistant Professor of Urology
Emory University School of Medicine
Atlanta, GA

The Emory Clinic, Building B
1365 Clifton Road NE, Room 6512
Atlanta, GA 30322

Pamela T. Prescott, M.D., M.P.H.
Associate Professor
University of California at Davis
Division of Endocrinology
4150 V Street, PSSB, G400
Sacramento, CA 95758

Tom Prindiville, M.D.
University of California at Davis
Division of Gastroenterology
PSSB – 3500
4150 V Street
Sacramento, CA 95817

John D. Puskas, M.D.
Associate Professor of Cardiothoracic Surgery
Emory University School of Medicine
Medical Office Tower
550 Peachtree Street
Atlanta, GA 30308

Charles L. Raison, M.D.
Assistant Professor of Psychiatry
Dept. of Psychiatry & Behavioral Services
1639 Pierce Drive, Suite 4000
Atlanta, GA 30322

Hugh W. Randall, M.D.
Leach Professor of Gynecology and Obstetrics
Emory University School of Medicine
20 Linden Avenue
Atlanta, GA 30308

Sunil S. Rayan, M.D.
Resident in Vascular Surgery
Emory University School of Medicine
Woodruff Memorial Building
101 Woodruff Circle, Room 5105
Atlanta, GA 30322

V. Seenu Reddy, M.D., M.B.A.
Resident in Cardiothoracic Surgery
Emory University School of Medicine
Atlanta, GA

The Emory Clinic, Building A
1365 Clifton Road NE, Room 2223
Atlanta, GA 30322

Dustin L. Reid, M.D.
Resident in Plastic and Reconstructive Surgery
Emory University School of Medicine
Atlanta, GA

Paces Plastic Surgery
3200 Downwood Circle
The Palisades, Suite 640
Atlanta, GA 30327

John M. Rhee, M.D.
Assistant Professor of Orthopedic Surgery
Emory University School of Medicine
Atlanta, GA

Emory Orthopedic Center
59 Executive Park South
Atlanta, GA 30329

James Roberson, M.D.
Professor of Orthopedic Surgery and Chairman
Department of Orthopedics
Emory University School of Medicine
Atlanta, GA

Emory Orthopedic Center
59 Executive Park South
Atlanta, GA 30329

Eve Rodler, M.D.
Assistant Professor of Medicine
Robert Wood Johnson School of Medicine
3 Cooper Plaza, Suite 220
Camden, NJ 08103

Lorenzo Rossaro
Professor and Chief
Univ. of California Davis Medical Ctr.
Department of Internal Medicine
2315 Stockton Blvd, Housestaff
Facility, 2nd floor
Sacramento, CA 05918

Atef A. Salam, M.D.
Professor of Surgery
Emory University School of Medicine
Atlanta, GA

The Emory Clinic, Building A
1365 Clifton Road NE, Room 3314
Atlanta, GA 30322

Tarek A. Salam, M.D.
Professor of Surgery
Ain Shams Medical School
Cairo, Egypt

The Emory Clinic, Building A
1365 Clifton Road NE, Room 3314
Atlanta, GA 30322

Brett S. Sanders, M.D.
Resident in Orthopedic Surgery
Emory University School of Medicine
Atlanta, GA

Emory Orthopedic Center
59 Executive Park South
Atlanta, GA 30329

Scott L. Schissel, M.D., Ph.D.
Clinical Fellow, Pulmonary & Critical Care Medicine
Brigham and Women's Hospital
Harvard Medical School
45 Francis Street
Boston, MA 02115

Brennan A. Scott, M.D.
Gastroenterologist
Palo Alto Medical Foundation
795 EI Camino Real
Palo Alto, CA 94301

Daniel L. Serna, M.D.
Resident in Cardiothoracic Surgery
Emory University School of Medicine
Atlanta, GA

The Emory Clinic, Building A
1365 Clifton Road NE, Room 3314
Atlanta, GA 30322

Alonzo T. Sexton II, M.D.
Resident in Orthopedic Surgery
Emory University School of Medicine
Atlanta, GA

Emory Orthopedic Center
59 Executive Park South
Atlanta, GA 30329

C. Diane Song, M.D.
Assistant Professor of Ophthalmology
Emory University School of Medicine
The Emory Clinic, Building B
The Eye Center
1365 Clifton Road NE, Room 45411
Atlanta, GA 30322

Nathan O. Spell, III
Assistant Professor
Emory University
1525 Clifton Road
Atlanta, GA

James P. Steinberg, M.D.
Associate Professor of Medicine
Division of Infectious Diseases
Emory Crawford Long Hospital
550 Peachtree St., Rm 5.4412
Atlanta, GA 30308

Neil Stollman, M.D.
Associate Clinical Professor of Medicine
Division of Gastroenterology
University of California, San Francisco
90 Oakmont Avenue
Piedmont, CA 94610

Steve Szczerba, M.D.
Resident in Plastic and Reconstructive Surgery
Emory University School of Medicine
Atlanta, GA

Paces Plastic Surgery
3200 Downwood Circle
The Palisades, Suite 640
Atlanta, GA 30327

Madhav Thambisetty, M.D., Ph.D.
Clinical Research Fellow and
Honorary Specialist Registrar
Section of Old Age Psychiatry & Dept. of Neurology
Institute of Psychiatry at the Maudsley
King's College London
Box P070
De Crespigny Park
Denmark Hill
London SE5 8AF

Vinod H. Thourani, M.D.
Resident in Cardiothoracic Surgery
Emory University School of Medicine
Atlanta, GA

The Emory Clinic, Building A
1365 Clifton Road NE, Room 2223
Atlanta, GA 30322

Dwayne Thwaites, M.D.
Resident in Urology
Emory University School of Medicine
The Emory Clinic, Building B
1365 Clifton Road NE
Atlanta, GA 30322

Nomi Traub, M.D.
Assistant Professor of Medicine
Emory University School of Medicine
49 Jesse Hill Jr. Drive
Atlanta, GA 30303

Gary A. Tuma, M.D.
Resident in Plastic and Reconstructive Surgery
Emory University School of Medicine
Atlanta, GA

Paces Plastic Surgery
3200 Downwood Circle
The Palisades, Suite 640
Atlanta, GA 30327

J. David Vega, M.D.
Associate Professor of Cardiothoracic Surgery
Emory University School of Medicine
Atlanta, GA

The Emory Clinic, Building A
1365 Clifton Road NE, Room 2212
Atlanta, GA 30322

Giri Venkatraman, M.D.
Assistant Professor of Otolaryngology
Emory University School of Medicine
Atlanta, GA

The Emory Clinic, Building A
1365 Clifton Road NE, Room 2311
Atlanta, GA 30322

Robert M. Walker, M.D.
Emory University School of Medicine
Atlanta, GA

Clyde Watkins, M.D.
Assistant Professor of Medicine
Emory University School of Medicine
49 Jesse Hill Jr. Drive
Atlanta, GA 30303

Victor J. Weiss, M.D.
Clinical Assistant Professor of Surgery
University of Mississippi School of Medicine
Cardiovascular Surgical Clinic
501 Marshall St., Suite 100
Jackson, MS 39202

Howard Weitz, M.D., F.A.C.P., F.A.C.C.
Professor of Medicine
Vice-Chairman for Education
Jefferson Medical College
Thomas Jefferson University Hospital
Philadelphia, PA

Neil H. Winawer, M.D.
Associate Professor of Medicine
Emory University School of Medicine
49 Jesse Hill Jr. Drive
Atlanta, GA 30303

Ted Wun, M.D., F.A.C.P.
Associate Professor of Medicine
VA Northern California Health Care System
4501 X Street, Suite 3016
Sacramento, CA 95817

John W. Xerogeanes, M.D.
Assistant Professor of Orthopedic Surgery
Emory University School of Medicine
Atlanta, GA

Emory Orthopedic Center
59 Executive Park South
Atlanta, GA 30329

Seth A. Yellin, M.D.
Assistant Professor of Otolaryngology
Emory University School of Medicine
Director
Emory Facial Center
993-C Johnson Ferry Rd, Suite 315
Atlanta, GA 30342

Jane Y. Yeun, M.D., F.A.C.P.
Associate Professor
University of California at Davis Medical Center
Nephrology Division
4150 V Street, Suite 3500
Sacramento, CA 95817

Y. Jonathan Zhang, M.D.
Resident in Neurosurgery
Emory University School of Medicine
Atlanta, GA

The Emory Clinic
1365 Clifton Road NE, Room B6501
Atlanta, GA 30322

Shanta M. Zimmer, M.D.
Senior Associate
Emory University School of Medicine
Division of Infectious Disease
Atlanta VAMC
1670 Clairmont Road
Research 5A161
Decatur, GA 30030

Preface

As "they" say, time flies. It has been over 25 years since we began work on the first edition of *Medical Management of the Surgical Patient*. It is hard to believe that so much time has passed and that there have been so many changes in the practice of medicine. In 1977, coronary bypass surgery was just beginning to be a common procedure, angioplasty was in its infancy and there was no such thing as endoscopic surgery. No one had any idea that AIDS was about to enter the scene. If anyone has said that peptic ulcer disease was an infectious disease, he would have been laughed at and no one was talking about the morals and ethics of medical care. Things have changed!

It seems to us that there is something special about a fourth edition. Getting a first or second edition done isn't easy, but not unusual. A third edition is a "tipping point," it means that the book is of some real use. A fourth edition affirms a book as a standard.

And we certainly hope that is the case. We have gathered in this volume a large group of experts in perioperative care. There are two nationally known conferences in perioperative medicine: Thomas Jefferson and University of California, Davis. Many of our authors are experts from those institutions. Those of us at Emory have been working on these problems since 1977. We have also asked physicians at other institutions to help us on topics where their expertise was demonstrated.

Virtually every chapter has been entirely rewritten. We have again tried to make *Medical Management of the Surgical Patient* a usable, well-documented reference book; there are other excellent handbooks. As in previous additions, we have added new chapters to fill in some gaps.

Introduction

The interchange between physicians discussing a patient's case has been mentioned in written history since ancient Greece. From the time of Hippocrates, physicians have been encouraged to seek consultation on difficult cases when they were in doubt. They were urged not to be jealous of one another but to realize their own limitations and to use the knowledge of their colleagues to help. "Nor, among physicians, do those who treat by diet envy those who employ surgery, but they even call each other into consultation and commend one another." It is clear, however, that there were disagreements in those days: "Physicians who meet in consultation must never quarrel or jeer at one another." There were also "wretched quarrelsome consultations at the bedside of the patient, with no consultant agreeing with another, fearing he might acknowledge a superior."

Over the next 25 centuries, consultation has had its ups and downs. Much of what was written had to do with the etiquette and ethics of the interaction. In medieval Europe, little changed from ancient times. Physicians were encouraged to ask colleagues for help if needed and to refrain from criticizing each other in front of non-physicians.

In the fourteenth century, patients were warned against consulting large numbers of doctors because there would be "endless disagreements and different suggestions" and "the patients [would] suffer from lack of care." The doctor could call in another physician for consultations, but the treatment should be administered by the one knowing the most about the case. Physicians, curiously enough, were warned about consulting with other physicians. "It is better if he have good excuses that he may refuse their demands. He may feign an injury, or illness, or some other likely excuse. But if he accepts their demands let him make a covenant for his work and make it beforehand ... Clearly advise the other leech that he will give no definite answer in any case until he has seen the sickness and the symptoms of the patient." At least the last is sound advice.

The seventeenth and eighteenth centuries brought out the best and the worst in physicians. In Italy, Julius Caesar Claudinius wrote, "There is no part of a Physician's Office more illustrious than Consultation, because by it alone unlearned physicians are known from the Learned .... And there is nothing that brings greater advantage to the Sick." Contrast this with the following: "On December 28, 1750, Drs. John Williams and Parker Bennett, of Jamaica, having become involved in a wrangle about their respective views on bilious fever, came to blows, and, the next day, proceeded to a desperate hand-to-hand combat with swords and pistols, which ended fatally for both. It is said that Johann Peter Frank was so disgusted with the behavior of doctors in consultation that he advised the calling in of the police on all such occasions." Again, in contrast to the brutish behavior in the British colony, John Gregory wrote that "consultation, when required, is to be conducted in a gentlemanly manner. The chief concern is to be the relief of the patient's suffering and not personal advancement. That is, the duty to one's patients takes precedence over personal and professional differences."

During the eighteenth century, there had been (and would continue to be) a great deal of competition between practitioners. At the turn of the nineteenth century, there was much activity in writing about the ethics of medicine, most of which was aimed at avoiding the harmful effect of this competition. Two men in particular bear mention – Johann Stieglitz and Thomas Percival.

In 1798, Stieglitz addressed the problem of the profession's internal difficulties and the distrust they engendered in the public. Many practitioners were afraid to admit their need for help and thus avoided consultation with more knowledgeable physicians. He encouraged consultation for the good of the patient while exhorting the

Medical Management of the Surgical Patient: A Textbook of Perioperative Medicine, ed. M. F. Lubin, R. B. Smith, T. F. Dobson, N. Spell, H. K. Walker. 4th edn. Published by Cambridge University Press. © Cambridge University 2006.

consultants to treat the consulting physicians as colleagues and with respect that would only improve the public's view of the profession.

In 1803, Percival published *Medical Ethics*, a few years after he had been requested to write on the subject by his fellow physicians. Much of the book was devoted to the etiquette of professional interaction, and consultation was addressed in much the same manner as in centuries past: consultation should be obtained to help the patient; no jealousy, competition, or patient stealing should be tolerated; conflict in front of patients was to be avoided at all costs. It is a tribute to the relative timelessness of Percival's work that much of it was used almost verbatim in the AMA Codes of Ethics in 1847, 1911, and 1912.

In the late 1800s, another problem surfaced in England. A great gap had appeared between the eminent consultants and general practitioners. Although the former, because of superior knowledge and prestige, were able to command high fees from wealthy clients, they apparently continued to see less well-to-do patients for the same fees that were being charged by the general practitioners. This attracted business to the consultants but left the ordinary physicians with much less work and poor incomes. The result, as could have been anticipated, was ill feeling between the groups. The conflict was of such consequence that the *British Medical Journal* in 1872 was moved to comment entirely against the "great consultants," who they believed should charge higher fees. This would decrease the burden of the overworked consultants and distribute the workload and the income in a more reasonable manner.

There was great fear among the general practitioners of sending their patients to consultants, because often these patients remained in the care of the more prestigious men whose care was considered better and whose fees were identical. Thus, the patients had no incentive to return to their practitioners. Therefore, in 1886, the Association of General Practitioners was established to try to regulate the relations between these opponents.

In the United States, meanwhile, another problem was developing. In the mid-1800s, many states repealed their laws regulating medicine, resulting in a large influx of quacks and cults. Because of this, a code of ethics restricting competition among doctors was adopted by the medical profession. This code condemned practitioners who did not have orthodox training, who claimed secret medications, and, importantly for consultants, who offered special abilities. (They may have actually had special abilities.) Although the code did much to discourage unqualified practitioners, as medical practice moved into the twentieth century, it allowed ill feeling to exist between

general practitioners and a growing group of medical "specialists."

A number of other negative results surfaced. Because the code forbade consultations with unlicensed physicians, if a patient insisted on a consultation with an outsider, the legitimate physician was forced to withdraw from the case, leaving the patient in the hands of these unqualified people. The rules also provided an opportunity for exclusion of even qualified physicians, and in the late 1800s, women, blacks, and those who were trying to specialize were at times subjected to these consultation bans.

In the twentieth century, laws have again been passed reducing the numbers of unqualified practitioners. The International Code of Ethics encourages consultation in difficult cases. The attainment of equal status by osteopathic physicians is an interesting sidelight to these ancient struggles to protect patients and the profession.

Today, the problem is entirely different. In previous centuries, consultation was requested from a physician who, although similarly trained, was thought to be more knowledgeable overall. Even 60 years ago, in "uncomplicated" cases, consultation was generally considered unnecessary. The doctor who took care of the patient was the doctor who did the surgery, attended to preoperative and postoperative care, and continued to do the "primary care" long after.

For the past few decades, however, as medical knowledge has mushroomed and physicians have specialized and subspecialized, these tasks have been divided and subdivided. This division of labor has helped the great advances in medicine in the United States, but it also has created some special problems.

The proliferation in consultative medicine has allowed patients to have a large number of experts taking care of each separate part of an illness. The internist asks the cardiologist to consult on myocardial infarctions; the cardiologist asks the endocrinologist to consult on patients with diabetes; the surgeon asks the internist for help on patients with hypertension and congestive failure. Although this accumulation of expertise is impressive and would seem to lead to the best care possible, it can, and not infrequently does, lead to conflicting orders, incompatible medications, and conflicts between consulting physicians. Unfortunately, these conflicts are at times perceived by the patients and can cause unnecessary insecurity, fear, and anger.

These kinds of problems are common in the perisurgical patient who has complicating medical problems before surgery or who develops complications afterward. The surgeon frequently needs to have medical support to help with the complicated problems of preoperative and postoperative care. Unfortunately, the internist's knowledge of the surgical procedures, the recovery course, and complications is often scanty. This sets up a situation in which each physician has knowledge that the other needs to take optimal care of the patient.

The advantages of the primary care physician, although they should be obvious, have been lost in the tangle of subspecialization. This physician can be either the internist or the surgeon. The important concept is that the responsibility for the integration of therapies falls to that one physician because he or she is most familiar with all aspects of the patient's case. All other physicians must function as advisors (consultants) to the primary care provider.

The consultant's role can be a difficult one. It is imperative that the primary physician be aware of, and approve of, all therapy, and therefore feel free to accept and reject the advice of the consultant. Rejection is, thankfully, an unusual occurrence. Under ideal circumstances, it is best for the consultant to discuss all recommendations with the primary physician before they are written in the chart. In this way, information can be exchanged, theories can be discussed, and a mutually satisfactory plan of treatment can be formulated. This avoids the confusion, anger, and mistakes that can occur when the consultant must institute therapy without discussion; this should be done only in an emergency situation, when delay would cause harm to the patient.

Another area of potential difficulty for the consultant is in discussing plans and diagnoses with patients who are exquisitely sensitive to any discrepancy, real or perceived, between physicians. This can cause misunderstanding and anxiety for the patient, and can require an immense amount of explanation by the primary physician to re-establish the patient's trust, to help him or her understand what is happening, and to allay his or her fears.

In general, it is best for the consultant to communicate treatment plans through the primary physician. When asked, the consultant can give the patient the broad outline of possibilities to be presented to the primary physician. The consultant should always make it clear that the final decision about what is to be done will be made by the primary physician and the patient.

There seem to be five basic principles behind optimal patient care. The first is the one-patient/one-doctor principle of primary care, or the "final common pathway" to integrate therapies as discussed above. Second, the primary doctor and consultant should trust each other. There needs to be a feeling between them that each one is able to provide something important to the patient's care. Third, communication is indispensable. If the physicians take the time to talk to one another, confusion, irritation, anger, and mistakes can be avoided. The fourth principle is really a corollary of the third, and that is cooperation. It is the natural extension of communication: if two physicians can talk to each other and each one trusts the other's judgment and knowledge, they will be able to cooperate, even in areas of disagreement, in taking the best care of the patient.

The final principle that ties the others together is etiquette. As in all human interactions, the way people deal with each other may be as important as the content of the interaction. A brilliant consultation, handled in a brusque and rude manner may be no more useful than no consultation at all. Controversial or optimal therapies begun before consultation with the primary physician will make further interaction difficult. Finally, and worst of all, improper therapy instituted erroneously or because of inadequate information not only will harm the physicians' relationship but may harm the patient as well.

The art consultation is one that involves many aspects of interaction. The primary physician and the patient must feel that the consultant is concerned not only with the hard scientific facts of the patient's care from the specialist's viewpoint but with optimal overall management. The request for consultation is not a carte blanche for management; it is a request for advice in treating some part of the patient's illness. Thus, the consultant should feel like an invited guest in someone's house, not the master of ceremonies.

Part I

Medical management

Anesthesia management of the surgical patient

L. Reuven Pasternak

The Johns Hopkins University School of Medicine and Public Health, Baltimore, Maryland

Few aspects of healthcare involve as much simultaneous interaction by different physicians as the management of the patient undergoing surgery. At a minimum, the primary care provider, surgeon and anesthesiologist form a team of three physicians, all of whom bring a different perspective and expertise to the care of the patient. As the medical intensity of patients increases, there is also an increasing number of specialty physicians actively involved in this process.

The intersection of the primary care provider and the anesthesiologist first occurs when the surgeon schedules a patient for surgery. At that point the series of events that culminates in medical evaluation, anesthetic assessment, and perioperative management starts. This chapter will begin with that aspect of preparation of the patient for elective surgery. The greatest detail is spent in this area as this is where, by far, the greatest overlap of expertise and communication occurs. The remainder of the chapter will then briefly cover the standard issues involved in perioperative management. These comments are not so much geared to make the primary care provider an expert in the field but are more designed to provide some familiarity with the environment into which the patient is going. It is assumed that detailed information about anesthesia care is provided directly to the patient by the anesthesia provider and/or preoperative systems.

Preoperative evaluation: preparation for surgery

The importance of this phase of clinical management is indicated by its global nature. As the administration of anesthesia may involve a risk for the patient that equals or even exceeds that of the surgery itself, the preoperative evaluation is a crucial first step that may affect the clinical safety and organizational integrity of the entire surgical system. The preoperative assessment of the surgical patient for surgery poses a formidable challenge. While the relative merits of alternative surgical and anesthetic techniques has been extensively studied and reviewed in the literature and other forums, the issue of appropriate preoperative assessment has often remained ambiguous.

Several issues have combined to cause this previously simple process to become more complex.

- While the surgeon has retained the opportunity to examine and assess the patient before the scheduling of surgery, the anesthesiologist often does not have the same access to the patient that had previously existed with routine preoperative admissions.
- The selection of procedures by third party payers to be done on an outpatient and same day admission basis is generally determined on the presumed complexity of the procedure and not the patient's other underlying medical problems or potential issues associated with anesthesia. Consequently, the anesthesiologist is often asked to manage patients with complex medical conditions undergoing less complex surgery with little prior information.
- Organized health plans often seek to retain as much of the control of the process as possible, including determining when and where tests and consultations are to be done.
- Many hospitals and surgical units have yet to organize and develop preoperative evaluation units due to the expense of staff and space at a time when financial constraints are increasingly severe.
- There has been no consistent system for risk assessment to determine appropriate preoperative management.
- Multiple professional societies have developed specific and often contradictory guidelines on preoperative evaluation for their members.

Medical Management of the Surgical Patient: A Textbook of Perioperative Medicine, ed. M. F. Lubin, R. B. Smith, T. F. Dobson, N. Spell, H. K. Walker. 4th edn. Published by Cambridge University Press. © Cambridge University 2006.

To further compound the issues there are multiple strategies and guidelines for assessment of the patient undergoing surgery, often from organizations outside of the anesthesia community and, at times, with little input from anesthesiologists or consideration of anesthesia-related issues.

Philosophy

The purpose of the preoperative evaluation is to identify and reduce the risks associated with anesthesia and surgery. The preoperative evaluation is that portion of the general process that is designed to address issues related to the perioperative management of the surgical patient by anesthesiologists. All preoperative activities, including evaluation prior to the day of surgery, testing, and consultation, should be undertaken only on the reasonable expectation that they will enhance the safety, comfort and efficiency of the process for the patient, clinical staff, and overall system. Decisions concerning preoperative management should be associated with a consideration of how any aspect of the evaluation will affect the management and outcome of the perioperative process. Evaluations and interventions that do not have a demonstrated beneficial effect do not have value to the patient, clinician or manager and should not be undertaken on the basis of custom or convenience.

The preoperative evaluation is therefore a focused assessment to address issues relevant to the safe administration of anesthesia and performance of surgery. The use of this event to perform unrelated general medical screening and intervention should be undertaken only in association with appropriate primary and specialty care support. Only anesthesia staff may determine a patient's fitness for administration of anesthesia and appropriate anesthesia technique. The performance of a history and physical examination by other healthcare providers does not constitute a clearance for administration of anesthesia but provides information to the anesthesia staff to make that determination. Thus, internists and other specialists do not "clear" patients for surgery. Rather, they provide an assessment of the current health status of the patient, including whether the patient is as optimally managed as possible.

When evaluating patients for surgery, it should be remembered that the anesthesiologist has only a temporary but important relationship with the patient. Patients' continuing care, including assessment of new or acute exacerbations of chronic conditions, should be done by their primary care providers and associated consultants with whom they will have long-term relationships. Patients should be apprised of the fact that the preoperative evaluation is not a substitute for regular primary care. Requests by patients for performance of tests not deemed necessary for the performance of surgery or administration of surgery should also be referred to their primary healthcare source.

Risk classification

While the purpose of the preoperative evaluation is to reduce risk, current risk classification systems are ill-equipped to provide assistance with patient classification. The first attempt to quantify risks associated with surgery was undertaken by Meyer Saklad[1] in 1941 at the request of the American Society of Anesthesiology. This effort was the first by any medical specialty to stratify risk for its patients. Saklad's system did so based on mortality secondary to the associated preoperative medical condition. Type of anesthesia and nature of surgery were not considerations in this system and the divisions were based on empirical experience rather than on specific sets of data and reflect the techniques and standards of practice as of 50 years ago. Four preoperative risk categories were established ranging from category 1 (least likely to die) to category 4 (highest expectation of mortality).

The current American Society of Anesthesiology (ASA) classification system (Fig. 1.1) is a modification of this work, adding an additional fifth category for moribund patients undergoing surgery in a desperate attempt to preserve life. Numerous studies have demonstrated an association of mortality with ASA Classification independent of anesthetic technique.[2–14] However, these data have limited application as it relates to mortality as its sole outcome and is based on anesthetic techniques as practiced more than 20 years ago. Apfelbaum[15] and Meridy,[16] for example, have noted a lack of correlation between ASA status and cancellations, unplanned admissions and other perioperative complications in outpatient surgery.

Thus, while useful as a broad assessment of preoperative medical status, the current ASA Classification is limited in its ability to truly establish risk or serve as a basis for formulating clinical guidelines without an associated risk index for the surgical procedure. In addition, while concerning itself with the identification of risk, there is a remarkable lack of data delineating outcomes in ambulatory surgery and anesthesia. When the ASA Task Force on Preoperative Evaluation recently issued its recommendations for all preoperative assessment, it initially tried to do so using an evidence-based approach linking specific tests and interventions with designated outcomes. The

ASA Class 1

No organic, physiologic, biochemical, or psychiatric disturbance
The pathologic process for which the operation is to be performed is localized and does not entail
a systemic disturbance

ASA Class 2

Mild to moderate systemic disease disturbance caused either by the condition to be treated
surgically or by other pathologic processes

Well-controlled hypertension	Well-controlled diabetes mellitus
History of asthma	Mild obesity
Anemia	Age <1 year or >70 years
Cigarette use	Pregnancy

ASA Class 3

Severe systemic disturbance or disease from whatever cause, even though it may not be possible to
define the degree of disability with finality

Angina	Symptomatic respiratory disease
Status postmyocardial infarction	(e.g., asthma, COPD)
Poorly controlled hypertension	Massive obesity

ASA Class 4

Indicative of the patient with severe systemic disorders that are already life-threatening, not always
correctable by operation

Unstable angina	Debilitating respiratory disease
Congestive heart failure	Hepatorenal failure

ASA Class 5

The moribund patient who has little chance of survival but is submitted to operation in desperation

Modifier: Emergency operation (E): Any patient in one of the above classes who is operated upon as an
emergency is considered to be in poorer physical condition.

Fig. 1.1. American Society of Anesthesiology (ASA) classification system.

literature in this area for all of anesthesia was such that, of over 1200 articles identified in this area, fewer than 30 fit the criteria for use. Lack of information of sufficient scientific validity mandated that the guideline development had to yield to an advisory that was based on consensus opinion subject to further scientific investigation and validation using evidence-based studies at a future date. For purposes of risk stratification, the ASA advisory adopted a modification of the risk index system for patient medical severity and surgical severity as used by the other most commonly used algorithm for patient preoperative assessment, the AHA\ACC guidelines for preoperative assessment of the cardiac patient for non-cardiac surgery.[17]

Patient and procedure selection

The nature of patient and procedure selection is a function of medical status, surgical procedure and availability of appropriate postoperative assistance, ranging from home care to intensive care support. While elective surgical procedures are by definition not emergencies, many are nonetheless relatively urgent in nature. The delay of some procedures, such as biopsies for staging of oncology treatments, may unnecessarily delay and inappropriately compromise the care of the patient. Surgeons and anesthesiologists must make a judgment if delay will truly reduce the risk for the patient or merely postpone the inevitable task of dealing with a potentially difficult challenge in the operating room. Finally, while mandates for early discharge by regulatory and managed care groups are based almost wholly on postoperative physiologic status, patient comfort and availability of appropriate assistance at home should be a major consideration in this process. In these circumstances, it is anticipated that the primary care provider will provide insight about the medical status of the patient and assist with optimal stabilization prior to surgery. Advice as to type of anesthesia technique should be deferred to the anesthesia team, who will tailor their technique to the special needs of the patient.

Time of the evaluation

At the current time, over 60% of surgery performed in the United States is outpatient and another 10%–15% is performed on a same day admission basis. For this 70% of the nearly 30 million surgical procedures performed each year, the challenge of appropriate timing and content of the assessment is important and sometimes difficult. Initially, it was a common assumption that a preoperative visit prior to the day of surgery confers some added measure of safety and comfort for patients. On the basis of this assumption, patients were often asked to take the time and expense required to comply with such requirements while hospitals and anesthesiologists had to staff centers able to handle this demand.

Eventually, the literature called this practice into question. Fisher's study[18] demonstrated for outpatients and inpatients that prior preoperative evaluation by anesthesia staff reduced cancellations, tests, and consultations. This study was thus useful in demonstrating the need for a screening mechanism that allowed for patient assessment prior to the day of surgery. However, the assertion that these benefits could be obtained only in a system where all patients visited a preoperative evaluation center was not demonstrated. Some studies demonstrated that no preoperative evaluation visit prior to the day of surgery was necessary for healthy patients undergoing minor procedures.[19,20] Some of the most comprehensive work in this

area has been by Twersky et al.,[21] which indicates that patient evaluations on the day of surgery may be performed in a manner that is safe and effective. However, even in these studies, patients were not stratified by medical status or surgical procedure and were not relevant for the larger patient population managed by most anesthesiologists.

In discussions with major academic and private practice medical center directors, it has been observed by this author that the percentage of patients who required having an onsite visit prior averages about 25%–33%. The preoperative assessment must be a balance between patient convenience and the need to have information available in a timely fashion to allow for planning appropriate preoperative and perioperative management. While the ideal system may include a preoperative evaluation prior to the day of surgery for all patients, the logistics of patient schedules and their often otherwise healthy status makes this ideal impractical and, at times, unnecessary. This point is of significant concern to hospital preoperative evaluation staff who believe that resources may be inappropriately committed to patients with little need of those services to the detriment of others with more extensive medical and surgical issues and with waste of resources needed elsewhere.

The algorithm adopted by the ASA for preoperative evaluation (Fig. 1.2)[22] recognizes that there are categories of patients (health individuals for low-risk surgical procedures) for whom a preoperative assessment (consisting of information made available prior to the day of surgery for review) is sufficient. Similarly, there are some individuals for whom assessment prior to the day of surgery is mandated by their medical condition and/or planned surgery. It is difficult to provide a standard recommendation for how ambulatory surgical centers should place its patients into these categories; much depends on the ease of availability and validity of data provided prior to the day of surgery. What is uniformly recommended is that appropriate information should be made available to anesthesia staff prior to the day of surgery to allow for review and appropriate action. An example of conditions for which assessment by anesthesia directed staff prior to the day of surgery is provided in Fig. 1.2.

It is increasingly recognized that the role of the primary care provider is critical in this process. That individual is most familiar with the health status of the patient. Thus, while they are not in a position to "clear for anesthesia," they are in a position to provide the pertinent medical information prior to the day of surgery that would allow surgical systems staff to determine the need for any additional information or consultation.

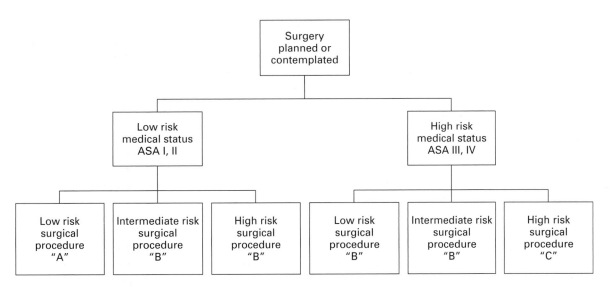

Low risk procedure: poses minimal physiologic stress and risk to the patient independent of medical condition (e.g., office based, minor surgery).

Medium risk procedure: moderate physiologic stress and risk with minimal blood loss, fluid shift or postoperative change in normal physiology.

High risk procedure: significant perioperative and postoperative physiologic stress.

"A": patient may have preoperative assessment on day of surgery on basis of available preoperative data.

"B": patient may require preoperative consultation, based on the nature of the patient's medical condition and planned procedure.

"C": patient should have preoperative consultation with anesthesia staff prior to the day of surgery.

Fig. 1.2. Illustrative algorithm for preoperative evaluation. Adapted from ASA task force on preoperative evaluation.

Laboratory testing

Laboratory and other diagnostic tests associated with preoperative evaluations represent one of the most costly issues associated with surgery. It is difficult to attach a precise dollar cost on this activity. However, it is conservatively estimated that at least 10% of the over $30 billion spent on laboratory testing each year is for preoperative evaluation. The traditional system of the protocol "battery of tests" evolved from a lack of clear definition of their role in preoperative screening, insufficient information on their utility, and a mistaken belief that voluminous information, no matter how irrelevant, enhanced the safety of care and reduced physician liability for adverse events. Protocol testing relieved physicians and their associates of the responsibility of decision making as an easier, though more costly, alternative to selective tests based on patients' individual health profiles.

At a time when the cost of care and the convenience of patients is a major concern, the role of tests as a screening device is rightfully diminishing. The patient history, physical examination, and judgment of the physician are replacing protocols as the basis for testing. While information about other aspects of the preoperative evaluation may be ambiguous, there is extensive literature and experience to support the selective use of testing which also confirms that the use of broad testing panels has a strong tendency to result in excessive testing. Laboratory testing, like all areas of medical intervention, should be undertaken on a "value-added" basis: a reasonable expectation that a potential issue exists that is relevant to anesthesia.

The utility of the preoperative test is based on several key considerations. The first issue is relevance. While some abnormalities are clearly of concern (e.g., cardiac and respiratory), others may have little or no effect on anesthetic plan and outcome and thus do not warrant thorough investigation in this format. The second issue is the prevalence of the condition in both symptomatic and asymptomatic patients. A low prevalence in asymptomatic patients indicates that screening is of little use. The third issue is that of test sensitivity and specificity. Low sensitivity permits false-negative results and patients at risk undergo anesthesia without appropriate preparation. Low specificity causes a large number of false-positives subjecting patients to additional testing, with coincident inconvenience, costs, and potential morbidity. Testing should therefore be done for conditions that are medically relevant using tests of high sensitivity and specificity. A final consideration is cost. Selection of alternative testing modalities should also take into consideration the financial and nonfinancial costs of testing with selection of the less costly approach where it does not compromise the quality of the information desired. Testing in the asymptomatic population should only be done in patients for whom the potential condition is significant and of reasonable prevalence with tests of reasonable sensitivity and specificity.

Attaching precise numbers to the above caveats is difficult and is the subject of cost–benefit and cost–effectiveness analysis for each of the tests concerned. While this has not been established for many of the routine diagnostic tests that we employ, it has been established in the medical, surgical, and anesthesia literature that the use of screening tests without specific indication is not appropriate. In a study of 19 980 tests on 1000 patients, Korvin et al.[23] encountered 2223 abnormal values of which 993 were initially considered to be unanticipated. Of these, 223 led to further evaluation and new diagnoses and in only one case was the diagnosis unrelated to other known medical issues and resulted in new patient care. This involved elevated liver studies in a male who had received halothane anesthesia and for whom the recommendation was made that this agent be avoided. Robbins and Mushlin,[24] in evaluating preoperative testing from a medical perspective, provide an excellent review of the sensitivity, specificity and consequent utility of a wide range of tests. Kaplan et al.[25] reviewed the records of 2000 patients undergoing elective surgery who received a routine battery of complete blood cell count, differential cell count, prothrombin time, partial thromboplastin time, platelet count, glucose level, and six channel chemistries. They found that 60% of these tests would not have been performed had they been done only on the basis of clinical indication and that, of these, only 0.22% revealed abnormalities that might have affected perioperative management. These findings were replicated by Turnbull and Buck,[26] in a review of 1010 otherwise healthy patients undergoing cholecystectomy,

who discovered 225 abnormal results in 5003 tests of which 104 were judged to be important and for whom only four patients might have derived some benefit.

In addition to protocols lacking critical review, another reason for excess testing often relates to a lack of communication between medical colleagues. A retrospective study by Kitz et al.[27] compared the use of chest X-rays, electrocardiograms, and chemistry panels in patients undergoing knee arthroscopy and diagnostic laparoscopy or laparoscopic tubal ligation. The groups were divided into patients electively admitted prior to the day of surgery and those who were outpatients. Both patient groups were healthy ASA I and II with tests ordered in the first group by the admitting surgeon and in the second by the anesthesiologist. Though medically similar, the groups had significantly different rates of testing with the higher test rate by surgeons attributable to their desire to not have cases canceled and lack of information from anesthesia staff about test indications.

Additional studies of specific tests have also confirmed the use of the history and physical as a basis for specific tests. Urinalysis, long a mainstay of testing and still required by law in some states, has been found to be of extremely limited use in patients without preexisting medical condition or positive physical findings.[28] Their use for prevention of postoperative surgical problems outside the realm of genitourinary surgery was addressed by Lawrence et al.[29] In a classic application of cost–benefit analysis, it was determined that routine urinalysis for all knee replacement surgery in the United States would cost $1 500 000 per wound prevented and not add to the safety or effectiveness of the surgery. Rucker et al.,[30] in a review of 905 routine chest X-rays for elective surgical procedures, determined that 368 had no risk factors by history and physical and that only one had a minor abnormality. Of the remaining 504 remaining patients, 22% (114) had serious abnormalities, virtually all of which would have been anticipated by the history and physical examination. Charpak et al.,[31] in a retrospective review of postoperative complications, found no circumstances in which absence of a chest X-ray in patients without prior pulmonary disease would have altered outcome or management, even when the complications were respiratory in nature. In both studies, no correlation was established between age and occurrence of positive chest X-rays in patients independent of coexisting positive history or physical examination. Similar findings are available for hemoglobin determinations,[32,33] serum chemistries,[34] and pulmonary function testing.[35]

In accordance with the philosophy that a test is undertaken because of a realistic possibility of adding valuable

General

Medical condition inhibiting ability to engage in normal daily activity

Medical conditions necessitating continual assistance or monitoring at home within the past six months

Admission within the past two months for acute or exacerbation of chronic condition

Cardiocirculatory

History of angina, coronary artery disease, myocardial infarction

Symptomatic arrhythmias

Poorly controlled hypertension (diastolic >110, systolic >160)

History of congestive heart failure

Respiratory

Asthma/COPD requiring chronic medication or with acute exacerbation and progression within past 6 months

History of major airway surgery or unusual airway anatomy

Upper and/or lower airway tumor or obstruction

History of chronic respiratory distress requiring home ventilatory assistance or monitoring

Endocrine

Insulin-dependent diabetes mellitus

Adrenal disorders

Active thyroid disease

Neuromuscular

History of seizure disorder or other significant CNS disease (e.g., multiple sclerosis)

History of myopathy or other muscle disorders

Hepatic

Any active hepatobiliary disease or compromise

Musculoskeletal

Kyphosis and/or scoliosis causing functional compromise

Temporomandibular joint disorder

Cervical or thoracic spine injury

Oncology

Patients receiving chemotherapy

Other oncology process with significant physiologic residual or compromise

Gastrointestinal

Massive obesity (>140% ideal body weight)

Hiatal hernia

Symptomatic gastroesophageal reflux

Fig. 1.3. Condition for which preoperative evaluation may be recommended prior to the day of surgery.

information, protocol screening without specific indication is not appropriate. In addition to lack of utility for the physician, such testing may, in fact, do harm to patients through unnecessary and potentially invasive interventions, heightened anxieties, and markedly increased costs that may place the physician in a position of having to explain proceeding with surgery in the face of incomplete or irrelevant data. As observed in the literature, there is little rationale for testing other than on the basis of specific indicators. Testing should be done only on an expectation of a finding that might have reasonable relevance for anesthesia and surgery based on:

- presence of a positive finding on the history and physical examination.
- need of the surgeon or other clinician for baseline values in anticipation of significant changes due to surgery or other medical interventions (e.g., chemotherapy).
- patient's inclusion in a population at higher risk for the presence of a relevant condition even though they may exhibit no individual signs of that condition themselves.

The associated recommendations are noted in Fig. 1.3. By this standard, patients less than 50 years of age without coexisting medical disease would require no preoperative testing, while patients greater than 50 years of age would require an electrocardiogram as per the anesthesiologist. Further testing is done on an individualized basis as indicated by history, physical, and nature of the surgical procedure. It is estimated conservatively that such testing at our institution could reduce preoperative testing by 70%.

Consultations

Specialty consultations should not be obtained on an automatic basis because of organ-specific problems but because there is a specific issue that remains to be addressed. For example, in some centers it is routine to require all patients with any cardiac risk factor to be seen by a cardiologist prior to surgery. These consultations often provide no new information or insight other than that which can be obtained by a review of existing records and a basic history and physical examination. At worst, these requests for consultation are at times taken as a request for suggestions concerning the perioperative management with recommendations made that are based on erroneous assumptions concerning the risks associated with anesthetic techniques. When indicated, requests for consultations should be specifically and narrowly worded to request the specialist's evaluation of the patient's clinical condition, and not to "clear for anesthesia."

Preparation of the patient on the day of surgery

N.p.o.

Preoperative fasting is aimed at reducing the risk of aspiration on induction of anesthesia and the risk of postoperative emesis. It had long been assumed that any gastric intake prior to surgery posed a major risk to the patient. This standard assumption, however, has been shown to be misleading. Some recent studies in adults demonstrate reduced and less acidic gastric contents when patients are given 150 ml of clear fluid 2 hours before surgery.[36] Scarr et al., in their study of 211 patients, found that patients who were permitted to have 150 ml of tea, coffee, apple juice, or water up to 3 hours before surgery had no difference in gastric volume or pH than those who were n.p.o. for the traditional 8-hour period. Schreiner et al.[37] evaluated this same issue in pediatric patients, comparing those with routine n.p.o. status with those allowed to take clear liquids up to 2 hours before surgery, with the only limitation in volume being the last intake (8 ounces). The study group taking oral fluids was found to be less anxious and less irritable at the time of induction, while not having any statistically significant difference in gastric volume or pH. Similarly, Sandhar et al.[38] evaluated oral intake of liquids (5 ml/kg) with and without ranitidine (2 mg/kg) and ranitidine alone up to 2 to 3 hours before surgery in patients 1 to 14 years of age. The use of fluids alone did not appear to place patients at risk, and the combination with ranitidine was found to be beneficial.

These findings increasingly suggest that the 8-hour n.p.o. rule for outpatients may be subjecting many low-risk individuals, especially children and the elderly, to unwarranted discomfort and that allowing clear liquids up to 2 to 3 hours before surgery may be preferable. Current recommendations retain the 8-hour n.p.o. rule for solids, but allow up to 150–200 cm³ of liquid 2 hours before surgery. From a practical standpoint, however, the ability to convey this in instructions is sometimes difficult for the patient to follow, and it sometimes remains simpler to require a full 8-hour n.p.o. period prior to surgery except for sips of liquids required for medication or for special circumstances on an individualized basis.

Preoperative medication

It is generally recommended that patients take their routine medications prior to, and on the day of, surgery. Exceptions to this recommendation include diuretics, oral hypoglycemic agents, anticoagulants, and insulin. Anticoagulants will usually need to be withheld per instructions of the surgeon. Insulin should be brought by the patient to the hospital or surgical facility on the day of surgery with one-third to one-half of the usual dose administered after testing for blood glucose levels and the start of an i.v. to prevent against hypoglycemia. For this reason, it is strongly recommended that insulin-dependent diabetics be scheduled as early on the schedule as possible to protect against wide swings in their glucose levels prior to surgery.

At times, a compassionate primary care physician may prescribe sedation to be taken by the patient prior to arrival for an outpatient or same day admission procedure. This practice should be discouraged as the patient may not be in appropriate condition to work with the anesthesiologist who must also then cope with an exogenous agent in determining and obtaining informed consent for an appropriate anesthetic plan.

Perioperative management

As with all other aspects of management, the perioperative care of the ambulatory surgery patient requires scrupulous attention to issues of safety, comfort, convenience, and efficiency. Selection of anesthetic technique must thus ensure a cooperative patient for the surgeon. The anesthesiologist must use a method that ensures rapid induction and emergence from anesthesia, with the patient feeling little discomfort in the recovery period and thus allowing for a reasonably quick discharge. The margin for error is considerably smaller in outpatient procedures, since often little time is available to stabilize a patient during the perioperative period if one discovers excessive or insufficient depth of anesthesia.

As with any procedure, the anesthetic technique is discussed with the patient and a notation made in the record of this fact. This discussion constitutes informed consent and is increasingly being conducted with the same formality as the surgical consent. Just as the surgeon is required to state potential complications and potential unplanned interventions that may occur, patients should be advised of alternative plans that may ensue. These plans are usually in the form of general anesthesia in the event that other techniques are insufficient for the procedure's successful completion. At times, patients for whom general anesthesia is contraindicated may have a procedure performed with sedation or a regional technique. In these circumstances, both surgeon and patient should be fully aware that an attempt to perform the procedure one way does not constitute open clearance to proceed under all circumstances. Also, if the initial effort is unsuccessful, the surgery should be discontinued and performed in a different setting.

On occasion, primary care providers advise patients, suggest appropriate anesthetic techniques and agents and at times place these suggestions in the medical record. While done with the best of intention, this practice often prejudices the discussion between the anesthesiologist and the patient and may cause undo confusion and distress on the day of surgery. Accordingly, the primary care

provider is discouraged from this practice. Instead, patient concerns and preferences, if any, should be noted with discussion of technique and agents left to the discussion between the anesthesiologist and patient.

Monitoring and anesthesia equipment

A fully operational anesthesia system includes pulse oximetry, capnography, ECG, blood pressure measurement, and precordial or esophageal stethoscope. The provision of anesthesia services in any location, whether inside or outside of the operating room, requires the availability of these modalities of monitoring as a minimum standard of care. Within the operating room, the ability to monitor inspiratory and expiratory inhalation agents is proving to be of significant value in modifying anesthetic technique to allow for smooth induction and rapid emergence.

Monitored sedation

Monitored sedation, when possible, often provides the safest, most comfortable, and most efficient anesthetic management. It is especially desirable in patients whose medical condition (e.g., major cardiorespiratory disease and difficult airways) makes them relatively more difficult candidates for general anesthesia. Whereas regional and general anesthesia may provide deep anesthesia over a large body area and allow leeway to both anesthesiologist and surgeon, monitored sedation requires scrupulous technique by both. Common procedures using these techniques include carpal tunnel repair; other hand procedures; cataract extraction and lens implanting; significant dermatologic procedures; and some hernia repairs.

Procedures that can often be performed by experienced surgeons in this way include breast biopsies, inguinal hernia repairs, limited superficial procedures on the skin and subcutaneous tissue, ophthalmic procedures such as cataract extraction, and procedures on distal portions of extremities to a local block by the surgeon. Surgery performed with local anesthesia thus requires a technique that is limited, is amenable to local infiltration, is performed rapidly, and does not require excessive doses of either local anesthesia or sedation. Surgical skill is critical; attempts to perform such invasive procedures as tonsillectomy and laparoscopy with sedation and local anesthesia is fraught with potential disaster in the hands of anyone but the most skilled surgeon.

With some surgeons, patient sedation may not be required. In general, however, sedation allows a patient to achieve a more relaxed state and permits a more pleasant and rapid completion of the procedure. A wide array of drugs is employed. The standard technique that has generally worked well involves the use of a benzodiazepine with a short-acting narcotic, replacing the past practice of relying on barbiturates. Midazolam's tendency to cause less postoperative drowsiness than diazepam, combined with its faster onset of action and less vein-irritating nature, has made midazolam the mainstay of current technique. Contrary to much conventional wisdom, the retrograde amnesia associated with midazolam is minimal and instead is marked by the patient's impaired ability to integrate events into long-term memory after its administration.[39–41]

Administration of short-acting narcotics, such as fentanyl (1 to 2 mcg/kg), can supplement the sedative nature of the midazolam, with the anesthesiologist checking closely for any impaired or compromised ventilation. Alfentanil (10 to 20 mcg/kg) is also effective and provides more rapid onset and shorter duration of action than fentanyl. As with all procedures, varying levels of stimulation occur, usually associated with initial and subsequent injections of local anesthetic into the surgical site. Administration of 25 to 50 mg of a short-acting barbiturate or 10 to 20 mg of propofol immediately before anesthesia induction may preclude the need for larger doses of longer-acting agents. Frequent need for such medication, however, indicates the need for deeper sedation.

An alternative and increasingly popular approach to sedation involves the intravenous use of propofol, a rapid-onset, short-acting hypnotic. After an initial dose of 1 mg/kg, increments of 0.25 mg/kg up to a total dose of 2.5 mg are used to achieve sedation. A continuous infusion of 20 mcg/kg is then used to maintain sedation, adjusting to the patient's level of sedation and vital signs. When using this technique, one must remember that propofol is a hypnotic and not an analgesic. Therefore its success depends even more on appropriate local anesthetic use than with a benzodiazepine or hypnotic, although propofol has the advantage of faster onset and cessation of action.

A critical point to remember is that the surgeon administers the local agent to provide anesthesia. Patient discomfort that persists despite sedation in the unstimulated state may indicate the need for more local anesthetic infiltration or alteration of technique. In some individuals, "light" sedation with local anesthesia may not be satisfactory. While light sedation is designed to provide a calming influence, these individuals may proceed to what is known as "deep" sedation. When used, deep sedation carries many of the risks of general anesthesia and, at times, may be more problematic. Patients receiving deep sedation have a profound alteration of consciousness and may

not be able to cooperate with a surgeon's request to remain still, at times becoming agitated. The patient's airway muscles also become relaxed, causing potential airway obstruction and desaturation of blood oxygen content. When this occurs, general anesthesia may be preferred as a means of protecting the airway and providing a situation permitting the surgeon to complete the procedure.

Regional anesthesia

Regional anesthesia offers a potentially major benefit for patients undergoing procedures on the extremities. Although this is especially true for those patients for whom general anesthesia may provide a significant risk, regional anesthesia also provides advantages for the general patient population. The most frequently cited criticisms of regional anesthesia, other than spinal, is the time that is needed to place and establish a block, usually 20 to 30 minutes, and the perceived risk of failure and need to switch to general anesthesia.

In assessing the usefulness of regional anesthesia, one must consider recovery time and the patient's postoperative comfort. In a review of 543 brachial plexus blocks, Davis[42] found a success rate of 93% for anesthesiologists performing such blocks regularly. Bowe et al.[43] and Baysinger et al.[44,45] demonstrated that brachial plexus anesthesia for carpal tunnel release and upper extremity procedures did not significantly differ from general anesthesia in total OR and recovery room time. However, the incidence of postoperative nausea, emesis, and pain requiring medication was less than half that found in patients who had general anesthesia.

Similar findings have been shown for arthroscopy of the knee with the patient under epidural or spinal anesthesia, and administration of narcotic by this route for prolonged analgesia.[46–49] As with brachial plexus blockade, the incidence of nausea, emesis, and postoperative pain were significantly less than with general anesthesia. Parnas et al.[48] demonstrated a frequency of pain of 20.3% vs. 27.0% in patients under regional and general anesthesia, respectively, but found significantly less nausea and emesis (4.1% vs. 16.5%, respectively). Bowe et al.[46] found an even greater difference in postoperative pain (27% vs. 65% for regional vs. general) and nausea with emesis (1.5% vs. 25% for regional vs. general). In all studies, neither OR nor recovery times were significantly different between these two groups. Of interest is the additional finding of Randel et al.[49] that epidural anesthesia results in a decreased recovery time of 123 minutes, compared with 164 minutes for general anesthesia.

Epidural anesthesia has been found to provide significant benefit and safety for peripheral vascular, urologic, gynecologic, and arthroscopic surgery.[49–51] Randel et al.[49] showed that the additional time required for placement of the block should be compensated for by reduced time to oral intake, ambulation, voiding, and discharge. Although the incidence of moderate to severe headache was less than with either general or spinal anesthesia, patients undergoing epidural anesthesia did have a higher incidence of moderate to severe backache.

Spinal anesthesia usually offers the benefit of a more rapidly achieved and intense block than that achieved with epidural anesthesia. The risk of spinal headache and subsequent distress used to be a major issue. Three aspects of spinal headache were of concern, especially in the ambulatory setting: (a) its occurrence 2 to 3 days postoperatively, after routine follow-up has already been accomplished; (b) it incapacitates the patient for several days thereafter; and (c) the potential need for readmission or further intervention with a blood patch. Advocates of spinal anesthesia point out the low incidence of postoperative spinal headache as a justification for its use. Some advocates, such as Mulroy,[50] have maintained that alteration in technique and appropriate patient selection can reduce the incidence to well under 1% or less and assert that maintenance of a recumbent position does not help avoid headache[52,53] and may simply delay its onset. The use of 27-gauge needles and use of Greene "pencil point" or Whitacre side-port needles has reduced the incidence of postdural puncture headaches to less than 1%. The decreasing costs and clinical advantages of the 27-gauge Whitacre is increasingly making it the standard for spinal anesthesia.

The use of spinal anesthesia is still relatively contraindicated in patients with pre-existing back pain or injury unless it presents a clear advantage in the patient at risk for general anesthesia.

A final but important consideration in this area is the increasing use of regional anesthesia to supplement general anesthesia for postoperative analgesia. This situation usually arises in the administration of caudal anesthetics to pediatric patients undergoing urologic or lower extremity procedures. The most significant of these has been the use of caudal anesthesia in the pediatric population undergoing genitourinary and lower extremity procedures. It is noteworthy that caudal anesthesia has found widespread favor in alleviating the discomfort associated with inguinal hernia repairs, orchiopexies, and other procedures.[38,54] Although the delayed discharge associated with caudal anesthesia has been the principal objection to its use, usually by surgeons, the use of 0.125%

bupivacaine has diminished the incidence of postoperative urinary retention while maintaining equivalent analgesia[51] to the point that this consideration should no longer prevent its use.

Local infiltration with anesthetics is also useful in diminishing postoperative pain. Placing local anesthetics into the wound is an increasingly popular technique. Casey et al.[55] found that simple instillation of 0.25% bupivacaine was as effective as a more elaborate ilioinguinal or iliohypogastric block with bupivacaine for patients having inguinal hernia repair. Studies have also found a significant reduction in postoperative pain in patients having bilateral tubal ligation, with injection of 5 ml of 1% etidocaine into the banded portion of the tube.[56] Narchi et al.[57] obtained similar results in patients undergoing laparoscopy, with 80 ml of 0.5% lidocaine or 0.5% bupivacaine applied to the right subdiaphragmatic area. Studies are currently evaluating instillation of local anesthetics and narcotics in the knee joint for arthroscopy. Such techniques require close cooperation and communication between the surgeon and anesthesiologist.

General anesthesia

When required, general anesthesia remains a safe and effective manner to achieve the goals of anesthesia. Principal problems associated with the otherwise successful general anesthetic are somnolence, nausea and emesis, postoperative pain, and associated delays in discharge and, in ambulatory surgery, possible admission. As the number of procedures performed with sedation and regional anesthesia increases, general anesthesia may be required less frequently. Nonetheless, it remains a mainstay of anesthetic practice, and considerable progress has been made to reduce the problems just listed.

Before the introduction of propofol, sodium pentothal or thiopental were accepted as the mainstays for induction. Considerable evidence now shows that propofol offers distinct advantages. Sampson et al.,[58] in an analysis of the two agents, compared 4 mg/kg of thiopental with 2.5 mg/kg of propofol followed by 100% O_2 for outpatient procedures. The recovery time until patients were comfortable postoperatively was considerably better for the patients receiving propofol than for those receiving thiopental. These findings of reduced recovery time, less nausea, and greater postoperative alertness have also been consistently reported in other studies. Anecdotal information from practitioners also note patient emergence marked by greater satisfaction, at times bordering on a transient pleasant euphoria. Marais et al.[59] and Sung et al.,[60] in separate studies indicative of future

(These tests are those required for administration of anesthesia and are not intended to limit those required by surgeons for issues specific to their surgical management)

Age 50 or less and no existing comorbidity
No tests required

Electrocardiogram

Age 50 or older	Current or past circulatory disease
Hypertension	Diabetes mellitus (age 40 or older)
Current or past significant cardiac disease	Renal, thyroid or other metabolic disease

Chest X-ray
Asthma or COPD that is debilitating or with change of symptoms or acute episode within past
6 months
Cardiothoracic procedure

Serum chemistries

Renal disease	Diuretic therapy
Adrenal or thyroid disorders	Chemotherapy

Urinalysis

Diabetes mellitus	Recent genitourinary infection
Renal disease	Metabolic disorder involving renal function
Genito-urologic procedure	

Complete blood count
Hematological disorder
Vascular procedure
Chemotherapy

Coagulation studies
Anticoagulation therapy
Vascular procedure

Pregnancy testing
Patients for whom pregnancy might complicate the surgery
Patients of uncertain status by history

Fig. 1.4. Recommended laboratory testing.

cost–benefit analyses, also found that propofol, by decreasing patient stay and postoperative symptoms, was also effective in reducing costs. Because of its application on a near universal basis for sedation and general anesthesia, propofol is the most commonly used anesthetic agent in virtually all parts of the world today.

The availability of newer agents has altered perspectives on optimal maintenance of general anesthesia. Specifically, propofol; the short-acting neuromuscular agents atracurium, vecuronium, mivacurium and rocuronium; the short-acting narcotics fentanyl, alfentanil, sufentanil, and remifentanil; and newer inhalation agents desflurane and sevoflurane are allowing new approaches to general anesthesia in the outpatient.

Before the availability of these agents, the major issue was whether an inhalation technique or a balanced technique with narcotics and nitrous oxide (N_2O) was optimal. In assessing volatile agents, little has been found to differentiate among them as to postoperative drowsiness, headache, myalgia, or nausea and vomiting[61–63] and perioperative stability. However, the introduction of short-acting hypnotics and narcotics, such as propofol and alfentanil, has assisted in the development of total intra-venous anesthesia (TIVA) as a means of providing general anesthesia. In two studies, propofol in a continuous infusion of 12 mg/kg/h was compared with enflurane[64] and enflurane and isoflurane. In both instances, patients receiving propofol had significantly less nausea and emesis, less recovery time, and less need for intervention for these problems in the recovery room. Although one study has found that narcotics do not enhance TIVA,[65] many strongly advocate the continuous infusion of pro-pofol and narcotics in combination.

Conclusions

The interaction of primary care providers and anesthesiol-ogists is one of the most critical for the safety, efficiency, and comfort of patients. These individuals bring different perspectives and expertise to the care of the patient under-going surgical procedures. It is increasingly important for each to have a better understanding of the issues involved in chronic patient care and perioperative management at a time when the healthcare system is placing more demands on physicians and the systems in which they work.

REFERENCES

1. Saklad, M. Grading of patients for surgical procedures. *Anesthesiology* 1941; **2**: 281–284.
2. Brown, D. L. Anesthetic risk: a historical perspective. In Brown, D. L. (ed.) *Risk and Outcome in Anesthesia.* Philadelphia: J. B. Lippincott Co., 1988.
3. Derrington, M. C. & Smith, G. A review of anesthetic risk, morbidity, and mortality. *Br. J. Anaesth.* 1987; **59**: 815–833.
4. Farrow, S. C., Fowkes, F. G. R., Lunn, J. N., Robertson, I. B., & Samuel, P. Epidemiology in anaesthesia II: Factors affecting mortality in hospital. *Br. J. Anaesth.* 1982; **54**: 811–816.
5. Fowkes, S. C., Fowkes, F. G. R., Lunn, J. N., Robertson, I. B., & Samuel, P. Epidemiology in anaesthesia III: factors affecting mortality in hospitals. *Br. J. Anaesth.* 1982; **54**: 811–816.
6. Goldstein, A. & Keats, A. S. The risk of anesthesia. *Anesthesiology* 1970; **33**: 130–143.
7. Lunn, J. N., Farrow, S. C., Fowkes, F. G. R., Robertson, I. B., & Samuel, P. Epidemiology in anaesthesia I: Anaesthetic prac-tice over 20 years. *Br. J. Anaesth.* 1982; **54**: 803–809.
8. Lunn, J. N., Hunter, A. R., & Scott, D. B. Anesthesia-related surgical mortality. *Anaesthesia* 1983; **38**: 1090–1096.
9. Vacanti, C. J., VanHouten, R. J., & Hill, R. C. A statistical analy-sis of the relationship of physical status to postoperative mor-tality in 68,388 cases. *Anesth. Analg.* 1970; **49**: 564–566.
10. Keats, A. S. Anesthesia mortality in perspective. *Anesth. Analg.* 1990; **70**: 113–119.
11. Rao, T. L. K., Jacobs, K. H., & El-Etr, A. A. Reinfarction following anesthesia in patients with myocardial infarction. *Anesthesiology* 1983; **59**: 499–505.
12. Dripps, R. D., Lamont, A., & Eckenhoff, J. E. The role of anesthesia in surgical mortality. *J. Am. Med. Assoc.* 1961; **178**: 261–266.
13. Marx, G. F., Mateo, C. V., & Orkin, L. R. Computer analysis of postanesthetic deaths. *Anesthesiology* 1973; **39**: 54–58.
14. Carter, D. C. & Campbell, D. Evaluation of the risks of surgery. *Br. Med. Bull.* 1988; **44**: 322–340.
15. Apfelbaum, J. L. Preoperative evaluation, laboratory screen-ing, and selection of adult surgical outpatients in the 1990s. *Anesthesiol. Rev.* 1990; **17**: 4–12.
16. Meridy, H. W. Criteria for selection of ambulatory surgical patients and guidelines for anesthetic management: a retro-spective study of 1553 cases. *Anesth. Analg.* 1982; **61**: 921–926.
17. Fleisher, L. A. Applying the new AHA\ACC perioperative car-diovascular evaluation guidelines to the elderly outpatient. 2002. SAMBA.
18. Fischer, S. P. Development and effectiveness of an anesthesia preoperative evaluation clinic in a teaching hospital. *Anesthesiology* 1996; **85**: 196–206.
19. Arellano, R., Cruise, C., & Chung, F. Timing of the anesthetist's preoperative outpatient interview. *Anesth. Analg.* 1989; **68**: 645–648.
20. Rosenblatt, M. A., Bradford, C., Miller, R., & Zahl, K. A preopera-tive interview by an anesthesiologist does not lower preopera-tive anxiety in outpatients. *Anesthesiology* 1989; **71**: A926.
21. Twersky, R. S., Frank, D., & Lebovits, A. Timing of preoperative evaluation for surgical outpatients – does it matter? Part II. *Anesthesiology* 1990; **73**: A1.
22. *American Society of Anesthesiologists Task Force on Preoperative Evaluation.* Practice Advisory for Preoperative Evaluation. *Anesthesiology* 2002; **96**: 485–496.
23. Korvin, C. C., Pearce, R. H., & Stanley, J. Admissions screening: clinical benefits. *Ann. Intern. Med.* 1975; **83**: 197–203.
24. Robbins, J. A. & Mushlin, A. I. Preoperative evaluation of the healthy patient. *Med. Clin. North Am.* 1979; **63**: 1145–1156.
25. Kaplan, E. B., Sheiner, L. B., Boeckman, A. J. *et al.* The useful-ness of preoperative laboratory testing. *J. Am. Med. Assoc.* 1985; **253**: 3576–3581.
26. Turnbull, J. M. & Buck, C. The value of preoperative screening investigations in otherwise healthy individuals. *Arch. Intern. Med.* 1987; **147**: 1101–1105.
27. Kitz, D. S., Slusarz-Ladden, C., & Lecky, J. H. Hospital resources used for inpatient and ambulatory surgery. *Anesthesiology* 1988; **69**: 383–386.
28. Zilva, J. F. Is unselective urine biochemical urine testing cost effective? *Br. Med. J.* 1985; **291**: 323–325.
29. Lawrence, V. A., Gafni, A., & Gross, M. The unproven utility of the preoperative urinalysis: economic evaluation. *J. Clin. Epidemiol.* 1989; 1185–1191.
30. Rucker, L., Frye, B. D., & Staten, M. A. Usefulness of chest roentgenograms in preoperative patients. *J. Am. Med. Assoc.* 1983; **250**: 3209–3211.

31. Charpak, Y., Blery, C., Chastang, C., Szatan, M., & Fourgeaux, B. Prospective assessment of a protocol for selective ordering of preoperative chest X-rays. *Can. J. Anaesth.* 1988; **35**: 259–264.

32. Hackman, T. & Steward, D. J. What is the value of preoperative hemoglobin determinations in pediatric outpatients? *Anesthesiology* 1989; **71**: A1168.

33. O'Conner, M. E. & Drasner, K. Preoperative laboratory testing of children undergoing elective surgery. *Anesth. Analg.* 1990; **70**: 176–180.

34. Bold, A. M. & Currin, B. Use and abuse of clinical chemistry in surgery. *Br. Med. J.* 1965; **2**: 1051–1052.

35. Zibrak, J. D., O'Donnell, C. R., & Marton, K. Indications for pulmonary function testing. *Ann. Intern. Med.* 1990; **112**: 763–771.

36. Baram, D., Smith, C., & Stinson, S. Intraoperative topical etidocaine for reducing postoperative pain after laparoscopic tubal ligation. *J. Reprod. Med.* 1990; **35**: 407.

37. Baughman, V. L., Becker, G. L., Ryan, C. M. *et al.* Effectiveness of triazolam, diazepam, and placebo as preanesthetic medications. *Anesthesiology* 1989; **71**: 196.

38. Baysinger, C. L. *et al.* Brachial plexus blockade and general anesthesia for carpal tunnel release in ambulatory patients. *Proceedings of the Fifth Annual SAMBA Conference*, Baltimore, 1990 (abstract).

39. Boldt, H. J. The management of laparotomy patients and their modified after-treatment. *NY Med. J.* 1907; **85**: 145.

40. Bowe, E. A., Baysinger, C. L., Sykes, L. A., & Bowe, L. S. Subarachnoid blockade versus general anesthesia for knee arthroscopy in outpatients. *Anesthesiology* 1990; **73**: A45.

41. Carbat, P. A. T. & van Crvel, H. Lumbar puncture headache: controlled study on the preventive effect of 24 hours bed rest. *Lancet* 1981; **1**: 1133.

42. Carter, J. A., Dye, A. M., & Cooper, G. M. Recovery after daycase anesthesia: the effect of different inhalational anaesthetic agents. *Anaesthesia* 1985; **40**: 545.

43. Casey, W. F., Rice, L. J., Hannallah, R. S. *et al.* A comparison between bupivacaine instillation versus ilioinguinal/iliohypogastric nerve block for postoperative analgesia following inguinal herniorrhaphy in children. *Anesthesiology* 1990; **72**: 637.

44. Cope, D. K., Sison, G. F., Wood, M. A., Cooper, W. N., & Patrissi, G. A. Impaired learning and recall after IV sedation: implications for outpatients. *Anesth. Analg.* 1990; **70**: S69.

45. Davis, W. J. Outpatient brachial plexus anesthesia. *Anesthesiology* 1990; **73**: A25.

46. Forrest, J. B., Rehder, K., Goldsmith, C. H. *et al.* Multicenter study of general anesthesia. *Anesthesiology* 1990; **72**: 252.

47. Ghoneim, M. M. & Mewaldt, S. P. Benzodiazepines and human memory: a review. *Anesthesiology* 1990; **72**: 926.

48. Lerman, J., Christensen, S. K., & Farrow-Gillespie, A. C. Effects of metoclopramide and ranitidine on gastric fluid pH and volume in children. *Anesthesiology* 1988; **69**(3A): A748.

49. Marais, M. L. *et al.* Reduced demands on recovery room resources with propofol (Diprivan) compared with thiopental-isoflurane. *Anesthesiol. Rev.* 1989; **16**: 29.

50. Mingus, M. L. *et al.* Droperidol dose-response in out-patients following alfentanil-nitrous oxide anaesthesia. *Proceedings of the Fifth Annual SAMBA Conference, Baltimore*, 1990 (abstract).

51. Mulroy, M. F. Is spinal anesthesia appropriate for outpatient? *SAMBA Newslett.* 1989; **4**: 1.

52. Narchi, P., Lecoq, G., Fernandez, H., & Benhamon, D. *et al.* Intraperitoneal local anesthetics and scapular pain following daycase laparoscopy. *Anesthesiology* 1990; **73**: A5.

53. Pandit, S. K., Kothary, S. P., Pandit, U. A. *et al.* Dose–response study of droperidol and metoclopramide as antiemetics for outpatient anesthesia. *Anesth. Analg.* 1989; **68**: 798.

54. Pandit, S. K., Kothary, S. P., Randel, G. I., & Levy, L. Recovery after outpatient anesthesia: propofol versus enflurane. *Anesthesiology* 1988; **69**: A565.

55. Parnas, S. M. *et al.* A prospective evaluation of epidural versus general anesthesia for outpatient arthroscopy. *Proceedings of the Fifth Annual SAMBA Conference*, Baltimore, 1990 (abstract).

56. Philip, B. K. Supplemental medication for ambulatory procedures under regional anesthesia. *Anesth. Analg.* 1985; **64**: 1117.

57. Randel, G. I., Levy, L., Kothary, S. P., Brousseau, M., & Pandit, S. K. Epidural anesthesia is superior to spinal or general for outpatient knee arthroscopy. *Anesthesiology* 1989; **71**: A769.

58. Raybould, D., Bradshaw, E. G. Premedication for day case surgery. *Anaesthesia* 1987; **42**: 591.

59. Rice, L. J., Pudimat, M. A., Hannallah, R. S. Timing of caudal block placement does not affect duration of postoperative analgesia in pediatric ambulatory surgical patients. *Anesthesiology* 1988; **69**: A771.

60. Rice, L. J., Binding, R. R., Vaughn, G. C., Thompson, R., & Newman, K. Intraoperative and postoperative analgesia in children undergoing inguinal herniorrhaphy: a comparison of caudal bupivacaine 0.125% and 0.25%. *Anesthesiology* 1990; **73**: A3.

61. Sampson, I. H. *et al.* Comparison of propofol and thiamylal for induction and maintenance of anaesthesia for outpatient surgery. *Br. J. Anaesth.* 1988; **61**: 707.

62. Sandhar, B. K. *et al.* The effect of oral liquids and ranitidine on gastric fluid volume and pH in children undergoing outpatient surgery. *Anesthesiology* 1989; **71**: 327.

63. Schreiner, M. S., Triebwasser, A., & Keon, T. P. Ingestion of liquids compared with preoperative fasting in pediatric outpatients. *Anesthesiology* 1990; **72**: 593.

64. Sung, Y. F., Reiss, N., & Tillette, T. The differential cost of anesthesia and recovery with propofol-nitrous oxide anesthesia versus thiopental-nitrous oxide. *Proceedings of the Fifth Annual SAMBA Conference, Baltimore*, 1990 (abstract).

65. Thornberry, E. A. & Thomas, T. A. Posture and post-spinal headache. *Br. J. Anaesth.* 1988; **60**: 195.

2

Nutrition

Joseph D. Ansley

Emory University School of Medicine, Department of Surgery, Atlanta, GA

The nutritional status of surgical patients and the metabolic response to injury are recognized as important factors in wound healing, postoperative complications, infection, and the overall recovery from surgical procedures.[1] Providing appropriate nutritional support to surgical patients can be difficult, however, because surgical disease and surgical procedures often do not allow the normal oral intake of the nutritionally complete diet that is needed to maintain adequate muscle mass, visceral proteins, and metabolism. Inadequate intake may result from obstructive lesions of the gastrointestinal tract, malabsorption, anorexia related to cancer or other debilitating conditions, postoperative ileus, or the necessity for prolonged bowel rest. A major advance in resolving the problem of inadequate nutritional intake was made by Dudrick and colleagues,[2] who developed a concentrated total parenteral nutrition (TPN) solution that could be administered through the large-caliber, high-flow central veins. This significant development has been followed by more than three decades of clinical application and additional nutritional research leading to many refinements in the composition of the solutions and to a new understanding of nutritional processes in health and disease.[3–5]

The increased knowledge and interest in nutrition resulting from the development of TPN techniques has stimulated many other nutrition-related activities and specialized research. Some of the most active and productive areas include the biochemical response to traumatic stress,[4] advances in body composition research,[5] the importance of the enteral route of nutrient administration,[6] and the potential for enhancement of the immune system with specialized diets.[7] The processes and knowledge of nutritional support that evolved from parenteral nutrition techniques have resulted in a return to the use of the gastrointestinal tract as the primary method for providing nutrition for surgical or medical patients. The methods of delivery and the dietary compounds in use today have been refined so that enteral nutrition can and should be used in most surgical patients in the perioperative period.[8,9] Enteral nutrition is less costly, more physiologic, and associated with fewer metabolic or infectious complications than TPN.[10,11]

Assessment of nutritional status

The decision to use specialized nutritional support should be based on nutritional evaluations of patients in conjunction with assessments of the expected course of the surgical diseases or procedures. Patients who are well nourished or only mildly malnourished are unlikely to require specialized nutritional support unless they are unable to resume adequate oral intake within 7 to 10 days. Patients who are moderately malnourished can benefit from nutritional support if they will have an inadequate intake for more than 3 to 5 days. Patients who are severely malnourished may benefit from specialized nutritional support for 7 to 14 days before operation. If the urgency of the procedure precludes preoperative therapy, nutritional support should be instituted within 1 to 3 days after operation. (Table 2.1)[9]

The nutritional status should be assessed using clinical information from patients' histories and physical examinations supplemented by anthropometric measurements, visceral protein measurements, and immunologic tests when available.[12] In patients with the marasmic form of protein-calorie malnutrition that is associated with starvation, clinical evaluation based on carefully performed histories and physical examinations may be sufficient for nutritional assessment.[13] A history of weight loss greater than 10% over 3 months is significant and has been shown to be of important prognostic value when it is associated with some evidence of physiologic impairment such as weakness, fatigue, or malaise.[14]

Medical Management of the Surgical Patient: A Textbook of Perioperative Medicine, ed. M. F. Lubin, R. B. Smith, T. F. Dobson, N. Spell, H. K. Walker.
4th edn. Published by Cambridge University Press. © Cambridge University 2006.

Table 2.1. Indications for nutritional intervention in the perioperative period[a]

- Inadequate nutrient intake for 7–10 days in previously well-nourished patient
- Inadequate nutrient intake for 5 days in previously well-nourished or mildly malnourished patient with acute stress
- Inadequate nutrient intake for 3 days in moderate or severely malnourished patient
- Weight loss of over 10% of preillness weight
- Preoperative supplementation for 7 to 14 days in severely malnourished patient if surgery can be safely delayed
- Therapeutic bowel rest

Note:

[a] Significant cardiopulmonary, electrolyte, and acid–base problems should be corrected first in acutely stressed patients to provide an optimal and safe metabolic state for nutrient assimilation.

Table 2.2. Nutritional assessment

	Malnutrition severity		
	Mild	Moderate	Severe
Weight loss (%)	<10	10–20	>20
Albumin (g/dl)	<3.5	<3.0	<2.0
Transferrin (mg/dl)	<220	<170	<100
Prealbumin (mg/dl)	<17	<12	<7
Total lymphocyte count (cells/mm^3)	<2000	<1500	<1000

Common equations for nutritional assessment

Nitrogen balance = 24-h protein intake/6.25 − (24-h urine urea nitrogen + 4)

Modification of the Harris–Benedict equation for basal energy expenditure (in kcal)

Women: 655 + (9.6 × weight (in kg)) + (1.7 × height (in cm)) − (4.7 × age (in years))

Men: 66 + (13.7 × weight) + (5 × height) − (6.8 × age)

Ideal body weight estimation

Women: 100 lb + 5 lb for each inch over 60

Men: 106 lb + 6 lb for each inch over 60

Anthropometric tests have been important for nutritional assessment in clinical research studies and for determining the prevalence of malnutrition but may not be helpful in the evaluation of individual patients.[15,16] Preoperative immunologic testing with delayed hypersensitivity skin tests (in combination with other laboratory tests, such as measurement of the albumin level) has been used as a prognostic indicator of postoperative sepsis and death.[17] Because such testing is relatively non-specific by itself, however, and because there is a 48-hour delay in obtaining results, it is not often used in the evaluation of individual patients. The creatinine-to-height ratio also has been shown to be a sensitive indicator of protein-calorie undernutrition in studies of hospitalized surgical patients[18] and patients with cancer.[19] It requires careful 24-hour urine collection in patients who are stable and is less useful for the evaluation of acutely stressed patients.

Measurement of the visceral proteins (albumin, transferrin, and prealbumin) and determination of the total lymphocyte count are the most useful laboratory tests in diagnosing and classifying the nutritional status in patients with the hypoalbuminemic form of protein-calorie malnutrition. This type of malnutrition is seen most often in hospitalized patients today. It is less clinically recognizable than the marasmic form of malnutrition because weight loss may not be present despite severe depletion of the visceral protein stores.[20] When evaluating visceral protein values, those obtained before surgical intervention, significant stress, or the administration of intravenous fluid or blood have greater prognostic value. Albumin particularly,[21] and transferrin and prealbumin to a lesser degree are decreased with fluid hydration and the acute stress of trauma.[22] The shorter half-life of prealbumin may make

it potentially more useful in demonstrating an early response to nutritional therapy. From a practical standpoint, most hospitalized patients can be properly assessed from a careful history and physical examination combined with measurement of one or more of the visceral proteins (Table 2.2).

Once the need for nutritional support has been determined, calorie and protein requirements must be assessed based on energy expenditure and level of stress. The Harris–Benedict equation for basal energy expenditure (BEE; see Table 2.2) is reliable for initial therapy when the correct stress level modifier is used (1.2 × BEE for mild stress to 1.75 × BEE for moderate to severe stress).[23] More specific energy requirements can be determined using indirect calorimetry[24] to measure oxygen consumption when the study is performed by trained personnel and and the information obtained is interpreted properly.[25] Protein requirements can be estimated from patient weight and level of stress, using 0.8 g/kg for maintenance, 1.5 g/kg for moderate stress, and 2 g/kg for severe stress. Nitrogen balance studies are useful in monitoring patient response to therapy. The 24-hour urine urea nitrogen excretion is used most commonly for this determination, with the addition of a factor of 4 for unmeasured urine nitrogen and extrarenal nitrogen loss. Total urinary nitrogen determination provides a more specific value for nitrogen excretion but is not performed by all clinical laboratories.[26]

Indications for perioperative nutritional support

Although specialized nutritional support is considered important in patients who cannot meet their nutrient requirements by oral intake, the specific questions of when, to whom and how to provide this support remains controversial. An early meta-analysis of perioperative parenteral nutrition from reports published through 1986 did not indicate a benefit for unselected patients undergoing major surgery, but did suggest that nutritional support would be helpful in subgroups at high risk, such as severely malnourished patients.[27] Another study that randomly assigned patients to receive TPN or standard nutrition before operation reached a similar conclusion. The study showed similar rates of major postoperative complications in both groups but more infectious complications in those patients receiving TPN who were well nourished or only mildly malnourished before operation. In contrast, patients receiving TPN who were severely malnourished before operation had fewer non-infectious complications and were the only subgroup to benefit from the nutritional therapy.[28] A later economic analysis from the same trial, however, found that there was no decrease in the cost of care for any subgroup of patients receiving TPN.[29]

Another appraisal of this controversy reviewed both perioperative enteral nutritional and perioperative TPN, and concluded that perioperative nutritional support in properly selected groups of patients with overt malnutrition can be medically effective and reduce morbidity and mortality.[30] In a more recent meta-analysis of TPN compared to standard care in critically ill patients there was no effect on mortality but there was an association with lower complication rates in malnourished patients.[31]

These studies should not be used to negate the value of perioperative nutritional support but to indicate that patients should be selected for such therapy based on careful perioperative nutritional assessment and consideration of the expected stress factors related to the disease or procedure and the expected time before adequate oral nutrition can be provided. In addition, patients should receive the method and type of nutritional support that is associated with the fewest complications and the lowest cost while providing the most effective and physiologic nutritional repletion.

Methods of nutritional support

Enteral nutrition

Nutritional support should be given through the gastrointestinal tract whenever possible because of the benefits

Table 2.3. Types of enteral nutrition formulas

Oral supplements

Palatable clear liquid type diet with added protein, minerals and vitamins. Fat free. Use to supplement clear liquid diet for short period of time. Not nutritionally complete.

Examples: Boost Breeze, NuBasics

Palatable full liquid type diet with intact protein, carbohydrate, fat, minerals, and vitamins. Low residue and lactose free and considered nutritionally complete.

Examples: Boost, Ensure, NuBasics

Enteral tube feeding

Intact protein, lactose free, low residue, low to moderate osmolality, nutritionally complete diet.

Examples: Osmolite, Isocal, Nutren, Isosource

Intact protein, lactose free, low residue, moderate to high osmolality, nutritionally complete diet.

Examples: Magnacal, Nutren 2.0, TwoCal HN, Nova Source 2.0

Intact protein, lactose free, low osmolality, with added fiber nutritionally complete diet.

Examples: Jevity, Ultracal

Protein as peptides and free amino acids, lactose free, low residue, low to moderate osmolality nutritionally complete diet.

Examples: Crucial, Peptamen, Subdue, Optimental

Protein as free amino acids, lactose free, low residue, low fat with high osmolality.

Examples: Vivonex TEN

Intact protein with supplemental arginine, omega-3 fatty acids and nucleotides.Lactose free, low residue nutritionally complete diet.

Examples: Impact, Crucial

Intact protein, low-carbohydrate, calorically dense with eicosapentaenoic acid and gamma-linolenic acid and antioxidants to modulate the inflammatory response in critically ill patients with ARDS.

Example: Oxepa

Low or high protein, low or high calorie variations of the diets above are available to help meet the various needs of most patients.

of maintaining gastrointestinal structure and function in enhancing the utilization of nutrients, and because such nutrition is easier and safer to administer and costs less.[9] This can often be accomplished with oral supplements in conscious patients who are capable of swallowing adequate amounts of one of the many nutritional formulas that are available (Table 2.3). Consultation with a dietitian who is knowledgeable regarding the many types of formulas available is important to obtain patient compliance and ensure that the formula used is nutritionally complete and meets patient needs.

If oral supplementation is not possible or adequate in amount, other methods of enteral tube feeding should be used (Table 2.4). Most medical and surgical patients can

Table 2.4. Methods of enteral nutritional support

Oral supplements
  Nutritionally complete
  Modular
Enteral feeding with small-bore tube (8 or 10 french)
  Nasogastric
  Nasoduodenal
  Nasojejunal
Gastrostomy
  Percutaneous endoscopic gastrostomy
  Percutaneous radiologic gastrostomy
  Surgical gastrostomy
Jejunostomy
  Percutaneous gastrojejunostomy
  Surgical needle catheter jejunostomy
  Surgical 14F to 16F tube jejunostomy
Parenteral feeding
  Peripheral intravenous
  Central intravenous
Combined enteral and parenteral feeding

Table 2.5. Complications of enteral feeding

Mechanical (tube-related) complications
Erosions of nares, otitis media, oropharyngeal erosions: incidence decreased by use of small-bore flexible feeding tubes properly placed and affixed to patient's cheek.
Occlusion of tube: incidence decreased by use of mechanical pumps, frequent irrigation of tube with water, and use of prepared commercial formulas.
Pulmonary aspiration: incidence decreased by elevation of head of bed, use of small-bore feeding tubes, frequent checks for increased gastric residual, and use of jejunostomy feedings in patients at high risk for aspiration.
Incorrect placement of feeding tube: obtain radiograph to verify position of tube in gastrointestinal tract before initiating feeding and verify enteric contents frequently by checking residual volume.

Gastrointestinal complications
Abdominal pain, cramping, nausea, and diarrhea: incidence decreased by slow, stepwise progression in formula infusion rate or concentration; may require change in formula type; also may be related to concomitant medications, particularly antibiotics.
Small bowel necrosis: associated with use of vasopressors for hypotension, inadequate resuscitation, or rapid advancement of tube feeding rate. Must assess patient frequently when feeding into the jejunum.

Metabolic complications
Less frequent than with parenteral nutrition, but patient needs to be monitored for glucose intolerance and electrolyte abnormalities, with particular attention to the need for free water.

be fed through nasogastric or nasoenteric tubes using small catheters and appropriate feeding solutions.[32,33] These enteral feeding tubes usually can be placed successfully by experienced personnel and have been associated with less discomfort and fewer complications than have large-bore nasogastric tubes used for decompression of the stomach (Table 2.5). In conscious patients with no history of swallowing difficulties or gastroesophageal reflux and for whom the head of the bed can be elevated 30 degrees, flexible small-bore nasogastric feeding tubes can be used to infuse the nutrient solution into the stomach. In patients who are thought to be a higher risk for gastroesophageal reflux and possible pulmonary aspiration, nasoduodenal or nasojejunal tubes should be placed. Some techniques use stylets in the feeding tube, which may help in directing the end of the tube into the duodenum.[34] In other techniques, patients are positioned with their right sides down to allow peristalsis to carry the weighted end of the tube into the duodenum and jejunum. Stimulation of gastric peristalsis with metoclopramide or erythromycin has also improved the rate of successful enteral placement of these tubes in some studies.[35] When these techniques are not successful, manipulation under fluoroscopy by an experienced radiologist or endoscopic manipulation by an endoscopist can facilitate proper tube placement into the duodenum.

If prolonged enteral feeding is anticipated, newer procedures that have been developed using endoscopic or radiologic techniques that can be used for the placement of percutaneous gastrostomy or gastrojejunostomy feeding tubes.[33] Surgeons should also consider intraoperative placement of feeding tubes if patients are not expected to be able to resume adequate oral intake within an appropriate length of time after operation or if they have preexisting moderate or severe malnutrition. If enteral feeding is believed to be a temporary measure, surgeons can have the anesthetist place a nasoenteric tube into the stomach which is then manually placed in the duodenum or jejunum by the surgeon.

Surgeons may also consider placing a Stamm gastrostomy tube or feeding jejunostomy tube for prolonged enteral feeding. In constructing a jejunostomy, either the needle catheter technique[36] or the Witzel technique using a 14F to 16F catheter maybe used. With the latter technique, the catheter is less likely to be occluded by the feeding solution and should last longer.[37]

Enteral feeding formulas have been developed that vary in caloric density, protein complexity and content, fat content, osmolarity, and cost. Most patients will benefit

Table 2.6. Protocol for enteral tube feeding

Nasogastric route: Use small-bore, flexible tube (8F preferred); obtain radiograph after placement to confirm position.

Elevate head of bed at least 30 degrees.

Use feeding pump for continuous feeding.

Begin with full-strength formula at 25 to 30 ml/h and, if tolerated, increase by 25 to 30 ml/h at 12-hour intervals until desired total volume is reached.[a]

Check gastric residuals every 4 hours; if greater than 100 ml, hold feeding and repeat at hourly intervals until residuals are less than 100 ml before resuming feeding.

Irrigate with 30 to 50 ml of water after each residual check or after any medications are given. (If patient requires additional free water, use greater volumes of water for irrigation.)

If patient experiences diarrhea or intestinal cramping, slow rate of feeding or decrease concentration of formula.

Note:

[a] When using hypertonic formulas or feeding into the jejunum with a nasojejunal or jejunostomy tube, diluting the formula to one-half or three-quarter strength may improve tolerance initially. The concentration can then be increased after the desired volume is reached.

from one of the standard prepared enteral feeding formulas (see Table 2.3). These ready-to-use formulas are polymeric, containing intact protein, complex carbohydrates, long- and medium-chain triglycerides, vitamins, and trace elements. They are low in residue and lactose-free. Those formulas are isotonic or slightly hypertonic, with a choice of normal or high nitrogen content, and can be obtained with a caloric content of 1 to 2 kcal/ml. These polymeric formulas are usually tolerated as well as, or better than, the more expensive elemental or peptide-based formulas.[38,39]

Over the past decade specialized enteral diets have become available which may enhance immune function in certain clinical situations. These diets are supplemented with one or more of the immunonutrients (arginine, glutamine, nucleotides, and omega-3 fatty acids). There remains controversy as to what concentration and what combination of these immunonutrients is most effective and some concern that in some subgroups of septic critically ill patients they may be harmful[40] so they should be used with close monitoring.

These solutions can be administered into the stomach beginning at a rate of 25 to 30 ml/h and increasing by the same amount every 12 to 24 hours until the final desired volume that meets patient needs is reached. If abdominal cramping, diarrhea, or elevated gastric residuals develop, feeding is stopped and resumed later at a lower rate or at a lower concentration of formula (Table 2.6). The efficiency

Table 2.7. Complications of total parenteral nutrition

Mechanical (catheter-related) complications

Pneumothorax

Hydrothorax

Arterial injury

Arteriovenous fistula

Cardiac arrhythmias

Air embolism

Vein thrombosis

Pulmonary embolism

Decrease incidence with proper technique of catheter insertion and management. Initial chest radiograph to confirm proper position and detect pneumothorax or pleural fluid. Daily clinical examination with repeated radiograph as indicated.

Sepsis

Bacterial

Fungal

Decrease incidence with proper sterile technique of catheter insertion and catheter care protocol for dressing changes and intravenous tubing changes. Maintain line for total parenteral nutrition only.

Metabolic complications

Hyperglycemia or hypoglycemia

Electrolyte abnormality

Acid-base disorder

Azotemia

Hyperphosphatemia or hypophosphatemia

Hypermagnesemia or hypomagnesemia

Elevated liver test from hepatic steatosis

Essential fatty acid, vitamin, or trace element deficiency

Decrease incidence with careful adjustments of total parenteral nutrition formula and careful monitoring of fluid balance and laboratory values. Avoid excess dextrose. Obtain blood levels for essential fatty acids, vitamins, and trace elements when total parenteral nutrition is continued for a prolonged time.

of enteral feeding has been shown to be improved by the use of a protocol for progression of the rate or concentration of the formula.[41] If the feeding tube is in the jejunum, a similar protocol is followed except that it may be necessary to start with more dilute, half-strength formula to improve tolerance. After the desired volume is obtained, the concentration may be increased to three-quarter strength formula and then to full-strength formula in a stepwise manner. It usually takes 3 to 5 days to reach the desired volume of the nutrient formula with either technique.

The most common complication of enteral feeding that interferes with provision of the desired nutrient volume is diarrhea (See Table 2.7). This can usually be controlled by adjusting the rate of concentration of the solution. Adjustments in the formula type may be necessary because some patients are more tolerant of the peptide-based formulas or the peptide/elemental formulas. Other patients tolerate enteral feeding better when fiber is included in the formula.[42] In addition, medications, particularly those containing sorbitol that are given with the tube feeding and antibiotics, can cause diarrhea. Antibiotic-associated diarrhea frequently results from bacterial over-growth with *Clostridium difficile*, which requires specific therapy with oral metronidazole in most cases or oral vancomycin in resistant cases.[43] If adjustments in the formula type, osmolarity, or fiber content do not correct the excessive diarrhea (more than three stools per day) and the results of stool cultures and C difficile titers are negative, antidiarrheal medications may be instituted cautiously using kaolin-pectin first and then paregoric or lopermide if necessary.[44] Another particularly severe complication of feeding into the small bowel beyond the duodenum is that of small bowel necrosis. This particular problem is difficult to predict or recognize but is usually associated with the use of vasopressors, inadequate resuscitation, or rapid advancement of tube feeding rates.[45]

Peripheral parenteral nutrition

If the gastrointestinal tract cannot or should not be used for nutritional support, parenteral nutrition is indicated. Patients who require maintenance nutritional therapy for only a short time and in whom fluid volume tolerance is not a concern can be given peripheral parenteral nutrition.[46] Fifteen hundred to 1800 kcal can be provided, along with 50 to 70 mg of protein, electrolytes, and vitamins in 2.5 to 3 l of intravenous fluid per day. Most of the calories given are derived from a 20% lipid emulsion that provides 1000 kcal/500 ml; additional calories are provided by 5% dextrose solution. The protein and electrolyte solution should have an osmolarity less than 900 and is better tolerated in the peripheral venous system when it is given simultaneously with the lipid emulsion via a Y-connector or as an all-in-one solution of dextrose, protein, electrolyte and lipid emulsion. Also for short-term nutritional support a commercially prepared peripheral nutrition solution containing 3% amino acids, 3% glycerol as a lower osmolar energy source (replacing glucose), and electrolytes can be given simultaneously with a lipid emulsion in patients. In a study of patients who had undergone major trauma or surgery it was found that the glycerol caused no adverse effects and that nitrogen balance was maintained near equilibrium over a period of 5 days.[47]

These peripheral parenteral nutrition solutions may also be used to supplement enteral nutrition when only a low volume or concentration of enteral feeding is tolerated that does not meet patient requirements. Using this approach, patients gain the benefits of the trophic effect of enteral feeding on the intestine and are ensured of receiving adequate total nutrition.

Total parenteral nutrition

If enteral feeding cannot be used because of an inadequately functioning gastrointestinal tract or if nutritional requirements exceed the amount that can be given by peripheral vein, TPN is indicated. Hyperosmolar concentrated feeding solutions containing dextrose, amino acids, minerals, vitamins, and trace elements can be infused into a large caliber, high-flow central vein. Techniques for cannulation of the central veins are well described and have low complication rates in experienced hands[48]. The procedure should be performed in a sterile manner using caps, masks, gowns, gloves, and appropriate skin preparation and draping. The potential technical complications are pneumothorax, arterial puncture, arterio-venous fistula, poor catheter placement, and air embolism which should be explained to patients, along with the potential for later catheter sepsis and appropriate consent should be obtained. The infraclavicular subclavian vein approach is preferred by most physicians because of the greater ability to maintain an intact sterile dressing in this area compared to the neck, where movement is more frequent. Strict maintenance of this hyperalimentation line using specific guidelines for catheter care,[49,50] dressing changes,[51] line changes,[52] and nursing care[50] are important to reduce technical complications, and catheter sepsis. The use of multiple-lumen intravenous catheters for TPN has been controversial but appears to be safe if a standard protocol is followed, maintaining only one lumen for the hyperalimentation fluid.[53] Catheter sepsis is a major problem in patients receiving TPN. When it occurs, the catheter should be removed and central venous access obtained at a different site with a new catheter. Because some patients receiving TPN may have other potential sources of sepsis, it may be acceptable to change the catheter over a guide wire in patients with difficult venous access. The catheter tip is cultured to determined whether infection is present and the intravenous site is moved to a new area only if the culture results are positive.

Parenteral solutions

The ability to adjust the concentration of the solution given through a central venous catheter provides greater flexibility in the volume that can be administered and in the amounts of dextrose, amino acids, minerals, vitamins,

Table 2.8. Parenteral nutritional requirements

Water	1 ml/kcal
Calories	25–35 kcal/kg/d
Carbohydrate	4 mg/kg/min/d
	50%–60% total calories
Fat	20–30% total calories
Protein	0.8–2.0 g/kg/d
Essential fatty acids	4% total calories
Minerals	
Na^+	60–120 meq/d
K^+	60–100 meq/d
Cl^-	60–120 meq/d
Mg^{2+}	8–10 meq/d
Ca^{2+}	200–400 mg/d
Phosphorus	300–400 mg/d
Trace elements	
Zinc	2.5–4.0 mg/d
Copper	0.5–1.5 mg/d
Chromium	10.0–15.0 µg/d
Manganese	0.1–0.8 mg/d
Selenium	20.0–40.0 µg/d
Vitamins	
Fat-soluble	
A	3330.0 IU
D	200.0 IU
E	10.0 IU
K	5.0 mg/wk
Water-soluble	
B_1	3.0 mg
B_2	3.6 mg
Pantothenic acid	15.0 mg
Niacin	40.0 mg
B6	4.0 mg
Biotin	60.0 µg
Folic acid	400 µg
B_{12}	5.0 µg
C	100.0 mg

Table 2.9. Total parenteral nutrition formula for a 24-hour period

Volume	2000 ml
Dextrose	300 g
Protein	100 g
Sodium	70 meq
Potassium	80 meq
Calcium	9 meq
Magnesium	10 meq
Phosphorus	24 mM
Chloride	70 meq
Acetate	207 meq
MVI-12	10 ml
MTE-4	3 ml
Phytonadione	1 mg
Kilocalories from	
Dextrose	1020 (3.4×300)
Protein	400 (4.0×100)
Total	1420
If 20% lipid emulsion (300 ml) added	600 (2×300)
Total	2020

Acetate content varies with different amino acid solutions used.

Adjustments in the amount of protein, electrolytes, and minerals are necessary for special disease states such as renal insufficiency and hepatic insufficiency.

MVI-12 contains recommended amounts of fat-soluble and water-soluble vitamins except vitamin K (phytonadione), which is added separately.

MTE-4 contains the trace elements zinc 5 mg. Copper 1 mg, manganese 0.5 mg, and chromium 10 µg. Selenium 20 µg is recommended for long-term total parenteral nutrition.

Protein sources include 8.5% to 10% amino acid solutions such as Travasol, Aminosyn, and Freamine-III. These are mixed in pharmacies with the components listed above.

and trace elements that can be included in the formula (Table 2.8). This flexibility is limited primarily by the pharmacologic properties of the individual components: their stability in solution and potential incompatibilities that can lead to precipitation. Calcium, phosphorus, and magnesium in particular precipitate if their concentrations are not compatible. It is essential that pharmacists experienced with nutritional support and the compounding of nutrient solutions determine that a formula meets patient needs and supervise the proper compounding of these solutions under sterile conditions to ensure their safety and effectiveness.

Most patients who receive TPN require a balanced-fuel formula, with 20% to 30% of calories from fat, 15% to 20% from protein and 50% to 65% from dextrose (Table 2.9). The lipid emulsion can be given as a separate infusion either peripherally or centrally, although many hospitals combine all the ingredients into one container for infusion over 24 hours. This total nutrient admixture system may be time-saving and cost-effective from the pharmacy and nursing standpoint. There does not appear to be an increased risk of infection even though an inline bacterial filter is not used with this method.[54] It is especially important that all the components and concentrations of this total nutrient admixture solution be compatible, however, because any precipitation that occurs will be obscured by the lipid emulsion.

Monitoring

Monitoring of the clinical status and laboratory values is important for patients receiving TPN to allow metabolic

Table 2.10. Recommended monitoring for parenteral nutrition

Parameter	Frequency
Weight	Daily
Intake and output	On each shift daily
Vital signs	On each shift daily
Blood tests	
Glucose Electrolytes Blood urea nitrogen Creatinine	Daily until stable, then every other day
Calcium Phosphorus Magnesium	Daily until stable then twice a week
Alkaline phosphatase Bilirubin	Twice a week
Hemoglobin Triglycerides Albumin Prealbumin	Once a week
24-hour urine for urine urea nitrogen to determine nitrogen balance	Once a week

abnormalities to be recognized and corrected.[55] Patient weight, intake, output, and vital signs must be observed closely each day. The blood glucose level should be determined using a chemstrip or urine glucose test every 6 hours (or more often) as indicated. Serum electrolyte, phosphorus, magnesium, calcium, creatinine, and blood urea nitrogen levels should be obtained daily for the first 3 or 4 days until they are stable and then every other day or twice a week thereafter. Liver enzymes and serum triglyceride levels should be measured on a weekly basis. A 24-hour urine collection for urine urea nitrogen or total urine nitrogen should be performed so that a nitrogen balance can be calculated weekly (Table 2.10).

Any abnormal test results should be addressed by changing the quantity or concentration of TPN ingredients and in some instances to totally deleting a component. The most common adjustment made is alteration of the dextrose content to correct hyperglycemia; the amount of dextrose can be decreased or insulin can be added to the solution. Recent studies have shown that intensive insulin therapy to maintain the blood glucose in a normal range can reduce morbidity and mortality in critically ill patients in the surgical critical care unit.[56] Other changes in electrolyte and mineral content (particularly potassium, phosphorus, and magnesium) are often necessary because of the increase in metabolic processes, which may result in rapid utilization of these components. The lipid emulsion should be deleted in patients who develop hypertriglyceridemia until their levels return to normal. If triglyceride levels remain high, the lipid emulsion can be given slowly over a 24-hour period once a week to supply essential fatty acids.

When giving the TPN solution, a steady infusion rate should be maintained; if the volume given falls behind, no attempt should be made to catch up. If the solution runs out or if intravenous access is lost, a solution of 5% or 10% dextrose should be infused to prevent the potential danger of hypoglycemia.

During the early experience with TPN, it was generally believed that patients should be fed as much solution as possible. In recent years, however, the potential dangers of overfeeding have been recognized increasingly. One of these problems is hepatic steatosis, which is related in most cases to excessive caloric intake, primarily with dextrose.[57,58] Another potential problem of overfeeding with excess dextrose is the associated increase in CO_2 production, which may interfere with the weaning of patients from artificial ventilation and adds an additional physiologic stress.[59]

Some patients receiving prolonged hyperalimentation develop liver test abnormalities that do not respond to adjustments in the amount of dextrose and total calories administered. These patients may benefit from the use of a cyclic hyperalimentation protocol in which the total nutritional requirement is given over 12 to 16 hours and no intravenous nutrition is provided for the remaining 8 to 12 hours. This method is suggested to improve fat mobilization and visceral protein synthesis in the liver by simulating the physiologic meal profile of nutrients.[60] This cyclic hyperalimentation is used in many patients who are receiving hyperalimentation at home. In addition to the potential metabolic benefits, it also has the psychological benefit of freeing patients from the infusion apparatus for a certain period.

In patients with specific disease conditions, the amount of nutrients in the parenteral solution must be altered to prevent possible toxicity from excessive protein or minerals. Protein, potassium, phosphorus, magnesium, and trace elements often need to be restricted in patients with acute renal insufficiency, and blood levels should be monitored closely to prevent toxicity. In patients who are undergoing dialysis, greater amounts of protein and minerals can be given but blood levels still must be observed closely. Optimal non-protein calories can be given with concentrated dextrose and lipid emulsions in limited volumes if fluid restriction is necessary.

Patients with hepatic insufficiency need to be monitored for protein intolerance and electrolyte abnormalities. Most patients with liver disease tolerate standard proteins at maintenance levels with an appropriate amount of non-protein calories. In patients with hepatic encephalopathy who do not respond to medical therapy, it may be necessary to use a liver-specific mixture of amino acids with lower aromatic and higher branched-chain amino acids, although the benefit remains controversial.[61]

Patients with cancer are frequently malnourished and may require nutritional support after surgical procedures or during radiotherapy or chemotherapy, but they may not restore lean body mass efficiently. Preoperative nutritional therapy may reduce the risk of postoperative complications in properly selected patients who are malnourished but are not terminal and are expected to respond to therapy.[62]

Recent experimental work has examined specific nutrient substances that may improve the efficiency of nutritional repletion in acutely stressed patients. Glutamine supplementation of parenteral nutrition formulas improved nitrogen balance in patients undergoing bone marrow transplantation in one study[63] and may improve the recovery of the intestine from starvation atrophy.[64]

Nutritional support teams

As the provision of nutritional support has become more complex during the past two decades, many hospitals have established nutritional support teams to improve efficiency and reduce complications. These teams bring together the expertise of several different specialty areas. In addition to physicians, the teams should include clinical pharmacists, nurse clinicians with the interest in direct patient care and infection control, registered dietitians, and others with a special interest in the assessment of nutritional states and the provision of optimal nutrient repletion. A decrease in metabolic and technical complications has been demonstrated when a nutrition support team either provides consultative services or takes over the complete care and provision of nutritional therapy. All members of the team should participate in the evaluation and treatment of patients and in the development of protocols for provision of care. In addition, members can inform their colleagues on the team of new scientific developments and products in their areas of expertise within the expanding field of nutritional support.

REFERENCES

1. Cuthbertson, D. The metabolic response to injury and its nutritional implications: retrospect and prospect. *J. Parenteral Enteral Nutr.* 1979; **3**: 108.
2. Dudrick, S., Wilmore, D., Vars, H., & Rhoads, J. Long-term total parenteral nutrition with growth, development, and positive nitrogen balance. *Surgery* 1968; **64**: 134.
3. Moore, F. Energy and the maintenance of the body cell mass. *J. Parenteral Enteral Nutr.* 1980; **4**: 228.
4. Gilder, H. Parenteral nourishment of patients undergoing surgical or traumatic stress. *J. Parenteral Enteral Nutr.* 1986; **10**: 88.
5. Hill, G. Body composition research: implications for the practice of clinical nutrition. *J. Parenteral Enteral Nutr.* 1992; **16**: 197.
6. Kudsk, K., Croce, M., Fabian, T. *et al.* Enteral versus parenteral feeding: effects on septic morbidity after blunt and penetrating abdominal trauma. *Ann. Surg.* 1992; **215**: 503.
7. Suchner, U., Kuhn, K., & Furst, P. The scientific basis of immunonutrition. *Proc. Nutrit. Soc.* 2000; **59**: 553.
8. McClave, S., Lowen, C., & Snider, H. Immunonutrition and enteral hyperalimentation of critically ill patients. *Dig. Dis. Sci.* 1992; **37**: 1153.
9. A.S.P.E.N. Board of Directors and Clinical Guidelines Task Force. Guidelines for the use of parenteral and enteral nutrition in adult and pediatric patients. J. Parenteral Enteral Nutr. 2002; 26.
10. Heymsfield, S., Bethal, R., Ansley, J. *et al.* Enteral hyperalimentation: an alternative to central venous hyperalimentation. *Ann. Intern. Med.* 1979; **90**: 63.
11. Parrish, C. Enteral feeding: the art and the science. *Nutr. Clin. Pract.* 2003; **18**: 76.
12. Blackburn, G., Bistrian, B., Maini, B. *et al.* Nutritional and metabolic assessment of the hospitalized patient. *J. Parenteral Enteral Nutr.* 1977; **1**: 11.
13. Baker, J., Detsky, A., Wesson, D. *et al.* Nutritional assessment: a comparison of clinical judgment and objective measurements. *N. Engl. J. Med.* 1982; **306**: 969.
14. Windsor, J. & Hill, G. Weight loss with physiologic impairment: basic indicator of surgical risk. *Ann. Surg.* 1988; **207**: 290.
15. Bistrian, B., Blackburn, G., Hallowell, E. *et al.* Protein status of general surgical patients. *J. Am. Med. Assoc.* 1974; **230**: 858.
16. Bistrian, B., Blackburn, G., Vitale, J. *et al.* Prevalence of malnutrition in general medical patients. *J. Am. Med. Assoc.* 1976; **235**: 1567.
17. Christou, N., Tellado-Rodriguez, J., Chartrand, L. *et al.* Estimating mortality risk in preoperative patients using immunologic, nutritional, and acute-phase response variables. *Ann. Surg.* 1989; **210**: 69.
18. Bistrian, B., Blackburn, G., Sherman, M. *et al.* Therapeutic index of nutritional depletion in hospitalized patients. *Gynecol. Obstet.* 1975; **141**: 512.
19. Nixon, D., Heymsfield, S., Cohen, A. *et al.* Protein-caloric undernutrition in hospitalized cancer patients. *Am. J. Med.* 1980; **68**: 683.
20. McClave, S., Mitoraj, T., Thielmeier, K. *et al.* Differentiating subtypes (hypoalbuminemic vs. marasmic) of protein-calorie

malnutrition: incidence and clinical significance in a university hospital setting. *J. Parenteral Enteral Nutr.* 1992; **16**: 337.

21. Dahn, M., Jacobs, L., Smith, S. *et al.* The significance of hypoalbuminemia following injury and infection. *Am. Surg.* 1985; **51**: 340.

22. Sun, X., Iles, M., & Weissman, C. Physiologic variables and fluid resuscitation in the postoperative intensive care unit patient. *Crit. Care Med.* 1993; **21**: 555.

23. Van Way, III C. Variability of the Harris–Benedict equation in recently published textbooks. *J. Parenteral Enteral Nutr.* 1992; **16**: 566.

24. Cortes, V. & Nelson, L. Errors in estimating energy expenditure in critically ill surgical patients. *Arch. Surg.* 1989; **124**: 287.

25. McClave, S., Lowen, C., Kleber, M. *et al.* Clinical use of the respiratory quotient obtained from indirect calorimetry. *J. Parenteral Enteral Nutr.* 2003; **27**: 21.

26. Konstantinides, F., Boehm, K., Radmer, W. *et al.* Pyrochemiluminescence: real time, cost-effective method for determining total urinary nitrogen in clinical nitrogen balance studies. *Clin. Chem.* 1988; **34**: 2518.

27. Detsky, A., Baker, J., O'Rourke, K. *et al.* Perioperative parenteral nutrition: a meta-analysis. *Ann. Intern. Med.* 1987; **107**: 195.

28. The Veterans Affairs Total Parenteral Nutrition Cooperative Study Group. Perioperative total parenteral nutrition in surgical patients. *N. Engl. J. Med.* 1991; **325**: 525.

29. Eisenberg, J., Glick, H., Buzby, G. *et al.* Does perioperative total parenteral nutrition reduce medical care costs? *J. Parenteral Enteral Nutr.* 1993; **17**: 201.

30. Campos, A. & Mequid, M. A critical appraisal of the usefulness of perioperative nutritional support. *Am. J. Clin. Nutr.* 1992; **55**: 117.

31. Heyland, D., MacDonald, S., Keefe, L. *et al.* Total parenteral nutrition in the critically ill patient – a meta-analysis. *J. Am. Med. Assoc.* 1998; **280**: 2013.

32. Bethal, R., Jansen, R., Heymsfield, S. *et al.* Nasogastric hyperalimentation through a polyethylene catheter: an alternative to central venous hyperalimentation. *Am. J. Clin. Nutr.* 1979; **32**: 1112.

33. Vanek, V. Ins and outs of enteral access. Part I: Short-term enteral access. *Nutr. Clin. Pract.* 2002; **17**: 275.

34. Caulfield, K., Page, C., & Pestana, C. Technique for intraduodenal placement of transnasal enteral feeding catheters. *Nutr. Clin. Pract.* 1991; **6**: 23.

35. Kalliafas, S., Choban, P., Ziegler, D. *et al.* Erythromycin facilitates postpyloric placement of nasoduodenal feeding tubes in intensive care unit patients: randomized, double-blinded, placebo-controlled trial. *J. Parenteral Enteral Nutr.* 1996; **20**: 385.

36. Moore, F., Moore, E., Jones, T. *et al.* TEN versus TPN following abdominal trauma: reduced septic morbidity. *J. Trauma* 1989; **29**: 916.

37. Weltz, C., Morris, J., & Mullen, J. Surgical jejunostomy in aspiration risk patients. *Ann. Surg.* 1992; **215**: 140.

38. Ford, E., Hull, S., Jennings, L. *et al.* Clinical comparison of tolerance to elemental or polymeric enteral feedings in the postoperative patient. *J. Am. Coll. Nutr.* 1992; **11**: 11.

39. Mowatt-Larssen, C., Brown, R., Wojtysiak, S. *et al.* Comparison of tolerance and nutritional outcome between a peptide and a standard enteral formula in critically ill, hypoalbuminemic patients. *J. Parenteral Enteral Nutr.* 1992; **16**: 20.

40. Heyland, D. Immunonutrition in the critically ill patient: putting the cart before the horse. *Nutr. Clin. Pract.* 2002; **17**: 267.

41. Chapman, G., Curtas, S., & Meguid, M. Standardized enteral orders attain caloric goals sooner: a prospective study. *J. Parenteral Enteral Nutr.* 1992; **16**: 149.

42. Guenter, P., Settle, R., Perlmutter, S. *et al.* Tube feeding-related diarrhea in acutely ill patients. *J. Parenteral Enteral Nutr.* 1991; **15**: 277.

43. Fekety, R. & Shah, A. Diagnosis and treatment of clostridium difficile colitis. *J. Am. Med. Assoc.* 1993; **269**: 71.

44. Eisenberg, P. Causes of diarrhea in tube-fed patients: a comprehensive approach to diagnosis and management. *Nutr. Clin. Pract.* 1993; **8**: 119.

45. Mcclave, S. & Chang, W. Feeding the hypotensive patient: does enteral feeding precipitate or protect against ischemic bowel? *Nutr. Clin. Pract.* 2003; **18**: 279.

46. Payne-James, J. & Khawaja, H. First choice for total parenteral nutrition: the peripheral route. *J. Parenteral Enteral Nutr.* 1993; **17**: 468.

47. Waxman, K., Day, A., Stellin, G. *et al.* Safety and efficacy of glycerol and amino acids in combination with lipid emulsion for peripheral parenteral nutrition support. *J. Parenteral Enteral Nutr.* 1992; **16**: 374.

48. Grant, J. *Handbook of Total Parenteral Nutrition.* Philadelphia: W. B. Saunders, 1992: 107–117.

49. Sitzman, J., Townsend, T., Siler, M. *et al.* Septic and technical complications of central venous catheterization: a prospective study of 200 consecutive patients. *Ann. Surg.* 1985; **202**: 766.

50. Williams, W. Infection control during parenteral nutrition therapy. *J. Parenteral Enteral Nutr.* 1985; **9**: 735.

51. Hoffman, K., Weber, D., Samsa, G. *et al.* Transparent polyurethane film as an intravenous catheter dressing: a meta-analysis of the infection risks. *J. Am. Med. Assoc.* 1992; **267**: 2072.

52. Cobb, D., High, K., Sawyer, R. *et al.* A controlled trial of scheduled replacement of central venous and pulmonary artery catheters. *N. Engl. J. Med.* 1992; **327**: 1062.

53. Pemberton, L., Lyman, B., Lander, V. *et al.* Sepsis from triple- vs single-lumen catheters during total parenteral nutrition in surgical or critically ill patients. *Arch. Surg.* 1986; **121**: 591.

54. Campos, A., Palazzi, M., & Meguid, M. Clinical use of total nutritional admixtures. *Nutrition* 1990; **6**: 347.

55. Weinsier, R., Bacon, J., & Butterworth, C. Central venous alimentation: a prospective study of the frequency of metabolic abnormalities among medical and surgical patients. *J. Parenteral Enteral Nutr.* 1982; **6**: 421.

56. Van den Berghe, G., Woutens, P., Weekers, F. *et al.* Intensive insulin therapy in critically ill patients. *N. Engl. J. Med.* 2001; **345**: 1359.

57. Leaseburge, L., Winn, N., & Schloerb, P. Liver test alterations with total parenteral nutrition and nutritional status. *J. Parenteral Enteral Nutr.* 1992; **16**: 348.

58. Buchmiller, C., Kleiman-Wexler, R., Ephgrave, K. *et al.* Liver dysfunction and energy source: results of a randomized clinical trial. *J. Parenteral Enteral Nutr.* 1993; **17**: 301.

59. Askanzi, J., Rosenaum, S. H., Heyman, A. I. *et al.* Respiratory changes induced by the large glucose loads of total parenteral nutrition. *J. Am. Med. Assoc.* 1980; **243**: 1444.

60. Maini, B., Blackburn, G., Bistrian, B. *et al.* Cyclic hyperalimentation: an optimal technique for preservation of visceral protein. *J. Surg. Res.* 1976; **20**: 515.

61. Kanematsu, T., Koyangi, N., Matsumata, T. *et al.* Lack of preventive effect of branched chain amino acid solution on postoperative hepatic encephalopathy in patients with cirrhosis: a randomized prospective trial. *Surgery* 1988; **104**: 482.

62. Barrera, R. Nutritional support in cancer patients. *J. Parenteral Enteral Nutr.* 2002; **26**: 563.

63. Ziegler, T. R., Young, L. S., Benfell, K. *et al.* Clinical and metabolic efficacy of glutamine supplemented parenteral nutrition after bone marrow transplantation: a randomized, double-blind, controlled study. *Ann. Intern. Med.* 1992; **116**: 821.

64. Inoue, Y., Grant, J. P., & Snyder, P. J. Effect of glutamine-supplemented total parenteral nutrition on recovery of the small intestine after starvation atrophy. *J. Parenteral Enteral Nutr.* 1993; **17**: 165.

3

Preoperative testing

Nomi L. Traub

Overview and historical perspective

The goal of preoperative medical evaluation of patients should be reduction of intraoperative and perioperative morbidity and mortality. A review of the literature suggests this is best acccomplished by a meticulous preoperative history and physical exam. The data gleaned from the history and physical, combined with information about the planned procedure, form the basis for selection of medically indicated preoperative tests.

Routine preoperative testing for all patients, rather than indicated testing for selected patients, came into vogue with the advent of multiphasic screening in the 1960s. The alluring notion that routine testing would lead to the discovery and treatment of unsuspected abnormalities, thereby decreasing perioperative complications, has not been realized. Large-scale routine testing leads to the discovery of numerous minor abnormalities, usually of no importance to surgical care. Further evaluation of these abnormal values may incur additional cost, potential harm to patients from more invasive investigations, and often unnecessary surgical delays.

During the 1970s and 1980s, multiple investigators focused attention on the usefulness and cost-effectiveness of screening laboratory tests. In a landmark article in 1985, Kaplan et al.[1] assessed the value of routine laboratory screening of preoperative patients. He and coworkers studied a random sample of 2000 patients who underwent tests before elective surgery in an academic medical center. They set criteria for test indications and "action limits" for test results. Action limits were defined as abnormalities that would be expected to trigger a response from the surgical team, not simply results that fell outside the normal range as defined by the laboratory. For example, a hematocrit of 34% in an elderly woman is outside the normal range in the laboratory but generally is not investigated by the surgical team. The lower action limit for hematocrit in this study was set at 30%.

Kaplan's group found there was no indication for about 60% of the preoperative tests that were performed. Only 3.4% (96 tests) of the results of the entire group of tests fell outside their action limits; 0.36% (ten tests) of the total number of tests were in the group that would not have been ordered and 0.14% (four tests) were of potential significance. Despite the potential significance of four of the tests, none was acted on. No changes were made in patient care, and no complications resulted from the abnormalities.

In another study, McKee and Scott[2] evaluated 400 patients admitted for elective surgery. Although 16% of the preoperative tests performed on these patients revealed some abnormality, only 0.013% caused a change in management. Thirteen cases of anemia were addressed; only one complication occurred in this group. None of the biochemical tests required attention. Among 323 electrocardiograms performed, there were 101 abnormalities, only 2 of which warranted any action. One silent myocardial infarction was detected and the patient's procedure was delayed 6 months; digoxin toxicity was noted in another patient and the drug dosage was decreased before surgery. Three hundred and twenty seven chest radiographs were done; 121 were abnormal but only 4 required action. The authors did not indicate the nature of the radiographic abnormalities nor the indications for action in this study.

A third retrospective study of preoperative laboratory screening was done by Narr and colleagues[3] at the Mayo Clinic. These investigators evaluated all patients in ASA class I (healthy patients) who were admitted for elective surgery. The routine tests performed included a complete blood count and measurement of creatinine, electrolytes, aspartate aminotransferase, and glucose levels. Only 160 (4%) of 3782 patients had abnormal test results. The

Medical Management of the Surgical Patient: A Textbook of Perioperative Medicine, ed. M. F. Lubin, R. B. Smith, T. F. Dobson, N. Spell, H. K. Walker. 4th edn. Published by Cambridge University Press. © Cambridge University 2006.

history and physical examination anticipated thirty of these. Forty-seven patients underwent further assessment due to abnormal laboratory values; only ten patients were treated for any abnormality. Treatments included oral potassium supplementation in one patient, oral iron in three patients, insulin therapy in one patient, and advice to lose weight in five patients with hyperglycemia. No surgical procedure was delayed and there were no adverse outcomes due to test results. As a result of the study, the Mayo Clinic abolished the requirement for preoperative laboratory testing for healthy patients under 40 years old.

In 1997, Narr and colleagues[4] published a follow-up to their original study, reviewing the course of 1044 patients who underwent anesthesia and surgery without preoperative testing. These were predominantly young, healthy patients. Ninety-seven percent of the patients had an ASA physical status of I or II, and 93% were under 50 years old. No deaths or major perioperative morbidity occurred.

The authors reviewed all laboratory testing done intraoperatively and postoperatively. In adult patients, there were two abnormal intraoperative laboratory results. One was a hemoglobin of 8 gm/dl in a patient who had excessive blood loss during sinus surgery. No transfusion was administered. The second was a right bundle branch block on an EKG of a 19-year-old patient with a wide QRS complex on the cardiac monitor. No further assessment of the problem occurred. One abnormal laboratory test was found in an adult postoperatively. A 30-year-old complained of an irregular heartbeat after a meniscectomy, and had PVCs on his EKG. Further evaluation revealed a soft diastolic murmur, and he was subsequently diagnosed with rheumatic heart disease.

The authors concluded that no laboratory test done intraoperatively or postoperatively changed medical or surgical management significantly. They postulated that patients assessed as healthy by history and physical may safely undergo anesthesia and surgery without preoperative laboratory tests. In their institution, the availability of rapid intraoperative and postoperative laboratory tests allows prompt reaction to abnormalities that may unexpectedly arise.

A systematic review, sponsored by the National Health Service in the UK, and published by Munro et al. in 1997,[5] reviewed the then available evidence on the value of routine preoperative testing in healthy, asymptomatic adults (all were case series). This rigorous review concluded that preoperative tests produce a wide range of abnormalities, even in healthy individuals. The clinical significance of these abnormalities is uncertain and rarely leads to changes in management. The authors summarized that the power of preoperative tests to predict adverse

outcomes in asymptomatic patients is weak. They reflected that perhaps routine preoperative tests might be beneficial in asymptomatic elderly patients, though there was no evidence supporting this.

In response to the limited data in elderly patients, Dzankic et al.[6] studied 544 consecutive patients over 70 years old, who underwent noncardiac surgery. The majority of the patients were ASA class II and III, and the mean age was 78 years. Preoperative tests obtained included Na^+, K^+, creatinine, glucose, hemoglobin, and platelet count. Preoperative risk factors and laboratory tests were examined for association with the occurrence of postoperative adverse outcomes. The predefined adverse outcomes were cardiovascular, pulmonary, renal, hepatic, gastrointestinal, neurologic, infectious, thromboembolic or surgical complications, reoperation, and death.

The overall in-hospital mortality rate of the group was 3.7% and 20% (110 patients) developed at least one postoperative complication. The percentage of abnormal preoperative laboratory results in patients with ASA <II was 3.6%, vs. 9.6% in patients with ASA >II. Overall, there was a low prevalence of abnormal electrolytes or platelet counts. Though the prevalence of abnormal creatinine, glucose, and hemoglobin was higher, abnormal values were not predictive of adverse postoperative outcomes. By multivariate analysis, only ASA class and surgical risk independently predicted adverse outcomes. The most common adverse outcomes were cardiac and neurologic complications. Based on this study, it seems as though even geriatric patients should undergo selective laboratory testing based on history and physical findings, rather than routine testing, based on age criteria. Geriatric surgical patients with few comorbidities (ASA I-II) likely resemble the general population in terms of prevalence of laboratory abnormalities.

In January 2000, Schein et al.[7] published the results of the first large, multicenter randomized trial of routine preoperative testing. Patients undergoing 19 557 cataract surgeries were randomly assigned to either a testing or no-testing group. Routine preoperative tests in the testing group included EKG, complete blood count, electrolytes, BUN, creatinine, and glucose. The cumulative rate of medical events in the two groups was the same (31.3 events per 1000 operations). Hypertension and arrhythmia (mostly bradycardia) were the two most common events that occurred in patients undergoing cataract surgery. Despite the advanced age and the likely presence of coexisting illnesses in these patients, preoperative testing did not alter perioperative morbidity and mortality. Obviously, the small surgical risk associated with cataract surgery makes these results difficult to generalize to other procedures.

In summary, routine batteries of preoperative tests in asymptomatic patients rarely lead to changes in perioperative management or to improved outcomes. Multiple case-series, whether retrospective or prospective, report similar findings, as did a systematic review of the evidence. Studies in which preoperative tests were withheld show no adverse changes in morbidity or mortality as a result of the omission of tests.

The following section reviews the data about specific tests – the prevalence of abnormalities in studies, whether these abnormalities influence management, and the rationale and indications for specific testing. In some of the studies cited, indicated and routine tests were not differentiated from each other. The prevalence of abnormalities, therefore, may be overestimated, since it is calculated with the inclusion of patients with signs and symptoms, not just asymptomatic individuals.

Hemoglobin

The prevalence of anemia (defined as Hb <10 g/dl in some studies, and Hb out of the reference range in others) found in studies of routine preoperative screening ranges from 0.3%–10.5%.[1,3,6,8,9] Rates of anemia increase with increasing age and higher ASA classification.[6,9] Routine tests rarely lead to a change in management (only 0.1–0.2% of the tests influenced management).[1,3,8]

In orthopedic patients undergoing procedures associated with significant blood loss, lower preoperative baseline hemoglobin levels predict the subsequent need for postoperative transfusion.[10] Several guidelines recommend a baseline preoperative hemoglobin for any surgery in which significant blood loss is expected.[11,12,20] In this scenario, routine testing may facilitate use of autologous transfusions or erythropoietin to avoid allogeneic transfusions.

Indications for preoperative hemoglobin testing include history of anemia, or physical findings of anemia, renal insufficiency, malignancy, anticoagulant use, or use of myelosuppressive drugs.

White blood cell count

Multiple studies show that the prevalence of unexpected abnormalities in white blood cell counts is less than 1%.[1,8,13,14] Only Turnbull's study[8] addresses the impact of routine white blood cell count on patient management and no patient's management was altered. Routine screening of white blood cell count is not recommended.

Indications for preoperative white blood cell count testing include a history of a myeloproliferative disorder, signs or symptoms of infection, or a high risk of leukopenia from drugs or underlying disease.

Platelet count

The prevalence of platelet count abnormalities in multiple studies of routine preoperative testing is less than 2%.[1,3,6,8,13–15] Rohrer's study[16] identified 8% of preoperative platelet counts as abnormal, but all were minimally elevated, and none influenced clinical management. No other study of routine platelet counts found an impact on patient management. Routine preoperative platelet counts are not recommended.

Indications for a platelet count include suspicion of a bleeding disorder, known myeloproliferative disease, or recent chemotherapy.

Complete blood counts

Since routine preoperative testing of hemoglobin or hematocrit is recommended in cases of expected blood loss, it is preferable to order a hemoglobin/hematocrit rather than a complete blood count. Smetana[17] points out that many institutions combine hemoglobin/hematocrit with white blood cell count and platelet count. Though minor abnormalities in white blood cell count or platelet count may turn up, they are unlikely to affect surgical outcome and usually surgery can proceed. Smetana recommends repeat testing to ascertain the abnormalities and consideration of a prudent workup if abnormalities persist.

Coagulation tests

Numerous studies of routine prothrombin time testing show abnormalities in 1% or less of patients.[1,8,9,14–16] Studies of partial thromboplastin time testing reveal a higher rate of abnormalities, ranging from 0.3–16.3%.[1,8,9,14–16,18,19] Studies evaluating the effect of these abnormalities on the perioperative management reveal a change in management in less than 1% of cases.[5] When performed routinely, abnormalities of these tests of hemostasis do not predict intraoperative or postoperative bleeding.[5] Routine testing of hemostasis with prothrombin time and partial thromboplastin time are not recommended. History and physical seem to be a better screening tool for hemostatic disorders.

Indications for testing include suspicion or history of a bleeding disorder, use of anticoagulants, chronic liver disease or malnutrition.

Chemistry testing

Electrolytes

Most studies examine sodium and potassium levels and some do not separate the individual tests on a six-factor automated multiple analysis. The prevalence of abnormal results of sodium testing is low, 0.5%–1.2%.[6,8,14,15] and does not lead to changes in management or adverse outcomes. The prevalence of abnormal potassium levels ranges from 0.2%–9%.[3,6,8,14,15] In the past, mild degrees of preoperative hypokalemia were corrected due to concerns that hypokalemia predisposed patients to life-threatening arrhythmias. Current anesthesia literature does not support the policy of correcting mild hypokalemia perioperatively.[20] Several studies suggest that there is no relationship between potassium levels and perioperative arrhythmias.[21,22] A routine measurement of electrolytes preoperatively is not recommended.

Indications for testing include a history of renal insufficiency, use of diuretics, digoxin, ACE inhibitors, angiotensin receptor blockers, or other medications leading to electrolyte abnormalities, or a history of endocrinopathy predisposing to abnormalities.

Renal function tests

The prevalence of abnormal creatinine (defined variably as >1.5–2.0 mg/dl) in studies of preoperative testing ranges from 0.2–12%.[6,8,14,15,23] Though older literature reveals infrequent changes in management based on findings of abnormal renal function, more recent data[23,24] correlate renal insufficiency with postoperative complications. Smetana and Macpherson[17] calculate the positive likelihood ratio for abnormal renal function tests as 3.3, (based on outcome data from nine trials) meaning that an abnormal test has some clinical usefulness in predicting adverse outcomes. Since moderate renal insufficiency can be a marker for adverse events but clinically unsuspected, it may be reasonable to routinely evaluate asymptomatic older patients, particularly those undergoing major surgical procedures. Though there is no clear consensus, routine measurement of creatinine is recommended in patients over 50 years old.

Indications for testing include a history of renal disease, diabetes, hypertension, congestive heart failure, use of diuretics, ACE inhibitors, angiotensin-receptor blockers, NSAIDS, and major surgical procedures.

Glucose

The prevalence of abnormal glucose values found during routine preoperative testing ranges from 1.1%–8%.[1,3,6,8,14,15] The majority of abnormal results are in patients with known diabetes. Less than 1% of these abnormal values influence perioperative management. Though established diabetes requiring treatment influences operative complication risk, there is no evidence that discovering unsuspected diabetes preoperatively changes outcome. Routine preoperative measurement of serum glucose is not recommended.

Indications for testing include a history of diabetes or corticosteroid use.

Hepatic profile

Only a few of the case-series evaluating routine preoperative testing examine hepatic tests, and the systematic review published in 1997[5] does not include data on hepatic tests. The prevalence of abnormal SGOT or alkaline phosphatase in retrospective studies ranges from 0.3%–3.5%.[3,9,14] The finding of abnormal hepatic tests influences perioperative management in less than 0.1% of cases. Routine measurement of hepatic profiles is not recommended.

Albumin levels may help in risk assessment preoperatively, though correction of low levels does not clearly alter risk. A low albumin level preoperatively is a risk factor for postoperative respiratory failure, and for mortality.[25,26] The National Veterans Affairs Surgical Risk Study[26] showed that albumin was the strongest predictor of morbidity and mortality within thirty days of surgery. In this study of 54 215 non-cardiac surgery cases, a decrease in serum albumin from 4.6 gm/dl to 2.1 gm/dl was associated with an increase in mortality from 1% to 29%. Albumin infusion is not thought helpful in reducing risk.

Indications for hepatic testing include patients with cirrhosis, jaundice, signs of portal hypertension, or malnutrition. An argument can be made for measurement of albumin in patients about to undergo major surgery, to aid in risk assessment.

Urinalysis

Though the urinalysis has multiple components, studies focus mainly on the detection of pyuria, which could conceivably be treated prior to surgery to prevent complications. The prevalence of urinary abnormalities (variably defined in studies) ranges from 2.4%–39%.[8,13,27,28] Only 1%–2% influence management preoperatively, which generally involves treatment of a presumed or proven urinary tract infection. Most other urinary abnormalities are not acted upon, and often pyuria is ignored as well.

Lawrence and Kroenke[27] reviewed the usefulness of preoperative urinalysis in 1988. They retrospectively studied 200 non-prosthetic knee procedures. Fifteen percent of the routine urinalyses were abnormal, but only 29% of those were addressed. There were no differences in rates of wound infection between patients with normal and abnormal results of urinalysis. However, as wound infection was a rare outcome, the study had inadequate power to be conclusive.

Routine urinalysis is not recommended.

Electrocardiography

The theoretical rationale for obtaining a preoperative EKG is to detect unsuspected cardiac conditions that increase the risk of perioperative cardiac complications. The original Goldman index[29] found two electrocardiographic factors that predicted complications – rhythm other than sinus or PACs, and greater than five PVCs per minute documented any time before surgery. Both these factors are possible to detect clinically. In Goldman's analysis of 1001 patients, other electrocardiographic findings, such as old myocardial infarction by electrocardiography, ST-segment or T-wave changes, and bundle-branch blocks, were insignificant variables for prediction of cardiac risk. The data collected for the revised cardiac risk index proposed by Lee et al.[23] indicate that Q waves confer cardiovascular risk. In Lee's study,[23] preoperative ST–T wave changes were not associated with worse outcomes, nor were abnormal rhythms on EKG.

Multiple studies reveal a fairly high rate of abnormalities on routine preoperative EKGs, ranging from 4.6%–31.7%.[5] The prevalence of abnormalities increases with age, with cardiovascular risk factors, and ASA status.[30–33] Many of the abnormalities are not clinically significant. In their systematic review, Munro et al.[5] concluded that only findings from 0%–2.2% of EKGs lead to a change in management.

Tait et al.[31] studied the efficacy of routine preoperative EKGs in predicting perioperative cardiovascular complications. In a retrospective chart review of 573 patients (ASA class I and II) undergoing elective surgery, Tait found much higher rates of EKG abnormalities in patients

with cardiovascular risk factors than those without. (51% vs. 26.1%) However, there was no difference in the prevalence of perioperative events between the group with normal EKGs and the group with abnormal EKGs. Additionally, healthy male and female patients who had EKGs based solely on their age had a similar prevalence of abnormal EKGs and perioperative events to patients of all ages without cardiovascular risk factors. He concluded that routine EKG screening for patients without cardiovascular risk factors is not valuable, and that chronological age alone may not be a useful criteria for screening.

Tait's results echo those of Gold et al.,[34] who retrospectively evaluated 751 patients undergoing ambulatory surgery. In these relatively healthy (primarily ASA class I or II) patients, 43% of EKGs were abnormal. In this study, increasing age and ASA status, as well as male sex, were correlated with a higher likelihood of an abnormal preoperative EKG. The authors used lenient criteria to define adverse cardiovascular events and to judge the potential usefulness of the preoperative EKG. Despite these lenient criteria, there were only 12 (1.6% of the patients) cardiovascular complications and the authors believed that a preoperative EKG might have been clinically useful in half the cases. Five of these six cases occurred in patients over the age of 60. The authors concluded that routine preoperative EKGs were not useful in relatively healthy patients under age 60.

Ashton et al.[35] evaluated preoperative and postoperative EKGs in 206 men undergoing transurethral prostate resection. Serum CK and CKMBs were obtained preoperatively and in the morning of the first three postoperative days. Twenty one percent of patients developed postoperative EKG abnormalities. T wave changes were the most common; none developed new Q waves or left bundle branch block. Only one patient suffered a perioperative myocardial infarction within the first three days, confirmed by CKMB elevation. This patient had no codable changes on postoperative EKGs. In this study, the predictive value of postoperative EKG changes for the presence of infarction was zero. The predictive value of an unchanged EKG for the absence of infarction was 99.4%. Only one of the patients who had postoperative EKG changes had a cardiac event in the year following surgery. The authors concluded that routine perioperative EKGs are of little value when the incidence of perioperative infarction is low. This study refuted the idea of the potential value of a preoperative EKG as a baseline.

Though the evidence that preoperative EKGs affect adverse outcomes is slim, many experts recommend an EKG in men over 40 years of age, and women over 50 years of age and in patients with cardiovascular risk factors. In light of the data reviewed above, it seems reasonable to raise the age threshold for routine preoperative EKGs to 60 years, in patients without other cardiovascular risk factors. Due to the high rate of EKG abnormalities in patients over age 60 years, a "baseline" EKG may be pragmatic, though the value of a baseline has not been studied. EKGs are unnecessary prior to minor procedures, such as cataract surgery.

Indications for EKG are a history of cardiac disease, or abnormal cardiac findings on clinical examination.

Chest radiography

The rationale for obtaining a preoperative chest radiograph is to identify unsuspected abnormalities that would lead to a cancellation of surgery or modification of anesthetic technique. Another possible rationale is to establish a baseline that may be helpful if a postoperative complication occurs. Multiple studies of preoperative chest radiographs find a fairly high rate of abnormalities (approximately 20%), but that few of these abnormalities alter perioperative management. Younger, asymptomatic patients have fewer abnormalities.

Roizen[20] provides a fairly extensive list of the reported case-series of preoperative chest radiographs. He concludes that a routine chest radiograph is not warranted for any asymptomatic person, without risk factors, who is less than 75 years old.

One of the larger, more recent studies, published by Silvestri[36] in 1999, examined 6111 patients undergoing elective surgery in twenty Italian hospitals. One thousand and sixteen patients (18.3% of the patients) had an abnormal chest radiograph, which influenced anaesthetic management in 313 (5.1% of the patients). Using multivariate analysis, the factors predicting the usefulness of the preoperative chest radiograph were male sex, age over 60 years, ASA class > III, respiratory diseases, and the presence of two or more coexisting diseases.

Archer et al.[37] reviewed the literature (1966–1992) on routine preoperative chest radiography in North American and European populations. Abnormalities were found in 10% of 14 390 patients. However, only 1.3% of patients had unsuspected abnormalities. The majority of the abnormalities were known or suspected based on the history and physical examination. Findings influenced management in only 0.1% of patients.

Blery et al.[38] retrospectively evaluated a protocol for selective preoperative testing in 3866 consecutive surgical patients. In the protocol, the indication for a chest radiograph was the presence of cardiovascular or pulmonary disease. They reviewed the cases of 2765 patients who did not have preoperative chest radiographs to evaluate whether there had been adverse consequences. In the opinion of the anesthetists involved, there were two cases (0.1% of patients) who may have suffered from the omission of a chest radiograph.

Overall, there is no consensus on the value of routine chest radiography. It seems reasonable to recommend a routine preoperative chest radiograph at age 60, though the age cutoff is somewhat arbitrary.

Chest radiography is indicated in patients with cardiopulmonary disease by history or evidence of cardiopulmonary disease by physical exam.

Pulmonary function tests

In 1990, The American College of Physicians developed a position paper[39] on the evidence-based use of preoperative pulmonary function tests. They recommend the use of spirometry and arterial blood gas analysis for patients being considered for lung resection. In this scenario, pulmonary function tests identify patients at high risk for life-threatening pulmonary complications after the procedure. Data are less conclusive for other surgical procedures. The position paper notes that it may be prudent to perform arterial blood gas analysis and spirometry in patients with a history of tobacco use and dyspnea, prior to coronary artery bypass graft or abdominal surgery.

Kroenke et al.[40] examined pulmonary complications in a group of patients with severe COPD (FEV1 < 50% predicted) undergoing surgery (excluding lung resection surgery). There were no pulmonary complications in the majority of procedures (76 of 107 procedures). The type and duration of surgery influenced the risk of complications. Complications occurred more often after coronary artery bypass graft or major abdominal surgeries. Six deaths occurred, and all but one were in patients undergoing coronary artery bypass graft.

In another retrospective study, Kroenke[41] examined the effect of COPD on pulmonary complications, in patients undergoing thoracic and major abdominal surgery. He compared a cohort of 26 patients with severe COPD with 52 patients with mild-moderate COPD and 52 patients without COPD. All the patients underwent thoracic or major abdominal surgery. Patients with severe COPD had higher rates of complications but spirometry was not an independent predictor of complications. Age, ASA class, abnormal chest radiograph, and the administration of perioperative bronchodilators were associated with higher rates of complications.

The above studies, published after the position paper in 1990, support the premise of the position paper. Routine pulmonary function tests should not be ordered solely for risk assessment prior to high-risk surgeries, with the exception of lung resection surgery.

Review of previous tests

Macpherson and colleagues[42] examined the utility of repeated preoperative testing in patients who had undergone laboratory tests within a year before elective surgery. They retrospectively evaluated results of laboratory tests done on 1109 patients who had elective surgery. The specific laboratory tests they analyzed were the complete blood count; sodium, potassium, and creatinine levels; and the prothrombin time and partial thromboplastin time. They found that about half the tests performed at the time of hospital admission for surgery duplicated tests done during the previous year. If the prior tests were normal, only 0.4% repeat values were outside a range considered acceptable for surgery. Most of these abnormalities were predictable from a patient's history. These authors recommended that previous normal tests within four months of surgery need not be repeated if there were no indication for retesting.

Summary

Few preoperative tests should be ordered routinely, based on the predominantly retrospective data from case series reviewed in this chapter. There are clearly still substantial areas of uncertainty in the literature due to the lack of randomized prospective trials, and the relatively low number of adverse perioperative events that occur. This ambiguity leads to various recommendations for preoperative testing by different authorities. Most authorities concur that preoperative testing should stem from information obtained through the history and physical examination, and should be pursued only if the outcome will likely influence management.

Based on the data, there is a consensus that young, healthy patients require no routine testing. In older patients with underlying diseases, the likelihood of abnormal tests is higher, and more liberal use of testing may be indicated. There is a growing trend in the literature that chronological age alone should not determine the use of preoperative testing, and that physiological age, based on comorbidities and overall health practices is probably a more important determinant of surgical outcome.

Currently, there is no clear substitute for a meticulous history and physical examination, combined with clinical judgment, when ordering preoperative testing.

REFERENCES

1. Kaplan, E. B., Sheiner, L. B., Boeckmann, A. J. *et al.* The usefulness of preoperative laboratory screening. *J. Am. Med. Assoc.* 1985; **253**: 3576–3581.
2. McKee, R. F. & Scott, E. M. The value of routine preoperative investigations. *Ann. R. Coll. Surg. Engl.* 1987; **69**: 60–162.
3. Narr, B. J., Hansen, T. R., & Warner, M. A. Preoperative laboratory screening in healthy Mayo patients: cost effective elimination of tests and unchanged outcomes. *Mayo. Clin. Proc.* 1991; **66**: 155–159.
4. Narr, B. J., Warner, M. E., Scroeder, D. R. *et al.* Outcomes of patients with no laboratory assessment before anesthesia and a surgical procedure. *Mayo. Clin. Proc.* 1997; **72**: 505–509.
5. Munro, J., Booth, A., & Nicholl, J. Routine preoperative testing: a systematic review of the evidence. *Health Technol. Assessm.* 1997; **1**(12): 1–62.
6. Dzankic, S., Pastor, D., Gonzalez, C. *et al.* The prevalence and predictive value of abnormal preoperative tests in elderly surgical patients. *Anest. Analg.* 2001; **93**: 301–308.
7. Schein, O. D., Katz, J., Bass, E. B. *et al.* The value of routine preoperative medical testing before cataract surgery. *N. Engl. J. Med.* 2000; **342**: 168–175.
8. Turnbull, J. M. & Buck, C. The value of preoperative screening investigations in otherwise healthy individuals. *Arch. Intern. Med.* 1987; **147**: 1101–1105.
9. Sanders, D. P., McKinney, F. W., & Harris, W. H. Clinical evaluation and cost effectiveness of preoperative laboratory assessment on patients undergoing total hip arthroplasty. *Orthopedics* 1989; **12**: 1449–1453.
10. Faris, P. M., Spence, R. K., Larholt, K. M. *et al.* The predictive power of baseline hemoglobin for transfusion risk in surgery patients. *Orthopedics* 1999; **22**(suppl): s135–140.
11. Fischer, S. P. Cost effective preoperative evaluation and testing. *Chest* 1999; **115**: 96s–100s.
12. Poland, M. D. Practice Guideline for preoperative testing. *Wiscons. Med. J.* 1997; **96**(10): 48–51.
13. Johnson, H., Knee-Ioli, S., Butler, T. A. *et al.* Are routine tests necessary to evaluate ambulatory surgical patients? *Surgery* 1988; **104**: 639–645.
14. Perez, A., Planell, J., Bacardaz, C. *et al.* Value of routine preoperative tests: a muticenter study in four general hospitals. *Br. J. Anaesth.* 1995; **74**: 250–256.
15. Alsumait, B. M., Alhumood, S. A., Ivanova, T. *et al.* A prospective evaluation of preoperative screening laboratory tests in general surgery patients. *Med. Princip. Pract.* 2002; **11**: 42–45.
16. Rohrer, M. J., Michelotti, M. C., & Nahrwold, D. L. A prospective evaluation of the efficacy of preoperative coagulation testing. *Ann. Surg.* 1988; **208**: 554–557.

17. Smetana, G. W. & Macpherson, D. S. The case against routine preoperative laboratory testing. *Med. Clin. N. Am.* 2003; **87**: 7–40.

18. Macpherson, C., Jacobs, P., & Den, D. Abnormal perioperative haemorrhage in asymptomatic patients is not predicted by laboratory testing. *S. Afr. Med. J.* 1993; **83**: 106–108.

19. Suchman, A. & Mushin, A. How well does the activated partial thromboplastin time predict postoperative hemorrhage? *J. Am. Med. Assoc.* 1986; **256**: 750–753.

20. Roizen, M. F., Foss, J. F., & Fischer, S. J. Preoperative evaluation. In Miller, R. D., ed. *Anesthesia*, 5th edn. Philadelphia: Churchill Livingstone, 2000: 824–883.

21. Hirsch, I. A., Tomlinson, D. L., Slogoff, S. *et al.* The overstated risk of preoperative hypokalemia. *Anesth. Analg.* 1988; **67**: 131–136.

22. Nally, B. R., Dunbar, S. B., Zellinger, M. *et al.* Supraventricular tachycardia after coronary artery bypass grafting surgery and fluid and electrolyte variables. *Heart Lung* 1996; **25**: 31–36.

23. Lee, T. H., Marcantonio, E. R., Mangione, C. M. *et al.* Derivation and prospective validation of a simple index for prediction of cardiac risk of major noncardiac surgery. *Circulation* 1999; **100**: 1043–1049.

24. Higgins, T. L., Estafanous, F. G., Loop, F. D. *et al.* Stratification of morbidity and mortality outcome by preoperative risk factors in coronary artery bypass patients. A clinical severity score. *J. Am. Med. Assoc.* 1992; **267**: 2344–2348.

25. Arozullah, A., Daley, J., Henderson, W. *et al.* Multifactorial risk index for predicting postoperative respiratory failure in men after noncardiac surgery. *Ann. Surg.* 2000; **232**: 243–253.

26. Gibbs, J., Cull, W., Henderson, W. *et al.* Preoperative serum albumin level as a predictor of operative mortality and morbidity: results from the National VA Surgical Risk Study. *Arch. Surg.* 1999; **134**: 36–42.

27. Lawrence, V. A. & Kroenke, K. The unproven utility of preoperative urinalysis. *Arch. Int. Med.* 1988; **148**: 1370–1373.

28. Adams, J. G. Jr., Weigelt, J. A., & Poulos, E. Usefulness of preoperative laboratory assessment of patients undergoing elective herniorrhaphy. *Arch. Surg.* 1992; **127**: 801–804.

29. Goldman, L., Caldera, D. L., Nussbaum, S. R. *et al.* Multifactorial index of cardiac risk in noncardiac surgical procedures. *N. Engl. J. Med.* 1977; **297**: 845–850.

30. Goldberger, A. L. & O'Konski, M. Utility of the routine electrocardiogram before surgery and on general hospital admission. *Ann. Int. Med.* 1986; **105**: 552–557.

31. Tait, A. R., Parr, H. G., & Tremper, K. K. Evaluation of the efficacy of routine preoperative electrocardiograms. *J. Cardioth. Vasc. Anesth.* 1997; **11**: 752–755.

32. McClean, G. & McCoy, E. Routine pre-operative electrocardiography. *Br. J. Clin. Pract.* 1990; **44**: 92–95.

33. Seymour, D. G., Pringle, R., & Maclennan, W. J. The role of the routine pre-operative electrocardiogram in the elderly surgical patient. *Age and Ageing* 1983; **12**: 97–104.

34. Gold, B. S., Young, M. L., Kinman, J. L. *et al.* The utility of preoperative electrocardiograms in the ambulatory surgical patient. *Arch. Int. Med.* 1992; **152**: 301–305.

35. Ashton, C. M., Tjomas, J., Wray, N. P. *et al.* The frequency and significance of ECG changes after transurethral prostate resection. *J. Am. Geriatr. Soc.* 1991; **39**: 575–580.

36. Silvestri, L., Maffessanti, M., Gregori, D. *et al.* Usefulness of routine pre-operative chest radiography for anaesthetic management: a prospective multicentre pilot study. *Europ. J. Anaesth.* 1999; **16**: 749–760.

37. Archer, C., Levy, A. R., & McGregor, M. Value of routine preoperative chest X-rays: a meta-analysis. *Can. J. Anaesth.* 1993; **40**: 1022–1027.

38. Blery, C., Charpak, Y., Szatan, M. *et al.* Evaluation of a protocol for selective ordering of preoperative tests. *Lancet* 1986; **1**: 139–141.

39. American College of Physicians. Position paper: preoperative pulmonary function testing. *Ann. Intern. Med.* 1990; **112**: 793–794.

40. Kroenke, K., Lawrence, V. A., Theroux, J. F. *et al.* Operative risk in patients with severe obstructive pulmonary disease. *Arch. Int. Med.* 1992; **152**: 967–973.

41. Kroenke, K., Lawrence, V. A., Theroux, J. F. *et al.* Postoperative complications after thoracic and major abdominal surgery in patients with and without obstructive lung disease. *Chest* 1993; **104**: 1445–1451.

42. Macpherson, D. S., Snow, R., & Lofgren, R. P. Preoperative screening: value of previous tests. *Ann. Int. Med.* 1990; **113**: 969–973.

4

Chronic medications around the time of surgery

Nathan O. Spell, III

Division of General Medicine, Emory University School of Medicine, Atlanta, Georgia

Introduction

Physicians caring for patients in the perioperative period face decisions about what to do with chronic medications. This chapter will provide recommendations for continuing or stopping common medications around surgery. It is organized by type of medication and medical condition being treated, but medications are covered only once when used to treat multiple conditions. See Table 4.1 for a summary of recommendations made in this chapter. For information on medications not found in this chapter or elsewhere in this book, a useful search strategy is to enter keywords "preoperative care" or "perioperative care" and the particular medication name or category into an online medical information search vehicle such as PubMed or OVID.

General considerations

Informed decisions about medications around surgery can enhance patient safety and optimize the outcome of the surgery. With the goal of keeping chronic illnesses stable, one could argue to make no changes in a patient's medications. However, each medication may carry particular risks for the surgical patient and adds to the complexity of care. Since the chance of an adverse drug reaction or drug–drug interaction increases exponentially with the number of medications,[1] safety should be improved by reducing the number of medications the patient uses around surgery. Inexpensive or free software for hand-held computers and personal digital assistants (PDAs) allows for rapid search for known drug-drug interactions at the bedside.

Complicating judgments regarding medication use is the state of our knowledge about perioperative effects of

Table 4.1. Summary of recommendations for chronic medications taken before surgery

Medications usually continued	Medications usually stopped
Beta adrenergic blockers	Aspirin and antiplatelet drugs
Calcium channel blockers, nitrates	NSAIDs (unselective and COX-2 inhibitors)
Antiarrhythmics	Diuretics
Bronchodilators and other drugs for obstructive lung diseases	Lipid lowering drugs
	Estrogens and SERMs
Thyroid hormone	Dopamine receptor agonists
Antithyroid drugs	Monoamine oxidase (MAO) inhibitors
Insulin	Herbal products
Corticosteroids	
Anticonvulsants	
Carbidopa/levodopa	
Drugs for myasthenia gravis	
Selective serotonin reuptake inhibitors (SSRIs)	
Tricyclic antidepressants (TCAs)	
Antipsychotic drugs	
Benzodiazepines	
Opioid analgesics	

medications. For some medications (beta-blockers, for example) there is a body of well-controlled research addressing perioperative safety and benefits. This is the exception rather than the rule. Therefore, many of the recommendations presented here are derived from general consensus and expert opinion, where they exist. For each patient, then, the advice given will depend upon the balance of these and additional factors unique to the surgery and to the patient (see Table 4.2).

Medical Management of the Surgical Patient: A Textbook of Perioperative Medicine, ed. M. F. Lubin, R. B. Smith, T. F. Dobson, N. Spell, H. K. Walker. 4th edn. Published by Cambridge University Press. © Cambridge University 2006.

Table 4.2. Factors affecting perioperative medication decisions

Related to the surgery	Related to the patient	Related to the medication
Type of anesthesia	Age	Known or anticipated
Duration of procedure	Cardiovascular risk	perioperative risks
Emergent vs. elective surgery	Comorbid medical illnesses	Risk of withdrawal effects
Anticipated blood loss	Medication allergies	Drug–drug interactions
Impact of surgical site bleeding	Variable drug metabolism	Drug–disease interactions
Particular organ-specific risks	Patient desires	Availability of alternative
of the surgery	Duration of NPO status	medications and
	Hypotension	routes of delivery
	Postoperative organ dysfunction	

Medication categories

Antiplatelet agents (aspirin, clopidogrel and ticlopidine)

Aspirin and clopidogrel (Plavix) are commonly used for prevention of myocardial infarction (MI) and ischemic stroke. Both have been shown to increase postoperative bleeding and need for blood product transfusion.[2,3] Low-dose aspirin (40–325 mg a day) permanently inhibits platelet cyclooxygenase with little effect on systemic prostaglandins.[4] Clopidogrel and ticlopidine (Ticlid) inhibit platelet aggregation through actions on adenosine diphosphate receptors.[4] With aspirin and clopidogrel, the effect is abolished by normal replacement of the platelet pool over about a week after discontinuation. Ticlopidine has a steady-state half-life of 4–5 days,[4] so stopping it for 3–4 weeks may be necessary to restore platelet function. If the surgical bleeding risk is small or if the patient is at high risk for postoperative MI, one may choose to continue the drugs.[5,6] When increased bleeding risk is a large concern and these agents have been recently used, effects on platelet function may be assessed with a bleeding time or platelet function assays. Platelet transfusion, if necessary, can reverse the bleeding tendency.

Non-steroidal anti-inflammatory drugs (NSAIDs)

NSAIDs are used chronically for pain relief and anti-inflammatory effects; several are available over-the-counter. These drugs reversibly inhibit cyclooxygenase (COX). Non-selective NSAIDs inhibit platelet aggregation, though usually less effectively and for shorter duration than aspirin. Within 1–3 days of discontinuation, anti-platelet effects are minimal. The selective COX-2 inhibitors have negligible antiplatelet effects.[4]

NSAIDs may be used to good effect for postoperative pain management, though with this caution. Vasodilating prostaglandins are critically important for maintenance of renal medullary blood flow, especially for patients with impaired renal function or decreased effective renal blood flow due to bleeding, hypotension or the effects of angiotensin converting enzyme (ACE) inhibitors and diuretics. Since NSAIDs inhibit these prostaglandins,[4] decreased renal clearance and renal injury may occur in postoperative patients at risk. Patients with no contraindications may be given NSAIDs immediately after surgery.

Antihypertensive medications

Diuretics are usually recommended to be discontinued on the day of surgery.[5] The rationale is twofold: avoidance of hypokalemia and maintenance of intravascular volume. Patients who are volume depleted are more likely to suffer hypotension at induction of anesthesia or with blood loss and are more susceptible to ischemic renal injury. When recognized, volume depletion and electrolyte disturbances should be corrected. If needed for antihypertensive effect or volume control, diuretics may be resumed as soon as the patient is able to take oral medication. Intravenous (i.v.) forms are easily administered when necessary.

Most other antihypertensive medications should be administered without interruption in the perioperative period, unless contraindicated by individual patient circumstances. Several categories deserve special mention. Beta adrenergic blockers have been shown to have cardioprotective effects when administered just before and continuing after surgery in patients of intermediate cardiac risk.[7] Extrapolating from this evidence, beta-blockers should be continued in patients who take them regularly. Intravenous forms are available when the patient is unable to take oral medications, but i.v. administration requires closer monitoring and is inherently riskier than oral dosing. Though less of a problem for the most commonly used preparations, patients taking older short-acting beta-blockers such as propranolol are at risk of rebound hypertension if the medication is abruptly discontinued. Centrally acting adrenergic drugs such as clonidine, guanabenz, guanfacine and methyldopa may also result in significant rebound hypertension if discontinued.[8] Clonidine is available in a transdermal patch that can easily be used through surgery. Conversion from oral to transdermal clonidine may be considered in the week before surgery for patients who are not likely to resume oral intake right away after surgery.

Calcium channel blockers are generally continued through surgery.[8] i.v. Diltiazem and verapamil are available, if necessary, and may be useful for treatment of atrial arrhythmias and hypertension. Because of reports of transient ischemic episodes and other adverse events when immediate release nifedipine has been used for hypertensive urgencies and emergencies,[9] avoid it for treatment of postoperative hypertension. Long-acting or slow-release dihydropyridines can be safely continued perioperatively.

Angiotensin converting enzyme (ACE) inhibitors and angiotensin receptor blockers (ARBs) are assuming a larger role in the treatment of hypertension. These drugs act by reducing the amount (ACE inhibitors) or activity (ARBs) of angiotensin II, a potent endogenous vasoconstrictor.[4] Within the kidney, the physiologic effect of these drugs is to reduce the transglomerular filtration pressure and effective renal blood flow. Renal artery stenosis, intravascular volume depletion or hemorrhage, hypotension, or concomitant use of diuretics or NSAIDs increases the risk that ACE inhibitors or ARBs may contribute to postoperative renal dysfunction. ACE inhibitors and ARBs may also increase the incidence of a hypotensive response to anesthetic induction.[10,11] For these reasons and others, some authorities[12] recommend holding these drugs in the perioperative period. However, these medications are very useful in the management of acute hypertensive episodes[9] and Pigott *et al.* reported no advantage to withholding ACE inhibitors in patients with normal left ventricular function undergoing cardiac surgery.[13] There is inadequate evidence at this time to recommend for or against routine continuation in the perioperative period.

Antianginal medications

Because unstable angina greatly increases surgical risks, antianginal medications should be continued.[12] Beta-blockers and calcium channel-blockers are discussed above. Nitrates are available in a variety of forms: oral,

transdermal and i.v. If a patient is using an oral form requiring multiple daily doses, conversion to a once daily form of isosorbide mononitrate or to a transdermal patch will provide coverage through the surgery. For patients expected to be unable to take oral medications for more than the day of surgery, the transdermal patch may be optimal. i.v. Nitroglycerin may be necessary for postoperative unstable angina treatment in the intensive care unit.

Digoxin

A substantial number of patients still take digoxin, though its use is declining. If a patient requires digoxin for management of atrial arrhythmia or for stability of congestive heart failure, continuation is probably best. However, some patients may have questionable indications for digoxin, prompting reconsideration of its use. Since the toxic threshold for digoxin is low, measuring the serum level preoperatively is advised.[1] Perioperative events, including drug interactions, acidosis, hypoxia, electrolyte disturbances and catecholamine surges, increase the potential for digoxin-mediated proarrhythmia.[4] Appropriate monitoring of serum chemistries, oxygen status and renal function (digoxin is cleared through the kidneys) can alert the physician to problems as they develop. In patients with normal renal function, the half-life of digoxin is nearly 2 days, so missing a dose does not pose a significant risk. If necessary, i.v. digoxin may be administered for patients unable to take it by mouth.

Antiarrhythmic medications

Medications used to treat serious cardiac arrhythmias should be continued.[8] Most antiarrhythmic medications have the potential to cause arrhythmia, also. For the patient who will be unable to take oral medications for an extended period, it may be wise to consult the patient's cardiologist for advice about converting to an i.v. form for prophylaxis or for treatment of arrhythmias as they occur. Amiodarone has an i.v. form available for treatment of acute arrhythmias; but since the drug has a very long half-life, the patient who has achieved a steady state before surgery will have continued therapeutic effect even if they cannot take oral medication for an extended period.[8]

Lipid-lowering medications

Most lipid-lowering agents – niacin, fibric acid derivatives (gemfibrozil and fenofibrate) and HMG-CoA reductase inhibitors or "statins" (atorvastatin, fluvastatin, lovastatin, pravastatin and simvastatin) – predispose patients to myositis and rhabdomyolysis, particularly when used in combination or when levels rise through drug interactions. These medications should be discontinued before surgery[4] and may be resumed when the patient is stable and able to eat postoperatively. Bile acid sequestrants such as colestipol, cholestyramine, and colesevelam (WelChol) may cause troublesome gastrointestinal side effects and may bind other drugs in the gut. Since there is no apparent reason to continue these drugs, they may be stopped before surgery and resumed at discharge.

Pulmonary medications

Inhaled bronchodilators such as ipratroprium and beta-adrenergic agonists, cromolyn and inhaled corticosteroids should be continued to support stability of chronic lung diseases.[14] The oral leukotriene inhibitors (montelukast, zafirlukast and zileuton) likewise should be continued. Theophylline has been supplanted by more effective medications in most patients with asthma, COPD and emphysema. In the patient for whom theophylline remains effective, continue the medication.[14] However, theophylline has significant potential for toxic side effects and for drug interactions. If it is continued, measuring the preoperative serum theophylline level and being observant for signs of toxicity is advised.[15]

Estrogens and selective estrogen receptor modulators (SERMs)

Estrogens increase the risk of venous thromboembolism, and deep vein thrombosis and pulmonary embolism remain significant risks of major surgery. Oral contraceptives increase this risk 2–4-fold[16] compared with women not taking these compounds. In vitro assays of coagulation suggest that several weeks are necessary for coagulation activity to return to baseline following withdrawal of oral contraceptives.[17] Postmenopausal hormone replacement has been shown to increase the risk of postoperative thromboembolism.[18] Since the risk of venous thromboembolism remains elevated for weeks to months after orthopedic surgery of the lower extremities[19] and major abdominal or pelvic surgery, the conservative recommendation is to discontinue these medications 30 days before and for 90 days after elective surgery.[20] The SERMs raloxifene (Evista) and tamoxifen (Nolovadex) increase the risk of thromboembolism similarly to estrogen.[21,22]

Stopping estrogens and SERMs perioperatively should improve patient safety through reduction of thromboembolism risk. However, this benefit must be balanced against the effects of withdrawal for the individual patient.

The risks of pregnancy for the woman off her oral contraceptives may be greater than the expected benefit. A woman with severe menopausal symptoms may be quite uncomfortable without hormone replacement. A woman with breast cancer may have an increased chance of disease progression while off tamoxifen for 4 months. Discussion of the recommendations with the patient will inform the best judgment in each case.

Thyroid medications

Thyroid hormone replacement is easily and safely continued with once daily oral levothyroxine. Its long half-life of 6–7 days[4] minimizes any risk of missing a dose or two. For the patient with prolonged inability to take or absorb oral medication, i.v. replacement is available.

If recent-onset thyrotoxicosis has been controlled with antithyroid medications, it is important to continue these drugs to promote safety in the perioperative period. Propylthiouracil and methimazole are available only as oral preparations. An advantage of methimazole is once daily dosing once the thyroid activity is controlled. For the patient unable to take medication by mouth for a prolonged period, a nasogastric or percutaneous gastrostomy tube may be necessary.[23] Should thyrotoxicosis develop, beta-blockers are useful to manage the cardiovascular effects.

Diabetic medications

For patients requiring insulin (juvenile-onset and some adult-onset diabetic patients), continuation of insulin is necessary. Since patients are usually kept "n.p.o." before surgery, short-acting insulin is not given preoperatively except as necessary to manage significant hyperglycemia. Long-acting insulin doses are usually reduced by one third to one half.[5] Close monitoring of the glucose level is necessary except for brief surgery under local anesthesia, with supplemental insulin given as needed. For long surgical cases and for patients with labile glucose values, a continuous insulin infusion with close monitoring and adjustment may be the best approach. Oral medications are usually held the day of surgery and may be resumed once the patient is stable and begins eating postoperatively.[24]

Corticosteroids

If used chronically, systemic corticosteroids are continued through surgery. Depending upon the frequency and dose, pulse or "stress-dose" steroids may be needed perioperatively. This topic is discussed elsewhere in this book.

Anticonvulsants

Treatment for seizure disorders should continue through surgery.[8] If the patient is unable to resume oral medication immediately or develops breakthrough seizures, i.v. anticonvulsants are available. Anticonvulsants are also used for other conditions, such as adjunctive treatment of migraine headaches, neuropathic pain and psychiatric disorders. In these situations the patient may simply resume medication when able to tolerate oral forms.

Antiparkinson medications

Medications used to treat Parkinson's disease have many side effects and potential for drug interactions, especially with sympathomimetic agents that may be necessary in the perioperative state. However, muscle rigidity in Parkinson's disease can complicate ventilator weaning and inhibit participation in treatment. Carbidopa/levodopa (Sinemet and Sinemet CR), the most commonly used drug, is recommended to be continued the morning of surgery and resumed as soon as possible afterward.[8] Dopamine receptor agonists (bromocriptine, pergolide, pramipexole, ropinirole) have been recommended to be withheld the day of surgery but resumed afterward as soon as the patient is able to do so.[25] Selegiline, a monoamine oxidase (MAO) inhibitor, may be continued only with extreme caution as described in a following section.

Medications for myasthenia gravis

As with muscle rigidity in Parkinson's disease, muscle weakness from myasthenia gravis may impair the patient's recovery from surgery. Pyridostigmine or neostigmine should be taken by the patient the morning of surgery and continued as soon as the patient is able to resume oral intake. During the time the patient is "n.p.o.," i.v. preparations may be carefully titrated to the desired effect (usually about 1/30th of the oral dose is given every 4–6 hours).[25]

Antidepressants

In general, if antidepressant medication is essential for the patient, it may be continued in the perioperative period. Selective serotonin reuptake inhibitors (SSRIs) have few serious adverse effects except the serotonin syndrome when combined with drugs having MAO inhibitor activity.[4] Tricyclic antidepressants (TCAs) are used for depression and for neuropathic pain and act by blocking reuptake of norepinephrine and serotonin at the synaptic junction. TCAs may increase the effects of sympathomimetic agents given during or after surgery and may have proarrhythmic and conduction effects in the heart.[4] Anticholinergic side effects, such as delirium, ileus, and sedation, are also common with TCAs. There is no consensus, but most authorities do not suggest stopping TCAs since serious adverse effects seem to be rare.[1,4,5] If the patient does not have serious depression, it may be best to follow the advice of Holleran and taper off the medication several days in advance of surgery.[26]

Monoamine oxidase (MAO) inhibitors are much less commonly used for depression than SSRIs and TCAs. Serious adverse effects of MAO inhibitors include a potentially fatal interaction with meperidine (Demerol) and severe hypertension resulting from coadministration of sympathomimetic agents, among many other drug–drug interactions.[5,26] Most authorities therefore recommend tapering MAO inhibitors off at least 2 weeks before surgery.[1,13,26] The opposite conclusion is offered by Smith *et al.*, who suggest that with great care and collaboration with an experienced anesthesiologist, MAO inhibitors may be safely continued.[8] This latter approach may be attempted in selected severely depressed patients for whom the MAO inhibitors have been the only effective treatment and will be necessary when surgery is urgent and there is not time to taper off the MAO inhibitor.

Other psychiatric medications and opiates

Antipsychotic agents appear to be safe around the time of surgery and are usually continued.[26] A potentially serious reaction is the neuroleptic malignant syndrome, manifest by hyperthermia, muscle rigidity, and autonomic dysregulation. This syndrome may be difficult to distinguish clinically from malignant hyperthermia caused by anesthetic agents, but the latter entity occurs less often with current anesthetics.

Lithium, a standard treatment in bipolar disorder, alters sodium transport in neurons. It is cleared through the kidneys and has a relatively low therapeutic ratio. Adverse effects include potentiation of neuromuscular blockade, delirium, coma and cardiac arrhythmias.[14,26] Diuretics and changes in renal function may cause serum levels to rise.[4] There is no consensus on whether to stop or to continue lithium perioperatively, and a similar risk/benefit judgment must be individualized as with MAO inhibitors. If it is continued, the serum lithium level should be checked before surgery and monitored afterward if the situation warrants (for instance, change in renal function or if new medications are introduced).[15]

Benzodiazepines, when used chronically, may result in physiological and psychological dependence. Withdrawal symptoms such as insomnia, anxiety and panic attacks, delirium, hypertension and tachycardia may occur from abrupt discontinuation.[14] Continuation of the medication on the patient's usual schedule is the safest step. i.v. or i.m. benzodiazepines are easily administered when necessary.

Opioid analgesics (morphine, codeine, hydrocodone, etc.), as with benzodiazepines, may cause withdrawal symptoms if not continued through surgery. Patients who take these drugs chronically may also develop tolerance, requiring higher than usual doses to achieve adequate pain relief after surgery.[14]

Antiretroviral medications

Drug therapy for patients with the human immunodeficiency virus (HIV) and the acquired immunodeficiency syndrome (AIDS) typically involves a large number of medications in order to maximally suppress viral replication and to prevent emergence of drug resistance.[27] Disruptions to therapy are undesirable but may be unavoidable with surgery, depending upon the length of time a patient cannot adequately take oral medication. If the patient is expected to resume eating and taking medications the day of surgery, it is best to continue. But, if the patient is not able to eat or develops significant renal or hepatic dysfunction, all antiretroviral agents should be stopped. Resumption of an antiretroviral regimen will depend upon the patient's unique situation and may best be determined in consultation with the physician providing ongoing care for the infection.

Herbal medications

A substantial proportion of patients undergoing surgery are current users of alternative medicine.[28] Herbal products may have significant adverse effects in the perioperative period, including bleeding, hypertension, arrhythmias, sedation, and hepatic toxicity.[29] Complex adverse interactions with traditional medications are also possible. To minimize the risk of known and unknown adverse drug events, a consensus is developing to stop herbal medications several weeks before surgery.[15,30]

REFERENCES

1. Cygan, R. & Waitzkin, H. Stopping and restarting medications in the perioperative period. *J. Gen. Intern. Med.* 1987; **2**(4): 270–283.

2. Ley, S. J. Quality care outcomes in cardiac surgery: the role of evidence-based practice. *AACN Clin. Issues* 2001; **12**(4): 606–617.

3. Taggart, D. P., Siddiqui, A., & Wheatley, D. J. Low dose preoperative aspirin therapy, postoperative blood loss, and transfusion requirements. *Ann. Thorac. Surg.* 1990; **50**(3): 424–428.

4. *Mosby's Drug Consult*. St. Louis: Mosby, Inc, 2002.

5. Kroenke, K., Gooby-Toedt, D., & Jackson, J. L. Chronic medications in the perioperative period. *South Med. J.* 1998; **91**(4): 358–364.

6. Merritt, J. C. & Bhatt, D. L. The efficacy and safety of perioperative antiplatelet therapy. *J. Thromb. Thrombolysis* 2002; **13**(2): 97–103.

7. Mangano, D. T., Layug, E. L., Wallace, A. *et al.* Effect of atenolol on mortality and cardiovascular morbidity after noncardiac surgery. *N. Engl. J. Med.* 1996; **335**(23): 1713–1720.

8. Smith, M. S., Muir, H., & Hall, R. Perioperative management of drug therapy, clinical considerations. 1996; *Drugs* **51**(2): 238–259.

9. Cherney, D. & Straus, S. Management of patients with hypertensive urgencies and emergencies. *J. Gen. Intern. Med.* 2002; **17**(12): 937–945.

10. Brabant, S. M., Bertrand, M., Eyraud, D. *et al.* The hemodynamic effects of anesthetic induction in vascular surgical patients chronically treated with angiotensin II receptor antagonists. *Anesth. Analg.* 1999; **89**(6): 1388–1392.

11. Coriat, P., Richer, C., Douraki, T. *et al.* Influence of chronic angiotensin-converting enzyme inhibition on anesthetic induction. *Anesthesiology* 1994; **81**(2): 299–307.

12. Roizen, M. F. Anesthetic implications of concurrent diseases. In Miller, R. D., ed. *Anesthesia*, 5th edn. Philadelphia: Churchill Livingstone, 2000: 903–1015.

13. Pigott, D. W., Nagle, C., Allman, K. *et al.* Effect of omitting regular ACE inhibitor medication before cardiac surgery on haemodynamic variables and vasoactive drug requirements. *Br. J. Anaesth.* 1999; **83**(5): 715–720.

14. Heard, S. O. & Stevens, D. S. Preanesthetic evaluation. In Kirby, R. R. & Gravenstein, N., eds. *Clinical Anesthesia Practice*. Philadelphia: W. B. Saunders, 1994: 5–9.

15. Spell, N. O. Stopping and restarting medications in the perioperative period. *Med. Clin. North Am.* 2001; **85**(5): 1117–1128.

16. Williams, R. G. & Yardley, M. P. Oral contraceptive therapy and the surgical management of ENT patients: a review of current clinical practice. *Clin. Otolaryngol.* 1990; **15**(6): 525–528.

17. Bonnar, J. Coagulation effects of oral contraception. *Am. J. Obstet. Gynecol.* 1987; **157**: 1042–1048.

18. Grady, D., Wenger, N. K., Herrington, D. *et al.* Postmenopausal hormone therapy increases risk for venous thromboembolic disease. The Heart and Estrogen/progestin Replacement Study. *Ann. Intern. Med.* 2000; **132**(9): 689–696.

19. Merli, G. J. Duration of deep vein thrombosis and pulmonary embolism prophylaxis after joint arthroplasty. *Med. Clin. North Am.* 2001; **85**(5): 1101–1107.

20. New Zealand Guidelines Group. Best practice evidence-based guideline for the appropriate prescribing of hormone

replacement therapy. Wellington (NZ): New Zealand Guidelines Group; 2001 May.

21. Cummings, S. R., Eckert, S., Krueger, K. A. *et al.* The effect of raloxifene on risk of breast cancer in postmenopausal women: results from the MORE randomized trial. Multiple Outcomes of Raloxifene Evaluation. *J. Am. Med. Assoc.* 1999; **281**(23): 2189–2197.

22. Haynes, B. & Dowsett, M. Clinical pharmacology of selective estrogen receptor modulators. *Drugs Aging* 1999; **14**(5): 323–336.

23. Guarnieri, K. M. & McKeon, B. P. Drug metabolism, reactions, and interactions in the surgical patient: prevention of medication-induced morbidity. In Goldmann, D. R., Brown, F. H., & Guarnieri, D. M., eds. *Perioperative Medicine*, 2nd edn. New York: McGraw-Hill, 1994: 479–490.

24. Hoogwerf, B. J. Postoperative management of the diabetic patient. *Med. Clin. North Am.* 2001; **85**(5): 1213–1228.

25. Bell, R. D. & Merli, G. J. Perioperative assessment and management of the surgical patient with neurologic problems. In Merli, G. J. & Weitz, H. H., eds. *Medical Management of the Surgical Patient*, 2nd edn. Philadelphia: W. B. Saunders, 1998: 283–311.

26. Holleran, D. K. & Ziring, B. S. Medical evaluation of the patient with psychiatric illness. In Merli, G. J. & Weitz, H. H., eds. *Medical Management of the Surgical Patient*, 2nd edn. Philadelphia: W. B. Saunders, 1998: 351–358.

27. Yarchoan, R. & Broder, S. Treatment of HIV infection and AIDS. In Goldman, L. & Bennett, J. C., eds. *Cecil Textbook of Medicine*, 21st edn. Philadelphia: W. B. Saunders, 2000: 1933–1941.

28. Tsen, L. C., Segal, S., Pothier, M. *et al.* Alternative medicine use in presurgical patients. *Anesthesiology* 2000; **93**(1): 148–151.

29. Ang-Lee, M. K., Moss, J., & Yuan, C. S. Herbal medicines and perioperative care. *J. Am. Med. Assoc.* 2001; **286**(20): 208–216.

30. Cheng, B., Hung, C. T., & Chiu, W. Herbal medicines and anaesthesia. *Hong Kong Med. J.* 2002; **8**(2): 123–130.

5

Ethical considerations in the surgical patient

Carl C. Hug, Jr.[1] and Kathleen Kinlaw[2]

[1]Emory University Hospital, Atlanta, GA
[2]Health Science Ethics, Emory University, Atlanta, GA

In the long tradition of medical ethics, many theories and frameworks for ethical analysis of issues and situations have been developed. Four primary principles[1] have been identified as most relevant for making clinical decisions:

Beneficence: promoting good, acting in the best interests of the patient

Non-maleficence: avoiding harm by action or omission

Autonomy: respecting patients' rights to make decisions about their health care

Justice: fair and equitable treatment that reflects what the patient is due.

These principles can be instrumental in the ethical analysis of clinical situations in which the best option for patient care is not clear. Each is considered *prima facie*, a principle that is to be honored unless it is in conflict with an equal or greater principle, in which case the relative weight of each principle will have to be decided. For example, determining whether aggressive interventions and continuing life-supporting measures are in the best interest of the patient will have to be weighed against the suffering that they engender and the patient's autonomous expression of their wishes to avoid certain procedures. In the USA, high priority is placed on patient autonomy in healthcare decisions. Many of the ethical issues covered in this chapter illustrate the emphasis on patient autonomy.

Patient autonomy

This refers to the patient's right to make decisions about his/her own health, including the right to accept or to forego treatments. Information about the state of health and disease, indications for treatment, treatment alternatives with the relative benefits and risks of each, and the consequences of refusing treatment is necessary for the patient to make prudent decisions.

Case analysis

Jonsen *et al.*[2] have developed a practical method for analyzing situations for individual patients. They identify four major topics for consideration in any decision about medical interventions.

Medical indications

These include the diagnosis and prognosis of the disease with and without treatment, alternative treatments, goals and probabilities of success for each, and balance of benefits and complications.

Patient preferences

These include the patient's decision-making capacity, how well informed the patient is, and the patient's understanding of the information. Central to this topic is respect for the patient's values and goals. If the patient is unable to make decisions, is the surrogate using appropriate standards in accordance with previously expressed wishes and advance directives in the best interest of the patient? Within ethical and legal boundaries, is the patient's right to choose being respected?

Quality of life

This includes the likelihood for returning the patient to his or her normal or usual level of function; physical, mental, and social deficits that are likely if the treatment succeeds

Medical Management of the Surgical Patient: A Textbook of Perioperative Medicine, ed. M. F. Lubin, R. B. Smith, T. F. Dobson, N. Spell, H. K. Walker. 4th edn. Published by Cambridge University Press. © Cambridge University 2006.

or if it fails and their acceptability/unacceptability to the patient; conditions that would make the patient's continued life undesirable; plans for comfort and palliative care if treatment is foregone. Are the likely outcomes aligned with previously expressed wishes and advance directives? Is the patient's right to choose being respected to the extent possible in regard to ethical principles and the law?

Contextual features

These include family, financial, religious, cultural and other patient-related issues that might influence the decision as well as provider, institutional, legal, scientific, or resource allocation issues that could impact the decision.

In deciding whether or not an intervention is medically indicated, it is important to keep in mind that at least one of the following goals of medicine mentioned by Jonsen et al.[3] should be realistically achievable:
  (i) promotion of health and prevention of disease
  (ii) relief of symptoms, pain, and suffering
 (iii) cure of disease
  (iv) prevention of untimely death
  (v) improvement of functional status or maintenance of compromised status
  (vi) education and counseling of patients regarding their condition and prognosis
 (vii) avoidance of harm to the patient.
The goals of treatment need to be reassessed regularly and continually evaluated against scientific and clinical evidence so that the healthcare team and family reach a consensus on realistic goals of intervention.

The importance of providing a realistic prognosis

Presently, medical schools and residency training programs do a very good job in teaching the intricacies of diagnosis and therapy, but there appears to be little emphasis placed on prognostic estimation and communication of those estimates to the patient, especially when the prognosis is poor with or without treatment. An overly optimistic prognosis is dangerous because it may cause a patient and family to be unprepared for disabilities and death, and it makes them reluctant to accept limitations on aggressive, futile care that is not medically appropriate. Overly pessimistic prognoses may produce undue anxiety and loss of hope.[4] The physician's challenge is to communicate the facts clearly and accurately, to manage the reactions of the patient and family members to those facts, and to guide them to an appropriate balance of optimism and pessimism.

For a thorough discussion of prognosis, see the book by Nicholas A. Christakis, M.D., a physician and sociologist, who has written *Death Foretold: Prophecy and Prognosis in Medical Care.*[4] It details the challenges of dealing with uncertainty and offers practical approaches to managing them.

The American Council for Graduate Medical Education (ACGME) and the American Board of Medical Specialties (ABMS) have joined together to assist medical schools and residency training programs in the development of educational protocols designed to achieve the six competencies and to implement the 13 assessment tools that have been defined by the Outcome Project conducted by the ACGME with the support of the Robert Wood Johnson Foundation. Two of the six competencies, professionalism and communication, relate directly to the professional and ethical obligations of physicians to their patients in terms of providing realistic prognoses and offering reasonable alternatives of curative, restorative and palliative care.[5]

Consent to and refusal of treatment

The right of a patient to be fully informed prior to consenting to medical treatment has been clearly established ethically and legally. Informed consent can be defined as the willing acceptance of a medical intervention by a patient after adequate disclosure and understanding of the nature of the intervention, its risks, benefits and alternatives. In medical practice the concept of informed consent has evolved from that of gaining the patient's consent or authorization for the proposed intervention based solely on the physician's recommendation, to informed consent based on adequate disclosure of relevant information, to making sure that the patient understands the information disclosed before providing authorization for the procedure.[6]

Fundamental to informed consent is the requirement that the patient has the capacity to make a decision, that is, to understand the medical decision (i.e., the benefits and risks of the proposed diagnostic or therapeutic intervention and their alternatives) and to make his or her own choices. Decision-making capacity determinations are typically made by the attending physician, sometimes in consultation with a psychiatrist if capacity is in doubt. Competency, the more global assessment of an individual's ability to manage his or her own life decisions, is a legal concept. As physicians and others interact with patients, they gain insight as to their mental capacity and, barring obvious deficiencies, the patients are presumed to be competent unless legal proceedings determine otherwise.

Assessments of decision making capacity[7–9] should include:

(i) the patient's ability to understand relevant information, including comprehension, recall (verbalization), and retention of information as well as an understanding of causal relationships and probabilities;

(ii) the patient's ability to appreciate their medical situation and its implications, including the alternatives, risks and benefits of each alternative, and the likely consequences;

(iii) the ability to reason, to deliberate, to reach a conclusion based on the information provided;

(iv) the ability to express a choice and to recognize one's power to make that choice.

The stress of dealing with pain or other symptoms as well as the influence of medications may impact decision-making capacity. However, medications to relieve pain and other symptoms may actually assist the distressed patient in retaining decision-making capacity. Decision-making capacity should be evaluated specifically for the medical decision facing the patient. In other words: can this patient understand and make a choice about the specific intervention under consideration? A patient with limitations in some areas of life (e.g., inability to manage one's fiscal affairs; a psychiatric diagnosis; frailty in advanced age) may still have the decision-making capacity needed to make a decision about the medical procedure he or she is facing.

In addition to assessing the patient's capacity to consent, the physician has an ethical obligation to make reasonable efforts to assure that all relevant information has been disclosed and that the patient comprehends that information. The history of medicine, ethics, and health law has confirmed the right of the patient to give informed consent to accept or to refuse treatment.[10]

Physicians are responsible for:

(i) being knowledgeable, competent information-givers who disclose information relevant to patient's ability to consent,

(ii) assessing and assuring the patient's understanding of the information,

(iii) assuring that the patient's consent is voluntary and free from controlling influences, and

(iv) obtaining authorization or consent in a way that respects within reason the patient's need for time to make the decision and for reassessing such authorization periodically during longer-term interventions.[11]

Physicians may act without the patient or a surrogate's consent in emergencies. Utilizing the concept of "therapeutic privilege," the ability to withhold information that is felt to be harmful to a patient needs to be carefully examined. Health teams may feel compelled to consider withholding information based on beneficence and on non-maleficence. However, physicians should be cautious about making assumptions about what information the patient can handle. Alternatively, patients may be asked to help determine how much information they wish to receive. Mrs. Jones, do you wish to know as much as possible about your test results? Where limited information is requested, patients may be able to identify alternative decision makers whom they wish to involve in decision making.

Right to refuse treatment

Healthcare teams are often ethically troubled when patients do not agree to the recommended course of treatment. Refusal of treatment by an adult, who has decision-making capacity and is well informed, should be respected, even if that refusal leads to serious harm to the individual. The right to refuse treatment is ethically supported by the principle of autonomy and has been supported in multiple US legal jurisdictions. Refusal of treatment by an adult patient with decision-making capacity based on religious beliefs is also generally supported ethically and legally. If no third parties are affected by the refusal of treatment (e.g., a dependent child will be left without a caregiver), religiously based refusals should be honored. Where the physician feels strongly about the compelling reasons for treatment, the physician can certainly continue to discuss the reasons for refusal with the patient and try to persuade the patient to reconsider the decision. Manipulation or coercion are not ethically permissible. A physician who objects to the decision not to treat based on personal or professional values can seek to have the care of the patient transferred to another physician. However, staying with patients and families through discussions of decisions such as refusal of life-sustaining treatments can provide a powerful occasion for developing mutual understanding and respect which will carry over to other healthcare decisions.[12]

End-of-life care

In November 2002, the Last Acts organization, funded by the Robert Wood Johnson Foundation, released the report, "Means to a better end: a report on dying in America today."[13] The report assessed how well each of the 50 states was doing in providing end-of-life care, utilizing such indicators as the status of advance care planning, where deaths occurred (e.g., home vs. acute care settings), time spent in intensive care units, pain management, and utilization of hospice services. The report concluded "that Americans, at best, have no better than a fair chance of finding good care for their loved ones or for themselves when facing a life-threatening illness."

Despite recent surveys indicating that, on average, more that 70% of Americans wish to die at home; only 25% of Americans actually do so. Approximately 50% of Americans age 65 and older die in hospitals and 20% to 25% die in nursing homes.[13]

Do not resuscitate decisions

From the perspectives of medicine, ethics, and law, a patient suffering pulmonary and/or cardiac arrest is presumed to choose cardiopulmonary resuscitation (CPR) and it should be performed unless, and until, there is direct evidence that the patient previously has decided to forego CPR (i.e., DNR status). Most states have laws clarifying when and by what process resuscitative procedures may be withheld. Most healthcare organizations have established do not resuscitate (DNR) policies in compliance with state laws and Joint Commission on Accreditation of HealthCare Organizations (JCAHO) guidelines. Many states have laws and protocols for the honoring of "prehospital" DNR orders outside of medical facilities.[14]

There are two general justifications for refraining from CPR.

(i) The patient has clearly expressed his or her wish that CPR not be performed.

(ii) It is judged clinically by physicians that CPR would be medically ineffective or inappropriate.

DNR orders should be written after a careful conversation with the patient or surrogate and should reflect the patient's preferences or the surrogate's reflections on the patient's previously expressed wishes and on what would be in the patient's best interests. The conversation should be clearly documented in the progress notes of the patient's medical record. All members of the health care team should be informed of the DNR status and, where applicable, appropriate wristbands should be attached and posting on the medical chart cover and elsewhere should occur.

Patients or surrogates may, of course, change their minds at any time regarding DNR orders. Physicians should revisit the decision if and when improvement in the patient's condition occurs. Some institutions have a policy mandating review of DNR orders on a regular basis.

Meaning of DNR

There are two acronyms in use: DNR – do not resuscitate; DNAR – do not attempt to resuscitate. We prefer the acronym "DNR" to emphasize what it does and doesn't mean. DNR means that, in the case of spontaneous respiration ceasing and/or the heart beat stopping, measures such as artificial ventilation, chest compressions, electrical defibrillation, and resuscitative doses of epinephrine and other drugs routinely administered according to CPR protocol, will not be employed. DNR also means "do not relax" in the sense that all other types of care will continue at their current level. This includes both life-supporting measures agreed upon by the patient and physician, and most especially, all measures of prevention of pain, anxiety and other forms of suffering. In fact, life-supporting on-going measures can be increased, or added to, in the presence of an existing DNR status.[15]

Managing patients with DNR directives under emergency conditions

Emergency-care providers operate under the rules and laws mandating presumption of a patient's desire to be resuscitated unless and until there is solid evidence to the contrary, such as a living will or communication with a credible healthcare proxy who states that the patient's wishes are not to be resuscitated. Depending on state law and EMS (Emergency Medical Service) standards, a wrist band or other notification worn by the patient may be accepted under some conditions by emergency medical providers. Most states require a clear statement of DNR status along with the name(s) and contact number(s) of the person(s) who can verify the patient's wishes. In the presence of valid DNR, CPR should not be initiated, or if it is in progress, it should be stopped.

Many states allow the honoring of DNR orders outside of hospital and DNR orders maybe "portable," that is, honored by EMT personnel en route from one site to another and by the medical and nursing staff at the receiving institution.

Managing patients with DNR directives for elective interventions

If a patient with a DNR order is to undergo anesthesia and surgery, the question of maintenance of the DNR order during the perioperative period arises. The American College of Surgeons issued a statement: recommending "required reconsideration" of prior DNR orders.[16] A new conversation with the patient or surrogate decision maker should occur, emphasizing that there is added risk for a life-threatening event during the operation, but many such events are transient and correctable. Patients and families need to understand that surgical and anesthetic management of the patient during surgery usually necessitates use of certain procedures (e.g., tracheal intubation, mechanical ventilation, resuscitative drugs) that are components of CPR. Physicians and hospital personnel should work with the patient and family to reconsider the DNR decision during this time, rather than make an assumption either to suspend the DNR order or to maintain the order without the consent of the patient or the surrogate. The American Society of Anesthesiologists Ethical Guidelines suggest four options for managing DNR status during and immediately after invasive, risky interventions that can lead to cardiopulmonary arrest.[17]

Suspension of DNR

This is necessary for certain procedures during which it is routine standard practice to employ one or more life supporting techniques (e.g., open heart surgery). Generally speaking, the suspension is for the period of time of the procedure per se and continuing through the usual expected time for recovery from drugs used to provide anesthesia, analgesia and sedation. It also includes the usual time required for recovery from the acute insult of the intervention. Some institutions mandate suspension of DNR status for any intervention because there is concern (a) about the risks of malpractice claims and suits, and (b) the possibility that an anesthesiologist or anesthetist may hold back on the administration of anesthetic and analgesic drugs for fear of being responsible for the patient's death, and this creates the risk of patient suffering due to awareness, anxiety, and pain during and after the intervention. However, for palliative procedures in patients who are facing imminent death with a DNR status, we and many others believe that automatic suspension of DNR is inappropriate. (See goal-directed CPR below.)

Maintenance of DNR status

This may be appropriate for some patients who are undergoing palliative interventions for a terminal condition near the end of life.

Modification of DNR status

The patient and/or the proxy for healthcare decisions may choose to negotiate with the physicians about suspending certain types of resuscitative measures during an intervention. For example, if it is to be done under general anesthesia during which it is routine to assist or support breathing mechanically with or without an endotracheal tube, this provision of DNR should be suspended. On the other hand, if ventricular fibrillation is not expected or is rare under the conditions of the intervention, the patient may continue to refuse electrical defibrillation.

Goal-directed CPR

Under this method of management, the patient assents to the judgment of the physicians involved in the intervention. Temporary, easily reversible events (e.g., hypotension, bradycardia) would be treated as long as the specific goals of the intervention are achievable and unacceptable disabilities are unlikely. Should the latter become apparent after the resuscitative measures are undertaken, they can simply be discontinued according to the wishes and advance directives of the patient.[18]

In regard to palliative interventions, it should be noted that, while the physician accepts responsibility for a complication, a laudable thing to do, it does not create the obligation to reverse the complication and its consequences. The occurrence of an iatrogenic complication during a palliative intervention does not give the physicians the right to perform corrective interventions without the patient's consent or to override the patient's decision.[19] If the physician is unsure about what to do, especially if she or he is young and inexperienced, consultation with colleagues, and particularly with a senior mentor, is appropriate in order to validate the decision and also to provide support for the decision in case of later recrimination by the patient or anyone else.

Most patients receiving palliative (comfort) care have accepted the conclusion that they will die of their disease. In most cases they have already decided that they do not want to be resuscitated should their breathing and/or circulation stop, and a DNR status has been established through their living will, a physician's order, and statements to their next of kin or proxy for healthcare decisions.

Advance directives

Advance directives refer to any expression by a patient that is intended to guide care, should the patient lose his or her decision-making capacity. Directives are a part of the advance care planning process that emphasizes communication about patient preferences with loved ones and healthcare professionals. This concept is founded ethically on the intent to protect the patient's autonomy, the ability of the patient to govern or make decisions about their own care. Ideally, advance care planning allows for the patient to "think through" and to communicate their values and preferences to their surrogate, family members and physicians that should facilitate informed decision making should the patient no longer be able to guide his or her care. Such planning can catalyze family discussion and may minimize dissent at later times when difficult decisions need to be made.

The federal Patient Self Determination Act of 1990 requires all healthcare facilities receiving Medicare and Medicaid funding to ask all patients whether they have advance directive documents and, if not, whether they wish to receive information about advance planning and to prepare such documents.[20] There are two primary types of legally recognized advance directives.

(i) The Living Will is a document that allows an individual to indicate in writing the interventions she/he would want and not want if she/he is no longer able to make decisions. Forty-seven states and the District of Columbia have laws recognizing living wills.[21]

(ii) Durable Power of Attorney for Health Care (or a medical power of attorney) is a more comprehensive document. It allows an individual to appoint another person (usually called an "agent" or "healthcare proxy" or "surrogate") to make healthcare decisions should the individual lose decision-making capacity. All 50 states have laws which recognize these powers.[21]

Published studies estimate that about 15% of the US population currently has advance directives.[22]

The utilization of advance directive documents is somewhat controversial in actual practice. The documents must be readily available and family members may not know where they are kept, or even that they exist. Unless the documents are physically present, they cannot be honored. Even when directives are available, they may not contain enough specific information to help surrogates or healthcare professionals make decisions in the immediate context. At the present time, legal directives are also "state specific," meaning that institutions may not be willing to allow a directive to be implemented unless it follows the statutory format recognized in the state where the facility is located. Several groups are now working to create a universal form of advance directive that can easily be recognized and honored across state lines.

There is some evidence that directives are less likely to be honored if either the treating physician or family disagrees with the patient's preferences expressed in the directive.[23] Communication about the documents, in advance, is essential for surrogates to feel empowered to act on behalf of the patient and for clinicians to understand the patient's wishes. Discussions with physicians and other healthcare professionals sparked by the writing of an advance directive may be more important than the information recorded in a living will.

Philosophically, it can be questioned whether any written directive will accurately reflect the wishes of the person when the need to implement the directive actually arises. Patients may change their preferences as a chronic illness progresses or at the point when a medical problem arises. Though perhaps imperfect, advance care planning does provide the opportunity to consider one's own values and to communicate them to clinicians and loved ones. Ideally, one's thinking should be revisited regularly and the written and verbal directives revised accordingly.

Therapeutic trials, including surgery and other interventions

Medicine has been described as the science of uncertainty and the art of probability. It is impossible to know with certainty the outcome of any treatment prospectively, whether or not it will be successful, whether or not complications will occur. There is always a statistically based benefit-to-burden ratio, and the burdens include complications of the intervention or lack of its success leading to more or less permanent disabilities and death. At this point in history, statistical estimates of risks apply to selected groups of patients and cannot be used with certainty to predict the outcome for any individual patient. The teaching point remains: "Never say never or always in medicine."

In the face of these uncertainties, the physician nevertheless has an obligation to provide the patient with a realistic assessment based on group data, statistical estimates, and the physician's personal experience with patients in similar circumstances.[4] The only way to determine whether or not a treatment will be successful or not and whether complications will occur or not, is to do a therapeutic trial. In considering such a trial, it is wise for the patient to answer two questions:[24] (a) What are your (realistic) goals for the proposed intervention? (b) What bad (realistic) outcomes, including more or less permanent disabilities and death, are unacceptable to you? The goals have to be realistically achievable by the intervention, and from the patient's point of view, they may range from full restoration of independent function to something as simple as being able sit in a chair and communicate with grandchildren and other family members and friends.

In regard to potential disabilities, most patients do not have any notion of their impact on the quality of everyday life. When they begin to appreciate the practical consequences of confinement to a wheelchair, they may consider this degree of disability to be unacceptable. The chronic weakness, fatigue and depression associated with every-other-day hemodialysis may be intolerable. Even though it takes time, the physician has an obligation to help the patient to understand the potential consequences of a lack of success or the occurrence of complications of the intervention.

From the physician's point of view, the benefit-to-burden ratio must be acceptable, and each physician has to decide what is acceptable for him/herself. It should be noted that, as a group, physicians tend to overestimate the burdens of disabilities compared to patients' estimates.[25] Also, patients often change their opinion about the burdens of disabilities as they experience them and learn to make adjustments to them (e.g., the initial depression and ultimate optimism of paraplegics over time).

In ethical terms, "the moral burden of proof often should be heavier when the decision is to withhold than when it is to withdraw treatments".[26] "Only after starting treatments will it be possible in many cases, . . . to balance prospective benefits and burdens."[26]

In the case of a surgical trial, the defined benefits must outweigh the disabilities in terms of their importance to the patient, but not in terms of their statistical chance of occurrence. For example, given a completely unacceptable existing state of chronically poor health, it would be appropriate for the patient to choose a 25% chance of improvement even though the risks of death and disability are considerably higher. The ethical basis of this is the Principle of Double Effect in which the improved health condition is intended and the risks of complications and death are recognized and accepted, but not intended.[27] A therapeutic trial, even with a high risk of death, is not euthanasia or physician-assisted suicide.

In practical terms, a surgical trial includes a period of time after the intervention to determine what the likely outcome will be for the patient. In the presence of progressive improvement, continuation of life-supporting measures is indicated. However, the patient, healthcare proxy, family members and friends and the physicians providing care must be willing to discontinue futile therapies, including life-supporting measures if the patient is unlikely to realize his/her stated goals, deterioration of health status is progressive, and multiple organ systems failure ensues. ". . . trial interventions coupled with hard-nosed clinical realism, may appropriately balance the possibilities for good or ill . . . ."[28]

If the physician believes that the benefit-to-burden ratio is unacceptable in the face of a patient's or family members' demands for an intervention for whatever reason, therapeutic trial or not, the physician must follow his/her own beliefs and refuse to provide or to participate in the intervention. If she/he is in the midst of an ongoing therapeutic relationship with the patient, the options are to offer an alternative treatment, to refer the patient to another physician, or if futile, to appeal to an institutional mechanism for dealing with futile (medically non-indicated) interventions. [See medically inappropriate (futile) interventions below.]

Methods for assessment of the patient's condition and prognosis

Over the years, particularly in the 1980s and 1990s, scoring systems[29,30] have been developed in an attempt to express severity of illness numerically as a means of summarizing and publicizing data, conducting clinical research, measuring and comparing outcomes of treatments, and in the last 10–15 years especially, to provide an objective measure of the benefits of healthcare expenditures. Clinical scoring systems combined with laboratory measures have been correlated individually (univariate analysis) and collectively (multivariate analysis) with outcomes (e.g., benefits of treatment, progression of disease). Such correlations have been elaborated into mathematical models intended to assess the risks of morbidity and mortality and to predict short and long-term outcomes for precisely defined groups of patients (e.g., patients undergoing percutaneous cardiac interventions (PCI) or cardiac surgery). Although some of the scoring systems have proven to be quite reliable in predicting outcomes for a particular group of patients more or less precisely characterized, none has been able to predict the outcome for any individual patient. There is always residual uncertainty even with the most elaborate mathematical models. (Hence, the necessity of undertaking an individual patient's therapeutic trial as discussed above.) Also, the number of variables entered into most models is large and the equations for the model are quite sophisticated and too complicated for use by a physician standing at the patient's bedside. A few attempts have been made to utilize such models to enhance the individual physician's clinical judgment in making treatment or non-treatment decisions for individual patients, but little success has been realized to date (e.g., see SUPPORT, study to understand prognosis and preferences for outcomes and risks of treatments[31]).

Table 5.1a. Definitions of organ system failure (French definition when different)[32]

If the patient had one or more of the following during a 24-hour period (regardless of values), organ system failure (OSF) existed on that day.

Cardiovascular failure (presence of one or more of the following):
Heart rate ≤ 54/min
Mean arterial blood pressure ≤ 49 mmHg (systolic blood pressure < 60 mmHg)
Occurrence of ventricular tachycardia and/or ventricular fibrillation
Serum pH ≤ 7.24 with a P_aCO_2 of ≤ 49 mmHg

Respiratory failure (presence of one or more of the following):
Respiratory rate ≤ 5/min or ≥ 49/min
$P_aCO_2 \geq 50$ mmHg
$A_aDO_2 \geq 350$ mmHg $A_aDO_2 = 713\ F_IO_2 - P_aCO_2 - P_aO_2$
Dependent on ventilator or CPAP on the second day of OSF (e.g., not applicable the initial 24 hours of OSF).

Renal failure (presence of one or more of the following):
Urine output ≤ 479 ml/24 hours or ≤ 159 ml/8 hours.
Serum BUN ≥ 100 mg/100 ml (*>36 micromoles/l*)
Serum creatinine ≥ 3.5 mg/100 ml (*>310 micromoles/l*)

Hematologic failure (presence of one or more of the following):
WBC ≤ 1000/mm^3
Platelets $\leq 20\,000$/mm^3
Hematocrit $\leq 20\%$

Neurologic failure
Glasgow Coma Score ≤ 6 (in absence of sedation)

As an intensive care physician, I find it useful to employ a rather simple, easily remembered correlation between the dysfunction of one or more organ systems (Table 5.1a) and in-hospital mortality that was elaborated by Knaus and Wagner in 1989.[32] The basis of their correlations was the precise definition of each organ system's failure and the impact of failure of one or more organ systems on 5248 patients in 13 USA and 27 French hospitals. With the failure of three or more organ systems over a 7-day period, 103 of 105 patients died in-hospital, and one has to wonder about the outcome, particularly the quality of life, of the two survivors who were discharged from hospital (Table 5.1b). This simple correlation has been very useful to me as an intensive care physician in (a) organizing my clinical impressions, (b) documenting the patient's status and likely outcome in the medical record, and (c) communicating prognosis and discussing options with the family members and friends of the patient. It has been particularly useful in supporting the decision of the healthcare proxy and family members to forego major new interventions, to establish a DNR status, and to withdraw life support.

Table 5.1b. Multiple organ dysfunction

Number of organs	Days	Mortality
1	1	20/40%
1	7	25/50%
>3	1	80%[a]
>3	7	~100%[a]

Note:
[a] no difference $</>$ 65 years.
Source: ($n = 2843 + 2405$) Knaus & Wagner, 1989.[32]

Patient preferences

In the USA today, an analogy has been drawn between medical practice and the auto repair business. The attitude seems to be: "If it's broke, fix or replace it." Some physicians act and are viewed as technicians.[33] From the patient's point of view, someone else pays for the care, no limits should be set (or nobody knows how to set them), and there is always the hope for a miracle. Physicians have financial incentives to treat disease but not withhold services when there is a questionable indication of their medical appropriateness. These perspectives stand in stark contrast to what has been found by surveys of USA citizens.

Most citizens prefer to die peacefully and with dignity at home, wish to avoid pain and suffering, wish to avoid dependence on machines, family members and others, and wish to avoid depleting financial resources of the family and their estates. However, few prospectively define wishes or formulate advance directives. Death is a feared and taboo subject for discussion among the healthy. As Morrie Schwartz said in Tuesdays with Morrie,[34] "Everyone knows they are going to die, but nobody believes it … If we did, we would do things differently."

The issues of social justice, particularly about criteria for access to or denial of medical care, particularly when the cost-to-benefit ratio is very high, will have to be solved by society at large, and cannot and should not be decided by the individual physician taking care of an individual patient. The physician–patient interactions should focus on functional goals and accumulating disabilities with chronic disease and age, and on functional outcome in terms of quality of life of interventions. Patients and their family members need to be informed not only about the chances of success and the risks of death of an intervention, but about the intermediate, more-or-less permanent, disabilities that can occur and their implications for long-term care facilities and the associated costs, especially when the quality of life of the patient is unacceptably poor.[35]

Withholding and withdrawing treatment

The AMA Council on Ethical and Judicial Affairs defines life-sustaining treatment as "any treatment that serves to prolong life without reversing the underlying medical disease."[36] Foregoing life-sustaining treatment is ethically, medically, and legally permissible under certain circumstances. Support for the concept comes from multiple medical, nursing, and ethics organizations, as well as from the 1983 President's Commission for the Study of Ethical Problems in Medicine and Biomedical and Behavioral Research.[37–40] One national survey from 1994–1995 indicates that 75% of ICU deaths occurred following a decision to withhold or withdraw some type of life-sustaining treatment.[41]

As discussed earlier, respect for patient autonomy requires physicians to respect the patient's own decision to withhold or withdraw interventions if the patient has the capacity to decide. If the patient can no longer speak for him/herself, physicians turn first to advance directives and, if those are absent, to surrogate decision makers. Surrogates are ethically and legally given the right to represent the patient, either through substituted judgment – indicating their knowledge of what the patient would have wanted in the current circumstance – or determining what they believe to be in the best interests of the patient. Surrogate decisions should be honored unless the clinician believes the decision is not what the patient would have wanted or could not "reasonably be judged to be in the patient's best interests."

There is no ethically significant difference between withholding and withdrawing treatment from a patient. If important reasons exist to consider withholding an intervention in the first place, but the decision is made to begin treatment, the same rationale would support withdrawing treatment at a later time. Beginning treatment may be permissible and desirable if one anticipates gaining new information that will clarify a decision later in caring for the patient. Removal of treatment should be considered if the patient's condition indicates that continuation of that treatment no longer benefits the patient. In their text, *Clinical Ethics*, ethics professor Albert Jonsen, physician professor Mark Siegler, and legal professor William Winslade conclude that, if we can not advance the interests of the patient and no goal of medicine is achievable, no duty to treat exists.[42] Merely sustaining cardiopulmonary function (i.e., organic life) is not a goal of medicine; often it is only prolonging death.

Futility

Multiple attempts have been made to define the controversial concept of what constitutes a medically futile intervention. Some have attempted stricter definitions such as: an intervention that has no pathophysiologic rationale (Dr. Bernard Lo) or an intervention that merely prolongs the dying process. Others, like Dr. Laurence Schneiderman, attempted a quantitative definition, claiming that a treatment that has been unsuccessful in the last 100 cases should be considered "futile." Most professional association guidelines that discuss futile treatment include the idea that these treatments provide no medical benefit to the patient, based on the patient's own medical goals.[43]

Yet, there is a sense, even if no consensus definition can be found, that there ought to be limits to treatments that will not meet reasonable medical goals for the patient or will impose unreasonable pain and suffering on the patient. Often at conflict ethically in these decisions is respect for patient autonomy – as implemented by a surrogate decision maker – and respect for professional integrity of clinicians who object to continuing treatment that is perceived to violate professional duty. Communication that identifies the common interests of all involved and focuses on patient goals and values is essential and may lead to resolution.

Where consensus cannot be reached, the AMA Council on Ethical and Legal Affairs recommends that all health care institutions have a medical futility policy that provides for a "fair process" approach to decision making.[44] Such an approach would support such steps as a standing body including patient and public representatives; an accessible, published process; inclusion of second opinions and external review; support for and inclusion of surrogate decision makers throughout; and exploration of patient transfer options. If the process ends with a recommendation against continued treatment, "the intervention … need not be provided." An example of such a process exists in the Guidelines on Medically Inappropriate Interventions, jointly agreed to by Houston-area hospitals.[45] (In fact the AMA policy draws heavily on the Houston experience.) The Houston guidelines were codified in Texas state law in 1999 under the Texas Health and Safety Code (166.046), which allows for life-sustaining treatment to be withdrawn 10 days after the patient or surrogate receives a written explanation of the decision that treatment is considered "medically inappropriate." The state of Virginia also has a state medical futility statute (Virginia Code – Health Decisions Act 54.1–2990) stating that physicians are not required to provide treatment felt to be "medically or ethically inappropriate." There have been two cases to date testing the futility statute in Virginia. One case (Baby K in 1994) supported continued treatment of a child with anencephaly based on the preemption of the futility statute by the federal EMTALA (Emergency Medical Treatment and Active Labor Act). The other case (Bryan vs. Rectors and Visitors of the University of Virginia 1996) clarified that EMTALA only required stabilization of the patient in respiratory distress, not continued treatment. Further legal tests in Virginia and Texas are expected in attempts to clarify futility statutes.[46]

The American Medical Association's Council on Ethical and Judicial Affairs indicates that physicians are not ethically obligated to deliver care that, in their best professional judgment, will not have a reasonable chance of benefiting their patients. Patients should not be given treatments simply because they demand them. Denial of treatment should be justified by reliance on openly stated ethical principles and acceptable standards of care . . . not on the concept of "futility," which cannot be meaningfully defined.[43]

Comfort care/palliative care and hospice

Diane Meier, Director of the Center to Advance Palliative Care, defines palliative care as "interdisciplinary care that aims to relieve suffering and improve quality of life for patients with advanced illness and their families."[47] The Joint Commission (JCAHO) standard on care at the end-of-life[48] reflects a multidimensional understanding of palliative care, as does the World Health Organization's definition of palliative care:[49]

- provides relief from pain and other symptoms,
- affirms life and regard dying as a normal process,
- neither hastens nor postpones death,
- integrates psychological and spiritual care,
- supports the patient's living as actively as possible until death,
- utilizes an interdisciplinary team approach,
- provides a support system for the family,
- enhances quality of life,
- is compatible with life-prolonging therapies.

Palliative care can be "offered simultaneous with all other appropriate medical treatment."[47] Central to this concept is that palliative care can, and should, be offered early in the course of treatment, rather than be seen as a care

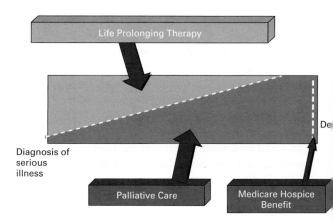

Fig. 5.1. Palliative care's place in the course of illness.[47]

alternative that is only offered after curative treatment has been exhausted. Figure 5.1 demonstrates that palliative care begins at the point of diagnosis with serious illness and is provided along with life-supporting interventions. Through the course of illness, the proportion of interventions of a palliative nature is likely to increase as life-supporting interventions are continued. If restorative interventions are not successful, the patient may reach a point beyond which palliative care alone is provided until the patient dies.

At present, resources to provide palliative care support in acute care settings to patients, families and healthcare teams is limited. In 2000, the American Hospital Association conducted a self-reported study of US hospitals that indicated that 14% of hospitals have programs providing specialized palliative services; 23% report having hospice programs, and 42% offer programs to educate staff about pain management.[50]

When a patient and family are ready to move away from restorative therapies and the healthcare team believes that life expectancy is 6 months or less, patients become eligible for hospice care. Hospice care can be provided in the patient's home, a hospice facility, or in a long-term care facility. Hospice benefits may include physicians, nurses, chaplains, and social services; physical and occupational therapy; medical supplies and equipment; respite care, outpatient prescription medications for pain, and other symptoms. Since 1982, reimbursement for hospice care has been a Medicare benefit. Although the number of Medicare patients choosing hospice has increased dramatically over the last two decades, the average length of stay has decreased from 70 days in 1983 to 59 days in 1998,[51] and 36 days more recently.[13]

The multidisciplinary benefits of hospice care cannot be fully realized by the patient and family if referrals to hospice care are made too close to death. Patients and families require time to make the decision to forego curative interventions in favor of hospice care. Physician willingness to discuss options for end-of-life care can have a positive influence on patients and families.

Current literature suggests that many physicians do not feel well informed about end-of-life care options. In one study of oncologists and other oncology program physicians by Von Roenn *et al.*,[52] the findings were:

- 86% of respondents thought that the majority of patients were under-medicated,
- 49% rated pain control in their own practice as fair to very poor,
- 73% evaluated their own training in pain management as fair to very poor.

In a 1998 survey of oncologists by the American Society of Clinical Oncology[53] less than one-third of respondents indicated their training was very helpful in introducing hospice or palliative care, coordinating end-of-life care or communicating with patients near the end of life.

The direct discussion of care options, including the option of having the remaining time of life focused on comfort and time with loved ones rather than on restorative interventions, may be one of the most significant and remembered events in the patient–family–physician relationships.

Palliative care in hospitals increases appropriate referrals to hospice care at home or in nursing homes, improves continuity of care as the patient is transferred to a new venue, and supports patients and families at a difficult time. Palliative care may also lower expenditures by hospitals and payers by reducing hospital and ICU lengths of stay and direct costs (e.g., laboratory fees, drugs). Diane Meier, Director of the Center to Advance Palliative Care, has reviewed several palliative care programs utilizing patient/family satisfaction variables and cost-savings factors at Mt. Sinai Hospital in New York City, Kaiser Permanente hospitals, the Ireland Cancer Center, Virginia Commonwealth University and University of Michigan.[54–57]

Delivering bad news

Bad news comes in the form of a serious diagnosis with a poor prognosis, complications of therapy, less than successful outcomes of interventions, and death itself, especially when it is unanticipated. No one likes to deliver bad news, but physicians have the obligation to tell the truth

Table 5.2. Delivering bad news

- Compose message – accuracy, consistency
- Plan meeting – who, when, setting
- Understand your own biases, feelings
- Language – concern, empathy, verbal, body
- Acknowledge strong reactions, discuss them
- Tolerate silence
- Achieve common understanding
- Follow-up – chart, care team, family

and to disclose the facts, as they are known. At the present time, few physicians have been trained in the skills of delivering bad news, and they are not comfortable doing so for a number of reasons including their reluctance to give up, their view of death as a medical failure, and their lack of preparation for and inability to control the highly variable reactions of patients and family members. Some suggestions for planning and executing the delivery of bad news are shown in Table 5.2. More detailed discussions of the do's and don'ts can be found in textbooks.[58]

Disclosure of medical errors

Beginning with the publication of *To Err is Human*, by the Institute of Medicine in 2000, there has been an increasingly intense focus on medical errors, how to prevent them, and what should be done when they occur.[59] Disclosure of errors to patients and their families is of particular concern. On one hand, there is trepidation about malpractice suits and increasingly larger awards to plaintiffs. On the other, there is the ethical obligation to tell the truth. Moreover, there is accumulating evidence that attempts to hide errors are responsible for increasing the numbers of suits and driving up punitive payouts to injured patients.

An increasing number of institutions are adopting full disclosure policies because they are facing mandates to do so from federal and state governments, JCAHO, ethical obligations, and consumer activism.[60,61] It is being recognized that the wall of silence that has characterized medical misadventures, undermines trust, ignores patient autonomy, stifles safety advancement, and exacerbates the legal, economic and public relations problems related to subsequent discovery of non-disclosure. Ignoring or denying culpability is known to increase malpractice risks because most patients and their families sense that something has gone wrong, and the failure to have mistakes disclosed to them by the healthcare providers sends them in anger to seek legal counsel and to initiate a claim

Table 5.3. Serious reportable events

- Surgical: wrong operation, foreign object retained, unexpected death
- Products, devices: contamination, unintended use, air embolism
- Patient protection: missing, +/− suicide, discharge to wrong person
- Care errors: meds, bld rxn, gluc, pressure ulcers (OB, peds)
- Environment: restraints, fall, burn, shock
- Criminal: assault, abduction, impersonator

or suit. The major serious reportable events are listed in Table 5.3.

Several points bear special emphasis. The accurate and complete reporting of facts is required, but speculation about the mechanism of injury and who may be responsible should be avoided, because in the early period after a misadventure the complete facts are not yet fully known or integrated. Coincidence-in-time is not proof of a cause-and-effect relationship. There are numerous cases in which a complication has been attributed to someone's action when it is ultimately demonstrated beyond doubt that the particular action did not contribute to the injury. Therefore, avoid the "blame game."

It is very important for the physicians, nurses and others involved in the patient's care to have a common understanding of the facts and to maintain a consistent message which is often difficult to do because, as the message is passed from one person to another in a series of individuals, the message changes and the person initiating it doesn't recognize it when it comes back to him/her. Physicians can make mistakes of judgments, and despite their best efforts, their skills may fail them occasionally. It is both appropriate and laudable for them to acknowledge an error or mistake and, in most cases, the patient and family members see the concerned and apologetic physician as being a human being who is not deserving of punishment. They will greatly appreciate the physician's efforts to minimize the consequences of the mistake and to keep them informed in ongoing discussions, which enhance the physician-patient relationship and reduce the feelings of anger, abandonment and irresponsibility that lead them to seek legal consultation.

Definition of death

There are two basic definitions of death. Irreversible cessation of circulatory and respiratory function defined as a lack of heartbeat and spontaneous breathing, is the most widely understood and accepted definition of death.[62,63]

However, a second definition is needed because drugs and machines can support the circulation and breathing, making it impossible to rely on the traditional vital signs. Also, concerns about the limited supply of organs for transplantation, and the benefit of harvesting organs during or immediately after cessation of the circulation of oxygenated blood has supported the development of a neurological definition widely referred to as "brain death." A 1981 Presidential Commission formulated the Uniform Determination of Death Act which has been adopted by 31 states as a legally acceptable means of determining death, which under this definition is characterized as the irreversible cessation of all brain functions including those of the neocortex, brain stem and all other brain regions.[64,65] It does not include irreversible coma or a persistent vegetative state.

The neurological definition remains controversial for metaphysical, cultural, legal, and even medical reasons.[65] The basic problem is that the term death applies to whole organisms and not to the loss of function in any single organ, even the brain. The neurological definition is not accepted by all cultures, religions, and governments. It leads to questions such as: when is a person really dead? Is brain death a separate type of death that occurs before "real" death? The fetus continues to live and can be born of a brain-dead mother. A brain-dead child continues to grow. All of this creates a suspicion that death is "malleable" and can be adjusted for utilitarian purposes (e.g., organ donation), which contributes to ambivalence among those facing a decision about organ donation.[62,63]

There are specific clinical criteria for brain death (Table 5.4), and these criteria must be met in the opinion of two physicians (usually neurologists) completing independent evaluations of the patient separated by some time interval. There are also a number of confirmatory tests for the determination of brain death (Table 5.4).[64]

Once brain death has been declared, the common practice today is to inform the patient's family of the fact and to move them to the realization that aggressive support measures are no longer appropriate. Then the questions of what they would like to happen before cardiopulmonary death occurs (e.g., time for other family members to arrive, organ donation) are addressed. Physicians may be prepared to discontinue the support measures at any time on the basis of them being medically inappropriate, but it is appropriate to allow some time to accommodate the patient's previously expressed wishes and the family's reasonable requests.

Table 5.4. Clinical criteria for brain death

Absence of:
- motor responses
- pupillary responses to light
- corneal reflexes
- caloric responses
- gag reflex
- coughing during tracheal suctioning
- respiratory drive at a $PaCO_2 \geq 60$ mmHg or 20 mmHg above patient's baseline

Pupils at dilation midpoint (4–6 mm)

Confirmatory tests
- cerebral angiography
- EEG
- transcranial Doppler
- cerebral scintigraphy

Other points to be considered are: biological activity persists for a time after heart beat and breathing stop; the same is true of the brain which cannot exert its sensing and controlling functions. Should brain death be defined as "total brain necrosis?" Many clinicians believe that permanent unconsciousness negates personhood. Without the potential for thought, the basis of personal identity is lost. Death is a process, a chain of events, before which the patient is fully alive and at the end of which the patient is fully dead. Dying in days or weeks is not the same as "dead." A rigid definition of death is the irreversible cessation of all integrated functioning of the human organism as a whole – mental and physical.

Physicians and other healthcare personnel should be aware of these issues as they address family members and friends of patients who cannot recover independent function and for whom continuing life support measures appear medically futile. Morrie Schwartz on the subject of "Tuesdays with Morrie," said to Ted Koppel on Nightline, "For me, Ted, living means I can be responsive to the other person. It means I can show my emotions and my feelings. Talk to them. Feel with them … When that is gone, Morrie is gone."[66] Physicians and patients may believe that we should prolong a life that is, or can be, meaningful, but that it is quite different from prolonging death with its associated suffering. We need to be prepared to discuss these concerns openly with our patients and their families.

Summary

In this chapter, we have attempted to address succinctly the most frequently encountered ethical issues that relate directly to the patient facing a surgical operation or other major intervention. Because these interventions entail potential benefits for the patient as well as risks of disability and death, decisions to proceed are often complicated and careful communication with patient and family is vital. Working to establish common goals based on informed understanding and appreciation for values and beliefs will often help everyone involved reach a consensus about how care of the patient will proceed. Ethical considerations are central to the clinical management of our patients.

REFERENCES

1. Beauchamp, T. L., Childress, J. F. *et al. Principles of Bioethics.* 5th edn. New York: Oxford University Press, 2001.
2. Jonsen, A. R., Siegler, M., Winslade, W. J. *et al. Clinical Ethics,* 5th edn. New York: McGraw-Hill, 2002: 1–2.
3. Jonsen, A. R., Siegler, M., Winslade, W. J. *et al. Clinical Ethics,* 5th edn. New York: McGraw-Hill, 2002: 15–18.
4. Christakis, N. A. *et al. Death Foretold; Prophecy and Prognosis in Medical Care.* Chicago: University of Chicago Press, 1999; xiii–xvi.
5. ACGME Outcomes Project; see www.ACGME.org
6. Beauchamp, T. L., Childress, J. F. *et al. Principles of Biomedical Ethics,* 5th edn. New York: Oxford University Press, 2001: 77–79.
7. Appelbaum, P. S., Grisso, T. *et al.* Assessing patient's capacities to consent to treatment. *N. Engl. J. Med.* 1988; **319**(25): 1635–1638.
8. Appelbaum, P. S., Grisso, T. *et al.* The MacArthur Treatment Competency Study, I: mental illness and competence to consent to treatment. *Law Hum. Behav.* 1995; **19**: 105–126.
9. Venesy, B. A. *et al.* A clinician's guide to decision making capacity and ethically sound medical decisions. *Am. J. Phys. Med. Rehabil.* 1994; **73**(3): 219–226.
10. National Commission for the Protection of Human Subject of Biomedical and Behavioral Research. The Belmont Report (Washington, D.C.:DHEW Publication 0578–0012; 1978). Salgo v. Stanford University Board of Trustees, 154 Cal. App. 2d560; 1957. Canterburg v. Spence, 464 F.2d 772 (D.C. Cir. 1972).
11. Beauchamp, T. L., Childress, J. F. *et al. Principles of Biomedical Ethics,* 5th edn. New York: Oxford University Press, 2001: 79–80.
12. Jonsen, A. R., Siegler, M., Winslade, W. J. *et al. Clinical Ethics,* 5th edn. New York: McGraw-Hill 2002: 69–73.
13. Last Acts: "Means to a Better End: A Report on Dying in America". November 2002; 3, 14, 72–73. www.rwif.org.
14. Sabatino, C. P. *et al.* Survey of state EMS-DNR laws and protocols. *J. Law, Med. Ethics* 1999; **27**(4): 297–315.
15. AMA Council on Ethical and Legal Affairs: Opinion no. 2.22. Do-not-resuscitate orders. In *Code of Medical Ethics, Current*

Opinions, Chicago: American Medical Association, 1999: 67–69. Also see: Guidelines for the appropriate use of do-not-resuscitate orders. *J. Am. Med. Assoc.* 1991; **265**: 1868–1871.

16. Statement of the American College of Surgeons on Advance Directives by Patients: "Do not resuscitate" in the operating room. *Am. Coll. Surg. Bull.* 1994; **79**(9): 29.

17. American Society of Anesthesiologists: Ethical guidelines for the anesthesia care of patients with do-not-resuscitate orders or other directives that limit treatment. ASA Standards, Guidelines and Statements, www.ASAhq.org.

18. Truog, R. D., Waisel, D. B., Burns, J. P. *et al.* DNR in the OR; a goal-directed approach. *Anesthesiology* 1999; **90**: 289–295.

19. Casarett, D., Ross, L. F. *et al.* Overriding a patient's refusal of treatment after an iatrogenic complication. *N. Engl. J. Med.* 1997; **336**: 1908–1910.

20. Federal Patient Self-Determination Act 1990; 42 U.S.C. 1395 cc(a). www.fha.org.

21. Last Acts. Means to a better end: a report on dying in America today. November 18, 2002; 9–10 www.rwjf.org.

22. Schwartz, C. E. *et al.* U Mass End of Life Working Group: Early intervention in planning end-of-life care with ambulatory geriatric patients. *Arch. Int. Med.* 2002; **162**: 1611–1618.

23. Kinlaw, K., Trotochaud, K., Thompson, N. *et al.* End of Life Care Practices: A Survey of Organizational Members of the Health Care Ethics Consortium of Georgia. January 2001; 11–12.

24. Hug, C. C. Jr. *et al.* End-of-life issues and the anesthesiologist. In Lowenstein, E., ed. *Medical Ethics, Int. Anesth. Clin.* 2001; **39**(3): 35–52 (see 44–47).

25. Leplege, A., Hunt, S. *et al.* The problem of quality of life in medicine. *J. Am. Med. Assoc.* 1997; **278**: 47–50.

26. Beauchamp, T. L., Childress, J. F. *et al. Principles of Biomedical Ethics*, 5th edn. New York: Oxford University Press, 2001: 122.

27. Beauckamp, T. L., Childress, J. F. *et al. Principles of Biomedical Ethics*, 5th edn. New York: Oxford University Press, 2001: 128–32.

28. Ware, S., Milch, R., Weaver, W. L. *et al.* Care of dying patients. In McCullough, L., Jones, J. W., & Brody, B. A., eds. *Surgical Ethics*, New York: Oxford University Press, 1998: 182.

29. Knaus, W. A., Draper, E. A., Wagner, D. P. *et al.* APACHE II. A severity of disease classification system. *Crit. Care Med.* 198; **13**: 818–829.

30. Goldman, L., Caldera, D. L., Nussbaum, S. R. *et al.* Multifactorial index of cardiac risk in non-cardiac surgical procedures. *N. Engl. J. Med.* 1977; **297**: 845–850.

31. The SUPPORT Principal Investigators: A controlled trial to improve care for seriously ill hospitalized patients; The study to understand prognoses and preferences for outcomes and risks of treatment (SUPPORT). *J. Am. Med. Assoc.* 1995; **274**: 1591–1598.

32. Knaus, W. A., Wagner, D. P. *et al.* Multiple systems organ failure: epidemiology and prognosis. *Crit. Care Clin.* 1989; **5**: 221–32.

33. Hug, C. C. Jr. *et al.* Rovenstine Lecture: Patient values, Hippocrates, science and technology: what we (physicians) can do versus should do for the patient. *Anesthesiology* 2000; **93**: 556–564.

34. Albom, M. *et al. Tuesdays with Morrie, An Old Man, a Young Man, and Life's Greatest Lesson.* New York: Doubleday; 1997; 80–81.

35. Walter, L. C., Brand, R. J., Counsell, S. R. *et al.* Development and validation of a prognostic index for 1-year mortality in older adults after hospitalization. *J. Am. Med. Assoc.* 2001; **285**: 2987–2994.

36. AMA Council on Ethical and Judicial Affairs: Opinion no. 2.20, Withholding or withdrawing life-sustaining medical treatment. In *Code of Medical Ethics, Current Opinions*, Chicago: AMA 1998: 45–61.

37. The President's Commission for the Study of Ethical Problems in Medicine and Biomedical and Behavioral Research. *Deciding to Forego Life-Sustaining Treatment.* Washington, DC: US Government Priority Office, 1983.

38. *Guidelines on Termination of Life-Sustaining Treatment and the Care of the Dying.* Briarcliff Manor, NY: The Hasting Center, 1987.

39. Task Force on Ethics of the Society of Critical Care Medicine. Censuses Report on the Ethics of Foregoing Life-Sustaining Treatments in the Critically Ill. *Crit. Care Med.* 1990; **18**: 1435–1439.

40. American Nurses Association. *Foregoing Nutrition and Hydration, and Promotion of Comfort and Relief of Pain in Dying Patients.* Available at: http//www.nursingworld.org/readroom/position/ethics. Accessed 3–19–03.

41. Prendergrast, T. J., Claessens, M. T., Luce, J. M. *et al.* A national survey of end of life care for critically ill patients. *Am. J. Respir. Crit. Care Med.* 1998; **158**: 1163–1167.

42. Jonsen, A. *et al.*, ibid, pp. 129–130.

43. Futility Reference(s). For example, American College of Emergency Physicians. Nonbeneficial ("Futile") Emergency Medical Interventions. March 1998, reaffirmed October 2002. Available at www.acep.org/sitemap/ to policy statements. Accessed 3–19–03. American Medical Association. Council on Ethical and Judicial Affairs. E-2.035 Futile Care. June 1994.

44. AMA Council on Ethical and Judicial Affairs: Opinion no.2.037, Medical futility in end-of-life care. In *Code of Medical Ethics, Current Opinions*, Chicago: AMA, 1999: 10.

45. Halevy, A., Brody, B. A. *et al.* For the Houston City-Wide Task Force on Medical Futility: a multi-institution collaborative policy on medical futility. *J. Am. Med. Assoc.* 1996; **276**: 571–574.

46. Futility Court Cases: In re Baby K, 16 F.3d 590 (4th Cir.), cert. denied, 115 S. Ct. 91, 1994. Bryan vs. Rectors and Visitors of the University of Virginia, 95 F. 3d 349 (4th Cir.) 1996.

47. Meier, D. Presentation available at www.capc.org/content/287/287.ppt. Accessed 3–19–03.

48. Joint Commission for the Accreditation of Healthcare Organizations. Chapter 3, Patients Rights and Organization Ethics, Standards R1.1.2.8-R1.1.2.9, 2002.

49. World Health Organization. Definition of Palliative Care. 1990. Available at www5.who.int/cancer. Accessed 3–19–03.

50. Means to a Better End (see prior reference[13]), page 21.

51. General Accounting Office report GAO/HEHS-00–182 Medicare: More Beneficiaries Use Hospice but for Fewer Days of Care, September 2000.

52. Von Roenn, J. H., Cleeland, C. S., Gonin, R. *et al.* fcp:// @fc.LearnLink.Emory.Edu,%232400015/MailBox/Physician attitudes and practice in cancer pain management. A survey from the Eastern Cooperative Oncology Group. Physician attitudes and practice in cancer pain management. A survey from the Eastern Cooperative Oncology Group. *Ann. Intern. Med.* 1993; **119**(2): 121–126.

53. Foley, K. M. & Gelband, H., eds. National Cancer Policy Board, Institute of Medicine and National Research Council. *Improving Palliative Care for Cancer.* Washington, DC: National Academy Press, 2001; 289.

54. Meier, D. *et al.* Palliative Care in Hospitals: Making the Case. Presentation available at www.capc.org/content/287/ 287.ppt. Accessed 3–19–03.

55. Cassel, J. B., Smith, T. J., Coyne, P. J. *et al.* A high-volume, specialist, standardized care palliative care unit generates revenue sufficient to cover end of life care costs. ASCO annual program abstract 2002. Available at abstracts at http:// www.asco.org/ac, www.asco.org/ac. Accessed 3–19–03.

56. Lilly, C. M., DeMeo, D. L., Sonna, L. A. *et al.* An intensive communication intervention for the critically ill. *Am. J. Med.* 2000; **109**(6): 469–475.

57. Campbell, M. L., Frank, R. R. *et al.* Experience with an end-of-life practice at a university hospital. *Crit. Care Med.* 1997; **25**(1): 197–202.

58. Buckman, R. *et al. How to Break Bad News: A Guide for Health Care Professionals.* Baltimore: Johns Hopkins Press, 1992.

59. Kohn, K. T., Corrigan, J. M., Donaldson, M. S., eds. for the Committee on Quality of Health Care in America, Institute of Medicine. *To Err is Human: Building a Safer Health System.* Washington, DC: National Academy Press, 1999 vs 2000.

60. Leape, L. L. *et al.* Reporting of adverse events. *N. Engl. J. Med.* 2002; **37**: 1633–1638.

61. Flynn, E., Jackson, J. A., Lindgren, K. *et al. Shining the Light on Errors: How Open Should We Be?* Oak Brook, IL: University HealthSystem Consortium, 2002.

62. Younger, S. J., Arnold, R. M., Schapiro, R., eds. *The Definition of Death: Contemporary Controversies.* Baltimore, MD: Johns Hopkins University Press, 1999.

63. Wijdicks, E. F. M. ed. *Brain Death.* Philadelphia, PA: Lippincott, Williams and Wilkins 2001.

64. Wijdicks, E. F. M. *et al.* The diagnosis of brain death. *N. Engl. J. Med.* 2001; **344**: 1215–1221.

65. Capron, A. M. Brain death – well settled yet still unresolved. *N. Engl. J. Med.* 2001; **344**: 1244–1246.

66. Albom, M. *et al. Tuesdays with Morrie, An Old Man, A Young Man, and Life's Greatest Lesson.* New York: Doubleday, 1997: 162.

Cardiology

6

Cardiovascular disease

Howard Weitz

Thomas Jefferson University Hospital, Philadelphia, PA

General overview

A team approach to patients with cardiovascular disease who undergo non-cardiac surgery is the ideal way to expedite perioperative care. It is essential to assess patients' risk of cardiac complications and to identify those risk factors that may be reversed or ameliorated if time allows before surgery. The most likely cardiovascular problems that patients may encounter in the perioperative period should also be anticipated and an approach to these problems planned in advance. For the patient who undergoes surgery on an emergency basis, preoperative evaluation may be limited to those components that are critical and essential for the surgical procedure. In these circumstances the consultant may well perform a more detailed evaluation in the postoperative period. For many patients the preoperative evaluation is their only opportunity for medical assessment. The consultant should bear this in mind and consider the preoperative evaluation visit as an opportunity for assessment of general cardiovascular risk and development of a plan for cardiac risk reduction.

The physicians who are responsible for preoperative cardiac risk assessment and perioperative care vary according to locale. In many regions, family physicians, general internists, or cardiologists perform these duties. In other areas, these tasks are performed by surgeons or anesthesiologists. The selection of anesthetic agents as well as their means of administration is typically the domain of anesthesiologists; however, it is essential that surgeons and medical consultants understand the basic cardiovascular and hemodynamic effects of anesthesia.

Anesthesia considerations

Physiologic response to anesthesia and surgery

Anesthesia and surgery are accompanied by physiologic responses to preserve homeostasis. In the patient with compensated heart disease these normal responses may precipitate decompensation. Catecholamine production increases in response to the stress of surgery, leading to increases in myocardial oxygen demand as well as increased afterload that may provoke myocardial ischemia in the patient with coronary artery disease. In addition, several perioperative factors may lead to decreased myocardial oxygen delivery. Hypoventilation and atelectasis may reduce arterial oxygen saturation. Anemia decreases myocardial oxygen delivery. Volume depletion or perioperative hypotension may result in coronary artery hypoperfusion. Sodium and water retention are increased in response to aldosterone secretion in an effort to maintain intravascular volume. In the patient with impaired ventricular function and/or "fixed" cardiac output (e.g., critical aortic stenosis, severe left ventricular dysfunction), this may result in congestive heart failure.

Cardiovascular effects of anesthetic agents

Inhalation agents

Inhalation agents all produce dose-dependent myocardial depression. Nitrous oxide is the least depressant and, because its use is associated with an increase in peripheral vascular resistance, systemic blood pressure is maintained. Halothane, rarely used in adults because of idiosyncratic hepatotoxicity, produces the greatest degree of

Medical Management of the Surgical Patient: A Textbook of Perioperative Medicine, ed. M. F. Lubin, R. B. Smith, T. F. Dobson, N. Spell, H. K. Walker.
4th edn. Published by Cambridge University Press. © Cambridge University 2006.

myocardial depression of all the inhaled agents. All inhalational agents cause decreases in blood pressure. For halothane and enflurane it is direct myocardial depression in conjunction with decreased cardiac output and stroke volume that result in the blood pressure decrease. For isoflurane, sevoflurane, and desflurane the associated blood pressure decrease is caused by a reduction in systemic vascular resistance with peripheral vasodilation. This may result in hypotension in the patient who is concurrently receiving vasodilators (nitrates, hydralazine, and nifedipine) or is intravascularly volume depleted. Treatment of hypotension in this setting should be with fluid administration. The depressant effects of inhalational anesthetics may be accentuated in patients with abnormal hearts.[1] Desflurane is associated with sympathetic activation and is therefore of limited use in patients with cardiac disease. Sevoflurane appears to be similar to isoflurane and safe in the patient with ischemic heart disease. It has been described as having a more stable effect on heart rate than the other inhaled agents.

Intravenous anesthetic agents

Thiopental is the prototypical intravenous barbiturate intravenous anesthetic agent. Its cardiac effects during non-cardiac surgery can be significant. It leads to venous dilatation with a reduction in preload as well as myocardial depression. These physiologic responses may result in an increase in heart rate. It should be used with caution therefore in the patient with decreased preload (e.g., hypovolemia) receiving vasodilator medications as well as in the patient in whom increased heart rate would be detrimental, e.g., the patient with ischemia.

Opioids are commonly used in anesthesia to blunt the sympathetic response to intubation and surgical manipulation. Sufentanil and fentanyl are the most commonly used agents of this class. They serve to prevent increases in intraoperative myocardial oxygen demand by maintenance of cardiac output and preventing increases in heart rate.[2]

Propofol is commonly used for induction and maintenance of general anesthesia and for sedation during regional anesthesia. It is particularly well suited for use in outpatient surgery because of its short duration of action and antiemetic properties. Its use may be associated with hypotension, especially after bolus administration.[3]

Spinal anesthesia

Spinal anesthesia is relatively contraindicated in patients with "fixed" cardiac output (e.g., critical aortic stenosis, severe left ventricular dysfunction) because these patients are unable to augment cardiac output in response to the vasodilation and subsequent hypotension that often accompany this technique.

Regional vs. general anesthesia

Several studies have found no difference between the effects of regional and general anesthesia on cardiovascular morbidity or mortality. There are several unique settings in which one modality may be preferable. Regional anesthesia produces less respiratory and cardiac depression than general anesthesia, and its use may be advantageous in the patient with left ventricular dysfunction, congestive heart failure, or pulmonary disease. Some have suggested that, in certain high risk groups (e.g., those who undergo vascular surgery), epidural analgesia along with general anesthesia is associated with a lower risk of perioperative cardiac complication than general anesthesia alone. In a meta analysis of 141 randomized trials involving 9559 patients general anesthesia was compared to neuraxial blockade, e.g., spinal or epidural anesthesia. In 60 of these trials patients received both general anesthesia and neuraxial blockade. Neuraxial blockade, with or without general anesthesia was associated with a 44% decreased incidence of deep vein thrombosis, a 55% decreased incidence of pulmonary embolus, and a 33% decreased incidence of myocardial infarction. Overall mortality was reduced by approximately 33% in patients receiving neuraxial blockade. The conclusion of the authors was that neuraxial blockade lowers the risk of postoperative complications and mortality and may do so by altering the "stress response" to surgery.[4] While these findings support the use of neuraxial blockade, further research is needed to assess the degree of benefit and to determine whether the improved outcomes in this analysis are a result of neuraxial blockade or are a response to avoidance of general anesthesia.

A meta-analysis of 17 studies (1173 patients) has been performed to assess the response on cardiac outcome in patients who receive postoperative epidural analgesia. In this analysis it was demonstrated that patients who received epidural analgesia for at least 24 hours following surgery had a 5.3% reduction in postoperative myocardial infarction. Postoperative epidural analgesia however had no effect on the incidence of postoperative mortality.[5] In terms of specific surgical procedures and non-cardiac outcomes, non-randomized trials yield some evidence that peripheral vascular graft patency is enhanced if regional anesthesia is utilized and continued in the immediate postoperative period and return of bowel function is quicker in colonic surgery when epidural anesthesia is used.[6]

Table 6.1. Multifactorial index of cardiac risk in non-cardiac surgery[a]

Risk factor	Points
History	
Myocardial infarction within 6 months	10
Age >70 years	5
Physical examination	
S3 or jugular venous distension	11
Significant aortic stenosis	3
Electrocardiogram	
Rhythm other than sinus or sinus plus atrial premature beats on preoperative electrocardiogram	7
>5 ventricular premature contractions per minute at any time prior to surgery	7
Medical status	
Poor general medical status, i.e.,	3
potassium <3.0 meq/l or HCO_3 < 20 meq/l	
BUN > 50 mg/dl or Cr > 3.0 mg/dl, pO_2 < 60 mm Hg or	
pCO_2 > 50 mm Hg, evidence of abnormal liver function	
patient bedridden	
Surgical procedure	
Abdominal, thoracic, aortic surgery	3
Emergency operation	4
Total	53

Note:

[a] From Goldman, L., Caldera, D. L., Nussbaum, S. R., *et al.* Multifactorial index of cardiac risk in noncardiac surgical procedures. *N. Engl. J. Med.* **297**: 845–850, 1977.

Assessment of cardiac risk

In 1977 a multifactorial risk factor index was defined by Goldman and associates (Table 6.1) to identify the high-risk surgical patient preoperatively as well as to delineate cardiovascular risk factors that could be corrected prior to surgery in an effort to decrease cardiovascular morbidity and mortality associated with non-cardiac surgery.[7] Nine clinical or historical features, the majority of which were reversible, were found to be associated with an increased incidence of perioperative complications. The factors were assigned "risk points" by multivariate analysis, enabling a preoperative estimate of total cardiac risk and determination of the likelihood of life-threatening complications (e.g., myocardial infarction, pulmonary edema, ventricular tachycardia, and cardiac death). Patients were stratified into four risk classes based on their total accumulated risk points. Risk determined with the original multifactorial cardiac risk index has been integrated with

the type of surgery to estimate the probability of cardiac complications in non-cardiac surgery.

The multifactorial risk index has been validated in prospective studies stratifying unselected, consecutive patients who undergo non-cardiac surgery. It has been less reliable when used to risk stratify selected patient subgroups particularly those with or at high risk for coronary artery disease and those who are to undergo major vascular surgery. This index as well as others that were developed contemporaneously were derived from relatively small numbers of patients and predated significant change in anesthesia and surgery. They have therefore not maintained their clinical relevance.[8]

A more recent modification of the multifactorial index has been developed for use with stable patients undergoing major non-cardiac surgery and has been shown to perform well as a tool to predict the probability of major cardiac complications.[9] This index uses six readily available clinical factors to place the preoperative patient into one of four risk groups:

- high risk type of surgery (intraperitoneal, intrathoracic, or suprainguinal vascular)
- history of ischemic heart disease
- history of congestive heart failure
- history of cerebrovascular disease
- diabetes requiring treatment with insulin prior to surgery
- renal insufficiency with preoperative serum creatinine >2.0 mg/dl.

Rates of major cardiac complication (myocardial infarction, pulmonary edema, ventricular fibrillation or primary cardiac arrest, and complete heart block) with 0, 1, 2, or ≥3 of these factors were 0.4%, 0.9%, 7%, and 11%, respectively.

To facilitate preoperative risk assessment of patients with cardiovascular disease, a consensus guideline was developed by a consensus panel of the American College of Cardiology and the American Heart Association.[10] The panel acknowledged that the number of evidence-based trials pertaining to perioperative cardiovascular evaluation and therapy was limited and therefore the guidelines are based on a large part from studies not directly derived from non-cardiac surgery and on expert opinion. The guideline initially published in 1996 and revised in 2002 seeks to identify and define those clinical situations in which preoperative testing and intervention may improve patient perioperative outcome. One of their themes is that cardiac intervention is rarely necessary to lower the risk of surgery.

These guidelines employ a strategy that requires assessment of clinical predictors, functional status, surgery specific risk, and history of prior coronary evaluation and or treatment. The preoperative history and physical examination should focus on identifying the presence of clinical predictors including the presence of cardiovascular disease and its treatment. A goal of the guideline is the identification of the patient at increased risk who would benefit, in the long term, from medical therapy or coronary artery revascularization.

Clinical predictors (Table 6.2) have, in a large part, been identified from the risk indices that have been developed since the initial multifactorial index of 1977. The consensus committee suggested that these risk predictors be categorized into three groups: major predictors (acute MI (documented MI less than 7 days previously), recent MI (MI more than 7 days but less than 30 days prior to surgery), unstable or severe angina, evidence of a large ischemic burden as determined by symptoms or non-invasive testing, decompensated congestive heart failure, significant arrhythmia (supraventricular arrhythmia with uncontrolled ventricular rate, symptomatic arrhythmia in the presence of underlying heart disease, high degree atrioventricular block, and severe valvular heart disease), intermediate predictors (mild angina, prior myocardial infarction (more than 30 days prior to surgery), compensated or prior congestive heart failure, diabetes mellitus, renal insufficiency (serum $Cr \geq 2.0\,g/dl$)), and minor (advanced age, rhythm other than sinus, abnormal electrocardiogram, low functional capacity, history of stroke, and uncontrolled systemic hypertension).

Functional capacity has been shown to be a predictor with poor functional capacity a marker for subsequent cardiac events.[11,12] Poor functional capacity, even when not a result of cardiac causes, was empirically postulated in the 1996 initial ACC/AHA preoperative evaluation guideline to be a risk for perioperative cardiac complication. There is now evidence to support that postulate. In a series of 600 patients who underwent non-cardiac surgery it has been shown that perioperative myocardial ischemia and cardiovascular events were more common in patients unable to walk four blocks or climb two flights of stairs.[13] It may be quantitated by evaluating the patient's daily activity. Perioperative cardiac risk is increased in patients unable to reach or exceed an aerobic demand of 4 METS (metabolic equivalents) during normal activity. Energy expenditures of eating, dressing, walking and other low level activities range from 1–4 METS. More vigorous activity, e.g., climbing a flight of stairs, brisk walking, playing golf is equivalent to 4–10 METS. Strenuous activity like tennis and swimming exceeds 10 METS.

Surgery specific risk is determined by the type of surgery and its associated hemodynamic stress (Table 6.3). High

Table 6.2. Clinical predictors of increased perioperative cardiovascular risk (myocardial infarction, congestive heart failure, death)[a]

Major

Unstable coronary syndromes
    Acute MI (documented MI less than 7 days previously)
    Recent (greater than 7 days but less than or equal to 30 days) myocardial infarction with evidence of important ischemic risk by clinical symptoms or non-invasive study
    Unstable or severe[a] angina (Canadian class III or IV)[b]
Decompensated congestive heart failure
Significant arrhythmias
    High grade atrioventricular block
    Symptomatic ventricular arrhythmias in the presence of underlying heart disease
    Supraventricular arrhythmias with uncontrolled ventricular rate
Severe valvular disease

Intermediate

Mild angina pectoris (Canadian class I or II)
Previous myocardial infarction by history or pathologic Q waves
Compensated or prior congestive heart failure
Diabetes mellitus
Renal insufficiency (serum $Cr > 2.0\,mg/dl$)

Minor

Advanced age
Abnormal electrocardiogram (left ventricular hypertrophy, left bundle branch block, ST–T abnormalities)
Rhythm other than sinus (e.g., atrial fibrillation)
Low functional capacity (e.g., inability to climb one flight of stairs with a bag of groceries)
History of stroke
Uncontrolled systemic hypertension

Notes:
[a] May include "stable" angina in patients who are usually sedentary.
[b] From Compare, L. Grading of angina pectoris. *Circulation* 1976; **54**: 522–523. Reproduced from Eagle, K. A., Berger, P. B., Calkins, H. *et al*. ACC/AHA guideline update for perioperative cardiovascular evaluation for noncardiac surgery: a report of the American College of Cardiology/American Heart Association Task Force on Practice Guidelines (Committee to Update the 1996 Guidelines on Perioperative Cardiovascular Evaluation for Noncardiac Surgery.) 2002. American College of Cardiology website. Available at http://www.acc.org/clinical/guidelines/perio/dirIndex.htm.

risk procedures are those with a reported cardiac risk greater than 5%. They include emergent major operations particularly in the elderly, aortic and major vascular surgery, peripheral vascular surgery, anticipated prolonged surgical procedures associated with large fluid shifts or blood loss. Intermediate risk procedures are those

Table 6.3. Cardiac risk stratification for non-cardiac surgical procedures

High (reported cardiac risk often >5%)
Emergent major operations, particularly in the elderly
Aortic and other major vascular surgery
Peripheral vascular surgery
Anticipated prolonged surgical procedures associated with
    large fluid shifts or blood loss

Intermediate (reported cardiac risk <5%)
Carotid endarterectomy
Head and neck surgery
Intraperitoneal and intrathoracic surgery
Orthopedic surgery
Prostate surgery

Low[a] (reported cardiac risk <1%)
Endoscopic procedures
Superficial procedures
Cataract surgery
Breast surgery

Note:
[a] Do not generally require further preoperative cardiac testing.
Reproduced from Eagle, K. A., Berger, P. B., Calkins, H. *et al.* ACC/AHA guideline update for perioperative cardiovascular evaluation for noncardiac surgery: a report of the American College of Cardiology/American Heart Association Task Force on Practice Guidelines (Committee to Update the 1996 Guidelines on Perioperative Cardiovascular Evaluation for Noncardiac Surgery.) 2002. American College of Cardiology website. Available at http://www.acc.org/clinical/guidelines/perio/dirIndex.htm.

associated with a risk less than 5% but greater than 1%. They include carotid endarterectomy, head and neck surgery, intraperitoneal and intrathoracic surgery, orthopedic surgery, prostate surgery. Low-risk procedures are those associated with a cardiac risk less than 1%. They include endoscopic procedures, superficial procedures, cataract surgery, and breast surgery.

After the patient's clinical predictors, functional capacity and surgery specific risk are identified and a six-step algorithm guides decision making regarding further cardiac testing and/proceeding to surgery (Fig. 6.1).

1. *Is the surgery an emergency?* If so, the patient should proceed to surgery without delay for further preoperative evaluation. We typically treat patients in this group as if they did have coronary artery disease, if they have coronary artery disease risk factors, or if their functional capacity is poor and coronary disease could be occult (i.e., asymptomatic) due to decreased activity. The patient's cardiac risk profile as well as overall medical state should be assessed in the postoperative period. If the surgery is not an emergency, we then ask:

2. *Has the patient had coronary artery revascularization within the past 5 years?* If the patient has had coronary artery revascularization with coronary artery bypass surgery within the past 5 years or coronary artery angioplasty from 6 months to 5 years previously and has not had symptoms or signs of myocardial ischemia, retrospective data suggest that the risk of perioperative myocardial infarction is low.[14,15] The consensus guideline states that, for this patient group, further preoperative cardiac testing is usually not necessary. We take into consideration the patient's daily activity when answering this question, realizing that for the patient who is sedentary, progression of coronary artery disease may be occult because their physical activity is not strenuous enough to provoke symptoms of ischemia. For the patient who has undergone coronary angioplasty with placement of a non-drug eluting intracoronary stent, it is recommended that non-cardiac surgery be delayed until the patient's mandatory antiplatelet regimen is completed, which is typically 4 weeks following stent implantation. This is to avoid the risk of major hemorrhage if surgery is performed while the patient is receiving aggressive antiplatelet therapy as well as to prevent premature termination of antiplatelet therapy which would dramatically increase the stent thrombosis risk. For most patients who have undergone coronary stent placement, this approach would delay non-cardiac surgery for at least 4–6 weeks following intracoronary stent placement. By that time, stents are generally endothelialized and a course of post-stent placement antithrombotic therapy is completed.[16,17] For the patient who has undergone placement of a coated drug-eluting stent, the period of dual antiplatelet therapy after stenting is even longer and should similarly be completed before non-cardiac surgery is performed.

3. *Has the patient undergone a coronary evaluation within the past 2 years?* If the patient has had coronary assessment with either coronary angiography or non-invasive myocardial perfusion imaging with favorable results and has not experienced a change in clinical status or symptoms since that evaluation, the guideline suggests that repeat coronary testing prior to non-cardiac surgery is usually unnecessary.

4. *Does the patient have an unstable coronary syndrome or a major clinical predictor of risk?* In this patient group non-cardiac surgery is usually delayed unless it is an emergency. For the patient who has an unstable coronary syndrome, coronary angiography is often performed to define coronary anatomy and a coronary revascularization procedure performed if indicated. For the patient with severe valvular heart disease,

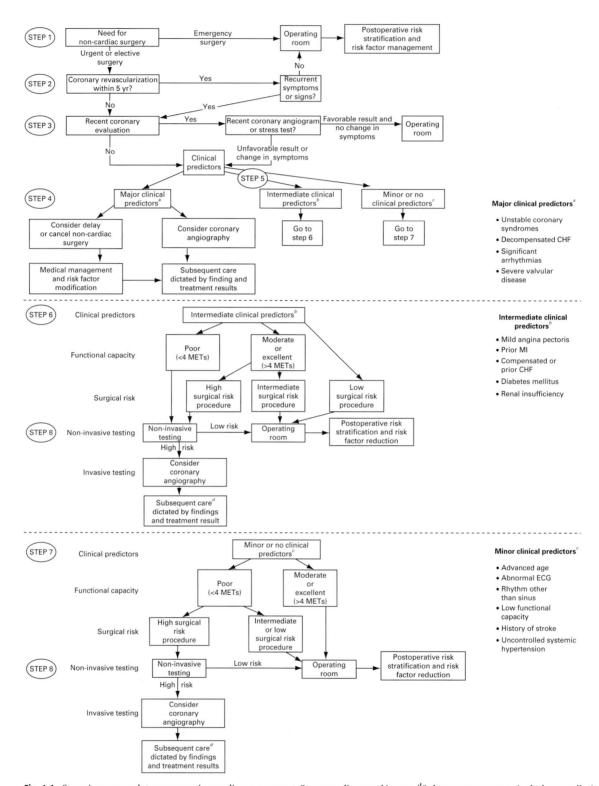

Fig. 6.1. Stepwise approach to preoperative cardiac assessment. Steps are discussed in text. [d]Subsequent care may include cancellation or delay of surgery, coronary revascularization followed by non-cardiac surgery, or intensified care. CHF indicates congestive heart failure. Reproduced from Reference 10.

evaluation is performed to assess whether valve repair or replacement is indicated. For the patient with decompensated congestive heart failure or significant arrhythmias, stabilization of these problems should be undertaken before non-emergency non-cardiac surgery is performed.

5. *Does the patient have intermediate predictor of risk?* The risk of perioperative cardiac complication for the patient with one or more of the intermediate predictors of risk (mild angina pectoris, prior myocardial infarction (MI more than 30 days prior to surgery), compensated or prior congestive heart failure, diabetes mellitus, or renal insufficiency (serum $Cr \geq 2.0$) is determined by consideration of the patient's functional capacity, risk attributed to the specific surgical procedure, and in selected cases the results of preoperative cardiac stress testing. Functional capacity is quantitated by assessing the patient's activities of daily living and expressing that activity in terms of metabolic equivalents (MET). Perioperative cardiac risk has been shown to be increased in patients with poor exercise tolerance, e.g., those who are unable to carry out activity of 4 METS during their daily activities.[13] Cardiac risk is increased even if the inability to perform this degree of activity is due to a non-cardiac cause, i.e., osteoarthritis. As defined by the Duke Activity Status Index, activities that utilize 4 METS include performing light work around the house and climbing a flight of stairs (Fig. 6.2).[18] In practice, the ACC/AHA guideline suggests that those patients with intermediate clinical predictors and poor functional capacity (inability to perform 4 METS) undergo non-invasive cardiac testing prior to surgery. Patients in this group, whose non-invasive testing reveals low risk of myocardial ischemia, then proceed to surgery, while those whose cardiac testing reveals the presence of significant myocardial

ischemia are considered at higher perioperative risk. It is this latter group that is considered for coronary angiography to assess whether they are candidates for coronary artery revascularization. In this group the clinician may suggest cancellation of the patient's non-cardiac surgery to allow for reversing the patient's treatable risk factors. For the patient with moderate functional capacity, i.e., capability of performing 4 or more METS activity, non-invasive cardiac testing is only performed if they are to undergo a high-risk surgical procedure. Those who undergo an intermediate risk or low risk procedure proceed to surgery without preoperative non-invasive cardiac testing.

6. *Does the patient have minor or no clinical predictors?* If a high risk surgical procedure is planned and the patients' functional capacity is poor, non-invasive cardiac testing is recommended to distinguish between the high risk patient with abnormal non-invasive testing in contrast to the patient whose non-invasive cardiac testing did not reveal evidence of inducible myocardial ischemia. The latter patient is deemed low risk and proceeds to surgery. The patient with minor or no clinical predictors with poor functional capacity who undergoes an intermediate or low risk surgical procedure is considered low risk as would the patient with moderate or better functional capacity. They would proceed to surgery without preoperative non-invasive cardiac testing.

A shortcut to aid in the decision to employ non-invasive testing has been proposed (see Table 6.4). Non-invasive testing is recommended in the patient with intermediate clinical predictors who has either poor functional capacity (less than 4 METS) or is to undergo a high risk procedure. In the absence of intermediate risk predictors, non-invasive testing is considered if the surgical risk is high and the functional capacity is low.

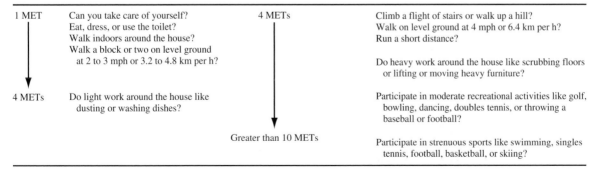

Fig. 6.2. Duke Activity Score. Estimated energy requirements for various activities. MET indicates metabolic equivalent. Reproduced from Reference 10.

Table 6.4. Shortcut to non-invasive testing in preoperative evaluation

1. Intermediate clinical predictors present (Canadian class 1 or 2 angina, prior MI based on history or ECQ Q waves, compensated or prior heart failure, or diabetes)
2. Poor functional capacity (less than 4 METS)
3. High surgical risk procedure (major operation, aortic repair or peripheral vascular surgery, prolonged surgical procedure with large fluid shifts or blood loss

Source: Non-invasive testing performed if any two of the following present. (From ACC/AHA 2002 Guideline).

Risk assessment prior to vascular surgery

Major vascular surgery presents a special challenge for preoperative assessment. Patients with major vascular disease have been demonstrated to have an increased prevalence of coronary artery disease. If their vascular disease or other comorbid conditions result in physical inactivity, the patient with major vascular disease may have no symptoms of myocardial ischemia despite the presence of significant coronary artery disease because of their limited activity.

Advanced age, a history of diabetes, myocardial infarction, angina, or congestive heart failure have been validated as risk factors for cardiac complication in vascular surgery. The absence of any of these factors was shown by L'Italien to be associated with only a 3% incidence of perioperative cardiac complication, while presence of one or two of these factors was associated with an 8% risk. If three or more risk factors were present, the risk of perioperative cardiac complication or death was 18%.[19] In a database review of vascular surgery patients, Paul found that the presence of these risk markers correlated with the likelihood of underlying coronary artery disease. The absence of any of these risk factors predicted a low likelihood of severe coronary artery disease while the presence of three or more of these factors was linked to a high incidence of left main or triple vessel coronary artery disease.[20]

The American College of Cardiology/American Heart Association *Guideline for Perioperative Cardiac Evaluation Prior to Noncardiac Surgery* classifies aortic, major vascular, and peripheral vascular surgery as high risk with surgery specific risk of cardiac complication greater than 5%. Carotid endarterectomy is classified as an intermediate risk procedure with risk of cardiac complication at less than 5%. The preoperative evaluation of these patients proceeds as it would for non-vascular surgery. The patient who has undergone a recent coronary angiogram or stress test with favorable results is estimated to be at favorable cardiac risk and proceeds to the operating room. For the patient who does not meet these criteria, their clinical predictors aid in the determination of their risk. For the patient with major predictors, aorta, major vascular, or carotid surgery is delayed until these predictors can be reversed. If their risk predictor is unstable or if there is severe myocardial ischemia, this patient typically requires coronary angiography with coronary revascularization, if indicated, prior to aorta surgery. For the patient with a critical carotid artery stenosis who requires coronary artery bypass surgery, we often perform simultaneous carotid and coronary artery revascularization to decrease the risk of stroke in the period during coronary artery bypass surgery. For patients with intermediate predictors, the high risk nature of aorta, other major vascular and peripheral vascular surgery necessitates non-invasive testing of myocardial perfusion (e.g., dipyridamole thallium imaging) to aid in risk assessment. A result suggestive of significant myocardial ischemia usually leads to a delay of surgery to allow for coronary angiography with myocardial revascularization if indicated. The patient with minimal or no ischemia proceeds to surgery. For the patient with minimal or no predictors, functional capacity is useful to aid in risk stratification prior to aorta surgery. Those with poor functional capacity require non-invasive testing of myocardial perfusion to further assess risk while those with good functional capacity able to perform 4 METS or more activity are deemed to be at low cardiac risk and undergo surgery. It is important to realize that the above approach pertains to the patient undergoing elective aorta repair or major vascular surgery. The guideline suggests that patients who require emergency surgery proceed to surgery without delay and that their cardiac status be closely observed in the perioperative period.

Risk assessment prior to transplant surgery

In many instances transplantation surgery is performed in patients with significant medical comorbidities. The patient who undergoes kidney transplantation is at least at intermediate risk of cardiac complication because of renal insufficiency. Many of these patients also have diabetes mellitus which contributes to their risk of complication. A retrospective review of 2694 patients who underwent renal transplantation identified age >50 and pre-existing heart disease especially in diabetics as risk factors that significantly increased the risk of perioperative cardiac complication.[21] In 176 patients who underwent kidney or kidney–pancreas transplant the occurrence of postoperative cardiac complications correlated with the presence of reversible myocardial perfusion defects on preoperative dipyridamole thallium imaging.[22] For the patient who undergoes liver transplantation dobutamine stress echocardiography has been shown to have utility in the prediction of postoperative cardiac complications.[23,24]

Elderly patients

In the elderly patient who undergoes surgery the cardiovascular response to surgery may be affected by the presence of preexisting heart disease as well as by normal physiologic changes of the cardiovascular system that accompany aging. Many physiologic changes that occur in response to aging have a significant effect on the cardiovascular response to surgery. The resting heart rate and the heart rate response to stress decrease.[25] Because cardiac output is a function of heart rate and stroke volume, output increases in elderly patients in response to stress primarily by increasing the left ventricular end-diastolic volume.[26] In patients with left ventricular dysfunction, decreased ventricular compliance, or intravascular volume overload, this compensatory response may result in congestive heart failure. Baroreceptor responsiveness decreases with increased age and may cause exaggerated hypotension after intravascular volume loss or with the administration of vasodilators or diuretics. The incidence of sick sinus syndrome and other cardiac conduction disorders is also increased, and occult conduction disorders may be unmasked when β-blockers or calcium channel antagonists are used in the perioperative period. Other cardiovascular changes that may affect cardiac function in the perioperative period are left ventricular hypertrophy with associated decreased left ventricular compliance, elevated left ventricular end-diastolic pressure, and subsequent interstitial edema. In this situation, which often results from long-standing hypertension, left ventricular hypertrophy may cause diastolic left ventricular dysfunction. Drug metabolism is altered in the elderly. Renal function declines and cardiovascular drugs cleared by the kidney (e.g., digoxin, enalapril) may have increased half-lives. Hepatic blood flow also decreases, leading to delayed metabolism of agents such as lidocaine, propranolol, and verapamil.[27]

Age has been demonstrated to be a risk factor for perioperative cardiovascular complication. Patients older than 70 years old have been shown to have a higher rate of major perioperative complications and mortality after non-cardiac surgery as well as a longer length of hospital stay. In a study of surgical patients aged 80 or older the overall postoperative mortality rate was 4.6%; 25% of the patients developed one or more adverse postoperative events.

Neurological and cardiovascular complications were the leading cause of morbidity. Risk factors for development of a postoperative complication were preoperative history of neurologic disease, particularly preoperative dementia, as well as preoperative history of congestive heart failure and arrhythmia.[7,28–30] In a study of 513 surgical patients aged 70 or older, 386 had at least one abnormality on the preoperative electrocardiogram. The presence of abnormalities on preoperative ECGs, however, was not associated with an increased risk of postoperative cardiac complications (OR = 0.63). Abnormalities on preoperative ECGs are common but are of limited value in predicting postoperative cardiac complications in older patients undergoing non-cardiac surgery. These results suggest that obtaining preoperative ECGs based on an age cutoff alone may not be indicated, because ECG abnormalities in older people are prevalent but non-specific and less useful than the presence and severity of comorbidities in predicting postoperative cardiac complications.[31]

Prevention of perioperative myocardial ischemia, and myocardial infarction

Evidence to support the use of beta blockers to decrease the incidence of myocardial ischemia and infarction related to non-cardiac surgery is based upon several small studies. Mangano, in a study of 200 patients with coronary artery disease or coronary disease risk factors, found a long-term benefit of atenolol when given prior to, and for several days following, surgery. In this study, myocardial ischemia was reduced by 50% in the atenolol-treated group during the first 48 hours following surgery. There was no difference between groups in terms of non-fatal or fatal myocardial infarction during the first week following surgery; however, during the 2-year follow-up period, the mortality rate was 10% in patients given atenolol and 21% in controls.[32] Based on this study, the American College of Physicians guideline on preoperative evaluation recommends the use of atenolol for patients with known coronary artery disease or significant coronary artery disease risk factors.[33] Raby, in a small pilot study, demonstrated that strict perioperative heart rate control with beta blockers, when tailored to an individual's ischemic threshold (determined by preoperative continuous ambulatory ischemia monitoring), was associated with a reduction of postoperative myocardial ischemia during the 48 hours following surgery.[34]

Two studies are of particular importance in deciding who should receive perioperative prophylactic β-blockers in the perioperative period. Poldermans and Boersma reported on a cohort of 1351 patients who underwent elective vascular surgery.[35,36] Clinical risk factors, as well as quantitation of inducible myocardial ischemia using dobutamine stress echocardiography, were used to risk stratify patients. Clinical risk factors tabulated for each patient were: age $\geq$70, current angina, prior myocardial infarction, congestive heart failure, prior cerebrovascular event, diabetes mellitus and renal insufficiency with Cr > 2.0. For patients with fewer than three risk factors, those who received perioperative β blockers (bisoprolol 5–10 mg/day beginning at least 1 week prior to surgery and continued for 30 days following surgery with the bisoprolol titrated to heart rate <80 bpm) had a lower incidence of cardiac complications (0.8%) than those who did not receive β-blockers (2.3%). In patients with three or more risk factors, those whose preoperative dobutamine stress echo revealed no inducible ischemia or ischemia in four or less left ventricular segments (of a total of 16 segments), perioperative β-blockers were effective in decreasing the incidence of cardiac complication, 2.3% vs. 10.6%. In the highest risk group, those with three or more risk factors and inducible ischemia involving five or more left ventricular segments β-blockers were ineffective in decreasing cardiac complications. Based on this evidence, we attempt to utilize perioperative β-blockers in all patients with known cardiovascular disease or at increased cardiac risk as predicted by the clinical risk factors listed above. We attempt to initiate β-blockers at least 1 week prior to surgery, realizing that in many patients the realities of surgery lead to identification of these patients at time periods considerably less than 1 week prior to surgery, and continue for at least 30 days following surgery. Many patients whom we identify as requiring these agents in the perioperative period have indications for long-term β-blocker use. We attempt to titrate the β-blocker to a heart rate of 60–70 bpm. Particular care must be taken to avoid excessive bradycardia when patients are treated with peri-operative beta blockers.

There is no evidence that intraoperative nitrates or calcium channel antagonists are of benefit to prevent intraoperative myocardial ischemia.[37,38] Prophylactic nitrates may actually be harmful if they lead to excessive preload reduction with subsequent hypotension.

Alpha-2 adrenoceptor agonists (clonidine, dexmedetomide, mivazerol) have been studied to assess whether reducing central sympathetic activity is effective in decreasing perioperative myocardial ischemia. There is evidence that they reduce myocardial ischemia and/or myocardial infarction following vascular surgery.[42] Pending results of large-scale trials, these agents cannot be recommended to decrease myocardial ischemia and infarction in the perioperative period.

In a study of 300 patients with known coronary artery disease or high risk for coronary artery disease who underwent abdominal, thoracic, or vascular surgery, maintenance of perioperative normothermia led to a decreased incidence of perioperative morbid events (unstable angina, cardiac arrest, myocardial infarction) (6.3% morbid events in the hypothermic group vs. 1.4% morbid events in the normothermic group) as well as a decrease in episodes of ventricular tachycardia.[39]

No prospective, randomized studies have been conducted to evaluate the efficacy of preoperative coronary artery revascularization in reducing perioperative risk prior to non-vascular surgery. A protective effect of previous coronary artery bypass surgery has been suggested. Pooled data from studies that used historical control subjects reveal that, of 2000 patients who underwent noncardiac surgery, the rate of postoperative infarction was significantly lower in those who underwent previous coronary artery bypass surgery (0%–1.2%) than in those who did not (1.1% to 6%).[37] In addition to the perioperative benefit, Hertzer noted a late benefit that he attributed to perioperative coronary revascularization. In a group of patients who underwent coronary artery bypass surgery before aortic aneurysm repair, survival 5 years after aneurysm surgery was similar to that of patients with trivial coronary disease.[40]

In other studies, the overall benefit of preoperative myocardial revascularization has been less clear. Data from the Coronary Artery Surgery Study (CASS) reveal higher perioperative mortality in non-randomized patients who underwent non-cardiac surgery without preceding coronary surgery (2.4%) than in those who had preceding coronary surgery (0.9%). The operative mortality for coronary artery bypass surgery was 1.4%. Therefore, the combination of coronary surgery followed by noncardiac surgery was no less risky than was non-cardiac surgery alone in medically treated patients.[41] In a subsequent analysis of the CASS registry database, Eagle found that, in patients with known coronary artery disease, noncardiac surgery (involving the thorax, abdomen, vasculature, head and neck) was associated with increased risk of perioperative cardiac complication, which was reduced in patients with prior CABG. It was also demonstrated that the protection afforded by CABG was sustained for at least 6 years following the coronary revascularization procedure. In a study of elective coronary artery revascularization prior to vascular surgery, coronary revascularization was found to not be of benefit in reducing overall perioperative mortality in patients with stable coronary artery disease if treated with beta blockers, aspirin and statins in the absence of left main coronary artery disease, aortic stenosis and severe left ventricular dysfunction. The American College of Cardiology/American Heart Association consensus-based guidelines for preoperative cardiovascular evaluation prior to non-cardiac surgery recommend that the individual patient's perioperative and long-term risk be considered when deciding whether or not to perform coronary artery bypass surgery prior to non-cardiac surgery. They advocate that coronary artery bypass surgery be performed prior to non-cardiac surgery in patients who meet established criteria for coronary bypass, i.e., left main coronary stenosis, three-vessel coronary artery disease in conjunction with left ventricular dysfunction, two-vessel coronary disease when one of the vessels is the left anterior descending coronary artery with a severe proximal stenosis, and myocardial ischemia despite a maximal medical regimen. The guidelines highlight that coronary artery bypass grafting should be performed in the above patients prior to high or intermediate risk non-cardiac surgery when long-term outcome would be improved by the coronary surgery.

It has been suggested that percutaneous transluminal coronary angioplasty reduces perioperative cardiac morbidity when it is performed to alleviate myocardial ischemia before non-cardiac surgery. The few studies that have assessed this technique, however, were non-randomized and based on historical controls.[42,43] Because there may be elastic recoil and plaque disruption at the site of the coronary angioplasty, it has been recommended, based on theoretical grounds, to delay elective non-cardiac surgery for several days to allow for stabilization of the coronary endothelium.

For the patient who has undergone coronary angioplasty with placement of an intracoronary stent, it is recommended that non-cardiac surgery be delayed until the patient's mandatory antiplatelet regimen is completed, which is typically a 4-week regimen of clopidogrel and aspirin following stent implantation with continued long-term aspirin. This is to avoid the risk of major hemorrhage if surgery is performed while the patient is receiving aggressive antiplatelet therapy as well as to prevent premature termination of antiplatelet therapy which would dramatically increase the stent thrombosis risk.[17] For most patients who have undergone coronary stent placement, this approach would delay non-cardiac surgery for at least 5–6 weeks following intracoronary stent placement. By that time, stents are generally endothelialized and a course of post-stent placement antithrombotic therapy is completed.[16,17] For the patient who has undergone placement of a drug-eluting stent, the period of dual antiplatelet therapy after stenting is even longer and should similarly be completed before non-cardiac surgery is performed, e.g. 3 months for a sirulimus-coated stent and 6 months for a paclitaxel-coated stent. This focused approach serves to reduce the risk of stent thrombosis in those patients whose antiplatelet agents would be prematurely discontinued, and bleeding in those who would undergo surgery while still receiving their antiplatelet regimen.[44,44a]

For patients with chronic stable angina it is important to continue their antianginal therapy in the perioperative period. Beta-blockers are continued to the time of surgery. For prolonged effect, a long-acting preparation (i.e., nadolol or atenolol) may be given on the morning of surgery. If patients are unable to resume oral intake 24 hours after surgery, β-blockers may be given intravenously (e.g., propranolol, 0.5 to 2 mg every 1 to 6 hours). Parenteral metoprolol or esmolol may also be used. Oral β-blocker therapy is resumed as soon as possible after surgery.

Patients who are receiving long-term antianginal treatment with calcium channel antagonists are usually given a long-acting oral preparation on the morning of surgery. If they are unable to resume oral intake 24 hours after surgery, we generally add intravenous or topical nitrates to the regimen. The only calcium channel antagonists available for intravenous use are verapamil and diltiazem. Because their effect is primarily antiarrhythmic when they are given intravenously, we do not use these agents as primary anti-ischemic therapy for patients who are unable to take oral medications.

Management of cardiac medications in the perioperative period

Perioperative continuation of patient's long-term cardiac medications is often challenging. Many oral medications have no parenteral substitutes. The stress of surgery may render patients' long-term cardiac medical regiments inadequate during the perioperative period. Finally, few controlled studies have evaluated the use of cardiac medications during and after non-cardiac surgery. Several guidelines are helpful in attempting to maintain patients' long-term medical therapeutic regimens in the perioperative period.

Beta-adrenergic blockers are used in the treatment of myocardial ischemia, arrhythmias, hypertension, and left ventricular systolic dysfunction. Patients who receive β-blockers on a long-term basis should be given oral doses on the morning of their surgical procedure. Long-acting agents such as atenolol and sustained release metoprolol provide β-blockade for as long as 24 hours. Patients' long-term β-blocker regimens are then restarted 24 hours after surgery if oral intake has resumed. For patients whose gastrointestinal tracts are not functional at that time, the administration of intravenous β-blockers (e.g., propranolol, 0.5 to 2 mg every 4 to 6 hours) is begun and continued until the usual long-term oral β-blocker is tolerated. This regimen is often effective for patients who are receiving β-blockers for coronary artery disease or cardiac arrhythmias but may require alteration in patients who take these drugs for hypertension or congestive heart failure. For the patient with hypertension, labetalol (a test dose of 2.5 to 5.0 mg intravenously, then an infusion of 20 to 80 mg) may also be given by intravenous infusion at 2 mg/min until the blood pressure is controlled or until a total of 300 mg has been given. The short-acting intravenous β-blocker esmolol (at a loading infusion of 500 µg/kg per min for 1 minute followed by a continuous infusion of 50 µg/kg per min) may also be used to control blood pressure in the postoperative period. Patients whose blood pressures are not controlled with these agents may require supplemental antihypertensive agents in addition to intravenous β-blockers until oral medications are resumed. For patients receiving β-blockers as treatment for chronic congestive heart failure, we try to avoid discontinuation of β-blockers in the perioperative period unless the patient develops deterioration of their clinical status as manifest by hypoperfusion or requires intravenous positive inotropic agents. In these cases we temporarily discontinue the β-blocker but reinstitute it as soon as the patient is stabilized in an effort to reduce the risk of significant deterioration.

Nitrates are commonly used by patients with ischemic heart disease. Patients who are stable receiving nitrates on a long-term basis typically are given their oral nitrate preparations on the morning of the surgical procedure. Topical nitroglycerine ointment (0.5–2 inches) is then applied every 8 hours until oral nitrates are resumed. This approach helps to maintain a "nitrate-free" period to decrease the risk of development of nitrate vasotolerance. Nitrates may cause excessive preload reduction and hypotension, which may be exacerbated by intravascular volume depletion and by the simultaneous use of other vasodilator medications or anesthetic agents. In some patients, hypotension may occur unpredictably with the initial administration of nitrates. For this reason, we recommend that the initiation of nitrates, given to decrease the likelihood of perioperative myocardial ischemia, be administered well before surgery. Intravenous nitroglycerine should be considered when nitrates are used to treat perioperative myocardial ischemia.

Intravenous nitroprusside is effective in controlling perioperative hypertension but the need for continuous blood pressure monitoring, and the risk of cyanate toxicity, makes its use impractical for more than a few days. Intravenous methyldopa and enalaprilat, given three to four times daily, are effective in controlling postoperative hypertension, are well tolerated, and may be used without continuous blood pressure monitoring in stable patients. They are useful adjuncts for controlling hypertension in the perioperative period.

Intravascular volume depletion may occur in patients receiving long-term diuretic therapy and places them at risk of hypotension when anesthetic agents that produce vasodilation are administered. Intravascular volume depletion is suggested by the presence of orthostatic changes in the blood pressure and heart rate and should be corrected with fluid administration, before surgery if possible. Patients who take diuretics may also have hypokalemia or hyperkalemia from potassium-sparing agents. Serum potassium levels should be checked in these patients before surgery. It has been suggested that a chronic serum potassium level of 3 mmol/l or higher is acceptable for anesthesia and surgery, and that chronic asymptomatic hypokalemia as low as 2.5 mmol/l may be adequate in patients who are at low risk for cardiac complications.[45] Hypokalemia has been shown to increase the incidence of cardiac arrhythmias in patients taking digoxin; therefore, perioperative hypokalemia should be corrected in this patient group.

Calcium channel antagonists are used to treat angina, hypertension, and arrhythmias. Sustained release preparations of the calcium channel antagonists that patients have been using may be given on the morning of surgery in an effort to achieve effective drug levels for the next 24 hours. Patients who are capable of oral intake the day after surgery may resume oral calcium channel antagonists. Problems exist, however, in substituting appropriate parenteral formulations for patients who cannot resume oral calcium channel antagonists at this time. The few calcium channel antagonists that are available for parenteral administration often have their primary effect on the cardiac conduction system rather than in treating hypertension or angina. Intravenous verapamil has potent negative chronotropic effects and can induce heart block. Intravenous diltiazem is indicated primarily to control the ventricular response in patients with atrial fibrillation and to convert paroxysmal supraventricular tachycardia to sinus rhythm in patients who have atrioventricular nodal reentrant tachycardia. There is no parenteral preparation of nifedipine or amlodipine.

In patients who receive calcium channel antagonists for their antianginal effects, topical or intravenous nitrates may be substituted until oral intake resumes. In patients who take calcium channel antagonists for hypertension, intravenous alpha methyl dopa or enalaprilat is often effective until oral medications are resumed.

Digitalis glycosides may be given orally on the morning of surgery and then intravenously on a daily basis until patients' long-term oral regimens are resumed. The intravenous administration of these agents increases their bioavailability by as much as 20%, and the maintenance parenteral dose may have to be reduced appropriately.

Angiotensin-converting enzyme inhibitors are used to treat hypertension and left ventricular systolic dysfunction. Enalaprilat is the only agent of this class available for parenteral administration and is given intravenously every 6 hours.

The abrupt withdrawal of centrally acting antihypertensive agents, which may occur in the perioperative period, may result in a "discontinuation syndrome" characterized by sympathetic overactivity and rebound hypertension.[46] Symptoms may resemble those of pheochromocytoma. Clonidine is the prototype drug of this class. The discontinuation syndrome may occur 18 to 72 hours after clonidine is withdrawn but rarely occurs in patients who receive less than 1.2 mg of clonidine daily. This syndrome may be aggravated by the simultaneous use of β-blockers, which may block peripheral vasodilatory β-receptors, leaving vasoconstrictor α-receptors unopposed.[47] The syndrome may be terminated by resumption of clonidine therapy. If that is not possible because patients cannot resume oral intake, rebound hypertension may be controlled with intravenous nitroprusside or labetalol. Clonidine withdrawal syndrome may be prevented by slow tapering of clonidine before surgery. For patients in whom this is not feasible, transdermal clonidine may be given in the perioperative period. The transdermal clonidine requires about 48 hours to achieve therapeutic drug levels. Therefore, it should be given well in advance of surgery and at its initiation be administered simultaneously with oral clonidine for about 48 hours. The transdermal preparation maintains therapeutic clonidine levels for as long as 7 days.

Clopidogrel is a thienopyridine antiplatelet agent administered along with aspirin typically for 2–4 weeks to patients who have had bare metal coronary stenting or 3 to 6 months following placement of a drug-eluting stent depending on the type of stent used. There is evidence that a beneficial effect on the reduction of stent thrombosis may exist with up to 9 months of post-stent placement clopidogrel use.[48] It is also used in the treatment of patients with acute coronary syndromes.[49] Clopidogrel may increase the risk of bleeding during or immediately following major surgery. Because its effect on platelets and bleeding may last for 5 days, many surgeons request at least a 5-day period between the discontinuation of clopidogrel and subsequent major surgery.

Perioperative invasive cardiac monitoring

Invasive pulmonary artery pressue monitoring is often used in patients who are at increased risk for myocardial infarction during and after operation in an effort to diagnose and treat perioperative myocardial ischemia. Indications for perioperative pulmonary monitoring are ill-defined. Myocardial ischemia decreases left ventricular compliance and increases left ventricular end-diastolic pressure, left atrial pressure, pulmonary capillary wedge pressure, and pulmonary artery pressure. If it is extensive, myocardial ischemia may also reduce cardiac output. These hemodynamic consequences may occur before myocardial ischemia is apparent on standard electrocardiographic monitoring or manifest as abnormalities of cardiac hemodynamics.

Although it is attractive in theory, invasive pulmonary artery pressure monitoring has suboptimal sensitivity and specificity for the detection of perioperative myocardial ischemia. Numerous perioperative situations (e.g., intravascular volume overload, increased afterload) may result in increased pulmonary artery capillary wedge pressure without associated myocardial ischemia. Similarly, myocardial ischemia may be present without changes in pulmonary artery capillary pressure.

The indication for use of pulmonary artery catheters in the perioperative period is unclear. A multicenter, randomized, controlled clinical trial comparing perioperative therapy guided by pulmonary artery catheter derived data vs. standard care in high risk (American Society of Anesthesiologists (ASA) class III or IV risk) patients 60 years of age or older found no mortality benefit to therapy directed by pulmonary artery catheter.[50] It has been our approach to assess the need for invasive hemodynamic monitoring on an individual basis. Intuitive indications for invasive hemodynamic monitoring are: anticipation of fluid shifts in the patient with left ventricular dysfunction or fixed cardiac output; major vascular surgery in the patient with left ventricular dysfunction; and surgery in the patient with recent myocardial infarction or unstable angina.

REFERENCES

1. Park, K. W. Cardiovascular effects of inhalational anesthetics. *Int. Anesth. Clin.* 2002; **40**: 1–14.

2. Wiklund, L. & Rosenbaum, S. Anesthesiology, Part 1. *N. Engl. J. Med.* 1997; **337**: 1132–1141.

3. Higgins, T. L., Yarad, J. P., Estafanous, F. G., Coyle, J. P., Ko, H. K., & Goodale, D. B. Propofol versus midazolam for intensive care unit sedation after coronary artery bypass graft. *Crit. Care Med.* 1994; **22**: 1415–1423.

4. Rodgers, A., Walker, N., Schug, S. *et al.* Reduction of postoperative mortality and morbidity with epidural or spinal anesthesia: results from overview of randomised trials. *BMJ* 2000; **321**: 1493.

5. Beattie, W. S., Badner, N. H., & Choi, P. Epidural analgesia reduces postoperative myocardial infarction: a meta analysis. *Anesth. Analg.* 2001; **93**: 853–858.

6. Breen, P. & Park, K. General anesthesia versus regional anesthesia. *Int. Anesth. Clin.* 2002; **40**: 61–71.

7. Goldman, L., Caldera, D. L., Nussbaum, S. R. *et al.* Multifactorial index of cardiac risk in noncardiac surgical procedures. *N. Engl. J. Med.* 1978; **297**: 845.

8. Detsky, A. S., Abrams, H. B., McLaughlin, J. R. *et al.* Predicting cardiac complications in patients undergoing noncardiac surgery. *J. Gen. Intern. Med.* 1986; **1**: 211–219.

9. Lee, T. H., Marcantonio, E., Mangione, C. M. *et al.* Derivation and prospective validation of a simple index for prediction of cardiac risks of major noncardiac surgery. *Circulation* 1999; **100**: 1043–1049.

10. Eagle, K., Berger, P. B., Calkins, H. *et al.* ACC/AHA guideline update for perioperative cardiovascular evaluation for noncardiac surgery: a report of the American College of Cardiology/American Heart Association Task Force on Practice Guidelines (Committee to Update the 1996 Guidelines on Perioperative Cardiovascular Evaluation for Noncardiac Surgery). American College of Cardiology website 2002. Available at http://www.acc.org/clinical/guidelines/peris/dirindex.htm.

11. Weiner, D. A., Ryan, T., McCabe, C. H. *et al.* Prognostic importance of a clinical profile and exercise test in medically treated patients with coronary artery disease. *J. Am. Coll. Cardiol.* 1984; **3**: 772–779.

12. Nelson, C. L., Herndon, J. E., Mark, D. B., Pryor, D. B., Califf, R. M., & Hlatky, M. A. Relation of clinical and angiographic factors to functional capacity as measured by the Duke Activity Status Index. *Am. J. Cardiol.* 1991; **68**: 973–975.

13. Reilly, D. F., McNeely, M. J., Doerner, D. *et al.* Self-reported exercise tolerance and the risk of serious perioperative complications. *Arch. Intern. Med.* 1999; **159**: 2185–2192.

14. Mahar, L. J., Steen, P. A., Tinker, J., Vlietstra, R. E., Smith, H. C., & Pluth, J. R. Perioperative myocardial infarction in patients with coronary artery disease with and without aorta-coronary artery bypass grafts. *J. Thorac. Cardiovasc. Surg.* 1978; **76**: 772–779.

15. Eagle, K. A., Rihal, C. S., Mickel, M. C., Holmes, D. R., Foster, E. D., & Gersh, B. J. Cardiac risk of noncardiac surgery: influence of coronary disease and type of surgery in 3368 operations. CASS Investigators and University of Michigan Heart Care Program. Coronary Artery Surgery Study. *Circulation* 1997; **96**: 1882–1887.

16. Wilson, S., Fasseas, P., Orford, J. *et al.* Clinical outcome of patients undergoing noncardiac surgery in the two months following coronary stenting. *J. Am. Coll. Cardiol.* 2003; **42**: 234–240.

17. Kaluza, G. L., Joseph, J., Lee, J. R., Raizner, M. E., & Raizner, A. E. Catastrophic outcomes of noncardiac surgery soon after coronary stenting [comment]. *J. Am. Coll. Cardiol.* 2000; **35**: 1288–1294.

18. Hlatky, M. A., Boineau, R. E., Higginbitham, M. B. *et al.* A brief self administered questionnaire to determine functional capacity (the Duke Activity Status Index). *Am. J. Cardiol.* 1989; **64**: 651–654.

19. L'Italien, G. J., Paul, S. D., Hendel, R. C. *et al.* Development and validation of a Bayesian model for perioperative cardiac risk assessment in a cohort of 1,081 vascular surgical candidates. *J. Am. Coll. Cardiol.* 1996; **27**: 779–786.

20. Paul, S. D., Eagle, K. A., Kuntz, K. M., Young, J. R., & Hertzer, N. R. Concordance of preoperative clinical risk with angiographic severity of coronary artery disease in patients undergoing vascular surgery. *Circulation* 1996; **94**: 1561–1566.

21. Humar, A., Kerr, S. R., Ramcharan, T., Gillingham, K. J., & Matas, A. J. Perioperative cardiac morbidity in kidney transplant recipients: incidence and risk. *Clin. Transpl.* 2001; **15**: 154–158.

22. Mistry, B. M., Bastani, B., Solomon, H. *et al.* Prognostic value of dipyridamole thallium-201 screening to minimize perioperative cardiac complications in diabetics undergoing kidney or kidney–pancreas transplantation. *Clin. Transpl.* 1998; **12**: 130–135.

23. Plotkin, J. S., Benitez, R. M., Kuo, P. C. *et al.* Dobutamine stress echocardiography for preoperative cardiac risk stratification in patients undergoing orthotopic liver transplantation. *Liver Transpl. Surg.* 1998; **4**: 253–257.

24. Donovan, C. L., Marcovitz, P. A., Punch, J. D. *et al.* Two-dimensional and dobutamine stress echocardiography in the preoperative assessment of patients with end-stage liver disease prior to orthotopic liver transplantation. *Transplantation* 1996; **61**: 1180–1188.

25. Rosberg, B. & Wulff, K. Hemodynamics following normovolemic hemodilution in elderly patients. *Acta Anaesthesiol. Scand.* 1981; **25**: 402–406.

26. Rodeheffer, R., Gerstenblith, G., Becker, L. *et al.* Exercise cardiac output is maintained with advancing age in healthy human subjects: cardiac dilatation and increased stroke volume compensate for a diminished heart rate. *Circulation* 1984; **69**: 203–213.

27. Wenger, N. K. Cardiovascular disease in the elderly. *Curr. Probl. Cardiol.* 1992; **17**: 618–624.

28. Polanczyk, C. A., Marcantonio, E., Goldman, L. *et al.* Impact of age on perioperative complications and length of stay in patients undergoing noncardiac surgery. *Ann. Intern. Med.* 2001; **134**: 637–643.

29. Leung, J. M., Dzankic, S. Relative importance of preoperative health status versus intraoperative factors in predicting postoperative adverse outcomes in geriatric surgical patients. *J. Am. Geriatr. Soc.* 2001; **49**: 1080–1085.

30. Liu, L. L. & Leung, J. M. Predicting adverse postoperative outcomes in patients aged 80 years or older. *J. Am. Geriatr. Soc.* 2000; **48**: 405–412.

31. Liu, L. L., Dzankic, S., & Leung, J. M. Preoperative electrocardiogram abnormalities do not predict postoperative cardiac complications in geriatric surgical patients. *J. Am. Geriatr. Soc.* 2002; **50**: 1186–1191.

32. Mangano, D. T., Layug, E. L., Wallace, A., & Tateo, I. Effect of atenolol on mortality and cardiovascular morbidity after noncardiac surgery. *N. Engl. J. Med.* 1996; **335**: 1713.

33. Palda, V. A. & Detsky, A. S. Perioperative assessment and management of risk from coronary artery disease. *Ann. Intern. Med.* 1997; **127**: 313–328.

34. Raby, K. E., Brull, S. J., Timimi, F. *et al.* The effect of heart rate control on myocardial ischemia among high risk patients after vascular surgery. *Cardiovasc. Anesth.* 1999; **88**: 477–482.

35. Boersma, E., Poldermans, D., Bax, J. J. *et al.* Predictors of cardiac events after major vascular surgery: role of clinical characteristics, dobutamine echocardiography, and β-blocker therapy. *JAMA* 2001; **285**: 1865–1873.

36. Poldermans, D., Boersma, E., Bax, J. J. *et al.* The effect of bisoprolol on perioperative mortality and myocardial infarction in high risk patients undergoing vascular surgery. *N. Engl. J. Med.* 1999; **341**: 1789–1794.

37. Thomson, I. R., Mutch, W. A., & Culligan, J. D. Failure of intravenous nitroglycerine to prevent intraoperative myocardial ischemia during fentanyl-pancuronium anesthesia. *Anesthesiology* 1984; **61**: 385–393.

38. Slogoff, S. & Keats, A. S. Does chronic treatment with calcium entry blocking drugs reduce perioperative myocardial ischemia? *Anesthesiology* 1988; **68**: 676–680.

38a. Wijeysundera, D., Naik, S., & Beattie, W. S. Alpha-2 adrenal antagonists to prevent cardio-vascular complications. A meta-analysis. *Am. J. Med.* 2003; **114**: 742–752.

39. Frank, S., Fleisher, L., Breslow, M. *et al.* Perioperative maintenance of normothermia reduces the incidence of morbid events. *J. Am. Med. Assoc.* 1997; **227**: 1127–1134.

40. Hertzer, N. R., Young, J. R., Beven, E. *et al.* Late results of coronary bypass in patients with infrarenal aortic aneurysms: the Cleveland Clinic experience. *Ann. Surg.* 1987; **205**: 360–367.

41. Foster, E., Davis, K., & Carpenter, J. Risk of noncardiac operation in patients with defined coronary artery disease: the Coronary Artery Surgery Study (CASS) Registry experience. *Ann. Thorac. Surg.* 1986; **41**: 42.

41a. McFalls, E., Ward, H., Morhz, T. *et al.* Coronary artery revascularization before elective major vascular surgery, *N. Engl. J. Med.* 2004; **351**: 2795–2804.

42. Huber, K., Evans, M., Bresnahan, J. *et al.* Outcome of noncardiac operations in patients with severe coronary artery disease successfully treated preoperatively with coronary angioplasty. *Mayo Clin. Proc.* 1992; **67**: 15–21.

43. Allen, J., Helling, T., & Hartzler, G. Operative procedures not involving the heart after percutaneous transluminal coronary angioplasty. *Surg. Gynecol. Obstet.* 1991; **173**: 285–288.

44. Kaluza, G. L., Joseph, J., Lee, J. R., Raizner, M. E., & Raizner, A. E. Catastrophic outcomes of noncardiac surgery soon after coronary stenting. *J. Am. Coll. Cardiol.* 2000; **35**: 1288–1294.

44a. Weitz, H. H. When can a patient receiving a drug-eluting stent undergo non-cardiac surgery? *Cleveland Clin. J. Med.* 2005; **79**: 818–820.

45. Restrick, L. J., Huddy, N., & Hoffbrand, B. I. Diuretic induced hypokalemia: much ado about nothing? *Postgrad. Med. J.* 1992; **68**: 318–320.

46. Houston, M. C. Abrupt cessation of treatment in hypertension: consideration of clinical features, mechanisms, prevention, and management of the discontinuation syndrome. *Am. Heart J.* 1981; **102**: 415.

47. Bailey, R. & Neale, T. Rapid clonidine with blood pressure overshoot exaggerated by beta blockade. *BMJ* 1976; **1**: 942–943.

48. Mehta, S. R., Yusuf, S., Peters, R. J. *et al.* Effects of pretreatment with clopidogrel and aspirin followed by long-term therapy in patients undergoing percutaneous coronary intervention: the PCI-CURE study. *Lancet* 2001; **358**: 527–533.

49. Yusuf, S., Zhao, F., Mehta, S. R., Chrolavicius, S., Tognoni, G., & Fox, K. K. Effects of clopidogrel in addition to aspirin in patients with acute coronary syndromes without ST segment elevation. *N. Engl. J. Med.* 2001; **345**: 494–502.

50. Sandham, J. D., Hull, R. D., Brant, R. F. *et al.* A randomized controlled trial of the use of pulmonary-artery catheters in high risk surgical patients. *N. Engl. J. Med.* 2003; **348**: 5–14.

Arrhythmias and conduction abnormalities

Incidence and clinical significance of perioperative arrhythmias

Cardiac arrhythmias are common in the perioperative period. They are usually clinically insignificant. In one study using continuous electrocardiographic monitoring, 84% of patients were documented to have at least transient arrhythmias during their hospitalization for surgery. Only 5% of these arrhythmias were clinically important.[1] In another study Kuner and associates noted a 62% incidence of one or more transient arrhythmias in the perioperative period. The dysrhythmias were primarily supraventricular, most commonly wandering atrial pacemaker, isorhythmic atrioventricular (AV) dissociation, nodal rhythm, and sinus bradycardia. Ventricular premature contractions were common but paroxysmal ventricular tachycardia was rare.[2] The Multicenter Study of General Anesthesia reported a 70.2% incidence of tachycardia, bradycardia, or dysrhythmia in more than 17 000 patients who underwent a variety of surgical procedures. Adverse outcomes as a result of these dysrhythmias were reported in only 1.6% of the patients.[3,4]

In a study of men who underwent non-cardiac surgery and had known coronary artery disease or significant risk factors for coronary artery disease, O'Kelly found that frequent or major ventricular arrhythmias (more than 30 ventricular premature contractions per hour or ventricular tachycardia) occurred in 44% of the patients who were monitored (21% before operation, 16% during operation, and 36% after operation). Preoperative ventricular arrhythmias were associated with the occurrence of intraoperative and postoperative arrhythmias. These arrhythmias were largely benign, and sustained ventricular tachycardia or ventricular fibrillation did not occur.[5]

Multifactorial risk indices identified preoperative ventricular premature contractions and rhythms other than sinus rhythm as markers of risk in non-cardiac surgery. We currently believe that ventricular premature contractions and related ventricular ectopy are markers of risk when they occur in the presence of ischemic or structural heart disease. The American College of Cardiology/American Heart Association *Practice Guideline on Perioperative Cardiovascular Evaluation for Noncardiac Surgery* classifies symptomatic ventricular arrhythmias in the presence of underlying heart disease, supraventricular arrhythmias with uncontrolled ventricular rate, and high-grade atrioventricular block in the presence of underlying heart disease as major clinical predictors of increased perioperative cardiovascular risk. This guideline classifies preoperative rhythm other than sinus rhythm (e.g., atrial fibrillation) as a minor risk factor.[6,7]

We look for evidence of structural or ischemic heart disease, metabolic derangements, and electrolyte abnormalities when arrhythmias or conduction abnormalities are identified prior to surgery. We do not consider preoperative ventricular premature contractions or complex ventricular arrhythmias in the absence of heart disease or metabolic or electrolyte abnormality to be significant risk factors. Patients with atrial premature contractions and supraventricular arrhythmias that occur without the development of hemodynamic instability are also not considered to be at increased risk. While the presence of atrial fibrillation is a minor risk factor for cardiac complication, a challenge in the perioperative period is adjustment of anticoagulation regimens for those patients who are receiving long-term anticoagulant therapy. Patients with chronic atrial fibrillation may be treated with medications to control the ventricular response or with medications to maintain sinus rhythm. Care is required to maintain these medications or appropriate substitutes in the perioperative period.

Risk factors for, and etiology of, perioperative arrhythmias and conduction abnormalities

In a study of patients who underwent non-cardiac surgery and developed supraventricualr arrhythmias in the perioperative period, Polanczyk identified the following preoperative correlates for the development of perioperative arrhythmia: male sex (odds ratio (OR), 1.3 (95% CI, 1.0 to 1.7)), age 70 years or older (OR, 1.3 (CI, 1.0 to 1.7)), significant valvular disease (OR, 2.1 (CI, 1.2 to 3.6)), history of supraventricular arrhythmia (OR, 3.4 (CI, 2.4 to 4.8)) or asthma (OR, 2.0 (CI, 1.3 to 3.1)), congestive heart failure

(OR, 1.7 (CI, 1.1 to 2.7)), premature atrial complexes on preoperative electrocardiography (OR, 2.1 (CI, 1.3 to 3.4)), American Society of Anesthesiologists class III or IV (OR, 1.4 (CI, 1.1 to 1.9)), and type of procedure: abdominal aortic aneurysm (OR, 3.9 (CI, 2.4 to 6.3)) or abdominal (OR, 2.5 (CI, 1.7 to 3.6)), vascular (OR, 1.6 (CI, 1.1 to 2.4)), and intrathoracic (OR, 9.2 (CI, 6.7 to 13)) procedures.[8] Multiple studies have shown that the only consistent independent risk factor for postoperative atrial fibrillation is age ≥ 60.[8–10]

Sinus tachycardia is common in the perioperative period and often results from catecholamine release precipitated by stress, pain, or anxiety. Hypovolemia or anemia may cause sinus tachycardia as a compensatory response to increase cardiac output. Less common but ominous causes of sinus tachycardia are perioperative congestive heart failure and myocardial infarction. The anesthetic agent ketamine may cause sinus tachycardia as a result of central sympathetic stimulation. Hypercarbia and hypoxemia resulting from inadequate ventilation may cause sinus tachycardia as well as ventricular tachycardia.

Bradycardia is seen frequently during hospitalization for surgery and has numerous causes. Narcotics, with the exception of meperidine, may cause bradycardia by producing central vagal stimulation.[11] Anticholinesterases which are administered to antagonize the effect of nondepolarizing neuromuscular blocking agents may result in bradycardia.[12] An imbalance between sympathetic and parasympathetic tone may be produced in patients undergoing spinal or epidural anesthesia if cardiac stimulating sympathetic fibers are anesthetized. This can occur if the spinal cord is anesthetized at the level of the sympathetic ganglia (T-1 to T-4) or if spinal anesthesia is placed two to six segments distant from this region because the anesthetic agent may migrate or ascending preganglionic sympathetic fibers in the paravertebral chain may be blocked. Unopposed parasympathetic (vagal) activity may occur and lead to peripheral vasodilation and hypotension in addition to bradycardia.[13]

Reflex bradycardia occasionally associated with heart block and sinus arrest, may occur during surgical procedures (Table 6.5). It is usually caused by a reflex arc whose efferent limb is the vagus nerve. In addition to bradycardia, this vagally mediated reflex may result in peripheral vasodilation and hypotension. Anesthetic agents such as vecuronium, atacurium, halothane, fentanyl, and succinylcholine may predispose to this reflex.[14] It can be prevented by premedication with an anticholinergic agent such as atropine. If reflex bradycardia does occur, it often can be terminated by discontinuing the procedure or administering anticholinergic agents.

Table 6.5. Reflex bradycardia during surgery

Surgical procedure	Afferent reflex pathway	Ref
Abdominal manipulation	Celiac plexus	63
Mesenteric traction	?	64
Liver biopsy	Hepatic, celiac plexus	65
Laparoscopy	Parasympathetic stimulation from peritoneal stimulation	66
Ocular stimulation (Oculocardiac reflex)	Parasympathetic fibers in the ciliary nerves and the ophthalmic nerve run to the trigeminal nerve which is adjacent to the nucleus ambiguous, which is the origin of the vagus	14
Maxilla or zygoma stimulation	Trigeminal nerve	67
Neurosurgery (tentorium stimulation)	Ophthalmic nerve innervates tentorium; reflex similar to oculocardiac reflex	68
Laryngoscopy	Laryngeal stimulation	69
Blepharoplasty	Same as oculocardiac reflex	14

In O'Kelly's study of perioperative ventricular arrhythmias, the presence of preoperative ventricular ectopy was the most significant predictor of intraoperative and postoperative ventricular arrhythmias. Other risk factors were history of congestive heart failure and history of cigarette smoking. Additional causes of perioperative arrhythmias include hypoxia, hypercarbia, and acute hypokalemia.[5]

Arrhythmias may be precipitated by medications used specifically during ophthalmic surgery as a result of systemic absorption of eye drops. Ophthalmic atropine has been reported to cause supraventricular tachycardia and atrial fibrillation, timolol and pilocarpine eye drops have been reported to cause bradycardia.[15,16]

Patients with preoperative cardiac arrhythmias

If atrial fibrillation is detected during the initial preoperative evaluation, we often delay non-emergency surgery and evaluate the patient in a manner similar to our approach to that for the patient with newly diagnosed atrial fibrillation not going to surgery. We attempt to identify precipitating causes. An echocardiogram is performed to evaluate for the presence of structural cardiac abnormalities. Electrolytes as well as thyroid function are assessed. Since the AFFIRM Trial found that, in patients with persistent or recurrent atrial fibrillation, rhythm control was not superior in terms of mortality to rate control with antithrombotic therapy, our approach in newly diagnosed atrial fibrillation is to assess the need for restoration of sinus rhythm vs. rate control of atrial fibrillation; to evaluate the patient's need for antithrombotic therapy to prevent stroke; and to appropriately control ventricular response of the atrial fibrillation.[17] If the patient is unstable (e.g., pulmonary edema, unstable angina) urgent cardioversion may have to be performed. If the patient is stable, our approach is to slow the ventricular rate with A–V nodal blocking agents (e.g., diltiazem, verapamil, esmolol, metoprolol, propranolol). Up to two-thirds of patients will spontaneously convert to sinus rhythm within 24 hours of the onset of atrial fibrillation.[18] If we are unable to determine the duration of the patient's atrial fibrillation, we initiate warfarin anticoagulation to decrease the likelihood of systemic embolism. When cardioversion is planned, we either perform cardioversion after 3 weeks of therapeutic warfarin therapy or, as an alternate approach, transesophageal echocardiography is performed and cardioversion is attempted if there is no evidence of left atrial thrombi. In both approaches warfarin is continued with maintenance of INR 2.0–3.0 for three to four weeks following conversion. We then plan surgery to occur after completion of this warfarin course.

For the patient with chronic atrial fibrillation who receives long-term anticoagulation, there are no clear guidelines for the management of anticoagulation in the perioperative period. A consensus recommendation from the American College of Chest Physicians states that: for patients with a low risk of thromboembolism (e.g., atrial fibrillation and no history of prior stroke) warfarin is stopped approximately 4 days before surgery and restarted immediately following surgery; for patients at intermediate risk of thromboembolism, warfarin is stopped 4 days prior to surgery and the patient is then covered with low dose heparin 5000 μ sc beginning 2 days before surgery or with a prophylactic dose of low molecular weight heparin, and then LMWH is begun along with warfarin therapy after surgery; for patients at high risk of thromboembolism (e.g., prior history of thromboembolism, mechanical cardiac valve in the mitral position) warfarin is stopped 4 days before surgery, therapy with full dose low molecular weight heparin is begun when INR falls below the therapeutic level, low molecular weight heparin is stopped 12 to 24 hours prior to surgery and then restarted along with warfarin as soon as possible following surgery. An alternative approach in this group is to begin continuous intravenous heparin when the INR falls below the therapeutic range, discontinuing the heparin 5 hours prior to surgery and restarting as soon as possible following surgery along with warfarin. Heparin is continued until the INR rises to the therapeutic range.[19]

Patients are commonly found to have asymptomatic ventricular ectopy at the time of preoperative evaluation. When significant ventricular ectopy (e.g., frequent ventricular premature contractions, non-sustained ventricular tachycardia) is identified, we search for a metabolic cause such as hypoxia or hypokalemia. If none is identified, we then search for the presence of underlying structural cardiac disease and perform an echocardiogram to evaluate left ventricular function. We frequently perform an exercise stress test or vasodilator myocardial imaging to investigate the possibility that myocardial ischemia is playing a role, although this is controversial in patients without symptoms of ischemic disease. In the patient with normal left ventricular function and no evidence of inducible myocardial ischemia, asymptomatic ventricular ectopy is usually benign. Patients with severe left ventricular dysfunction or inducible myocardial ischemia as a cause of ventricular ectopy are at increased risk of death. These patients are further evaluated in terms of the reversibility of their cardiac dysfunction. For the patient with left ventricular dysfunction (ejection fraction $\leq$30%) secondary to ischemia, prophylactic placement of a cardiac defibrillator is considered.

Special consideration must be given to patients who take the antiarrhythmic agent, amiodarone. This drug is used to treat serious ventricular arrhythmias and, in low doses, to treat supraventricular tachycardia and atrial fibrillation. One side effect of this drug is chronic pulmonary interstitial disease. Acute life-threatening pulmonary complications such as the adult respiratory distress syndrome have been observed in patients undergoing cardiac, as well as noncardiac, surgery while receiving amiodarone. Respiratory failure has been reported 16 to 72 hours after surgery, unrelated to the dose of amiodarone. Amiodarone levels persist in the body for weeks after its use has been discontinued and amiodarone-related postoperative adult respiratory distress syndrome has been observed in patients who stopped taking the drug 6 days before surgery. The cause of this complication is speculative and may be linked to oxidative lung injury induced by high concentrations of inspired oxygen in the perioperative period. This acute amiodarone pulmonary toxicity should be kept in mind for the patient receiving amiodarone who develops perioperative adult respiratory distress syndrome.

Identification and treatment of specific disorders of cardiac rate and rhythm

The guiding principle in the treatment of perioperative cardiac arrhythmias is that the cause of the arrhythmia should be treated and reversed if possible. In the setting of an unstable or life-threatening tachyarrhythmia, cardioversion is frequently utilized to restore regular rhythm while the cause of the arrhythmia is being identified and treated.

Common causes of perioperative arrhythmias are catecholamine release; alterations in automomic tone; electrolyte abnormalities (e.g., acute hypokalemia, hyperkalemia); acid–base disturbances (e.g., acidosis, alkalosis); anemia; and acute volume depletion. Less commonly, myocardial ischemia is the cause of serious cardiac arrhythmias or conduction abnormalities. Indications for the treatment of perioperative arrhythmias include hemodynamic instability, myocardial ischemia, and myocardial infarction, or the suspicion that these deleterious consequences may occur if the arrhythmia persists.

Sinus tachycardia

Sinus tachycardia is the most common perioperative rhythm abnormality and is almost always benign. It is characterized by a heart rate between 100 and 160 beats/minute. The electrocardiogram demonstrates a regular rhythm with a normal P wave before each QRS complex. The QRS complex is normal unless patients have myocardial ischemia, aberrant ventricular conduction, or conduction abnormalities. The most common causes of sinus tachycardia are pain, hypovolemia, anemia, hypoxia, fever, and hypercarbia. Treatment is directed at the inciting factor. Patients with coronary artery disease may develop myocardial ischemia as a result of increased heart rate and increased myocardial oxygen demand. Beta-adrenergic blockers may be beneficial in this instance to decrease the heart rate and alleviate myocardial ischemia while the underlying cause of the sinus tachycardia is being treated.

Atrial premature contractions

Atrial premature contractions are of minor clinical significance but may be harbingers of supraventricular tachycardia or atrial fibrillation. They arise in the atria at a site other than the sinus node and therefore, are represented on the electrocardiogram by a P wave that has a different configuration and occurs earlier in the cardiac cycle than does a normal P wave. Atrial premature contractions typically produce a normal QRS complex. If the premature contraction arrives at the ventricular conduction tissue when it is still refractory and has not fully repolarized, it may result in no QRS complex or one that is abnormal as a result of aberrant ventricular conduction. The aberrant QRS complex is usually of right bundle branch block morphology because the refractory period of the right bundle is longer than that of the left bundle.

Atrial flutter and atrial fibrillation

There are no evidence-based guidelines for the treatment of atrial fibrillation that occurs following non-cardiac surgery. The American College of Cardiology/American Heart Association/European Society of Cardiology *Guidelines for the Management of Patients with Atrial Fibrillation* provide recommendations for treatment of atrial fibrillation that occurs in relation to cardiac surgery. The guideline does not address atrial flutter or fibrillation that occurs as a result of non-cardiac surgery.[20] Our recommendations are adapted in large part from our approach to atrial flutter and atrial fibrillation in the non-surgical setting. We treat perioperative atrial flutter and atrial fibrillation in similar fashion.

Hemodynamic instability and the presence of myocardial ischemia or congestive heart failure dictate the treatment that should be employed for postoperative atrial flutter or atrial fibrillation. If atrial fibrillation causes the patient to be unstable, the immediate goal is to restore sinus rhythm, usually by direct current (DC) cardioversion. If the arrhythmia is well tolerated, the initial plan should be to control the ventricular rate. If patients remain in atrial flutter or fibrillation and are hemodynamically stable, conversion to sinus rhythm may be attempted under elective conditions.

Digoxin has traditionally been the agent of choice for controlling the ventricular rate in either atrial fibrillation or atrial flutter. Unfortunately, it has a slow onset of action and may have significant side effects[21]. Digoxin's main role is as an adjunct to a β-blocker or a calcium channel blocker for additional rate control. Digoxin is still the drug of first choice for ventricular rate control in patients in atrial fibrillation with decompensated heart failure because of the drug's positive inotropic effect. Acute rate control is now easily achieved with continuous intravenous infusion of diltiazem. Verapamil and esmolol are also available as continuous infusion agents[22]. It is our preference that, when patients are switched from continuous intravenous medications to oral medications, β-blockers

be used (if it is possible to do so) because of the long-term beneficial effects of β-blockers in patients with ischemic heart disease.

The treatment of persistent atrial fibrillation after surgery has not been standardized; different centers have different approaches. The basic decision is whether it is best to aggressively pursue rhythm control or whether it is preferable to employ a rate control strategy. One study of cardiac surgery patients with postoperative atrial fibrillation treated with a rate control strategy noted that 90% of their patients were in sinus rhythm at 4 weeks.[23] We prefer that all patients with either frequent paroxysms or persistent atrial fibrillation have systemic anticoagulation for several weeks following surgery if they have a low risk for bleeding. After that period, the patient's risk for recurrent atrial fibrillation is reassessed and a decision about long-term therapy can be made.

For patients at high risk for developing bleeding complications and those in whom ventricular rate control is difficult, a rhythm control approach is frequently undertaken. In such patients, we usually restore sinus rhythm with direct current electrical countershock. Most antiarrhythmic medications have only moderate efficacy in terminating atrial fibrillation. However, Ibutilide, a Class III antiarrhythmic medication is effective in terminating atrial flutter of recent onset.[24,25] Ibutilide can also be used to lower the atrial defibrillation threshold, an approach that allows a higher success rate for electrical cardioversion.[26] The shorter the duration of the atrial fibrillation, the better is the success rate of cardioversion. However, it should be noted that new onset atrial fibrillation has a high spontaneous conversion rate to sinus rhythm.[27]

Because of the known increased risk of acute thromboembolic complication following cardioversion we do not perform pharmacological or electrical cardioversion if atrial fibrillation or flutter has persisted for more than 24 to 48 hours.[28] If a rhythm control approach is undertaken, antiarrhythmic medications are usually initiated to prevent the recurrence of atrial fibrillation if the patient reverts to sinus rhythm spontaneously. It is our preference to use a class III antiarrhythmic medication, either sotalol or amiodarone, in patients with structural heart disease. On occasion, a class I-A agent such as quinidine can be used if bradycardia prevents the use of sotalol or amiodarone.[29] Evidence-based data regarding the use of dofetilide (a relatively new class III anti-arrhythmic agent) in the management of postoperative atrial fibrillation have not yet been reported.[30] We do not use class I-C drugs such as propafenone or flecainide in patients with ischemic heart disease; however, we frequently use them in patients without ischemic heart disease.[31]

We prefer to discontinue anti-arrhythmic medications 4 to 8 weeks after surgery unless the patient is at high risk for recurrent atrial fibrillation. No large randomized studies have been performed evaluating the risk–benefit ratio of systemic anticoagulation, or comparing rhythm control to rate control for the management of post-operative atrial fibrillation. Therefore, an individual approach is required in the management of these conditions.

Of all non-cardiac surgical procedures, thoracic surgery is probably most often complicated by the onset of post-operative atrial fibrillation. The peak incidence of atrial fibrillation that accompanies thoracic surgery is between postoperative days 2 and 4. The mechanism for thoracic surgery-induced atrial fibrillation is unclear. The pulmonary veins in non-surgical patients have been found to be a trigger zone for the onset of atrial fibrillation as well as an important factor to sustain atrial fibrillation once it starts.[32] Manipulation of the pulmonary veins may play a role in the occurrence of atrial fibrillation following thoracic surgery. It is important to note that digoxin is particularly ineffective in the control of ventricular response to atrial fibrillation that follows thoracic surgery.[33,34]

Paroxysmal supraventricular tachycardia

Paroxysmal supraventricular tachycardia (PSVT) is characterized by the sudden onset of a rapid regular rhythm with rates between 150 and 250 beats/min. The most common mechanism requires two different electrical pathways, one to conduct faster than the other. With atrioventricular nodal re-entrant tachycardia (AVNRT), the most common type of PSVT, a premature atrial complex that is blocked in the fast pathway and redirected through the slow pathway typically triggers the tachycardia. The electrical impulse, after proceeding down the slow pathway, re-enters the fast pathway in retrograde fashion. It then travels back, in antegrade fashion toward the ventricles and again re-enters the fast pathway to travel back to the atria in retrograde fashion. In AVNRT this circuit is found in the AV node. Re-entrant PSVT that utilizes an accessory pathway outside of the AV node (e.g., Wolff–Parkinson–White syndrome) is called atrioventricular re-entrant tachycardia (AVRT). On occasion, an atrial tachycardia or atrial flutter will have the 12-lead ECG pattern of PSVT.

The management of PSVT is identical, regardless of whether the mechanism is AVNRT or AVRT. If patients are unstable hemodynamically, have angina or congestive heart failure because of the tachycardia, immediate synchronized DC cardioversion should be performed. PSVT is usually responsive to DC cardioversion with 50 J

monophasic shock. If a 50 J monophasic shock does not restore sinus rhythm, shocks at higher energy levels should be administered (i.e., 100 J, 200 J).[35] If the QRS complex is wide and the rhythm has not been definitely proven to be supraventricular, it should be treated as ventricular tachycardia. If patients are stable hemodynamically during PSVT, vagal maneuvers or medical therapy may suffice to terminate the arrhythmia. Vagal maneuvers slow conduction through the AV node by increasing parasympathetic tone. These maneuvers terminate the arrhythmia by disrupting the re-entrant circuit that is necessary to sustain the tachycardia. The most effective vagal maneuver is the Valsalva maneuver (54% termination rate). However, the Valsalva maneuver may be impossible to perform in the perioperative period, either because of the inability of patients to cooperate or because of the high sympathetic tone.[36] Carotid sinus massage has a success rate of 17% using the right carotid and 5% using the left, and may be the easiest vagal maneuver in the perioperative period to perform. It must be performed while using electrocardiographic monitoring; intravenous atropine and other antiarrhythmic drugs should be available in the event that advanced heart block or another arrhythmia occurs. Carotid sinus massage should not be used in elderly patients or in those with carotid bruits or known cerebrovascular disease because of the risk of inducing a stroke. If vagal maneuvers are unsuccessful or contraindicated and patients remain stable hemodynamically, intravenous adenosine should be administered. This agent is the initial drug of choice for the conversion of hemodynamically stable PSVT and is successful in more than 90% of cases. Adenosine should be given as a 6 mg rapid infusion over 1 to 3 seconds. If conversion is not achieved after 1 or 2 minutes, an additional 12 mg rapid infusion should be given. If the rhythm does not convert with the use of adenosine, rate control with dilhazem or beta blockers is recommended.[37] If patients become hemodynamically unstable during attempts at conversion to sinus rhythm using medical therapy, DC cardioversion should be performed promptly. In one of the few studies of PSVT in the postsurgical patient, adenosine had only a 44% successful conversion rate, and arrhythmia recurrences were common (52% of patients).[38] The high recurrence rate of PSVT suggests that many patients will require suppressive therapy while they are critically ill.

Multifocal atrial tachycardia

Multifocal atrial tachycardia (MAT) is an automatic arrhythmia characterized by an atrial rate greater than

100 beats/minute with organized, discrete, non-sinus P-waves with at least three different forms in the same electrocardiographic lead.[39] It is usually associated with severe pulmonary disease and often accompanies critical illness. When the onset of MAT occurs in the perioperative period, respiratory failure, pneumonia, and congestive heart failure are common causes. Therapy centers on treating the pulmonary, cardiac, or other acute illness that led to the onset of the arrhythmia.[40] When MAT persists despite these maneuvers, additional medical therapy may be indicated if the arrhythmia is hemodynamically significant (i.e., contributing to hypotension, congestive heart failure, or myocardial ischemia). Intravenous magnesium may be helpful for patients with hypomagnesemia or hypokalemia. Beta-blockers may be effective in decreasing the ventricular rate but must be used with extreme caution, if at all, in patients with reversible airways disease or severe acute congestive heart failure. For patients with bronchospastic lung disease calcium channel blockers or amiodarone may be used instead of β-blockers. It serves to decrease the tachycardia rate by decreasing the degree of atrial ectopy. Digitalis preparations are rarely effective in the treatment of MAT. Aminophylline, even at therapeutic levels, may aggravate the tachycardia by increasing the atrial rate and the number of ectopic atrial beats. MAT is usually resistant to DC cardioversion.

Ventricular premature contractions and non-sustained ventricular tachycardia

No specific medical therapy is indicated for patients who develop asymptomatic, hemodynamically insignificant ventricular premature contractions, or non-sustained ventricular tachycardia in the perioperative period. The cause of these dysrhythmias should be determined and the provoking factors corrected if possible. Common causes of acute ventricular arrhythmias in the perioperative period include acute myocardial ischemia, hypoxia, hypokalemia, and hypomagnesemia. Right heart catheters may cause ventricular irritability and ectopy as a result of trauma to the right ventricular outflow tract in patients who require these devices to aid in hemodynamic monitoring during the perioperative period. This should resolve on repositioning or removal of the monitoring catheter.

No well-studied data are available regarding the treatment of symptomatic or hemodynamically significant non-sustained ventricular tachycardia that develops acutely in the perioperative period. It is our approach to conduct an immediate search for a reversible etiology. We occasionally initiate medical antiarrhythmic therapy with intravenous β-blockers, lidocaine, or procainamide.

Sustained ventricular tachycardia and ventricular fibrillation

Patients who develop sustained ventricular tachycardia or ventricular fibrillation in the perioperative period should be treated according to the Advanced Cardiac Life Support protocol. Patients who have ventricular fibrillation or hemodynamically unstable ventricular tachycardia should undergo immediate DC cardioversion. For the patient with normal left ventricular function and hemodynamically stable ventricular tachycardia, an alternate approach to cardioversion is intravenous procainamide or amiodarone. For the patient with left ventricular dysfunction, amiodarone is the antiarrhythmic agent of choice. If these agents are ineffective in restoring normal rhythm, DC cardioversion should be performed. Readers are referred to the *Advanced Cardiac Life Support Guidelines* for further information.

Wide-complex tachycardia of unknown type

Supraventricular tachycardia occasionally may be accompanied by aberrant ventricular conduction, resulting in a wide QRS complex. Although criteria have been established to aid in the identification of the arrhythmia, a definite diagnosis is often elusive. A 12-lead ECG should be obtained. If atrial–ventricular dissociation is present (e.g., loss of a 1:1 relationship between P wave and QRS complex) the ECG is highly specific for ventricular tachycardia. We treat the patient with perioperative wide-complex tachycardia of unknown type in the manner recommended by *2005 American Heart Association Guidelines*.[37] For the hemodynamically stable patient with preserved left ventricular function we utilize intravenous amiodarone 150 mg over 10 minutes with the dose repeated as needed to a maximum dose of 2.2 g/24 h. If these agents are ineffective, or if the patient develops hemodynamic instability, synchronized cardioversion should be used.

Perioperative conduction abnormalities

In the perioperative period, sinus bradycardia and a Mobitz I type of second-degree AV block are common. Mobitz I AV block is a progressive prolongation of the PR interval until a P-wave is not conducted to the ventricles. The P-wave that follows is conducted to the ventricles with a PR interval that is shorter than the PR interval that was associated with the last conducted P-wave. These conduction abnormalities usually result from enhanced vagal tone and, if they are hemodynamically significant, they typically respond to 0.5 to 1 mg of intravenous atropine.

A Mobitz II type of second-degree AV block (a fixed PR interval with P-wave conduction to the ventricles blocked on a constant [e.g., 2:1, 3:1, 4:1] or variable basis) is usually caused by diffuse disease of the conduction system distal to the AV node. Many patients with this conduction disturbance are at high risk for progression to complete heart block, and a means of providing temporary-demand cardiac pacing should be quickly available in the event that this occurs. New-onset Mobitz II AV block in the perioperative period should initiate a search for myocardial ischemia or myocardial infarction.

Third-degree AV block occurs when no atrial impulses reach the ventricles. An associated ventricular rate of 40 to 60 beats per minute with normal appearing QRS complexes suggests that the escape rhythm is originating at the level of the AV node. This type of heart block may result from enhanced vagal tone; medications that depress AV nodal conduction (e.g., β-blockers, digitalis) and, less commonly, AV nodal ischemia. It is often reversible and may respond to the administration of intravenous atropine or the discontinuation of offending pharmacologic agents. If complete heart block is associated with a ventricular escape rate of 20 to 40 beats per minute and the QRS complex is wide, the escape rhythm is originating from the ventricles. This strongly suggests the presence of extensive conduction system disease and warrants the placement of a cardiac pacemaker.

Chronic bifascicular block (i.e., right bundle–branch block with either left anterior hemiblock or left posterior hemiblock, or left bundle–branch block) rarely progresses to advanced hemodynamically significant heart block in the perioperative period.[43–45] The preoperative insertion of temporary pacemaker therefore, is not indicated, in general, for this patient group. Possible exceptions are patients with pre-existing left bundle–branch block who are undergoing perioperative pulmonary artery catheterization. Transient right bundle–branch block, which is well tolerated in normal patients, may occur in as many as 5% of patients who undergo pulmonary artery catheterization.[46] Transient complete heart block has been reported in patients with pre-existing left bundle–branch block who have developed acute right bundle–branch block related to this procedure.[47,48] Given the potential for this significant complication, a method for pacing the left ventricle should be available in the event that complete heart block develops in this clinical setting. A temporary pacemaker should be inserted before surgery if patients meet the criteria for permanent pacemaker implantation and if a permanent pacing device has not yet been implanted (Table 6.6).

Table 6.6. Selected indications for implantation of cardiac pacemakers

Third-degree or advanced second-degree AV block associated with:
  Symptomatic bradycardia
  Documented asystole >3 seconds or escape rate less than 40 beats per minute in an awake symptom-free person
Second-degree AV block, regardless of site or type, with: symptomatic bradycardia; bifascicular block with intermittent complete heart block with symptomatic bradycardia; symptomatic bifascicular block with intermittent type II second-degree AV block; sinus node dysfunction with documented symptomatic bradycardia
Following acute myocardial infarction:
  Persistent second-degree AV block in the His–Purkinje system with bilateral bundle–branch block or third-degree AV block within or below the His–Purkinje system.
  Persistent and symptomatic second- or third-degree AV block.

Source: Adapted from Gregoratus, G. *et al.* 2002[49]

Long QT syndrome

The long QT syndrome is a heterogeneous group of disorders characterized by a prolonged QT interval when corrected for heart rate, malignant ventricular arrhythmias (classically the torsades de pointes form of ventricular tachycardia), and the risk of sudden death. It is most commonly acquired as a result of a drug or metabolic abnormality (see Table 6.7). It may also occur as a congenital form inherited as a result of either autosomal dominant or recessive genetic mutations. To date, seven different genetic defects which encode for abnormal cardiac ion channels have been identified that may result in long QT syndrome.

The approach to patients in the perioperative period depends on whether the long QT is congenital or acquired. Congenital long QT syndrome is adrenergic dependent and ventricular arrhythmias are typically provoked by sympathetic stimulation (i.e., pain, physical exertion). Long-term treatment with β-blockers, permanent pacing, or left cervicothoracic sympathectomy is frequently effective.[49] ICD implantation is recommended for selected patients in whom syncope, sustained ventricular arrhythmias, or aborted sudden cardiac death has occurred despite this standard therapy. ICD implantation as primary treatment should be considered in the patient in whom aborted sudden cardiac death is the initial presentation of the long QT syndrome and in those patients with long QT who have a strong family history of sudden cardiac death.[50]

Table 6.7. Selected causes of acquired long QT syndrome

Antiarrhythmic drugs
Type IA agents (e.g., quinidine, procainamide, disopyramide)
Type III agents (Amiodarone, Sotalol)

Non-cardiac drugs
Phenothiazines
Tricyclic antidepressants
Haloperidol
Selective serotonin reuptake inhibitors (SSRI)
Antibiotics (e.g., erythromycin, azithromycin, clarithromycin, ampicillin, trimethoprin-sulfamethoxazole, ketoconazole, itraconazole)

Metabolic and electrolyte disorders
Hypokalemia
Hypomagnesemia
Nutritional disorders (starvation, liquid protein diets)

Central nervous system disorders
Subarachnoid hemorrhage
Intracerebral hemorrhage
Head trauma
Encephalitis

For patients with congenital long QT syndrome, we provide perioperative β-blockade to blunt the adrenergic response to the surgery. Beta-blockers also shift the rate-adjusted QT interval to the normal range, which may contribute to their efficacy. We attempt to avoid anesthetics that may prolong the QT interval (e.g., succinylcholine, propofol, enflurane, or halothane).[51] Although isoflurane has been demonstrated to prolong the QT interval in normals, it shortens the QT interval in those with long QT syndrome and has been proposed as an acceptable anesthetic agent for this patient group.[52] Thiopental has also been reported to prolong the QT interval in normals but has no effect on the QT duration in patients with long QT syndrome.[53] Finally we minimize sympathetic stimulation and provide adequate sedation to blunt the adrenergic response to surgery.

In patients who have acquired long QT syndrome, we discontinue administration of the offending drug or correct the metabolic or electrolyte abnormality before undertaking surgery.

Despite these measures, malignant ventricular arrhythmias may still occur in the patient with long QT in the perioperative period. The treatment for ventricular ectopy is the same for idiopathic and acquired long QT syndrome. Intravenous magnesium sulfate, 2 g given over 1–2 minutes, with a followup dose 15 minutes later if required is often effective in restoring regular rhythm. Immediate ventricular pacing should be used if magnesium sulfate is ineffective. Pacing at rates of 70–80 beats per minute may shorten the QT interval and decrease the dispersion of refractoriness of the cardiac conduction system. Intravenous isoproterenol may be used cautiously to increase the heart rate and suppress ventricular arrhythmia until temporary ventricular pacing is achieved. If these methods are unsuccessful in restoring the patients baseline stable rhythm, DC cardioversion should be considered.

Cardiac conduction issues in the patient with a cardiac transplant who requires non-cardiac surgery

Cardiac physiology is altered after cardiac transplantation. Because the transplanted heart is denervated, cardiac reflexes mediated by the autonomic nervous system are blunted or absent. As a result, heart rate abnormalities may be seen in the perioperative period. The resting heart rate is higher than normal but the heart rate response to stress is less than that of an innervated heart. When the heart rate does increase as a result of stress, it does so gradually in response to circulating catecholamines. Reflex tachycardia does not occur in response to vasodilation or volume loss. The effect of certain cardiac drugs on cardiac conduction is altered. Agents that affect the heart indirectly through their action on the autonomic nervous system are generally ineffective. Therefore, the chronotropic effect of atropine is absent, as is the AV nodal inhibitory effect of digoxin. The antiarrhythmic efficacy of β-blockers and calcium channel antagonists (e.g., verapamil, diltiazem) is unchanged. The transplanted heart becomes overly sensitive to adenosine, and reduced doses (i.e., one-third to one-half lower than those given to patients with intact cardiac innervation) should be used when this drug is administered to control arrhythmias.[54,55]

Bradyarrhythmias following acute spinal cord injury

Acute injury to the cervical spinal cord is frequently accompanied by clinically significant bradyarrhythmias and, in some cases, hypotension. Acute autonomic dysfunction is thought to be the cause. Sympathetic nerves exit the spinal cord in preganglionic fibers at the first through fourth thoracic levels. With a complete cervical spinal cord lesion, sympathetic control from higher centers is interrupted. Parasympathetic control, which is mediated by the vagus nerve, is unaffected by spinal cord interruption. The clinical picture, therefore is one of unopposed parasympathetic activity in the setting of markedly reduced sympathetic activity. Sympathetic stimulation with low-dose isoproterenol has been used in several patients for the treatment of clinically significant bradyarrhythmias. These cardiovascular abnormalities have been demonstrated to resolve within 14 to 30 days following acute cervical spinal cord injury. The reason for resolution is not known but may be related to adaptive sympathetic disinhibition (i.e., loss of reflex sympathetic inhibitory control from higher centers or increase in the number and function of adrenergic receptors).[56,57]

Management of permanent cardiac pacemakers

While most pacemakers are implanted as treatment of bradyarrhythmias or conduction system abnormalities, other indications for pacemakers include treatment of heart failure in the patient with severe left ventricular dysfunction (bi-ventricular pacemaker), neurocardiogenic syncope, long QT syndrome, and selected patients with hypertrophic cardiomyopathy. It is important to know the indication that led to implantation of the patient's pacemaker and whether or not they are pacemaker dependent.

There is no industry-wide standard regarding pacemaker programming, estimation of battery reserve, etc. It is therefore important that the type of pacemaker and the name of its manufacturer be identified prior to surgery. If the patients or their physicians are unable to provide this information, it may be identified by chest X-ray, which reveals radio opaque identification markers on the pacemaker generator. The pacemaker should be tested and its settings recorded.

While pacemaker problems are uncommon in the perioperative period, one series identified a pacemaker abnormality (e.g., inhibition, acceleration, change in pacing mode) in 13% of pacemaker patients.[58]

The most significant pacemaker problem in the perioperative period is alteration of pacemaker function inhibition resulting from electrocautery-induced electromagnetic interference (EMI). If the pacemaker interprets EMI as the patients electrical heart activity, the pacemaker may be inhibited. If the patient has a dual chamber pacemaker and EMI is sensed only by the atrial sensing circuitry, the ventricular pacing channel may pace at the pacemaker upper rate limit. Some pacemakers respond to the "noise" of EMI by pacing in an asynchronous (fixed rate) mode. Some older pacemakers may respond to EMI by reprogramming. The pacemaker response to the electrical interference of electrocautery may be obtained from the pacemaker manufacturer. This alteration of pacemaker function may be prevented by avoiding the application of electrocautery directly over the pacemaker pulse generator and by keeping the electrocautery current path, which is from electrode tip to ground plate, as far away as possible from the pulse generator. The pacemaker should be programmed to the asynchronous (fixed rate mode) so that it does not inhibit in response to EMI. Many pacemakers will operate in an asynchronous mode if a magnet is applied to the skin over the pulse generator and, while that has been a common approach to perioperative pacemaker management, it is important to realize that a number of new pacemakers have a programmable option that prevents this pacemaker response to magnet application.

Since the early 1990s many pacemakers have "rate-adaptive" systems devised to facilitate a change in heart rate response to a change in the desired cardiac output. Various biologic parameters have been used to trigger heart rate responses. The most common include sensation of vibration at the pulse generator site as a manifestation of perceived patient physical activity and respiratory rate as determined by a minute ventilation sensor. The adaptive rate system may therefore sense surgical-induced vibration or shivering, which commonly occurs upon recovery from anesthesia, and inappropriately pace at a high rate. Similarly, intraoperative hyperventilation may also lead to the pacemaker generating a heart rate more rapid than actually desired if the pacemaker adaptive rate sensor is linked to the patient's minute ventilation. For these reasons the rate-responsive feature should be deactivated during surgery.

For patients who require placement of central venous catheters or right heart pulmonary artery catheters, care should be taken to avoid tangling these catheters in the pacemaker leads. Newly placed pacemaker leads are at risk of becoming dislodged by right heart catheter insertion. For the patient who requires external defibrillation, electrical discharge to their pacemaker will be minimized if the defibrillator paddles are placed in an anteroposterior position.[59]

It should be noted that many of the new pacemakers have a programmable option that would make magnet application ineffective. For this reason, knowledge of the patient's pacemaker dependency state and programming of the device may be required. Some pacemakers respond to magnet application only with a brief period of asynchronous pacing. Therefore, it is recommended that continuous telemetry be available during the surgical procedure.

There is no industry-wide standard response to either electromagnetic interference or magnet application. It is therefore important that data regarding the individual pacemaker response to electromagnetic interference and magnet application be obtained from the pacemaker manufacturer. However, in general the recommendations outlined above will be effective.

Management of automatic implantable cardioverter defibrillators (AICDs)

Automatic implantable cardioverter defibrillators (AICD) are used for secondary prevention for the patient who has survived sudden cardiac death and are effective in the primary prevention of sudden cardiac death for the patient with prior myocardial infarction and advanced left ventricular dysfunction (ejection fraction $\leq$30%).[60] The number of AICD implants is expected to increase significantly in this latter group as it is estimated that, in the USA, 3 million to 4 million patients have coronary heart disease and advanced left ventricular dysfunction with 400 000 new cases each year.[61,62]

Electrocautery may affect AICDs in the same manner as it does pacemakers; the electromagnetic signal produced by electrocautery may be interpreted as intrinsic cardiac events. This phenomenon can lead to inhibition of pacing. In addition, if the electrocautery induced electromagnetic interference is interpreted by the AICD as a rapid ventricular rate, the AICD may deliver unnecessary and undesired shocks. While the frequency of such an occurrence is small, the results of AICD shock delivered during a surgical procedure can be devastating. Therefore, it is recommended that AICDs be deactivated before surgery if the use of electrocautery is a possibility. Continuous electrocardiographic monitoring and advanced cardiac life support, including an external defibrillator, should be available during the time that the AICD is deactivated. The AICD should be deactivated by one of two techniques. Either a magnet may be placed over the AICD for the duration of electrocautery, or the device can be deactivated with the use of the programmer. Magnet application over the pulse generator will disable the device from detecting tachyarrhythmias. For most AICDs, magnet application only deactivates the device temporarily, but some AICDs can be permanently deactivated with magnet application. Magnet application will not affect pacing functions of the AICD. Therefore, electrocautery may inhibit pacing from an AICD. It should be remembered that most patients with AICDs have significant left ventricular dysfunction with ischemic heart disease. These patients require close observation during the perioperative period.

REFERENCES

1. Marchlinski, F. Arrhythmias and conduction disturbances in surgical patients. In Goldman, D., ed. *Medical Care of the Surgical Patient*, Philadelphia: J. B. Lippincott, 1982: 59–77.

2. Kuner, J., Enescu, V., & Utsu, F. Cardiac arrhythmias during anesthesia. *Dis. Chest* 1967; **52**: 580–587.

3. Forrest, J. B., Cahalan, M., Rehder, K. *et al.* Multicenter study of general anesthesia. II. Results. *Anesthesiology* 1990; **72**: 262–268.

4. Forrest, J. B., Rehder, K., Cahalan, M. K., & Goldsmith, C. H. Multicenter study of general anesthesia. III. Predictors of severe perioperative adverse outcomes [published erratum appears in Anesthesiology 1992 Jul; 77(1): 222] [see comments]. *Anesthesiology* 1992; **76**(1): 3–15.

5. O'Kelly, B., Browner, W. S., Massie, B., Tubau, J., Ngo, L., & Mangano, D. T. Ventricular arrhythmias in patients undergoing noncardiac surgery. The Study of Perioperative Ischemia Research Group. [comment]. *J. Am. Med. Assoc.* 1992; **268**(2): 217–221.

6. Goldman, L., Caldera, D. L., Nussbanm, S. R. *et al.* Multifactorial index of cardiac risk in noncardiac surgical procedures. *N. Engl. J. Med.* 1978; **297**: 845.

7. Eagle, K. A., Berger, P. B., Calkins, H. *et al.* ACC/AHA guideline update for perioperative cardiovascular evaluation for noncardiac surgery – executive summary: a report of the American College of Cardiology/American Heart Association Task Force on Practice Guidelines (Committee to Update the 1996 Guidelines on Perioperative Cardiovascular Evaluation for Noncardiac Surgery). *J. Am. Coll. Cardiol.* 2002; **39**(3): 542–553.

8. Polanczyk, C. A., Goldman, L., Marcantonio, E. R., Orav, E. J., & Lee, T. H. Supraventricular arrhythmia in patients having noncardiac surgery: clinical correlates and effect on length of stay. *Ann. Intern. Med.* 1998; **129** (4): 279–285.

9. Amar, D., Zhang, H., Leung, D., Roistacher, N., & Kadish, A. Older age is the strongest predictor of postoperative atrial fibrillation. *Anesthesiology* 2002; **96**(2): 352–356.

10. Sebel, P. S. & Bovill, J. G. *Opioid analgesics in cardiac anesthesia.* In Kaplan, J. A., ed. *Cardiac Anesthesia*, Orlando: Grune & Stratton, 1987: 67–123.

11. Marymount, J. H. & O'Connor, B. S. *Postoperative cardiovascular complications.* In Veder, J. S. & Spiess, B. D. *Post Anesthesia Care*, Philadelphia: W. B. Saunders, 1992: 42.

12. Underwood, S. M. & Glynn, C. J. Sick sinus syndrome manifest after spinal anesthesia. *Anaesthesia* 1988; **43**: 307–309.

13. Doyle, D. J. & Mark, P. W. Reflex bradycardia during surgery. *Can. J. Anaesth.* 1990; **37**: 219–222.

14. Merli, G. J., Weitz, H., Martin, J. H. *et al.* Cardiac dysrhythmias associated with ophthalmic atropine. *Arch. Intern. Med.* 1986; **146**: 45–47.

15. Mishra, P., Calvey, T. N., Williams, N. E. *et al.* Intraoperative bradycardia and hypotension associated with timolol and pilocarpine eye drops. *Br. J. Anaesth.* 1983; **55**: 897–899.

16. The Atrial Fibrillation Follow-up Investigation of Rhythm Management (AFFIRM) Investigators. A comparison of rate control and rhythm control in patients with atrial fibrillation. *N. Engl. J. Med.* 2002; **347**: 1825–1833.

17. Falk, R. Atrial fibrillation. *N. Engl. J. Med.* 2001; **344**: 1067–1078.

18. Ansell, J., Hirsh, J., Dalen, J. *et al.* Managing oral anticoagulant therapy. *Chest* 2001 **119**: 22S–38S.

19. Fuster, V., Ryden, L. E., Asinger, R. W. *et al.* ACC/AHA/ESC guidelines for the management of patients with atrial fibrillation: a report of the American College of Cardiology/American Heart Association Task Force on Practice Guidelines and the European Society of Cardiology Committee for Practice Guidelines and Policy Conferences (Committee to Develop Guidelines for the Management of Patients with Atrial Fibrillation). *J. Am. Coll. Cardiol.* 2001; **38**: 1266.

20. Tisdale, J. E., Padhi, I. D., Goldberg, A. D. *et al.* A randomized, double-blinded comparison of intravenous diltiazem and digoxin for atrial fibrillation after coronary artery bypass surgery. *Am. Heart J.* 1998; **135**: 739–747.

21. Balser, J. R., Martinez, E. A., Winters, B. D. *et al.* Beta-adrenergic blockade accelerates conversion of postoperative supraventricular tachyarrhythmias. *Anesthesiology* 1998; **89**: 1052–1059.

22. Myers, M. G. & Alnemri, K. Rate control for atrial fibrillation following coronary artery bypass surgery. *Can. J. Cardiol.* 1998; **14**: 1363–1366.

23. Volgman, A. S., Carberry, P. A., Stambler, B. *et al.* Conversion efficacy and safety of intravenous ibutilide compared with intravenous procainamide in patients with atrial flutter or fibrillation. *J. Am. Coll. Cardiol.* 1998; **31**: 1414–1419.

24. Stambler, B. S., Wood, M. A., Ellenbogen, K. A., Perry, K. T., Wakefield, L. K., & Vanderlugt, J. T. Efficacy and safety of repeated intravenous doses of ibutilide for rapid conversion of atrial flutter or fibrillation. Ibutilide Repeat Dose Study Investigators. *Circulation* 1996; **94**: 1613–1621.

25. Oral, H., Souza, J. J., Michaud, G. F. *et al.* Facilitating transthoracic cardioversion of atrial fibrillation with ibutilide pretreatment. *N. Engl. J. Med.* 1999; **340**: 1849–1854.

26. Danias, P. G., Caulfield, T. A., Weigner, M. J., Silverman, D. I., & Manning, W. I. Likelihood of spontaneous conversion of atrial fibrillation to sinus rhythm. *J. Am. Coll. Cardiol.* 1998; **31**: 588–592.

27. Laupacis, A., Albers, G., Dalen, J., Dunn, M. I., Jacobson, A. K., & Singer, D. E. Antithrombotic therapy in atrial fibrillation. *Chest* 1998; **114**: 579S–589S.

28. Salerno, D. M. Quinidine. Worse than adverse? *Circulation* 1991; **84**: 2196–2198.

29. Torp-Pedersen, C., Moller, M., Bloch-Thomsen, P. E. *et al.* Camm, A. J. Dofetilide in patients with congestive heart failure and left ventricular dysfunction. Danish Investigations of Arrhythmias and Mortality on Dofetilide Study Group. *N. Engl. J. Med.* 1999; **341**: 857–865.

30. Reiffel, J. A. Drug choices in the treatment of atrial fibrillation. *Am. J. Cardiol.* 2000; **85**: 12D–19D.

31. Haissaguerre, M., Jais, P., Shah, D. C. *et al.* Spontaneous initiation of atrial fibrillation by ectopic beats originating in the pulmonary veins. *N. Engl. J. Med.* 1998; **339**: 659–666.

32. Ritchie, A. J., Whiteside, M., Tolan, M., & McGuigan, J. A. Cardiac dysrhythmia in total thoracic oesophagectomy. A prospective study. *Eur. J. Cardiothor. Surg.* 1993; **7**: 420–422.

33. Amar, D., Roistacher, N., Burt, M. E. *et al.* Effects of diltiazem versus digoxin on dysrhythmias and cardiac function after pneumonectomy. *Ann. Thorac. Surg.* 1997; **63**: 1374–1381.

34. Guidelines 2000 for Cardiopulmonary Resuscitation and Emergency Cardiovascular Care. Part 6. Advanced Cardiovascular Life support. Section 2: Defibrillation. The American Heart Association in collaboration with the International Liaison Committee on Resuscitation. *Circulation* 2000; **8** Suppl: I90–194.

35. Mehta, R., Wafa, S., Ward, D. E., & Camm, A. J. Relative efficacy of various physical manoeuvres in the termination of junctional tachycardia. *Lancet* 1988; **1**: 1181–1185.

36. Guidelines 2000 for Cardiopulmonary Resuscitation and Emergency Cardiovascular Care. Part 6: Advanced Cardiovascular Life Support: Section 5: Pharmacology I: Agents for Arrhythmias. *Circulation* 2000; **102**(Suppl. I).

37. 2005 American Heart Association Guidelines for cardiopulmonary resuscitation and emergency cardiovascular care. Part 7.3. Management of symptomatic bradycardia and tachycardia. *Circulation* 2005; **112** (Suppl. I): IV 67–77.

38. Kastor, J. A. Multifocal atrial tachycardia. *N. Engl. J. Med.* 1990; **322**: 1713–1717.

39. Scher, D. L. & Arsura, E. L. Multifocal atrial tachycardia: mechanisms, clinical correlates, and treatment. *Am. Heart. J.* 1989; **118**: 574–580.

40. Habibzadeh, M. A. Multifocal atrial tachycardia: a 66 month follow-up of 50 patients. *Heart Lung* 1980; **9**: 328–335.

41. Guidelines 2000 for Cardiopulmonary Resuscitation and Emergency Cardiovascular Care. Part 6: Advanced Cardiovascular Life Support: Section 7: Algorithm Approach to ACLS Emergencies: Section 7A: Principles and Practice of ACLS. The American Heart Association in collaboration with the International Liaison Committee on Resuscitation. *Circulation* 2000; **102**(8Suppl): 1136–1139.

42. Berg, G. R. & Kotler, M. N. The significance of bilateral bundle branch block in the preoperative patient. A retrospective electrocardiographic and clinical study in 30 patients. *Chest* 1971; **59**: 62–67.

43. Belloci, F., Santarelli, P., DiGennaro, M., Ansalone, G., & Fenici, R. The risk of cardiac complications in surgical patients with bifascicular block. *Chest* 1980; **77**: 343–348.

44. Gauss, A., Hubner, C., Radermacher, P., Georgieff, M., & Schutz, W. Perioperative risk of bradyarrhythmias in patients with asymptomatic chronic bifascicular block or left bundle branch block: does an additional first degree atrioventricular block make any difference? *Anesthesiology* 1998; **88**: 679–687.

45. Sprung, C. L., Pozen, R. G., Rozanski, J. J. *et al.* Advanced ventricular arrhythmias during bedside pulmonary artery catheterization. *Am. J. Med.*, 1982; **72**: 203–208.

46. Abernathy, W. S. Complete heart block caused by the Swan–Ganz catheter. *Chest* 1974; **65**: 349.

47. Thomson, I. R., Dalton, B. C., Lappas, D. G. *et al.* Right bundle-branch block and complete heart block caused by the Swan–Ganz catheter. *Anesthesiology* 1979; **51**: 359–362.

48. Gregoratos, G., Abrams, J., Epstein, A. E. *et al.* ACC/AHA/NASPE Guideline Update for Implantation of Cardiac Pacemakers and Antiarrhythmia Devices: a Report of the American College of Cardiology/American Heart Association Task Force on Practice Guidelines (ACC/AHA/NASPE Committee on Pacemaker Implantation), 2002.

49. Groh, W., Silka, M. J., Oliver, R. P., Halperin, D, McAnulty, J. H., & Kron, J. Use of implantable cardioverter – defibrillator in the congenital long QT syndrome. *Am. J. Cardiol.* 1996; **78**: 703–706.

50. Richardson, M. G., Roark, G. L., & Helfaer, M. A. Intraoperative epinephrine-induced torsades de pointes in a child with long-QT syndrome. *Anesthesiology* 1992; **76**: 647–649.

51. Medak, R. & Benumof, J. L. Perioperative management of the prolonged QT interval syndrome. *Br. J. Anaesth.* 1983; **55**: 361–364.

52. Wilton, N. C. & Hantler, C. B. Congenital long QT syndrome: changes in QT interval during anesthesia with thiopental vecuronium fentanyl and isoflurane. *Anesth. Analg.* 1987; **66**: 357–360.

53. Ellenbogen, K. A., Thames, M. D., DiMarco, J. P. *et al.* Electrophysiological effects of adenosine in the transplanted human heart: evidence of supersensitivity. *Circulation* 1990; **81**: 821–828.

54. O'Connell, J. B., Bourge, R. C., Costanzo-Nordin, M. R. *et al.* Cardiac transplantation: recipient selection, donor procurement, and medical follow-up: a statement for health professionals from the Committee on Cardiac Transplantation of the Council on Clinical Cardiology, American Heart Association. *Circulation* 1992; **86**: 1061–1079.

55. Lehmann, K. G., Kane, J. G., Piepmeier, J. M. *et al.* Cardiovascular abnormalities accompanying acute spinal cord injury in humans: incidence, time course and severity. *J. Am. Coll. Cardiol.* 1987; **10**: 46–52.

56. Leaf, D. A., Bahl, R. A., & Adkins, R. H. Risk of cardiac dysrhythmia in chronic spinal cord injury patients. *Paraplegia* 1997; **31**(9): 571–575.

57. Trankina, M. F., Black, S., & Gibby, G. Pacemakers: perioperative evaluation, management, and complications (abstr.). *Anesthesiology* 2000; **93**(3A): A–1193.

58. Senthuran, S., Toff, W. D., Vuylsteke, A., Solesbury, P. M., & Menon, D. K. Implanted cardiac pacemakers and defibrillators in anaesthetic practice. *Br. J. Anaesth.* 2002; **88**(5): 627–631.

59. Moss, A. J., Zareba, W., Hall, J. *et al.* Prophylactic implantation of a defibrillator in patients with myocardial infarction and reduced ejection fraction. *N. Engl. J. Med.* 2002; **346**: 877–883.

60. Cohn, J. N., Bristow, M. R., Chien, K. R. *et al.* Report of the National Heart, Lung, and Blood Institute Special Emphasis Panel on Heart Failure Research. *Circulation* 1997; **95**: 766–770.

61. Myerburg, R. J. Sudden cardiac death: exploring the limits of our knowledge. *J. Cardiovasc. Electrophysiol.* 2001; **12**: 369–381.

62. Rocco, A. G. & Vandan, L. D. Changes in circulation consequent in manipulation during abdominal surgery. *J. Am. Med. Assoc.* 1957; **164**: 14–18.

63. Seltzer, J. L., Ritter, D. E., Starsnic, M. A. *et al.* The hemodynamic response to traction on the abdominal mesentery. *Anesthesiology* 1985; **63**: 96–99.

64. Sullivan, S. & Watson, W. C. Acute transient hypotension as complication of percutaneous liver biopsy. *Lancet* 1974; **1**: 389–390.

65. Doyle, D. J. & Mark, P. W. Laparoscopy and vagal arrest. *Anaesthesia* 1989; **44**: 433.

66. Robideaux, V. Oculocardiac reflex caused by midface disimpaction. *Anesthesiology* 1978; **49**: 433.

67. Hopkins, C. S. Bradycardia during neurosurgery: a new reflex? *Anaesthesia* 1988; **43**: 157–158.

68. Podolakin, W. & Wells, D. G. Precipitous bradycardia induced by laryngoscopy in cardiac surgical patients. *Can. J. Anaesth.* 1987; **34**: 618–621.

69. Matarasso, A. The oculocardiac reflex in blepharoplasty surgery. *Plast. Reconstr. Surg.* 1989; **83**: 243–250.

Valvular heart disease

Mitral stenosis

Mitral stenosis in adults is usually a result of rheumatic fever. Rheumatic valvulitis causes scarring of the mitral valve leaflets, with fusion of the commissures as well as subvalvular apparatus. With the reduced incidence of rheumatic fever in developed countries, non-rheumatic causes of mitral valve stenosis should be considered. In the elderly idiopathic calcification of the mitral valve annulus with extension to the mitral valve, leaflets may result in functional mitral stenosis. Rare causes of mitral stenosis are systemic lupus erythematosus, rheumatoid arthritis, and carcinoid syndrome.

In normal adults, the mitral valve area is 4 to 5 cm^2. Mitral stenosis is critical when the valve area is reduced to 1 cm^2 or less. As mitral valve leaflet fusion progresses, left atrial pressure increases to maintain left ventricular filling, and a diastolic transvalvular pressure gradient exists between the left atrium and ventricle. Increased left atrial pressure leads to increased pulmonary vascular pressure. Conditions that decrease diastolic filling time (e.g., tachycardia) as well as those that increase cardiac blood flow across the mitral valve (e.g., physical exercise, fever) further increase left atrial and pulmonary vascular pressure. The pressure gradient across the mitral valve is proportional to the square of the transvalvular flow rate. Therefore, modest increases in transvalvular flow result in significant increases in the pressure gradient.[1] The onset of atrial fibrillation with the loss of the atrial contribution to ventricular filling as well as decreased diastolic filling time associated with a rapid heart rate may also lead to increased left atrial pressure. Pulmonary hypertension occurs as mitral stenosis progresses. Although pulmonary venous and arterial hypertension is usually reversible after mechanical correction of mitral stenosis, advanced disease is often associated with mitral regurgitation, hypertrophy of the pulmonary vasculature, and an irreversible component of pulmonary hypertension. Right ventricular pressure overload may occur as a consequence of pulmonary hypertension.

The clinical findings of mitral stenosis result from inability of the left atrium to empty normally and from pulmonary venous and arterial hypertension. Symptoms such as exertional dyspnea may occur when the mitral valve area decreases to less than 2.5 cm^2. Rest symptoms such as orthopnea and paroxysmal nocturnal dyspnea occur when the valve area is less than 1.5 cm^2. Fatigue resulting from decreased cardiac output characterizes late disease. Hoarseness may occur and is caused by compression of the left recurrent laryngeal nerve by the enlarged left atrium and pulmonary artery. Atrial fibrillation commonly accompanies mitral stenosis and is the result of persistently elevated left atrial pressure and left atrial dilatation as well as involvement of the left atrium by rheumatic carditis. Atrial fibrillation with rapid ventricular response may lead to pulmonary edema due to the decreased diastolic filling time that occurs when heart rate increases. Patients with atrial fibrillation are at high risk for intracardiac thrombus formation with subsequent systemic embolization. The risk of embolization increases with increased size of the left atrium and atrial appendage as well as with decreased cardiac output.

Physical findings of mitral stenosis include an accentuated first heart sound that decreases in intensity as stenosis worsens and a high pitched opening snap heard after the second heart sound that is caused by opening of the stenotic but pliable mitral valve. As mitral stenosis progresses, left atrial pressure rises and the interval between the second heart sound and the opening snap shortens. When valve mobility is lost, the opening snap disappears. A low pitched diastolic rumble is heard at the apex and its duration correlates with the severity of stenosis. Patients

in whom sinus rhythm is preserved may have presystolic accentuation of the murmur.

Transthoracic echocardiography is essential in patient evaluation. It confirms the diagnosis, identifies the etiology (e.g., leaflet fusion of rheumatic mitral valve stenosis, mitral annulus calcification in the elderly), allows for estimation of valve orifice area, and with the use of Doppler techniques facilitates an approximation of the transvalvular pressure gradient. Echocardiography may also facilitate identification of mitral regurgitation which coexists in as many as 40% of patients with mitral stenosis, as well as other valve lesions. Though not indicated in every patient with mitral stenosis, transesophageal echocardiography is an effective tool to determine the presence or absence of left atrial thrombi, the presence of which would be a contraindication to restoration of sinus rhythm in the mitral stenosis patient who is in atrial fibrillation.

Therapy is based on the severity of symptoms. Patients with minimal symptoms often respond to diuretics; those with atrial fibrillation respond to control of the ventricular response with digoxin, β-blockers, or calcium channel antagonists. Survival is decreased when symptoms are more than mild. Therefore, patients with New York Heart Association functional class II symptoms and moderate or severe stenosis (mitral valve area $\leq$1.5 cm^2 or mean gradient $\geq$5 mm Hg) may be considered for mitral balloon valvotomy if they have suitable mitral valve morphology (i.e., valve with minimal calcification, good leaflet mobility, little involvement of the subvalvular apparatus, and minimal or no valve regurgitation). Balloon mitral valvotomy is contraindicated in patients with left atrial thrombi. The prognosis is poor for patients who have New York Heart Association functional class III or IV symptoms and evidence of severe mitral stenosis if left untreated. They should be considered for treatment with either balloon valvotomy or valve replacement.[2] Percutaneous balloon mitral valvuloplasty or mitral valve replacement is only indicated prior to non-cardiac surgery if the patient otherwise meets the indications for interventional treatment of their mitral stenosis irrespective of the non-cardiac surgery.[3]

Intravascular volume status and heart rate are key factors that require attention in patients undergoing noncardiac surgery. Volume overload must be avoided because further increases in left atrial pressure may result in pulmonary edema. Conversely, excessive volume depletion or preload reduction may decrease left ventricular filling pressure and cardiac output. Perioperative tachycardia may impair left ventricular filling and can be treated with β-blockers, calcium channel antagonists, or digoxin in patients who have atrial fibrillation with rapid ventricular response. Because of the significant hemodynamic alterations that occur with relatively small volume shifts in patients with severe mitral stenosis, invasive hemodynamic monitoring of the pulmonary capillary wedge pressure should be considered if perioperative volume changes are anticipated. Infective endocarditis prophylaxis for indicated procedures is necessary.

Mitral stenosis increases the risk of embolism in the patient with atrial fibrillation. Many of these patients are chronically anticoagulated with warfarin. For the patient who undergoes surgery, care should be taken to minimize the time that the patient will be not anticoagulated in the perioperative period. Strategies include performing surgery without stopping anticoagulation in the patient in whom perioperative bleeding is unlikely, e.g., cataract surgery; stopping warfarin 48–72 hours prior to surgery so that surgery may be performed when the INR is ≤1.5 with warfarin resumed within 24 hours of surgery. For the patient at significantly increased risk of embolism, e.g., the patient with mitral stenosis and atrial fibrillation who is elderly, has left ventricular dysfunction or history of prior embolism or hypertension, we often stop the warfarin several days prior to surgery and treat with heparin when the INR becomes subtherapeutic. Heparin is discontinued several hours prior to surgery and restarted as soon as possible following surgery. Warfarin is then restarted. Heparin is discontinued when the INR is therapeutic. An alternative approach, though not studied in prospective randomized trials and not approved by the US Food and Drug Administration for this indication, is to use low molecular weight heparin as "bridge" anticoagulation rather than continuous unfractionated heparin. For this purpose enoxaparin can be given at 1 mg/kg subcutaneously every 12 hours after warfarin is withheld and INR decreases below therapeutic range. Low molecular weight heparin should be stopped 12 hours prior to surgery and resumed when hemostasis is stable in the postoperative period. Warfarin is restarted in the postoperative period and low molecular weight heparin discontinued when INR is therapeutic.[4]

Mitral regurgitation

Mitral regurgitation may be caused by one or more abnormalities of the structures that comprise the mitral valve apparatus: the anterior and posterior valve leaflets, chordae tendineae, papillary muscles, and mitral valve annulus. It may also result from poor alignment of a structurally normal valve apparatus or from mitral annular dilation, both of which are caused by left ventricular dysfunction or dilation. Common causes of mitral apparatus dysfunction are myxomatous degeneration of the mitral valve leaflets or chordae, infective endocarditis that may involve the valve leaflets, coronary artery disease with myocardial ischemia resulting in papillary muscle dysfunction, or rheumatic valve disease. Less common but clinically significant causes of mitral regurgitation include mitral annular calcification (usually limited to the elderly) and distortion of the mitral valve apparatus as a result of systolic anterior motion of the mitral valve in the setting of hypertrophic cardiomyopathy. Degeneration of the mitral valve may be seen in patients receiving long-term hemodialysis as well as those with the antiphospholipid antibody syndrome.

The pathophysiology of mitral regurgitation depends on whether the regurgitation occurs on an acute or chronic basis. Acute mitral regurgitation is characterized by sudden increase in left atrial volume and pressure as blood is ejected back into the left atrium during systole. This acute volume overload will also result in decreased cardiac output and acute pulmonary edema. The patient with chronic mitral regurgitation develops ventricular dilatation slowly which helps to accommodate significant increases in blood volume without significant increases in left ventricular end-diastolic pressure. Thus pulmonary congestion is initially prevented. Although patients may be stable for long periods, chronic left ventricular volume overload eventually leads to left ventricular dysfunction with decreased ejection fraction, decreased cardiac output, elevated left ventricular filling pressure, and pulmonary congestion.

The total left ventricular ejection fraction (forward and regurgitant) is increased in patients with preserved left ventricular function and should be greater than normal (55%). A "normal" ejection fraction (50%–55%) in the patient with severe mitral regurgitation gives the appearance that ventricular function is preserved but in reality is evidence of significant left ventricular dysfunction.

In otherwise healthy persons, the sudden onset of fulminant heart failure with the presence of an apical holosystolic murmur strongly suggests acute mitral regurgitation resulting from chordal rupture. Congestive heart failure in patients with inferior wall myocardial infarctions indicates the possibility of papillary muscle dysfunction. Sudden respiratory distress after a febrile illness suggests acute mitral regurgitation caused by ruptured chordae or valve leaflet perforation due to infective endocarditis.

In the presence of acute mitral regurgitation, patients usually have sinus tachycardia and a non-displaced hyperdynamic left ventricular apical impulse. An apical systolic murmur begins with S1 but often ends before S2 as left atrial and left ventricular pressures equalize and valvular regurgitation ceases. In chronic mitral regurgitation, the left ventricular apical impulse is displaced because of left ventricular dilatation. A holosystolic blowing murmur is heard at the apex and radiates to the axilla. A third heart sound is common and does not necessarily indicate the presence of left ventricular dysfunction. It may occur solely as a result of early diastolic filling.[5] A left parasternal lift and accentuated pulmonic component of the second heart sound suggest coexistent pulmonary hypertension.

Echocardiography is an essential diagnostic study for evaluation of the patient with mitral regurgitation. It provides a measure of the degree of regurgitation as well as an estimate of left ventricular chamber size and function. It usually leads to the identification of the component of the mitral valve apparatus that is responsible for the mitral regurgitation. If tricuspid regurgitation is present, echo-doppler techniques can be used to measure the pressure gradient between the right ventricle and the right atrium and enable an estimate of pulmonary artery systolic pressure.

When surgical correction of mitral regurgitation is performed, it is desirable to repair rather than replace the valve. Valve repair is associated with lower periopera-tive mortality and better preservation of left ventricular function and, if sinus rhythm is maintained, freedom from the use of warfarin, which is necessary in the patient with a mechanical valve prosthesis. Patients with mitral valve calcification and scarring as well as those with severe myxomatous degeneration and destruction of the valve and chordae are usually not candidates for valve repair.

Left ventricular function is a major determinant of postoperative survival. Non-invasive measurements of ventricular function, ejection fraction and ventricular dimension determined by echocardiography guide the timing of operation. In the patient with severe chronic mitral regurgitation normal ejection fraction should be $\geq$60%. An ejection fraction less than 60% is indicative of a reduced long-term survival. For the patient with severe asymptomatic mitral regurgitation, mitral valve surgery should be performed if there is evidence of left ventricular dysfunction, e.g., left ventricular ejection fraction <60%. Left ventricular end systolic dimension should be <45 mm in the patient with normal left ventricular function. Therefore, for the patient with asymptomatic severe mitral regurgitation, surgery should be considered when the left ventricular end systolic dimension exceeds this value. Surgery is considered in the asymptomatic patient with severe mitral regurgitation and preserved left ventric-ular function if the patient has had recent onset of episodic or chronic atrial fibrillation or has evidence of pulmonary hypertension (pulmonary artery systolic pressure >50 mm Hg at rest or >60 mmHg with exercise). In the symptomatic patient with severe mitral regurgita-tion, surgery should be performed as long as the ejection fraction is greater than 30% (LVEF <30% in the patient with severe left ventricular dysfunction is indicative of severe left ventricular dysfunction).[2,6] When the left ven-tricular ejection fraction is <30% operative, mortality increases significantly. In this high risk group surgery should only be considered if it is highly likely that mitral valve repair will be performed.[7]

The status of left ventricular function is a major deter-minant of perioperative complications in patients with mitral regurgitation who undergo non-cardiac surgery. We believe that patients with chronic severe mitral regur-gitation should undergo non-invasive assessment of left ventricular function before non-cardiac surgery. If the ejection fraction is not greater than normal, as would be expected, we are particularly vigilant regarding fluid administration and volume shifts in an effort to avoid the development of congestive heart failure. Patients with mitral regurgitation tolerate afterload reduction well in the perioperative period. Agents that increase afterload (e.g., vasopressors) increase the amount of regurgitant blood, and their uses should be avoided if possible. Infective endocarditis prophylaxis for indicated proce-dures is necessary.

Mitral valve prolapse

Mitral valve prolapse (MVP) is a condition in which one or both mitral valve leaflets extend above the mitral annular plane during systole and prolapse into the left atrium. The degree of valve abnormality varies greatly, ranging from relatively normal valves with only intermittent prolapse to markedly abnormal valve structures with valve leaflet thickening, redundancy, and regurgitation. MVP occurs in about 3% of the population.

Most persons with MVP are asymptomatic. Some have symptoms that are unrelated to the valve abnormality. These symptoms may be associated with autonomic dys-function and include chest pain, palpitations, dizziness, and symptoms of panic.[8,9]

The diagnosis is usually made on hearing the classic mid-systolic click and, in patients with mitral regurgitation, a mid to late systolic murmur. Conditions that decrease the size of the left ventricle (i.e., the Valsalva maneuver, dehydration) cause the valve to prolapse earlier, in which case the click is heard closer to S1 and the intensity and duration of the murmur may be increased. The diagnosis is confirmed by transthoracic echocardiography.

The risk of infective endocarditis is the greatest concern for patients with MVP who are undergoing non-cardiac surgery. The risk of developing endocarditis, in the setting of bacteremia, has been estimated to be 1 in 1400 in patients who have MVP and mitral regurgitation, 35 times greater than in those who have MVP without valve regurgitation.[10] Patients who require endocarditis prophylaxis in the setting of procedures associated with bacteremia include those with the characteristic click-murmur of MVP with mitral regurgitation, those with an isolated click and echocardiographic evidence of MVP with MR, and those with an isolated click without murmur but who have echocardiographic evidence of risk factors for endocarditis, e.g., mitral leaflet thickening, elongated chordae, left atrial enlargement, and left ventricular dilatation.[11–13]

It has been suggested that patients with MVP have a slightly higher incidence of cardiac arrhythmias. The etiology is unclear and the risk of serious arrhythmias is low. These arrhythmias often respond to cessation of caffeine, alcohol or other stimulants. Beta-adrenergic blockers may be used if these maneuvers are not successful.[14] Patients who have dizziness associated with MVP often have decreased blood volume.[15] The onset of this symptom in the perioperative period should prompt an assessment of volume status and the administration of fluids if indicated.

Aortic regurgitation

Aortic regurgitation may be caused by processes that affect the aortic valve leaflets (e.g., rheumatic fever, infective endocarditis, congenital bicuspid aortic valve) or the aortic root and valve-supporting structures (aortic dissection, systemic hypertension, cystic medial necrosis, Marfan's syndrome). Eighty percent of cases that come to medical attention are chronic.

Chronic aortic regurgitation is accompanied by left ventricular dilatation and a gradual, progressive increase in left ventricular end-diastolic volume with only an initial slight increase in left ventricular end-diastolic pressure. The dilated left ventricle facilitates the rapid return of blood back to the ventricle during diastole, resulting in decreased peripheral arterial diastolic pressure. Left ventricular stroke volume, composed of both forward and regurgitant blood flow, is increased. The heart rate usually remains normal. This compensation often permits patients to remain asymptomatic even with severe aortic regurgitation. This combination of increased stroke volume and decreased diastolic blood pressure explains several of the classic physical findings of chronic aortic regurgitation:

wide pulse pressure, water-hammer pulse (brisk pulse upstroke with rapid collapse), de Musset's sign (head bobbing during systole related to increased stroke volume), and Quincke's pulse (visible nail bed capillary pulsations).

Acute aortic regurgitation, in contrast, is characterized by the abrupt regurgitation of blood into a normal left ventricle leading to a sudden increase in left ventricular volume and marked elevation of left ventricular end-diastole pressure. Compensatory mechanisms do not occur as in chronic aortic regurgitation. The heart rate increases, cardiac output decreases, and peripheral vasoconstriction occurs. The wide pulse pressure of chronic aortic regurgitation is not present and systolic blood pressure may decrease. Acute heart failure and pulmonary edema are common. Because of the absence of chronic compensation, the classic physical findings of chronic aortic regurgitation are not present.

Acute aortic regurgitation may rapidly progress to intractable heart failure. Therefore, it is an indication for urgent aortic valve replacement. In contrast, chronic aortic regurgitation may be associated with minimal or no symptoms for years.

Aortic valve replacement is indicated for patients with acute severe aortic regurgitation. For the patient with chronic aortic regurgitation the indications for surgery vary based on the presence of symptoms. Surgery is indicated for the patient with New York Heart Association functional class III, IV symptoms, severe aortic regurgitation and normal left ventricular systolic function (ejection fraction $\geq 50\%$). Patients with New York Heart Association functional class III, III, IV symptoms with mild-to-moderate left ventricular dysfunction (ejection fraction 25%–49%) should also undergo aortic valve replacement. The risks of surgery increase markedly when ejection fraction is less than 25%, but the benefit of surgery often outweighs that risk. For patients with asymptomatic severe aortic regurgitation aortic valve replacement is indicated in the setting of left ventricular dysfunction (ejection fraction <50%). Aortic valve replacement is also suggested for patients with severe left ventricular dilatation (left ventricular end-systolic dimension >55 mm) even in the absence of symptoms.[2]

In non-cardiac surgery operative risk correlates more closely with the status of left ventricular function than with the degree of aortic valve regurgitation. Vasopressors that raise peripheral vascular resistance may increase the degree of regurgitation and when used must be done so with caution. Bradycardia is associated with increased diastolic filling time which raises the magnitude of regurgitant volume by lengthening the period during which regurgitation may occur. In contrast to patients with aortic stenosis, patients with aortic regurgitation typically tolerate vasodilation well, often with an increase in cardiac output. Caution must be exercised to prevent excessive decreases in already lowered diastolic pressure in an effort to preclude reductions in coronary artery perfusion pressure. Infective endocarditis prophylaxis for indicated surgical procedures is necessary.

Aortic stenosis

In adults, clinically significant aortic stenosis is usually the result of degenerative calcification of otherwise normal tricuspid aortic valves. When aortic stenosis manifests in adults younger that 50 years old, it is usually a result of calcification and fusion of a congenital bicuspid aortic valve. Even when it is severe, aortic stenosis remains clinically silent for many years. The onset of symptoms indicates that patients are at risk for sudden cardiac death. In patients with untreated symptomatic aortic stenosis, the occurrence of angina or syncope indicates a potential survival of only 2 to 3 years. The onset of congestive heart failure is more ominous and suggests the likelihood of death within 1 to 2 years. Sudden death is rare in those with asymptomatic, hemodynamically severe aortic stenosis (i.e., aortic gradient greater than 50 mm Hg and aortic valve area $\leq 1.0\,\mathrm{cm}^2$).

The classic physical findings of significant aortic stenosis are a low-amplitude and slow-rising carotid pulse pressure (pulsus parvus and tardus), a sustained apical impulse, a crescendo–decrescendo harsh systolic murmur heard at the second right intercostal space radiating to the carotids and precordium, an S4, and diminished intensity of the aortic component of the second heart sound. As the degree of aortic obstruction increases, the systolic murmur peaks later in systole and the intensity of the aortic component of the second heart sound decreases and may disappear.

The absence of these classic findings does not rule out the presence of critical aortic stenosis. The intensity of the heart murmur may decrease as the left ventricle fails. The carotid pulse findings may be altered in elderly patients with non-compliant peripheral vasculatures. Transthoracic echocardiography is essential to estimate the degree of aortic stenosis more precisely and to quantitate left ventricular function.

Adults with critical aortic stenosis (e.g., aortic valve area $\leq 1.0\,\mathrm{cm}^2$) should undergo aortic valve replacement once they experience symptoms (e.g., angina, presyncope, syncope, congestive heart failure) or manifest evidence of left ventricular dysfunction even without symptoms. Fifty percent of adults with critical aortic stenosis and angina have significant coronary artery disease that may require revascularization at the time of aortic valve replacement.

Survival after aortic valve replacement is excellent and patients with left ventricular dysfunction often experience marked improvement in ventricular function following surgery.

Because the risk of aortic valve replacement exceeds the risk of sudden death in patients with asymptomatic critical aortic stenosis with normal left ventricular function, aortic valve replacement is not performed until the patient develops symptoms or left ventricular function. An exception is for the patient with asymptomatic critical aortic stenosis who requires coronary artery bypass surgery; aortic valve replacement at the time of coronary artery bypass surgery is recommended.

Balloon aortic valvuloplasty has been described as a non-surgical means of decreasing the degree of aortic obstruction in aortic stenosis. The immediate and long-term results of this procedure have been disappointing. Although the aortic valve area following this procedure may be increased up to 60%, many patients with critical aortic stenosis still have significant aortic stenosis after the procedure. Mortality or major morbidity occurs in as many as 13% of patients who undergo balloon aortic valvuloplasty, and aortic valve restenosis occurs in 50% of patients within 6 months. This modality has a limited role in patients with aortic stenosis who require non-cardiac surgery. It may be considered for those patients with critical aortic stenosis and either congestive heart failure or hypotension who require urgent non-cardiac surgery. It may also be considered before non-cardiac surgery in patients with hemodynamic compromise as a result of critical aortic stenosis who are not candidates for aortic valve replacement.[16,17]

Aortic stenosis was the only valvular heart disease abnormality found by Goldman to be associated with an increased risk of perioperative cardiac complication or death.[18] Patients with critical aortic stenosis have a 13% cardiac perioperative mortality, compared to an overall cardiac mortality of 1.9%. Other studies that have examined the multifactorial risk index have confirmed aortic stenosis to be a risk factor for perioperative cardiac complications.[19,20] O'Keefe reported a small series of patients with moderate or critical aortic stenosis who underwent elective non-cardiac surgery. Although no deaths occurred, 10% of the patients had significant perioperative hypotension that was transient in all but one case. Local anesthesia was used in about half the cases and was not associated with any cardiac complications. Subsequent observations of patients with severe aortic stenosis indicate that their adverse event rate in relation to non-cardiac surgery is similar to patients without aortic stenosis. This overall lower than expected complication rate was attributed to effective preoperative identification of aortic stenosis as well as careful peri-operative anesthesia monitoring and management.[21,22]

One of the hemodynamic consequences of severe aortic stenosis is a "fixed" cardiac output resulting from left ventricular outflow tract obstruction. Patients are unable to increase cardiac output in response to the stress of surgery and there is decreased left ventricular compliance related to left ventricular hypertrophy. Patients become dependent on adequate preload. Hypovolemia and the vasodilation that may accompany spinal anesthesia or vasodilators are tolerated poorly and may result in profound hypotension. The onset of atrial fibrillation with loss of the atrial contribution to ventricular filling may lead to severe hemodynamic compromise.

We believe that the perioperative approach to patients with aortic stenosis must be individualized and based on the severity of the aortic stenosis, patients' symptoms, left ventricular function, and the anticipated hemodynamic demands of the surgical procedure. All patients with aortic stenosis should receive bacterial endocarditis prophylaxis if indicated. Patients with asymptomatic critical aortic stenosis who have preserved left ventricular function are monitored closely during the perioperative period. Invasive hemodynamic monitoring is used if the surgical procedure is associated with significant fluid shifts or changes in preload or afterload. Patients with symptomatic critical aortic stenosis or aortic stenosis associated with severe left ventricular dysfunction should undergo aortic valve replacement before non-cardiac surgery if possible. If the non-cardiac surgery cannot be delayed or if the patients are not candidates for aortic valve replacement, the risks and benefits of aortic valvuloplasty are considered. If patients are not candidates for aortic balloon valvuloplasty and surgery is absolutely necessary, it is performed under the guidance of invasive hemodynamic monitoring. The use of vasodilators and anesthetic techniques that may cause vasodilation are avoided if possible.

A unique clinical association that may result in the need for non-cardiac surgery in the patient with severe aortic stenosis is bleeding from gastrointestinal dysplasia (Heyde's syndrome). In this syndrome bleeding often ceases after aortic valve replacement. While the cause of this relationship is unknown, there have been case reports of deficiency of von Willebrand factor that has normalized after aortic valve replacement.[23]

Treatment of patients with prosthetic heart valves

The major concerns for the patient with a prosthetic heart valve who undergoes non-cardiac surgery are the management of anticoagulation for the patient with a mechanical valve and the need for endocarditis prophylaxis.

Few trials describe the rates of prosthetic valve thrombosis in patients who are not receiving anticoagulants. Overall, the risk of valve thrombosis or thromboembolism is higher in patients with valve prostheses in the mitral position. Although data are scant, the incidence of valve thrombosis is probably greater in patients who are not receiving anticoagulants and who have tilting disc valves (e.g., Bjork–Shiley) and are lower in patients with leaflet valves (e.g., St. Jude).[24] Guidelines of the American College of Chest Physicians recommend that for patients in whom the risk of thromboembolism is high without anticoagulation (e.g., mechanical valve in the mitral position, Bjork–Shiley valve, thrombosis, or embolus in the past year, or three or more of the following risk factors: atrial fibrillation, previous embolism at any time, hypercoagulable condition, or mechanical prosthesis and left ventricular ejection fraction less than 30%) that warfarin be withheld prior to surgery and continuous full dose intravenous heparin be initiated when the INR (international normalized ratio) becomes subtherapeutic. Heparin is discontinued 4–6 hours prior to surgery and then resumed as soon as is feasible following surgery. Warfarin is resumed at the patient's maintenance dose when oral intake is resumed and heparin discontinued when the INR reaches therapeutic range.[25] For patients whose risk of valve thromboembolism is lower, warfarin is usually discontinued 48–72 hours before surgery with the goal of an INR ≤ 1.5 at the time of surgery. It is resumed as soon as possible during the 24 hours following surgery. If the patient is unable to take oral medications at that time, continuous full dose intravenous heparin is begun and continued until warfarin is restarted. For patients at low risk of bleeding during surgery while anticoagulated (e.g., cataract surgery, superficial procedures) a recommendation of the American College of Cardiology/American Heart Association Guidelines for the management of patients with valvular heart disease is to briefly reduce the INR to the low or subtherapeutic range prior to surgery and resume the patient's maintenance dose of warfarin following the procedure.[26] Dental extractions can be safely performed on patients at a therapeutic level of anticoagulation.[27] While low molecular weight heparin has been described in observational reports of small numbers of patients to be an alternative approach for anticoagulation to "bridge" the period of cessation of anticoagulation for the patient who is maintained on warfarin chronically and requires its discontinuation in the perioperative period, there are no data supporting this approach for the patient with a mechanical heart valve.[28]

Bacterial endocarditis prophylaxis (Tables 6.8, 6.9, 6.10, 6.11)[29]

Bacterial endocarditis prophylaxis is indicated for patients with specific cardiac structural abnormalities who are at risk for bacteremia resulting from the disruption of mucosal surfaces colonized with bacteria. It is estimated that, even if endocarditis prophylaxis were completely effective, less than 10% of cases of bacterial endocarditis could be prevented. Reasons include the fact that the organisms targeted by currently recommended antibiotic regimens, *Streptococcus viridans* and *Enterococcus*, account for only 50% of all cases of endocarditis, and only 25% of patients with *Streptococcus viridans* and 40% of those with *Enterococcus endocarditis* develop their infection after procedures for which prophylaxis would have been given. Only half of all patients with endocarditis have a cardiac condition that would have made them candidates for antibiotic prophylaxis.

Antibiotic prophylaxis is recommended for those with high-risk cardiac lesions (e.g., prosthetic cardiac valves), most congenital cardiac lesions (e.g., bicuspid aortic valve, patent ductus arteriosus, cyanotic congenital heart lesions), a previous history of bacterial endocarditis even in the absence of structural heart disease, rheumatic and other acquired valvular lesions, mitral valve prolapse in the presence of the characteristic click-murmur of MVP with mitral regurgitation, those with an isolated click and echocardiographic evidence of MVP with MR, and those with an isolated click without murmur but who have echocardiographic evidence of risk factors for endocarditis, e.g., mitral leaflet thickening, elongated chordae, left atrial enlargement, and left ventricular dilatation,[11–13] and the patient hypertrophic cardiomyopathy with left ventricular outflow tract obstruction. Endocarditis prophylaxis is not recommended for patients with isolated atrial septal defects of the secundum type, an innocent or physiologic systolic murmur, previous rheumatic fever without valve abnormality, or a cardiac pacemaker. It is also not indicated in the patient who has undergone surgical repair of a ventricular septal defect without residua more than 6 months earlier, or previous coronary artery bypass surgery.

Antibiotic prophylaxis is indicated for procedures during which transient bacteremia is expected. These include specific dental, oropharyngeal, respiratory tract, genitourinary, gastrointestinal, gynecologic, obstetric, and general surgical procedures. Prophylactic antibiotic regimens are directed specifically toward the most likely infecting organism, which is *S. viridans* in dental and upper respiratory tract procedures and *Enterococcus* in genitourinary and gastrointestinal procedures.

Table 6.8. Procedures and endocarditis prophylaxis

Endocarditis prophylaxis recommended
Respiratory tract
Tonsillectomy and/or adenoidectomy
Surgical operations that involve respiratory mucosa
Bronchoscopy with a rigid bronchoscope

Gastrointestinal tract [a]
Sclerotherapy for esophageal varices
Esophageal stricture dilation
Endoscopic retrograde cholangiography with biliary obstruction
Biliary tract surgery
Surgical operations that involve intestinal mucosa

Genitourinary tract
Prostatic surgery
Cystoscopy
Urethral dilation

Endocarditis prophylaxis not recommended
Respiratory tract
Endotracheal intubation
Bronchoscopy with a flexible bronchoscope, with or without biopsy [b]
Tympanostomy tube insertion

Gastrointestinal tract
Transesophageal echocardiography [b]
Endoscopy with or without gastrointestinal biopsy [b]

Genitourinary tract
Vaginal hysterectomy [b]
Vaginal delivery [b]
Cesarean section

In uninfected tissue
Urethral catheterization
Uterine dilatation and curettage
Therapeutic abortion
Sterilization procedures

Insertion or removal of intrauterine devices
Other
    Cardiac catheterization, including balloon angioplasty
    Implanted cardiac pacemakers, implanted defibrillators, and coronary stents
    Incision or biopsy of surgically scrubbed skin
    Circumcision

Notes:
[a] Prophylaxis is recommended for high-risk patients; it is optional for medium-risk patients.
[b] Prophylaxis is optional for high-risk patients.
Source: From Dajani, A., Taubert, K., Wilson, W. *et al.* Prevention of bacterial endocarditis. *Circulation* 1997; **96**: 358.

Table 6.9. Dental procedures and endocarditis prophylaxis

Endocarditis prophylaxis recommended[a]

Dental extractions

Periodontal procedures including surgery, scaling and root planing, probing, and recall maintenance

Dental implant placement and reimplantation of avulsed teeth

Endodontic (root canal) instrumentation or surgery only beyond the apex

Subgingival placement of antibiotic fibers or strips

Initial placement of orthodontic bands but not brackets

Intraligamentary local anesthetic injections

Prophylactic cleaning of teeth or implants where bleeding is anticipated

Endocarditis prophylaxis not recommended

Restorative dentistry[b] (operative and prosthodontic) with or without retraction cord[c]

Local anesthetic injections (non-intraligamentary)

Intracanal endodontic treatment; postplacement and buildup

Placement of rubber dams

Postoperative suture removal

Placement of removable prosthodontic or orthodontic appliances

Taking of oral impressions

Fluoride treatments

Taking of oral radiographs

Orthodontic appliance adjustment

Shedding of primary teeth

Notes:

[a] Prophylaxis is recommended for patients with high- and moderate-risk cardiac conditions.

[b] This includes restoration of decayed teeth (filling cavities) and replacement of missing teeth.

[c] Clinical judgment may indicate antibiotic use in selected circumstances that may create significant bleeding.

Source: From Dajani, A., Taubert, K., Wilson, W. *et al.* Prevention of bacterial endocarditis. *Circulation* 1997; **96**: 358.

Table 6.10. Prophylactic regimens for dental, oral, respiratory tract, or esophageal procedures

Situation	Agent	Regimen
Standard general prophylaxis	Amoxicillin	Adults: 2.0 g; children: 50 mg/kg orally 1 h before procedure
Unable to take oral medications	Ampicillin	Adults: 2.0 g i.m. or i.v.; children: 50 mg/kg i.m. or i.v. within 30 min before procedure
Allergic to penicillin	Clindamycin or	Adults: 600 mg; children: 20 mg/kg orally 1 h before procedure
	Cephalexin[a] or cefadroxil[a] or	Adults: 2.0 g; children: 50 mg/kg orally 1 h before procedure
	Azithromycin or clarithromycin	Adults: 500 mg; children: 15 mg/kg orally 1 h before procedure
Allergic to penicillin and unable to take oral medications	Clindamycin or	Adults: 600 mg; children: 20 mg/kg i.v. within 30 min before procedure
	Cefazolin[a]	Adults: 1.0 g; children: 25 mg/kg i.m. or i.v. within 30 min before procedure

Notes:

i.m. indicates intramuscularly, and i.v., intravenously.

[a] Cephalosporins should not be used in individuals with immediate-type hypersensitivity reaction (urticaria, angioedema, or anaphylaxis) to penicillins.

Source: From Dajani, A., Taubert, K., Wilson, W. *et al.* Prevention of bacterial endocarditis. *Circulation* 1997; **96**: 358.

Table 6.11 Prophylactic regimens for genitourinary/gastrointestinal (excluding esophageal) procedures

Situation	Agents[a]	Regimen[b]
High-risk patients	Ampicillin plus gentamicin	Adults: ampicillin 2.0 g i.m. or i.v. plus gentamicin 1.5 mg/kg (not to exceed 120 mg) within 30 min of starting procedure; 6 h later, ampicillin 1 g i.m./i.v. or amoxicillin 1 g orally
		Children: ampicillin 50 mg/kg i.m. or i.v. (not to exceed 2.0 g) plus gentamicin 1.5 mg/kg within 30 min of starting the procedure; 6 h later, ampicillin 25 mg/kg i.m./i.v. or amoxicillin 25 mg/kg orally
High-risk patients allergic to ampicillin/amoxicillin	Vancomycin plus gentamicin	Adults: vancomycin 1.0 g i.v. over 1–2 h plus gentamicin 1.5 mg/kg i.v./i.m. (not to exceed 120 mg); complete injection/infusion within 30 min of starting procedure
		Children: vancomycin 20 mg/kg i.v. over 1–2 h plus gentamicin 1.5 mg/kg i.v./i.m.; complete injection/infusion within 30 min of starting procedure
Moderate-risk patients	Amoxicillin or ampicillin	Adults: amoxicillin 2.0 g orally 1 h before procedure, or ampicillin 2.0 g i.m./i.v. within 30 min of starting procedure
		Children: amoxicillin 50 mg/kg orally 1 h before procedure, or ampicillin 50 mg/kg i.m./i.v. within 30 min of starting procedure
Moderate-risk patients allergic to ampicillin/amoxicillin	Vancomycin	Adults: vancomycin 1.0 g i.v. over 1–2 h complete infusion within 30 min of starting procedure
		Children: vancomycin 20 mg/kg i.v. over 1–2 h; complete infusion within 30 min of starting procedure

Notes:
i.m. indicates intramuscularly, and i.v., intravenously.
[a] Total children's dose should not exceed adult dose.
[b] No second dose of vancomycin or gentamicin is recommended.
Source: From Dajani, A., Taubert, K., Wilson, W. *et al.* Prevention of bacterial endocarditis. *Circulation* 1997; **96**: 358.

REFERENCES

1. Gorlin, R. & Gorlin, S. G. Hydraulic formula for calculation of the area of stenotic mitral valve, other cardiac valves and central circulatory states. *Am. Heart J.*, 1951; **41**: 1–29.
2. Anonymous. Guidelines for the management of patients with valvular heart disease: executive summary. A report of the American College of Cardiology/American Heart Association Task Force on Practice Guidelines (Committee on Management of Patients with Valvular Heart Disease). *J. Am. Coll. Cardiol.* 1998; **32**: 1486–1588.
3. Eagle, K. A., Berger, P. B., Calkins, H. *et al.* ACC/AHA guideline update for perioperative cardiovascular evaluation for noncardiac surgery – executive summary: a report of the American College of Cardiology/American Heart Association Task Force on Practice Guidelines (Committee to Update the 1996 Guidelines on Perioperative Cardiovascular Evaluation for Noncardiac Surgery). *J. Am. Coll. Cardiol.* 2002; **39**(3): 542–553.
4. Spandorfer, J. The management of anticoagulation before and after procedures. *Med. Clin. N. Am.* 2001; **85**(5): 1109–1116.
5. Folland, E. D., Kriegel, B. J., & Henderson, W. G. Implications of third heart sounds in patients with valvular heart disease: the Veterans Affairs Cooperative Study on Valvular Heart Disease. *N. Engl. J. Med.* 1992; **327**: 458–462.
6. Otto, C. M. Evaluation and management of chronic mitral regurgitation. *N. Engl. J. Med.* 2001; **345**(10): 740–746.
7. Otto, C. M. Timing of surgery in mitral regurgitation. *Heart* 2003; **89**: 100–105.
8. Gaffney, F. A., Karlsson, E. S., & Campbell, W. Autonomic dysfunction in women with mitral valve prolapse syndrome. *Circulation* 1979; **59**: 894–901.
9. Fontana, M. E., Sparks, E. A., Bondonlas, H., & Wooley, C. F. Mitral valve prolapse and the mitral valve prolapse syndrome. *Curr. Probl. Cardiol.* 1991; **16**: 309–375.
10. MacMahon, S. W., Hickey, A. J., & Wilcken, D. E. Risk of infective endocarditis in mitral valve prolapse with and without precordial systolic murmurs. *Am. J. Cardiol.* 1987; **59**: 105–108.

11. Clemens, J. D., Horwitz, R. I., Jaffe, C. C., Feinstein, A. R., & Stanton, B. F. A controlled evaluation of the risk of bacterial endocarditis in persons with mitral-valve prolapse. *N. Engl. J. Med.* 1982; **307**: 776–781.

12. Marks, A. R., Choong, C. Y., Sanfilippo, A. J., Ferre, M., & Weyman, A. E. Identification of high-risk and low-risk subgroups of patients with mitral valve prolapse. *N. Engl. J. Med.* 1989; **320**: 1031–1036.

13. Babuty, D., Cosnay, P., & Breuillac, J. C. Ventricular arrhythmia factors in mitral valve prolapse. *Pacing Clin. Electrophysiol.* 1994; **17**: 1090–1099.

14. Devereux, R. B., Kramer-Fox, R., & Kligfield, P. Mitral valve prolapse: causes, clinical manifestations, and management. *Ann. Intern. Med.* 1989; **111**: 305–317.

15. Hayes, S. N., Holmes, D. R., & Nishimura, R. A. Palliative percutaneous aortic balloon valvuloplasty before noncardiac surgery. *Mayo Clin. Proc.* 1989; **64**: 753–757.

16. Cribier, A. & Letac, B. Percutaneous balloon aortic valvuloplasty in adults with calcific aortic stenosis. *Curr. Opin. Cardiol.* 1991; **6**: 212.

17. Goldman, L., Caldera, D. L., Nussbaum, S. R. *et al.* Multifactorial index of cardiac risk in noncardiac surgical procedures. *N. Engl. J. Med.* 1978; **297**: 845.

18. Detsky, A. S., Abrams, H. B., & McLaughlin, J. R. Predicting cardiac complications in patients undergoing noncardiac surgery. *J. Gen. Intern. Med.* 1986; **1**: 211–219.

19. Zeldin, R. A. Assessing cardiac risk in patients who undergo noncardiac surgical procedures. *Can. J. Surg.* 1984; **27**: 402–404.

20. Torsher, L. C., Shub, C., Rettke, S. R., & Brown, D. L. Risk of patients with severe aortic stenosis undergoing noncardiac surgery. *Am. J. Cardiol.* 1998; **81**; 448–452.

21. Raymer, K. & Yang, H. C. Patients with aortic stenosis: cardiac complications in noncardiac surgery. *Can. J. Anaesth.* 1998; **45**: 855–859.

22. Warkentin, T. E., Moore, J. C., & Morgan, D. G. Gastrointestinal angiodysplasia and aortic stenosis. *N. Engl. J. Med.* 2002; **347**: 858–859.

23. Harker, L. A. Antithrombotic therapy following mitral valve replacement. In Duran, C. *Recent Progress in Mitral Valve Disease*, Butterworth: London, 1984: 340–345.

24. Salem, D. N., Dandelin, H. D., Levine, H. J., Pauker, S. G., Eckman, M. H., & Riff, J. Antithrombotic therapy in valvular heart disease. *Chest* 2001; **119**: 207S–219S.

25. Bonow, R. O., Cardabello, B., de Leon, A. C. *et al.* ACC/AHA Guidelines for the Management of Patients With Valvular Heart Disease. Executive Summary. A report of the American College of Cardiology/American Heart Association Task Force on Practice Guidelines (Committee on Management of Patients with Valvular Heart Disease). *J. Heart Valve Dis.* 1998; **7**(6): 672–707.

26. McIntyre, H. Management during dental surgery of patients on anticoagulants. *Lancet* 1966; **2**: 99–100.

27. Spandorfer, J. The management of anticoagulation before and after procedures. *Med. Clin. N. Am.* 2001; **85**(5): 1109–1116.

28. Dajani, A. S., Taubert, K. A., Wilson, W. *et al.* Prevention of bacterial endocarditis. Recommendations by the American Heart Association. *Circulation* 1997; **96**: 358.

29. Molavi, A. Endocarditis: recognition, management, and prophylaxis. *Cardiovasc. Clin.* 1992; **23**: 139–174.

7

Postoperative chest pain and shortness of breath

Geno J. Merli[1] and Michael F. Lubin[2]

[1]Jefferson Medical College, Philadelphia, PA
[2]Emory University School of Medicine, Atlanta, GA

Chest pain and shortness of breath are frequently encountered medical problems in the postoperative period. The time at which they appear after surgery is important in determining their cause. This chapter reviews the possible causes for these presenting symptoms.

Myocardial infarction

Chest pain in the postoperative period is always worrisome because of the possibility of myocardial infarction (MI). This concern is well founded. Mortality rates are 30% to 50% for a first postoperative MI and even higher for subsequent MIs in the perioperative period. Although no data are available concerning specific treatment in this situation, standard therapy for MI is likely to be helpful.

The incidence of postoperative MI approaches zero in patients who have no history of, or possess risk factors for, ischemic heart disease compared to 6% in those with a history of ischemic heart disease. The incidence of postoperative MI has been reported to peak between 3 and 5 days after surgical procedures.[1] More recently, this at risk period has been found to occur as early as 24 to 48 hours after surgery.[2,3]

Two groups of patients appear to be at greatest risk for postoperative MIs and probably sustain the largest number of postoperative MIs as well: those with clinically diagnosed coronary artery disease and those with significant peripheral vascular disease.[4] Diagnosing postoperative MI can be difficult. Incisional pain, gastrointestinal or respiratory complications, and sedative and pain medications may obscure symptoms. Pain typical of MI is commonly absent when MI occurs after surgery; many patients do not have chest pain. In Becker's study,[3] only 40% of patients had chest pain as a presenting complaint and in Charlson's study,[2] only 30% of patients with electrocardiographic (ECG) changes experienced chest pain.

Because chest pain does not occur in many patients, physicians must be aware of several other symptoms and signs that suggest the possibility of MI, including new or worsening heart failure, hypotension, arrhythmias, and even altered mental status, particularly in the elderly.

Patients' histories take just a few minutes to elicit and may be life-saving if either MI or ischemia is present. Chest pain does not always occur but is still a common symptom. Ischemic pain is generally described as heavy or pressing, or as a constriction in the substernal area. It may be spread over a large area of the chest and is rarely localized. The pain may radiate down the left arm or both arms. It is not influenced by position and may be associated with nausea, vomiting, weakness, diaphoresis, and, at times, the urge to defecate. The physical examination also can be helpful. The presence of overt heart failure with distended neck veins, rales, and an S_3 gallop in patients without other causes of heart failure is strong evidence of a postoperative MI. A new arrhythmia is also suggestive.

The ECG can provide helpful information but may also cause confusion. It cannot be emphasized too strongly that the absence of ECG changes in patients with chest pain does not rule out the diagnosis of cardiac ischemia or infarction. Many patients with acute MIs initially have normal ECGs, and many postoperative patients have ECG changes in the absence of MIs. If the ECG is normal, unchanged, or reveals non-specific changes, clinicians must evaluate the possibility of MI on the basis of patients' histories, physical examinations, and other findings (i.e., hypotension, arrhythmias). In the final analysis, it is important for good patient care to transfer those with suspicious findings to an intensive care area to rule out the possibility of MI.

Medical Management of the Surgical Patient: A Textbook of Perioperative Medicine, ed. M. F. Lubin, R. B. Smith, T. F. Dobson, N. Spell, H. K. Walker.
4th edn. Published by Cambridge University Press. © Cambridge University 2006.

Measurement of the creatine phosphokinase or CPK-MB levels also may be helpful. Newer tests like troponin I and II are also helpful. Although enzyme changes can be informative, these are basically retrospective tests and patients must be observed before the results become available. In addition, in Charlson's study,[2] many patients with mildly to moderately elevated levels, including CPK-MB levels above 5% had no symptoms or signs of MI and no ECG changes. It appears that some patients with elevated CPK-MB levels after surgery do not have MIs. Badner and colleagues[5] used several criteria, including daily clinical assessments, ECGs, and measurements of CK levels, CK-MB fractions, and troponin T, to prospectively study postoperative myocardial infarction in patients with known ischemic heart disease. A diagnosis was made when the total CK was greater than 174 U/l, with the presence of two of the following: (a) CK-MB greater than 5%, (b) new Q waves greater than 0.04 per second in duration and greater than 1 mm deep in at least two contiguous leads, (c) troponin T greater than 0.2 g/l, or (d) a positive pyrophosphate scan. According to these criteria, the peak incidence of postoperative myocardial infarction occurred during the first postoperative night, with a rapid decrease in incidence thereafter. Chest pain was an uncommon symptom, and more than 50% of cases were non-Q wave events. This chapter raises the issue that postoperative myocardial infarction may occur because of prolonged ischemia rather than thrombotic occlusion of a coronary artery.

All levels of information should be correlated in making the diagnosis of postoperative MI. Patients with suggestive symptoms, signs, and ECG changes clearly have MIs, whereas those without clear cut findings should have CK-MB and troponin levels along with serial ECGs and more non-invasive or invasive testing as clinically indicated. If the diagnosis of myocardial infarction is confirmed, the treatment modalities with antithrombotic and thrombolytic agents would carry significant risk for major bleeding in the face of recent surgery. Berger and colleagues[6] reported on the benefit of primary angioplasty in such cases.

Pulmonary embolism

Pulmonary embolism is another serious cause of chest pain and is one of the leading causes of death in postoperative patients who either have not received venous thromboembolism prophylaxis or were prescribed ineffective modalities. Episodes of pulmonary embolism usually occur between 3 and 7 days after surgery. Patients not receiving venous thromboembolism prophylaxis with risk factors such as previous deep venous thrombosis or

pulmonary embolism, long procedures, or older age who are undergoing high-risk operations such as orthopedic procedures have the greatest risk for the development of proximal clot with its associated higher incidence of pulmonary embolism.[7]

The most clear-cut cause of chest pain in patients with pulmonary embolism is pulmonary infarction which occurs in less than 10% of cases. The pain is pleuritic (i.e., sharp or sticking pain that increases with respiration and is usually unaffected by position). Patients with pulmonary infarction often have hemoptysis. Many patients who have pulmonary embolism but do not have pulmonary infarction also have chest pain, which also may be pleuritic in nature. Chest pain with other characteristics, including pressure and squeezing pain also occur.

Physical examinations in patients with documented pulmonary embolism may be entirely normal except for the findings of tachycardia. Auscultation of the heart may reveal an increased component of the second heart sound. A pleural rub can be noted on auscultation over the lung area where the underlying pulmonary infarction has occurred. In addition, crackles may be heard over the involved lung segments.

The diagnosis of postoperative pulmonary embolus is addressed in more detail in Chapter 17, but some basic principles are mentioned here. Laboratory examination may be helpful. The ECG often shows only a sinus tachycardia; the QRS axis may be shifted more commonly to either the right, but may be shifted to the left. Arterial blood gas levels usually, but not always, reveal significant hypoxia and a respiratory alkalosis with a low P_{CO_2}. The chest radiograph may show basilar atelectasis but this is common in postoperative patients. If pulmonary infarction has occurred, there may be a dense infiltrate. It is important that pulmonary infarction be differentiated from a new bacterial pneumonia. Significant fever, cough, and sputum production point toward a diagnosis of pneumonia, although these may occur with pulmonary embolism as well.

Gastroesophageal reflux

Gastroesophageal reflux is a common medical problem and a frequent cause of esophagitis in the postoperative period. The condition may be exacerbated by prolonged recumbency, abdominal surgery, medications, and by the use of a nasogastric tube. It is a common cause of postoperative chest pain.

Substernal burning with water brash or regurgitation is common after surgery. These symptoms may occur at any time after operation, and gastroesophageal reflux should be suspected in patients with previous symptoms and in those with prior histories of the problem. There are other causes of esophagitis, including diabetes, malnutrition, acquired immunodeficiency syndrome, and debility. Drugs such as calcium antagonists, sedatives, and anticholinergic agents decrease lower esophageal sphincter pressure and may exacerbate gastroesophageal reflux in the postoperative period.[8]

Pericarditis

Pericarditis is an infrequent cause of chest pain in the postoperative period. It is seen mainly in patients undergoing cardiopulmonary bypass procedures. The characteristic pain of pericarditis is sharp, stabbing, and located in the mid-chest. It may be exacerbated by changes in position, especially lying down or twisting the trunk, and is usually relieved by sitting up and leaning forward. On physical examination, there is often an audible pericardial rub, although many patients have a brief rub or none at all. The rub may have one, two, or three components.

Pericarditis is usually an expected postoperative complication after cardiac surgery. It is usually seen immediately after the procedure and results from direct pericardial irritation. The postpericardiotomy syndrome generally occurs 1 to 3 weeks after the procedure and is probably immunologically mediated. Pericarditis may also occur in the postoperative period in patients with acute or chronic renal failure.

Shortness of breath

Shortness of breath is another common postoperative complaint. It may be associated with many conditions, ranging from benign problems such as anxiety to life-threatening problems such as heart failure. A discussion of pulmonary causes of shortness of breath is presented in Chapter 17.

The symptom of shortness of breath must be differentiated from the physiologic derangement of hypoxia. Although they commonly occur together, either may be present without the other. In patients with emphysema or restrictive lung disease, for example, the resting P_aO_2 may be relatively normal. Shortness of breath is common in such patients because the work involved in breathing with stiff lungs is greatly increased. In young patients with pneumonia, however, a significant degree of hypoxia may be present without any shortness of breath because the work of breathing may not be increased appreciably in young, otherwise healthy patients.

Congestive heart failure

Congestive heart failure (CHF) occurs at two distinct times after surgery. Seventy percent of patients who have postoperative CHF develop pulmonary edema within the first hour after reversal of anesthesia. Intraoperative fluid overload is the cause in most cases, although postoperative hypertension, anesthetic-induced myocardial dysfunction, and termination of positive-pressure ventilation are also important factors.[9] Congestive heart failure also occurs 24 to 48 hours after surgery because of the mobilization of interstitial fluid,[10] although most cases of postoperative congestive heart failure result from volume overload, myocardial ischemia or infarction, and in some patients the withdrawal from long-term heart failure medications.[11]

Supraventricular tachycardia

Perioperative arrhythmias are common and occur in as many as 80% of patients during anesthesia and surgery.[12] These arrhythmias are not usually significant and include a wandering atrial pacemaker, atrioventricular dissociation, nodal rhythm, and sinus bradycardia. Under 5% of perioperative arrhythmias are clinically important. Supraventricular tachycardia must be considered as a postoperative cause for shortness of breath. Narrow-complex supraventricular tachycardia, atrial fibrillation, and atrial flutter are the most important considerations. Appropriate intervention to correct the hemodynamic changes induced by these rhythms is necessary.

REFERENCES

1. Goldman, L., Caldera, D., Nussbaum, S. *et al.* Multifactorial index of cardiac risk in noncardiac surgical procedures. *N. Engl. J. Med.* 1977; **297**: 845–850.
2. Charlson, M. E., MacKenzie, C. R., Ales, K. L. *et al.* The postoperative electrocardiogram and creatine kinase: implications for diagnosis of myocardial infarction after non-cardiac surgery. *J. Clin. Epidemiol.* 1989; **42**: 25–34.
3. Becker, R. C. & Underwood, D. A. Myocardial infarction in patients undergoing noncardiac surgery. *Clevel. Clin. J. Med.* 1987; **54**: 25–28.

4. Ashton, C. M., Petersen, N. J., Wray, N. P. *et al.* The incidence of perioperative myocardial infarction in men undergoing noncardiac surgery. *Ann. Intern. Med.* 1993; **118**: 504–510.

5. Badner, N., Knill, R., Brown, J., Novick, T., & Gelb, A. Myocardial infarction after non-cardiac surgery. *Anesthesiology* 1998; **88**: 572–578.

6. Berger, P., Bellot, V., Bell, M. *et al.* An immediate invasive strategy for the treatment of acute myocardial infarction early after noncardiac surgery. *Am. J. Cardiol.* 2001; **87**: 1100–1102.

7. Geerts, W. H., Heit, J. A., Clagett, G. P. *et al.* Prevention of venous thromboembolism. *Chest* 2001; **119**(Suppl): 132S–175S.

8. Gordon, S., Chatzinoff, M., & Peiken, S. Medical care of the surgical patient with gastrointestinal disease. *Med. Clin. North Am.* 1987; **71**: 433–452.

9. Cooperman, L. & Price, H. Pulmonary edema in the operative and postoperative period: a review of 40 cases. *Ann. Surg.* 1970; **172**: 883–891.

10. Charlson, M., MacKenzie, R., Gold, J. *et al.* Risks for postoperative congestive heart failure. *Surg. Gynecol. Obstet.* 1991; **172**: 95–104.

11. Weitz, H. Perioperative cardiac complications. *Med. Clin. North Am.* 2001; **85**: 1151–1169.

12. Goldman, L. Supraventricular tachyarrhythmias in hospitalized adults after surgery. *Chest* 1978; **73**: 450–454.

Hypertension

8

Perioperative management of hypertension

Craig R. Keenan

Department of Medicine, University of California, Davis, CA

Perioperative management of hypertension

Hypertension affects an estimated 50 million persons in the USA, including 25% of adults and more than 50% of individuals over age 65 years.[1] Thus, many surgeons, anesthesiologists, primary care physicians, and consultants will care for surgical patients with hypertension. Hypertension can increase surgical risk, and it often causes end-organ damage of the brain, heart, and kidneys, with important implications for surgical risk and perioperative management. The essentials of diagnosis, evaluation, and treatment of hypertension have been detailed in recent reviews.[2] This chapter concentrates on the preoperative risk assessment of hypertensive patients and on the perioperative management of hypertension.

Hemodynamic response to anesthesia

A discussion of perioperative hypertension requires a basic understanding of the physiologic responses to anesthesia in normotensive and hypertensive patients. There are four main periods during anesthesia: the induction, intubation, maintenance, and recovery periods. During induction, most patients have a fall in blood pressure. During laryngoscopy and intubation, the sympathetic nervous system is activated and blood pressure and heart rate rise. With deepening anesthesia, a decline in mean arterial pressure and heart rate occur due to the effects of pharmacologic agents, a decrease in sympathetic nervous system activity, and loss of the baroreceptor reflex. During recovery from anesthesia around the time of extubation, blood pressure and heart rate slowly increase in the first 15 minutes, and are accompanied by general arousal.

Patients with untreated hypertension can have exaggerated responses during all of these phases.[3–5] During the induction phase, blood pressure declines more precipitously in patients with hypertension. During laryngoscopy and intubation, the blood pressure and heart rate can increase to a much greater degree, due to a significant increase in plasma catecholamines as compared to normotensive patients. In the maintenance phase, hypertensive patients are more likely to have blood pressure lability, with episodes of both hypertension and hypotension. Finally, during recovery hypertensive patients can have exaggerated arousal responses with large increases in blood pressure and heart rate.

Preoperative risk assessment of hypertensive patients

In determining the operative risk of hypertension, the complexity of studying hypertension as an independent risk factor must be recognized, given its intimate link to coronary artery disease (CAD), chronic renal disease, cerebrovascular disease, left ventricular hypertrophy (LVH), and systolic and diastolic congestive heart failure (CHF). Many patients have hypertension without these target organ diseases, but many others have overt or previously unrecognized end-organ disease. These conditions all increase perioperative risk above that of hypertension alone. Thus, the perioperative risk assessment in the hypertensive patient entails determining the risks of hypertension itself plus the risks of any concomitant end organ disease.[6]

Risks of hypertension

Of patients with chronic hypertension, only 25% have their blood pressure controlled on medications, 39% are on

Medical Management of the Surgical Patient: A Textbook of Perioperative Medicine, ed. M. F. Lubin, R. B. Smith, T. F. Dobson, N. Spell, H. K. Walker. 4th edn. Published by Cambridge University Press. © Cambridge University 2006.

medications but uncontrolled, and 36% are unaware that they have hypertension and are untreated.[1] Thus, three-quarters of hypertensive patients being evaluated for surgery will have uncontrolled hypertension. The most significant and well-studied surgical risks of hypertension are perioperative cardiovascular events, specifically myocardial infarction (MI) and death. Other recognized risks include renal failure, stroke, and CHF. No randomized, controlled trials have evaluated the independent effects of hypertension on operative risk, so observational studies provide almost all of our information on this subject.

Goldman and colleagues' classic study of cardiac risk for non-cardiac surgery prospectively evaluated 1001 consecutive patients in the mid-1970s.[7,8] In the subset of 676 patients undergoing non-emergent surgery, there were 179 patients with preoperative hypertension, including 79 patients with adequate treatment (blood pressure <160/90 mm Hg), 40 with inadequate treatment (>160/90 mm Hg), and 77 with blood pressure >160/90 mm Hg on no therapy.[9] Only 5 patients had severe hypertension, defined as a diastolic blood pressure between 111 and 119 mm Hg, and 19 patients had isolated systolic hypertension >160 mm Hg. In multivariate analyses, pre-existing hypertension was associated with postoperative hypertension in 25% of patients and with intraoperative hypotension requiring a fluid challenge or adrenergic agent for correction in 20%–30% of patients.[10] These associations were independent of the level of preoperative blood pressure control. Preoperative hypertension, however, was *not* an independent predictor of perioperative cardiac complications such as myocardial infarction or death.

In a larger and more recent study, Forrest and colleagues evaluated data on 17 201 patients from a major randomized trial of inhalation agents for general anesthesia.[11] Severe adverse outcomes, most of which were cardiovascular or respiratory complications, were reported in 847 patients. Multivariate analyses demonstrated that a history of hypertension was associated with the development of tachycardia, bradycardia, and postoperative hypertension, but not with severe cardiopulmonary events or death. Other multivariate analyses similarly have found no independent association between hypertension and severe perioperative cardiac complications.[12,13]

Most studies of perioperative risk have not distinguished between systolic and diastolic hypertension. A recent observational study found that isolated systolic hypertension (ISH), defined as a systolic blood pressure >140 mm Hg with diastolic pressure <90 mm Hg, was associated with a 30% increased risk of the combined endpoint of left ventricular dysfunction, cerebrovascular events, renal failure, and death after coronary bypass surgery.[14] Of note, 89% of these patients had a systolic pressure <170 mm Hg. This study suggests that ISH, even when not severe, may increase the risk of cardiovascular events. Nonetheless, other authors argue that the degree of ISH has not been shown to increase the risk of surgery (though it may increase perioperative ischemia) and do not recommend delaying surgery based on ISH alone.[15] More prospective studies on a diverse population of surgical patients with ISH are needed to determine the true risk.

Others more directly examined intraoperative hemodynamics and myocardial ischemia in hypertensive patients. Prys-Roberts and colleagues recorded the cardiovascular responses to anesthesia in 7 normotensive patients, 15 patients with treated hypertension, and 7 patients with untreated hypertension.[5] This non-randomized, non-blinded study found that patients with preoperative diastolic blood pressures >110 mm Hg, regardless of pharmacologic treatment, commonly developed arrhythmias and/or severe intraoperative hypotension with associated myocardial ischemia. Patients with better-controlled hypertension behaved similarly to normotensive patients, with no hypotensive or ischemic events.[5] Stone and colleagues evaluated surgical patients without overt CAD, and with treated and untreated mild to moderate hypertension (between 160/90 and 200/100 mm Hg).[16] They detected intraoperative myocardial ischemia in 11 of 39 untreated hypertensive patients and in 4 of 7 patients with hypertension treated with diuretics, but in none of 44 patients taking atenolol. Despite the fact that intraoperative ischemia was observed, no patients in either study suffered perioperative myocardial infarction or death. The small numbers of patients involved in these trials limit any significant conclusions.

Intraoperative hemodynamic instability and myocardial ischemia, however, have been associated with postoperative renal failure, CHF, cerebrovascular events, MI, and cardiac death. Charlson *et al.* found that prolonged intraoperative hemodynamic hypotension and/or hypertension is associated with increased risk of cardiac death, ischemia, and infarction.[17] Preoperative and intraoperative myocardial ischemia, often associated with hemodynamic instability, predicts postoperative myocardial infarction in coronary bypass patients.[18,19] And patients undergoing vascular surgery were found to have a 2.7-fold increased risk of postoperative cardiac events if they had intraoperative ischemia.[20]

Perioperative risks of end-organ diseases related to hypertension

Hypertension is a major risk factor for CAD, and CAD definitely increases perioperative cardiac risk.[7,8,13,20,21] Browner and colleagues found that concomitant hypertension was associated with increased in-hospital myocardial ischemia and death for patients undergoing non-cardiac surgery who had known CAD or high risk for CAD.[22] In patients surviving the initial hospitalization, hypertension was not independently associated with the occurrence of major cardiovascular events in the following 2 years.[23] The same group of patients were monitored for myocardial ischemia with continuous electrocardiograms before, during, and after surgery.[24] A history of hypertension, left ventricular hypertrophy, diabetes, CAD, and digoxin use were independent predictors of postoperative myocardial ischemia in a multivariate model. In turn, postoperative myocardial ischemia has been associated strongly with severe cardiovascular complications.[25]

Many patients have undiagnosed CAD. Up to 25% of MIs are unrecognized (or "silent"). Patients with unrecognized MI, however, have the same risks of recurrent MI and death as those with established CAD.[26] Thus, a significant number of hypertensive patients may show evidence of unrecognized MI as evidenced by pathologic Q waves on a routine ECG. At a minimum, such patients need careful evaluation of their cardiac risk as outlined in recent guidelines.[27]

CHF may result from systolic or diastolic dysfunction in hypertensive patients. The presence of CHF is an independent predictor of major perioperative cardiac complications and of postoperative CHF itself.[7,8,13,28] CHF is a syndrome, and many of the underlying causes are important surgical risk factors, such as CAD or severe aortic stenosis. Thus, identifying the underlying cause before surgery is very important if at all possible. At a minimum, treatment should be optimized prior to surgery.

Hypertension is a risk factor for both chronic renal insufficiency and cerebrovascular disease. A serum creatinine > 3.0 mg/dl was an independent predictor of cardiac risk in Goldman's original cardiac risk study.[7] The Revised Cardiac Risk Index from 1999, which revised Goldman's work, found that a serum creatinine > 2.0 mg/dl is an independent risk factor for major cardiac complications around non-cardiac surgery.[13] Similarly, a history of transient ischemic attack or stroke was also an independent predictor of major cardiac complications.[13]

The presence of LVH on the preoperative electrocardiogram (ECG), with or without ST segment depression, has an increased risk of perioperative myocardial infarction and cardiac death in 405 patients undergoing major vascular surgery.[29] As mentioned above, LVH in patients with CAD or at high risk for CAD is an independent predictor of postoperative ischemia.[24]

The Revised Cardiac Risk Index for major non-cardiac surgery,[13] found six independent predictors of major cardiac complications: high-risk surgery, history of ischemic heart disease, history of CHF, history of cerebrovascular disease, preoperative treatment with insulin, and serum creatinine >2.0 mg/dl. In a prospective validation study of this index, rates of major cardiac complications for patients with 0, 1, 2, or ≥3 of these factors were 0.5%, 1.3%, 4%, and 9%, respectively.[13] Hypertensive patients with end-organ damage are likely to have two or more of these predictors and are at significantly increased risk for perioperative cardiac events.

Summary of perioperative risks

Observational data indicate that hypertension does not independently predict perioperative adverse cardiac events. The studies, however, have small numbers of patients with severe hypertension. Severely hypertensive patients have significant hemodynamic instability and intraoperative myocardial ischemia, factors that are strongly associated with adverse events in other studies. Thus, patients with severe hypertension (>180/110 mm Hg) are felt to have significant perioperative cardiovascular risk. Patients with only mild to moderate hypertension, who are well represented in the cohort studies, have much less hemodynamic instability and ischemia, and do not show the increased risk. ISH systolic hypertension, even if mild, may increase surgical risk, but further study of its risks and the effects of therapy needs to be done. Lastly, hypertensive patients often have end organ damage leading to CAD, CHF, LVH, cerebrovascular disease, and renal insufficiency, all of which independently increase cardiac risk.

Preoperative evaluation of the hypertensive patient

A recommended preoperative evaluation of patients with existing or newly discovered hypertension is outlined in Table 8.1. The first step is a thorough history, including questioning the patient about diseases associated with hypertension, including CHF, CAD, renal failure, and cerebrovascular disease. Ask specifically about symptoms of these conditions, including chest pain, paroxysmal nocturnal dyspnea, orthopnea, and edema. Knowing about

Table 8.1. Recommended preoperative evaluation of hypertensive patients

History
Medical conditions: CAD, CHF, cerebrovascular disease, renal disease
Prior surgeries and complications. History of excessive bleeding
Social history: functional status, smoking, alcohol and drug intake
Review of systems: chest pain, shortness of breath, dyspnea, exertional
    capacity, edema, orthopnea, paroxysmal nocturnal dyspnea, paroxysmal
    sweating and/or headache

Allergies
General allergies and prior adverse reactions to anesthetic agents

Medications
Prescription and over the counter agents

Physical exam
Emphasis on cardiopulmonary exam: evidence of CHF

Laboratory and other tests
Electrolytes, blood urea nitrogen, creatinine
12-lead electrocardiogram

Other tests, if indicated by history or examination
Chest radiograph
Tests for myocardial ischemia
    exercise electrocardiography or echocardiography, pharmacologic stress
    nuclear imaging or echocardiography
Echocardiogram (suspected CHF or severe valvular disease)
Serum-free metanephrines (suspected pheochromocytoma)

these conditions and optimizing them prior to surgery are important goals. Patients should also be asked about symptoms of pheochromocytoma, including episodic headache, sweating, and tachycardia. This disease is discussed further below.

A complete list of allergies and medications, including over the counter preparations, is essential. Always ask about prior anesthetic adverse reactions and for symptoms of abnormal bleeding. The physical examination should include careful measurement of the blood pressure, and should focus on the cardiac and pulmonary exams. Look carefully for evidence of LVH or CHF, including a third or fourth heart sound, a displaced or sustained point of maximal impulse, an elevated jugular venous pressure, pulmonary crackles, and peripheral edema.

All patients with hypertension should get a preoperative 12-lead ECG to look for evidence of prior MI and LVH, which have important implications for cardiac risk. This ECG serves as a baseline tracing for comparison in the event of suspected ischemic events in the perioperative period. A chest X-ray should be performed if the history or physical examination suggests new or active cardiac or pulmonary disease.

Serum electrolytes, urea nitrogen, and creatinine should be measured prior to surgery to assess baseline renal

function and potassium levels. This is particularly important for patients taking antihypertensives known to cause hypokalemia or hyperkalemia, including thiazide and loop diuretics, potassium-sparing diuretics, angiotensin converting enzyme inhibitors, and angiotensin II receptor blockers. Hypokalemia can contribute to perioperative ileus and can potentiate the effect of non-depolarizing muscle relaxants. Although the data are not definitive, hypokalemia likely predisposes surgical patients to cardiac dysrhythmias.[30,31] Hyperkalemia can also cause life-threatening arrhythmias. Perioperative use of depolarizing neuromuscular blocking agents can cause acute rises in serum potassium levels of approximately 0.5 meq/l.[32] Thus, both hypokalemia and hyperkalemia need to be identified and corrected prior to surgery.

Lastly, all patients with hypertension need an explicit consideration of perioperative cardiac risks using current guidelines.[27,33] Based upon this consideration, further preoperative cardiac testing may be indicated.

Secondary hypertension

Secondary causes of hypertension must be considered when evaluating any patient with elevated blood pressure, including renal artery stenosis, primary hyperaldosteronism, Cushing's syndrome, sleep apnea, hypothyroidism, primary hyperparathyroidism, alcohol or other substance abuse, primary renal disease, and pheochromocytoma. With the exception of pheochromocytoma and hypothyroidism, patients with secondary hypertension do not appear to be at increased risk at the time of surgery. They nonetheless carry the same risks as patients with essential hypertension, including those related to uncontrolled blood pressure and end organ diseases. Surgery need not be postponed for diagnosis if blood pressure is reasonably controlled.

Hypothyroid patients undergoing surgery have increased rates of CHF, neuropsychiatric problems, and gastrointestinal hypomotility.[34] These patients are more susceptible to intraoperative hypotension, delayed recovery from anesthesia, hypoventilation, and increased sensitivity to anesthetic agents.[35] It seems prudent to delay elective procedures to allow treatment to a euthyroid state, especially with severe hypothyroidism.

Surgery in patients with unrecognized pheochromocytoma is extremely dangerous due to catecholamine release triggered by perioperative events, with a mortality rate approaching 80% in reported cases.[36] Thus, all patients should be asked about symptoms of pheochromocytoma, including the classic triad of episodic headaches, sweating, and tachycardia. Most patients with pheochromocytoma

Table 8.2. Classification of blood pressure severity[2]

Category	Systolic BP (mm Hg)	Diastolic BP (mm Hg)
Normal	<120	<80
Prehypertension	120–139	80–89
Hypertension		
Stage 1	140–159	90–99
Stage 2	≥160	≥100

will have two of these symptoms, which unfortunately are present in many patients without the disorder. Half of the patients have classic paroxysmal hypertension and most of the rest have persistent blood pressure elevations. Because pheochromocytoma can be a familial disorder, obtaining a family history is important.

The diagnosis of pheochromocytoma is challenging. Testing for plasma free metanephrines has a sensitivity of 99%.[37,38] The specificity of this test is only 89% and the prevalence of pheochromocytoma is very low (0.5 % to 4 %), so false-positive tests will be common. However, this test is a good initial screen for the rare preoperative patient who has signs and symptoms suggestive of pheochromocytoma, since it is crucial to identify the disorder prior to surgery. If it is normal, it essentially excludes pheochromocytoma. Given the high false-positive rate, further testing must be done to distinguish true-positives from false-positives unless metanephrine levels are very high. Although recommendations vary, a recent NIH Conference recommends plasma metanephrines and catecholamines as the next diagnostic step.[38] If either is positive, this should be followed by a glucagon stimulation test or clonidine suppression test. A diagnosis of pheochromocytoma by biochemical testing is followed by localizing imaging tests and surgical removal of the tumor. In the rare case when a patient has known pheochromoctyoma and surgery is emergent, specific interventions, including alpha-blockade and aggressive fluid management are used to treat patients in the perioperative period.[39]

Perioperative management of hypertension

Management of preoperative blood pressure

Hypertension management in surgical patients depends upon the urgency of the planned surgery and the severity of hypertension. The Seventh Report of the Joint National Committee on High Blood Pressure classifies hypertension severity as outlined in Table 8.2.[2] As noted above,

patients with severe hypertension (>180/110 mm Hg) are at increased operative risk for hemodynamic instability, arrhythmia, and myocardial ischemia. Thus, elective surgery should be delayed and oral antihypertensive therapy instituted or adjusted to control the blood pressure prior to surgery. The optimal duration of control prior to surgery is not known, but the adverse vascular system changes associated with severe hypertension can take 6–8 weeks to reverse. Thus, some recommend that control be maintained for several weeks prior to surgery.[6] This has not been prospectively studied, but is reasonable in situations where a delay of surgery will not cause harm. If a patient has severe hypertension and requires emergent surgery, treatment with intravenous antihypertensive agents can be started immediately and continued intraoperatively and postoperatively. For blood pressures <180/110 mm Hg, delaying surgery will not reduce risk, and patients can proceed to surgery. If time permits, however, getting improved control of mild to moderate hypertension by adjusting a patient's oral antihypertensive regimen is recommended.

Perioperative management of antihypertensive medications

In the late 1960s, some authors recommended that patients on chronic antihypertensive therapy have their medications withheld prior to surgery because of concerns about interactions with anesthetic agents and adverse cardiac effects.[40] Since then, however, it has become very clear that most antihypertensive medications should be continued up until the time of surgery to maintain blood pressure control and avoid adverse events. This includes taking the medications on the morning of surgery with small sips of water. Failure to do so can lead to withdrawal syndromes, severe perioperative hypertension, hemodynamic instability, ischemia, and death.[41–44] A discussion of specific agents follows.

Beta-blocking agents

Beta-blockers are beneficial during and after surgery. They reduce myocardial ischemia in normotensive and hypertensive patients, reduce arrhythmias during surgery, reduce mortality after non-cardiac and cardiac surgeries, and reduce hemodynamic fluctuations associated with recovery from anesthesia, laryngoscopy, and surgical stimuli.[45–53] Acute cessation of beta-blockers can cause a withdrawal syndrome that can lead to severe hypertension, myocardial ischemia and infarction, and death in surgical and non-surgical patients.[54–56] Beta-blocker withdrawal in non-surgical patients with hypertension has been associated with a transient fourfold increase in the risk of CAD.[57] Thus, there are many compelling reasons to continue beta-blockers perioperatively. For those unable to take oral medications postoperatively, intravenous beta-blockers should be substituted.

Clonidine

Clonidine, a central-acting α-2 adrenergic agonist, also has proven benefits in the perioperative period. In addition to its antihypertensive and sympatholytic properties, it also has sedative and analgesic effects. Studies have shown that *de novo* administration of clonidine or mivazeril (a newer α-2 agonist) in the perioperative period decreases myocardial ischemia, reduces anesthesia requirements, reduces postoperative pain medication requirements, reduces postanesthetic shivering, blunts the stress response to surgery, and improves perioperative hemodynamics.[58–65] Some studies, but not all, show that it may prolong the duration of anesthesia.[66–68] Patients on chronic clonidine therapy are likely to realize some of these benefits as well.

Like β-blockers, oral and transdermal clonidine have a well-recognized withdrawal syndrome, which can lead to hypertensive crisis, perioperative hemodynamic instability, arrhythmias, and myocardial ischemia.[42–44,55,69–71] This syndrome can start as early as 12 hours after the last dose. Thus, clonidine should be continued up until the time of surgery and resumed in the immediate postoperative period. If it is anticipated that a patient will be unable to take oral medications by 12 hours after surgery, oral clonidine can be converted to a transdermal patch preoperatively. As it can take 48–72 hours to get therapeutic drug levels after placing a patch, the conversion should be started 3 days prior to the surgery, while tapering the oral dose of clonidine to 50% on day 2 and 25% on day 3. The dose relationship between oral and transdermal therapy is not always equivalent, so a 0.1 mg per day patch is used first, except in patients on large oral doses, in which case one may start with a 0.2 mg or 0.3 mg per day patch.[72] Others have successfully used clonidine crushed and suspended in sorbitol or saline for rectal administration in the perioperative period.[73]

Angiotensin-converting enzyme inhibitors

Angiotensin-converting enzyme inhibitors (ACEI) prevent the formation of angiotensin II, a potent vasoconstrictor. The use of these agents has expanded greatly due to their demonstrated benefits for patients with hypertension, CHF, chronic renal failure, diabetic nephropathy, or CAD. ACEI discontinuation does not lead to a withdrawal syndrome, and the more commonly used long-acting ACEI can have lasting effects for 18–24 hours after the last dose. In several small studies, ACEI therapy has been shown to increase the risk of hypotension during anesthetic induction and increase pressor requirements after coronary artery bypass surgery (CABG).[74–80] To study this issue further, Coriat and colleagues randomized 51 vascular surgery patients on chronic ACEI therapy with enalapril or captopril to continue the ACEI on the morning of surgery or to withhold it for 12–24 hours preoperatively.[74] Among patients continued on the ACEI, 76% had severe hypotension during anesthetic induction that required ephedrine for correction, compared to only 20% of the patients in whom the ACEI was withheld. Importantly, no significant increase in preoperative blood pressure was seen in patients that had their ACEI held. Other perioperative events were not studied. Similarly, Pigott *et al.* randomized 40 patients on chronic ACEI therapy undergoing CABG.[81] There was no difference in hypotension on induction, but patients who held their ACEI did require more vasodilators postoperatively for blood pressure control, while those who continued the ACEI had lower mean arterial pressures, but did not require more vasoconstrictors. These two small studies do not give a clear answer as to whether ACEI should be held prior to surgery, and there is no clear consensus on this issue. If the ACEI is continued on the day of surgery, the anesthetist must be particularly vigilant for severe hypotension.

Angiotensin II receptor blockers

Angiotensin receptor blockers (ARB), which block the vasoconstrictive action of angiotensin II, are now commonly used for hypertension, CHF, chronic renal insufficiency, and diabetic nephropathy. Like ACEI, ARB have also been shown to cause significant hypotension with anesthetic induction.[82] In some cases, the hypotension is refractory to conventional pressor therapy with phenylephrine and ephedrine, and terlipressin has been necessary to maintain blood pressure.[82]

To evaluate the benefits of withholding ARB prior to surgery, Bertrand and colleagues evaluated whether holding chronic ARB for 24 hours prior to vascular surgery would reduce this hemodynamic instability.[83] Thirty-seven patients on chronic ARB therapy were randomized to hold the ARB on the day prior to surgery or to take the ARB 1 hour before anesthesia. When the ARB was held, there were significantly fewer patients with intraoperative hypotension. When hypotension did develop, the episodes were of shorter duration, were less refractory to therapy, and required lesser amounts of vasoactive drugs to maintain blood pressure. There was no difference seen in preoperative or postoperative blood pressure control. Thus, the available data indicate that it is reasonable for patients on chronic ARB therapy to withhold the drug on the day of surgery to prevent significant hypotension, although there is no clear consensus on this issue.

Diuretic agents

Diuretics are common and effective antihypertensive agents. Their use in surgical patients carries two major risks. One is the development of hypokalemia (from kaliuretic agents) or hyperkalemia (from potassium-sparing agents), with inherent risks of arrhythmias and ileus. The other is intravascular volume depletion, which can combine with the systemic vasodilation of anesthetic agents to cause hypotension intraoperatively. It is reasonable to withhold diuretics on the morning of surgery to decrease the risk of hypotension, but the clinician must carefully monitor patients' volume status and potassium levels in the perioperative period. Intravenous furosemide can be used in patients unable to resume their oral dosing.

Calcium-channel blockers

Calcium-channel blockers (CCBs) cause vasodilation by inhibiting intracellular transport of calcium through specific calcium channels. Although there is no significant rebound hypertension with discontinuation, some patients on CCBs for angina can infrequently develop coronary vasospasm or recurrent angina.[84–86] Because CCBs inhibit platelet aggregation, there is some concern about an increase in perioperative bleeding. One prospective observational study of 161 patients undergoing hip fracture surgery found that patients on CCBs had a significant twofold risk of receiving a transfusion.[87] A retrospective study of patients undergoing CABG also suggested increased transfusion requirements.[88] This data, however, needs to be validated in larger studies before recommending discontinuation of CCBs for this reason.

Thus, CCBs should be continued in the perioperative period for blood pressure control, as long as there is no hypotension or severe bradycardia. Given the lack of a significant withdrawal syndrome, other parenteral medications can be used in the place of CCBs for patients unable to take the oral preparations postoperatively. Patients who have been on CCBs for angina pectoris or vasospastic angina should be continued on them or observed very carefully for evidence of worsening angina. An intravenous CCB, nicardipine, is available for use in the perioperative period.

Other agents

Occasionally, patients will be taking older antihypertensive agents. Withdrawal syndromes and adverse outcomes have been associated with methyldopa, guanabenz, reserpine, and hydralazine.[41,43] Thus, these agents should be continued in the perioperative period. If patients are unable to take oral medications postoperatively, hydralazine and methyldopa can be administered parenterally. Reserpine and guanabenz do not have parenteral preparations, and thus tapering off of these medications prior to surgery can be considered. Many other antihypertensive agents with better side effect and dosing profiles can be used in their place.

Minoxidil is a potent vasodilator that can lead to significant volume retention and reflex tachycardia. Thus, beta-blockers and diuretics are often coadministered with this drug. One case series has reported rebound hypertension with rapid discontinuation of minoxidil in children,[89] and patients on this agent usually have severe hypertension. Thus, it should be continued in the perioperative period whenever possible. There is no parenteral preparation of minoxidil.

Newly diagnosed hypertension

Making a new diagnosis of hypertension during a preoperative evaluation is common. The preoperative risk assessment, evaluation, and initial blood pressure goals are the same as those outlined above. All patients should start lifestyle modifications.[2] Patients with severe hypertension (BP > 180/110) need pharmacologic therapy for preoperative blood pressure control. All other patients that do not reach their goal blood pressure with lifestyle modifications alone should be started on medication, with most patients requiring two or more agents to achieve their goals.[2]

The recommended first-line antihypertensive agents for most patients are thiazide-type diuretics.[2] Meta-analysis has shown that low-dose diuretics prevent stroke, CHF, CAD, and death, while β-blockers prevent stroke and CHF.[90] One recent major randomized trial compared a thiazide diuretic (chlorthalidone) to an α-blocker (doxazosin), an ACEI (lisinopril), and a dihydropyridine CCB (amlodipine) as first-line therapy for hypertension.[91] No difference between the groups was found for the primary endpoint of fatal CAD or non-fatal MI. Chlorthalidone-treated patients had lower rates of CHF than the other agents, and patients in the lisinopril group had higher rates of cardiovascular disease (defined as CAD, stroke, CHF, or peripheral arterial disease) and stroke as compared to chlorthalidone. Another recent trial that randomized patients to first-line therapy with either a diuretic (hydrochlorothiazide) or an ACEI (enalapril) gave contrasting results. It found that patients on enalapril had borderline significant reductions in a combined endpoint of death or cardiovascular events, and that this benefit was restricted to male patients. Given these results, it is reasonable to start a thiazide diuretic as first-line therapy in most hypertensive patients without comorbid conditions, although ACEI can be considered for men.

Comorbid conditions may dictate using other agents as first-line therapy. Diabetes with proteinuria, non-diabetic renal insufficiency, and systolic CHF are all indications for an ACEI, or an ARB if they cannot tolerate the ACEI. CAD, especially a history of MI, is an indication for β-blocker therapy.[2] Patients with a normal LVEF who are at higher risk for CAD (i.e., with diabetes or peripheral arterial disease plus another cardiac risk factor) have a reduction of mortality, CAD events, and stroke when treated with ramipril. Given the recognized benefits of β-blockers in the perioperative period, they are an excellent first choice for patients who will be started on therapy shortly before their surgery, particularly if they have other cardiovascular risk factors.

Use of β-blockers in hypertensive patients to reduce operative risk

Studies of the perioperative use of β-blockers in patients with, or at high risk for, CAD show significant reductions in ischemia, MI, and death.[48,51,52,92–94] Given these proven benefits, β-blockers should be given to these high-risk patients around the time of surgery unless contraindicated. The criteria for entry into Mangano's classic study of perioperative atenolol were the presence of CAD (MI, typical angina, or atypical angina with positive stress test) or high risk for CAD, defined by the presence of two or more risk factors, including hypertension, age >65 years, cholesterol >240 mg/dl, diabetes mellitus, or current tobacco use.[48] Many hypertensive patients are candidates for perioperative atenolol therapy based on this study. Other authors recommend a different set of criteria for the use of β-blockers using Lee's Revised Cardiac Index that does not include hypertension itself as a criterion.[95] Given their cardiac risks, all hypertensive patients should be screened against these criteria. Those meeting the criteria should be strongly considered for the use of perioperative β-blockade to reduce their operative risk.

Postoperative hypertension

As they emerge from anesthesia, many patients develop mild elevations in blood pressure and heart rate due to generalized arousal. A small subset of patients will have severe elevations in blood pressure, termed postoperative

hypertension (POH). Its onset is usually during the first 10–30 minutes after the end of anesthesia and most episodes are transient, although prolonged episodes do occur and present a greater risk for complications.[96] For all patients admitted to the recovery room, the incidence of POH is about 3%,[96] but incidences vary greatly from 3%–80% depending upon the population of patients being studied. Reported rates are much higher after CABG, aortic valve surgery, carotid endarterectomy, intracranial surgery, abdominal aortic aneurysm resections, and radical neck dissection. Pre-existing hypertension is a major risk factor for the development of POH.[9,11] POH has been associated with stroke, myocardial ischemia and infarction, hemorrhage and hematoma at the surgical site, disruption of surgical anastamoses, renal failure, arrhythmias, and death. Thus, monitoring for the development of POH and rapid correction when it occurs is important to reduce adverse outcomes.

Some POH episodes can be avoided by continuing blood pressure medications up until the day of surgery to avoid antihypertensive withdrawal, as discussed above. Many other factors can contribute to POH, including pain, anxiety, hypercarbia, hypoxia, volume overload, hypothermia, and bladder distension. The initial step in evaluating patients with POH is to look for these factors and correct them. If the hypertension persists, antihypertensive therapy should be instituted, usually with rapid-acting intravenous preparations.

Medications for postoperative hypertension

Since many POH events are of short duration and because hypotension can occur with the use of long-acting medications, the ideal antihypertensive agent for POH has a rapid onset, a short duration of action, an available intravenous preparation, and an easily titratable action. Many drugs have been used for POH, and Table 8.3 summarizes commonly used agents. These are the same drugs used for hypertensive emergencies. The choice of drug depends upon characteristics of the patient, the surgical procedure, and the experience of the treating clinicians with specific agents. Information about the drugs and considerations for specific disease states are discussed below.

Nitroprusside is the prototypical agent, with a rapid and easily titratable action. Although it is very effective, nitroprusside can cause several important adverse effects, and thus must be monitored closely. Nitroprusside can cause cyanide or thiocyanate toxicity, especially in patients with hepatic and renal failure, even at "safe" infusion rates.[97] Doses over 4 μg/kg per min can lead rapidly to cyanide toxicity. Thiocyanate levels and cyanide levels must be

Table 8.3. Intravenous medications for postoperative hypertension

Agent	Mechanism	Dose	Onset	Duration	Adverse effects and comments
Labetalol	β-blocker and α-blocker	20 mg i.v. over 2 minutes then 10–80 mg i.v. every 10 minutes to max 300 mg/24 h; or 0.5–2 mg/min i.v. infusion	5–10 min	3–6 h	Bradycardia, hyperkalemia, heart failure, heart block, bronchospasm, hypotension, nausea, severe hepatocellular injury. Reduce dose in hepatic insufficiency
Esmolol	β-blocker	Load 500 µg/kg i.v. over 1 minute, then 50–300 µg/kg/min i.v. infusion	1–2 min	10–30 min	Bradycardia, heart block, heart failure, bronchospasm, hypotension
Nitroprusside	Vasodilator	0.25–10 µg/kg/min i.v. infusion	Seconds	1–10 min	Thiocyanate and cyanide toxicity, hypotension, headache, nausea, vomiting, methemoglobinemia, rebound hypertension, coronary steal. Can raise intracranial pressure. Doses over 4 µg/kg/min can rapidly lead to toxicity
Nitroglycerin	Vasodilator	5–100 µg/min i.v. infusion	2–5 min	3–5 min	Headache, hypotension, reflex tachycardia, methemoglobinemia. Can develop tachyphylaxis. Best used in patients with myocardial ischemia
Nicardipine	Calcium channel blocker	Start 5 mg/h i.v. infusion, increase by 1–2.5 mg/h increments every 15 minutes (max 15 mg/h). Once at goal BP, reduce to 3 mg/h, titrate as needed. Usual dose 2–15 mg/h i.v.	1–5 min	3 h	Hypotension, tachycardia, headache, flushing, edema. Reduce dose in hepatic insufficiency
Enalaprilat	ACE inhibitor	1.25 mg i.v. every 6 h. Max dose 5 mg every 6 h for up to 36 h	30 min–4 h	6 h	Hypotension, renal insufficiency, angioedema. Response can be variable. Can be converted to oral therapy. Need to lower start dose in renal insufficiency to 0.625 mg every 6 hours
Fenoldopam	Dopamine receptor agonist	No bolus. 0.03–1.6 µg/kg/min i.v. infusion. Adjust at 15 min intervals	5–15 min	10 min–4 hr	Hypotension, tachycardia, headache, nausea, elevated intraocular pressure, flushing, contraindicated in sulfite sensitivity. Can increase GFR and urinary output in patients with renal insufficiency. Safety of concomitant use with β-blockers not clear

monitored closely with prolonged use. Patients on nitroprusside can develop coronary steal and reflex tachycardia, which can be detrimental to patients with CAD. Patients can also develop rebound hypertension when the drug is discontinued. Thus, alternative agents should be considered for patients with CAD, renal failure, or hepatic insufficiency.

Other less commonly used vasodilators include hydralazine, diazoxide, and nitroglycerine. All vasodilators can lead to reflex tachycardia, increased myocardial oxygen consumption, and myocardial ischemia. Hydralazine is less predictable than other agents, but can be used in pregnant women. Nitroglycerin is effective but less potent than nitroprusside. Patients on nitroglycerin have better coronary blood flow than those on nitroprusside, so it is a good choice in patients with myocardial ischemia and hypertension.

Labetalol is a combined α- and β-blocker that is given by either parenteral bolus dosing or continuous infusion. It can be converted easily to pill form when the patient resumes oral intake. It has proven efficacy and safety in POH.[98–110] Major side effects include postural hypotension, bronchospasm, bradycardia, and exacerbation of heart failure in patients with reduced left ventricular function. Life-threatening hyperkalemia can develop in patients with advanced renal failure,[111–113] so alternative agents may be more appropriate for such patients.

Esmolol is a short-acting β-blocker that can be used effectively in the perioperative period.[106,110,114,115] As with labetalol, esmolol can cause bradycardia, heart block, and worsening heart failure in patients with left ventricular dysfunction.

Fenoldopam is a newer selective dopamine agonist that is powerful and effective in treating hypertensive emergencies and POH.[116] It can increase intraocular pressure, and is thus contraindicated in patients with glaucoma. Reflex tachycardia is common, especially at high doses. Neither rebound hypertension nor tachyphylaxis has been reported. Fenoldopam may be preferable in patients with renal insufficiency. In studies comparing it to nitroprusside for severe hypertension, patients on fenoldopam had improvements in glomerular filtration rates, sodium excretion, and urinary output which were not seen in the nitroprusside-treated patients.[117,118]

Nicardipine is a fast-acting dihydropyridine CCB which has been effective in treating POH, and has few major side effects.[103,119–124] Because it can cause reflex tachycardia, it may be beneficial to use it in combination with a β-blocker in patients with CAD to prevent demand ischemia. Nifedipine, another dihydropyridine CCB, has been recommended in the past, but sublingual and oral capsules should not be used given their risk for severe, unpredictable falls in blood pressure. Such hypotensive episodes are linked to serious adverse events, including cerebrovascular ischemia, myocardial ischemia and infarction, conduction disturbances, and death.[125] Parenteral isradipine has been effective, but is not available in the United States.

Enalaprilat is the only available parenteral ACEI. Its onset of action can be delayed for up to 6 hours, especially after the first dose, so it is best used as an adjunctive agent for POH or hypertensive emergencies. It can be converted easily to oral enalapril once a patient resumes oral medications.

Intracranial surgery

Intraoperative and postoperative hypertension, but not pre-existing hypertension, are significant risk factors for intracranial hemorrhage after craniotomy.[126] After neurosurgery, patients have disturbed cerebral blood flow autoregulation, and hypertension can cause increases in cerebral blood flow, elevations in intracranial pressure, cerebral edema, and cerebral hemorrhage.[127] Antihypertensive agents used to treat POH can cause cerebral vasodilatation and subsequent increases in cerebral blood volume, which can cause a rise in intracranial pressure.[127] Drugs that cause cerebral vasodilation (e.g., sodium nitroprusside, nitroglycerine, hydralazine, and calcium channel blockers) can theoretically cause this adverse effect. Esmolol and labetalol do not increase cerebral blood flow, and thus are potentially beneficial in this setting. Both have been used to control blood pressure after intracranial surgery, and labetalol has been shown to improve intracranial pressure and cerebral perfusion pressure when added to nitroprusside.[106,107,114] Enalaprilat has also been effective in a small number of patients after removal of intracranial tumors.[128] Another small study that compared adding nicardipine or labetalol to enalaprilat showed that patients in the nicardipine arm had more hypotension, bradycardia, tachycardia, and treatment failures.[103] This study did not look at cerebral edema or bleeding complications. In general, aggressive management of blood pressure after craniotomy is recommended, and labetalol or esmolol have a theoretic advantage over other agents.

Coronary artery bypass surgery

POH is very common after CABG, affecting 30%–80% of patients. Left untreated, it is associated with hemorrhage, rupture of sutures, stroke, and myocardial ischemia. Many different antihypertensive agents have been used successfully, including sodium nitroprusside, nitroglycerine, β-blockers, α-blockers, ACEI, and CCB. Although nitroprusside has been commonly used, there is concern over its safety, as mentioned above. Nitroprusside can contribute to myocardial ischemia, and nitroglycerine and nitroprusside both can lead to intrapulmonary shunting and worsened arterial oxygenation. Indeed, changing from these agents to labetalol improves oxygenation in patients with high oxygen requirements after bypass surgery.[129] Labetalol can cause myocardial depression and other agents may be better in patients with reduced left ventricular function.

Carotid endarterectomy

POH very commonly complicates carotid endarterectomy (CEA) surgery, affecting up to 60% of patients. Two large retrospective studies found that 78%–80% of patients who developed POH had preoperative hypertension.[130,131] Additionally, Asiddao found that patients with poorly controlled preoperative hypertension (>170/95 mm Hg) were more likely to develop severe POH than patients with controlled preoperative blood pressures.[130] These and

Table 8.4 Goals of hypertension therapy[2]

Category	Goal (mm Hg)
Uncomplicated hypertension	<140/90
Hypertension in diabetes mellitus	<130/80
Hypertension in renal disease	<130/80
Preoperative blood pressure	<180/110
Ideal	<140/90
For CEA	<140/90

other studies also show that patients who develop POH are much more likely to develop both transient and permanent neurologic complications.[130–134] The treatment of POH after CEA requires rapid-acting intravenous agents. Published studies report successful use of sodium nitroprusside, nicardipine, and labetalol.[102,135,136] Thus, patients undergoing elective CEA need good blood pressure control prior to surgery to potentially reduce their risk of adverse events, and all patients must be monitored closely for POH. If POH develops, aggressive treatment is indicated to prevent serious neurologic complications.

Postoperative treatment of chronic hypertension

Patients can resume their usual antihypertensive medications as soon as they are able to take oral medications. Some patients will have a modest decline in blood pressure after major surgery, and may require less antihypertensive medication. Blood pressure returns to preoperative values within 2–4 weeks of surgery. The optimal duration of β-blocker therapy for reduction of cardiac risk is not known,[95] but should probably be continued for the duration of the hospitalization at a minimum. Many patients with a history of MI or angina should be continued on β-blockers indefinitely for cardiac risk reduction. Blood pressure goals for antihypertensive therapy are listed in Table 8.4, and are dependent upon comorbid conditions.[2] Most hypertensive patients are undertreated.[1] Thus, close follow-up with a regular provider after surgery is crucial to monitor and adjust medications for optimal treatment and the prevention of end-organ disease.

Summary

Hypertension is extremely common in surgical patients. Preoperative assessment requires an assessment of the risks of hypertension itself and the risks of concomitant end-organ diseases. All patients need an explicit assessment of cardiac risk and consideration of perioperative

β-blocker therapy. In general, patients with mild to moderate hypertension can proceed to surgery, while patients with severe hypertension should have procedures delayed if possible to allow preoperative control of blood pressure. Postoperative hypertension is common, especially after intracranial surgery, CEA, and CABG. POH can have significant complications and may require intravenous antihypertensive therapy for control and prevention of severe complications. After surgery, close follow-up and control of blood pressure is essential to prevent long-term complications.

REFERENCES

1. Association AH. 2002 Heart and Stroke Statistical Update. Available at: http://www.american heart.org/downloadable/heart/10148328094661013190990123HS_State_02.pdf. Access verified January 23, 2003. 2002.

2. The sixth report of the Joint National Committee on prevention, detection, evaluation, and treatment of high blood pressure. *Arch. Intern. Med.* 1997; **157**: 2413–2446.

3. Wolfsthal, S. D. Is blood pressure control necessary before surgery? *Med. Clin. North Am.* 1993; **77**: 349–363.

4. Prys-Roberts, C., Greene, L. T., Meloche, R., & Foex, P. Studies of anaesthesia in relation to hypertension. II. Haemodynamic consequences of induction and endotracheal intubation. *Br. J. Anaesth.* 1971; **43**: 531–547.

5. Prys-Roberts, C., Meloche, R., & Foex, P. Studies of anaesthesia in relation to hypertension. I. Cardiovascular responses of treated and untreated patients. *Br. J. Anaesth.* 1971; **43**: 122–137.

6. Fleisher, L. A. Preoperative evaluation of the patient with hypertension. *J. Am. Med. Assoc.* 2002; **287**: 2043–2046.

7. Goldman, L., Caldera, D. L., Nussbaum, S. R. *et al.* Multifactorial index of cardiac risk in noncardiac surgical procedures. *N. Engl. J. Med.* 1977; **297**: 845–850.

8. Goldman, L., Caldera, D. L., Southwick, F. S. *et al.* Cardiac risk factors and complications in non-cardiac surgery. *Medicine (Baltimore)* 1978; **57**: 357–370.

9. Goldman, L. & Caldera, D. L. Risks of general anesthesia and elective operation in the hypertensive patient. *Anesthesiology* 1979; **50**: 285–292.

10. Goldman, L. Cardiac risks and complications of noncardiac surgery. *Ann. Intern. Med.* 1983; **98**: 504–513.

11. Forrest, J. B., Rehder, K., Cahalan, M. K., & Goldsmith, C. H. Multicenter study of general anesthesia. III. Predictors of severe perioperative adverse outcomes. *Anesthesiology* 1992; **76**: 3–15.

12. Detsky, A. S., Abrams, H. B., McLaughlin, J. R. *et al.* Predicting cardiac complications in patients undergoing non-cardiac surgery. *J. Gen. Intern. Med.* 1986; **1**: 211–219.

13. Lee, T. H., Marcantonio, E. R., Mangione, C. M. *et al.* Derivation and prospective validation of a simple index for

prediction of cardiac risk of major noncardiac surgery. *Circulation* 1999; **100**: 1043–1049.

14. Aronson, S., Boisvert, D., & Lapp, W. Isolated systolic hypertension is associated with adverse outcomes from coronary artery bypass grafting surgery. *Anesth. Analg.* 2002; **94**: 1079–1084, table of contents.

15. Prys-Roberts, C. Isolated systolic hypertension: pressure on the anaesthetist? *Anaesthesia* 2001; **56**: 505–510.

16. Stone, J. G., Foex, P., Sear, J. W., Johnson, L. L., Khambatta, H. J., & Triner, L. Risk of myocardial ischaemia during anaesthesia in treated and untreated hypertensive patients. *Br. J. Anaesth.* 1988; **61**: 675–679.

17. Charlson, M. E., MacKenzie, C. R., Gold, J. P. *et al.* The preoperative and intraoperative hemodynamic predictors of postoperative myocardial infarction or ischemia in patients undergoing noncardiac surgery. *Ann. Surg.* 1989; **210**: 637–648.

18. Slogoff, S. & Keats, A. S. Does perioperative myocardial ischemia lead to postoperative myocardial infarction? *Anesthesiology* 1985; **62**: 107–114.

19. Slogoff, S. & Keats, A. S. Further observations on perioperative myocardial ischemia. *Anesthesiology* 1986; **65**: 539–542.

20. Raby, K. E., Barry, J., Creager, M. A., Cook, E. F., Weisberg, M. C., & Goldman, L. Detection and significance of intraoperative and postoperative myocardial ischemia in peripheral vascular surgery. *J. Am. Med. Assoc.* 1992; **268**: 222–227.

21. Ashton, C. M., Petersen, N. J., Wray, N. P. *et al.* The incidence of perioperative myocardial infarction in men undergoing noncardiac surgery. *Ann. Intern. Med.* 1993; **118**: 504–510.

22. Browner, W. S., Li, J., & Mangano, D. T. In-hospital and long-term mortality in male veterans following noncardiac surgery. The Study of Perioperative Ischemia Research Group. *J. Am. Med. Assoc.* 1992; **268**: 228–232.

23. Mangano, D. T., Browner, W. S., Hollenberg, M., Li, J., & Tateo, I. M. Long-term cardiac prognosis following noncardiac surgery. The Study of Perioperative Ischemia Research Group. *J. Am. Med. Assoc.* 1992; **268**: 233–239.

24. Hollenberg, M., Mangano, D. T., Browner, W. S., London, M. J., Tubau, J. F., & Tateo, I. M. Predictors of postoperative myocardial ischemia in patients undergoing noncardiac surgery. The Study of Perioperative Ischemia Research Group. *J. Am. Med. Assoc.* 1992; **268**: 205–209.

25. Mangano, D. T., Browner, W. S., Hollenberg, M., London, M. J., Tubau, J. F., & Tateo, I. M. Association of perioperative myocardial ischemia with cardiac morbidity and mortality in men undergoing noncardiac surgery. The Study of Perioperative Ischemia Research Group. *N. Engl. J. Med.* 1990; **323**: 1781–1788.

26. Sheifer, S. E., Manolio, T. A., & Gersh, B. J. Unrecognized myocardial infarction. *Ann. Intern. Med.* 2001; **135**: 801–811.

27. Eagle, K. A., Berger, P. B., Calkins, H. *et al.* ACC/AHA guideline update for perioperative cardiovascular evaluation for noncardiac surgery – executive summary. A report of the American College of Cardiology/American Heart Association Task Force on Practice Guidelines (Committee to Update the 1996 Guidelines on Perioperative Cardiovascular Evaluation for Noncardiac Surgery). *Circulation* 2002; **105**: 1257–1267.

28. Charlson, M. E., MacKenzie, C. R., Gold, J. P., Ales, K. L., Topkins, M., & Shires, G. T. Risk for postoperative congestive heart failure. *Surg. Gynecol. Obstet.* 1991; **172**: 95–104.

29. Landesberg, G., Einav, S., Christopherson, R. *et al.* Perioperative ischemia and cardiac complications in major vascular surgery: importance of the preoperative twelve-lead electrocardiogram. *J. Vasc. Surg.* 1997; **26**: 570–578.

30. Wahr, J. A., Parks, R., Boisvert, D. *et al.* Preoperative serum potassium levels and perioperative outcomes in cardiac surgery patients. Multicenter Study of Perioperative Ischemia Research Group. *J. Am. Med. Assoc.* 1999; **281**: 2203–2210.

31. Hirsch, I. A., Tomlinson, D. L., Slogoff, S., & Keats, A. S. The overstated risk of preoperative hypokalemia. *Anesth. Analg.* 1988; **67**: 131–136.

32. Koide, M. & Waud, B. E. Serum potassium concentrations after succinylcholine in patients with renal failure. *Anesthesiology* 1972; **36**: 142–145.

33. Palda, V. A. & Detsky, A. S. Perioperative assessment and management of risk from coronary artery disease. *Ann. Intern. Med.* 1997; **127**: 313–328.

34. Ladenson, P. W., Levin, A. A., Ridgway, E. C., & Daniels, G. H. Complications of surgery in hypothyroid patients. *Am. J. Med.* 1984; **77**: 261–266.

35. Edwards, R. Thyroid and parathyroid disease. *Int. Anesth. Clin.* 1997; **35**: 62.

36. Sellevold, O. F., Raeder, J., & Stenseth, R. Undiagnosed phaeochromocytoma in the perioperative period. Case reports. *Acta Anaesthesiol. Scand.* 1985; **29**: 474–479.

37. Lenders, J. W., Pacak, K., Walther, M. M., *et al.* Biochemical diagnosis of pheochromocytoma: which test is best? *J. Am. Med. Assoc.* 2002; **287**: 1427–1434.

38. Pacak, K., Linehan, W. M., Eisenhofer, G., Walther, M. M., & Goldstein, D. S. Recent advances in genetics, diagnosis, localization, and treatment of pheochromocytoma. *Ann. Intern. Med.* 2001; **134**: 315–329.

39. Kinney, M. A., Narr, B. J., & Warner, M. A. Perioperative management of pheochromocytoma. *J. Cardiothorac. Vasc. Anesth.* 2002; **16**: 359–369.

40. Crandell, D. The anesthetic hazards in patients on antihypertensive therapy. *J. Am. Med. Assoc.* 1961; **179**: 495–500.

41. Katz, J. D., Croneau, L. H., & Barash, P. G. Postoperative hypertension: a hazard of abrupt cessation of antihypertensive medication in the preoperative period. *Am. Heart J.* 1976; **92**: 79–80.

42. Bruce, D. L., Croley, T. F., & Lee, J. S. Preoperative clonidine withdrawal syndrome. *Anesthesiology* 1979; **51**: 90–92.

43. Houston, M. C. Abrupt cessation of treatment in hypertension: consideration of clinical features, mechanisms, prevention and management of the discontinuation syndrome. *Am. Heart J.* 1981; **102**: 415–430.

44. Brodsky, J. B. & Bravo, J. J. Acute postoperative clonidine withdrawal syndrome. *Anesthesiology* 1976; **44**: 519–520.

45. Prys-Roberts, C. Interactions of anaesthesia and high pre-operative doses of beta-receptor antagonists. *Acta Anaesthesiol. Scand. Suppl.* 1982; **76**: 47–53.

46. Prys-Roberts, C., Foex, P., Biro, G. P., & Roberts, J. G. Studies of anaesthesia in relation to hypertension. V. Adrenergic beta-receptor blockade. *Br. J. Anaesth.* 1973; **45**: 671–681.

47. Ferguson, T. B., Jr., Coombs, L. P., & Peterson, E. D. Preoperative beta-blocker use and mortality and morbidity following CABG surgery in North America. *J. Am. Med. Assoc.* 2002; **287**: 2221–2227.

48. Mangano, D. T., Layug, E. L., Wallace, A., & Tateo, I. Effect of atenolol on mortality and cardiovascular morbidity after non-cardiac surgery. Multicenter Study of Perioperative Ischemia Research Group. *N. Engl. J. Med.* 1996; **335**: 1713–1720.

49. Magnusson, J., Thulin, T., Werner, O., Jarhult, J., & Thomson, D. Haemodynamic effects of pretreatment with metoprolol in hypertensive patients undergoing surgery. *Br. J. Anaesth.* 1986; **58**: 251–260.

50. Pasternack, P. F., Grossi, E. A., Baumann, F. G. *et al.* Beta blockade to decrease silent myocardial ischemia during peripheral vascular surgery. *Am. J. Surg.* 1989; **158**: 113–116.

51. Poldermans, D., Boersma, E., Bax, J. J., *et al.* Bisoprolol reduces cardiac death and myocardial infarction in high-risk patients as long as 2 years after successful major vascular surgery. *Eur. Heart J.* 2001; **22**: 1353–1358.

52. Poldermans, D., Boersma, E., Bax, J. J. *et al.* The effect of bisoprolol on perioperative mortality and myocardial infarction in high-risk patients undergoing vascular surgery. Dutch Echocardiographic Cardiac Risk Evaluation Applying Stress Echocardiography Study Group. *N. Engl. J. Med.* 1999; **341**: 1789–1794.

53. Low, J. M., Harvey, J. T., Prys-Roberts, C., & Dagnino, J. Studies of anaesthesia in relation to hypertension. VII: Adrenergic responses to laryngoscopy. *Br. J. Anaesth.* 1986; **58**: 471–477.

54. Goldman, L. Noncardiac surgery in patients receiving propranolol. Case reports and recommended approach. *Arch. Intern. Med.* 1981; **141**: 193–196.

55. Hart, G. R. & Anderson, R. J. Withdrawal syndromes and the cessation of antihypertensive therapy. *Arch. Intern. Med.* 1981; **141**: 1125–1127.

56. Shammash, J. B., Trost, J. C., Gold, J. M., Berlin, J. A., Golden, M. A., & Kimmel, S. E. Perioperative beta-blocker withdrawal and mortality in vascular surgical patients. *Am. Heart J.* 2001; **141**: 148–153.

57. Psaty, B. M., Koepsell, T. D., Wagner, E. H., LoGerfo, J. P., & Inui, T. S. The relative risk of incident coronary heart disease associated with recently stopping the use of beta-blockers. *J. Am. Med. Assoc.* 1990; **263**: 1653–1657.

58. Buggy, D., Higgins, P., Moran, C., O'Donovan, F., & McCarroll, M. Clonidine at induction reduces shivering after general anaesthesia. *Can. J. Anaesth.* 1997; **44**: 263–267.

59. Dorman, B. H., Zucker, J. R., Verrier, E. D., Gartman, D. M., & Slachman, F. N. Clonidine improves perioperative myocardial ischemia, reduces anesthetic requirement, and alters hemodynamic parameters in patients undergoing coronary artery bypass surgery. *J. Cardiothorac. Vasc. Anesth.* 1993; **7**: 386–395.

60. Dorman, T., Clarkson, K., Rosenfeld, B. A., Shanholtz, C., Lipsett, P. A., & Breslow, M. J. Effects of clonidine on prolonged postoperative sympathetic response. *Crit. Care Med.* 1997; **25**: 1147–1152.

61. Ellis, J. E., Drijvers, G., Pedlow, S. *et al.* Premedication with oral and transdermal clonidine provides safe and efficacious postoperative sympatholysis. *Anesth. Analg.* 1994; **79**: 1133–1140.

62. Goyagi, T., Tanaka, M., & Nishikawa, T. Oral clonidine premedication reduces induction dose and prolongs awakening time from propofol-nitrous oxide anesthesia. *Can. J. Anaesth.* 1999; **46**: 894–896.

63. Howie, M. B., Hiestand, D. C., Jopling, M. W., Romanelli, V. A., Kelly, W. B., & McSweeney, T. D. Effect of oral clonidine premedication on anesthetic requirement, hormonal response, hemodynamics, and recovery in coronary artery bypass graft surgery patients. *J. Clin. Anesth.* 1996; **8**: 263–272.

64. Stuhmeier, K. D., Mainzer, B., Cierpka, J., Sandmann, W., & Tarnow, J. Small, oral dose of clonidine reduces the incidence of intraoperative myocardial ischemia in patients having vascular surgery. *Anesthesiology* 1996; **85**: 706–712.

65. Zalunardo, M. P., Zollinger, A., Spahn, D. R., Seifert, B., & Pasch, T. Preoperative clonidine attenuates stress response during emergence from anesthesia. *J. Clin. Anesth.* 2000; **12**: 343–349.

66. Goyagi, T., Tanaka, M., & Nishikawa, T. Oral clonidine premedication reduces the awakening concentration of isoflurane. *Anesth. Analg.* 1998; **86**: 410–413.

67. Bellaiche, S., Bonnet, F., Sperandio, M., Lerouge, P., Cannet, G., & Roujas, F. Clonidine does not delay recovery from anaesthesia. *Br. J. Anaesth.* 1991; **66**: 353–357.

68. Higuchi, H., Adachi, Y., Arimura, S., Ogata, M., & Satoh, T. Oral clonidine premedication reduces the awakening concentration of propofol. *Anesth. Analg.* 2002; **94**: 609–614; table of contents.

69. O'Connor, D. E. Accelerated acute clonidine withdrawal syndrome during coronary artery bypass surgery. A case report. *Br. J. Anaesth.* 1981; **53**: 431–433.

70. Kaukinen, S., Kaukinen, L., & Eerola, R. Preoperative and postoperative use of clonidine with neurolept anaesthesia. *Acta Anaesthesiol. Scand.* 1979; **23**: 113–120.

71. Schmidt, G. R. & Schuna, A. A. Rebound hypertension after discontinuation of transdermal clonidine. *Clin. Pharm.* 1988; **7**: 772–774.

72. Bernstein, J. S. Transdermal clonidine therapy for the perioperative period. *Anesthesiology* 1986; **65**: 451.

73. Johnston, R. V., Nicholas, D. A., Lawson, N. W., & Wallfisch, H. K., Arens, J. F. The use of rectal clonidine in the perioperative period. *Anesthesiology* 1986; **64**: 288–290.

74. Coriat, P., Richer, C., Douraki, T. *et al.* Influence of chronic angiotensin-converting enzyme inhibition on anesthetic induction. *Anesthesiology* 1994; **81**: 299–307.

75. Colson, P., Saussine, M., Seguin, J. R., Cuchet, D., Chaptal, P. A., & Roquefeuil, B. Hemodynamic effects of anesthesia in patients chronically treated with angiotensin-converting enzyme inhibitors. *Anesth. Analg.* 1992; **74**: 805–808.

76. Ryckwaert, F. & Colson, P. Hemodynamic effects of anesthesia in patients with ischemic heart failure chronically treated with

angiotensin-converting enzyme inhibitors. *Anesth. Analg.* 1997; **84**: 945–949.

77. Kataja, J. H., Kaukinen, S., Viinamaki, O. V., Metsa-Ketela, T. J., & Vapaatalo, H. Hemodynamic and hormonal changes in patients pretreated with captopril for surgery of the abdominal aorta. *J. Cardiothorac. Anesth.* 1989; **3**: 425–432.

78. McCarthy, G. J., Hainsworth, M., Lindsay, K., Wright, J. M., & Brown, T. A. Pressor responses to tracheal intubation after sublingual captopril. A pilot study. *Anaesthesia* 1990; **45**: 243–245.

79. Yates, A. P. & Hunter, D. N. Anaesthesia and angiotensin-converting enzyme inhibitors. The effect of enalapril on peri-operative cardiovascular stability. *Anaesthesia* 1988; **43**: 935–938.

80. Tuman, K. J., McCarthy, R. J., O'Connor, C. J., Holm, W. E., & Ivankovich, A. D. Angiotensin-converting enzyme inhibitors increase vasoconstrictor requirements after cardiopulmonary bypass. *Anesth. Analg.* 1995; **80**: 473–479.

81. Pigott, D. W., Nagle, C., Allman, K., Westaby, S., & Evans, R. D. Effect of omitting regular ACE inhibitor medication before cardiac surgery on haemodynamic variables and vasoactive drug requirements. *Br. J. Anaesth.* 1999; **83**: 715–720.

82. Brabant, S. M., Bertrand, M., Eyraud, D., Darmon, P. L., & Coriat, P. The hemodynamic effects of anesthetic induction in vascular surgical patients chronically treated with angiotensin II receptor antagonists. *Anesth. Analg.* 1999; **89**: 1388–1392.

83. Bertrand, M., Godet, G., Meersschaert, K., Brun, L., Salcedo, E., & Coriat, P. Should the angiotensin II antagonists be discontinued before surgery? *Anesth. Analg.* 2001; **92**: 26–30.

84. Gottlieb, S. O., Ouyang, P., Achuff, S. C. *et al.* Acute nifedipine withdrawal: consequences of preoperative and late cessation of therapy in patients with prior unstable angina. *J. Am. Coll. Cardiol.* 1984; **4**: 382–388.

85. Engelman, R. M., Hadji-Rousou, I., Breyer, R. H., Whittredge, P., Harbison, W., & Chircop, R. V. Rebound vasospasm after coronary revascularization in association with calcium antagonist withdrawal. *Ann. Thorac. Surg.* 1984; **37**: 469–472.

86. Subramanian, V. B., Bowles, M. J., Khurmi, N. S., Davies, A. B., O'Hara, M. J., & Raftery, E. B. Calcium antagonist withdrawal syndrome: objective demonstration with frequency-modulated ambulatory ST-segment monitoring. *Br. Med. J. (Clin. Res. Ed)* 1983; **286**: 520–521.

87. Zuccala, G., Pahor, M., Landi, F. *et al.* Use of calcium antagonists and need for perioperative transfusion in older patients with hip fracture: observational study. *BMJ* 1997; **314**: 643–644.

88. Mychaskiw, G., 2nd, Hoehner, P., Abdel-Aziz, A. *et al.* Preoperative exposure to calcium channel blockers suggests increased blood product use following cardiac surgery. *J. Miss. State Med. Assoc.* 2000; **41**: 752–756.

89. Makker, S. P. & Moorthy, B. Rebound hypertension following minoxidil withdrawal. *J. Pediatr.* 1980; **96**: 762–766.

90. Psaty, B. M., Smith, N. L., Siscovick, D. S. *et al.* Health outcomes associated with antihypertensive therapies used as first-line agents. A systematic review and meta-analysis. *J. Am. Med. Assoc.* 1997; **277**: 739–745.

91. Major outcomes in high-risk hypertensive patients randomized to angiotensin-converting enzyme inhibitor or calcium channel blocker vs diuretic: The Antihypertensive and Lipid-Lowering Treatment to Prevent Heart Attack Trial (ALLHAT). *J. Am. Med. Assoc.* 2002; **288**: 2981–2997.

92. Raby, K. E., Brull, S. J., Timimi, F. *et al.* The effect of heart rate control on myocardial ischemia among high-risk patients after vascular surgery. *Anesth. Analg.* 1999; **88**: 477–482.

93. Wallace, A., Layug, B., Tateo, I. *et al.* Prophylactic atenolol reduces postoperative myocardial ischemia. McSPI Research Group. *Anesthesiology* 1998; **88**: 7–17.

94. Urban, M. K., Markowitz, S. M., Gordon, M. A., Urquhart, B. L., & Kligfield, P. Postoperative prophylactic administration of beta-adrenergic blockers in patients at risk for myocardial ischemia. *Anesth. Analg.* 2000; **90**: 1257–1261.

95. Auerbach, A. D., & Goldman, L. Beta-blockers and reduction of cardiac events in noncardiac surgery: scientific review. *J. Am. Med. Assoc.* 2002; **287**: 1435–1444.

96. Gal, T. J. & Cooperman, L. H. Hypertension in the immediate postoperative period. *Br. J. Anaesth.* 1975; **47**: 70–74.

97. Patel, C. B., Laboy, V., Venus, B., Mathru, M., & Wier, D. Use of sodium nitroprusside in post-coronary bypass surgery. A plea for conservatism. *Chest* 1986; **89**: 663–667.

98. Chauvin, M., Deriaz, H., & Viars, P. Continuous i.v. infusion of labetalol for postoperative hypertension. Haemodynamic effects and plasma kinetics. *Br. J. Anaesth.* 1987; **59**: 1250–1256.

99. Cosentino, F., Vidt, D. G., Orlowski, J. P., Shiesley, D., & Little, J. R. The safety of cumulative doses of labetalol in perioperative hypertension. *Cleve. Clin. J. Med.* 1989; **56**: 371–376.

100. Cruise, C. J., Skrobik, Y., Webster, R. E., Marquez-Julio, A., & David, T. E. Intravenous labetalol versus sodium nitroprusside for treatment of hypertension postcoronary bypass surgery. *Anesthesiology* 1989; **71**: 835–839.

101. Dimich, I., Lingham, R., Gabrielson, G., Singh, P. P., & Kaplan, J. A. Comparative hemodynamic effects of labetalol and hydralazine in the treatment of postoperative hypertension. *J. Clin. Anesth.* 1989; **1**: 201–206.

102. Geniton, D. J. A comparison of the hemodynamic effects of labetalol and sodium nitroprusside in patients undergoing carotid endarterectomy. *AANA J.* 1990; **58**: 281–287.

103. Kross, R. A., Ferri, E., Leung, D. *et al.* A comparative study between a calcium channel blocker (Nicardipine) and a combined alpha-beta-blocker (Labetalol) for the control of emergence hypertension during craniotomy for tumor surgery. *Anesth. Analg.* 2000; **91**: 904–909.

104. Leslie, J. B., Kalayjian, R. W., Sirgo, M. A., Plachetka, J. R., & Watkins, W. D. Intravenous labetalol for treatment of postoperative hypertension. *Anesthesiology* 1987; **67**: 413–416.

105. Malsch, E., Katonah, J., Gratz, I., & Scott, A. The effectiveness of labetalol in treating postoperative hypertension. *Nurse Anesth.* 1991; **2**: 65–71.

106. Muzzi, D. A., Black, S., Losasso, T. J., & Cucchiara, R. F. Labetalol and esmolol in the control of hypertension after intracranial surgery. *Anesth. Analg.* 1990; **70**: 68–71.

107. Orlowski, J. P., Shiesley, D., Vidt, D. G., Barnett, G. H., & Little, J. R. Labetalol to control blood pressure after cerebrovascular surgery. *Crit. Care Med.* 1988; **16**: 765–768.

108. Orlowski, J. P., Vidt, D. G., Walker, S., & Haluska, J. F. The hemodynamic effects of intravenous labetalol for postoperative hypertension. *Cleve Clin. J. Med.* 1989; **56**: 29–34.

109. Prys-Roberts, C. & Dagnino, J. Continuous i.v. infusion of labetalol for postoperative hypertension. *Br. J. Anaesth.* 1988; **60**: 600.

110. Singh, P. P., Dimich, I., Sampson, I., & Sonnenklar, N. A comparison of esmolol and labetalol for the treatment of perioperative hypertension in geriatric ambulatory surgical patients. *Can. J. Anaesth.* 1992; **39**: 559–562.

111. Arthur, S. & Greenberg, A. Hyperkalemia associated with intravenous labetalol therapy for acute hypertension in renal transplant recipients. *Clin. Nephrol.* 1990; **33**: 269–271.

112. McCauley, J., Murray, J., Jordan, M., Scantlebury, V., Vivas, C., & Shapiro, R. Labetalol-induced hyperkalemia in renal transplant recipients. *Am. J. Nephrol.* 2002; **22**: 347–351.

113. Hamad, A., Salameh, M., Zihlif, M., Feinfeld, D. A., & Carvounis, C. P. Life-threatening hyperkalemia after intravenous labetalol injection for hypertensive emergency in a hemodialysis patient. *Am. J. Nephrol.* 2001; **21**: 241–244.

114. Gibson, B. E., Black, S., Maass, L., & Cucchiara, R. F. Esmolol for the control of hypertension after neurologic surgery. *Clin. Pharmacol. Ther.* 1988; **44**: 650–653.

115. Gray, R. J., Bateman, T. M., Czer, L. S., Conklin, C., & Matloff, J. M. Comparison of esmolol and nitroprusside for acute post-cardiac surgical hypertension. *Am. J. Cardiol.* 1987; **59**: 887–891.

116. Murphy, M. B., Murray, C., & Shorten, G. D. Fenoldopam: a selective peripheral dopamine-receptor agonist for the treatment of severe hypertension. *N. Engl. J. Med.* 2001; **345**: 1548–1557.

117. Shusterman, N. H., Elliott, W. J., & White, W. B. Fenoldopam, but not nitroprusside, improves renal function in severely hypertensive patients with impaired renal function. *Am. J. Med.* 1993; **95**: 161–168.

118. Elliott, W. J., Weber, R. R., Nelson, K. S. *et al.* Renal and hemodynamic effects of intravenous fenoldopam versus nitroprusside in severe hypertension. *Circulation* 1990; **81**: 970–977.

119. Goldberg, M. E., Clark, S., Joseph, J. *et al.* Nicardipine versus placebo for the treatment of postoperative hypertension. *Am. Heart J.* 1990; **119**: 446–450.

120. Efficacy and safety of intravenous nicardipine in the control of postoperative hypertension. IV Nicardipine Study Group. *Chest* 1991; **99**: 393–398.

121. Halpern, N. A., Alicea, M., Krakoff, L. R., & Greenstein, R. Postoperative hypertension: a prospective, placebo-controlled, randomized, double-blind trial, with intravenous nicardipine hydrochloride. *Angiology* 1990; **41**: 992–1004.

122. Halpern, N. A., Sladen, R. N., Goldberg, J. S. *et al.* Nicardipine infusion for postoperative hypertension after surgery of the head and neck. *Crit. Care Med.* 1990; **18**: 950–955.

123. van Wezel, H. B., Koolen, J. J., Visser, C. A. *et al.* Antihypertensive and anti-ischemic effects of nicardipine and nitroprusside in patients undergoing coronary artery bypass grafting. *Am. J. Cardiol.* 1989; **64**: 22H–27H.

124. Vincent, J. L., Berlot, G., Preiser, J. C., Engelman, E., Dereume, J. P., & Khan, R. J. Intravenous nicardipine in the treatment of postoperative arterial hypertension. *J. Cardiothorac. Vasc. Anesth.* 1997; **11**: 160–164.

125. Grossman, E., Messerli, F. H., Grodzicki, T., & Kowey, P. Should a moratorium be placed on sublingual nifedipine capsules given for hypertensive emergencies and pseudo-emergencies? *J. Am. Med. Assoc.* 1996; **276**: 1328–1331.

126. Basali, A., Mascha, E. J., Kalfas, I., & Schubert, A. Relation between perioperative hypertension and intracranial hemorrhage after craniotomy. *Anesthesiology* 2000; **93**: 48–54.

127. Van Aken, H., Cottrell, J. E., Anger, C., & Puchstein, C. Treatment of intraoperative hypertensive emergencies in patients with intracranial disease. *Am. J. Cardiol.* 1989; **63**: 43C–47C.

128. Tohmo, H. & Karanko, M. Enalaprilat controls postoperative hypertension while maintaining cardiac function and systemic oxygenation after neurosurgery. *Intens. Care Med.* 1995; **21**: 651–656.

129. Wood, G. Effect of antihypertensive agents on the arterial partial pressure of oxygen and venous admixture after cardiac surgery. *Crit. Care Med.* 1997; **25**: 1807–1812.

130. Asiddao, C. B., Donegan, J. H., Whitesell, R. C., & Kalbfleisch, J. H. Factors associated with perioperative complications during carotid endarterectomy. *Anesth. Analg.* 1982; **61**: 631–637.

131. Towne, J. B. & Bernhard, V. M. The relationship of postoperative hypertension to complications following carotid endarterectomy. *Surgery* 1980; **88**: 575–580.

132. Lehv, M. S., Salzman, E. W., & Silen, W. Hypertension complicating carotid endarterectomy. *Stroke* 1970; **1**: 307–313.

133. Hans, S. S., & Glover, J. L. The relationship of cardiac and neurological complications to blood pressure changes following carotid endarterectomy. *Am. Surg.* 1995; **61**: 356–359.

134. Wong, J. H., Findlay, J. M., & Suarez-Almazor, M. E. Hemodynamic instability after carotid endarterectomy: risk factors and associations with operative complications. *Neurosurgery* 1997; **41**: 35–41; discussion 41–43.

135. Dorman, T., Thompson, D. A., Breslow, M. J., Lipsett, P. A., & Rosenfeld, B. A. Nicardipine versus nitroprusside for breakthrough hypertension following carotid endarterectomy. *J. Clin. Anesth.* 2001; **13**: 16–19.

136. Skudlarick, J. L. & Mooring, S. L. Systolic hypertension and complications of carotid endarterectomy. *South Med. J.* 1982; **75**: 1563–1565, 1567.

Pulmonary

9

Perioperative pulmonary risk evaluation and management for non-cardiothoracic surgery

Michelle V. Conde, Ahsan M. Arozullah,[1] and Valerie A. Lawrence

University of Texas Health Science Center at San Antonio; San Antonio, Texas
[1]University of Illinois College of Medicine, Chicago, Illinois

Introduction

Pulmonary complications are among the most common causes of postoperative morbidity and mortality.[1-4] In one study of patients undergoing abdominal surgery, pulmonary complications were more frequent than cardiac complications and were associated with significantly longer hospital stays.[5] A cohort study of almost 9000 patients undergoing hip fracture repair showed that serious cardiac and pulmonary complications occurred at similar rates (2% and 3%, respectively) and were associated with similar mortality rates.[6] Additionally, a prospective study of patients, age 70 years, examined predictors of mortality up to 3 years following non-cardiac surgery and found that postoperative pulmonary complications were an independent predictor of decreased long-term survival.[7] These findings confirm the relative clinical importance of the incidence and associated morbidity and mortality of postoperative pulmonary complications.

The true incidence of pulmonary complications depends on the criteria used to define complications and on the type of surgery. The incidence ranged from as low as 5% to as high as 80% for upper abdominal procedures in some series.[2,3] In other series, the reported incidence of complications following upper abdominal surgery and thoracic surgery varied from 20% to 40%,[1] doubling in cigarette smokers,[8,9] and approaching 70% in patients with chronic obstructive pulmonary disease (COPD).[10] The criteria used to define complications in different studies have a significant impact on these estimates.[11] Some authors do not report any criteria for complications and others include clinically unimportant microatelectasis or arterial blood gas changes without clinical correlates as complications.[11]

There are different types of postoperative pulmonary complications, each with different clinical implications.

Atelectasis (from the Greek *ateles*, meaning imperfect, plus *ekatasis*, meaning expansion) occurs in essentially all patients who undergo general anesthesia. In most patients undergoing abdominal surgery, changes of microatelectasis develop routinely and do not delay recovery or discharge from hospital.[12] In high-risk patients, microatelectasis may progress to pneumonia, although atelectasis is not a prerequisite for pneumonia. Microatelectasis may also progress to diffuse, clinically detectable atelectasis that can involve an entire lobe or lung. Other pulmonary complications include retained tracheobronchial secretions; bronchospasm; bronchitis; pneumonia; pleural effusions; hypercapnia; and respiratory failure requiring mechanical ventilation. Small pleural effusions are frequently seen following abdominal surgery and resolve spontaneously in a few days.[13,14] Thromboembolic complications belong to a different pathophysiological family and are covered elsewhere.

Respiratory physiology during and after surgery

Many physiologic changes affect the respiratory system in the perioperative period. Characteristic alterations that occur in surgical patients undergoing general anesthesia include monotonous shallow breathing with loss of spontaneous deep breaths; decreased vital capacity and functional residual capacity (FRC) by 50% to 60% and 30%, respectively; increased work of breathing; and ventilation–perfusion mismatch.[15] Diaphragmatic dysfunction may also contribute to decreases in vital capacity and functional residual capacity in operations with incision sites near the diaphragm, e.g., abdominal aortic aneurysm repair, thoracic surgery, and upper abdominal surgery. Although not clearly understood, reflex inhibition of diaphragm function during manipulation of viscera close

Medical Management of the Surgical Patient: A Textbook of Perioperative Medicine, ed. M. F. Lubin, R. B. Smith, T. F. Dobson, N. Spell, H. K. Walker. 4th edn. Published by Cambridge University Press. © Cambridge University 2006.

to the diaphragm, mediated by afferent vagal nerves, may result in mechanical failure of the diaphragm.[15] Postoperative pain and splinting and depression of mucociliary transport in clearing respiratory secretions also contribute to the development of postoperative pulmonary complications. These physiologic changes may not be clinically significant or may progress to overt complications in those patients with poor pulmonary reserve.

Premature closing capacity and/or decreased FRC pose a risk for the development of postoperative pulmonary complications.[16] Closing capacity is the volume at which the dependent airways begin to close. In young healthy persons, this occurs below functional residual capacity (FRC), which is the volume of air remaining in the lungs after a normal tidal exhalation. In certain circumstances, however, the closing volume occurs prematurely or FRC is decreased. Because of the increased closing capacity to FRC ratio, airway closure may occur before completion of a normal tidal volume breath, resulting in ventilation/perfusion mismatch. Non-pulmonary factors contributing to an increased closing capacity to FRC ratio include the supine position, sedative or narcotic drugs, obesity, increased abdominal girth (e.g., ileus, pneumoperitoneum, ascites), bindings around the chest and abdomen, incisional pain, muscle weakness, poor nutrition, immobility, and excessively high concentrations of oxygen for prolonged periods. Pulmonary factors contributing to an altered closing capacity to FRC ratio include interstitial edema, loss of surfactant with air space instability, airway obstruction due to inflammation with swelling of bronchial and interbronchial tissue, constriction of bronchial smooth muscle, and retained secretions. The ventilation/perfusion mismatch may lead to atelectasis and hypoxemia.

The preoperative assessment

The most effective preoperative pulmonary evaluation assesses operative risk as a function of the patient's clinical profile and procedure-related risk. If the history and physical examination suggest significant pulmonary or cardiac disease, further diagnostic tests may be indicated. Once risk factors have been identified, the management plan can focus on minimizing risks and preventing complications. Some risk factors may not be modifiable prior to surgery while others may provide targets for risk reduction. Although internists do not make recommendations on anesthesia or surgical technique, information from the preoperative examination will influence the operating team's decisions.

The clinical profile

General health status/functional status

Poor general health status and functional status predict increased pulmonary risk.[17–19] Using overall general clinical impression, the American Society of Anesthesiologists (ASA) Physical Status Classification scheme classifies the impact of systemic disease on functional activity and mortality.[20] Class II or higher is associated with increasing pulmonary risk.[17] Other studies extend the observation of poor general health and decreased functional status as a significant predictor. In one prospective study of patients undergoing high-risk surgery, patients who were unable to climb more than two flights of stairs, regardless of etiology, had increased cardiopulmonary complications.[21] Partially dependent or fully dependent functional status, again, irrespective of etiology, can confer approximately a twofold increase in the development of postoperative respiratory failure and a 1.8- to 2.8-fold increase in postoperative pneumonia.[18]

Obesity

Obesity is often associated with reduced lung volumes and an increased closing capacity to functional residual capacity ratio. In combination with anesthesia, these physiologic changes may result in worsened ventilation–perfusion mismatch.[22] The evidence on obesity's predisposition to increase postoperative pulmonary complication risk is mixed, however. Several studies reported obesity as a risk factor in the development of postoperative pulmonary complications; however, most studies did not control for other comorbid conditions, as shown in a critical review of the impact of obesity on postoperative pulmonary complications.[17] Two often cited studies of abdominal operations found obesity (BMI $> 25\,\mathrm{kg/m^2}$[23] and BMI $\geq 27\,\mathrm{kg/m^2}$)[24] to be a significant, independent risk factor; however, the definitions used for postoperative pulmonary complications in these studies were broad and included atelectasis. In the first study,[23] atelectasis clearly comprised the majority of pulmonary complications (87.5%) and the same may well have been true in the other study.[24] Atelectasis is extremely common after abdominal operations and in neither study was there an attempt to define clinically important atelectasis. A high prevalence of atelectasis and potentially clinically unimportant atelectasis may have overestimated the strength of obesity as a risk factor for significant postoperative pulmonary complications. Other studies showed no increased postoperative pulmonary complication risk in obese patients compared with non-obese patients undergoing laparoscopic cholecystectomy[25] or gastric bypass,[26] cardiac,[27] or thoracic surgeries.[28] In a large cohort of almost 3000 patients undergoing elective non-cardiac surgery, there was no associated increase in postoperative pulmonary complications among patients with BMI $\geq 30\,kg/m^2$ vs. patients with BMI $20\,kg/m^2$ to $29\,kg/m^2$ after adjusting for several factors, including smoking history and comorbid diseases.[29] Thus, the balance of evidence suggests that obesity is not an independent risk factor for significant postoperative pulmonary complications.

Tobacco use

Cigarette smoking is associated with an increase in tracheobronchial secretions and depressed mucociliary clearance.[30] It is a well-established risk factor for postoperative pulmonary complications.[17-19,24,31] In patients undergoing abdominal surgery, smoking is associated with an increased relative risk for postoperative pulmonary complications of 1.4 to 4.3.[17] Smoking history ≥ 20–40 pack years,[32,33] even in the absence of chronic bronchitis or airflow obstruction, is associated with a higher incidence of postoperative pulmonary complications compared with non-smokers.

Pre-existing respiratory disease

Clinicians should seek diverse information regarding pulmonary symptoms and disease: history of obstructive lung disease (e.g., bronchitis, emphysema, or asthma); amount of sputum production; airway disease, e.g., cystic fibrosis, bronchiectasis, or recurrent pneumonias, particularly in the same lung region; obstructive sleep apnea; environmental or occupational exposure; prior surgery and associated respiratory difficulty; old chest injuries; and use of pulmonary or cardiac medications.

COPD

The incidence of postoperative pulmonary complications is increased among patients with COPD. The degree of risk attributable to COPD is difficult to estimate, however, because many relevant studies were retrospective or poorly designed, and the diagnosis of COPD was based on variable criteria.[11] In general, the relative risks range from 2.7–4.7.[17]

Preoperative sputum production

Preoperative sputum production is also a risk factor for postoperative pulmonary complications.[34-36] It has been variably defined, with one study defining it as sputum production for 3 or more months of the year.[34] In another study, preoperative sputum production of greater than 60 ml in 24 hours identified patients who were at higher risk for postoperative pulmonary complications.[36]

Asthma

It is important to document a history of asthma because intravenous agents used in induction have varying risk for inducing wheezing;[37] however, patients with well-compensated asthma are not at substantially increased risk for developing postoperative pulmonary complications. As an example, in 706 patients with asthma undergoing surgery with modern anesthesia techniques, the frequency of bronchospasm was only 1.7%; two patients developed intraoperative laryngospasm.[38] These complications were not associated with significant morbidity. There were no in-hospital deaths or episodes of pneumonia or pneumothorax.

Obstructive sleep apnea

In a case-control study of patients undergoing hip or knee replacement, obstructive sleep apnea was associated with an increased risk in the development of postoperative acute hypercapnea.[39] This complication was most often seen in the first 24 hours postoperatively.

Chest radiographs

The evidence is clear that routine screening preoperative chest radiographs in healthy individuals rarely identifies abnormalities that are new, delay surgery, or change the perioperative management plans. In a meta-analysis of studies of routine chest radiography in North American or European populations, 14 390 preoperative chest radiographs were reviewed.[40] Abnormalities were found in 10% of routine preoperative radiographs. In only 1.3% of radiographs were the abnormalities unexpected, changing perioperative management in only 0.1% of cases. A subsequent systematic review of the value of routine preoperative testing showed that preoperative chest radiographs led to a change in clinical management in only 0%–2.1% of patients.[41] Age >60 was identified as predicting an abnormal chest radiogram, although the specific clinical impact of these radiographic abnormalities was unclear.[42] Using multivariate analysis, one prospective multicenter study identified male gender, age >60 years, ASA class ≥ 3, and presence of respiratory diseases to be significantly related to the probability of a useful preoperative chest radiograph,[43] with utility determined by the anesthesiologist's affirmative response to the question, "did the preoperative chest radiograph alter the anesthetic management?"

The continued use of routine preoperative chest radiographs in healthy individuals is a significant waste of health care resources. Preoperative chest radiographs should be obtained only to answer specific questions and provide usable information that will affect perioperative management. Specifically, it is reasonable to obtain preoperative chest radiographs in patients with underlying cardiac or pulmonary disease or for evaluation of new or changing cardiac or pulmonary disease on the basis of signs or symptoms.

Arterial blood gases

Older studies reported hypercapnea as a strong risk factor for postoperative pulmonary complications.[10,44] In these studies, patients with hypercapnea also had severe obstruction by spirometry. It was not clear if hypercapnea provided additional predictive value to the clinical history and physical examination. Subsequently, a systematic review[45] of blinded studies examining risk factors for postoperative pulmonary complications identified 3 studies[35,46,47] that evaluated the utility of hypercapnea as an independent predictor. None of these three studies found hypercapnea to be independently associated with an increased risk of postoperative pulmonary complications.

Less information is available for the risk attributable to hypoxemia. As with hypercapnea, older studies reported hypoxemia as a risk factor for postoperative pulmonary complications;[47–49] however, small sample sizes and lack of demonstrated added value to the clinical evaluation limited these studies. Hypoxemia as an independent risk factor for postoperative pulmonary complications is not evaluated in any large series.

In general, arterial blood-gas analyses should not be used to identify patients for whom the risk of surgery is prohibitive as there is no clear threshold that absolutely precludes necessary surgery. In patients with marginal lung function, preoperative arterial blood gas analysis may provide useful baseline information for perioperative management.

Pulmonary function testing

Although the history and physical examination are the cornerstones of the preoperative evaluation, pulmonary function testing, which can include spirometry, lung volumes, and diffusion capacity, is often used to document the presence of respiratory dysfunction and to measure its severity. Spirometry is used most often and has many virtues: it accurately diagnoses the presence and severity of obstructive lung disease and is non-invasive and fairly inexpensive. On average, groups of patients with worse pulmonary function have higher group rates of postoperative pulmonary complications; however, spirometry's yield in providing added value to the clinical examination in predicting individual operative prognosis is unclear.[11] An older critical appraisal of 22 studies evaluating the predictive value of spirometry for postoperative pulmonary complications after laparotomy found the

evidence to be conflicting and the methodology of most studies significantly flawed.[11] The methodological flaws included poor standardization, inadequate blinding of observers, selection bias, inadequate control for cointerventions, and inclusion of questionable clinical outcomes such as microatelectasis. The investigators concluded that spirometry's ability to predict individual operative prognosis was unproved.

More recently, a critical review showed that spirometry has, at best, variable predictive value in predicting postoperative pulmonary complications; and in the few studies that evaluated clinical findings and spirometric results, clinical findings were more predictive than spirometric results.[17] Lawrence et al. showed that abnormal results of lung examination (decreased breath sounds, prolonged expiration, rales, wheezes, or rhonchi), abnormal chest radiograph, cardiac morbidity, and overall comorbidity predicted postoperative pulmonary complications while spirometric results did not.[46] Barisione et al. did show that pulmonary function testing results were predictive of postoperative pulmonary complications; however, they were weakly predictive compared with the history of chronic mucous hypersecretion, which was a stronger independent predictor.[34]

No single spirometric variable consistently correlates with risk and there is no spirometric value that absolutely contraindicates non-cardiothoracic surgery. Many patients with poor spirometric function can be navigated successfully through surgery, as evidenced by a study of postoperative complications in patients with severe obstructive lung disease, defined as forced expiratory volume in 1 second, <50% of predicted.[50] Using explicit criteria for minor and major pulmonary complications, investigators examined 89 patients with severe chronic obstructive lung disease undergoing 107 operations of various types. Six deaths and two cases of non-fatal ventilatory failure occurred; but five of the six deaths occurred in patients undergoing coronary artery bypass grafting compared with one death after 97 non-cardiac operations. ASA class, type of procedure, and duration of surgery performed better in predicting postoperative pulmonary complications than spirometry. Additionally, in a retrospective cohort study with controls, Kroenke et al. showed that, while patients with severe COPD ($FEV_1 < 50\%$ predicted) did have a higher incidence of major pulmonary complications, this occurred only in patients undergoing coronary artery bypass grafting.[51] The subset of patients with severe COPD undergoing non-cardiothoracic surgery had a similar incidence of postoperative pulmonary complications compared with patients who had mild to moderate COPD and patients without COPD. In both studies, the authors concluded that severe lung disease as defined by spirometry was not an absolute contraindication to necessary non-cardiothoracic surgery.

In cases where spirometry did predict postoperative complications, the complications were usually successfully treated and did not cause additional complications. Warner *et al.* evaluated 135 smokers with an FEV_1 0.9 ± 0.2 l undergoing abdominal surgery and compared their clinical course to 135 smokers undergoing abdominal surgery without airway obstruction on spirometry.[52] In this study, a decreased FEV_1 predicted the development of postoperative bronchospasm; however, bronchospasm was successfully treated in all cases and did not prolong hospitalization. The duration of endotracheal intubation or stay in the intensive care were not affected. Definite pneumonia developed postoperatively in five patients with airway obstruction whereas only one patient without airway obstruction developed postoperative pneumonia; however, the authors noted that the frequency of pneumonia in both groups was insufficient for statistical comparison. Thus, spirometric results did not appear to add additional benefit in managing complications, unless it prompted physicians to have a lower threshold for recognizing and treating bronchospasm early. This potential benefit of spirometry has not been rigorously evaluated. Finally, an economic analysis concluded that overutilization of routine PFTs for assessing preoperative pulmonary risk for abdominal surgery was wasteful and that reduced use could generate substantial savings without compromising patients' outcomes.[53]

In summary, routine preoperative spirometry, even in the high-risk setting of upper abdominal surgery, rarely contributes additional, useful information to the clinical history and physical information for predicting postoperative pulmonary complications in individual patients. Preoperative spirometry is indicated for further diagnostic evaluation of patients with unexplained dyspnea or chronic cough. Preoperative spirometry may also be indicated for those patients with chronic obstructive pulmonary disease or asthma in whom airflow obstruction is not optimally managed.

Procedure-related risk factors

Surgical site, laparoscopic approach, and duration of anesthesia

There are several procedure-related risk factors that are important in the development of postoperative pulmonary complications, including surgical site, laparoscopic approach, and duration of anesthesia. The strongest procedure-related risk factor is the type of surgery. Incisions closest to the diaphragm are associated with the greatest risk for postoperative pulmonary complications.[17–19] Thus, cardiothoracic surgery, abdominal aortic aneurysm repairs, and upper abdominal operations are associated with the highest risk. A systematic review comparing the effectiveness of laparoscopic cholecystectomy versus open cholecystectomy showed that laparoscopic cholecystectomy was associated with less deterioration in postoperative pulmonary function (e.g., pulmonary function testing results, for example); however, no definitive conclusion could be reached for clinically significant postoperative pulmonary complications.[54] Duration of anesthesia 2 to 6 hours or longer is a consistent risk factor cited in the literature.[35,45,47,50,55]

Route of anesthesia

Epidural or spinal anesthesia may attenuate the surgical stress response and have beneficial effects on cardiac and pulmonary status;[56] however, several studies have reached mixed conclusions.[18,57–60] A systematic review of 141 trials randomizing 9559 patients to spinal or epidural anesthesia (with or without general anesthesia) vs. general anesthesia alone showed that spinal or epidural anesthesia was associated with a 39% reduction in postoperative pneumonia, 59% reduction in respiratory depression, and nearly a one-third reduction in 30-day mortality.[61] Decreased incidence of deep venous thrombosis, pulmonary embolism, myocardial infarction, renal failure, and transfusion requirements were also associated with spinal or epidural anesthesia. Many of the trials included in the meta-analysis were published before 1991, with samples of less than 50 patients. Changes in anesthesia techniques since 1991 may affect these results. Additionally, the spinal/epidural anesthesia group included patients who also received general anesthesia. While this meta-analysis showed that spinal or epidural anesthesia (with or without general anesthesia) was associated with decreased postoperative pulmonary complication risk and improved 30-day mortality, it may be difficult to isolate the effect of general anesthesia alone vs. epidural or spinal anesthesia alone on postoperative complications, given the increasing frequency of combined techniques and postoperative epidural analgesia.[62]

Long-acting neuromuscular blocking agents

Another procedure-related risk factor is the use of pancuronium, a long-acting neuromuscular blocking agent. Compared with intermediate-acting agents, pancuronium is associated with a higher incidence of postoperative pulmonary complications. A prospective, randomized trial comparing the incidence of postoperative pulmonary complications following the use of pancuronium compared with two intermediate-acting agents (atracurium and vecuronium) showed that the incidence of residual neuromuscular blockade was increased in the pancuronium group.[63] Those patients in the pancuronium group who developed residual neuromuscular blockade were four times more likely to develop postoperative pulmonary complications.

Postoperative nasogastric tube placement

A systematic review of blinded studies identified postoperative nasogastric tube placement as a predictor for postoperative pulmonary complications.[45] Nasogastric tube placement impairs the cough reflex and provides a more direct pathway for oro-pharyngeal bacteria to the lungs, thus potentially increasing respiratory tract infections. In one multivariate analysis of factors associated with postoperative pulmonary complications, postoperative nasogastric tube placement was the most powerful predictor;[35] however, the sample size and rate of postoperative pulmonary complications may not have been large enough to examine other potentially important risk factors and the predictive model has not been validated in other settings.

Risk indices

Previous risk indices developed for predicting postoperative pulmonary complications were limited to specific types of surgery,[64,65] relatively small sample sizes,[64] and lacked validation in independent settings.[24,35,64,65] Arozullah et al. recently developed two risk indices, postoperative respiratory failure risk index and postoperative pneumonia risk index, utilizing secondary analyses of a large surgical cohort of veterans.[18,19] The respiratory failure index was developed using a cohort of 81 719 patients from 44 Veterans Affairs Medical Centers and the Pneumonia Index was developed using 160 805 patients from 100 Veterans Affairs Medical Centers. Both indices were validated on separate cohorts similar in size to the original development cohorts. These risk indices included risk factors related to the patient's general health/nutritional, respiratory, neurological, fluid, and immune status as well as risk factors related to the operation and anesthesia. There were a high number of risk factors consistent between the two indices.

Consistent with previous studies,[17] the most powerful predictor in these risk indices was the surgical site, with abdominal aortic aneurysm repair, thoracic surgery, and upper abdominal surgery associated with the highest risks. These risk indices confirmed other previously established risk factors, including functional status, tobacco use, and COPD. They also identified additional risk factors including neurosurgical, vascular, and neck procedures;

elevated or very low blood urea nitrogen; preoperative blood transfusion >4 units; impaired sensorium; history of cerebrovascular accident; steroid use for a chronic condition; and increased alcohol intake. Furthermore, patients undergoing general anesthesia were at an increased risk compared with patients in whom spinal anesthesia or other anesthesia techniques were used. In contrast to the conflicting findings of previous studies regarding age,[17] each decade above age ≥ 50 was associated with increasing risk for postoperative respiratory failure and pneumonia. The effect of body mass index and spirometry on risk for respiratory failure or pneumonia was not evaluated during the development of the risk indices.

The major strength of these risk indices is that the large sample size enabled the investigators to examine many potential risk factors simultaneously and to validate their findings in independent samples. The main limitation is the use of chart review data from primarily male veterans, resulting in limited generalizability to other populations, particularly women. Nonetheless, these validated risk indices allow for a scoring system and risk class assignment that predict the risk of postoperative respiratory failure and postoperative pneumonia in a sizeable portion of the population. Table 9.1 displays the associated odds ratio for each risk factor. Table 9.2 displays the scoring system and risk classification.

Using blinded and independent comparisons of preoperative variables and postoperative outcomes, another prediction model rigorously evaluated the accuracy of the preoperative history and physical examination in predicting pulmonary complications.[33] Two hundred and seventy-two consecutive patients were referred for evaluation. Among the exclusion criteria were history of sleep apnea, intrathoracic surgery, and coexisting debilitating medical problems likely to preclude participation (e.g., cognitive impairment). Postoperative pulmonary complications were explicitly defined as respiratory failure, pneumonia, and atelectasis requiring bronchoscopy. Significant, independent predictors and their respective odds ratios (OR) for the development of these complications were: age ≥ 65 (OR, 1.8), smoking ≥ 40 pack–years (OR, 1.9), and maximum laryngeal height $= 4$ cm (OR, 2.0). Maximum laryngeal height is the distance from the suprasternal notch to the thyroid cartilage measured in end-expiration. In patients with obstructive lung disease, hyperinflation of the lung fields can expand the ribcage outwards and upwards, thus reducing laryngeal height. $FEV_1 < 1$ l/min, $FVC < 1.5$ l/min, and $Pco_2 \leq 45$ mm Hg were found to predict the development of postoperative pulmonary complications; however, no adjustment was made for clinical variables and not all patients underwent

Table 9.1. Comparison of the risk factors included in the postoperative pneumonia and respiratory failure risk indices[b]

Risk factors	Postoperative pneumonia risk index (Odds ratio (95% CI))	Point value	Respiratory failure risk index (Odds ratio (95% CI))	Point value
Type of surgery				
AAA repair[a]	4.29 (3.34–5.50)	15	14.3 (12.0–16.9)	27
Thoracic	3.92 (3.36–4.57)	14	8.14 (7.17–9.25)	21
Upper abdominal	2.68 (2.38–3.03)	10	4.21 (3.80–4.67)	14
Neck	2.30 (1.73–3.05)	8	3.10 (2.40–4.01)	11
Neurosurgery	2.14 (1.66–2.75)	8	4.21 (3.80–4.67)	14
Vascular	1.29 (1.10–1.52)	3	4.21 (3.80–4.67)	14
Emergency surgery	1.33 (1.16–1.54)	3	3.12 (2.83–3.43)	11
General anesthesia	1.56 (1.36–1.80)	4	1.91 (1.64–2.21)[c]	—
Age				
≥80 years	5.63 (4.62–6.84)	17	—	—
70–79 years	3.58 (2.97–4.33)	13	—	—
60–69 years	2.38 (1.98–2.87)	9	—	—
50–59 years	1.49 (1.23–1.81)	4	—	—
≤50 years	1.00 (referent)	—	—	—
≥70 years	—	—	1.91 (1.71–2.13)	6
60–69 years	—	—	1.51 (1.36–1.69)	4
≤60 years	—	—	1.00 (referent)	—
Functional status				
Totally dependent	2.83 (2.33–3.43)	10	1.92 (1.74–2.11)	7
Partially dependent	1.83 (1.63–2.06)	6	1.92 (1.74–2.11)	7
Independent	1.00 (referent)	—	1.00 (referent)	—
Albumin				
<3.0 g/dl	—	—	2.53 (2.28–2.80)	9
≥3.0 g/dl	—	—	1.00 (referent)	—
Weight loss >10% (Within 6 months)	1.92 (1.68–2.18)	7	1.37 (1.19–1.57)[c]	—
Chronic steroid use	1.33 (1.12–1.58)	3	—	—
Alcohol >2 drinks/day (Within 2 weeks)	1.24 (1.08–1.42)	2	1.19 (1.07–1.33)[c]	—
Diabetes – insulin treated	—	—	1.15 (1.00–1.33)[c]	—
History of COPD	1.72 (1.55–1.91)	5	1.81 (1.66–1.98)	6
Current smoker				
Within 1 year	1.28 (1.17–1.42)	3	—	—
Within 2 weeks	—	—	1.24 (1.14–1.36)[c]	—
Preoperative pneumonia	—	—	1.70 (1.35–2.13)[c]	—
Dyspnea				
At rest	—	—	1.69 (1.36–2.09)[c]	—
On minimal exertion	—	—	1.21 (1.09–1.34)[c]	—
No dyspnea	—	—	1.00 (referent)	—
Impaired sensorium	1.51 (1.26–1.82)	4	1.22 (1.04–1.43)[c]	—
History of CVA	1.47 (1.28–1.68)	4	1.20 (1.05–1.38)[c]	—
History of CHF	—	—	1.25 (1.07–1.47)[c]	—
Blood urea nitrogen				
<8 mg/dl	1.47 (1.26–1.72)	4	1.00 (referent)	—
8–21 mg/dl	1.00 (referent)	—	1.00 (referent)	—
22–30 mg/dl	1.24 (1.11–1.39)	2	1.00 (referent)	—
>30 mg/dl	1.41 (1.22–1.64)	3	2.29 (2.04–2.56)	8

Table 9.1. (cont.)

Risk factors	Postoperative pneumonia risk index (Odds ratio (95% CI))	Point value	Respiratory failure risk index (Odds ratio (95% CI))	Point value
Preoperative renal failure	—	—	1.67 (1.23–2.27)[c]	—
Preoperative transfusion (>4 units)	1.35 (1.07–1.72)	3	1.56 (1.28–1.91)[c]	—

Notes:

[a] AAA – abdominal aortic aneurysm; COPD – chronic obstructive pulmonary disease; CVA – cerebrovascular accident; CHF – congestive heart failure.

[b] Adapted from *Med. Clin. N. Am.*, vol. 87, Arozullah, A. M., Conde, M. V., Lawrence, V. A., Preoperative evaluation for postoperative pulmonary complications, 153–173, 2003, with permission from Elsevier. Adapted from Arozullah, A. M. *et al.* Development and validation of a multifactorial risk index for predicting postoperative pneumonia after major non-cardiac surgery. *Ann. Intern. Med.* 2001; **135**: 847–857, and from Arozullah, A. M. *et al.* Multifactorial risk index for predicting postoperative respiratory failure in men after major non-cardiac surgery. *Ann. Surg.* 2000; **232**(2): 242–253, with permission.

[c] Risk factor was statistically significant in multivariable analysis, but was not included in the respiratory failure risk index.

Table 9.2. Risk class assignment by postoperative pneumonia and respiratory failure risk index scores[a]

Risk class	Postoperative pneumonia risk index (point total)	Predicted probability of pneumonia	Respiratory failure risk index (point total)	Predicted probability of respiratory failure
1	0–15	0.2%	0–10	0.5%
2	16–25	1.2%	11–19	2.2%
3	26–40	4.0%	20–27	5.0%
4	41–55	9.4%	28–40	11.6%
5	>55	15.3%	>40	30.5%

Note:

[a] Adapted from *Med. Clin. N. Am.*, vol. 87, Arozullah, A. M., Conde, M. V., Lawrence, V. A., Preoperative evaluation for postoperative pulmonary complications, 2003, 153–173, with permission from Elsevier. Adapted from Arozullah, A. M. *et al.* Development and validation of a multifactorial risk index for predicting postoperative pneumonia after major non-cardiac surgery. *Ann. Intern. Med.* 2001; **135**: 847–857, and from Arozullah, A. M. *et al.* Multifactorial risk index for predicting postoperative respiratory failure in men after major non-cardiac surgery. *Ann. Surg.* 2000; **232**(2): 242–253, with permission.

preoperative spirometry or arterial blood gas analysis. Nonetheless, this study adds to the literature in that it more precisely quantifies specific elements of the history and physical examination useful for predicting postoperative pulmonary complications.

Perioperative respiratory management

After careful preoperative evaluation, the prevention and treatment of postoperative pulmonary complications involve both preoperative and postoperative care. Perioperative respiratory management may include: smoking cessation; use of bronchodilators; clearance of secretions; provision of respiratory physiotherapy; administration of preoperative antibiotics; education of patients; use of breathing exercises, including incentive spirometry; and oxygen therapy.

Cessation of cigarette smoking

Increased tracheobronchial secretions and reduced mucociliary clearance can contribute to the development of postoperative pulmonary complications in patients who smoke. Abstinence from smoking may result in gradual improvement in mucociliary function and decreased upper-airway hypersensitivity.[66,67] Patients have fewer postoperative pulmonary complications if they stop smoking before surgery, but only when abstinence is sustained for 2 months. In a cohort study of 200 consecutive patients undergoing coronary artery bypass grafting, patients who smoked for 2 months or less prior to surgery had a fourfold increase in pulmonary complications compared to those abstaining for longer than 2 months (57.1% vs. 14.5%).[31] Those who abstained from smoking for more than 6 months had a rate similar to patients who never smoked. Similarly, in a retrospective study of 288 consecutive patients undergoing pulmonary surgery, the risk of developing postoperative pulmonary complications after abstinence for 10 weeks was similar to that in never-smokers.[68]

Smoking cessation prior to surgery also yields additional benefits. In a randomized trial of 120 hip and knee replacement patients, patients were randomized 6–8 weeks before surgery to an intervention of counseling and nicotine replacement vs. standard care with minimal information about risks of smoking and smoking cessation.[69] Patients in the intervention group had significantly fewer complications overall, fewer wound complications, trends toward fewer cardiac complications and need for second surgery, and significantly fewer hospital days. Of note, there were few pulmonary complications in both groups.

A paradoxical increase in pulmonary complications was reported in a few studies with short-term smoking abstinence of less than 4 to 8 weeks prior to surgery or even reduced tobacco use immediately before surgery;[31,68,70] however, the studies had important methodological flaws. In summary, preoperative smoking cessation of at least 2 months appears to be associated with reduced risk of perioperative complications. Shorter cessation times do not appear to reduce risk. Physicians can use the preoperative examination to counsel patients on the overall benefits of long-term smoking cessation, realizing that maximum benefit most likely occurs with at least 2 months of smoking abstinence prior to surgery.

Management of underlying pulmonary diseases

Respiratory infection

In otherwise healthy adults with an acute, uncomplicated viral upper respiratory infection (URI) awaiting elective surgery, the risk of postoperative pulmonary complications is unclear. Several studies in the pediatric literature showed that children undergoing an elective surgical procedure with an acute URI had an increased incidence of laryngospasm, bronchospasm, or oxygen desaturation,[71–75] while other studies reported minimal morbidity associated with anesthetizing a child with an acute, uncomplicated URI.[76–79] As an example, one prospective study of >1000 pediatric patients showed that there were no differences in the perioperative incidence of laryngospasm or bronchospasm between children with active upper respiratory infections (defined as ≥ 2 of the following: rhinorrhea, sore or scratchy throat, sneezing, nasal congestion, malaise, cough, or fever <38 °C), recent URIs (within 4 weeks of surgery), and asymptomatic children.[78] There was an increased incidence of breath holding >15 seconds and oxygen desaturation (oxygen saturation <90%) in children with active and recent URIs, though none were associated with any long-term adverse effects. No study clearly addresses this issue in adults, but clinical prudence has resulted in the traditional recommendation to postpone elective surgery for an episode of upper respiratory infection. Elective surgery should be delayed for the treatment of bacterial respiratory infections. There is no proven role for the use of prophylactic antibiotics in high-risk patients without an underlying, acute bacterial respiratory infection.

COPD

In order to ensure that patients with underlying COPD are at their best possible baseline before anesthesia is induced, bronchodilators should be given to patients with signs and symptoms of obstructive airway disease. Data suggest that many patients may respond to bronchodilator medication in the laboratory if they are tested with sufficient frequency.[80] Therefore, bronchodilators should not be withheld because of lack of reversibility on one test occasion. As recommended by the Global Initiative for Chronic Obstructive Lung Disease (GOLD) Guidelines, standard maintenance therapy for patients with COPD in the non-operative setting includes inhaled bronchodilator therapy for symptom management and long-acting bronchodilators if drug therapy is required on a regular basis.[81] In patients with moderate or severe COPD, combining bronchodilators with different mechanisms, such as a β_2-agonist and the anticholinergic agent ipratropium, will provide synergistic effects and a more sustained improvement in FEV_1. A subset of these patients may also benefit from the addition of inhaled glucocorticoid therapy.[81] Theophylline is effective in patients with stable COPD; however, it has a narrow therapeutic window and is burdened with serious side effects, including dysrhythmias, seizures, and even death. Warning symptoms of nausea or tremulousness may not precede the development of toxicity. Theophylline clearance also is altered by many other drugs and is influenced by the severity of illness. Theophylline should not be used in the perioperative period unless significant benefit is anticipated. It has not been studied whether therapy with theophylline or aminophylline, which improves diaphragmatic contractility, can improve diaphragmatic function after surgery and thereby reduce the incidence of pulmonary complications.

Concurrent β-blocker therapy

Perioperative β-blockers are effective in reducing cardiac events in patients with known coronary artery disease or risk factors for coronary artery disease who are undergoing non-cardiac surgery.[82] Traditionally, some physicians may have avoided β-blockers in patients with reactive airway disease or COPD. A recent meta-analysis, however, concluded that, in patients with mild to moderate reactive airway disease, cardioselective β-blocker use was not associated with adverse respiratory outcomes compared with placebo.[83] The average baseline FEV_1 in patients who received more than one dose of a cardioselective β-blocker was $1.81 \pm 0.13\,l$. In another systematic review, the use of cardioselective β-blockers in patients with COPD did not result in significant changes in FEV_1 or respiratory symptoms, even in those with severe COPD.[84] Of note, the studies included in the review were small and of short duration (<12 weeks). Cardioselective β-blocker therapy is not contraindicated in patients with stable, mild to moderate reactive airway disease or chronic airways obstruction.

Steroid stress coverage

Surgical stress may precipitate adrenal crisis in patients with a suppressed hypothalamic–pituitary–adrenal (HPA) axis from chronic corticosteroid therapy. Patients who are receiving greater than 20 mg/day of prednisone (or its equivalent) for more than 3 weeks or patients with clinical Cushing's syndrome should be given stress doses of corticosteroids.[85] It is unclear if HPA axis suppression occurs in patients taking fewer amounts of corticosteroids.

For elective surgery, a cosyntropin test can be performed prior to surgery to evaluate the HPA axis or steroids can be administered empirically. Numerous regimens are outlined in the literature and are based on anecdotal reports; no rigorous comparisons have been performed. For major elective procedures, one traditionally recommended regimen has been 100 mg of hydrocortisone given intravenously at midnight before or on the morning of surgery; then every 8 hours through the first postoperative day, followed by 50 mg every 8 hours on the second day, 25 mg every 8 hours on the third day; and then the elimination of one dose each day as long as the patient remains stable. For minor procedures, 50 mg of hydrocortisone may be given before surgery and then every 8 hours for two or three doses, followed by rapid tapering of the dosage.[86]

Salem *et al.*, however, questioned the need for such high doses of perioperative glucocorticoid coverage based on their review of the available data on cortisol secretion rates and major surgery.[87] They concluded that cortisol secretion in the first 24 hours after surgery rarely exceeded 200 mg. Thus, some experts now recommend the following regimen:[88] usual morning steroid dose and no additional replacement dose for minor surgical stress (e.g., inguinal herniorrhaphy). For moderate surgical stress, the usual morning steroid dose should be given followed by hydrocortisone 50 mg intravenously prior to procedure and hydrocortisone 25 mg every 8 hours for 24 hours postoperatively. The usual dose of corticosteroids is resumed thereafter. For major surgical stress, the usual morning steroid dose should be given followed by hydrocortisone 100 mg intravenously before induction of anesthesia and hydrocortisone 50 mg every 8 hours for 24 hours postoperatively. The dose is then tapered by half per day to maintenance level.

Lung expansion maneuvers

Lung expansion maneuvers are designed to provide maximal alveolar inflation, increase the ability to empty the lungs without premature airway closure, and thus, maintain a normal functional residual capacity. Lung expansion maneuvers include chest physiotherapy, incentive spirometry, intermittent positive pressure breathing (IPPB), and continuous positive airway pressure (CPAP). Chest physiotherapy consists of various combinations of deep breathing exercises, percussion and vibration, postural drainage, cough, suctioning, and mobilization. Physical therapists and respiratory therapists are usually well versed in breathing exercises, and their incorporation into perioperative care should be considered, especially in high-risk patients.

No single method has emerged as the procedure of choice. Incentive spirometry can decrease postoperative pulmonary complications by approximately 50%, particularly in high-risk patients undergoing upper abdominal surgery.[89,90] Incentive spirometry, deep breathing exercises, and intermittent positive pressure breathing are equally efficacious.[90] One recent systematic review of the effect of incentive spirometry on postoperative pulmonary complications concluded that current evidence did not support routine incentive spirometry for the prevention of pulmonary complications following cardiac or abdominal surgery.[91] Many of the studies included in the review, however, compared incentive spirometry to other lung expansion maneuvers and not to a pure control group. In most of the studies evaluated in the systematic review, there was no difference between incentive spirometry and other methods, with the exception of continuous positive airway pressure (CPAP). CPAP may be superior in patients with difficulty performing deep breathing exercises or using an incentive spirometer; however, CPAP is expensive and may cause patient discomfort, gastric distension, and barotrauma.[92]

The optimal duration and frequency of deep breathing exercises or incentive spirometry is unclear. One recommended regimen utilizes deep breathing exercises with or without an incentive spirometer (8–10 breaths with a 3- to 5-second inspiratory hold) every 1–2 hours while awake followed by forced expirations and coughing.[92,93] The frequency is decreased as the patient becomes more ambulatory. Another regimen utilizes 10 breaths over 15 minutes with an incentive spirometer four times a day postoperatively.[89] Given that some form of intervention is superior to no intervention and no particular technique is clearly superior, choosing techniques is probably not as important as is motivating patients, educating patients regarding the desired goals, initiating patient education preoperatively, and having experienced personnel (especially respiratory therapists and nurses) provide encouragement and supervision.[94,89,92]

Postoperative pain control

Postoperative pain contributes to shallow breathing and interferes with spontaneous deep breaths and coughing, resulting in decreased lung volumes and atelectasis. Similarly, narcotic analgesics may increase the risk of postoperative pulmonary complications; they reduce the ventilatory response to hypoxia and hypercapnia in healthy persons.[95] Judicious and adequate pain control, however, may improve deep breathing.

Epidural analgesia provides improved pain control over traditional parenteral opioid analgesia.[96–98] While previous studies have reached different conclusions regarding the effects of epidural analgesia compared with parenteral narcotics on postoperative pulmonary complications,[60,96–99] there is increasing evidence that postoperative epidural analgesia may decrease postoperative pulmonary complications compared with parenteral narcotics. In a meta-analysis, Ballantyne et al. showed that postoperative epidural analgesia reduced postoperative pulmonary morbidity.[100] There was a trend towards improved pulmonary morbidity with intercostal nerve blockade compared with systemic opioids. Moreover, in a randomized trial of (a) combined general anesthesia with intraoperative epidural anesthesia and postoperative epidural analgesia vs. (b) general anesthesia and postoperative parenteral narcotics, combined general anesthesia with epidural anesthesia/analgesia decreased the incidence of postoperative respiratory failure, although there were no differences in 30-day mortality or

Table 9.3. Risk factors for postoperative pulmonary complications[a]

Patient-related	Procedure-related
General health and Nutritional status	Incision near diaphragm
Age	Thoracic surgery
Low albumin	Upper abdominal surgery
Functional status	AAA repair
Weight loss > 10%	Other types of surgery
ASA Class	Neck surgery
Goldman class	Peripheral vascular surgery
Respiratory status	Neurosurgery
COPD history	Emergency surgery
Tobacco use	
Sputum production	Surgery technique
Pneumonia	Open vs. laparoscopic
Dyspnea	
OSA	Anesthesia duration >2 hours
Neurological status	Use of spinal/epidural anesthesia vs. general anesthesia
Impaired sensorium	
CVA history	
Fluid status	
CHF history	Use of long-acting neuromuscular blockade (pancuronium)
Renal failure	
Low or high BUN	
Preoperative blood transfusion	
Immune status	Pain control with parenteral narcotics vs. epidural analgesia
Chronic steroid use	
Alcohol use	
	Postoperative NG tube placement

Note:

Abbreviations: AAA, abdominal aortic aneurysm; ASA, American Society of Anesthesiologists; BUN, blood urea nitrogen; CVA – cerebrovascular accident; CHF – congestive heart failure; COPD, chronic obstructive pulmonary disease; OSA, obstructive sleep apnea; NG tube, nasogastric tube.

[a] Adapted from *Med. Clin. N. Am.*, **87**, Arozullah, A. M., Conde, M. V., Lawrence, V. A., Preoperative evaluation for postoperative pulmonary complications, 2003, 153–173, with permission from Elsevier.

cardiovascular events.[101] In this study of 915 high-risk patients undergoing major abdominal surgery, the incidence of respiratory failure was 23% in patients managed with epidural techniques compared with 30% in those managed with general anesthesia and postoperative parenteral narcotics.

Conclusions

There are numerous risk factors for postoperative pulmonary complications. Some risk factors may not be modifiable prior to surgery while others may provide targets for risk reduction. Table 9.3 summarizes risk factors for postoperative pulmonary complications. Although internists do not make recommendations on anesthesia or surgical technique, information obtained from the preoperative examination will influence the anesthesiology and surgical teams' decisions regarding the patient's intraoperative and postoperative care. Effective communication among the various specialists and an interdisciplinary approach is important in reducing postoperative pulmonary complication risk.

REFERENCES

1. Bartlett, R. H., Brennan, M. L., Gazzaniga, A. B., & Hanson, E. L. Studies on the pathogenesis and prevention of postoperative pulmonary complications. *Surg. Gynecol. Obstet.* 1973; **137**: 925–933.

2. Latimer, R. G., Dickman, M., Day, W. C., Gunn, M. L., & Schmidt, C. D. Ventilatory patterns and pulmonary complications after upper abdominal surgery determined by preoperative and postoperative computerized spirometry and blood gas analysis. *Am. J. Surg.* 1971; **122**: 622–632.

3. Pontoppidan, H. Mechanical aids to lung expansion in nonintubated surgical patients. *Am. Rev. Resp. Dis.* 1980; **122**: 109–119.

4. Garibaldi, R. A., Britt, M. R., Coleman, M. L., Reading, J. C., & Pace, N. L. Risk factors for postoperative pneumonia. *Am. J. Med.* 1981; **70**: 677–680.

5. Lawrence, V. A., Hilsenbeck, S. G., Mulrow, C. D., Dhanda, R., Sapp, J., & Page, C. P. Incidence and hospital stay for cardiac and pulmonary complications after abdominal surgery. *J. Gen. Intern. Med.* 1995; **10**: 671–678.

6. Lawrence, V. A., Hilsenbeck, S. G., Noveck, H., Poses, R. M., & Carson, J. L. Medical complications and outcomes after hip fracture repair. *Arch. Intern. Med.* 2002; **162**: 2053–2057.

7. Manku, K. & Leung, J. M. Prognostic significance of postoperative in-hospital complications in elderly patients. II. Long-term quality of life. *Anesth. Analg.* 2003; **96**: 590–594.

8. Collins, C. D., Darke, C. S., & Knowelden, J. Chest complications after upper abdominal surgery: their anticipation and prevention. *Bri. Med. J.* 1968; **1**: 401–406.

9. Laszlo, G., Archer, G. G., Darrell, J. H., Dawson, J. M., & Fletcher, C. M. The diagnosis and prophylaxis of pulmonary complications of surgical operation. *Br. J. Surg.* 1973; **60**: 129–134.

10. Stein, M., Koota, G. M., Simon, M., & Frank, H. A. Pulmonary evaluation of surgical patients. *J. Am. Med. Assoc.* 1962; **181**: 765–770.

11. Lawrence, V. A., Page, C. P., & Harris, G. D. Preoperative spirometry before abdominal operations. A critical appraisal of its predictive value. *Arch. Intern. Med.* 1989; **149**: 280–285.

12. Platell, C. & Hall, J. C. Atelectasis after abdominal surgery. *J. Am. Coll. Surg.* 1997; **185**: 584–592.

13. Light, R. W. & George, R. B. Incidence and significance of pleural effusion after abdominal surgery. *Chest* 1976; **69**: 621–625.

14. Nielsen, P. H., Jepsen, S. B., & Olsen, A. D. Postoperative pleural effusion following upper abdominal surgery. *Chest* 1989; **96**: 1133–1135.

15. Trayner, E. Jr. & Celli, B. R. Postoperative pulmonary complications. *Med. Clin. N. Am.* 2001; **85**: 1129–1139.

16. Wahba, R. M. Airway closure and intraoperative hypoxaemia: twenty-five years later. *Can. J. Anaesth.* 1996; **43**: 1144–1149.

17. Smetana, G. W. Preoperative pulmonary evaluation. *N. Engl. J. Med.* 1999; **340**: 937–944.

18. Arozullah, A. M., Khuri, S. F., Henderson, W. G., & Daley, J. Participants in the National Veterans Affairs Surgical Quality Improvement Development and validation of a multifactorial risk index for predicting postoperative pneumonia after major noncardiac surgery. *Ann. Intern. Med.* 2001; **135**: 847–857.

19. Arozullah, A., Daley, J., Henderson, W., & Khuri, S. Multifactorial risk index for predicting postoperative respiratory failure in men after noncardiac surgery. *Ann. Surg.* 2000; **232**: 243–253.

20. Cohen, M. M., Duncan, P. G., & Tate, R. B. Does anesthesia contribute to operative mortality? *J. Am. Med. Assoc.* 1988; **260**: 2859–2863.

21. Girish, M., Trayner, E., Jr., Dammann, O., Pinto-Plata, V., & Celli, B. Symptom-limited stair climbing as a predictor of postoperative cardiopulmonary complications after high-risk surgery. *Chest* 2001; **120**: 1147–1151.

22. Ray, C. S., Sue, D. Y., Bray, G., Hansen, J. E., & Wasserman, K. Effects of obesity on respiratory function. *Am. Rev. Resp. Dis.* 1983; **128**: 501–506.

23. Hall, J. C., Tarala, R. A., Hall, J. L., & Mander, J. A multivariate analysis of the risk of pulmonary complications after laparotomy. *Chest* 1991; **99**: 923–927.

24. Brooks-Brunn, J. A. Predictors of postoperative pulmonary complications following abdominal surgery. *Chest* 1997; **111**: 564–571.

25. Angrisani, L., Lorenzo, M., De Palma, G. *et al.* Laparoscopic cholecystectomy in obese patients compared with nonobese patients. *Surg. Laparosc. Endosc. Percutan. Tech.* 1995; **5**: 197–201.

26. Pasulka, P. S., Bistrian, B. R., Benotti, P. N., & Blackburn, G. L. The risks of surgery in obese patients. *Ann. Intern. Med.* 1986; **104**: 540–546.

27. Moulton, M. J., Creswell, L. L., Mackey, M. E., Cox, J. L., & Rosenbloom, M. Obesity is not a risk factor for significant adverse outcomes after cardiac surgery. *Circulation* 1996; **94**: II87–II92.

28. Dales, R. E., Dionne, G., Leech, J. A., Lunau, M., & Schweitzer, I. Preoperative prediction of pulmonary complications following thoracic surgery. *Chest* 1993; **104**: 155–159.

29. Thomas, E. J., Goldman, L., Mangione, C. M. *et al.* Body mass index as a correlate of postoperative complications and resource utilization. *Am. J. Med.* 1997; **102**: 277–283.

30. Wanner, A., Salathe, M., & O'Riordan, T. G. Mucociliary clearance in the airways. *Am. J. Resp. Crit. Care Med.* 1996; **154**: 1868–1902.

31. Warner, M. A., Offord, K. P., Warner, M. E., Lennon, R. L., Conover, M. A., & Jansson-Schumacher, U. Role of preoperative cessation of smoking and other factors in postoperative pulmonary complications: a blinded prospective study of coronary artery bypass patients. *Mayo Clin. Proc.* 1989; **64**: 609–616.

32. Dilworth, J. P. & White, R. J. Postoperative chest infection after upper abdominal surgery: an important problem for smokers. *Resp. Med.* 1992; **86**: 205–210.

33. McAlister, F. A., Khan, N. A., Straus, S. E. *et al.* Accuracy of the preoperative assessment in predicting pulmonary risk after non-thoracic surgery. *Am. J. Resp. Crit. Care Med.* 2003; **167**: 741–744.

34. Barisione, G., Rovida, S., Gazzaniga, G. M., & Fontana, L. Upper abdominal surgery: does a lung function test exist to predict early severe postoperative respiratory complication? *Europ. Resp. J.* 1997; **10**: 1301–1308.

35. Mitchell, C. K., Smoger, S. H., Pfeifer, M. P. *et al.* Multivariate analysis of factors associated with postoperative pulmonary complications following general elective surgery. *Arch. Surg.* 1998; **133**: 194–198.

36. Gracey, D. R., Divertie, M. B., & Didier, E. P. Preoperative pulmonary preparation of patients with chronic obstructive pulmonary disease: a prospective study. *Chest* 1979; **76**: 123–129.

37. Pizov, R., Brown, R. H., Weiss, Y. S. *et al.* Wheezing during induction of general anesthesia in patients with and without asthma. A randomized, blinded trial. *Anesthesiology* 1995; **82**: 1111–1116.

38. Warner, D. O., Warner, M. A., Barnes, R. D. *et al.* Perioperative respiratory complications in patients with asthma. *Anesthesiology* 1996; **85**: 460–467.

39. Gupta, R. M., Parvizi, J., Hanssen, A. D., & Gay, P. C. Postoperative complications in patients with obstructive sleep apnea syndrome undergoing hip or knee replacement: a case-control study. *Mayo Clin. Proc.* 2001; **76**: 897–905.

40. Archer, C., Levy, A. R., & McGregor, M. Value of routine preoperative chest X-rays: a meta-analysis. *Can. J. Anaesth.* 1993; **40**: 1022–1027.

41. Munro, J., Booth, A., & Nicholl, J. Routine preoperative testing: a systematic review of the evidence. *Health Tech. Assessm.* (*Winchester, UK*) 1997; **1**: 1–62.

42. Rucker, L., Frye, E. B., & Staten, M. A. Usefulness of screening chest roentgenograms in preoperative patients. *J. Am. Med. Assoc.* 1983; **250**: 3209–3211.

43. Silvestri, L., Maffessanti, M., Gregori, D., Berlot, G., & Gullo, A. Usefulness of routine pre-operative chest radiography for anaesthetic management: a prospective multicentre pilot study. *Europ. J. Anaesth.* 1999; **16**: 749–60.

44. Milledge, J. S. & Nunn, J. E. Criteria of fitness for anesthesia in patients with chronic obstructive lung disease. *Br. Med. J.* 1975; **3**: 670–673.

45. Fisher, B. W., Majumdar, S. R., & McAlister, F. A. Predicting pulmonary complications after nonthoracic surgery: a systematic review of blinded studies. *Am. J. Med.* 2002; **112**: 219–225.

46. Lawrence, V. A., Dhanda, R., Hilsenbeck, S. G., & Page, C. P. Risk of pulmonary complications after elective abdominal surgery. *Chest* 1996; **110**: 744–750.

47. Rao, M. K., Reilly, T. E., Schuller, D. E., & Young, D. C. Analysis of risk factors for postoperative pulmonary complications in head and neck surgery. *Laryngoscope* 1992; **102**: 45–47.

48. Fan, S. T., Lau, W. Y., Yip, W. C. *et al.* Prediction of postoperative pulmonary complications in oesophagogastric cancer surgery. *Br. J. Surg.* 1987; **74**: 408–410.

49. Vodinh, J., Bonnet, F., Touboul, C., Lefloch, J. P., Becquemin, J. P., & Harf, A. Risk factors of postoperative pulmonary complications after vascular surgery. *Surgery* 1989; **105**: 360–365.

50. Kroenke, K., Lawrence, V. A., Theroux, J. F., & Tuley, M. R. Operative risk in patients with severe obstructive pulmonary disease. *Arch. Intern. Med.* 1992; **152**: 967–971.

51. Kroenke, K., Lawrence, V. A., Theroux, J. F., Tuley, M. R., & Hilsenbeck, S. Postoperative complications after thoracic and major abdominal surgery in patients with and without obstructive lung disease. *Chest* 1993; **104**: 1445–1451.

52. Warner, D. O., Warner, M. A., Offord, K. P., Schroeder, D. R., Maxson, P., & Scanlon, P. D. Airway obstruction and perioperative complications in smokers undergoing abdominal surgery. *Anesthesiology* 1999; **90**: 372–379.

53. De Nino, L. A., Lawrence, V. A., Averyt, E. C., Hilsenbeck, S. G., Dhanda, R., & Page, C. P. Preoperative spirometry and laparotomy: blowing away dollars. *Chest* 1997; **111**: 1536–1541.

54. Downs, S. H., Black, N. A., Devlin, H. B., Royston, C. M. S., & Russell, R. C. G. Systematic review of the effectiveness and safety of laparoscopic cholecystectomy. *Ann. Roy. Coll. Surg. Engl.* 1996; **78**: 476.

55. Wong, D. H., Weber, E. C., Schell, M. J., Wong, A. B., Anderson, C. T., & Barker, S. J. Factors associated with postoperative pulmonary complications in patients with severe chronic obstructive pulmonary disease. *Anesth. Analg.* 1995; **80**: 276–284.

56. Buggy, D. J. & Smith, G. Epidural anaesthesia and analgesia: better outcome after major surgery? Growing evidence suggests so. *Br. Med. J.* 1999; **319**: 530–531.

57. O'Hara, D. A., Duff, A., Berlin, J. A. *et al.* The effect of anesthetic technique on postoperative outcomes in hip fracture repair. *Anesthesiology* 2000; **92**: 947–957.

58. Parker, M. J., Unwin, S. C., Handoll, H. H., & Griffiths, R. General versus spinal/epidural anaesthesia for surgery for hip fractures in adults. *Cochrane Database Syst. Rev.* [computer file] 2000: CD000521.

59. Pedersen, T., Eliasen, K., & Henriksen, E. A prospective study of risk factors and cardiopulmonary complications associated with anaesthesia and surgery: risk indicators of cardiopulmonary morbidity. *Acta Anaesth. Scand.* 1990; **34**: 144–155.

60. Yeager, M. P., Glass, D. D., Neff, R. K., & Brinck-Johnsen, T. Epidural anesthesia and analgesia in high-risk surgical patients. *Anesthesiology* 1987; **66**: 729–736.

61. Rodgers, A., Walker, N., Schug, S. *et al.* Reduction of post-operative mortality and morbidity with epidural or spinal anaesthesia: results from overview of randomised trials. *BMJ* 2000; **321**: 1493.

62. Lawrence, V. A. Predicting postoperative pulmonary complications: the sleeping giant stirs. *Ann. Inter. Med.* 2001; **135**: 919–921.

63. Berg, H., Roed, J., Viby-Mogensen, J. *et al.* Residual neuromuscular block is a risk factor for postoperative pulmonary complications. A prospective, randomised, and blinded study of postoperative pulmonary complications after atracurium, vecuronium and pancuronium. *Acta Anaesth. Scand.* 1997; **41**: 1095–1103.

64. Epstein, S. K., Faling, L. J., Daly, B. D., & Celli, B. R. Predicting complications after pulmonary resection. Preoperative exercise testing vs a multifactorial cardiopulmonary risk index. *Chest* 1993; **104**: 694–700.

65. Ondrula, D. P., Nelson, R. L., Prasad, M. L., Coyle, B. W., & Abcarian, H. Multifactorial index of preoperative risk factors in colon resections. *Dis. Colon Rectum* 1992; **35**: 117–122.

66. Buist, A. S., Sexton, G. J., Nagy, J. M., & Ross, B. B. The effect of smoking cessation and modification on lung function. *Am. Rev. Respir. Dis.* 1976; **114**: 115–122.

67. Camner, P. & Philipson, K. Some studies of tracheobronchial clearance in man. *Chest* 1973; **63**: 235–240.

68. Nakagawa, M., Tanaka, H., Tsukuma, H., & Kishi, Y. Relationship between the duration of the preoperative smoke-free period and the incidence of postoperative pulmonary complications after pulmonary surgery. *Chest* 2001; **120**: 705–710.

69. Moller, A. M., Villebro, N., Pedersen, P., & Tonnesen, H. Effect of preoperative smoking intervention on postoperative complications: a randomized clinical trial. *Lancet* 2002; **359**: 114–117.

70. Bluman, L. G., Mosca, L., Newman, N., & Simon, D. G. Preoperative smoking habits and postoperative pulmonary complications. *Chest* 1998; **113**: 883–889.

71. Olsson, G. L. Bronchospasm during anaesthesia. A computer-aided incidence study of 136,929 patients. *Acta Anaesth. Scand.* 1987; **31**: 244–252.

72. Olsson, G. L. & Hallen, B. Laryngospasm during anaesthesia. A computer-aided incidence study in 136,929 patients. *Acta Anaesth. Scand.* 1984; **28**: 567–575.

73. Cohen, M. M. & Cameron, C. B. Should you cancel the operation when a child has an upper respiratory tract infection? *Anesth. Analg.* 1991; **72**: 282–288.

74. Levy, L., Pandit, U. A., Randel, G. I., Lewis, I. H., & Tait, A. R. Upper respiratory tract infections and general anaesthesia in children. Peri-operative complications and oxygen saturation. *Anaesthesia* 1992; **47**: 678–682.

75. Rolf, N. & Cote, C. J. Frequency and severity of desaturation events during general anesthesia in children with and without upper respiratory infections. *J. Clin. Anesth.* 1992; **4**: 200–203.

76. Tait, A. R. & Knight, P. R. The effects of general anesthesia on upper respiratory tract infections in children. *Anesthesiology* 1987; **67**: 930–935.

77. Tait, A. R. & Knight, P. R. Intraoperative respiratory complications in patients with upper respiratory tract infections. *Can. J. Anaesth.* 1987; **34**: 300–303.

78. Tait, A. R., Malviya, S., Voepel-Lewis, T., Munro, H. M., Seiwert, M., & Pandit, U. A. Risk factors for perioperative adverse respiratory events in children with upper respiratory tract infections. *Anesthesiology* 2001; **95**: 299–306.

79. Tait, A. R., Voepel-Lewis, T., & Malviya, S. Perioperative considerations for the child with an upper respiratory tract infection. *J. Perianesthesia Nursing* 2000; **15**: 392–396.

80. Anthonisen, N. R. & Wright, E. C. Bronchodilator response in chronic obstructive pulmonary disease. *Am. Rev. Respir. Dis.* 1986; **133**: 814–819.

81. Pauwels, R. A., Buist, A. S., Calverley, P. M., Jenkins, C. R., & Hurd, S. S. The GSC. Global strategy for the diagnosis, management, and prevention of chronic obstructive pulmonary disease. NHLBI/WHO Global Initiative for Chronic Obstructive Lung Disease (GOLD) Workshop summary. *Am. J. Respir. Crit. Care Med.* 2001; **163**: 1256–1276.

82. Auerbach, A. D. & Goldman, L. Beta-Blockers and reduction of cardiac events in noncardiac surgery: scientific review. *J. Am. Med. Assoc.* 2002; **287**: 1435–1444.

83. Salpeter, S. R., Ormiston, T. M., & Salpeter, E. E. Cardioselective beta-blockers in patients with reactive airway disease: a meta-analysis. *Ann. Intern. Med.* 2002; **137**: 715–725.

84. Salpeter, S. S., Ormiston, T., Salpeter, E., Poole, P., & Cates, C. Cardioselective beta-blockers for chronic obstructive pulmonary disease. *Cochrane Database Syst. Rev.* 2002: CD003566.

85. Christy, N. P. Corticosteroid withdrawal. In Bardin, C. W., ed. *Current Therapy in Endocrinology and Metabolism.* New York: B. C. Decker, 1988: 113.

86. Lawrence, V. A. & Duncan, C. A. Perioperative respiratory management. In Lubin, M. F., Walker, H. K., & Smith III, R. B., eds. *Medical Management of the Surgical Patient.* Philadelphia: J. B. Lippincott; 1995: 122–126.

87. Salem, M., Tainsh, R. E., Jr., Bromberg, J., Loriaux, D. L., & Chernow, B. Perioperative glucocorticoid coverage. A reassessment 42 years after emergence of a problem. *Ann. Surg.* 1994; **219**: 416–425.

88. Welsh, G. A., Manzullo, E., & Orth, D. N. The surgical patient taking corticosteroids. In Rose B. D., ed. *UpToDate.* Waltham: UpToDate, 2005.

89. Celli, B. R., Rodriguez, K. S., & Snider, G. L. A controlled trial of intermittent positive pressure breathing, incentive spirometry, and deep breathing exercises in preventing pulmonary complications after abdominal surgery. *Am. Rev. Respir. Dis.* 1984; **130**: 12–15.

90. Thomas, J. A. & McIntosh, J. M. Are incentive spirometry, intermittent positive pressure breathing, and deep breathing

exercises effective in the prevention of postoperative pulmonary complications after upper abdominal surgery? A systematic overview and meta-analysis. *Phys. Ther.* 1994; **74**: 3–10.

91. Overend, T. J., Anderson, C. M., Lucy, S. D., Bhatia, C., Jonsson, B. I., & Timmermans, C. The effect of incentive spirometry on postoperative pulmonary complications: a systematic review. *Chest* 2001; **120**: 971–978.

92. Brooks-Brunn, J. A. Postoperative atelectasis and pneumonia. *Heart Lung* 1995; **24**: 94–115.

93. Hayden, S. P., Mayer, M. E., & Stoller, J. K. Postoperative pulmonary complications: risk assessment, prevention, and treatment. *Cleve. Clin. J. Med.* 1995; **62**: 401–407.

94. Chumillas, S., Ponce, J. L., Delgado, F., Viciano, V., & Mateu, M. Prevention of postoperative pulmonary complications through respiratory rehabilitation: a controlled clinical study. *Arch. Phys. Med. Rehab.* 1998; **79**: 5–9.

95. Weil, J. V., McCullough, R. E., Kline, J. S., & Sodal, I. E. Diminished ventilatory response to hypoxia and hypercapnia after morphine in normal man. *N. Engl. J. Med.* 1975; **292**: 1103–1106.

96. Jayr, C., Thomas, H., Rey, A., Farhat, F., Lasser, P., & Bourgain, J. L. Postoperative pulmonary complications. Epidural analgesia using bupivacaine and opioids versus parenteral opioids. *Anesthesiology* 1993; **78**: 666–676; discussion 22A.

97. Jayr, C., Mollie, A., Bourgain, J. L. *et al.* Postoperative pulmonary complications: general anesthesia with postoperative parenteral morphine compared with epidural analgesia. *Surgery* 1988; **104**: 57–63.

98. Hjortso, N. C., Neumann, P., Frosig, F. *et al.* A controlled study on the effect of epidural analgesia with local anaesthetics and morphine on morbidity after abdominal surgery. *Acta Anaesth. Scand.* 1985; **29**: 790–796.

99. Major, C. P., Jr., Greer, M. S., Russell, W. L., & Roe, S. M. Postoperative pulmonary complications and morbidity after abdominal aneurysmectomy: a comparison of postoperative epidural versus parenteral opioid analgesia. *Am. Surg.* 1996; **62**: 45–51.

100. Ballantyne, J. C., Carr, D. B., deFerranti, S. *et al.* The comparative effects of postoperative analgesic therapies on pulmonary outcome: cumulative meta-analyses of randomized, controlled trials. *Anesth. Analg.* 1998; **86**: 598–612.

101. Rigg, J. R., Jamrozik, K., Myles, P. S. *et al.* Epidural anaesthesia and analgesia and outcome of major surgery: a randomised trial. *Lancet* 2002; **359**: 1276–1282.

10

Acute lung injury (ALI) and the acute respiratory distress syndrome (ARDS)

Scott L. Schissel and Bruce D. Levy

Brigham and Women's Hospital and Harvard Medical School, Boston, MA

Introduction and definitions

Acute lung injury (ALI) is a devastating disorder caused by many underlying medical and surgical diseases; and, when complicated by severe hypoxemia, is termed the acute respiratory distress syndrome (ARDS).[1] In 1967, Ashbaugh and colleagues first described some key features of ARDS, including: (a) respiratory distress and tachypnea (b) severe hypoxemia (c) diffuse alveolar infiltrates on chest radiography and (d) decreased lung compliance, all occurring in the setting of an acute medical or surgical illness.[2] While this descriptive definition lacks specificity, it encompasses the fundamental concept that ALI is diffuse lung injury caused either by a direct (e.g., aspiration of gastric contents) or an indirect (e.g., sepsis) pulmonary insult.

In hopes of standardizing clinical care and research studies, attempts have been made to apply more strict criteria to the definition of ARDS. Murray and colleagues in 1988 proposed a comprehensive definition of ARDS, including details on: the severity of lung injury, the mechanism of lung injury, and the presence of non-pulmonary organ dysfunction.[3] Lung injury was quantified based on the severity of 4 parameters and termed the Lung Injury Score (LIS); it includes: (a) the ratio of the partial pressure of arterial oxygen to the fraction of inspired oxygen (P_aO_2/F_iO_2), (b) the level of positive end-expiratory pressure (PEEP) applied during mechanical ventilation, (c) the static lung compliance, and (d) the extent of alveolar infiltrates on chest radiographs. While the presence of non-pulmonary organ dysfunction and the mechanism of lung injury have important clinical consequences (see below), surprisingly, the extent of lung injury has little predictive value for the clinical course of ALI.[4–7] Thus, in 1994 the American–European Consensus Conference Committee recommended simpler definitions for both ALI and ARDS[5], requiring only 4 diagnostic criteria (Table 10.1).[1]

These current definitions have the advantages of being applied easily to both clinical work and research protocols and, given the P_aO_2/F_iO_2 of 300 or less for ALI, are more inclusive, identifying more patients who will likely benefit from new therapies.[7] Moreover, the National Institutes of Health study network on ARDS (including 10 medical centers and 75 intensive care units) has accepted these definitions, further standardizing ARDS research.[8]

Epidemiology

Incidence

Due to variability in its definition, the reported annual incidence of ARDS has ranged from 1.5 to 70 cases/100 000.[4,9,10] A recent Scandinavian population study employing the 1994 consensus definitions revealed annual incidences of ALI and ARDS of 31/100 000 and 13.5/100 000, respectively.[4] When considering the broader 1994 consensus definition, these numbers are in approximate agreement with the most recent US study revealing an annual ARDS incidence of ~8 cases/100 000.[9] From a more practical perspective, ~11% of all ICU admissions (including community and tertiary care centers) suffer from acute respiratory failure, with ~20% of these patients meeting criteria for ALI.[4] Thus, approximately 1 out of every 50 patients admitted to ICUs will suffer from ALI or ARDS!

Associated clinical disorders and risk factors

Although a large number of medical and surgical illnesses have been associated with the development of ARDS, it is easiest to classify the underlying disorders into Direct or Indirect injury to the lung, as reviewed by Ware and Matthay.[11] Most cases of ARDS (>80%) are caused by a

Medical Management of the Surgical Patient: A Textbook of Perioperative Medicine, ed. M. F. Lubin, R. B. Smith, T. F. Dobson, N. Spell, H. K. Walker. 4th edn. Published by Cambridge University Press. © Cambridge University 2006.

Table 10.1. Diagnostic criteria for ALI and ARDS[a]

Oxygenation	Onset	Chest radiograph	Absence of left atrial hypertension
ALI: $P_aO_2/F_iO_2 \leq 300$ mm Hg **ARDS**: $P_aO_2/F_iO_2 \leq 200$ mm Hg	Acute	Bilateral alveolar or interstitial infiltrates	PCWP ≤ 18 mm Hg *or* no clinical evidence of left atrial hypertension

Note:

[a] In 1994, the American–European Consensus Conference Committee proposed diagnostic criteria for ALI and ARDS.[1] These definitions are simple and easily applied to both clinical practice and research protocols.

Table 10.2. Common clinical disorders associated with ARDS[a]

Direct lung injury	Frequency (% of total ARDS cases)	Indirect lung injury	Frequency (% of total ARDS cases)
Pneumonia	33–46[b]	Sepsis	42[b]
Aspiration of gastric contents	10–12	Severe trauma	8.1–35
Pulmonary contusion	5–9	Multiple bone fractures	5.3–12
Near drowning	0.5–1.5	Flail chest	3
		Head trauma	3–9.1
		Burns	1.5
		Multiple transfusions	2.3–20
		Drug overdose	1.5–11
		Pancreatitis	3.6

Notes:

[a] The most common causes of direct and indirect lung injury with their estimated frequency of association with ARDS.[4,13]

[b] Overlap in cases involving pneumonia-induced sepsis.

Table 10.3. Estimated incidence of ARDS complicating specific surgical disorders[a]

Clinical condition	Incidence of ARDS (%)
Pulmonary contusion	21–25
Multiple fractures (≥ 2 long bones or unstable pelvic fracture)	≥ 11
Abdominal trauma (penetrating abdominal trauma index >15)	18
Hypertransfusion (>15 units in 24 hours)	21–35
Trauma or surgery complicated by hypertransfusion	50
Near-drowning	30

Note:

[a] The estimated incidence of ARDS in several conditions associated with surgery and trauma.[12,13]
Note the additive risk of ARDS when a surgical condition is complicated by the need for hypertransfusion.

relatively few number of clinical disorders (Table 10.2). The majority of ARDS cases (~45%) are seen in medical patients suffering from severe sepsis syndrome and/or bacterial pneumonia.[4,5,12,13] In contrast, primary surgical illnesses are identified as the cause of ARDS in only 8%–35% of ARDS cases.[4,12,13] Pulmonary contusion, multiple bone fractures (> two long bones or unstable pelvic fracture), and chest wall trauma are the most frequently reported surgical conditions in ARDS, whereas head trauma, near drowning, toxic inhalation, and burns are rare causes (Table 10.3).[4,13] Less frequent, but important,

additional conditions associated with ARDS include multiple transfusions (>10–15 units in 24 hours), aspiration of gastric contents, drug overdose, and severe pancreatitis.

Certain predisposing conditions, however, carry especially high risk for progression to ARDS. Sepsis is clearly the at-risk diagnosis most frequently associated with the development of ARDS, with some series reporting ALI/ARDS in up to 40% of sepsis cases.[5,13] In contrast, only ~25% of at-risk surgical and trauma patients (including abdominal trauma, multiple fractures, pulmonary contusion, near drowning, and requirement for hypertransfusion) develop ARDS.[13] The ARDS risk of specific surgical diagnoses, however, varies widely. For example, multiple fractures are complicated by ARDS in ~11% of cases; whereas near-drowning and trauma requiring multiple transfusions are associated with increased ARDS risks of ~30% and ~40%, respectively (Table 10.3).[5,12,13] Moreover, ARDS risk is markedly increased in patients suffering from more than one predisposing medical or surgical diagnosis; for example, the incidence of ARDS increases from 25% in patients with trauma to 56% in patients with trauma and sepsis.[5,13] Similar increased ARDS risk is observed in patients with multiple trauma risk factors.[13]

In addition to the underlying clinical disorder, several other clinical variables are predictive for the development of ARDS. Older age is one clear and reproducible risk factor. In a series of 271 trauma patients from Seattle, the incidence of ARDS in patients <30 years of age was 18% and in patients older than 60 years of age, 33%.[13] Chronic alcohol abuse is also an independent risk factor. In a series of 350 medical and surgical patients, ARDS developed in 20% of septic patients with no alcohol abuse history and in 52% with an alcohol abuse history; similarly, the ARDS incidence in trauma patients with and without a chronic alcohol abuse history was 34% and 22%, respectively.[12] While the mechanism(s) involved in this association are unknown, a contribution from occult liver dysfunction is plausible, especially given the role of the liver in several host-defense mechanisms[14] and the clear association between chronic liver disease and ARDS mortality (see below).[12]

Increased severity of critical illness is also associated with progression to ARDS. A study of 175 trauma patients by Moss and colleagues revealed a 2.5-fold increase in the relative risk of developing ARDS in patients with an acute physiology and chronic health evaluation (APACHE) II score of 16 or greater compared with those patients with scores less than 16.[12] Similarly, Hudson and colleagues reported ARDS incidences in trauma patients of 13% and 41% in patients with APACHE II scores of ≤9 and >20, respectively.[13] The correlation between severity of illness and development of ARDS is further established in trauma patients using the trauma-specific injury severity score (ISS). ARDS developed in no trauma patients with an ISS of ≤9 and in 25% of patients with an ISS >20.[13] Finally, severe metabolic acidosis and acidemia are also risk factors for developing ARDS. For example, in 259 drug overdose and aspiration patients, ARDS was threefold more likely to develop in those patients presenting with a serum pH less than 7.25. Similarly, a serum bicarbonate lower than 20 meq/l was also an independent risk factor

for ARDS in trauma patients.[13] Surprisingly, despite the number of non-pulmonary risk factors predictive for the development of ARDS, no pulmonary predictor has been identified, including a history of chronic lung disease.[4,13]

Mortality

Mortality in ARDS patients has historically been greater than 50%,[15–17] leading to significant frustration for critical care physicians and to marked suffering for patients and their families. While several published reports since 1990 indicate significant improvement in ARDS mortality,[4,6,7,17–19] enthusiasm must be tempered given the wide variability in these data.[6,7] Most encouraging is a report by Milberg and colleagues on a 900 patient ARDS cohort followed over 11 years at a single medical center (thereby minimizing variability); overall ARDS mortality from 1983 to 1989 was 67%, decreasing to 41% from 1990 to 1993.[17] Moreover, three additional reports since 1992, including over 600 ARDS patients, revealed mortality rates ranging from 41 to 47%.[4,18,19] In contrast, however, two modern series totaling over 350 ARDS patients revealed mortality rates from 58 to 65%,[6,7] raising some doubt regarding a true trend of decreasing ARDS mortality.

Nonetheless, if ARDS mortality is improving, then what are the possible reasons? Most deaths in ARDS patients are due to non-pulmonary causes, with sepsis and non-pulmonary organ failure accounting for greater than 80% of deaths.[15,16,19] Thus, improvement in ARDS survival may be attributable to advances in the care of septic/infected patients (e.g., improved antimicrobials) and in supporting patients through multiple organ failure. In partial support of this notion is Milberg and colleagues' observation that ARDS mortality from 1983 to 1993 was most significantly decreased in young septic patients, decreasing from 58% to 26%.[17]

More important than knowing overall mortality is understanding the risk factors for mortality in ARDS patients, as risk factor presence can help guide prognosis in individuals and identify ARDS subpopulations that may benefit from new or specialized therapies. Similar to the risk factors for developing ARDS, the predominant risk factors for ARDS mortality are non-pulmonary, with only a few primary pulmonary risk factors recently identified (Table 10.4).[18]

The foremost risk factor for ARDS mortality is advanced age.[4,17,19] Recently, Luhr and colleagues reported only an 18% mortality in ARDS patients younger than 45 years old compared to 60% in patients older than 75 years of age.[4] Several prior studies confirm this relationship, as Milberg and colleagues reported a threefold higher mortality in

Table 10.4. Risk factors for mortality in ARDS patients[a]

Non-pulmonary	Pulmonary
Advanced age	Increased pulmonary
Sepsis	dead space
Non-pulmonary organ failure	Decreased pulmonary
Pre-existing liver disease	static compliance
or cirrhosis	
Chronic alcohol abuse	
Elevated ISS and APACHE II score	
Immunocompromise	

Note:
[a] Non-pulmonary and pulmonary risk factors for mortality in ARDS. Note the relatively few pulmonary-specific risk factors.

ARDS patients with sepsis over the age of 60 compared with patients younger than 60 years old.[17] As with the risk for developing ARDS, different medical conditions predisposing to ARDS are associated with varied risks for mortality. Sepsis remains the diagnosis associated with the highest ARDS mortality.[7,19] Doyle and colleagues, for example, demonstrated a mortality odds ratio of 2.8 for ALI/ARDS patients presenting with sepsis.[7] In contrast, surgical and trauma ARDS patients, especially those without direct lung injury, have a markedly better survival rate than other ARDS patients.[12,17] Milberg and colleagues, for example, reported a 40% mortality for all ARDS patients, but only a 28% mortality in trauma patients with ARDS; moreover, this improved survival was observed over the entire 11-year study period.[17]

While perhaps intuitive, the presence and severity of non-pulmonary organ failure in the course of ARDS patients is a strong predictor of mortality.[7,15,16,19] In several studies including over 400 ARDS patients, non-survivors had an average of twice the number of organs failing compared to survivors.[15,16] More recently, Doyle and colleagues found that the presence of any non-pulmonary organ failure in 123 ALI/ARDS patients was most predictive of mortality, with an odds ratio of 8![7] Similarly, increased measures of overall systemic illness also correlate with mortality in ARDS. For example, Luhr and colleagues reported a proportional increase between ARDS mortality and the APACHE II score; APACHE II scores of 10 and 40 were associated with 90-day mortalities of 10% and 90%, respectively.[4] Thus, given the *systemic* inflammatory etiology and sequelae of lung injury (see below),[20,21] non-pulmonary organ dysfunction is likely a marker of the severity of systemic injury and thus a good predictor of mortality.

In addition to acquired organ failure, pre-existing organ dysfunction in ARDS patients is also a risk factor for increased mortality. In particular, chronic liver disease and cirrhosis is highly associated with poor outcomes.[4,6,7] Doyle and colleagues observed an odds ratio for mortality in cirrhotic ARDS patients of 5.2.[7] Moreover, Monchi and colleagues found in over 200 ARDS patients that cirrhosis was associated with a mortality odds ratio of 27; fivefold greater than any other risk factor.[6] The importance of normal liver function for ARDS recovery is further supported by the observation of Moss and colleagues that ARDS mortality is 1.5-fold greater in patients with a history of chronic alcohol abuse.[12] The hepatic mechanism(s) involved in protection and recovery from ARDS are unknown;[12] however, animal models of sepsis demonstrate a clear increase in inflammatory alveolar infiltrates and alveolar damage in the presence of liver injury.[14] Finally, other chronic diseases have been linked to increased ARDS mortality; most notably, chronic immunosuppression and chronic renal disease.[4]

ALI and ARDS are distinguished by the severity of hypoxemia (Table 10.1).[1] However, the degree of hypoxemia present early in the course of ALI and ARDS patients has no prognostic value.[4,6,7,18,19] The findings of Luhr and colleagues, in a study of 1200 patients with acute respiratory failure, dramatically illustrate this point, revealing equal mortality ($\sim$40%) in patients with acute respiratory failure, ALI, and ARDS.[4] Doyle *et al.* also found no mortality difference between two groups of lung injury patients with markedly different oxygenation, patients with a P_aO_2/F_iO_2 from 150–299 had equal mortality ($\sim$58%) to patients with a $P_aO_2/F_iO_2 < 150$.[7] Moreover, additional measures of lung injury and hypoxemia, including the level of PEEP used in mechanical ventilation, the respiratory compliance, the extent of alveolar infiltrates on chest radiography, and the lung injury score (a composite of all these variables) are of little value in predicting mortality from ARDS.[4,6,7] Most important for the clinician, therefore, is NOT to judge the severity and prognosis of lung injury patients based on respiratory parameters but, instead, to rely more on the non-pulmonary risk factors for disease progression and death discussed above. Hopefully, by doing so, more patients will be identified and receive care earlier in the course of ALI and ARDS.

Although respiratory parameters are, in general, of little benefit in risk stratifying ARDS patients, recent data suggest that increased pulmonary dead space and decreased pulmonary compliance may be useful independent predictors of mortality.[18] Pulmonary dead space is that volume of ventilated lung that does not participate in gas exchange with the pulmonary arterial circulation; or, in physiologic terms, it is that area of lung with an infinite ventilation to perfusion ratio. Thus, increased dead space leads to hypoventilation and an increase in the partial pressure of arterial carbon dioxide (P_aCO_2). Increased pulmonary dead space is a well-recognized feature of ARDS and likely occurs as a result of diffuse pulmonary vascular injury and microthrombosis.[22,23] Nuckton and colleagues were the first to study the relationship between pulmonary dead space and ARDS mortality. In their study of 179 ARDS patients, early elevated dead space was associated with increased mortality, with dead space being 18% higher in non-survivors compared to survivors.[18] Low pulmonary compliance indicates "stiff" lungs and is decreased in ARDS as a result of pulmonary edema and loss of surfactant.[22,24] In their study on dead space, Nuckton *et al.* also measured static compliance at uniform tidal volumes and reported a small, but significant, association between decreased lung compliance and increased ARDS mortality.[18] Surprisingly, no prior studies have demonstrated such a relationship; however, this may have been due to varying techniques in measuring respiratory compliance.[6] While further studies are needed to confirm these observations, it is exciting to speculate about the clinical utility of these and other, yet identified, pulmonary-specific predictors of ARDS outcome.

Clinical course and pathogenesis

Early or exudative phase

The natural history of ARDS is traditionally marked by three phases, each with characteristic clinical and pathologic features.[22,25,26] The first, named the early or exudative phase, generally encompasses the first 7 days of illness.[11,22,26] Clinically, this period represents the onset of respiratory symptoms after exposure to an ARDS risk factor. Although the onset of symptoms is usually rapid, ~12–36 hours after the initial underlying insult, symptoms can be delayed by 5–7 days.[13] Symptoms are non-specific, including dyspnea, tachypnea, and ultimately respiratory fatigue. Laboratory values are generally not helpful, but an arterial blood gas will confirm that the P_aO_2/F_iO_2 is less than 300 mmHg in ALI and 200 mmHg in ARDS.[1] Plain chest radiographs usually reveal multi-lobar, "fluffy" alveolar and interstitial opacities (Fig. 10.1). While these radiographic findings are characteristic, they are not specific for ARDS and are often indistinguishable from other common conditions, especially cardiogenic pulmonary edema.[27] Because the early presenting features of ARDS are non-specific, alternative pulmonary diagnoses should

be considered early in the course of illness. Some common alternative disorders include: congestive heart failure, diffuse infectious pneumonia, toxin injury (e.g., crack cocaine, heroin, radiation pneumonitis), and diffuse alveolar hemorrhage. Other important, but less common, alternative pulmonary disorders include: acute interstitial lung diseases (e.g., acute eosinophilic pneumonia, acute interstitial pneumonitis, bronchiolitis obliterans organizing pneumonia), acute immunologic injury (e.g., lupus pneumonitis, hypersensitivity pneumonitis, Goodpasture's syndrome), and neurogenic pulmonary edema.

Histologically, the exudative phase is marked by diffuse alveolar damage. Features include degeneration of both alveolar capillary endothelial cells and alveolar epithelial cells (type I pneumocytes), leading to loss of the normally tight alveolar barrier to fluid and macromolecules.[22,26] As a result, protein-rich edema accumulates, containing the pro-inflammatory cytokines interleukin-1, interleukin-8, and tumor necrosis factor.[21] In addition, condensed plasma proteins aggregate with cellular debris and dysfunctional pulmonary surfactant to form hyaline membrane whorls in alveolar septae. As demonstrated by computed tomography (CT) scans of ARDS patients (Fig. 10.2), this alveolar edema predominantly involves dependent portions of the lung, leading to marked consolidation and atelectasis.[25,28] The major physiologic effect of this pathobiology is a marked decreased in lung compliance, intrapulmonary shunt, and hypoxemia.[25] While it remains unknown how a

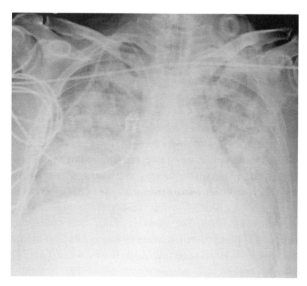

Fig. 10.1. Chest radiograph from an ARDS patient. This anteroposterior (AP) chest X-ray demonstrates the multilobar and symmetric air space opacities characteristic of the early or exudative phase of ARDS.

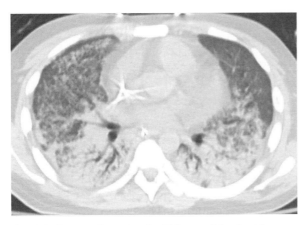

Fig. 10.2. Computed tomography (CT) scan of the chest from an ARDS patient. This chest CT scan image demonstrates the predominance of dependent alveolar edema and atelectasis in the early or exudative phase of ARDS.

diverse set of clinical disorders can cause extensive lung injury, ARDS is presumably initiated by injury to alveolar epithelial and endothelial cells.

In addition to alveolar injury, pulmonary vascular injury occurs early in ARDS and includes vascular obliteration by both microthrombi and fibrocellular proliferation.[23] These vascular injuries account for the moderate to severe pulmonary hypertension observed in ARDS. Moreover, loss of pulmonary arterial blood flow to ventilated portions of lung increases pulmonary dead space, explaining, in part, why even early ARDS patients can become hypercapneic.[18,25]

Intermediate or proliferative phase

The intermediate or proliferative phase of ARDS generally spans from day 7 to approximately day 21 of the disease.[22,26] Histologically, it marks the beginning of lung repair with organization of alveolar exudates and a change from neutrophil to lymphocyte-predominant infiltrates. In addition, type II pneumocytes proliferate along the alveolar basement membrane where they synthesize new surfactant and differentiate into new type I pneumocytes.[26] The proliferative phase is also the clinical point where patients may begin to recover rapidly. Unfortunately, some patients continue to have progressive lung injury and, ultimately, develop pulmonary fibrosis.[26,29] The mechanisms determining progression to fibrosis are unknown, yet the presence of type III procollagen peptide, a marker of pulmonary fibrosis, in alveoli at early stages of ARDS is associated with a protracted clinical course and increased mortality.[30]

Late or fibrotic phase

While most ARDS patients have excellent recovery of pulmonary function (see below),[31,32] the few with minimal recovery by 3–4 weeks enter the fibrotic phase of the disease.[22] This late phase is characterized by a transition from alveolar exudates and inflammation to extensive ductal and interstitial fibrosis. These fibrotic changes alter acinar architecture, leading to emphysema-like lesions and large bullae formation.[22,26] In addition, the pulmonary vascular bed undergoes intimal fibroproliferation leading to vascular occlusion and pulmonary hypertension.[23] The physiologic consequences of these pathologic changes include an increased risk for pneumothorax, altered lung compliance, and increased pulmonary dead space.[25] During this phase, patients often require long-term supplemental oxygen and/or ventilatory support. Given the morbidity in this group, it is not surprising that the presence of early pulmonary fibrosis is associated with increased mortality.[30,33]

Treatment and outcome in survivors

General principles

Any recent improvement in ARDS mortality is likely the result of general advances in the care of critically ill patients, as therapies aimed specifically at lung injury are either too new or have been unsuccessful. Thus, the initial approach to treating ARDS patients must include fastidious attention to: (a) recognition and treatment of the underlying at-risk diagnosis for ARDS (e.g., sepsis, pneumonia, trauma), (b) addressing ongoing fevers and infection, (c) minimizing procedures and their complications, (d) maintaining adequate nutrition and, (e) proper prophylaxis against: thromboembolism, gastrointestinal bleeding and injury, and central venous catheter infections. This section will focus on several new and promising ARDS-specific therapies and review several treatments of, as yet, unproven benefit.

Management of mechanical ventilation

Ventilator-induced lung injury

While mechanical ventilation can clearly prevent acute hypoxemic death, only recently appreciated is its potential to aggravate lung injury.[34] Nearly 30 years ago, Webb and Tierney demonstrated the potential harmful effects of high tidal volume (V_t) mechanical ventilation, observing marked alveolar edema and cellular damage in rats ventilated with high airway pressures and high tidal volumes.[35] More recently, Dreyfuss and colleagues, using

Table 10.5. Improved outcomes in ARDS with low tidal volume ventilation[a]

Clinical variable	Low tidal volume (6 cm³/kg)	Conventional tidal volume (12 cm³/kg)
Mortality	31%	40%
Off mechanical ventilation at hospital Day 28	66%	55%

Note:

[a] Mechanical ventilation of ARDS patients with a low tidal volume strategy markedly decreases ARDS mortality and leads to more rapid weaning from mechanical ventilation.[8] These findings support the use of tidal volumes of ~6 cm³/kg ideal body weight in ARDS patients.

torso-banding devices in rats to increase airway pressure but limit chest wall excursion and tidal volume, elegantly demonstrated that alveolar damage results from high tidal volume and *not* from high airway pressure.[36] Surprisingly, the alveolar edema and injury induced by high tidal volume ventilation can be completely prevented by applying positive end expiratory pressure (PEEP),[35,36] a maneuver that prevents alveolar collapse at end-expiration. Thus, at least in several animal models, ventilator-induced lung injury appears to require two processes: repeated alveolar over-distention and repeated *alveolar collapse.*

As described above, ARDS is a heterogeneous process, sparing areas of lung and leaving them with relatively normal compliance. Thus, the impact of ventilator-induced lung injury may be especially prominent in ARDS, where "normal" areas of lung are preferentially over-distended and injured. In fact, in animal models of acute lung injury, high tidal volume ventilation causes additional, synergistic alveolar damage.[37] As a result of these findings in animals, two important theories have emerged regarding mechanical ventilation in ARDS patients. The first is that ventilating ARDS patients with lower tidal volumes will result in less ventilator-induced lung injury and, in turn, improve clinical outcomes, the so-called "lung-protective" ventilation strategy. The second is that prevention of alveolar collapse at end-expiration, by addition of PEEP, will also reduce ventilator-induced lung injury, the so-called "open-lung" theory.[38]

Low tidal volume/lung-protective ventilation

While low-tidal volume ventilation has the theoretical benefit of reducing further lung injury, the principal risks associated with this strategy are respiratory acidosis and lower mean airway pressures, leading to possible alveolar collapse ("de-recruitment" of alveoli) and hypoxemia. Several clinical trials have examined the efficacy of low tidal volume ventilation in ARDS patients.[8,38–40] Both Stewart *et al.* and Brochard *et al.* randomized over 230 patients with ALI/ARDS to receive either conventional tidal volumes (~12 cm³/kg predicted body weight) or low tidal volumes

(~8 cm³/kg predicted body weight). In both studies, mortality was equivalent in patients receiving conventional and low tidal volume ventilation. Moreover, there were no differences in the duration of mechanical ventilation and length of intensive care unit stay between the two groups.[39,40] Importantly, patients in both studies assigned to low-tidal volume ventilation, compared to those assigned to conventional tidal volumes, had significantly higher P_aCO_2 values (so-called "permissive hypercapnia") and lower pH values. Although these data had cast early doubt on the validity of lung-protective ventilation, subsequent studies have yielded more promising results.[8,38]

In 2000, the National Institutes of Health acute respiratory distress syndrome network (ARDS Network) published a large-scale, randomized control trial comparing low-tidal volume (6 cm³/kg predicted body weight) ventilation to conventional tidal volume (12 cm³/kg predicted body weight) ventilation in over 800 ALI/ARDS patients.[8] Conventional tidal volume patients had their tidal volumes reduced only if the end-inspiratory plateau pressure exceeded 50 cm H_2O; in contrast, low tidal volume patients were permitted to reduce their tidal volumes to as low as 4 cm³/kg if the end-inspiratory plateau pressure exceeded 30 cm H_2O. Remarkably, mortality was significantly lower in the low-tidal volume patients compared to the conventional tidal volume patients, 31% and 40%, respectively. In addition, patients ventilated with low-tidal volumes spent significantly fewer days ventilator-dependent (Table 10.5). One strength of this study was its careful control for other respiratory variables. For example, all study patients were ventilated on volume-cycled assist control mode; and, there were no differences between the two groups in PEEP level, the P_aO_2/F_iO_2, or the absolute P_aO_2. In addition, respiratory acidosis in the low-tidal volume group was more aggressively treated than in prior studies.[40] In fact, the mean serum pHs in the low-tidal volume and conventional tidal volume groups were insignificantly different at 7.40 and 7.41, respectively; this was achieved by allowing the respiratory rate to increase to 35 breaths per minute in the low-tidal volume group and by initiating intravenous bicarbonate therapy for a serum $pH < 7.30$.[8] While further studies would be helpful to confirm the value of low-tidal volume ventilation, several attributes of the ARDS Network study strengthen its findings, including: the large size of the study (it included more patients than all prior studies combined), the "low-tidal volume" group achieved a lower mean tidal volume ($\sim$6 cm^3/kg) compared to this group in other studies ($\sim$8 cm^3/kg), and respiratory acidosis was better controlled than in prior studies.

Prevention of alveolar collapse with PEEP

In ARDS, the presence of alveolar and interstitial fluid and the loss of surfactant can markedly decrease lung compliance.[25] Thus, unless end-expiratory pressure is increased, significant alveolar collapse can occur at end-expiration. Repeated alveolar collapse not only impairs oxygenation, but may also contribute to ventilator-induced lung injury.[35,36] In most clinical settings, the amount of PEEP used is empirically set to minimize F_iO_2 and maximize P_aO_2,[8] with no assurance that the level of PEEP is adequate to prevent significant alveolar collapse at end-expiration. On most modern mechanical ventilators, however, it is possible to construct a static pressure–volume curve for the respiratory system. The lower inflection point on the curve represents alveolar opening (or "recruitment"); the pressure at this point is "optimal PEEP" for alveolar recruitment (Fig. 10.3).[34,38] Titration of the PEEP to the lower inflection point on the static pressure–volume curve, therefore, might improve oxygenation and

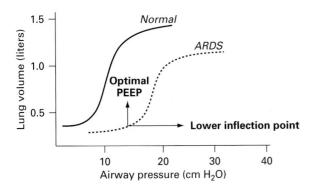

Fig. 10.3. Optimal PEEP in ARDS to prevent alveolar collapse at end-exhalation. Schematic static pressure–volume curves for the lung in a normal patient (*solid line*) and an ARDS patient (*dashed line*). The arrows mark the lower inflection point, where alveolar opening begins and therefore, the pressure where PEEP is optimal to prevent alveolar collapse at end-exhalation.

minimize lung injury. Again, this theory is referred to as the "open-lung" hypothesis.[38] In our experience, the lower inflection point on the static pressure–volume curve in ARDS is usually from 12–15 cm H_2O.

Several older studies have examined the efficacy of PEEP in preventing development of ARDS in at-risk patients; most studies were uncontrolled and yielded conflicting results.[41–43] In a randomized control trial, Pepe and colleagues assigned 92 patients at risk for developing ARDS to mechanical ventilation with and without 8 cm H_2O of PEEP. While the addition of PEEP increased P_aO_2, the PEEP and non-PEEP group had identical rates of ARDS and mortality.[44] Since, Amato and colleagues have reported on the clinical efficacy of a combined, low-tidal volume and "open-lung" ventilation strategy.[38] Fifty-three ARDS patients were randomized to either conventional mechanical ventilation, consisting of 12 cm^3/kg tidal volumes and PEEP set to minimize F_iO_2, *or* to lung-protective mechanical ventilation, consisting of 6 cm^3/kg tidal volumes with peak inspiratory pressures limited to 40 cm H_2O and the titration of PEEP to 2 cm H_2O above the lower inflection point on the static pressure–volume curve. In addition, alveolar "recruitment maneuvers" were frequently employed in the lung-protective group. These consisted of 40 second periods where respirations are held and the airway pressures are maintained at 35–40 cm H_2O; after, mechanical ventilation is continued at the prior or a higher PEEP level. Several favorable outcomes occurred in the lung protective group, including: markedly decreased 28-day mortality, increased rates of weaning from the ventilator, and higher values of P_aO_2. Overall mortality, however, was not different between the two groups; moreover, the small study size and the use of multiple interventions (low-tidal volumes, high PEEP, and recruitment maneuvers) preclude a definitive conclusion that high PEEP independently improves clinical outcomes in ARDS. Recently, the ARDS Network investigators conducted a trial in which 549 ARDS patients ventilated with low tidal volumes (6cm^3/kg) were randomly assigned to either low PEEP or high PEEP, otherwise ventilation parameters were similar between the two groups. PEEP was set by a pre-determined ratio of PEEP to FiO$_2$ specific for each group; the average PEEP levels were 8.3 and 13.2 cm H_2O for the low and high PEEP groups, respectively. There were no significant differences in mortality, ventilator-free days, length of ICU stay, or extent of organ failure between the low and high PEEP groups.[44a] Thus, these data do not support the use of higher PEEP added to a strategy of low tidal volume ventilation. In addition, high PEEP may have serious deleterious effects on other aspects of the patient. First, high levels of PEEP can cause alveolar pressure to exceed pulmonary capillary pressure, creating dead space and potentially increasing pulmonary blood flow through areas of shunt; this may cause both hypoxemia and hypercapnia. Second, excessive alveolar distending pressures may exacerbate ventilator-induced lung injury. And, finally, increased intrathoracic pressures will decrease cardiac pre-load and, in turn, may decrease systemic blood pressure and critical organ perfusion. Therefore, until more data becomes available on the clinical impact of low vs. high PEEP, it seems reasonable to set PEEP to minimize F_iO_2 and optimize P_aO_2 using parameters similar to those used by the ARDS Network in their study on low tidal volume ventilation (see below).[8]

Mechanical ventilation in the prone position

In 1974, Bryan speculated that placing mechanically ventilated ARDS patients into the prone position would improve dependent atelectasis, augment blood flow to ventral lung fields and, thereby, improve ventilation and perfusion matching.[45] Shortly after, several small case series demonstrated impressive improvements in arterial oxygenation after proning; typically, the P_aO_2 in nearly 80% of patients will rise 50–60 mmHg within 2 hours of proning.[46–49] And, although P_aO_2 will again fall when the patient is supine, re-proning results in reproducible gains in arterial oxygenation. While several potential mechanisms have been studied, it still remains unclear how prone positioning improves oxygenation. The following physiologic responses to proning likely contribute to improved arterial oxygenation: (a) decreased intrapulmonary shunt by opening of dependent, atelectatic lung,[49] (b) increased postural drainage of airway secretions, (c) decreased hydrostatic pressure in dependent and injured lung and, in turn, decreased interstitial edema.[50] Although several studies have verified the positive effects of proning on oxygenation,[47,49–51] until recently, no study has addressed the efficacy of prone positioning on important clinical outcomes.

In 2001, Gattinoni and colleagues randomized over 300 ALI/ARDS patients to supine or intermittent proned mechanical ventilation. While the P_aO_2/F_iO_2 increased by ~50 points in the prone position, both in-hospital and 6-month mortality were equivalent in the supine and proned groups. In a post-hoc analysis, however, the sickest quartile of patients (those with a $P_aO_2/F_iO_2 < 88$, simplified acute physiology (SAP) II score >49, or a tidal volume >12 cm^3/kg) had a lower 10-day mortality prone (20%) vs. supine (40%).[52] Thus, although prone positioning clearly improves arterial oxygenation, its effect on important clinical outcomes remains uncertain.

Moreover, unless the critical care team is experienced in proning, repositioning critically ill patients can be hazardous, leading to accidental endotracheal extubation, loss of central venous catheters, and orthopedic injury. Therefore, until further studies validate its efficacy, prone position ventilation should be reserved only for the most critically ill ARDS patients.

Other strategies in mechanical ventilation

Mechanical ventilation with low-tidal volume, high PEEP, and even prone positioning can be achieved with routine, widely available respiratory equipment. Several additional oxygenation and ventilation strategies, however, employing specialized technologies have been tested in ARDS patients, most with mixed or disappointing results. One such strategy is high frequency ventilation (HFV). By ventilating at extremely high respiratory rates (5–20 cycles per second), tidal volumes can be as low as 1–2 cm^3/kg but high mean airway pressures can be maintained, preventing alveolar collapse.[53–55] Early trials of HFV in adult ARDS patients revealed improved gas exchange but no obvious improvement in mortality.[54] A more recent trial randomizing 150 ARDS patients to HFV or conventional ventilation demonstrated both improved oxygenation and a trend toward improved survival in the HFV group.[55] While HFV has emerged as a safe alternative to conventional ventilation,[54,55] data from larger trials are required to prove HFV is clinically effective in ARDS.

Similarly, lung replacement therapy with extracorporeal membrane oxygenation (ECMO),[56] which provides a clear survival benefit in neonatal ARDS,[57,58] has yet to have proven survival benefit in adult ARDS.[59,60] To date, ECMO studies have enrolled several hundred adult ARDS patients who, otherwise, had an expected ≥80% mortality.[56] Despite these large numbers, studies have revealed no clear survival benefit when compared with internal or historical controls.[59,60] A large-scale randomized trial of modern ECMO in ARDS is under way in the UK and is scheduled for completion in 2003. Finally, ongoing research on partial liquid ventilation (PLV) has revealed some promising preliminary data in ARDS patients. The technique employs filling lungs to functional residual capacity (FRC) with perfluorocarbon, an inert, high density liquid that easily solubilizes oxygen and carbon dioxide.[61] In small trials in adult ARDS patients, PLV decreases physiologic shunt, improves static respiratory compliance, and has no obvious ill effects.[61,62] Again, no survival benefit was observed in these small trials,[62,63] but application of PLV to larger populations may prove it a beneficial strategy.

Recommendations

Until future studies confirm the efficacy of "adjunctive" ventilator therapies (e.g., high PEEP, prone positioning, HFV, ECMO, and PLV), we recommend the following evidence-based approach to mechanical ventilation in ARDS patients:[8]

- Calculate predicted body weight (PBW) in kilograms (kg)

  For men: PBW (kg) $= 50 + 2.3$(height (inches) $- 60$)

  For women: PBW (kg) $= 45.5 + 2.3$(height (inches) $- 60$)

- Ventilator mode

  Volume cycle, assist control

- Tidal volume (V_t)

  Initial V_t 8 cm^3/kg PBW

  Reduce to 6 cm^3/kg over 2–4 hours if ventilation adequate (see below)

  Goal inspiratory plateau pressures $<$30 cm H$_2$O; reduce V_t to as low as 4 cm^3/kg as needed (and permitted by ventilation) to achieve this goal

- P_aO_2 goal $= 55$–80 mmHg or pulse oximetry oxygen saturation 88%–95%

- Follow the F_iO_2 and PEEP applications used in the ARDS Network study group,[8] namely:

F_iO_2	0.3	0.4	0.4	0.5	0.5	0.6	0.7	0.7	0.7	0.8	0.9	0.9	0.9	1.0
PEEP	5	5	8	8	10	10	10	12	14	14	14	16	18	20–24

- Respiratory rate and acidosis management

  Goal arterial pH $= 7.30$–7.45

  If pH < 7.30, increase respiratory rate up to 35 breaths/minute

  If pH < 7.30 and the respiratory rate $= 35$, consider starting intravenous bicarbonate (or equivalent buffer)

If the above strategy fails and the patient is suffering from persistent hypoxemic respiratory failure, consider the following:

- neuromuscular blocking agents (if not already in use)
- prone position ventilation
- recruitment maneuvers (see *Management of Mechanical Ventilation*)
- HFV, ECMO, or PLV as part of a clinical research trial or in selected individuals.

Fluid management

Increased pulmonary vascular permeability and protein-rich alveolar edema are central features of ARDS.[21,22] In addition, impaired vascular integrity augments the normal increase in extravascular lung water that occurs with increasing left atrial pressure (Fig. 10.4). Maintaining a

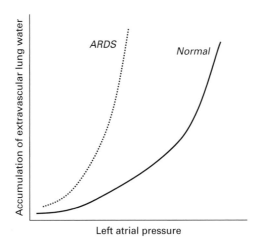

Fig. 10.4. Relationship between left atrial pressure and the accumulation of extravascular lung water. Schematic depicting the more rapid accumulation of extravascular lung water with increasing left atrial pressure in an ARDS patient (*dashed line*) compared to a normal patient (*solid line*).

normal or low left atrial filling pressure, therefore, should minimize pulmonary edema and improve arterial oxygenation and lung compliance. In fact, in several small studies of ARDS patients, aggressive fluid restriction and diuresis reduces extravascular lung water and improves pulmonary mechanics.[64,65] More important, however, are the findings by Humphrey *et al.* that reductions in pulmonary capillary wedge pressure (PCWP) are associated with improved clinical outcome in ARDS patients; in this retrospective study, patients with a drop in PCWP from a mean of 13 mmHg to 7 mmHg had a nearly threefold lower mortality and 30% shorter ICU stay compared to patients with a constant PCWP of 11–13 mmHg.[66] In addition, Mitchell *et al.* randomized ARDS patients to "conventional" fluid management or to goal-directed therapy aimed at reducing extravascular lung water and observed a sharp reduction in the total number of days on mechanical ventilation in the latter group (mean of 28 days vs. 9 days).[64] Thus, if there are no hemodynamic or renal contraindications, aggressive attempts at reducing left atrial filling pressures should be an important aspect of caring for ARDS patients.

Glucocorticoids

Increased levels of inflammatory cytokines and abundant neutrophils and macrophages are typical features of ARDS.[21,22] Thus, in an attempt to blunt inflammatory lung injury, several research groups and an untold number of individual clinicians have attempted to treat both early and late ARDS with glucocorticoids.[67] In 1987, Bernard *et al.*

reported the results of a randomized control trial of high-dose corticosteroids in 99 patients with early ARDS. Patients received either placebo or methylprednisolone at 30 mg/kg every 6 hours for only 24 hours. Through 6 weeks of follow-up, no differences in mortality, arterial oxygenation, or lung compliance were observed between the corticosteroid and placebo group.[68] In addition, similarly high doses (and brief courses) of methylprednisolone were also ineffective at preventing the development of ARDS in at-risk patients.[69] Unlike these disappointing results in early ARDS, Meduri and colleagues have reported on several studies demonstrating apparent excellent efficacy of glucocorticoids in treating the later, fibroproliferative stages of ARDS.[70–72] Most notable is a randomized trial of only 25 ARDS patients who, after continued clinical deterioration after 1 week of hospitalization, received either placebo or methylprednisolone at 2 mg/kg for 14 days, followed by tapering doses over the next 2 weeks.[72] Remarkably, the hospital mortality for the corticosteroid group was only 12%, but over 60% in the placebo group. Moreover, the P_aO_2/F_iO_2, lung injury score, and measure of non-pulmonary organ failure were all significantly better in the corticosteroid group.[72]

In short, these data are insufficient to determine the effectiveness of corticosteroids in either early or late ARDS. It is possible, for example, that longer courses and/or lower doses of corticosteroids will improve early ARDS outcomes, or that large-scale trials will prove corticosteroids to be ineffective in late ARDS. The ARDS Network is currently conducting a large-scale study of corticosteroids in ALI and ARDS and will, hopefully, clarify some of these lingering questions. Pending further data, corticosteroid use is not recommended in the care of early ARDS patients. If patients fail to improve after 1 week of supportive therapy and have no contraindications to corticosteroid therapy, consideration should be given to treating patients with corticosteroids at doses and durations used by Meduri and colleagues.[72]

Surfactant replacement therapy

Pulmonary surfactant is a lipid–protein complex secreted by type II pneumocytes that coats the surface of alveoli. It is composed primarily of phosphatidylcholine and has three surfactant-specific proteins. Surfactant reduces alveolar surface tension, thereby helping to prevent alveolar collapse at end-expiration. In addition, surfactant has antibacterial and immuno-regulatory activities.[24,73] The absence of pulmonary surfactant in neonates can lead to severe respiratory failure, named the respiratory distress syndrome (RDS).[24,74] Unlike RDS, adults with ARDS have

pulmonary surfactant but it contains abnormal phospholipid and protein, altering its surface tension-reducing properties.[75] Replacement therapy with exogenous surfactant has markedly reduced neonatal mortality in RDS.[74] To determine the efficacy of this therapy in ARDS, Anzueto et al. randomized over 700 ARDS patients to receive nebulized synthetic surfactant or placebo. Both mortality and arterial oxygenation were equivalent in the surfactant and placebo groups.[76] While these results are disappointing, the surfactant preparation in this study contained only lipid. In addition, the actual quantity of surfactant delivered to the lower airways was likely very small.[77] New investigations are underway testing more native surfactant preparations and efficient surfactant delivery systems.

Nitric oxide

In ARDS patients, arterial hypoxemia is largely due to pulmonary arterial perfusion through consolidated areas of lung, resulting in an intrapulmonary shunt. Nitric oxide, being an inhaled and locally acting pulmonary arterial vasodilator, increases perfusion to ventilated areas of lung, thereby reducing shunt and improving arterial oxygenation.[78] In 1993, Rossaint and colleagues first tested NO in ARDS patients; administration of 5–20 parts per million (ppm) of NO decreased pulmonary shunt and increased the P_aO_2/F_iO_2.[79] These positive preliminary findings led to several follow-up randomized clinical trials of NO in ARDS. Although NO clearly improves arterial oxygenation, it does not decrease mortality or increase success of ventilator weaning in ARDS patients.[80–82] Moreover, pulmonary arterial vasodilation is not always safe. For example, in patients with left-sided heart disease, increased pulmonary arterial blood flow can cause increased left ventricular preload and precipitate acute congestive heart failure. Thus, given its lack of efficacy, potentially dangerous side effects, and very high cost, inhaled NO cannot be recommended for the management of ARDS.

Other therapies

Inflammatory injury in ARDS is likely mediated, in part, by pro-inflammatory arachidonic acid metabolites such as thromboxane A_2 (TxA$_2$).[83,84] Moreover, progression to more severe lung injury may be blunted in some patients by endogenous anti-inflammatory eicosanoids, including prostaglandins E_1 (PGE$_1$) and E_2 (PGE$_2$).[85] In addition to glucocorticoids, therefore, several other anti-inflammatory therapies targeted specifically at these arachidonic acid

Table 10.6. Evidence-based recommendations for ARDS therapies[a]

Treatment	Recommendation
Mechanical ventilation:	
Low-tidal volume	A
High-PEEP or "open-lung"	C
Prone position	C
High frequency ventilation	C
ECMO	D
Minimize left atrial filling pressures	B
Glucocorticoids	C
Surfactant replacement	D
Inhaled nitric oxide	D
Other anti-inflammatory therapy (e.g., ketoconazole, PGE$_1$, NSAIDS)	D

Note:

[a] Based on current clinical evidence, several ARDS therapies have been assigned one of the following recommendation scores:

A = Good supportive clinical evidence: *Recommended therapy*

B = Supportive evidence, but limited clinical data: *Recommended therapy*

C = Indeterminate evidence: *Recommended only as alternative therapy*

D = Good evidence against efficacy of therapy: *Not recommended*

pathways have been tested in ARDS patients.[84] Unfortunately, none of these therapies, including ketoconazole (a thromboxane synthetase inhibitor),[86–88] cyclooxygenase inhibitors,[89] and PGE$_1$[85] has improved clinical outcomes in ARDS. A distinct class of arachidonate metabolites called lipoxins holds promise as a novel target for pharmacologic mimetics, as these compounds display potent counterregulatory properties that promote resolution of experimental pulmonary inflammation.[90] A more detailed understanding of these and other lipid mediators will hopefully elucidate mechanisms for lung repair and provide new therapies for ARDS.

Recommendations

The large number and varied clinical efficacy of ARDS therapies can make it difficult for clinicians to select a rational treatment plan for patients. In addition, the critical illness of ARDS patients can lead practitioners to unproven, and potentially harmful, therapies. Thus, while applying results of clinical trials to individual patients can be difficult, we advocate an ARDS treatment plan supported by clinical evidence. Table 10.6 lists the therapies discussed in this chapter and contains our summary recommendations regarding their use in ARDS.

Functional recovery in ARDS survivors

With improving ARDS survival, the functional recovery of ARDS survivors is an increasingly important issue for both patients and the healthcare system. Although ARDS patients can suffer profound and prolonged respiratory failure, it is encouraging that the majority of patients recover nearly normal lung function.[31,32] For example, Ghio *et al.* reported complete normalization of spirometry values and carbon monoxide diffusion capacities (DL$_{CO}$) in over a third of ARDS survivors 1 year after endotracheal extubation; moreover, most of the remaining patients were left with only mild abnormalities in their pulmonary function tests (Fig. 10.5).[31] In addition, patients recover most of their lung function by 6 months after lung injury.[32] Unlike mortality from ARDS, recovery of lung function is strongly associated with the extent of lung injury early in the disease. Low static respiratory compliance, high levels of required PEEP, longer durations of mechanical ventilation, and poor lung injury scores (LIS) are all associated

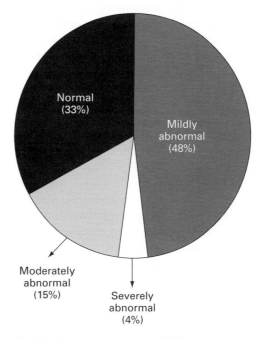

Fig. 10.5. Pulmonary function in ARDS survivors 1 year after recovery. Pulmonary function was tested using spirometry (measuring the forced expiratory volume at 1 second (FEV$_1$) and the forced vital capacity (FVC)) and by measuring the diffusion capacity for carbon monoxide (DLco). If the FEV$_1$, FVC, and DLco were all >80% of predicted values, pulmonary function was considered normal (*black*). If any of the three values were: 60%–79% predicted, 41%–59% predicted, or <40% predicted, then pulmonary function was considered mildly abnormal (*gray*), moderately abnormal (*stippled*), or severely abnormal (*white*), respectively.[31]

with worse pulmonary function recovery.[31,32] For example, McHugh *et al.* observed 30% lower FVC, DLco, and total lung capacity (TLC) values at 1 year of recovery in ARDS patients with an initial LIS >25 (severe) compared to those with a score <25 (limited).[32]

In addition to physiologic function, clinical function can also be impaired in ARDS survivors.[91,92] Poor recovery of lung function does not correlate with clinical functional recovery, including recovery from respiratory symptoms such as dyspnea, cough, and wheezing.[32] Davidson and colleagues compared 73 patients who had survived ARDS from either sepsis or trauma to control groups who had survived sepsis or trauma alone. Their findings revealed significantly worse scores in ARDS survivors compared to controls on subjective questionnaires examining a wide-range of physical, emotional, and respiratory symptoms.[91] Other studies have extended these findings, demonstrating significant rates of depression and even post-traumatic stress disorder in ARDS survivors.[92,93] From the perspective of caring for surgical patients, it is encouraging that survivors from trauma-induced ARDS have nearly 30% greater clinical functional recovery compared to patients surviving sepsis-induced ARDS.[91] Overall clinical recovery from ARDS is a complex process, involving important interactions between physical and psychosocial factors. A better understanding of mechanisms involved in recovery are essential to guide future therapies aimed at reducing long-term ARDS morbidity.

Concluding comments

The American–European Consensus Conference Committee definitions of ALI and ARDS identify lung injury as a common clinical disorder in critically-ill surgical patients. With general advances in critical care and the recent discovery of novel ARDS-specific therapies, mortality from this disease has decreased. Ongoing basic and clinical research will provide new potential therapies aimed at both prevention and lung repair, so that future patients will have less severe illness and improved survival and long-term recovery from ARDS.

REFERENCES

1. Bernard, G. R., Artigas, A., Brigham, K. L. *et al.* The American–European Consensus Conference on ARDS. Definitions, mechanisms, relevant outcomes, and clinical trial coordination. *Am. J. Respir. Crit. Care Med.* 1994; **149**(3 Pt 1): 818–824.

2. Ashbaugh, D. G., Bigelow, D. B., Petty, T. L. *et al.* Acute respiratory distress in adults. *Lancet* 1967; **2**(7511): 319–323.

3. Murray, J. F., Matthay, M. A., Luce, J. M. *et al.* An expanded definition of the adult respiratory distress syndrome. *Am. Rev. Respir. Dis.* 1988; **138**(3): 720–723.

4. Luhr, O. R., Antonsen, K., Karlsson, M. *et al.* Incidence and mortality after acute respiratory failure and acute respiratory distress syndrome in Sweden, Denmark, and Iceland. The ARF Study Group. *Am. J. Respir. Crit. Care Med.* 1999; **159**(6): 1849–1861.

5. Pepe, P. E., Potkin, R. T., Reus, D. H. *et al.* Clinical predictors of the adult respiratory distress syndrome. *Am. J. Surg.* 1982; **144**(1): 124–130.

6. Monchi, M., Bellenfant, F., Cariou, A. *et al.* Early predictive factors of survival in the acute respiratory distress syndrome. A multivariate analysis. *Am. J. Respir. Crit. Care Med.* 1998; **158**(4): 1076–1081.

7. Doyle, R. L., Szaflarski, N., Modin, G. W. *et al.* Identification of patients with acute lung injury. Predictors of mortality. *Am. J. Respir. Crit. Care Med.* 1995; **152**(6 Pt 1): 1818–1824.

8. The Acute Respiratory Distress Syndrome Network. Ventilation with lower tidal volumes as compared with traditional tidal volumes for acute lung injury and the acute respiratory distress syndrome. *N. Engl. J. Med.* 2000; **342**(18): 1301–1308.

9. Thomsen, G. E. & Morris, A. H. Incidence of the adult respiratory distress syndrome in the state of Utah. *Am. J. Respir. Crit. Care Med.* 1995; **152**(3): 965–971.

10. Villar, J. & Slutsky, A. S. The incidence of the adult respiratory distress syndrome. *Am. Rev. Respir. Dis.* 1989; **140**(3): 814–816.

11. Ware, L. B. & Matthay, M. A. The acute respiratory distress syndrome. *N. Engl. J. Med.* 2000; **342**(18): 1334–1349.

12. Moss, M., Bucher, B., Moore, F. A. *et al.* The role of chronic alcohol abuse in the development of acute respiratory distress syndrome in adults. *JAMA* 1996; **275**(1): 50–54.

13. Hudson, L. D., Milberg, J. A., Anardi, D. *et al.* Clinical risks for development of the acute respiratory distress syndrome. *Am. J. Respir. Crit. Care Med.* 1995; **151**(2 Pt 1): 293–301.

14. Matuschak, G. M., Pinsky, M. R., Klein, E. C. *et al.* Effects of D-galactosamine-induced acute liver injury on mortality and pulmonary responses to *Escherichia coli* lipopolysaccharide. Modulation by arachidonic acid metabolites. *Am. Rev. Respir. Dis.* 1990; **141**(5 Pt 1): 1296–1306.

15. Bell, R. C., Coalson, J. J., Smith, J. D. *et al.* Multiple organ system failure and infection in adult respiratory distress syndrome. *Ann. Intern. Med.* 1983; **99**(3): 293–298.

16. Montgomery, A. B., Stager, M. A., Carrico, C. J. *et al.* Causes of mortality in patients with the adult respiratory distress syndrome. *Am. Rev. Respir. Dis.* 1985; **132**(3): 485–489.

17. Milberg, J. A., Davis, D. R., Steinberg, K. P. *et al.* Improved survival of patients with acute respiratory distress syndrome (ARDS): 1983–1993. *JAMA* 1995; **273**(4): 306–309.

18. Nuckton, T. J., Alonso, J. A., Kallet, R. H. *et al.* Pulmonary dead-space fraction as a risk factor for death in the acute respiratory distress syndrome. *N. Engl. J. Med.* 2002; **346**(17): 1281–1286.

19. Suchyta, M. R., Clemmer, T. P., Elliott, C. G. *et al.* The adult respiratory distress syndrome. A report of survival and modifying factors. *Chest* 1992; **101**(4): 1074–1079.

20. Slutsky, A. S. & Tremblay, L. N. Multiple system organ failure. Is mechanical ventilation a contributing factor? *Am. J. Respir. Crit. Care Med.* 1998; **157**(6 Pt 1): 1721–1725.

21. Pugin, J., Verghese, G., Widmer, M. C. *et al.* The alveolar space is the site of intense inflammatory and profibrotic reactions in the early phase of acute respiratory distress syndrome. *Crit. Care Med.* 1999; **27**(2): 304–312.

22. Tomashefski, J. F., Jr. Pulmonary pathology of acute respiratory distress syndrome. *Clin. Chest Med.* 2000; **21**(3): 435–466.

23. Tomashefski, J. F., Jr., Davies, P., Boggis, C. *et al.* The pulmonary vascular lesions of the adult respiratory distress syndrome. *Am. J. Pathol.* 1983; **112**(1): 112–126.

24. Lewis, J. F. & Jobe, A. H. Surfactant and the adult respiratory distress syndrome. *Am. Rev. Respir. Dis.* 1993; **147**(1): 218–233.

25. Gattinoni, L., Bombino, M., Pelosi, P. *et al.* Lung structure and function in different stages of severe adult respiratory distress syndrome. *JAMA* 1994; **271**(22): 1772–1779.

26. Anderson, W. R. & Thielen, K. Correlative study of adult respiratory distress syndrome by light, scanning, and transmission electron microscopy. *Ultrastruct. Pathol.* 1992; **16**(6): 615–628.

27. Goodman, P. C. Radiographic findings in patients with acute respiratory distress syndrome. *Clin. Chest Med.* 2000; **21**(3): 419–433.

28. Puybasset, L., Cluzel, P., Chao, N. *et al.* A computed tomography scan assessment of regional lung volume in acute lung injury. The CT Scan ARDS Study Group. *Am. J. Respir. Crit. Care Med.* 1998; **158**(5 Pt 1): 1644–1655.

29. Zapol, W. M., Trelstad, R. L., Coffey, J. W. *et al.* Pulmonary fibrosis in severe acute respiratory failure. *Am. Rev. Respir. Dis.* 1979; **119**(4): 547–554.

30. Chesnutt, A. N., Matthay, M. A., Tibayan, F. A. *et al.* Early detection of type III procollagen peptide in acute lung injury. Pathogenetic and prognostic significance. *Am. J. Respir. Crit. Care Med.* 1997; **156**(3 Pt 1): 840–845.

31. Ghio, A. J., Elliott, C. G., Crapo, R. O. *et al.* Impairment after adult respiratory distress syndrome. An evaluation based on American Thoracic Society recommendations. *Am. Rev. Respir. Dis.* 1989; **139**(5): 1158–1162.

32. McHugh, L. G., Milberg, J. A., Whitcomb, M. E. *et al.* Recovery of function in survivors of the acute respiratory distress syndrome. *Am. J. Respir. Crit. Care Med.* 1994; **150**(1): 90–94.

33. Martin, C., Papazian, L., Payan, M. J. *et al.* Pulmonary fibrosis correlates with outcome in adult respiratory distress syndrome. A study in mechanically ventilated patients. *Chest* 1995; **107**(1): 196–200.

34. Tobin, M. Advances in mechanical ventilation. *N. Engl. J. Med.* 2001; **344**(26): 1986–1996.

35. Webb, H. H. & Tierney, D. F. Experimental pulmonary edema due to intermittent positive pressure ventilation with high inflation pressures. Protection by positive end-expiratory pressure. *Am. Rev. Respir. Dis.* 1974; **110**(5): 556–565.

36. Dreyfuss, D., Soler, P., Basset, G. *et al.* High inflation pressure pulmonary edema. Respective effects of high airway pressure, high tidal volume, and positive end-expiratory pressure. *Am. Rev. Respir. Dis.* 1988; **137**(5): 1159–1164.

37. Dreyfuss, D., Soler, P., & Saumon, G. Mechanical ventilation-induced pulmonary edema. Interaction with previous lung alterations. *Am. J. Respir. Crit. Care Med.* 1995; **151**(5): 1568–1575.

38. Amato, M. B., Barbas, C. S., Medeiros, D. M. *et al.* Effect of a protective-ventilation strategy on mortality in the acute respiratory distress syndrome. *N. Engl. J. Med.* 1998; **338**(6): 347–354.

39. Brochard, L., Roudot-Thoraval, F., Roupie, E. *et al.* Tidal volume reduction for prevention of ventilator-induced lung injury in acute respiratory distress syndrome. The Multicenter Trial Group on Tidal Volume reduction in ARDS. *Am. J. Respir. Crit. Care Med.* 1998; **158**(6): 1831–1838.

40. Stewart, T. E., Meade, M. O., Cook, D. J. *et al.* Evaluation of a ventilation strategy to prevent barotrauma in patients at high risk for acute respiratory distress syndrome. Pressure- and Volume-Limited Ventilation Strategy Group. *N. Engl. J. Med.* 1998; **338**(6): 355–361.

41. Weigelt, J. A., Mitchell, R. A., & Snyder, W. H., 3rd. Early positive end-expiratory pressure in the adult respiratory distress syndrome. *Arch. Surg.* 1979; **114**(4): 497–501.

42. Valdes, M. E., Powers, S. R., Jr., Shah, D. M. *et al.* Continuous positive airway pressure in prophylaxis of adult respiratory distress syndrome in trauma patients. *Surg. Forum* 1978; **29**: 187–189.

43. Schmidt, G. B., Bombeck, C. T., Bennett, E. J. *et al.* Continuous positive airway pressure in the prophylaxis of the adult respiratory distress syndrome (ARDS). *Langenbecks Arch. Chir.* 1975; Suppl: 439–442.

44. Pepe, P. E., Hudson, L. D., & Carrico, C. J. Early application of positive end-expiratory pressure in patients at risk for the adult respiratory-distress syndrome. *N. Engl. J. Med.* 1984; **311**(5): 281–286.

44a. The Acute Respiratory Distress Syndrome Network. Higher versus lower positive end-expiratory pressures in patients with the acute respiratory distress syndrome. *N. Engl. J. Med.* 2004; **351**(4): 327–336.

45. Bryan, A. C. Comments of a devil's advocate. *Am. Rev. Respir. Dis.* 1974; **110**: 143–144.

46. Piehl, M. A. & Brown, R. S. Use of extreme position changes in acute respiratory failure. *Crit. Care Med.* 1976; **4**(1): 13–14.

47. Langer, M., Mascheroni, D., Marcolin, R. *et al.* The prone position in ARDS patients. A clinical study. *Chest* 1988; **94**(1): 103–107.

48. Douglas, W. W., Rehder, K., Beynen, F. M. *et al.* Improved oxygenation in patients with acute respiratory failure: the prone position. *Am. Rev. Respir. Dis.* 1977; **115**(4): 559–566.

49. Pappert, D., Rossaint, R., Slama, K. *et al.* Influence of positioning on ventilation–perfusion relationships in severe adult respiratory distress syndrome. *Chest* 1994; **106**(5): 1511–1516.

50. Albert, R. K. Prone ventilation. *Clin. Chest Med.* 2000; **21**(3): 511–517.

51. Pelosi, P., Tubiolo, D., Mascheroni, D. *et al.* Effects of the prone position on respiratory mechanics and gas exchange during acute lung injury. *Am. J. Respir. Crit. Care Med.* 1998; **157**(2): 387–393.

52. Gattinoni, L., Tognoni, G., Pesenti, A. *et al.* Effect of prone positioning on the survival of patients with acute respiratory failure. *N. Engl. J. Med.* 2001; **345**(8): 568–573.

53. Slutsky, A. S. & Drazen, J. M. Ventilation with small tidal volumes. *N. Engl. J. Med.* 2002; **347**(9): 630–631.

54. Fort, P., Farmer, C., Westerman, J. *et al.* High-frequency oscillatory ventilation for adult respiratory distress syndrome – a pilot study. *Crit. Care Med.* 1997; **25**(6): 937–947.

55. Derdak, S., Mehta, S., Stewart, T. E. *et al.* High-frequency oscillatory ventilation for acute respiratory distress syndrome in adults: a randomized, controlled trial. *Am. J. Respir. Crit. Care Med.* 2002; **166**(6): 801–808.

56. Bartlett, R. H. Extracorporeal life support in the management of severe respiratory failure. *Clin. Chest Med.* 2000; **21**(3): 555–561.

57. Bartlett, R. H., Roloff, D. W., Cornell, R. G. *et al.* Extracorporeal circulation in neonatal respiratory failure: a prospective randomized study. *Pediatrics* 1985; **76**(4): 479–487.

58. O'Rourke, P. P., Crone, R. K., Vacanti, J. P. *et al.* Extracorporeal membrane oxygenation and conventional medical therapy in neonates with persistent pulmonary hypertension of the newborn: a prospective randomized study. *Pediatrics* 1989; **84**(6): 957–963.

59. Gattinoni, L., Pesenti, A., Mascheroni, D. *et al.* Low-frequency positive-pressure ventilation with extracorporeal CO_2 removal in severe acute respiratory failure. *JAMA* 1986; **256**(7): 881–886.

60. Morris, A. H., Wallace, C. J., Menlove, R. L. *et al.* Randomized clinical trial of pressure-controlled inverse ratio ventilation and extracorporeal CO_2 removal for adult respiratory distress syndrome. *Am. J. Respir. Crit. Care Med.* 1994; **149**(2 Pt 1): 295–305.

61. Wiedemann, H. P. Partial liquid ventilation for acute respiratory distress syndrome. *Clin. Chest Med.* 2000; **21**(3): 543–554.

62. Hirschl, R. B., Pranikoff, T., Wise, C. *et al.* Initial experience with partial liquid ventilation in adult patients with the acute respiratory distress syndrome. *JAMA* 1996; **275**(5): 383–389.

63. Bartlett, R. H., Croce, M., & Hirschl, R. B. A phase II randomized, controlled trial of partial liquid ventilation (PLV) in adult patients with acute hypoxemic respiratory failure (AHRF). *Crit. Care Med.* 1997; **25**(Suppl): A35.

64. Mitchell, J. P., Schuller, D., Calandrino, F. S. *et al.* Improved outcome based on fluid management in critically ill patients requiring pulmonary artery catheterization. *Am. Rev. Respir. Dis.* 1992; **145**(5): 990–998.

65. Bone, R. C. Treatment of adult respiratory distress syndrome with diuretics, dialysis, and positive end-expiratory pressure. *Crit. Care Med.* 1978; **6**: 136–139.

66. Humphrey, H., Hall, J., Sznajder, I. *et al.* Improved survival in ARDS patients associated with a reduction in pulmonary capillary wedge pressure. *Chest* 1990; **97**(5): 1176–1180.

67. Luce, J. M. Corticosteroids in ARDS. An evidence-based review. *Crit. Care Clin.* 2002; **18**(1): 79–89, vii.

68. Bernard, G. R., Luce, J. M., Sprung, C. L. *et al.* High-dose corticosteroids in patients with the adult respiratory distress syndrome. *N. Engl. J. Med.* 1987; **317**(25): 1565–1570.

69. Weigelt, J. A., Norcross, J. F., & Borman, K. R. Early steroid therapy for respiratory failure. *Arch. Surg.* 1985; **120**: 536–540.

70. Meduri, G. U., Belenchia, J. M., Estes, R. J. *et al.* Fibroproliferative phase of ARDS. Clinical findings and effects of corticosteroids. *Chest* 1991; **100**(4): 943–952.

71. Meduri, G. U., Chinn, A. J., Leeper, K. V. *et al.* Corticosteroid rescue treatment of progressive fibroproliferation in late ARDS. Patterns of response and predictors of outcome. *Chest* 1994; **105**(5): 1516–1527.

72. Meduri, G. U., Headley, A. S., Golden, E. *et al.* Effect of prolonged methylprednisolone therapy in unresolving acute respiratory distress syndrome: a randomized controlled trial. *J. Am. Med. Assoc.* 1998; **280**(2): 159–165.

73. Spragg, R. G. Surfactant replacement therapy. *Clin. Chest Med.* 2000; **21**(3): 531–541, ix.

74. Long, W., Thompson, T., Sundell, H. *et al.* The American Exosurf Neonatal Study Group I. Effects of two rescue doses of a synthetic surfactant on mortality rate and survival without bronchopulmonary dysplasia in 700- to 1350-gram infants with respiratory distress syndrome. *J. Pediatr.* 1991; **118**(4 (Pt 1)): 595–605.

75. Gregory, T. J., Longmore, W. J., Moxley, M. A. *et al.* Surfactant chemical composition and biophysical activity in acute respiratory distress syndrome. *J. Clin. Invest.* 1991; **88**(6): 1976–1981.

76. Anzueto, A., Baughman, R. P., Guntupalli, K. K. *et al.* Aerosolized surfactant in adults with sepsis-induced acute respiratory distress syndrome. Exosurf Acute Respiratory Distress Syndrome Sepsis Study Group. *N. Engl. J. Med.* 1996; **334**(22): 1417–1421.

77. MacIntyre, N. R., Coleman, R. E., Schuller, F. S. *et al.* Efficiency of the delivery of aerosolized artificial surfactant in intubated patients with the adult respiratory distress syndrome. *Am. J. Respir. Crit. Care Med.* 1994; **149**(Suppl.): A125.

78. Payen, D. M. Inhaled nitric oxide and acute lung injury. *Clin. Chest Med.* 2000; **21**(3): 519–529, ix.

79. Rossaint, R., Falke, K. J., Lopez, F. *et al.* Inhaled nitric oxide for the adult respiratory distress syndrome. *N. Engl. J. Med.* 1993; **328**(6): 399–405.

80. Dellinger, R. P., Zimmerman, J. L., Taylor, R. W. *et al.* Effects of inhaled nitric oxide in patients with acute respiratory distress syndrome: results of a randomized phase II trial. Inhaled Nitric Oxide in ARDS Study Group. *Crit. Care Med.* 1998; **26**(1): 15–23.

81. Lundin, S., Mang, H., Smithies, M. *et al.* Inhalation of nitric oxide in acute lung injury: results of a European multicentre study. The European Study Group of Inhaled Nitric Oxide. *Intens. Care Med.* 1999; **25**(9): 911–919.

82. Troncy, E., Collet, J. P., Shapiro, S. *et al.* Inhaled nitric oxide in acute respiratory distress syndrome: a pilot randomized

controlled study. *Am. J. Respir. Crit. Care Med.* 1998; **157**(5 Pt 1): 1483–1488.

83. Winn, R., Harlan, J., Nadir, B. *et al.* Thromboxane A2 mediates lung vasoconstriction but not permeability after endotoxin. *J. Clin. Invest.* 1983; **72**(3): 911–918.

84. Conner, B. D. & Bernard, G. R. Acute respiratory distress syndrome. Potential pharmacologic interventions. *Clin. Chest Med.* 2000; **21**(3): 563–587.

85. Abraham, E., Baughman, R., Fletcher, E. *et al.* Liposomal prostaglandin E1 (TLC C-53) in acute respiratory distress syndrome: a controlled, randomized, double-blind, multicenter clinical trial. TLC C-53 ARDS Study Group. *Crit. Care Med.* 1999; **27**(8): 1478–1485.

86. Slotman, G. J., Burchard, K. W., D'Arezzo, A. *et al.* Ketoconazole prevents acute respiratory failure in critically ill surgical patients. *J. Trauma* 1988; **28**(5): 648–654.

87. Yu, M. & Tomasa, G. A double-blind, prospective, randomized trial of ketoconazole, a thromboxane synthetase inhibitor, in the prophylaxis of the adult respiratory distress syndrome. *Crit. Care Med.* 1993; **21**(11): 1635–1642.

88. The ARDS Network. Ketoconazole for early treatment of acute lung injury and acute respiratory distress syndrome: a randomized controlled trial. *JAMA* 2000; **283**(15): 1995–2002.

89. Rinaldo, J. E. & Pennock, B. Effects of ibuprofen on endotoxin-induced alveolitis: biphasic dose response and dissociation between inflammation and hypoxemia. *Am. J. Med. Sci.* 1986; **291**(1): 29–38.

90. Levy, B. D., De Sanctis, G. T., Devchand, P. R. *et al.* Multipronged inhibition of airway hyper-responsiveness and inflammation by lipoxin A(4). *Nat. Med.* 2002; **8**(9): 1018–1023.

91. Davidson, T. A., Caldwell, E. S., Curtis, J. R. *et al.* Reduced quality of life in survivors of acute respiratory distress syndrome compared with critically ill control patients. *JAMA* 1999; **281**(4): 354–360.

92. Weinert, C. R., Gross, C. R., Kangas, J. R. *et al.* Health-related quality of life after acute lung injury. *Am. J. Respir. Crit. Care Med.* 1997; **156**(4 Pt 1): 1120–1128.

93. Stoll, C., Schelling, G., Bullinger, M. *et al.* Quality of life after prolonged intensive care treatment for acute lung failure. *Qual. Life Res.* 1995; **4**: 491–492.

11

Postoperative pulmonary complications

Eric G. Honig

Emory University School of Medicine, Atlanta, GA

Postoperative pulmonary complications are defined as pulmonary abnormalities occurring in the postoperative period that produce clinically significant identifiable disease or dysfunction that adversely affect the clinical course.[1] The incidence of these complications ranges from 2 to 100% in various series, depending on predisposing risk factors as well as the specific surgical procedure (Table 11.1).[2–4] Taken together, they are more common than postoperative cardiac complications, lead to longer hospital stays (22.7 vs. 10.4d),[5] and increase the relative risk of death to 14.9 (95% confidence limits 4.76–26.9), particularly due to pneumonia.[6]

Factors associated with an increased risk for postoperative pulmonary complications include the following:

- surgical site
- prolonged duration of surgery
- underlying lung disease
- smoking history (>20 pack years)
- obesity (BMI >25)
- poor nutritional status
- age >60 years
- ASA >3
- inadequate nurse staffing in postoperative care areas.

Patients should be evaluated preoperatively to identify these factors and efforts made to improve risk status. Preoperative respiratory assessment and management are discussed elsewhere.

The pathogenesis of pulmonary complications in the postoperative period has been well described.[7] Hypoventilation and reduced lung volumes beginning with anesthesia and surgery combine to produce atelectasis and predispose to respiratory tract infection. Immobility leads to higher risk of thromboembolic disease. Respiratory muscle dysfunction is common, especially following cardiac, chest, or upper abdominal operations. Cardiac surgeries are associated with a 10%–85%

Table 11.1. Incidence rates for postoperative pulmonary complications

Complication	Incidence (%)
Hypoxemia	10–40
Atelectasis	
Head and neck surgery	40
Cardiac surgery	100
Thoracotomy	37
Laparotomy	42
Pulmonary edema	2–20
Pneumonia	9–40
Deep venous thrombosis	5–28
Pulmonary embolism	2–5
Pleural effusion	
Cardiac surgery	20
Thoracotomy	75
Laparotomy	65

incidence of phrenic nerve dysfunction due to phrenic nerve injury, either by cold injury or by direct operative damage. Bilateral phrenic injury is seen in 2% of cases and can lead to ventilator dependence in patients with limited pulmonary reserve, especially during REM sleep. Dysfunction may last from 30 days up to 2 years. Thoracotomies with intercostal incisions may cause direct muscle injury with decreased respiratory muscle pressures for up to a month after surgery.

Reflex reduction in central phrenic nerve output secondary to vagal, splanchnic, or sympathetic afferent receptors frequently causes diaphragmatic dysfunction. Stimulation of GI viscera during surgical manipulation can cause cessation of diaphragmatic electrical activity.[8] Upper abdominal operations are associated with diaphragm dysfunction that may persist for 48 hours to

Medical Management of the Surgical Patient: A Textbook of Perioperative Medicine, ed. M. F. Lubin, R. B. Smith, T. F. Dobson, N. Spell, H. K. Walker. 4th edn. Published by Cambridge University Press. © Cambridge University 2006.

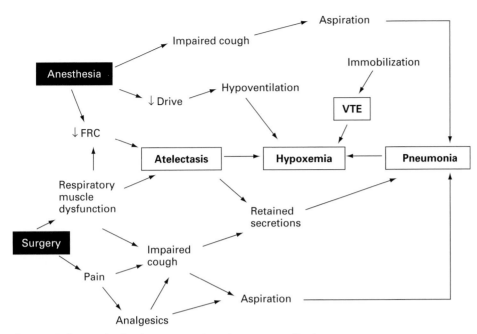

Fig 11.1. Pathogenesis of major postoperative pulmonary complications.

7 days after surgery. Patients adopt a rib cage-accessory muscle pattern of breathing which may predispose to basilar atelectasis. These changes are less dramatic after laparoscopic abdominal surgery.[9] Diaphragm dysfunction may be ameliorated by administration of theophylline or the respiratory stimulant doxapram.[10]

All these processes contribute to postoperative hypoxemia and can progress to respiratory failure in patients with limited respiratory reserve (Fig 11.1). Even with optimal preoperative and perioperative care, some patients will develop postoperative hypoxemia, atelectasis, pulmonary edema, pneumonia, pleural effusion or venous thromboembolism. This chapter covers their diagnosis and management.

Hypoxemia

Hypoxemia is common after surgery. It is defined as an arterial saturation less than 90% or a PaO_2 that is 75% or less of the preoperative value. Mild hypoxemia may be seen after up to 40% of surgeries and may be severe in 6%–7%. The largest drops are seen in the recovery room, but late desaturations are often seen on surgical wards through the second or third postoperative night and may be encountered as late as the fourth or fifth night. The frequency and severity of postoperative hypoxemia depends upon the surgical site, with thoracic and upper abdominal surgeries most severely affected. The average PaO_2 drops by 10%–30% immediately after surgery. In upper abdominal surgery, arterial oxygen typically decreases by 20%–30% in the first 48 hours after surgery. In non-abdominal, non-thoracic surgery it will decrease by 5%–10%. The risk of postoperative hypoxemia is further increased for obese patients, those requiring intravenous opioids for postoperative pain control, and for individuals with underlying chronic airflow obstruction.

Hypoxemia is multifactorial, resulting from anesthetic induced ventilation–perfusion mismatching and shunt, absorption atelectasis due to high intraoperative F_iO_2, airway tissue edema, secretions, the tongue falling into and obstructing the pharynx, alveolar hypoventilation due to residual anesthetic effect, decreased functional residual capacity (FRC), dependent airway closure, rapid shallow breathing, impaired cough, and mechanical ventilatory inefficiency due to incisional pain or restrictive bandages.[11]

Restrictive lung volume changes are thought to reflect the effects of general anesthesia and muscle relaxants in the supine patient. The decline in lung volumes begins during surgery and progresses for up to 4 days postoperatively. 20%–25% of basal lung tissue is collapsed in 85%–90% of patients. Intraoperative atelectasis can be briefly reversed by positive pressure breaths at 40 cm H_2O in almost all cases,[12] but it may take 2 weeks or more for lung volumes to return to baseline postoperatively. Total lung capacity (TLC) and each of its subdivisions decrease following thoracic and abdominal surgery, but not after operations on an extremity. Diminished TLC impairs cough effectiveness. There is a decline of 25%–50% in vital capacity (VC), residual volume (RV), functional residual capacity (FRC), tidal volume (VT) and in expiratory flow rates, such as forced expiratory volume in one second (FEV_1).

Persistent anesthetic or narcotic effects or a postoperative rebound in REM sleep may impair central control of ventilatory drive and upper airway patency. Mixed, central, and obstructive sleep apneas have been documented in many postoperative patients, with an average apnea–hypopnea index of 12 events/hour. Of these events 7%–25% were associated with oxygen desaturation.[13] Right to left intracardiac shunting through a patent foramen ovale may occur in patients with underlying pulmonary hypertension, particularly after pneumonectomy.[14] Hypoxemia may also be caused by any of the other postoperative pulmonary complications discussed below.

All postoperative patients should be monitored by pulse oximetry until oxygen saturation has returned to 93% or to their preoperative baseline. In high risk patients, monitoring may be needed for 5 days or more.[15] Supplemental oxygen should be administered as needed by a nasal cannula or face mask with appropriate caution for patients with severe chronic obstructive lung disease. Non-invasive or endotracheal positive pressure or mechanical ventilatory support may be required for refractory hypoxemic or hypercapnic respiratory failure.

Pulmonary edema

Pulmonary edema is an increase in extravascular lung water that forms when interstitial fluid accumulates faster than it can be drained by the pulmonary lymphatics. It is encountered in approximately 2%–20% of surgical patients, and is associated with an 11.9% case fatality rate. In the absence of medical comorbidity, incidence and mortality fall to 2.6% and 3.9%, respectively. In surgical patients, pulmonary edema is most often seen in patients with pre-existing cardiac disease.

Pulmonary edema may develop because of increased microvascular hydrostatic pressures or increased pulmonary capillary permeability. Less often, pulmonary edema forms because of structural stress failure of the pulmonary capillaries, or from reperfusion injury. Pulmonary edema causes an increase in pulmonary airway and vascular resistance, decreased FRC, V/Q mismatching, and an increased risk for lung infection. Shunt occurs when alveoli collapse or become filled by liquid.

Table 11.2. Appropriate intraoperative fluid replacement[16]

Source	Amount
Blood loss	Measured
Intraoperative evaporation	150 cm³/h
Insensible loss	25 cm³/h
Third space redistribution	200 cm³/h
Urine output	Measured (~70 cm³/h)
Tube drainage	Measured
Total	375 cm³/h + measured losses

Large volumes of fluids given during surgery characteristically re-enter the intravascular space on the third or fourth postoperative day causing increased pulmonary hydrostatic pressures. The amount of fluid that causes pulmonary edema varies with age, body weight, tissue turgor, cardiopulmonary and renal function, vasopressin levels, and size of the third space. Net retention of more than 2.2 l/d or more than 20% body weight increases the likelihood of pulmonary edema.[16] Administered fluids are often difficult to track because the fluid record appears in several different places in the chart. The surgeon is often unaware of the overall fluid status, and daily weights are frequently overlooked or not measured. Fluid replacement should be based on actual plus estimated intraoperative losses (Table 11.2).

A patient with underlying heart disease may develop congestive heart failure from volume overload or from a myocardial infarction during the surgery, producing pulmonary edema. Decreased plasma oncotic pressures may develop when protein from the intravascular compartment is lost into a third-space compartment, as with a postoperative ileus, or from the metabolic response to surgery. Pulmonary edema, however, rarely results from an isolated reduction in oncotic pressure.

Pulmonary edema or pulmonary hemorrhage secondary to upper airway obstruction has recently been described, occurring in 0.05%–0.1% of general anesthesias.[17] Pulmonary interstitial pressure tracks pleural pressure; in the presence of an obstructed upper airway, extreme negative pleural pressures can be generated. The fall in perimicrovascular pressure increases fluid filtration across the pulmonary vascular bed. When sufficiently severe, capillary stress failure may occur, leading to alveolar hemorrhage as well as to edema. Postobstructive edema can be severe, even fatal. It generally occurs shortly after extubation but may be seen as long as 36 hours postoperatively. Laryngospasm is often premonitory. When encountered, the jaw should be elevated and oxygen administered. Reintubation is often necessary. Resolution over 24 hours is the usual course.[18,19]

Toxic substances such as bacterial endotoxin, lysosomal enzymes, microemboli, fat emboli, or platelet aggregates released during surgery or from ischemic tissue may deposit in the pulmonary capillary bed and cause capillary endothelial injury. This damage produces capillary leak and permeability pulmonary edema.

Reperfusion pulmonary edema is seen in about 20% of lung transplants, resulting in increased ventilator dependence, length of stay, and raising mortality almost fourfold. Patients with pre-existing pulmonary hypertension are at greatest risk for this form of edema.[20]

The diagnosis of pulmonary edema is based on the clinical examination and on the roentgenographic picture, with bilateral râles, and a chest X-ray showing diffuse fluffy infiltrates. Hydrostatic edema commonly is associated with perihilar opacities in a butterfly-wing pattern, widening of the vascular pedicle, Kerley B lines, and with an enlarged cardiac silhouette. Jugular venous distention is common. Permeability edema tends to show patchy opacities with normal cardiac and vascular profiles.[21] Arterial blood gases show hypoxemia which may be severe. A Swan–Ganz catheter may be useful to the physician by measuring left-sided filling pressures to differentiate pulmonary edema caused by volume overload or a cardiac etiology from permeability pulmonary edema, but its use has not been shown to improve outcomes.

The treatment of pulmonary edema requires correction of underlying problems and scrupulous control of preload. A slightly negative fluid balance has been shown to improve survival in patients with pulmonary edema.[22] Reduction of intravascular and extracellular volume can be accomplished using potent diuretics such as furosemide, by hemodialysis, or by hemofiltration in patients with renal failure. Afterload reduction is essential in patients with impaired left ventricular systolic function. Left ventricular filling pressure should be maintained at the lowest level that does not produce a fall in cardiac stroke volume or a decrease in renal blood flow. This can normally be accomplished at pulmonary capillary wedge pressures of 10–14 mm Hg, but may need to be higher in the presence of an abnormally stiff left ventricle. Serum electrolytes should be followed closely to detect hypokalemia or hypernatremia from overdiuresis. Blood urea nitrogen and urine sodium are helpful indices of the adequacy of renal blood flow. Fluid balance should be monitored closely to avoid significant dehydration. Packed red cells may be given to anemic patients. Oxygen should be administered to all hypoxic patients. Positive pressure, through an endotracheal tube or by non-invasive mask ventilation, is useful in the treatment of pulmonary edema through alveolar recruitment, reduction of preload by reduction of venous return to the thorax, and by diminution of left ventricular afterload.

Atelectasis

Atelectasis is the collapse of a group of alveoli, a small lobule, a bronchopulmonary segment, a lobe, or rarely, a whole lung. It is one of the most common pulmonary complications in the post-operative patient. (Table 11.1) Atelectasis is clinically important because it leads to increased work of breathing, impaired gas exchange, and a predisposition to infection. Symptoms resulting from acute lobar collapse are in proportion to underlying lung diseases. An otherwise healthy person will have few symptoms from lobar collapse while a person with chronic lung disease can become significantly hypoxic and tachypneic. O'Donohue showed that clinically significant atelectasis occurs in 20% of patients undergoing upper abdominal surgery and 30% in thoracic surgery patients.[23] The evolution of atelectasis is described above. Microatelectasis, which is not radiographically visible but causes hypoxemia, is likewise common.

The diagnosis of atelectasis is based on the physical examination and on the chest roentgenogram. Tachypnea, râles, and absent, reduced, or bronchial breath sounds in dependent portions of the lungs, decreased resonance to percussion, and reduction in the movement of the ipsilateral diaphragm may be encountered. The presence or absence of fever does not reliably predict atelectasis.[24] The trachea may be shifted to the atelectatic side. There may be mild leukocytosis. The chest film may show increased density in a local segment, displacement of lobar fissures, elevation of the ipsilateral diaphragm, mediastinal shift towards the side of the collapse, hilar displacement, or compensatory hyperinflation of other lung segments. An air bronchogram indicates that the bronchus feeding the atelectatic segment is patent. It is sometimes difficult to differentiate between atelectasis and pneumonia, especially in the absence of bronchial obstruction. When atelectasis results from an obstructed bronchus, fremitus will be decreased and there will be dullness to percussion. Auscultation will show absent or decreased breath sounds.

The treatment of atelectasis is based on two principles. The lungs must be expanded with a transpulmonary pressure sufficient to open collapsed lung units, and stagnant secretions must be cleared. Supplemental oxygen may be necessary to treat hypoxemia. Various therapeutic maneuvers have been used to treat atelectasis. Treatment modalities include early mobilization, incentive spirometry, deep breathing exercises, yawning, coughing, chest physiotherapy, and nasal CPAP. Intermittent positive pressure breathing has been abandoned because of problems with barotrauma. Numerous studies have been done to compare different treatment modalities. Unfortunately, no consensus exists as to the best treatment options for atelectasis.[12]

Although 95% of hospitals in the United States use incentive spirometry to treat atelectasis after laparotomy and 71% after coronary artery bypass, meta-analyses have failed to document a consistent beneficial effect.[25] Benefit is seen only for intermediate risk patients; no advantage has been demonstrated for highest or lowest risk groups.[26] Among incentive spirometers, volumetric rather than flowmetric devices may be more effective and minimal imposed work of breathing appears to result in greater increments in inspiratory capacity. Utility of incentive spirometry may depend on adequate preoperative education and postoperative supervision, thereby negating any potential cost savings.

In most contemporary studies of postoperative patients, incentive spirometry combined with chest physiotherapy provides no better results than chest physiotherapy alone.[27,28] Chest physiotherapy generally consists of deep breathing exercises, chest percussion, and postural drainage where needed. Deep breathing is most effective when 5 sequential breaths are held at TLC for 5–6 seconds and repeated hourly during waking hours. For established atelectasis, positive pressure ventilation, delivered as PEEP, CPAP, or BiPAP at 10–15 cm H_2O appears to provide satisfactory therapeutic results.[29,30]

When an area of the lung is not ventilated, mucus secreted from the bronchi draining that area becomes thickened and impacted. This makes reexpansion of alveoli in that segment difficult. Chest physiotherapy and postural drainage will help to loosen and clear the mucus. Adequate hydration, along with the use of bronchodilators and mucolytic agents such as acetylcysteine or guaifenesin, may help to liquefy and mobilize secretions. Tracheal suctioning is used to remove mucus which cannot be removed by cough or other respiratory maneuvers. Adequate pain relief is crucial so that the patient can cough without discomfort. On the other hand, oversedation with narcotics can depress respiratory drive and cause shallow respirations, exacerbating the problem of atelectasis. Epidural analgesia appears to provide the best balance between pain relief and respiratory drive. Patient controlled infusions of analgesics may also provide an effective treatment.[31,32]

Often, conservative therapy, such as incentive spirometry, coughing, chest physiotherapy, bronchodilator

Table 11.3. Risk for nosocomial pneumonia among surgical patients[34]

High risk	Relative risk	Low risk
Abdominal aortic aneurysm	4.29	Ophthalmologic
Thoracotomy	3.94	Otorhinolaryngologic
Upper abdominal	2.68	Lower abdominal
Neck	2.3	GU
Neurosurgical	2.14	Extremity
Vascular	1.29	Peripheral vascular
Emergency	1.33	Spine and back

therapy, hydration and occasional mucolytic agent use and tracheal suctioning, will successfully reverse atelectasis in the first 24–48 hours. Occasionally, atelectasis must be treated by more aggressive measures. Fiberoptic bronchoscopy may be used to extract mucus plugs, instill mucolytic agents directly into affected areas and lavage the airways. If an air-bronchogram is present in the area of atelectasis, indicating patent central airways and suggestive of pneumonia, fiberoptic bronchoscopy is not likely to be helpful.[33] Selective air insufflation of atelectatic areas by a balloon tipped catheter introduced into the appropriate bronchus under fluoroscopic guidance or bronchoscopically may be effective in certain difficult cases. If adequate expansion cannot be accomplished with the above methods, endotracheal intubation and continuous mechanical ventilation may be needed.

Pneumonia

Epidemiology

Pneumonia is the second most common hospital-acquired infection and the leading cause of death from nosocomial infection. Hospital-acquired pneumonia is more common in surgical than medical populations.[34] Any procedure requiring general anesthesia involves increased risk for postoperative pneumonia. Relative risks of specific surgeries are summarized in Table 11.3.

Postoperative pneumonia occurs in up to 9%–40% of patients, the risk depending on the surgical procedure as well as patient-specific risk factors.

Burn patients, particularly those with inhalation injury are at the highest risk, 50% higher than cardiothoracic or neurosurgery patients, and nearly three times higher than medical patients.[35]

Although most published studies address nosocomial pneumonia in the ICU setting, more cases may be encountered on general care wards. Nosocomial pneumonia is four times more likely to be encountered in a surgical ward as in a corresponding medical area.[36,37] In the ICU, postoperative pneumonia is most often seen in the mechanically ventilated patient (ventilator-associated pneumonia, VAP). In the SICU, more than 80% of postoperative pneumonias are likely to be VAP. VAP is more likely (26%–40% prevalence) to be seen in a surgical ICU (SICU) than in a medical unit (15%–25% prevalence). The risk of VAP increases with the duration of mechanical ventilation by 1%–3% per day for at least the first 2 weeks of mechanical ventilation.[38]

A number of additional patient-related factors have been associated with increased risk for postoperative pneumonia. These include age, functional status, APACHE score, ethanol intake, tobacco abuse within the year prior to surgery, altered sensorium, malnutrition as evidenced by a low serum albumin, and recent transfusion of more than 4 units of packed red blood cells.

Morbidity and mortality

Postoperative pneumonia increases the cost of care and length of stay. Overall mortality may be increased tenfold compared to patients without postoperative pneumonia, although case fatality is generally lower in surgical patients than in medical patients hospitalized with pneumonia. VAP is associated with 6–21 times higher crude mortality rates, the highest rates (43%) associated with high risk organisms such as *Pseudomonas, Acinetobacter*, or methicillin-resistant *Staphylococcus aureus*. One-third of patients with VAP die of their pneumonia; twice as many die from their comorbidities.[39]

Pathogenesis

Nosocomial pneumonia arises from a variety of exposures including endogenous flora, other patients, hospital staff, the hospital environment, and surgical wound infection.[40] Common to most, however, is colonization of the oropharynx and upper airway by respiratory pathogens, followed by infection of the lower respiratory tract by aspiration. Colonization of the upper airway with hospital flora occurs within the first 72–96 hours of hospitalization and within a few hours after intubation. Underlying conditions associated with depressed sensorium or interventions that interfere with effective swallowing represent a particular risk for pneumonia.

Prevention

VAP is, to some extent, a preventable problem. Routine hand washing in between patients and the use of glove and gown barriers when examining patients with resistant infections are simple and effective interventions. The risk of aspiration can be minimized by keeping the patient in a semi-erect position and through avoidance of gastric over-distention. Small bore feeding tubes and postpyloric feeding tube placement may be helpful approaches. Nasotracheal tubes should be converted to orotracheal or to tracheostomy as quickly as possible. Oropharyngeal secretions should always be suctioned prior to deflation of an endotracheal tube cuff. Ventilator weaning and liberation should be pursued as expeditiously as possible. Continuous subglottic suction may emerge as an important preventive modality, but more experience is needed before a definitive recommendation can be made.

GI bleeding prophylaxis remains a controversial issue, especially regarding the relationship between gastric pH and the risk of oropharyngeal colonization and VAP. Antibiotics should be used in ventilated patients as sparingly as possible and discontinued or simplified as soon as the clinical situation permits. Neutropenic patients should receive appropriate antibiotic coverage along with GCSF. Chlorhexidine oral rinses may be helpful but should be restricted to high risk patients only. In the future, immune globulin, or specific vaccinations may find utility in the prevention of VAP.[41]

Management of postoperative pneumonia is based on the clinical context. Time since hospital admission and the prior administration of antibiotics as well as the nature of the patient's surgery are key considerations. For the first 72–96 hours of the hospital stay, the microbial flora in the upper airway is comprised of common community-acquired organisms. This is true of both general wards and intensive care units, whether the patient is intubated or not. Early-onset pneumonias are generally responsive to shorter courses of antibiotics and tend to be associated with a relatively lower mortality. The microbial flora seen in early pneumonias in surgical patients is the same as that encountered in community-acquired pneumonia in a medical setting. *Staphylococcus*, however, is frequent in neurosurgical and head-injured patients. When encountered early, and in the absence of prior antibiotics, it is almost always methicillin sensitive. Longer hospitalization and prior antibiotic use increases the likelihood of a methicillin-resistant isolate.

Many surgical patients receive antibiotics as part of their initial management, either as part of initial trauma resuscitation, or as preoperative wound prophylaxis. The use of antibiotics decreases the incidence of early onset pneumonias and virtually eliminates *H. influenzae* and *S. pneumoniae* as pathogens. Unfortunately, prior antibiotic use also increases the frequency of late onset pneumonias with a less-responsive and higher-risk bacterial flora. This is especially problematic with broad spectrum antibiotics, leading to the frequent isolation of resistance-prone organisms (e.g., *Pseudomonas, Acinetobacter baumanii*, methicillin-resistant *Staphylococcus aureus*). Patients with a shorter duration of preoperative hospitalization, such as those with trauma, are more likely to develop early type pneumonia while laparotomy patients tend to present with a late onset microbial spectrum.

Microbiology

Nosocomial pneumonia is polymicrobial in 40%–60% of cases. Bacteremia is seen in approximately 10%. Post-operative pneumonia differs from medical hospital-acquired pneumonia by an excess of *Staphylococcus* and aerobic gram-negative isolates.[42] There is considerable variation in the relative proportions of organisms reported in individual studies. Some of the variability may be attributable to a failure to distinguish among early and late, and antibiotic naïve and antibiotic exposed infections. A large series describing VAP in a mixed ICU population, however, is typical (Table 11.4).

Prior antibiotic use appears more important than timing in predicting the presence of resistant flora. Anaerobes are not frequently reported although they may be present in up to 20% of cases when specifically looked for. Nevertheless, expert consensus states that anaerobes may be safely ignored in the absence of necrotizing pneumonia or abscess formation.[44]

Diagnosis

Various criteria for the diagnosis of nosocomial and ventilator-associated pneumonia are presented below in Table 11.5. Infiltrates present prior to admission or before surgery are not considered as postoperative pneumonia. Refractory VAP is defined as VAP with failure to improve after 72 hours.

Clinical diagnosis of VAP is generally characterized by greater sensitivity than specificity. Requiring all clinical criteria (Table 11.5) to be met increases specificity, but sensitivity falls below 50%.

The chest roentgenogram is also sensitive but non-specific. Radiographic appearance can be influenced by respiratory phase, depth of inspiration and even ventilator mode. High rates of interobserver variability in interpretation are common. Most infiltrates in ventilated patients are not VAP; rather pulmonary edema, pulmonary hemorrhage, and focal atelectasis are more common.[45] Absence

Table 11.4. Microbial spectrum in VAP: organism (% isolated)[43]

Early onset, no antibiotics	Early onset, prior antibiotics
Enterobacteriaciae[a] (24.4)	Enterobacteriaciae[a] (20)
Hemophilus influenzae (19.5)	*Hemophilus influenzae* (10)
Methicillin-sensitive	Streptococcal species (25)
Staphylococcus aureus (14.5)	*Neisseria* (10)
Streptococcus pneumoniae (7.3)	*Pseudomonas* (20)
Other streptococcal species (17.1)	*Acinetobacter* (5)
Neisseria/Moraxella (12.2)	Methicillin-resistant
	Staphylococcus aureus (5)

Late onset, no antibiotics	Late onset, prior antibiotics
Enterobacteriaciae[a] (21.9)	*Pseudomonas* (21.7)
Streptococcus species (21.9)	*Acinetobacter* (13.2)
Methicillin-sensitive	Methicillin-resistant
Staphylococcus aureus (21.9)	*Staphylococcus aureus* (19.7)
Neisseria (12.5)	*Stenotrophomonas*
Hemophilus (3)	Enterobacter (15)
Pseudomonas (6.3)	*Streptococcus* species (9)
Acinetobacter (3.1)	Methicillin-sensitive
Methicillin-resistant	*Staphylococcus aureus* (5)
Staphylococcus aureus (5)	
Organism (% isolated)	

Note:

[a] Enterobacteriaciae (*E. coli, Enterobacter, Serratia, Proteus, Klebsiella*).

of an infiltrate, however, effectively excludes a diagnosis of VAP.[46] Specific microbiological sampling may be helpful when a high clinical suspicion and an abnormal chest film are both present.

The diagnostic approach to VAP is summarized in Fig. 11.2 and begins with examination of a Gram's stain of respiratory tract secretions. Available evidence suggests that invasive specimens (e.g., mini BAL, BAL, bronchoscopic brush) lead to better outcomes than simple sputa or blind endotracheal aspirates. If organisms are seen, antibiotics should be based upon the local antibiogram and subsequently modified based on culture results. If cultures are negative and clinical condition is unchanged, consideration should be given to discontinuing antibiotics. If no organisms are seen on Gram's stain, but the patient exhibits signs of SIRS or sepsis, empirical antibiotics should be started based on American Thoracic Society (ATS) recommendations[47] and the local antibiogram, modified as above by subsequent culture results. In the absence of findings of SIRS, antibiotics may be withheld and other sources of infection sought.[39,48,49]

Endotracheal suction specimens are evaluated in a manner similar to sputum, based on the number of

Table 11.5. Criteria for the diagnosis of ventilator-associated pneumonia

Source	Clinical[38,50]	Centers for Disease Control (CDC) criteria[51,52]	Clinical pulmonary infection score (CPIS)[53,54]	Tracheal suction[55]	Bronchoscopic protected brush specimen[56]	Bronchoalveolar lavage[57]
Criteria	New or progressive infiltrate beginning after intubation plus 2 of 3: 1. Temperature >38 °C 2. WBC > 10 000/ml 3. Purulent endotracheal secretions	1. Râles or dullness to percussion on physical examination of chest and any of the following: • New onset of purulent sputum or change in character of sputum • Isolation of organism from blood culture, transtracheal aspirate, bronchial brushing, or biopsy 2. Chest radiography showing new or progressive infiltrate, consolidation, cavitation, or pleural effusion and any of the following: • New onset of purulent sputum or change in character of sputum. • Isolation of organism from blood culture • Isolation of pathogen from specimen obtained by transtracheal aspirate bronchial brushing, or biopsy • Isolation of virus or detection of viral antigen in respiratory secretions • Diagnostic single antibody titer (IgM) or fourfold increase in paired serum samples (IgG) for pathogen • Histopathologic evidence of pneumonia	≥7 points Temperature (°C) 36.5–38.4 (0) 38.5–38.9 (1) ≥39 or ≤36 (2) Blood WBC $\times 10^3$/l ≥4 and ≤11 (0) <4 or >11 (1) Bands >0.5 (1) Daily tracheal secretion volume (0–4) Σ<14 (0) Σ≥14 (1) Purulence (1) P_aO_2/F_iO_2 ratio mm Hg >240 or ARDS (0) ≥240 no ARDS (2) Chest roentgenogram No infiltrate (0) Diffuse/patchy (1) Localized inflit (2) Semiquantitative culture (pathogens, 0–3 +) ≥1 + or no growth (0) >1+ (1) Culture matches Gram's stain (1)	Bacteria present on Gram's stain Culture > 10^5 cfu/ml	Culture > 10^3 cfu/ml	Culture > 10^4 cfu/ml with <1% squamous cells 2–25% intracellular organisms
Sensitivity (%)	48–100	68	72	Stain 94–100 Culture 38–82	33–100 (mean 67)	42–93 (mean 73)
Specificity (%)	12–91	97.8	85	Stain 14–38 Culture 67–100	50–100 (mean 95)	45–100 (mean 82)

Source: Modified from Welty-Wolf, 2001.[58]

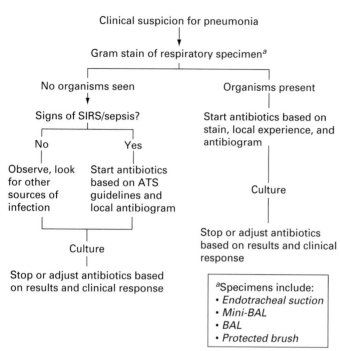

Clinical suspicion for pneumonia

Gram stain of respiratory specimen[a]

No organisms seen

Signs of SIRS/sepsis?

No — Observe, look for other sources of infection

Yes — Start antibiotics based on ATS guidelines and local antibiogram

Culture

Stop or adjust antibiotics based on results and clinical response

Organisms present

Start antibiotics based on stain, local experience, and antibiogram

Culture

Stop or adjust antibiotics based on results and clinical response

[a]Specimens include:
• Endotracheal suction
• Mini-BAL
• BAL
• Protected brush

Fig 11.2. Suggested algorithm for management of ventilator-associated pneumonia.

squamous epithelial cells and neutrophils. Diagnoses based on stains are more sensitive but less specific than those based on semiquantitative cultures, using a threshold of 10^5 or 10^6 cfu/ml. Absence of organisms on an adequate Gram's stain of endotracheal secretions makes significant pulmonary infection unlikely. Bronchoscopic specimens are somewhat less sensitive, but are associated with higher specificity than endotracheal aspirates.

In the absence of ongoing antibiotic therapy, negative cultures or lower bacterial concentrations than specified above are sufficient to exclude a clinically significant infection. Interpretation in the presence of antibiotics has not been standardized and remains problematic.[59]

Treatment

Prompt initiation of appropriate antibiotics within 12 hours of diagnosis leads to improved survival.[39,60] Modification of the antibiotic regimen based on culture results, however, fails to further improve on an initially good antibiotic choice or reverse the effects of a poor initial choice. While Gram's stain of an adequate respiratory tract specimen may help refine an initial antibiotic choice, culture results, which are not available for 24–48 hours, do not become available in sufficient time to improve outcome.[61] While invasive specimens do not necessarily improve survival, they are useful in eliminating

unnecessary antibiotics and reducing the overall duration of treatment.

The American Thoracic Society (ATS, 2001)[62] and Infectious Disease Society of America (IDSA, 2000)[63] have developed guidelines for the treatment of community-acquired pneumonia. These are applicable to patients with early onset pneumonia encountered in a ward setting or non-ventilated patients in the ICU. The ATS (1996)[47] guidelines for the management of hospital-acquired pneumonia are applicable for late pneumonias in similar settings. The ATS guidelines may be somewhat less useful in postoperative VAP because they do not address the surgical setting specifically.[61]

The most widely recommended approach to VAP is that each institution determines its own flora for the clinical scenarios shown above as well as the local sensitivity patterns for those organisms. Use of a locally derived algorithm can lead to correct therapy in as many as 94% of cases.[64] Hospital day, rather than ICU day, should be used to categorize by time, and antibiotic use within the past 15 days should be the basis for categorization. Monotherapy may be safely used for Group I (early pneumonia, no antibiotics).[44] As the probability of multiresistant organisms rises, combination therapy becomes more important and is obligatory for Group IV (late pneumonia, prior antibiotics) patients. Vancomycin or linezolid should be used as part of initial therapy for Group III and Group IV patients to cover the possibility of MRSA but can be safely withheld for Group I and II pneumonias or when an adequate Gram stain indicates the absence of Gram positive cocci.

An initial regimen should be modified once culture results become available. Any redundant or unnecessary antibiotics should be discontinued as soon as possible. All antibiotics should be stopped in the event of negative cultures.[65]

Duration of treatment has not been definitively determined. Too short a course of treatment will fail to eradicate the infection, leading to treatment failure, while too long a course will encourage resistant microorganisms to develop. The average duration of therapy, according to an expert panel, is about 10 days. This may be as short as 72 hours after clinical resolution in Group I–II patients, usually less than 7 days, but may be 14–21 days for Group IV patients. Failure to improve after 7 days should call for a reassessment of infections and their treatment.[66]

Aspiration

Aspiration is defined as inhalation of oropharyngeal or gastric contents into the larynx and lower respiratory tract. There are two separate aspiration syndromes, aspiration pneumonitis and aspiration pneumonia; clinicians commonly fail to distinguish the two, using antibiotics unnecessarily. Aspiration pneumonia is defined as inhalation of oropharyngeal secretions colonized by pathogens and is addressed above. It is important to note that, in the absence of severe periodontal disease or radiographic evidence of necrotizing pneumonia, anaerobes are only rarely present.[67]

Aspiration pneumonitis is chemical injury due to inhalation of sterile gastric contents. The major risk is depressed consciousness and is inversely related to the Glasgow Coma Score. It is a chemical burn, manifesting as wheezing, cough, dyspnea, and cyanosis, sometimes with hypotension. Severe aspiration injuries, associated with pH < 2.5 and aspirated volumes > 0.3 ml/kg (20–25 ml) may progress to ARDS. Aspiration may be clinically silent, manifesting only as a desaturation episode. The upper airway should be examined in the event of an aspiration episode and should be suctioned. Patients with depressed consciousness should be intubated. Empiric antibiotics are appropriate only for patients with small bowel obstruction or ileus and for pneumonitis that fails to resolve within 48 hours. Fluoroquinolones, piperacillin/tazobactam, or ceftriaxone provide adequate coverage in most cases. There is no benefit to the addition of systemic glucocorticoids.[68]

Venous thromboembolism

Epidemiology

Venous thromboembolism (VTE) is 10 to 100 times more frequent in the surgical setting than in a medical population, and may complicate 5%–28% of all operations.[69] Without adequate prophylaxis, deep venous thrombosis (DVT) is seen in 50% of hip replacements, 65% of knee replacements and half of all lower extremity trauma.[70] Quadriplegics have a threefold increased risk evident by day 5 postinjury with the greatest risk from days 21 through 90.[71] The incidence of perioperative VTE is reduced by some 80% in the presence of appropriate prophylaxis. Perioperative DVT prophylaxis is discussed elsewhere in this volume (see Chapter 17). Pulmonary embolism causes 5%–10% of all hospital deaths. It is found in 23.6% of surgical autopsies and is the attributable cause of death in 6.4% (27). VTE has a 20%–30% recurrence rate within 5–8 years without treatment. The risk of recurrence falls to 5%–8% with anticoagulant therapy. Approximately 6% of recurrent VTE episodes may be

fatal. There is a 2% rate of permanent disability due to chronic thrombophlebitis, chronic venous insufficiency, or to chronic thromboembolic pulmonary hypertension. Of all patients with PE 11% die within the first hour before treatment can be started. If PE remains unrecognized, 30% of initial survivors will die without further treatment. Mortality from PE complicated by shock, 10% of all cases, is 35%. The overall treated mortality for PE is 5%–8%, and is as low as 2% in patients without shock.[72]

The risk of perioperative VTE is determined by a number of patient-specific factors. The odds of VTE vary directly with age, but do not exclude patients under the age of 40 from risk. Malignancy and obesity are additive risks. As in a medical population, thrombophilia and hypercoagulable states may contribute to clotting risk. Inherited factors are present in up to 25% of the population. Of these, Factor V Leiden is the most common.[73] Screening does not improve perioperative outcomes, and is not recommended for surgical patients except for those with a positive family history of thrombophilia or recent personal history of unexplained DVT.[74] Acquired medical disorders, e.g., antiphospholipid antibody, myeloproliferative disorders, and nephrotic syndrome may increase individual risk. Clinical likelihood of VTE increases with the duration of preoperative immobilization, and with the duration, complexity, and location of the surgical procedure. Coronary artery bypass surgery, neurosurgery, joint replacement, and multiple trauma, especially skeletal are among the highest risk situations. More than half of postoperative pulmonary emboli are seen in the first 7 days after surgery.[75]

Each element of Virchow's triad is accentuated during the perioperative period. Stasis will be present in the bedbound patient preoperatively. During surgery, anesthesia and paralysis are associated with decreased venous blood flow. In the supine position, the right common iliac artery compresses the left common iliac vein, impeding venous drainage from the left leg. Tourniquets for lower extremity surgeries and increases in abdominal pressure during gas insufflation for laparoscopy will likewise compromise lower extremity blood flow.[69] In the postoperative period, immobilization is common. Blood flow is reduced to the ipsilateral side in joint replacement surgery. This can persist for as long as 1 week following knee replacement and for 6 weeks after total hip replacement.

Like trauma, surgical injury leads to increased coagulability. Levels of Antithrombin III, Protein S, and Protein C are reduced.[76] Tumor necrosis factor, von Willebrand factor and PAI-1 are all elevated postoperatively. The latter inhibits TPA and leads to a decrease in circulating plasmin activity. Surgical injury releases tissue factor into the circulation, activating the extrinsic coagulation pathway. In joint replacement surgery, methyl methacrylate glue has been shown to enhance coagulation when it gains access to the circulation. The net increase in thrombin generation may persist for as long as 5 weeks postoperatively.[77] Traumatic quadriplegics are at special risk due to venous valvular incompetence, loss of the skeletal muscle pump in the lower extremities, and impaired fibrinolysis. These patients are at particular risk in the first 2 weeks following injury, and clot formation may persist despite clinically adequate anticoagulation.[71] Deep venous thrombosis is commonly encountered adjacent to surgical sites, reflecting vascular torsion, compression, or interruption. DVT is 20 times more frequent in the ipsilateral leg in total hip replacements, is commonly seen in femoral vessels in hip replacement, and in popliteal vessels in knee replacement.

Diagnosis

Venous thromboembolism is an especially difficult diagnosis in the surgical patient because it is often clinically silent. Bedside diagnosis in this setting carries a sensitivity of 25% and a specificity of 33%.[78] In a medical population, 97% of patients with pulmonary embolism have dyspnea, tachycardia, or pleuritic chest pain. In a meta-analysis of six studies from 1976 through 1989 comprising 191 patients, 70%–100% of surgical pulmonary embolism is asymptomatic.[79] Of patients with documented postoperative DVT 13%–100% (average 40%–50%) had asymptomatic pulmonary emboli on lung scan.[80] Reliability of the bedside diagnosis of venous thromboembolism was often compromised by other postoperative issues, misinterpretation of premonitory signs such as syncope, and overconfidence in the efficacy of prophylactic measures.

This mandates a high level of suspicion on the part of the consulting physician and calls for an aggressive diagnostic workup when venous thromboembolism is considered. Because of the high rate of asymptomatic pulmonary emboli among surgical patients with documented DVT, both manifestations of VTE need to be evaluated in each patient. Preferred treatment options are summarized in Table 11.6.

DVT

The bedside diagnosis of DVT is notoriously unreliable. Calf pain has a sensitivity of 66%–91% with a specificity ranging from 3% to 87%. Calf tenderness has a sensitivity of 56%–82% and a specificity of 26%–74%. Calf swelling is 35%–97% sensitive and 8%–88% specific. Homans' sign is reported as 13%–48% sensitive and 39%–84% specific and

cannot be evaluated in the presence of bandages, casts, splints, or traction. Bedside findings can only suggest the need for further study.[81]

Contrast venography is the *de facto* gold standard for the diagnosis of DVT. It is infrequently used in contemporary practice because of the convenience of non-invasive modalities as well as problems with contrast allergy, venous access in the presence of edema, pain, possible phlebitis, and concern for precipitating renal failure.

Doppler or duplex ultrasound is currently a first-line diagnostic modality in DVT. It is 95% sensitive and 100% specific in symptomatic DVT patients. Accuracy falls above the inguinal ligaments and below the knee. Interpretation is operator dependent. Once again, the study is less reliable for the diagnosis of DVT in asymptomatic limbs, with 62% sensitivity and 97% specificity. Reliability is even lower for asymptomatic calf vein thrombosis with sensitivity of 33%–58%. Ultrasound is not suitable for the evaluation of recurrent or chronic DVT, and cannot be used in the presence of extreme obesity, edema, casts, and other immobilization devices.

CT venography has a sensitivity of 89%–100% and specificity of 92%–100% compared to Doppler ultrasound. It offers the advantage of visualization of abdominal and pelvic, as well as femoropopliteal thromboses, but is associated with increased radiation exposure and a cost 8 to 15 times higher than ultrasound studies.[82–85]

Magnetic resonance angiography is an attractive alternative in the setting of asymptomatic DVT. MRI has a reported sensitivity of 80%–100% and a specificity of 90%–100% for acute symptomatic proximal DVT. MRI is good for evaluation of celiac, iliac, calf, and bilateral venous disease, as well as for repeat examinations. Limitations include expense, patient claustrophobia, availability of reader expertise, and obesity. Of particular concern in the surgical setting is the absolute contraindication for metallic devices of any kind, including surgical clips and sutures.

Impedance plethysmography (IPG) has a reported sensitivity in symptomatic DVT of 65%–98% and a specificity of 83%–98%. A negative study is associated with a 1.5% risk of subsequent VTE and almost no risk of fatal pulmonary embolism. False-positive results may be seen with high intra-abdominal pressure in obesity or ascites, high central venous pressures, low arterial flow, and non-thrombotic outflow obstruction. IPG may be of limited value in evaluating calf vein DVT. IPG is of less value in surgical patients because thrombi tend to be smaller and non-occlusive and because of the higher frequency of asymptomatic cases. Diagnostic sensitivity has been reported as 12%–64% in hip surgery patients.

Radiolabeled fibrinogen studies have a sensitivity of 94% and a specificity of 91% but are not commonly used in current practice. Tc99 apcitide has a sensitivity of 67%–88% and a specificity of 73%–86% against contrast venography. Diagnostic performance is enhanced by comparison of 10-minute and 120-minute images.[86,87]

The standard approach for symptomatic DVT recommends duplex ultrasound or IPG. If initial studies are negative, serial studies should be obtained over a 7–14-day period. Contrast venography or MRI are recommended if clinical suspicion remains high. For the asymptomatic patient, ultrasound and IPG are considered unreliable. MRI or contrast venography may represent the best available choices.[81]

Pulmonary embolism

The clinical diagnosis of pulmonary embolism is also difficult. Tachypnea with acute respiratory alkalosis is the rule. Tachycardia is frequent. Arterial blood gases show abnormal A–aO$_2$ gradients in 85%–90% of cases, but a normal gradient does not rule out pulmonary embolism. The electrocardiogram is abnormal in 70%–87% of cases but findings are usually non-specific. S$_1$Q$_3$T$_3$ and right bundle branch block are seen in <20% of cases, and in up to 60% in patients with shock or syncope.

The plain chest roentgenogram is usually abnormal but, again, non-specific. Abnormal findings include pleural effusion, Hampton's hump, elevated hemidiaphragm, atelectasis and focal oligemia in involved segments, and Westermark's sign, present in 6% of patients.

D-dimer reflects breakdown of fibrin. ELISA (100% sensitivity) performs better than latex agglutination based tests (60%–67% sensitivity). A level below 500 micrograms per liter is thought to exclude the presence of DVT or PE. Absence of fibrin would be unexpected in the postoperative period, limiting the utility of this test in surgical patients. Because of diagnostic variability among various commercial test kits, measurement of D-dimer is not currently recommended as part of the standard evaluation. D-dimer is elevated after surgical procedures, especially in cancer patients, but higher levels have been reported in postoperative patients with VTE. In a surgical population the sensitivity of D-dimer is 100%, specificity 43%, positive predictive value 35% and negative predictive value 100%.[88] A low or negative D-dimer may therefore be of some value in the decision-making process.

The standard diagnostic evaluation for pulmonary embolism begins with radionuclide lung scanning (Fig. 11.3). For most situations, a perfusion scan alone will be adequate for diagnostic purposes. Prior clinical probability is central to interpretation; these probabilities will be higher for surgical patients than for otherwise comparable medical patients.

A negative perfusion scan effectively excludes a diagnosis of pulmonary embolism. For surgical patients with a compatible clinical picture, a high probability scan confirms the diagnosis and calls for immediate treatment. In the PIOPED study,[89] a large proportion (77%) of V/Q scans were indeterminate (intermediate or low probability), but 25% of these patients had pulmonary emboli demonstrated on angiography. Nondiagnostic results are more likely in the presence of pre-existing cardiopulmonary disorders.

In stable patients, a nondiagnostic nuclear scan should prompt evaluation of the lower extremities for the presence of DVT. Stability is defined as the absence of pulmonary edema, right ventricular failure, syncope, or tachyarrhythmia, a systolic blood pressure >90 mm Hg, and FEV$_1$ more than one liter, $P_aO_2 > 50$ mm Hg and $P_aCO_2 < 45$ mm Hg. In the presence of instability as defined above, pulmonary angiography is the next diagnostic step. Treatment can be withheld for a normal perfusion scan (98% sensitivity). Indeterminate scans with negative lower extremity DVT evaluations likewise need not be treated. The incidence of subsequent VTE is approximately 1.9%.[72,89,90]

Spiral CT has attracted considerable recent interest as an alternative screening study to V/Q imaging. Its proponents argue that there is a much lower proportion of nondiagnostic studies compared to radionuclide scanning with the added benefit of nonvascular diagnoses available from examination of the pulmonary parenchyma and pleural space. Sensitivity is reported between 60% and 100% with a specificity of 78%–97%. Spiral CT has high diagnostic reliability for large central clots (96% sensitivity, 92% specificity) but is less accurate for peripheral emboli, missing subsegmental emboli in 25%. Interobserver agreement is relatively poor for peripheral abnormalities, although subsegmental emboli were only reported in 6% of PIOPED cases. The risk of further thromboembolic events in the presence of a negative reading of a spiral CT study combined with a negative ultrasound examination of the lower extremities has been repeatedly shown to be less than 1%.[91,92] With these results, withholding anticoagulation in settings other than high prior probability may be an acceptable strategy.[93] The status of spiral CT is currently the subject of a large multicenter trial, and data pertaining specifically to surgical populations are needed before the role of the spiral CT can be reliably established.

Although contrast angiography is regarded as the gold standard for the diagnosis of pulmonary embolism, it

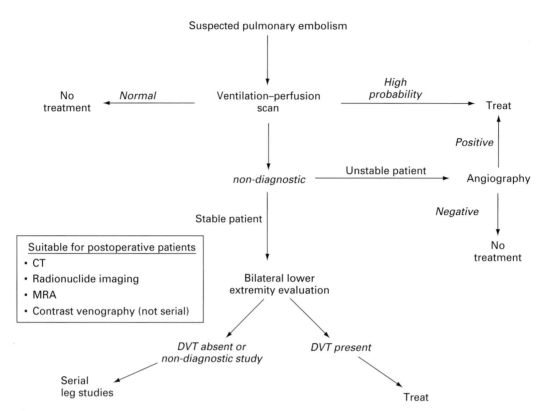

Fig 11.3. Suggested algorithm for approach to pulmonary thromboembolism in the postoperative setting. See text for abbreviations.

should be noted that reliability decreases for more peripheral clots. Interobserver agreement for subsegmental clots is on the order of 66%. Contrast pulmonary angiography is associated with a 4% complication rate and 0.2%–0.5% mortality. Renal failure occurs in 0.4% with elevation in creatinine in another 0.9%.[78,81]

Echocardiography is a potentially useful noninvasive modality. Direct visualization of central thrombus, right ventricular dilatation or dysfunction, paradoxical septal motion, and dilatation of the right pulmonary artery segment are all highly suggestive findings. Transthoracic echo is normal in 19% of pulmonary emboli. Transesophageal echo is capable of visualizing clot in 50%–60% of cases.

Treatment

Medical decision making in the management of postoperative VTE is difficult due to the lack of controlled trials on the subject. It demands a careful balance of the benefit of anticoagulation against the risk of exacerbating postoperative bleeding vs. the risk of untreated thromboembotic disease. Treatment should not be undertaken without face-to-face discussion with the primary surgical team.

Significant postoperative bleeding is seen in 3%–5% of surgeries. Bleeding may occur despite normal coagulation preoperatively. Half of these bleeding episodes require reexploration with consequent increased rates of wound infection, hospital stay, and resource consumption. Death occurs in approximately 3% of postoperative bleeds. Postoperative bleeding may occur due to a surgical problem and usually manifests as a specific bleeding site. This is seen in 30%–60% of reoperations. Medical bleeding presents as diffuse oozing, and is associated with worse outcomes. Causes of medical postoperative bleeding include prior medications, e.g., aspirin, NSAIDs, GlyIIb/IIIa inhibitors, coumadin, or intraoperative thrombolysis; coagulopathy due to thrombocytopenia, to factor deficiency, e.g., vitamin K-dependent factors, liver disease, transfusion washout, or DIC; to specific factor inhibitors acquired preoperatively or intraoperatively; or to increased fibrinolysis, e.g., due to clotted blood in the mediastinum after thoracotomy. The period of greatest risk for postoperative bleeding is in the first 24 hours, but bleeding can be seen as long as 10 days after surgery.[94–96]

The use of heparin increases the risk of postoperative bleeding. In a medical setting, the rate of major bleeding from unfractionated heparin is approximately 4%

(2.1%–9.5%).[97–99] Case fatality from major bleeding is approximately 3%. Among surgical patients, the risk of postoperative bleeding with heparin rises to 10.5%, and is usually major. Case fatality from major bleeds is similar to the medical population, 3%. Bleeding is typically seen at or near operative sites, in the thigh for hip replacement, or in the retroperitoneum for laparotomies. Other typical sites include intracranial, gastrointestinal, genitourinary, muscle, and abdominal wall.[100,101]

The rate of postoperative bleeding from heparin increases with increasing PTT. Risk of bleeding rises with heparin dose, with advancing age, and with associated comorbidities.[99] It should be noted, however, that the risk of recurrent thromboembolism exceeds the risk of bleeding due to overtreatment.[102]

Coumadin is not associated with increased bleeding risk in surgical settings, probably because the INR does not reach therapeutic levels for 72 hours after initiation.[103] Because of the varying half-lives of vitamin K dependent clotting factors, INR is unreliable in the first 3 days of treatment.[102,104,105]

Treatment for VTE is appropriate when clot is seen on contrast pulmonary angiogram, spiral CT, or in the presence of the high probability V/Q scan; when echocardiography reveals intracardiac thrombus or pulmonary artery clot; or when DVT is diagnosed by venography, ultrasound, or impedance or when there is high clinical suspicion for DVT or PE.[72,106]

VTE is treated with either unfractionated heparin (UFH) or with low molecular weight heparin (LMWH). LMWH is preferred for PE. Coumadin may be started at the same time. Heparin catalyzes Antithrombin III to inactivate Factors IIa, Xa, and IXa as well as V and VIII. The effective half-time of heparin varies directly with dose, usually between 30 and 150 minutes and is not affected by renal or hepatic failure. Heparin is dosed by weight and best administered by continuous infusion rather than by bolus. UFH is best administered intravenously, dosed by weight, and administered by continuous infusion. It is usually effective at doses of at least 18 units/kg per hour with an average daily dose in excess of 30 000 units. Heparin needs tend to be higher in the first few days of treatment. Heparin treatment is monitored using the activated partial thromboplastin time (aPTT). Target level is at least 1.5 times control, which loosely corresponds to serum heparin levels of approximately 0.3–0.7 IU/ml. Each individual laboratory should ideally correlate aPTT with heparin levels. Subtherapeutic aPTT is clearly associated with higher risk of recurrent VTE events; higher levels, however, do not consistently predict bleeding.[107]

Low molecular weight heparins (LMWH) are especially attractive preparations for DVT prophylaxis in surgical patients. LMWH have been shown to be clinically equivalent to unfractionated heparin in terms of efficacy. They may be associated with a lower bleeding risk. LMWH have a longer half-life than unfractionated heparin, a more predictable relationship of dose to anticoagulant effect, and may not require monitoring. LMWH are dosed by weight, although dosing has not been validated in patients weighing over 110 kg. Because LMWH are cleared by the kidneys, they are poorly suited for patients with a GFR < 30 ml/h. Monitoring should be done with Factor Xa levels targeted to 0.6–1.0 IU/ml 4 hours after dosing in patients with renal failure or morbid obesity. Although individual LMWH preparations have been shown to be effective in the treatment of VTE, they are not currently regarded as interchangeable. Anticoagulation by either unfractionated or low molecular weight heparin is contraindicated by craniotomy or eye surgery, and is ill-advised in the presence of active postoperative bleeding.[107]

Heparin induced thrombocytopenia (HIT) is a potentially serious complication of anticoagulant treatment, increasing the risk of postoperative bleeding as well as adding the risk of spontaneous arterial thrombosis. HIT is an antibody-mediated reaction directed against Platelet Factor 4 (PF-4). The risk of HIT is approximately 1% if heparin is administered for less than seven days and it is unusual after 14 days. Patients treated with UFH should have platelet counts at least every other day for two weeks or until UFH is stopped. Platelet monitoring is not required for patients receiving only LMWH. HIT should be suspected if there is a ≥50% drop in platelet count or if there is a new thrombotic event. If HIT is suspected, all heparin should be stopped and a HIT antibody panel obtained. Ultrasound examination of the lower extremities is recommended along with administration of a direct thrombin inhibitor such as lepirudin or argatroban. Consideration should be given to placement of a vena caval filter.[107a]

Significant bleeding associated with excess levels of unfractionated heparin can be reversed with protamine. It is dosed at 1 mg/100 U unfractionated heparin dosed against the amount of heparin infused over the previous several hours. For LMWH, protamine should be dosed at 1 mg/100 antifactor Xa units of LMWH. If bleeding persists, a second dose at 50% of the first, may be given. Activated Factor VII may be used in refractory cases. It is associated with significant side effects, including anaphylaxis, hypotension, and bradycardia. To minimize cardiovascular side effects, protamine should be administered slowly, over 1 to 3 minutes. Patients at risk for anaphylaxis

Table 11.6. Summary of preferred treatment options for surgical patients with VTE

	Low risk		High risk	
	<12 h	>12 h	<12 h	>12 h
Proximal DVT	Hold heparin, consider IVCF	Heparin/coumadin	IVCF	Heparin/coumadin
Submassive PE	IVCF	Heparin/coumadin	IVCF	Heparin/coumadin
Massive PE with shock	—	—	Clot extraction plus IVCF	Extraction or lysis; plus IVCF

from protamine should be pretreated with corticosteroids and antihistamines.[107]

Coumadin inhibits synthesis of Factors II, VII, IX and X as well as Proteins S and C. It takes several days for preformed factors to clear from plasma (VII first and II last). Initial loss of Proteins S and C lead to a hypercoagulable state when coumadin is started. It is therefore necessary to initiate coumadin concurrently with heparin. Coumadin is orally dosed at 5–10 mg per day. INR should first be checked after the first 2–3 doses, then daily until stable for 2 days, two or three times per week for 1 or 2 weeks and then monthly.[107b]

Thrombolytic treatment is indicated for pulmonary embolism with shock and for the treatment of painful lower extremity DVT with swelling and cyanosis (phlegmasia cerulea dolens). Thrombolytics afford three times more clot clearance than is afforded by heparin alone. Pulmonary vascular resistance is decreased by 35% compared to 4% by heparin alone. Caution is necessary in situations where bleeding risk is increased, such as in the postoperative patient. Current options for thrombolysis include streptokinase, urokinase, and TPA. Both streptokinase and urokinase increase plasminogen activity. Streptokinase is dosed at 250 000 units initially followed by 100 000 units per hour times 24. Urokinase is dosed at 400 IU/kg followed by 2200 IU/kg/h times 12. Heparin is held for both and resumed when aPTT is two times control. TPA is somewhat more specific for clot. It works by activating plasminogen bound to fibrin. TPA is dosed at 100 milligrams over 2 hours. Concurrent use of heparin is optional. Thrombolytic therapy is associated with improved 24-hour survival, but there is no difference in the degree of clot resolution at 7–30 days and no demonstrable advantage in survival to discharge. Thrombolytic therapy is associated with a worse bleeding risk than heparin preparations. The rate of bleeding seen with thrombolytic treatment of PE is greater than that encountered in the treatment of myocardial infarction. The risk of spontaneous intracranial hemorrhage is 2.1%, fatal in 1.6%. Because this is comparable to the 2% mortality for heparin treatment of PE in the absence of shock,

thrombolysis should not be considered in the absence of hemodynamic instability. There are anecdotal reports of the successful use of thrombolysis in the immediate postoperative period. These are associated with significant bleeding and high transfusion requirements, up to 20 units over a 24-hour period.[109–112]

Interruption of the inferior vena cava is generally accomplished noninvasively via the intravascular placement of an inferior vena cava filter device (IVCF), preferably below the level of the renal veins. While effective for the short term, the reduction in recurrent VTE events does not reach statistical significance after 2 years, with a rate of recurrent PE of 3.1%.[113] Side effects of IVCF placement include IVC thrombosis in 2%–30%, symptomatic IVC occlusion in 9%, and a rate of recurrent DVT of 20.8% vs. 11.6% in patients without filters. Indications for IVCF placement include inability to anticoagulate, persistence or recurrence of clot despite adequate anticoagulation, or after thrombectomy. Prophylactic placement of an IVCF in high-risk patients is also an accepted intervention.[81]

Clot extraction is a heroic intervention reserved for patients with massive hemodynamic compromise. Surgical thrombectomy is associated with 42% mortality in patients in shock, and 17% in those without. Interventional catheter extraction techniques have a reported 76% success rate, with an overall mortality of 17% in successful extractions. Successful thrombectomy by either approach should be followed by IVCF placement.[72,114]

Treatment choices must balance bleeding risk against the clinical syndrome encountered and must consider the patient's ability to withstand a recurrent event, especially pulmonary embolism. Patients in the first 12 hours after surgery are at the highest risk for anticoagulant induced bleeding. In this initial period, heparin can be delayed in low-risk patients with proximal DVT, but consideration should be given to IVCF placement. Submassive PE should be treated with IVCF. In the setting of nonmassive PE with adequate cardiopulmonary reserve, if non-invasive evaluation of the lower extremities is negative, withholding anticoagulation is a legitimate consideration. The rate of recurrent PE in the setting is comparable to those reported for IVCF.[90] Where possible, heparin should be withheld for that 12-hour period.[101] Beyond 12 hours, heparin is the first choice for both DVT and submassive PE.

For high-risk patients in the first 12 postoperative hours, IVCF placement is the preferred intervention for both proximal DVT and submassive PE. In the presence of PE with shock, clot extraction followed by filter placement is the preferred intervention. At 12 to 48 hours, risk of bleeding is somewhat reduced, but remains elevated. Most uncomplicated patients can be safely anticoagulated with heparin and coumadin. For laparotomy patients, coumadin should be withheld until postoperative ileus resolves and the patient is accepting oral medications. Thrombolysis again should be reserved for those patients in shock who are too unstable for surgical or catheter extraction, or when these techniques are unavailable. After 12 hours, LMWH is the treatment of choice for proximal DVT and for submassive PE. Clot extraction remains preferred to thrombolysis; in high-risk patients, either intervention should be followed by filter placement.

If anticoagulation is contraindicated by the presence of postoperative bleeding or by surgical site, filter placement is the approach of choice unless the patient has adequate cardiopulmonary reserve to withstand a recurrent VTE event and no DVT is demonstrable by serial non-invasive examination of the lower extremities. Beyond 48 hours postoperatively, VTE can be managed similarly to medical patients, although coagulation studies, platelet count, and hematocrit should be watched carefully. Heparin is continued until INR is ≥ 2 for two consecutive days. Duration of coumadin treatment depends on clinical setting. Isolated surgical VTE should be anticoagulated for 3–6 months. Recurrent VTE requires 1 year of treatment. VTE associated with conditions such as malignancy or thrombophilia require lifelong anticoagulation. Ongoing bleeding risk with coumadin anticoagulation is 1–2% per year.[72,81,105] Other complications of coumadin treatment include vascular purpura and skin necrosis. The latter is strongly associated with Protein C deficiency and cancer.[105]

Pleural effusion

Pleural effusion can be caused by many different problems associated with the postoperative state. Light and George[115] found pleural effusions in 49% of patients following abdominal surgery. Most effusions were small, less than 4 mm thick on decubitus films. Only 10% had more than 10 mm thickness. They observed that effusions were mostly ipsilateral to the side of the surgery, occurred

Table 11.7. Differential diagnosis of postoperative pleural effusions

Transudates	Exudates
CHF	Pneumonia
Hypervolemia	Pulmonary embolism (usually)
Ascites	Subphrenic abscess
Misplaced central venous catheter	Empyema
Pulmonary embolism (rarely)	Atelectasis
	Postpericardiotomy syndrome
	Diaphragmatic contusion

mostly in patients having upper abdominal surgery, and in patients who also had atelectasis.

Pleural effusions form when the rate of liquid accumulation exceeds the rate of drainage. Excessive hydrostatic or decreased oncotic pressures produce increased fluid filtration across the intact capillary walls and result in protein-poor transudates. Breakdown of normal formation–resorption mechanisms because of damage to pleural surface or blockage of lymphatics results in protein-rich exudates. The definition of an exudative pleural fluid is based on the presence of any one of the following criteria:

- pleural fluid total protein/serum total protein ratio greater than 0.5;
- pleural fluid LDH/serum LDH ratio greater than 0.6;
- pleural fluid LDH is greater than two-thirds upper normal for serum LDH.[116]

All three criteria must be absent to define a transudate. The differential diagnosis of postoperative pleural effusions is shown in Table 11.7.

Thoracentesis should be performed if a patient exhibits evidence of a pleural effusion on a chest roentgenogram and the fluid layers to a depth more than 10 mm on decubitus views. Smaller effusions can be followed with serial chest films and usually resolve spontaneously.

Transudates usually do not require drainage unless they cause respiratory compromise. In postoperative patients, transudates are most often due to congestive heart failure or volume overload. In this situation, correction of the underlying disorder is usually sufficient. Occasionally, a patient may have a recurrent transudative effusion causing respiratory compromise. In these cases, obliteration of the pleural space (pleurodesis) may be needed to prevent fluid collection. This is carried out by completely draining the fluid through a chest tube and instilling an inflammatory agent, usually talc or a tetracycline, causing symphysis of the visceral and parietal pleural leaves.

Pneumonia is among the most common causes of postoperative exudative effusions. Most parapneumonic effusions resolve with appropriate antibiotic treatment of the pneumonia but, bacteria may invade a sterile effusion and produce a complicated parapneumonic effusion or empyema. Parapneumonic effusions greater than 10 mm in depth should be tapped as early as possible to identify patients who may require drainage. Tube thoracostomy is needed if the fluid is thick pus, or reveals bacteria on Gram's stain, if the pH is less than 7.00, or if pleural fluid glucose is less than 40 mg/dl. If the fluid shows a pH above 7.20, glucose more than 40 mg/dl and pleural fluid LDH is less than 1000 IU/l, then chest tube drainage is not immediately necessary unless organisms are recovered. For intermediate values with pH 7.00–7.20, the thoracentesis should be repeated in 12–24 h.[117] Chest tube placement becomes advisable when deteriorating results are found on repeat thoracenteses. If drainage is delayed, a free effusion may organize into a gelatinous or fibrous peel that will likely go on to require an open thoracotomy or decortication for resolution.

Of coronary bypass patients 40–75% have small effusions, usually left-sided, and persistent at 30 days in 62%. These effusions are predominantly exudative, usually bloody, and generally do not require intervention. 0.78%–4% has large (more than 25% of the hemithorax) effusions that reach a maximum weeks to months after surgery. These late effusions are usually non-bloody, often lymphocytic exudates that are difficult to treat, requiring repeated thoracentesis, thoracostomy, pleurodesis, or rarely, pleurectomy. Conservative treatments should be tried first using NSAIDs or prednisone. These large, late onset effusions are thought to represent a forme fruste of Dressler's syndrome.[118,119]

Subphrenic abscess occurs in 1% of abdominal surgery patients, leading to an exudative pleural effusion that can occur 1–3 weeks postoperatively. Fluid exam usually reveals polymorphonuclear leukocytes. Pleural fluid white blood cell count may reach 50 000/mm^3, but the effusion rarely becomes infected. Management is to identify the abscess by thoracoabdominal CT or by liver–lung scanning, secure drainage, and treat with appropriate antibiotics.

Hemothorax, defined as a hematocrit at least 50% of that in peripheral blood, may be occasionally encountered in the postoperative period, either reflecting surgical bleeding, or from complications following tube or central venous catheter placement. All bloody effusions should therefore have a hematocrit measured. Hemothoraces may reflect local injury, or may be caused by translocation of abdominal blood. Coagulopathy or overanticoagulation may contribute to risk and severity. CT is often helpful in distinguishing hemothorax from a pleural effusion. Hemothoraces are characterized by a higher density than water and may show fibrous septation or loculation. Occasionally, pleural effusion and hemothorax coexist and can be identified by their different densities. The principal acute considerations are acute blood loss, and tension hemothorax. Definitive management is usually surgical. Management options include large bore thoracostomy, thoracoscopy, or surgical re-exploration. The latter is generally reserved for large blood collections, greater than 30% of the hemithorax. Long-term risks of unresolved hemothorax include infection, pleural effusion, and fibrothorax.[120]

Pulmonary emboli may cause either transudative or exudative effusions. Thoracentesis results are not specific for PE. Pleural fluid examination usually reveals a clear yellow fluid, but the effusion can be bloody. Pleural fluid glucose is normal and the differential may reveal either polymorphonuclear cells or mononuclear cells.

This chapter represents a revision of a chapter previously written by Dr. V. M. Patel and Dr. Honig.

REFERENCES

1. O'Donohue, W. J., Jr. Postoperative pulmonary complications. When are preventive and therapeutic measures necessary? *Postgrad. Med.* 1992; **91**: 167–170.
2. Sykes, L. A. & Bowe, E. A. Cardiorespiratory effects of anesthesia. *Clin. Chest Med.* 1993; **14**: 211–226.
3. Hedenstierna, G. Causes of gas exchange impairment during general anaesthesia. *Europ. J. Anaesth.* 1988; **5**: 221–231.
4. Wightman, J. A. A prospective survey of the incidence of postoperative pulmonary complications. *Br. J. Surg.* 1968; **55**: 85–91.
5. Lawrence, V. A., Hilsenbeck, S. G., Mulrow, C. D. *et al.* Incidence and hospital stay for cardiac and pulmonary complications after abdominal surgery. *J. Gen. Intern. Med.* 1995; **10**: 671–678.
6. Stephan, F., Boucheseiche, S., Hollande, J. *et al.* Pulmonary complications following lung resection: a comprehensive analysis of incidence and possible risk factors. *Chest* 2000; **118**: 1263–1270.
7. Bartlett, R. H., Brennan, M. L., Gazzaniga, A. B. *et al.* Studies on the pathogenesis and prevention of postoperative pulmonary complications. *Surg. Gynecol. Obstet.* 1973; **137**: 925–933.
8. Ford, G. T., Whitelaw, W. A., Rosenal, T. W. *et al.* Diaphragm function after upper abdominal surgery in humans. *Am. Rev. Respir. Dis.* 1983; **127**: 431–436.
9. Frazee, R. C., Roberts, J. W., Okeson, G. C. *et al.* Open versus laparoscopic cholecystectomy. A comparison of postoperative

pulmonary function. *Ann. Surg.* 1991; **213**: 651–653; discussion 653–654.

10. Siafakas, N. M., Mitrouska, I., Bouros, D. *et al.* Surgery and the respiratory muscles. *Thorax* 1999; **54**: 458–465.

11. Xue, F. S., Li, B. W., Zhang, G. S. *et al.* The influence of surgical sites on early postoperative hypoxemia in adults undergoing elective surgery. *Anesth. Analg.* 1999; **88**: 213–219.

12. Platell, C. & Hall, J. C. Atelectasis after abdominal surgery. *J. Am. Coll. Surg.* 1997; **185**: 584–592.

13. Rosenberg, J., Rasmussen, G. I., Wojdemann, K. R. *et al.* Ventilatory pattern and associated episodic hypoxaemia in the late postoperative period in the general surgical ward. *Anaesthesia* 1999; **54**: 323–328.

14. Durand, E., Bussy, E., & Gaillard, J. F. Lung scintigraphy in postpneumonectomy dyspnea due to a right-to-left shunt. *J. Nucl. Med.* 1997; **38**: 1812–1815.

15. Powell, J. F., Menon, D. K., & Jones, J. G. The effects of hypoxaemia and recommendations for postoperative oxygen therapy. *Anaesthesia* 1996; **51**: 769–772.

16. Arieff, A. I. Fatal postoperative pulmonary edema: pathogenesis and literature review. *Chest* 1999; **115**: 1371–1377.

17. McConkey, P. P. Postobstructive pulmonary oedema – a case series and review. *Anaesth. Intens. Care* 2000; **28**: 72–76.

18. Lathan, S. R., Silverman, M. E., Thomas, B. L. *et al.* Postoperative pulmonary edema. *South. Med. Assoc. J.* 1999; **92**: 313–315.

19. Schwartz, D. R., Maroo, A., Malhotra, A. *et al.* Negative pressure pulmonary hemorrhage. *Chest* 1999; **115**: 1194–1197.

20. King, R. C., Binns, O. A., Rodriguez, F. *et al.* Reperfusion injury significantly impacts clinical outcome after pulmonary transplantation. *Ann. Thorac. Surg.* 2000; **69**: 1681–1685.

21. Ely, E. W. & Haponik, E. F. Using the chest radiograph to determine intravascular volume status: the role of vascular pedicle width. *Chest* 2002; **121**: 942–950.

22. Mitchell, J. P., Schuller, D., Calandrino, F. S. *et al.* Improved outcome based on fluid management in critically ill patients requiring pulmonary artery catheterization. *Am. Rev. Respir. Dis.* 1992; **145**: 990–998.

23. O'Donohue, W. J., Jr. National survey of the usage of lung expansion modalities for the prevention and treatment of postoperative atelectasis following abdominal and thoracic surgery. *Chest* 1985; **87**: 76–80.

24. Engoren, M. Lack of association between atelectasis and fever. *Chest* 1995; **107**: 81–84.

25. Overend, T. J., Anderson, C. M., Lucy, S. D. *et al.* The effect of incentive spirometry on postoperative pulmonary complications: a systematic review. *Chest* 2001; **120**: 971–978.

26. Weindler, J. & Kiefer, R. T. The efficacy of postoperative incentive spirometry is influenced by the device-specific imposed work of breathing. *Chest* 2001; **119**: 1858–1864.

27. Crowe, J. M. & Bradley, C. A. The effectiveness of incentive spirometry with physical therapy for high-risk patients after coronary artery bypass surgery. *Phys. Ther.* 1997; **77**: 260–268.

28. Gosselink, R., Schrever, K., Cops, P. *et al.* Incentive spirometry does not enhance recovery after thoracic surgery. *Crit. Care Med.* 2000; **28**: 679–683.

29. Matte, P., Jacquet, L., Van Dyck, M. *et al.* Effects of conventional physiotherapy, continuous positive airway pressure and non-invasive ventilatory support with bilevel positive airway pressure after coronary artery bypass grafting. *Acta Anaesth. Scand.* 2000; **44**: 75–81.

30. Bohner, H., Kindgen-Milles, D., Grust, A. *et al.* Prophylactic nasal continuous positive airway pressure after major vascular surgery: results of a prospective randomized trial. *Langenbecks Arch. Surg.* 2002; **387**: 21–26.

31. Gust, R., Pecher, S., Gust, A. *et al.* Effect of patient-controlled analgesia on pulmonary complications after coronary artery bypass grafting. *Crit. Care Med.* 1999; **27**: 2218–2223.

32. Rigg, J. R., Jamrozik, K., Myles, P. S. *et al.* Epidural anaesthesia and analgesia and outcome of major surgery: a randomised trial. *Lancet* 2002; **359**: 1276–1282.

33. Marini, J. J., Pierson, D. J., Hudson, L. D. Acute lobar atelectasis: a prospective comparison of fiberoptic bronchoscopy and respiratory therapy. *Am. Rev. Respir. Dis.* 1979; **119**: 971–978.

34. Arozullah, A. M., Khuri, S. F., Henderson, W. G. *et al.* Development and validation of a multifactorial risk index for predicting postoperative pneumonia after major noncardiac surgery. *Ann. Intern. Med.* 2001; **135**: 847–857.

35. Anonymous. National Nosocomial Infections Surveillance (NNIS) System Report, Data Summary from January 1992–June 2001, issued August 2001. *Am. J. Infec. Contr.* 2001; **29**: 404–421.

36. Celis, R., Torres, A., Gatell, J. M. *et al.* Nosocomial pneumonia. A multivariate analysis of risk and prognosis. *Chest* 1988; **93**: 318–324.

37. Greenaway, C. A., Embil, J., Orr, P. H. *et al.* Nosocomial pneumonia on general medical and surgical wards in a tertiary-care hospital. *Infec. Contr. Hosp. Epidemiol.* 1997; **18**: 749–756.

38. Grossman, R. F. & Fein, A. Evidence-based assessment of diagnostic tests for ventilator-associated pneumonia. Executive summary. *Chest* 2000; **117**: 177S–181S.

39. Chastre, J. & Fagon, J. Y. Ventilator-associated pneumonia. *Am. J. Respir. Crit. Care Med.* 2002; **165**: 867–903.

40. Craven, D. E. Epidemiology of ventilator-associated pneumonia. *Chest* 2000; **117**: 186S–187S.

41. Kollef, M. H. The prevention of ventilator-associated pneumonia. *N. Engl. J. Med.* 1999; **340**: 627–634.

42. Montravers, P., Veber, B., Auboyer, C. *et al.* Diagnostic and therapeutic management of nosocomial pneumonia in surgical patients: results of the Eole study. *Crit. Care Med.* 2002; **30**: 368–375.

43. Trouillet, J. L., Chastre, J., Vuagnat, A. *et al.* Ventilator-associated pneumonia caused by potentially drug-resistant bacteria. *Am. J. Respir. Crit. Care Med.* 1998; **157**: 531–539.

44. Rello, J., Paiva, J. A., Baraibar, J. *et al.* International Conference for the Development of Consensus on the Diagnosis and Treatment of Ventilator-associated Pneumonia. *Chest* 2001; **120**: 955–970.

45. Singh, N., Falestiny, M. N., Rogers, P. *et al.* Pulmonary infiltrates in the surgical ICU: prospective assessment of predictors of etiology and mortality. *Chest* 1998; **114**: 1129–1136.

46. Wunderink, R. G. Radiologic diagnosis of ventilator-associated pneumonia. *Chest* 2000; **117**: 188S–190S.

47. Guidelines for the management of adults with hospital acquired, ventilar also coated, and healthcare-associated pneumonia. *Am. J. Respir. Crit. Care Med.* 2005; **171**: 388–416.

48. Fagon, J. Y., Chastre, J., Wolff, M. *et al.* Invasive and noninvasive strategies for management of suspected ventilator-associated pneumonia. A randomized trial [comment]. *Ann. Intern. Med.* 2000; **132**: 621–630.

49. Ost, D. E., Hall, C. S., Joseph, G. *et al.* Decision analysis of antibiotic and diagnostic strategies in ventilator-associated pneumonia. *Am. J. Respir. Crit. Care Med.* 2003; **168**: 1060–1067.

50. Andrews, C. P., Coalson, J. J., Smith, J. D. *et al.* Diagnosis of nosocomial bacterial pneumonia in acute, diffuse lung injury. *Chest* 1981; **80**: 254–258.

51. Garner, J. S., Jarvis, W. R., Emori, T. G. *et al.* CDC definitions for nosocomial infections, 1988. *Am. J. Infec. Cont.* 1988; **16**: 128–140.

52. Emori, T. G., Edwards, J. R., Culver, D. H. *et al.* Accuracy of reporting nosocomial infections in intensive-care-unit patients to the National Nosocomial Infections Surveillance System: a pilot study. *Infec. Cont. Hosp. Epidemiol.* 1998; **19**: 308–316.

53. Pugin, J., Auckenthaler, R., Mili, N. *et al.* Diagnosis of ventilator-associated pneumonia by bacteriologic analysis of bronchoscopic and nonbronchoscopic "blind" bronchoalveolar lavage fluid. *Am. Rev. Respir. Dis.* 1991; **143**: 1121–1129.

54. Wunderink, R. G. Clinical criteria in the diagnosis of ventilator-associated pneumonia. *Chest* 2000; **117**: 191S–194S.

55. Cook, D. & Mandell, L. Endotracheal aspiration in the diagnosis of ventilator-associated pneumonia. *Chest* 2000; **117**: 195S–197S.

56. Baughman, R. P. Protected-specimen brush technique in the diagnosis of ventilator-associated pneumonia. *Chest* 2000; **117**: 203S–206S.

57. Torres, A. & El-Ebiary, M. Bronchoscopic BAL in the diagnosis of ventilator-associated pneumonia. *Chest* 2000; **117**: 198S–202S.

58. Welty-Wolf, K. Ventilator-associated pneumonia. In MacIntyre, N. R. & Branson, R. D., eds. *Mechanical Ventilation.* Philadelphia: W. B. Saunders, 2001; 296–328.

59. Campbell, G. D., Jr. Blinded invasive diagnostic procedures in ventilator-associated pneumonia. *Chest* 2000; **117**: 207S–211S.

60. Lynch, J. P., 3rd. Hospital-acquired pneumonia: risk factors, microbiology, and treatment. *Chest* 2001; **119**: 373S–384S.

61. Fiel, S. Guidelines and critical pathways for severe hospital-acquired pneumonia. *Chest* 2001; **119**: 412S–418S.

62. Niederman, M. S., Mandell, L. A., Anzueto, A. *et al.* Guidelines for the management of adults with community-acquired pneumonia. Diagnosis, assessment of severity, antimicrobial therapy, and prevention. *Am. J. Respir. Crit. Care Med.* 2001; **163**: 1730–1754.

63. Bartlett, J. G., Dowell, S. F., Mandell, L. A. *et al.* Practice guidelines for the management of community-acquired pneumonia in adults. Infectious Diseases Society of America. *Clin. Infec. Dis.* 2000; **31**: 347–382.

64. Ibrahim, E. H., Ward, S., Sherman, G. *et al.* Experience with a clinical guideline for the treatment of ventilator-associated pneumonia. *Crit. Care Med.* 2001; **29**: 1109–1115.

65. Timsit, J. F., Chevret, S., Valcke, J. *et al.* Mortality of nosocomial pneumonia in ventilated patients: influence of diagnostic tools. *Am. J. Respir. Crit. Care Med.* 1996; **154**: 116–123.

66. Polk, H. C. & Mizuguchi, N. N. Multifactorial analyses in the diagnosis of pneumonia arising in the surgical intensive care unit. *Am. J. Surg.* 2000; **179**: 31S–35S.

67. Marik, P. E. & Careau, P. The role of anaerobes in patients with ventilator-associated pneumonia and aspiration pneumonia: a prospective study. *Chest* 1999; **115**: 178–183.

68. Marik, P. E. Aspiration pneumonitis and aspiration pneumonia. *N. Engl. J. Med.* 2001; **344**: 665–671.

69. Jackson, M. R. Diagnosis and management of venous thrombosis in the surgical patient. *Semin. Thromb. Hemost.* 1998; **24** Suppl 1: 67–76.

70. Muntz, J. E. Deep vein thrombosis and pulmonary embolism in the perioperative patient. *Am. J. Managed Care.* 2000; **6**: S1045–1052.

71. Miranda, A. R. & Hassouna, H. I. Mechanisms of thrombosis in spinal cord injury. *Hematol. – Oncol. Clin. N. Am.* 2000; **14**: 401–416.

72. Dalen, J. E. Pulmonary embolism: what have we learned since Virchow?: treatment and prevention. *Chest* 2002; **122**: 1801–1817.

73. Thomas, D. P. & Roberts, H. R. Hypercoagulability in venous and arterial thrombosis. *Ann. Intern. Med.* 1997; **126**: 638–644.

74. Wheeler, H. B. Should surgical patients be screened for thrombophilia? *Semin. Thromb. Hemost.* 1998; **24** Suppl. 1: 63–65.

75. Hauch, O., Jorgensen, L. N., Khattar, S. C. *et al.* Fatal pulmonary embolism associated with surgery. An autopsy study. *Acta Chir. Scand.* 1990; **156**: 747–749.

76. Kelsey, L. J., Fry, D. M., & VanderKolk, W. E. Thrombosis risk in the trauma patient. Prevention and treatment. *Hematol. – Oncol. Clin. N. Am.* 2000; **14**: 417–430.

77. Dahl, O. E. Mechanisms of hypercoagulability. *Thromb. Haemost.* 1999; **82**: 902–906.

78. Dalen, J. E. Pulmonary embolism: what have we learned since Virchow? Natural history, pathophysiology, and diagnosis. *Chest* 2002; **122**: 1440–1456.

79. Ryu, J. H., Olson, E. J., & Pellikka, P. A. Clinical recognition of pulmonary embolism: problem of unrecognized and asymptomatic cases. *Mayo Clin. Proc.* 1998; **73**: 873–879.

80. Monreal, M., Ruiz, J., Olazabal, A. *et al.* Deep venous thrombosis and the risk of pulmonary embolism. A systematic study. *Chest* 1992; **102**: 677–681.

81. Tapson, V. F., Carroll, B. A., Davidson, B. L. *et al.* The diagnostic approach to acute venous thromboembolism. Clinical practice guideline. American Thoracic Society. *Am. J. Respir. Crit. Care Med.* 1999; **160**: 1043–1066.

82. Begemann, P. G., Bonacker, M., Kemper, J. *et al.* Evaluation of the deep venous system in patients with suspected pulmonary embolism with multi-detector CT: a prospective study in comparison to Doppler sonography. *J. Comp. Assist. Tomogr.* 2003; **27**: 399–409.

83. Loud, P. A., Katz, D. S., Bruce, D. A. *et al.* Deep venous thrombosis with suspected pulmonary embolism: detection with combined CT venography and pulmonary angiography. *Radiology* 2001; **219**: 498–502.

84. Washington, L., Goodman, L. R., & Gonyo, M. B. CT for thromboembolic disease. *Radiol. Clin. N. Am.* 2002; **40**: 751–771.

85. Peterson, D. A., Kazerooni, E. A., Wakefield, T. W. *et al.* Computed tomographic venography is specific but not sensitive for diagnosis of acute lower-extremity deep venous thrombosis in patients with suspected pulmonary embolus. *J. Vasc. Surg.* 2001; **34**: 798–804.

86. Seabold, J. E. Radionuclide venography and labeled platelets in deep venous thrombosis. *Semin. Nucl. Med.* 2001; **31**: 124–128.

87. Taillefer, R. Radiolabeled peptides in the detection of deep venous thrombosis. *Semin. Nucl. Med.* 2001; **31**: 102–123.

88. Lippi, G., Veraldi, G. F., Fraccaroli, M. *et al.* Variation of plasma D-dimer following surgery: implications for prediction of postoperative venous thromboembolism. *Clin. Exp. Med.* 2001; **1**: 161–164.

89. The PIOPED Investigators. Value of the ventilation/perfusion scan in acute pulmonary embolism. Results of the prospective investigation of pulmonary embolism diagnosis (PIOPED). *JAMA* 1990; **263**: 2753–2759.

90. Stein, P. D., Hull, R. D., & Raskob, G. E. Withholding treatment in patients with acute pulmonary embolism who have a high risk of bleeding and negative serial noninvasive leg tests. *Am. J. Med.* 2000; **109**: 301–306.

91. Jett, J. R., Sloan, J. A., Midthun, D. E. *et al.* Outcomes after withholding anticoagulation from patients with suspected acute pulmonary embolism and negative computed tomographic findings: a cohort study. *Am. J. Respir. Crit. Care Med.* 2002; **165**: 508–513.

92. de Monye, W., Schiereck, J., Kieft, G. J. *et al.* Single-detector helical computed tomography as the primary diagnostic test in suspected pulmonary embolism: a multicenter clinical management study of 510 patients. *Ann. Intern. Med.* 2003; **138**: 307–314.

93. Fedullo, P. F. & Tapson, V. F. Clinical practice. The evaluation of suspected pulmonary embolism. *N. Engl. J. Med.* 2003; **349**: 1247–1256.

94. Scher, K. S. Unplanned reoperation for bleeding. *Am. Surg.* 1996; **62**: 52–55.

95. Hall, T. S., Brevetti, G. R., Skoultchi, A. J. *et al.* Re-exploration for hemorrhage following open heart surgery differentiation on the causes of bleeding and the impact on patient outcomes. *Ann. Thorac. Cardiovasc. Surg.* 2001; **7**: 352–357.

96. Dacey, L. J., Munoz, J. J., Baribeau, Y. R. *et al.* Reexploration for hemorrhage following coronary artery bypass grafting: incidence and risk factors. Northern New England Cardiovascular Disease Study Group. *Arch. Surg.* 1998; **133**: 442–447.

97. Zidane, M., Schram, M. T., Planken, E. W. *et al.* Frequency of major hemorrhage in patients treated with unfractionated intravenous heparin for deep venous thrombosis or pulmonary embolism: a study in routine clinical practice. *Arch. Intern. Med.* 2000; **160**: 2369–2373.

98. Douketis, J. D., Kearon, C., Bates, S. *et al.* Risk of fatal pulmonary embolism in patients with treated venous thromboembolism. *J. Am. Med. Assoc.* 1998; **279**: 458–462.

99. Levine, M. N., Raskob, G., Beuth, R. J. *et al.* Hemorrhagic complications of anticoagulant treatment. *Chest* 2004; **126**: 287S–310S.

100. Hull, R. D., Raskob, G. E., Rosenbloom, D. *et al.* Heparin for 5 days as compared with 10 days in the initial treatment of proximal venous thrombosis. *N. Engl. J. Med.* 1990; **322**: 1260–1264.

101. Kearon, C. & Hirsh, J. Management of anticoagulation before and after elective surgery. *N. Engl. J. Med.* 1997; **336**: 1506–1511.

102. Ginsberg, J. A., Crowther, M. A., White, R. H. *et al.* Anticoagulation therapy. *Hematology* 2001: 339–357.

103. Caliendo, F. J., Halpern, V. J., Marini, C. P. *et al.* Warfarin anticoagulation in the perioperative period: is it safe? *Ann. Vasc. Surg.* 1999; **13**: 11–16.

104. Bergqvist, D. & Lindblad, B. A 30-year survey of pulmonary embolism verified at autopsy: an analysis of 1274 surgical patients. *Br. J. Surg.* 1985; **72**: 105–108.

105. Ansell, J., Hirsh, J., Dalen, J. *et al.* Managing oral anticoagulant therapy. *Chest* 2001; **119**: 22S–38S.

106. Büller, H. R., Agnelli, G., Hull, R. D. *et al.* Antithrombotic therapy for venous thromboembolic disease. *Chest* 2004; **126**: 401S–428S.

107. Hirsh, J. & Raschke, R. Heparin and low-molecular-weight heparin: mechanisms of action, pharmacokinetics, dosing, monitoring, efficacy, and safety. *Chest* 2004; **126**: 188S–203S.

107a. Warkentin, T. E. & Greinacher, A. Heparin-induced thrombocytopenia: recognition, treatment and prevention. *Chest* 2004; **126**: 311S–337S.

107b. Ansell, J., Hirsh, J., Poller, L. *et al.* The pharmacology and management of the vitamin K antagonists, *Chest* 2004; **126**: 204S–233S.

108. Crowther, M. A., Berry, L. R., Monagle, P. T. *et al.* Mechanisms responsible for the failure of protamine to inactivate low-molecular-weight heparin. *Br. J. Haematol.* 2002; **116**: 178–186.

109. Hartmannsgruber, M. W., Trent, F. L., & Stolzfus, D. P. Thrombolytic therapy for treatment of pulmonary embolism in the postoperative period: case report and review of the literature. *J. Clin. Anesth.* 1996; **8**: 669–674.

110. Goldhaber, S. Z. Pulmonary embolism. *N. Engl. J. Med.* 1998; **339**: 93–104.

111. Dalen, J. E. The uncertain role of thrombolytic therapy in the treatment of pulmonary embolism. *Arch. Intern. Med.* 2002; **162**: 2521–2523.

112. Arcasoy, S. M. & Kreit, J. W. Thrombolytic therapy of pulmonary embolism: a comprehensive review of current evidence. *Chest* 1999; **115**: 1695–1707.

113. Decousus, H., Leizorovicz, A., Parent, F. *et al.* A clinical trial of vena caval filters in the prevention of pulmonary embolism in patients with proximal deep-vein thrombosis. Prevention du Risque d'Embolie Pulmonaire par Interruption Cave Study Group. *N. Engl. J. Med.* 1998; **338**: 409–415.

114. Aklog, L., Williams, C. S., Byrne, J. G. *et al.* Acute pulmonary embolectomy: a contemporary approach. *Circulation* 2002; **105**: 1416–1419.

115. Light, R. W. & George, R. B. Incidence and significance of pleural effusion after abdominal surgery. *Chest* 1976; **69**: 621–625.

116. Light, R. W. Useful tests on the pleural fluid in the management of patients with pleural effusions. *Curr. Opin. Pulm. Med.* 1999; **5**: 245–249.

117. Colice, G. L., Curtis, A., Deslauriers, J. *et al.* Medical and surgical treatment of parapneumonic effusions: an evidence-based guideline. *Chest* 2000; **118**: 1158–1171.

118. Light, R. W., Rogers, J. T., Cheng, D. *et al.* Large pleural effusions occurring after coronary artery bypass grafting. *Ann. Intern. Med.* 1999; **130**: 891–896.

119. Light, R. W. Pleural effusions after coronary artery bypass graft surgery. *Curr. Opin. Pulm. Med.* 2002; **8**: 308–311.

120. Light, R. W. & Broaddus, V. C. Pneumothorax, chylothorax, hemothorax, and fibrothorax. In Murray, J. F., Nadel, J. A., eds. *Textbook of Respiratory Medicine.* Philadelphia: Saunders, 2000; 2060–2063.

Gastroenterology

12

Peptic ulcer disease

John Affronti and Tommie Haywood

Emory Clinic, Atlanta, GA

Peptic ulcer disease is caused by defects in the gastrointestinal mucosa extending into the muscularis mucosa secondary to gastric acid and/or pepsin. Recent advances have provided a better understanding of peptic ulcer pathophysiology. The propensity for peptic ulcers is caused by the imbalance between digestive and protective factors. Since the discovery of the bacterium *Helicobacter pylori*, the medical management of peptic ulcer disease has changed dramatically. Most peptic ulcers fall into two etiologies: nonsteroidal anti-inflammatory drugs (NSAIDS) or *H. pylori*.

The clinical presentation of peptic ulcer disease is variable. Some patients with peptic ulcer disease have classic symptoms, while other patients may have ulcer symptoms and no identifiable ulcers (non-ulcer dyspepsia). Many patients with peptic ulcer disease have no symptoms.

Epidemiology

The annual incidence of peptic ulcer disease ranges from 0.1% to 0.3%. Several studies have shown the incidence of peptic ulcer disease in *H. pylori*-infected individuals to be about 1% per year, which is six to tenfold higher than *H. pylori*-negative individuals. Since the mid 1970s, the incidence of duodenal ulcer seems to be declining in the USA reflected by decreasing rate of hospitalization, surgery, and death. Rates of hospitalization for ulcer hemorrhage decreased slightly for duodenal ulcers but have increased for gastric ulcers. Death rates from peptic ulcer disease seem to be declining for younger men and increasing for the elderly. Estimates of ulcer prevalence must take into account the *H. pylori* status of the patient. Data from several sources suggests that the lifetime prevalence of peptic ulcer disease if 5%–10%, but in *H. pylori*-positive subjects, the lifetime prevalence increases to 10%–20%.

A minority of these patients develop symptoms requiring utilization of healthcare resources.

Pathogenesis

The regulation of acid and pepsin secretion is mediated by the balance of neural, endocrine, paracrine, and autocrine pathways of stimulation and inhibition. After the ingestion of a meal, acid and pepsin production is stimulated by gastrin release and vagally mediated stimulation of parietal cell acid production. Pepsinongen is secreted by chief cells in response to gastrin and histamine. In a low pH environment, the inactive pepsinogen in cleaved to the active pepsin. It has been shown that the average maximal acid secretory response (reflecting parietal cell mass) is greater in patients with duodenal ulcers than in normal subjects.[1,2]

Helicobacter pylori was discovered 20 years ago, and since then, the management of peptic ulcer disease has changed dramatically. *H. pylori* is the most common bacterium worldwide. The organism is uniquely adapted to colonize the human gastric mucosa and induce inflammation without invasion. *H. pylori* is responsible for the majority of gastric and duodenal ulcers. The lifetime risk of peptic ulcer disease in *H. pylori*-infected patients ranges from 3% in the USA to 25% in Japan. It has also been shown that eradication of *H. pylori* significantly lowers the recurrence rate of peptic ulcers. Effective antimicrobial regimens are available for the treatment of *H. pylori*.

The first line of defense against the acid–peptic environment is the mucus layer of the gastric and duodenal mucosa. This adherent mucus gel is an unstirred layer with a basic pH secondary to mucosal bicarbonate secretion – thus preventing pepsin diffusion to the mucosal surface. The mucosal secretion of bicarbonate provides a protective pH gradient. There is some speculation that

Medical Management of the Surgical Patient: A Textbook of Perioperative Medicine, ed. M. F. Lubin, R. B. Smith, T. F. Dobson, N. Spell, H. K. Walker. 4th edn. Published by Cambridge University Press. © Cambridge University 2006.

H. pylori may play a role in disrupting the integrity of the mucus barrier.[3]

Intrinsic epithelial cell protection against acid–peptic mucosal injury is a second-line defense. The specialized apical membrane of gastric mucosal cells serve as a barrier to acid back-diffusion. The barrier is regulated by endogenous growth factors such as transforming growth factor alpha. It is speculated that cells of the gastric mucosa may have intrinsic mechanisms of resisting oxidant injury via so-called "heat shock proteins."[4]

The third line of defense is the maintenance of mucosal blood flow, which provides processes that remove acid that has diffused across injured epithelium. Adequate mucosal blood flow is crucial for maintaining mucosal integrity and repairing any injury.

Prostaglandins play an important role in activating mucosal defense mechanisms. Prostaglandins are endogenous mediators of mucus production. NSAID-induced ulcers are associated with mucosal depletion of prostaglandin. This is suggested by findings that exogenous administration of prostaglandin enhances ulcer healing.[5] There are three putative mechanisms of how prostaglandins provide mucosal protection against acid-pepsin: (a) stimulation of mucosal bicarbonate secretion, (b) stimulation of mucus secretion, (c) increase in mucosal blood flow.

Cigarette smoking has been linked to occurrence, persistence, and recurrence of peptic ulcer disease. Not only are smokers at increased risk for both duodenal and gastric ulcers, but the risk of peptic ulcer disease may be related to the amount of cigarettes smoked.[6] The proposed mechanisms by which cigarette smoking causes peptic ulcer disease include increased duodenogastric bile reflux,[7] decreased duodenal pH,[8] reduced production of salivary epidermal growth factors, and decreased prostaglandin production.[9]

Dietary indiscretion as a culprit in causing or exacerbating peptic ulcer disease has yet to be proven with any convincing data. Caffeine has been shown to stimulate acid secretion and produce dyspepsia, but has not been shown to cause peptic ulcer disease.[10] Excessive alcohol use is associated with acute gastric hemorrhages. No evidence has shown that alcohol use causes gastritis or chronic peptic ulcer.[11,12] It is unknown whether alcohol ingestion stimulates excessive gastric production. Alcohol abuse interferes with patient compliance and ulcer healing.[13]

Clinical features

Classic ulcer pain is described as burning, gnawing abdominal pain, but can be vague or cramping. The term "dyspepsia" has been used to describe the symptom complex of epigastric discomfort, bloating, nausea, and anorexia. While the pain of duodenal ulcers has been described as vague, "hunger-like" and relieved with meals, the pain of gastric ulcers has been described as being more severe. Neither of these symptom categories has been proven to be sensitive or specific in the diagnosis of gastric versus duodenal ulcer. From 15%–44% of patients who are asymptomatic are found to have peptic ulcer at endoscopy.[14,15] Asymptomatic peptic ulcer disease is often present in patients taking NSAIDS. It is not uncommon for some patients to be free of heralding symptoms prior to presenting with ulcer hemorrhage or perforation.

Diagnostic techniques

The diagnosis of a peptic ulcer can be established by using endoscopy and directly visualizing the mucosa or from radiographic studies using contrast agents. Upper gastrointestinal series can detect about 70%–80% of gastric and duodenal ulcers.[16] With single-contrast radiographic studies, 50% of duodenal ulcers may be missed. Using double-contrast studies, 80%–90% of duodenal ulcers can be identified.[17,18] The sensitivity and specificity of radiographic contrast studies is technique and examiner dependent. Superficial lesions and lesions less the 0.5 cm are difficult to detect by radiography.

Guidelines for therapy

There are four important goals for peptic ulcer disease treatment: (a) to control and alleviate symptoms, (b) to promote healing, (c) to prevent recurrences, (d) to prevent complication such as hemorrhage, obstruction, or perforation. Most peptic ulcers slowly heal without therapy. Numerous clinical trials have contributed to our knowledge of the natural history of peptic ulcer disease. The majority of ulcer patients have had symptoms 2 or more years prior to presentation. Based on previous studies, in patients with no treatment for peptic ulcer disease, 40% of duodenal ulcers and 30% of gastric ulcers healed within 4 weeks.[19] However, the natural history of untreated peptic ulcer disease varies among patient population and geographical region of origin. Gastric ulcers spontaneously heal approximately 3 mm/week.[20] Therefore, larger ulcers take longer to heal. Numerous randomized, controlled trials have been performed to assess the efficacy of various therapies for healing duodenal ulcers. Full doses of histamine receptor antagonists or proton pump inhibitors are effective initial therapy of gastric ulcers. Proton pump inhibitors are the most potent alternative. Elimination of other potential offending agents such as cigarettes, nonsteroidal anti-inflammatory drugs, excessive alcohol use, and *H. pylori* also contribute to delay in ulcer healing. Recurrent peptic ulcers may be asymptomatic or symptomatic. Cure of *H. pylori* infection markedly reduced the recurrence of peptic ulcer disease. NSAID use, history of both gastric and duodenal ulcer, and prior history of ulcer complications predict ulcer recurrence. Finding a deformed duodenal bulb also predicts increased rate of ulcer recurrence and complication because scarring impairs quality of healing.[21]

Specific therapy of patients with peptic ulcer disease undergoing non-related surgery

Patients with acute ulcers requiring urgent surgery

Anti-ulcer medication such as histamine receptor antagonists or proton pump inhibitors should be administered immediately to patients with documented peptic ulcers who require emergent surgery. The route of administration is dependent on the patients ability to tolerate oral medications safely. The proton pump inhibitors are the most potent anti-ulcer medication. A single dose of omeprazole inhibits basal and stimulated gastric acid secretion by more than 90% over 24 hours. H^+/K^+-adenosine triphosphate is blocked irreversibly. Therefore, new proteins must be produced for gastric acid secretion. This effect of proton pump inhibitors makes them more potent anit-ulcer agents than histamine receptor antagonists. Intravenous pantoprazole is now available for patients that cannot tolerate oral proton pump inhibitors.

Complications of peptic ulcer disease such as hemorrhage or perforation are uncommon in the postoperative period, but have potential for grave outcome. Perioperative use of anti-ulcer medications is therefore recommended. Surgical procedures with high likelihood of hypotension, sepsis, uremia, respiratory failure, or neurologic complication increase the incidence of acute peptic ulcer disease. Neurosurgical,[22] aortic,[23] and cardiothoracic[24] surgery pose the highest risk for postoperative ulcer complications.

Patients with active ulcers who require elective surgery

Non-urgent surgery should be deferred, if possible, in patients with active ulcers. Either medically appropriate histamine receptor blocker or proton pump inhibitors should be administered to promote ulcer healing.

Lifestyle modifications should also be recommended to promote ulcer healing. Smoking cessation should be encouraged. No reliable evidence has yet proven diet to affect ulcer healing. Although the role of caffeine in causing ulcers or preventing the healing of peptic ulcer disease is controversial,[12] it should probably still be avoided.

Patients with chronic ulcer disease or history of recurrent ulcer disease who require surgery

Patients with a history of chronic or recurrent peptic ulcer disease or symptoms of peptic ulcer should be treated with histamine receptor blockers or proton pump inhibitors during surgery and the postoperative period. NSAIDS should be discontinued 7–10 days prior to surgery in these patients if there is no medical contraindication. The choice of utilizing histamine receptor antagonists vs. proton pump inhibitors should be tailored to the individual patient. In patients who have been on maintenance therapy for history of peptic ulcer disease, full dose anti-ulcer therapy should be provided in the pre- and postoperative period.

Drugs used to treat peptic ulcer disease

Histamine-2 receptor antagonists

There are four H2 receptor antagonists in the United States: cimetidine, ranitidine, famotidine, nizatidine. These agents inhibit acid production by blocking the parietal cell H2 receptor. These four agents are available orally, are easy to take, and have few side effects. Intravenous forms exist and are utilized in hospital patients who are unable to tolerate oral medications. H2RAs are well absorbed orally. After oral administration, peak serum concentration occurs 1 to 3 hours after dosing. The major route of elimination of H2RAs is renal. Therefore, doses of H2RAs should be adjusted in patients with renal failure. These drugs may be taken once or twice daily. Twice daily doses seem to suppress more daytime acid secretion. Doses taken daily in the evening appear to suppress nocturnal acid secretion by 90%.

Proton pump inhibitors

There are four available proton pump inhibitors in the United States: omeprazole, lansoprazole, pantaprazole, rabeprazole. These agents act by irreversibly inhibiting the H^+/K^+-ATPase (proton pump) effectively decreasing H^+ secretion. At recommended doses, proton pump inhibitors block 90% of daily acid secretion. With this decrease in gastric acidity, the G cells respond by secreting increased amounts of gastrin. Due to their potency and marked decrease in gastric acid production, these agents control symptoms and heal ulcers more rapidly than other anti-ulcer medication.

Sucralfate

Sucralfate appears to be as effective as H2RAs in healing uncomplicated duodenal ulcers.[25] Sucralfate is a sulfated polysaccharide complexed with aluminum hydroxide. It does not alter gastric acid or pepsin production. Also, it stimulates angiogenesis and granulation tissue formation. Sucralfate appears to be cytoprotective by binding to injured tissue, therefore decreasing exposure to acid and pepsin. Caution must be taken when sucralfate is administered with other medications as it may reduce their absorption – especially phenytoin and warfarin. Sucralfate occasionally causes constipation and nausea.

Antacids

Antacids effectively heal ulcers and are relatively safe. The mechanisms of action of antacids is unknown. These agents contain aluminum and magnesium hydroxide. Antacids must be taken in adequate amounts at specific times to neutralize gastric and duodenal acid. Different forms of antacids vary in potency, rate of acid neutralization, and rate of gastric emptying. Magnesium-containing antacids may contain large amounts of sodium, therefore caution must be taken in patients who are susceptible to sodium overload such as renal failure or congestive heart failure patients. Aluminum-containing antacid may cause phosphate depletion, constipation, and diarrhea. Antacids may also bind various drugs in the gut, so caution must be used when administered with other medications.

Prostaglandins

Prostaglandins not only inhibit acid secretion, but also enhance mucosal defense mechanisms. Prostaglandins, particularly of the E and I groups, inhibit the stimulation of parietal cell acid secretion by histamine. Only misoprostol has been approved in the United States for prevention of NSAID-induced gastric ulcers. The most frequent side effects of the prostaglandins are crampy abdominal pain and diarrhea. Misoprostol is contraindicated in women of childbearing age who are not taking contraceptives.

Bismuth

There are three forms of bismuth: colloidal bismuth subcitrate (CBS), bismuth subsalicylate (BSS, Pepto-Bismol), and ranitidine bismuth citrate (RBC). RBC have been approved in the USA for treatment of *H.pylori*-positive peptic ulcer. However, they are rarely used without adjuvant antibiotic therapy in *H. pylori* treatment. Bismuth does not inhibit or neutralize gastric acid or pepsin. Proposed mechanisms of bismuth ulcer healing includes binding to ulcer crater to protect injured tissue from acid, recruitment of macrophages to ulcer bed, and increase of mucosal prostaglandin, mucus, and bicarbonate production. Bismuth may cause black stools. Bismuth is renally excreted and should be avoided in patients with renal failure unless serum bismuth levels are measured.

REFERENCES

1. Lam, S. K. Pathogenesis and pathophysiology of duodenal ulcer. *Clin. Gastroenterol.* 1984; **13**: 447.
2. Blair, J. A. I., Feldman, M., Barnett, C. *et al.* Detailed comparison of basal and food-stimulated acid secretion rates and serum gastrin concentrations in duodenal ulcer patients and normal subjects. *J. Clin. Invest.* 1987; **79**: 582.
3. Sarosiek, J., Marshall, B. J., Peura, D. A. *et al.* Gastroduodenal mucus gel thickness in patients with *Helicobacter pylori*: A method for assessment of biopsy specimens. *Am. J. Gastroenterol.* 1991; **86**: 729.
4. Nakmura, K., Rokutan, K., Marui, N. *et al.* Induction of heat shock proteins and their implication in protection against ethanol-induced damage in cultured guinea pig gastric mucosal cells. *Gastroenterology* 1991; **101**: 161.
5. Poynard, T. & Pignon, J. P. *Acute Treatment of Duodenal Ulcer: Analysis of 293 Randomized Clinical Trials.* Paris: John Libbey Eurotext, 1989: 7.
6. Dippy, J., Rhodes, J., & Cross, S. Bile reflux in gastric ulcer: the effect of smoking, metoclopramide, carbenoxolone sodium. *Curr. Med. Res. Opin.* 1973; **1**: 569.
7. Murthy, S., Dinoso, V., Clearfield, H. *et al.* Simultaneous measurement of basal pancreatic, gastric acid secretion, plasma gastrin and secretion during smoking. *Gastroenterology* 1977; **73**: 758.
8. Murthy, S., Dinoso, V., & Clearfield, H. Acid pH changes in the duodenal bulb during smoking. *Gastroenterology* 1978; **75**: 1.
9. Quimby, G. Active smoking depresses prostaglandin synthesis in human gastric mucosa. *Ann. Intern. Med.* 1986; **104**: 616.
10. Tovey, F. I., Jayaraj, A. P., Lewin, M. R., & Clark, C. G. Diet: its role in the genesis of peptic ulceration. *Dig. Des.* 1989; **7**: 309.
11. Batterman, R. C. & Ehrenfeld, I. The influence of smoking upon the management of the peptic ulcer patient. *Gastroenterology* 1949; **12**: 575.

12. Permutt, R. P. & Cello, J. P. Duodenal ulcer disease in the hospitalized elderly patient. *Dig. Dis. Sci.* 1982; **27**: 1.

13. Reynolds, J. C. Famotidine therapy for active duodenal ulcers. *Ann. Intern. Med.* 1989; **111**: 7.

14. Ippoliti, A. F., Sturevant, R. A. L., Isenberg, J. I. *et al.* Climetidine versus intensive antacid therapy for duodenal ulcer. *Gastroenterology* 1978; **74**: 394.

15. Jorde, R., Bostad, L., & Burhol, P. G. Asymptomatic gastric ulcer: A follow-up study in patient with previous gastric ulcer disease. *Lancet* 1986; **1**: 119.

16. Montagne, J. P., Moss, A. A., & Margulis, A. R. Double-blind study of single and double contrast upper gastrointestinal examinations using endoscopy as control. *Am. J. Radiol.* 1978; **130**: 1041.

17. Levine, M. S. Role of the double-contrast upper gastrointestinal series in the 1990s [Review]. *Gastroenterol. Clin. North Am.* 1995; **24**: 289.

18. Glick, S. N. Duodenal ulcer. *Radiol. Clin. North Am.* 1994; **32**: 1259.

19. Steigmann, F. & Sulman, B. The time of healing gastric ulcers: implication as to therapy. *Gastroenterology* 1952; **20**: 20.

20. Massarrat, S. & Eisenmann, A. Factors affecting the healing rate of duodenal and pyloric ulcers with low-dose antacid treatment. *Gut* 1981; **22**: 97.

21. Van Deventer, G. M., Elashoff, J. D., Reddy, T. J. *et al.* A randomized study of maintenance therapy with ranitidine to prevent the recurrence of duodenal ulcer. *N. Engl. J. Med.* 1989; **320**: 113.

22. Chan, K. M., Mann, K. S., Lai, E. C. *et al.* Factors influencing the development of gastrointestinal therapy complications after neurosurgery: Results of multivariate analysis. *Neurosurgery* 1989; **25**: 378.

23. Kanno, H., Sakaguchi, S., & Hachiya, T. Bleeding peptic ulcer after abdominal aortic aneurysm surgery. *Arch. Surg.* 1991; **126**: 894.

24. Rosen, H. R., Vlatrakes, G. J., & Rattner, D. W. Fulminant peptic ulcer disease in cardiac surgical patients: pathogenesis, prevention, and management. *Crit. Care Med.* 1992; **20**: 354.

25. McCarthy, D. M. Sucralfate. *N. Engl. J. Med.* 1991; **325**: 1017–1025.

13

Liver disease

Enrique J. Martinez

Division Digestive Diseases and Nutrition, Emory University, Atlanta, GA

Introduction

Discussion of the medical management of the surgical patient is not complete unless one considers the key role that the liver plays in the body metabolism. The liver is the site of synthesis of many endogenous proteins that are involved in both the healing process as well as in the breakdown of the multitude of medications that patients receive. Unsuspected liver disease is estimated to occur in 1 in 700 otherwise healthy surgical candidates.[1,2] Some of these patients may be identified before surgery by abnormalities of blood work suggesting liver dysfunction. The degree of concern raised is dependent upon the degree and type of abnormality as well as the type of surgery. In the sections to follow we will examine these issues and attempt to provide a practical approach to the evaluation, risk assessment, and management of these patients.

Abnormal liver tests

The first order of evaluation of the abnormal liver tests is to determine their time of origin. Pre-existing abnormalities suggest non-operative factors and acute development of abnormalities later suggest operative or postoperative events. The role of a careful review of presurgical records and medical history taking cannot be overemphasized. Careful review of intraoperative and postoperative medical data complement the review process. Further diagnostic testing is dictated by review of this information.

Preoperative evaluation

While many blood tests may reflect liver diseases, we will focus on the enzymes aspartate aminotransferase (AST), alanine aminotransferase (ALT), bilirubin, and coagulation tests. Elevations of other factors such as gamma-glutamyltranspeptidase (GGT) or alkaline phosphatase may also detect underlying liver dysfunction, but their significance is directly proportional to the finding of other evidence of chronic hepatic dysfunction. Symptoms or physical stigmata of liver disease should be investigated if discovered on the preoperative evaluation. The clinical finding of jaundice is uncommon (<1%) in patients with normal livers, and as such raises the specter of more serious liver disease.[3]

Elevations of AST and ALT can be divided into mild (less than two to five times normal), moderate (five to ten times normal), and the severe (greater than ten times normal elevations).[3] Each of these categories has its own differential and infers its own degree of risk. Intuitively, one would expect corresponding surgical risk to be proportional to this enzyme level elevation; and studies support this conclusion.

Mild asymptomatic elevations of the liver enzymes are seen most frequently. Their differential includes medications, fatty liver, viral hepatitis, or chronic non-viral hepatitis. Few data are present to suggest that detection of these elevations in the absence of signs of diminished liver reserve, such as elevated prothrombin time or bilirubin levels, poses much risk to the patient undergoing surgery. While not preventing surgery, detection of any AST or ALT elevation should prompt evaluation as to the cause.

Moderate elevations of the liver enzymes suggest a greater degree of hepatic injury and greater susceptibility of the liver to a new injury. Common causes include medications, viral hepatitis, vascular injury, or chronic non-viral hepatitis. Careful drug history, particularly of new medications, becomes more critical as the degree of enzyme elevation worsens. Anesthetic agents in surgery can decrease oxygen delivery to the liver by decreasing

Medical Management of the Surgical Patient: A Textbook of Perioperative Medicine, ed. M. F. Lubin, R. B. Smith, T. F. Dobson, N. Spell, H. K. Walker. 4th edn. Published by Cambridge University Press. © Cambridge University 2006.

splanchnic blood flow and thereby worsen ischemic injury.[4,5] Since data on surgical mortality in patients with acute hepatitis are limited and variable,[6–8] whenever possible, elective surgery in these patients should be postponed to allow for further assessment of the course and etiology of the liver injury. If the surgery proceeds, careful observation of the postoperative course is necessary. Impaired functional reserve of the liver, as indicated by elevation of the prothrombin time or bilirubin, should raise even more concern.

Those patients with severe elevations of the liver enzymes represent a special subset. These patients are typically symptomatic, either directly related to the liver or to primary underlying disease processes. Severe elevations raise concern for acute viral hepatitis, vascular events, poor cardiac function, medications (particularly acetaminophen,) hepatic trauma, or malignancy. If the AST is >5000, one must consider acetaminophen (either alone or in combination with alcohol) as the etiology until proven otherwise to ensure treatment is not delayed. A recent review showed that AST elevation >3000 is associated with an operative mortality of 55%.[9] Ischemic hepatitis has been associated with a 75% mortality compared to a 33% mortality for other causes of severe elevations. Elective surgery should be clearly avoided in these patients.[9]

Recent onset of symptomatic illness in association with elevation of liver tests should prompt a thorough review of recent events. A typical presentation is new onset nausea and vomiting, suggesting an acute process that may continue to worsen in the near future. Given the uncertainty of the illness course, elective surgery should be postponed until the acute process is resolved or the risk is determined to be acceptable.

Stigmata of chronic liver disease, if found, raise further concern for surgical risk due to diminished functional liver reserve. Studies have suggested increased risk in symptomatic patients who have evidence of chronic disease.[10,11] The risk is determined by the type of surgery and the degree of preservation of liver function.[10] The mortality rates reported vary from 5%–67% and morbidity rates likewise vary from 7%–39%.[10] Risk stratification is performed using Child's classification system,[12–14] and Child's class A patients without decompensation do better than decompensated Child's C cirrhotics.

There are special considerations for abdominal surgery in cirrhotic patients. Umbilical hernias are a frequent occurrence, seen in 42% of patients with ascites vs. in 10% of those without.[15] If spontaneous rupture occurs, surgery is the only option and is associated with 14% mortality vs. 50% without surgery.[16–18] Another common upper abdominal surgery with substantial risk in the cirrhotic patient is cholecystectomy, which is associated with up to a 26% mortality rate and 25% morbidity rate.[19] For elective surgery in the earlier Child's A and B stages, laparoscopic cholecystectomy may be preferable to open cholecystectomy with a lower complication rate of 16% vs. 36%.[20–25] Advanced cirrhosis may make surgical treatment of recurrent cholecystitis untenable. In these cases, liver transplantation may be the only option. In the lower abdomen the repair of groin hernia appears to be better tolerated than umbilical hernia repair, even with ascites, with only 8% rate of recurrence.[26]

Operative and postoperative complications

Patients with liver disease, especially cirrhosis, are at an increased risk of postoperative complications. Up to a 30.1% incidence was noted in review by Ziser *et al.*[29] In decreasing frequency the following complications were noted: pneumonia (8%), ventilator dependence (7.8%), infection (7.5%), ascites decompensation (6.7%), and cardiac arrhythmia (5%). Postoperative deaths occurred 9.8% in hospital and 1.8% after discharge. The key aspect in the patient with liver disease is to be vigilant for these complications and to carefully review the operative record for evidence of any significant hypotension episodes, as superimposed hepatic ischemia increases risk of decompensation.

Intraoperative complications may include surgical injury such as inadvertent ligation of the hepatic artery or common bile duct during laparoscopic cholecystectomy. Either complication may result in the sudden rise of liver tests after surgery. Anesthetic injury is uncommon to see with current agents in use. Halothane previously had been associated with hepatitis in approximately 1 in 10 000 operations.[27,28]

The onset of acute viral hepatitis is uncommonly seen in the postoperative period. Blood transfusions are screened for the common viral entitities, but it is possible to see acute viral hepatitis develop from blood transfused from a subclinically infected donor. Appropriate diagnostic testing for viral hepatitis with the polymerase chain reaction should help detect this rare occurrence if other more likely causes have been excluded.

Postoperative medication-induced hepatitis

New and existing drugs have enormous potential for liver toxicity, and full discussion is beyond the scope of this chapter. If a patient develops abnormal liver tests only after surgery and the intraoperative record is unremarkable, one must look carefully at each individual medicine for its potential of causing the problem. Total parenteral nutrition (TPN) can cause cholestasis. If it must be continued, the patient may benefit from cycling TPN as a way to both stimulate appetite and reduce the time of hepatic exposure.[37]

Acetaminophen merits specific discussion due to its nearly ubiquitous presence in the hospital and its potential for serious toxicity. It is both an antipyretic and mild analgesic and is also part of the most common analgesic–narcotic pain medicines. The use in non-alcoholics of over 7.5 g a day as a single dose or of over 2 g a day in alcoholic patients can lead to significant toxicity.[30] One can easily imagine a scenario where a patient downplays alcohol consumption and then is given usual doses of an acetaminophen–narcotic analgesic and goes on to develop this toxicity. Sudden and dramatic elevations of AST/ALT (typically >5000) in surgical patients need to have acetaminophen toxicity excluded first due to its potential progression to liver failure if not detected. The use of acetylcysteine (Mucomyst) 140 mg/kg loading and then 70 mg/kg orally every 4 hours for 17 doses may have substantial impact and prevent a tragic situation from evolving. If not successful, orthotopic liver transplantation remains an option for patients who have not gone on to develop irreversible brain injury.

Onset of jaundice in the postoperative period is uncommon, occurring in <1% of patients, but is more common in patients with pre-existing liver disease. Since breakdown of hemoglobin liberates bilirubin, blood transfusion or resorption of hematoma may cause jaundice in patients with impaired liver function.[31] Other causes include impaired bile formation due to sepsis or to decreased hepatic blood flow from anesthetic agents or hypotension.[32–36] The time of occurrence of these events in usually within the first 10 days after the surgery with mild elevations of alkaline phosphatase along with the jaundice more than AST/ALT elevations. Mild elevations of bilirubin are usually benign and resolve as the patient recovers from the surgery or other event such as infection. The degree of bilirubin elevation is important to note, as a level greater than 6 mg/dl is associated with 46% mortality if this occurs in a patient with abdominal trauma and 86% mortality in a patient with intra-abdominal sepsis.[36] Typically, death in these patients comes from multiorgan system failure and is not from the acute liver injury.

Complications of liver disease

Ascites

The presence of ascites is an important sign of limited liver reserve. Mild to moderate ascites can be easily missed by experienced physicians in up to 50% cases.[37] If suspected but not confirmed by physical examination, body imaging allows the detection of as little as $100 \, cm^3$ of ascites. While it is important to note that liver disease will be the cause in 80%, the remaining will include a variety of causes, such as malignancy (12%), cardiac failure (5%), tuberculosis (2%), and pancreatic ascites (1%). The evaluation of ascites must include diagnostic paracentesis, as detection of a high serum ascites albumin gradient of >1.1 g/dl is helpful to categorize the etiology as being due to portal hypertension. Examples include cirrhosis, massive intrahepatic metastases, venoocclusive disorders, cardiac ascites, and myxedma. The finding of a low gradient raises concern about such processes as peritoneal carcinomatosis, tuberculous peritonitis, pancreatic ascites, renal failure, or serositis from collagen-vascular disorders.[38]

Detection of ascites from hepatic causes is important, as 2-year survival may be as low as 50%.[39] Its presence also marks the potential for development of spontaneous bacterial peritonitis, which accounts for 5%–10% of deaths in cirrhotics.[40,41] Studies of alcoholic liver disease have shown that 5-year survival decreases from 89% to 52% in patients who develop ascites, dropping even further to 32% if they continue to imbibe alcohol.[42] Ascites is felt to be a contributing factor in 50% of deaths in cirrhotic patients.[43] It is beyond the scope of this chapter to review the etiologies of ascites and, as such, our focus will be on important clinical issues of treatment.

Treatment of ascites ultimately will be needed in 90% of cases.[44,45] The stepwise approach to ascites begins with lifestyle modifications. In the decompensated patient bed rest helps to restore central venous volume, which in turn improves renal perfusion and diminishes renal sodium retention. Complete bed rest is practical only in the initial treatment of the hospitalized patient, as it runs counter to the goal of restoring the patient to prior function.

Because cirrhotic patients tend to have low urinary sodium excretion, control of their dietary intake becomes critical. Every gram of sodium ingested over the sodium excretion represents 200–300 ml of fluid retention.[46] While extremely low salt diets (<500mg) will cause fluid loss, they are rarely followed. It is more prudent to try a 2 g sodium diet. Should the serum sodium drop below 125 meq/l, fluid restriction to 1 liter per day may become necessary.

Bed rest and diet may work in up to 10% of patients, but the remaining 90% will need addition of diuretics for control. The goal of diuresis is to produce a 700–900 ml/day loss if no edema is present, and up to a 3 pound loss per day if peripheral edema is noted.[47,48] Spironolactone acts through direct antagonism of aldosterone at the level of the collecting duct, thus blocking sodium resorption and potassium excretion.[49] It may be efficacious as a single agent in up to 65% of patients.[50,51] Dosing should start at 50–100 mg per day and be titrated up to a maximum dose of 400 mg per day. Main limits to its use are severe hyperkalemia and painful gynecomastia. Other potassium-sparing diuretics are less effective.

If sprinolactone is not sufficient, addition of a loop diuretic may help in another 20% of patients. Dosing of furosemide at 20–40 mg/day is recommended with titration up to 160 mg/day. Other agents that work at the loop of Henle such as ethacrinic acid, bumetanide, or torasemide may be used. Theoretically, torasemide produces a greater natriuretic effect but is less often used in the USA.[52–54]

Resistance to loop diuretics may lead to introduction of metolazone. This drug functions at the cortical diluting segment and can lead to significant diuresis.[55] When used in combination with other diuretics, observe carefully for side effects such as hypokalemia and volume depletion.

Despite progressive use of diuretics, 10%–20% of patients will be refractory to medical management of their ascites.[56] This group can include failures of control with maximal doses or significant side effects from the medications at lower than maximal levels. Liver transplantation is the ultimate solution for this group; but due to organ shortages, options other than this may need to be considered.

Therapeutic paracentesis is the initial treatment of refractory ascites. It is used in up to 75% of all patients who have ascites and in 93% of refractory ascites patients.[57] When compared to diuretics alone, paracentesis proves more efficacious at eliminating ascites, decreases days in hospital and has fewer side effects.[58] The risk of paracentesis rises when greater than 5 l of fluid are removed without the use of plasma expanders.[59] Intravascular volume is felt to fall after 12–24 hours and, as such, use of longer-acting plasma expanders may be more beneficial. Albumin, hemaccel and dextran have different half-lives, with albumin having the longest at 21 days vs. 16 hours and 24 hours for the other two agents.[60] It is recommended to administer intravenous albumin, 6–8 g per liter of ascites removed, to minimize the renal side effects of large volume paracentesis.

Dependence on paracentesis despite optimal medical management warrants consideration of a more definitive treatment. Options include the peritoneovenous shunts (Denver, Leveen, Minnesota types) or transjugular intrahepatic portosystemic shunts (TIPS) to control the ascites. The peritoneovenous shunts are associated with a 10–60%

coagulopathy rate, generally subclinical.[61–64] If the majority of ascites is removed at the time of surgery, the coagulopathy appears to be dimished.[65–67] A major drawback is the 30%–40% shunt dysfunction rate seen from thrombosis, line kinks, or valve clogging.[65,66] A more serious complication is superior vena cava thrombosis in 2%–23%.[68,69] These shunts should be reserved for treatment of refractory ascites in the patient who is not a TIPS candidate.

The use of transjugular intrahepatic systemic shunts for refractory ascites is the mainstay of treatment for most cirrhotics who reach this point. The response rates vary from 50%–92% of patients, with lower response rates noted in patients with total bilirubin levels greater than 5 mg/dl.[70–75] Ochs et al. found, in one of the larger series, that TIPS successfully decreased the portal systemic gradient in 63% of cases. Of responders, 74% had complete remission of ascites, and partial remission occurred in another 18%.[71] Like surgical shunts, TIPS has potential for thrombosis in 10% and late malfunction of shunt in 32%. It is unclear at this time if the use of covered TIPS stents will result in a lower risk of these types of complications. The main issue to realize is that refractory ascites is a marker for end stage liver disease, as in these series there was a 58% cumulative 9-month mortality. Predictors of poor outcome include age >60 years at time of procedure and worsening total bilirubin levels post procedure.[76] The most disabling aspect of TIPS for refractory ascites is the high incidence (40%–50%) of encephalopathy associated with it. Recent trials are ongoing to assess benefit of total volume paracentesis vs. TIPS for the treatment of refractory ascites. Recently, a study by Allard et al. has started to demonstrate that TIPS placement improves some nutritional parameters in patients with refractory ascites.[77]

Discussion of the other complications of portal hypertension such as GI bleeding and encephalopathy are outside the scope of this chapter. It is worthwhile mentioning that one must be aware of the potential for encephalopathy to be aggravated in the cirrhotic patient in the postoperative period. Postoperative analgesia should be started at the lowest dose possible to relieve pain. Use shorter-acting agents first. One can always add more medication if necessary, whereas if the dose is too high, use of reversal agents will be needed. It is also important to limit acetaminophen to less than two grams a day in total. To achieve this, it is best to use non-acetaminophen containing narcotics so that their dose can be titrated independent of acetaminophen dosing. The use of sleep aids may also aggravate encephalopathy and should be avoided where possible, as many of the agents in common use have long half-lives which can be further prolonged in the cirrhotic patient. These issues are more critical once the patient is extubated to prevent the excess sedation complications which could lead to reintubation. Lactulose can reduce encephalopathy, given as an enema if oral or nasogastric access is unavailable. Gut decontaminants such as metronidazole or oral neomycin can be used if the patient has refractory encephalopathy, with caution for renal function changes being recommended with neomycin use.

REFERENCES

1. Schemel, W. H. Unexpected hepatic dysfunction found by multiple laboratory screening. *Anesth. Analg. (Cleve.)* 1976; **55**: 810.

2. Wataneeyawech, M. & Kelly, K. A. Jr. Hepatic diseases unsuspected before surgery. *NY State J. Med.* 1975; **75**: 1278.

3. Martinez, E. J. & Boyer, T. D. Preoperative and postoperative hepatic dysfunction. In Zakim, D., Boyer, T. D., eds. *Hepatology: A Textbook of Liver Disease*, Orlando: W. B. Saunders, 2002.

4. Ngai, S. H. Effects of anesthetics on various organs. *N. Engl. J. Med.* 1980; **302**: 564.

5. Cooperman, L. H. Effects of anesthesia on the splanchnic circulation. *Br. J. Anaesth.* 1972; **44**: 967.

6. Hardy, K. J. & Hughes, E. S. R. Laparotomy in viral hepatitis. *Med. J. Aust.* 1968; **1**: 710.

7. Strauss, A. A., Strauss, S. F., Schwartz, A. H. *et al.* Decompression by drainage of the common bile duct in subacute and chronic jaundice: A report of 73 cases with hepatitis or concomitant biliary duct infection as cause. *Am. J. Surg.* 1959; **97**: 137.

8. Bourke, J. B., Cannon, P., & Ritchie, H. D. Laparotomy for jaundice. *Lancet* 1967; **ii**: 521.

9. Johnson, R. D., O'Connor, M. L., & Kerr, R. M. Extreme serum elevations of aspartate aminotransferase. *Am. J. Gastroenterol.* 1995; **90**: 1244.

10. Friedman, L. S. & Maddrey, W. C. Surgery in the patient with liver disease. *Med. Clin. North Am.* 1987; **71**: 453.

11. Hargrove, M. D. Chronic active hepatitis possible adverse effect of exploratory laparotomy. *Surgery* 1970; **68**: 771.

12. Garrison, R. N., Cryer, H. M., Howard, D. A. *et al.* Clarification of risk factors for abdominal operations in patients with hepatic cirrhosis. *Ann. Surg.* 1984; **199**: 648.

13. Brown, M. W. & Burk, R. F. Development of intractable ascites following upper abdominal surgery in patients with cirrhosis. *Am. J. Med.* 1986; **80**: 879.

14. Chapman, C. B., Snell, A. M., & Rowntree, L. G. Decompensated portal cirrhosis. Report of 112 cases. *J. Am. Med. Assoc.* 1931; **97**: 237.

15. Chapman, C. B., Snell, A. M., & Rowntree, L. G. Decompensated portal cirrhosis. Report on one hundred and twelve cases. Clinical features of the ascitic stage of cirrhosis of the liver. *J. Am. Med. Assoc.* 1981; **97**: 237.

16. Leonetti, J. P., Aranha, G. V., Wilkinson, W. A. *et al.* Umbilical herniorrhaphy in cirrhotic patients. *Arch. Surg.* 1984; **119**: 442.

17. Yonemoto, R. H. & Davidson, C. S. Herniorrhaphy in cirrhosis of the liver with ascites. *N. Engl. J. Med.* 1956; **255**: 733.

18. Maniatis, A. G. & Hunt, C. M. Therapy for spontaneous umbilical hernia rupture. *Am. J. Gastroenterol.* 1995; **90**: 310.

19. Bloch, R. S., Allaben, R. D., & Wait, A. J. Cholecystectomy in patients with cirrhosis. *Arch. Surg.* 1985; **120**: 669.

20. Friel, C. M. Laparoscopic cholecystectomy in patients with hepatic cirrhosis: a five-year experience. *J. Gastrointest. Surg.* 1999; **3**: 286.

21. Yerdel, M. A., Tsuge, H., Mimura, H. *et al.* Laparoscopic cholecystectomy in cirrhotic patients: expanding indications. *Surg. Laparosc. Endosc.* 1993; **3**: 180.

22. Yerdel, M. A. Laparoscopic versus open cholecystectomy in cirrhotic patients: a prospective study. *Surg. Laprarosc. Endosc.* 1997; **7**: 483.

23. Sleeman, D. Laparascopic cholecystectomy in cirrhotic patients. *J. Am. Coll. Surg.* 1998; **187**: 400.

24. Gopalswamy, N. Risks of intra-abdominal nonshunt surgery in cirrhotics. *Dig. Dis.* 1998; **16**: 225.

25. D'Alburquerque, L. A. Laparoscopic cholecystectomy in cirrhotic patients. *Surg. Laparosc. Endosc.* 1995; **5**: 272.

26. Hurst, R. D. Management of groin hernias in patients with ascites. *Ann. Surg.* 1992; **216**: 696.

27. Farrell, G. C. Postoperative hepatic dysfunction. In Zakim, D., Boyer, T. D., eds. *Hepatology: A Textbook of Liver Disease*, 2nd edn. Philadelphia: W. B. Saunders Co., 1990: 869.

28. Farrell, G. C. Liver disease due to anaesthetic agents. In Farrell, G. C., ed. *Drug-Induced Liver Disease*. Edinburgh: Churchill Livingstone, 1994: 389.

29. Ziser, A., Plevak, D. J., Weisner, R. H. *et al.* Morbidity and mortality in cirrhotic patient undergoing anesthesia and surgery, *Anesthesiology* 1999; **90**: 42.

30. Farrell, G. C. Paracetamol-induced hepatotoxicity. In Farrell, G. C., ed. *Drug-Induced Liver Disease*. Edinburgh: Churchill Livingstone, 1994: 205.

31. LaMont, J. T. Postoperative jaundice. *Surg. Clin. North Am.* 1974; **54**: 637.

32. Gottlieb, J. E., Menashe, P. I., & Cruz, E. Gastrointestinal complications in critically ill patients: the intensivists' overview. *Am. J. Gastroenterol.* 1986; **81**: 227.

33. LaMont, J. T. & Isselbacher, K. J. Postoperative jaundice. *N. Engl. J. Med.* 1974; **288**: 305.

34. Schmid, M., Hefti, M. L., Gattiker, R. *et al.* Benign postoperative intrahepatic cholestasis. *N. Engl. J. Med.* 1965; **272**: 545.

35. Kantrowitz, P. A., Jones, W. A., Greenberger, N. J., & Isselbacher, K. J. Severe postoperative hyperbilirubinemia simulating obstructive jaundice. *N. Engl. J. Med.* 1967; **276**: 591.

36. te Boekhorst, T., Urlus, M., Doesburg, W. *et al.* Etiologic factors of jaundice in severely ill patients. A retrospective study in patients admitted to an intensive care unit with severe trauma

or with septic intra-abdominal complications following surgery and without evidence of bile duct obstruction. *J. Hepatol.* 1988; **7**: 111.

37. Cattau, E. L., Benjamin, S. B., Knuff, T. E., & Castell, D. O. The accuracy of the physical examination in the diagnosis of suspected ascites. *JAMA* 1982; **247**: 1164–1166.

38. Runyon, B. Ascites. In Schiff, L. & Schiff, E., eds. *Diseases of the Liver.* Philadelphia: J. B. Lippincott, 1993: 989.

39. Arroyo, V., Bernardi, M., Epstein, M., Henriksen, J. H., Schrier, R. W., & Rodes, J. Pathophysiology of ascites and functional renal failure in cirrhosis. *J. Hepatol.* 1988; **6**: 239–257.

40. Hoefs, J. L., Canawati, H. N., & Sapico, F. L. Spontaneous bacterial peritonitis. *Hepatology* 1982; **2**: 399–407.

41. Longmire-Cook, S. J. Pathophysiologic factors and management of ascites. *Surg. Gynecol. Obstet.* 1993; **176**: 191–202.

42. Powell, W. J. & Klatskin, G. Duration of survival in patients with Laennec's cirrhosis. *Am. J. Med.* 1968; **44**: 406–420.

43. Conn, H. O. Introduction to ASAIO workshop on peritoneovenous shunt in the management of ascites. *ASAIO Trans.* 1989; **35**: 160.

44. Longmire-Cook, S. J. Pathophysiologic factors and management of ascites. *Surg. Gynecol. Obstet.* 1993; **176**: 191–202.

45. Linas, S. L., Anderson, R. J., Miller, P. D., & Schrier, R. W. The rational use of diuretics in cirrhosis. In *The Kidney in Liver Disease.* 2nd edn., ed. M. Epstein. New York: Elsevier Biomedical, 1983: 555–567.

46. Stassen, W. N. & McCullough, A. J. Management of ascites. *Semin. Liver Dis.* 1985; **5**: 291–307.

47. Shear, L., Ching, S., & Gabuzda, G. J. Compartmentalization of ascites and edema in patients with hepatic cirrhosis. *N. Engl. J. Med.* 1970; **232**: 1391–1396.

48. Pockros, P. J. & Reynolds, T. B. Rapid diuresis in patients with ascites from chronic liver disease: the importance of peripheral edema. *Gastroenterology* 1986; **90**: 1827–1833.

49. Sansom, S. C. & O'Neill, R. G. Effects of mineralocorticoids on transport properties of cortical collecting duct basolateral membrane. *Am. J. Physiol.* 1986; **251**: F743–F757.

50. Fogel, M. R., Sawhney, V. K., Neal, E. A., Miller, R. G., Knauer, C. M., & Gregory, P. B. Diuresis in the ascitic patient: a randomized controlled trial of three agents. *J. Clin. Gastroenterol.* 1981; **3**: 73–80.

51. Perez-Ayuso, R. M., Arroyo, V., Planas, R. *et al.* Randomized comparative trial of efficacy of furosemide vs. Spironolactone in nonazotemic cirrhosis with ascites. *Gastroenterology* 1983; **84**: 961–968.

52. Laffi, G., Marra, F., Buzelli, G. *et al.* Comparison of the effects of torasemide and furosemide in nonazotemic cirrhotic patients with ascites: a randomized, double-blind study. *Hepatology* 1991; **13**: 1101–1105.

53. Broekhuysen, J., Deger, F., Douchamps, J., Ducarne, H., & Herchuelz, A. Torasemide, a new potent diuretic. Double-blind comparison with furosemide. *Europ. J. Clin. Pharmacol.* 1986; **31**: Suppl:29–34.

54. Dunn, C. J., Fitton, A., & Brogden, R. N. Torasemide. An update of its pharmacological properties and therapeutic efficacy. *Drugs* 1995; **49**: 121–142.

55. Epstein, M., Lepp, B. A., & Hoffman, D. S. Potentiation of furosemide by metolazone in refractory edema. *Curr. Ther. Res.* 1977; **21**: 656–660.

56. Gerbes, A. L. Medical treatment of ascites in cirrhosis. *J. Hepatol.* 1993; **12**: S4–S9.

57. Burroughs, A. K. Paracentesis for ascites in cirrhotic patients. *Gastroenterol. Int.* 1990; **2**: 120–123.

58. Gines, P., Arroyo, V., Quintero, E. *et al.* Comparison of paracentesis and diuretics in the treatment of cirrhotics with tense ascites. Results of a randomized trial. *Gastroenterology* 1987; **93**: 234–241.

59. Gines, P., Tito, L. I., Arroyo, V. *et al.* Randomized comparative study of therapeutic paracentesis with and without intravenous albumin in cirrhosis. *Gastroenterology* 1988; **94**: 1493–1502.

60. Gines, P. & Arroyo, V. Paracentesis in the management of cirrhotic ascites. *J. Hepatol.* 1993; **12**: S14–S18.

61. Greig, P. D., Langer, B., Blendis, L. M., Taylor, B. R., & Glynn, M. F. Complications after peritoneovenous shunting for ascites. *Am. J. Surg.* 1980; **139**: 125–131.

62. Starling, J. R. Peritoneovenous shunting in the management of malignant and cirrhotic ascites. *Wis. Med. J.* 1980; **79**: 25–29.

63. Rubinstein, D., McInnes, I., & Dudley, F. Morbidity and mortality after peritoneovenous shunt for refractory ascites. *Gut* 1985; **26**: 1070–1073.

64. Boyer, T. D. & Goldman, I. S. Treatment of cirrhotic ascites. *Adv. Intern. Med.* 1986; **31**: 3359–3377.

65. LeVeen, H. H., Vujic, I., d'Ovidio, N. G., & Hutto, R. B. Peritoneovenous shunt occlusion: etiology, diagnosis, therapy. *Ann. Surg.* 1984; **200**: 212–223.

66. Smadja, C. & Franco, D. The LeVeen shunt in the elective treatment of intractable ascites in cirrhosis. A prospective study on 140 patients. *Ann. Surg.* 1985; **201**: 488–493.

67. Greenlee, H. B., Stanley, M. M., & Reinhardt, G. F. Intractable ascites treated with peritoneovenous shunt (LeVeen). *Arch. Surg.* 1981; **116**: 518–524.

68. LeVeen, E. G. & LeVeen, H. H. The place of the peritoneovenous shunt in the treatment of ascites. *ASAIO Trans* 1989; **35**: 165–168.

69. Foley, W. J., Elliott, J. P. Jr., Smith, R. F., Reddy, D. J., Lewis, J. R. Jr., & Hageman, J. H. Central venous thrombosis and embolism associated with peritoneovenous shunts. *Arch. Surg.* 1984; **119**: 713–720.

70. Lebrec, D., Giuily, N., Hadengue, A. *et al.* Transjugular intrahepatic portosystemic shunt (TIPS) vs paracentesis for refractory ascites: results of a randomized trial. *J. Hepatol.* 1996; **25**: 135–144.

71. Ochs, A., Rossle, M., Haag, K. *et al.* The transjugular intrahepatic portosystemic stent shunt procedure for refractory ascites. *N. Engl. J. Med.* 1995; **332**: 1192–1197.

72. Benner, K. G., Sahagun, G., & Saxon, R. Selection of patients undergoing transjugular intrahepatic portosystemic shunt (TIPS) for refractory ascites. [Abstract]. *Hepatology* 1994; **20**: 114A.

73. Ferral, H., Bjarnason, H., & Wegrym, S. A. Refractory ascites: early experience in treatment with transjugular intrahepatics portosystemic shunt. *Radiology* 1993; **189**: 795–801.

74. Somberg, K., Lake, J. R., Tomlanovich, S. J., LaBerge, J. M., Feldstein, V., & Bass, N. M. Transjugular intrahepatic portal–systemic shunt in the treatment of refractory ascites: effect on clinical and hormonal response and renal function. *Hepatology* 1995; **1**: 709–716.

75. Quiroga, J., Sangro, B., Nunez, M. *et al.* Transjugular intra-hepatic portal–systemic shunt in the treatment of refractory ascites: effect on clinical, renal, humoral, and hemodynamic parameters. *Hepatology* 1995; **21**: 986–994.

76. Enrique, J., Martinez, E. J., & Jeffers, L. Self-limited viral hepatitis: A, E, CMV. EBV. In Wu, G. & Israel, J., eds. *Disease of the Liver and Bile Ducts: Diagnosis and Treatment.* Humana Press; 1998: 103–121.

77. Allard, J. P., Chau, J., Sandokji, K., Blendis, L. M., & Wong, F. Effects of ascites resolution after successful TIPS on nutrition in cirrhotic patients with refractory ascites. *Am. J. Gastroenterol.* 2001; **96**(8): 2442–2447.

14

Inflammatory bowel disease

Brennan A. Scott and Lorenzo Rossaro

University of California, Davis Medical Center Sacramento, CA

Introduction

Crohn's disease and ulcerative colitis are the major forms of idiopathic inflammatory bowel disease. These conditions are chronic and relapsing in nature and primarily affect the small and large intestine, but occasionally the oral cavity, esophagus, and stomach can be involved. The precise etiology of these disorders is unknown, but they are generally felt to develop from a complex interplay of genetic, environmental, and microbial factors.[1–3] There is generally no associated increase in mortality with inflammatory bowel disease, however there is often a high degree of morbidity, frequently requiring surgical intervention as part of the long-term treatment strategy. Although these diseases have many similarities, the indications for surgery and response to surgical therapy are quite different. In the majority of cases, clinical, radiological, and pathological findings will lead to the appropriate diagnosis; however in approximately 10% of cases, the distinction remains unclear and the patient is given a diagnosis of indeterminate colitis. It is imperative to have an accurate diagnosis prior to any planned surgical intervention in order to have the best possible outcome.

Crohn's disease

The incidence of Crohn's disease in the USA is estimated to be 5.8 cases per 100 000 person–years with a prevalence of 133 cases per 100 000 persons.[4] It presents in a bimodal fashion with a peak in the second and third decades of life, and another in the sixth decade. Most commonly (50%) there is involvement of both the small and large intestine, with 30% of cases being confined to the small bowel, and 20% with only colonic involvement.[5]

The most prominent clinical features of Crohn's disease are diarrhea, abdominal pain, and weight loss. Rectal bleeding, fever, and extraintestinal symptoms occur less frequently. It can be present in any luminal gastrointestinal location from mouth to anus, manifesting pathologically as a transmural inflammation. Features that are more specific for Crohn's disease are skip lesions (active disease separated by areas of normal tissue), small bowel involvement, and fistula formation. Non-caseating granulomas are felt to be fairly specific to Crohn's disease and are found in 15%–30% of biopsy samples and 70% of surgical specimens.[6–8] Deep linear ulcers or fissures, as well as small aphthoid erosions also favor the diagnosis of Crohn's disease.

Ulcerative colitis

The incidence of ulcerative colitis in the USA is estimated to be 7.6 cases per 100 000 person–years with a prevalence of 229 cases per 100 000 persons.[9] It presents in a similar bimodal fashion to Crohn's disease. Ulcerative colitis is more common in males than females while the opposite is true for Crohn's disease. It is a disease confined to the colon; however, in 15%–20% of cases there can be irregularities of the ileocecal valve and terminal ileum known as "backwash ileitis."[10] This is an important fact to consider because ulcerative colitis can be cured by colectomy while Crohn's disease generally cannot.

The clinical manifestation of ulcerative colitis is most commonly that of bloody diarrhea. The diarrhea may be small in volume and associated with tenesmus if the rectum is predominantly involved. Systemic symptoms such as fever, weight loss, malaise, and anemia are seen in proportion to the extent of disease, with patients having pancolitis

Medical Management of the Surgical Patient: A Textbook of Perioperative Medicine, ed. M. F. Lubin, R. B. Smith, T. F. Dobson, N. Spell, H. K. Walker. 4th edn. Published by Cambridge University Press. © Cambridge University 2006.

being the most severely affected. Extraintestinal manifestations of the disease involving the joints, skin, and eyes may be seen more commonly than in Crohn's disease that is limited to the small intestine. Endoscopically there is a granular appearing, edematous, friable mucosa extending proximally, and beginning in the rectum in the majority of cases. There is an abrupt demarcation between diseased and uninvolved mucosa. The inflammation is confined to the mucosa and submucosa in comparison to the transmural inflammation of Crohn's disease. Strictures, pseudopolyps, and ulcerations may be present, but fistulae are generally absent in ulcerative colitis. The microscopic appearance varies by disease severity and is not entirely specific to ulcerative colitis, but crypt distortion, crypt abscesses, mixed chronic and acute inflammation, and mucous depletion are often seen while granulomas are not.[11]

Indications for surgery in Crohn's disease

The majority of patients with Crohn's disease will require surgery at some point during the course of the disease.[12,13] Due to the recurrent nature and the extension of the disease, surgery is uncommonly curative and further operations are common. Because of the risk of serious long-term outcomes such as short-bowel syndrome, the decision to operate should be made carefully. Acute indications for surgery are complications such as perforation, abscess, uncontrollable hemorrhage, toxic megacolon, or bowel obstruction. Elective surgery may be performed for strictures, fistulae, malignancy, malnutrition, or poorly controlled disease despite aggressive medical management. Surgery should not be looked upon as a failure of treatment, but as an option for treating serious complications and conferring a better over-all well being when medical options cannot fully control active disease.

Indications for surgery in ulcerative colitis

In contrast to Crohn's disease, ulcerative colitis can be cured by surgery. Approximately one third of patients will eventually undergo colectomy for a variety of indications.[14] Emergent or urgent surgery is performed for hemorrhage, fulminant colitis, toxic megacolon, or perforation. Elective surgery may be performed for medically intractable disease, malnutrition, or dysplasia or malignancy found on surveillance colonoscopy. Although bleeding is common in ulcerative colitis and generally not severe, hemorrhage accounts for approximately 10% of emergency colectomies.[15]

Surgical options in inflammatory bowel disease

The type and extent of surgery performed will depend upon several factors. Different procedures will often be chosen for Crohn's disease as opposed to ulcerative colitis. The extent and activity of disease, as well as any existing complications or presence of dysplasia will also be important in choice of surgery.

In Crohn's disease the type of surgery performed can vary widely, as this disease can affect any portion of the gastrointestinal tract. Surgical procedures vary from a straightforward central venous catheter placement to complex abdominal and pelvic bowel procedures. Generally the diagnosis of Crohn's disease will be established prior to the patient entering the operating room; however if the patient's first presentation is an abscess or an acute abdomen, the diagnosis may be made at surgery. In a patient undergoing a surgical exploration for right lower quadrant pain who is found to have Crohn's disease, the surgeon may elect to resect the involved segment of bowel at that time in order to avoid the possible failure of medical therapy and the need for future surgery.[16] In addition to bowel resections, Crohn's patients may also commonly undergo stricturoplasty, or fistula resection. Surgery may be performed by laparotomy, laparoscopy, or laparoscopic-assisted bowel resection. For disease confined largely to the colon, an ileorectostomy may be the procedure of choice. In the case of toxic colitis it is common for an abdominal colectomy, ileostomy, and Hartman's pouch to be performed.[16]

When the decision to perform surgery for ulcerative colitis is made, the operation is generally curative. The surgical alternative chosen will be a variation of colectomy, with the type depending upon the circumstances. In the emergent situation the simplest procedure to perform is a subtotal colectomy with ileostomy. This option avoids a complicated pelvic dissection and leaves a rectal stump in place. Once the active disease has been controlled, these patients can undergo an ileal pouch-anal canal anastomosis. In patients undergoing elective proctocolectomy most will be candidates for a two-stage ileal pouch-anal anastomosis. The first stage includes a loop ileostomy that is taken down at a later date once the anastomosis and pouch have healed. In experienced hands, this procedure can be performed safely,[17] with good patient satisfaction and quality of life.[18] Crohn's disease, incompetent anal sphincter, distal rectal cancer, and inability of the pouch to reach the anal canal are contraindications to the procedure. Advanced age, obesity, previous small bowel resection, and indeterminant colitis are relative contraindications.[11] The alternative to ileal pouch-anal canal anastomosis is to leave an ileostomy in place. The Brooke ileostomy has been the standard surgery for ulcerative colitis for many years. In selected patients who would prefer not to have an external appliance, a continent ileostomy (Kock pouch) is an alternative. This procedure uses loops of small bowel to create a storage pouch with an intussuscepted valve.[19]

Preoperative care

Most surgery performed in patients with inflammatory bowel disease is elective or semi-elective, providing adequate time for careful preparation. The site and extent of disease should be well established before proceeding with surgery. A recent colonoscopy will provide important information about the disease activity in the colon; this should always include an examination of the terminal ileum when possible. In the evaluation of strictures and fistulae barium studies can be extremely valuable in defining precise anatomy. Abdominal and pelvic computed tomography scanning is important when an abscess is suspected.

The specific type of surgery planned should be discussed with the patient and family, with consideration of the potential for drains, stoma, short gut, and wound closure complications. The patient and family members should understand the goals of the procedure and be prepared emotionally for the potential outcomes, including disease recurrence.

As with any patient with chronic disease, inflammatory bowel disease patients are at risk for malnutrition. Whenever possible, the nutritional status of each patient should be assessed and addressed with enteral or parenteral nutrition where indicated. A detailed history and physical exam and serum albumin level are often sufficient for evaluation. Total parenteral nutrition (TPN) has not been shown to decrease mortality in surgical patients in general,[20] and the proper use of enteral and parenteral nutrition in inflammatory bowel disease patients remains controversial. Current data support the use for 5 to 14 days of preoperative TPN only in patients with severe malnutrition.[21] In situations that do not allow for complete nutritional evaluation and treatment, proper attention should be paid to hemoglobin, volume status, and electrolytes. In preparation for surgery patients should be on a clear liquid diet or *nil per os* 24 hours prior to surgery with an appropriate bowel preparation given the night before. Caution should be paid in feeding and ordering bowel preparations in patients suspected of having stenoses or strictures.

Consideration should be paid to the chronic medications taken by the patient. Antibiotics and 5-ASA compounds used for the treatment of active inflammatory bowel disease will likely become unnecessary for the patient undergoing surgical resection of diseased bowel and should be stopped. This does not apply to antibiotics being given for active infection or toxic colitis. The management of other immunosuppressive agents should be individualized to patient and circumstances. There are no trials specifically addressing the perioperative safety of azathioprine, 6-mercaptopurine, or methotrexate in inflammatory bowel disease patients. In the emergency setting the long half-life of these medications leaves no option. In patients in whom the surgery is expected to remove the diseased portion of bowel, it is expected that discontinuing these medications in the weeks prior to surgery or at the time of surgery would be reasonable. In the case where a surgery is unrelated to inflammatory bowel disease, or is not expected to remove all active sites of disease, it is generally prudent to continue these medications up to the time of surgery, provided that leukopenia is not present, and then resume them once bowel function has returned and the patient is tolerating oral medications. Discussing the planned surgery with the surgeon would also be useful to determine risks of poor wound or anastomotic healing. The risk of wound related and septic complications from perioperative steroid use remains somewhat controversial,[22–25] and is unlikely to have a major affect on outcome. The addition of intravenous cyclosporin to steroids in severe ulcerative colitis does not appear to increase the rate of perioperative complications in patients undergoing major abdominal surgery.[26]

Perioperative care

A major consideration in the perioperative or intraoperative care of patients with inflammatory bowel disease is the proper use of steroids. The normal daily production of cortisol by the adrenal glands is 15 to 20 mg per day, but in the perioperative period this may increase dramatically. Patients who have been on steroids for less than 3 weeks generally are not at high risk of adrenocortical suppression, but chronic steroid use has been shown to produce a blunted response to a corticotropin-releasing hormone stimulation test.[27] Patients should be assumed to have suppression of the hypothalamic-pituitary-adrenal axis if they have clinical Cushing's syndrome or have received more than 20 mg of prednisone equivalent daily for 3 consecutive weeks within the preceding year.[28] For these patients with suspected secondary adrenal insufficiency it is common to give 100 mg of hydrocortisone intravenously with the induction of anesthesia. This should be continued every eight hours for at least 24 hours, followed by a taper over the next 48 to 72 hours to the previous oral maintenance dose.[28] For patients with a less apparent risk of secondary adrenal suppression (i.e., 5–20 mg of prednisone equivalent per day for greater than 3 weeks within the preceding year), a more rapid taper may be used. If time permits, a preoperative cosyntropin stimulation test to measure adrenal responsiveness may be helpful to guide therapy.

Postoperative care

The postoperative care of the patient with inflammatory bowel disease should focus upon regaining bowel function, providing adequate nutrition, and reducing the risk of disease recurrence or related complications.

Endoscopic recurrence of Crohn's disease is seen in up to 70% of patients within one year and in 85% by the third year after bowel resection.[29] Clinical recurrence is seen in up to 60% of patients at five years and 94% after 15 years.[30] Recurrence is more common for patients who have ileocolonic disease. Many of these patients will undergo repeat surgery. There is data supporting the use of 5-aminosalicylates, metronidazole, and azathioprine/6-mercaptopurine in the prevention of postoperative recurrence of Crohn's disease,[31] but the decision to initiate or continue drug therapy or immunosuppression should be made carefully and on an individual basis. There is no data to support the use of glucocorticoids to prevent recurrence, and steroids should be tapered in the weeks following surgery. Smoking is associated with a higher surgical disease recurrence rate,[32] as is the presence of perforating disease,[33] juvenile onset of disease, and proximal small bowel disease.[34]

Knowledge of the patient's postoperative anatomy is important. Oral sulfasalazine and 5-ASA compounds will not come in contact with a Hartman's pouch, therefore topical or immunosuppressant therapies will need to be considered. Drugs that contain an azo-bond that needs cleavage by colonic bacteria will not be effective in patients who have had a colectomy.

Crohn's disease is a leading risk factor for developing short bowel syndrome. If 50% or less of the small bowel is removed, patients are usually able to maintain their nutritional status and are not at high risk of electrolyte and fluid loss, malabsorption, and other complications of short bowel syndrome. When patients have had 75% or more (approximately 450 cm) of their small bowel removed, care must be taken in the early postoperative period to maintain proper hydration, electrolyte balance,

and nutrition. In the immediate postoperative weeks profuse watery diarrhea is common, and it is during this time that intravenous hydration and nutrition are often crucial. Gastric hypersecretion may occur postoperatively due to hypergastrinemia and can be treated with H_2-receptor blockers or proton pump inhibitors.[35] Fluid loss from diarrhea may be slowed with loperamide hydrochloride, diphenoxylate, or other antidiarrheal medications. Once oral intake has resumed, fluid losses are best prevented with isotonic oral rehydrating fluids as both hypo- and hypertonic fluids can be detrimental. Enteral feeding should be initiated early to aid in intestinal adaptation. This process will occur over the following months, and will aid in symptom improvement. Factors that may influence the development and course of short bowel syndrome include not only the site and extent of bowel removed, but the presence or absence of an ileocecal valve, and the degree of intestinal adaptation.[11] Long-term sequelae of short bowel syndrome such as vitamin deficiencies, nephrolithiasis, and cholelithiasis should be anticipated early so that preventive and treatment strategies can be initiated.

Although controversial in the past, Crohn's disease has been shown to have a similar increased risk of colon cancer as ulcerative colitis when compared to the general population.[36] The need for colon cancer surveillance in these patients must not be overlooked.

Colectomy essentially cures ulcerative colitis. The immediate postoperative care of the colectomy patient with ulcerative colitis will be similar to other patients who have had major abdominal surgery, but there are some important follow-up issues to consider. The type of operation and amount of remaining colon or rectal tissue is important to take into consideration. Dysplasia and cancer can occur in the pouch[37–39] and rectal cuff mucosa[40–43] necessitating future surveillance. Recent reviews, however, have suggested that the incidence of dysplasia in ileal pouches performed for ulcerative colitis is rare.[44,45]

Summary

Surgery is often a necessary part of the treatment strategy for inflammatory bowel disease. Because Crohn's disease and ulcerative colitis are two distinct conditions that will respond differently to surgery, proper diagnosis is imperative when possible. Preoperative care should include recent laboratory, radiological, endoscopic, and clinical examinations to accurately determine disease location and activity. Attention should be paid to current medications, especially immunosuppressive agents, and special care should be taken in the use of perioperative steroids. The types of surgery performed vary widely depending upon disease state and complications; communication with the surgeon is important to assure appropriate attention to special considerations for each type of surgery. The preventive treatment of postoperative recurrence, malnutrition and other complications should be addressed early. The need for future endoscopic surveillance must not be overlooked when appropriate. A positive outcome is most likely when good preparation on the part of the patient, physician, and surgeon have taken place.

REFERENCES

1. Duerr, R. H. The genetics of inflammatory bowel disease. *Gastroenterol. Clin. North Am.* 2002; **31**: 63–76.
2. Farrell, R. J. & LaMont, J. T. Microbial factors in inflammatory bowel disease. *Gastroenterol. Clin. North Am.* 2002; **31**: 41–62.
3. Krishnan, A. & Korzenik, J. R. Inflammatory bowel disease and environmental influences. *Gastroenterol. Clin. North Am.* 2002; **31**: 21–39.
4. Loftus, E. V., Jr., Silverstein, M. D., Sandborn, W. J., Tremaine, W. J., Harmsen, W. S., & Zinsmeister, A. R. Crohn's disease in Olmsted County, Minnesota, 1940–1993: incidence, prevalence, and survival. *Gastroenterology* 1998; **114**: 1161–1168.
5. Steinhardt, H. J., Loeschke, K., Kasper, H., Holtermuller, K. H., & Schafer, H. European Cooperative Crohn's Disease Study (ECCDS): clinical features and natural history. *Digestion* 1985; **31**: 97–108.
6. Chambers, T. J. & Morson, B. C. The granuloma in Crohn's disease. *Gut* 1979; **20**: 269–274.
7. Haggitt, R. Differential diagnosis of colitis. In Goldman, H. A. H., Kaufman, N., ed. *Gastrointestinal Pathology*. Baltimore: Williams & Wilkins, 1988: 325–355.
8. Schmitz-Moormann, P., Pittner, P. M., Malchow, H., & Brandes, J. W. The granuloma in Crohn's disease. A bioptical study. *Pathol. Res. Pract.* 1984; **178**: 467–476.
9. Loftus, E. V., Jr., Silverstein, M. D., Sandborn, W. J., Tremaine, W. J., Harmsen, W. S., & Zinsmeister, A. R. Ulcerative colitis in Olmsted County, Minnesota, 1940–1993: incidence, prevalence, and survival. *Gut* 2000; **46**: 336–343.
10. Saltzstein, S. L. & Rosenberg, B. F. Ulcerative colitis of the ileum and regional enteritis of the colon, a comparative histopathologic study. *Am. J. Clin. Pathol.* 1963; **40**: 610.
11. Yamada, T., Alpers, D., Laine, L., Owyang, C., & Powell, D. *Textbook of Gastroenterology*. Philadelphia: Lippincott Williams & Wilkins, 1999.
12. Farmer, R. G., Hawk, W. A., & Turnbull, R. B., Jr. Indications for surgery in Crohn's disease: analysis of 500 cases. *Gastroenterology* 1976; **71**: 245–250.

13. Shorb, P. E., Jr. Surgical therapy for Crohn's disease. *Gastroenterol. Clin. North Am.* 1989; **18**: 111–128.
14. Wexner, S. D., Rosen, L., Lowry, A. *et al.* Practice parameters for the treatment of mucosal ulcerative colitis – supporting documentation. The Standards Practice Task Force. The American Society of Colon and Rectal Surgeons. *Dis. Colon Rectum* 1997; **40**: 1277–1285.
15. Robert, J. H., Sachar, D. B., Aufses, A. H., Jr., & Greenstein, A. J. Management of severe hemorrhage in ulcerative colitis. *Am. J. Surg.* 1990; **159**: 550–555.
16. Schraut, W. H. The surgical management of Crohn's disease. *Gastroenterol. Clin. North Am.* 2002; **31**: 255–263.
17. Pemberton, J. H., Kelly, K. A., Beart, R. W., Jr., Dozois, R. R., Wolff, B. G., & Ilstrup, D. M. Ileal pouch-anal anastomosis for chronic ulcerative colitis. *Long-term results. Ann. Surg.* 1987; **206**: 504–513.
18. Robb, B., Pritts, T., Gang, G. *et al.* Quality of life in patients undergoing ileal pouch-anal anastomosis at the University of Cincinnati. *Am. J. Surg.* 2002; **183**(4): 353–360.
19. Blumberg, D. & Beck, D. E. Surgery for ulcerative colitis. *Gastoenterol. Clin. North Am.* 2002; **31**: 219–235.
20. Heyland, D. K., Montalvo, M., MacDonald, S., Keefe, L., Su, X. Y., & Drover, J. W. Total parenteral nutrition in the surgical patient: a meta-analysis. *Can. J. Surg.* 2001; **44**: 102–111.
21. Sitrin, M. D. Perioperative nutrition support. In Bayless, T. M., Hanauer, S. B., eds. *Advanced Therapy of Inflammatory Bowel Disease*. Hamilton, Ontario: B. C. Decker, 2001: 449–451.
22. Cruse, P. J. & Foord, R. A five-year prospective study of 23,649 surgical wounds. *Arch. Surg.* 1973; **107**: 206–210.
23. Post, S., Betzler, M., von Ditfurth, B., Schurmann, G., Kuppers, P., & Herfarth, C. Risks of intestinal anastomoses in Crohn's disease. *Ann. Surg.* 1991; **213**: 37–42.
24. Manjoney, D. L., Koplewitz, M. J., & Abrams, J. S. Factors influencing perineal wound healing after proctectomy. *Am. J. Surg.* 1983; **145**: 183–189.
25. Ziv, Y., Church, J. M., Fazio, V. W., King, T. M., & Lavery, I. C. Effect of systemic steroids on ileal pouch-anal anastomosis in patients with ulcerative colitis. *Dis. Colon Rectum* 1996; **39**: 504–508.
26. Hyde, G. M., Jewell, D. P., Kettlewell, M. G., & Mortensen, N. J. Cyclosporin for severe ulcerative colitis does not increase the rate of perioperative complications. *Dis. Colon Rectum* 2001; **44**: 1436–1440.
27. Schlaghecke, R., Kornely, E., Santen, R. T., & Ridderskamp, P. The effect of long-term glucocorticoid therapy on pituitary-adrenal responses to exogenous corticotropin-releasing hormone. *N. Engl. J. Med.* 1992; **326**: 226–230.
28. Jabbour, S. A. Steroids and the surgical patient. *Med. Clin. North Am.* 2001; **85**: 1311–1317.
29. Rutgeerts, P., Geboes, K., Vantrappen, G., Beyls, J., Kerremans, R., & Hiele, M. Predictability of the postoperative course of Crohn's disease. *Gastroenterology* 1990; **99**: 956–963.
30. Greenstein, A. J., Sachar, D. B., Pasternack, B. S., & Janowitz, H. D. Reoperation and recurrence in Crohn's colitis and ileocolitis: crude and cumulative rates. *N. Engl. J. Med.* 1975; **293**: 685–690.

31. Rutgeerts, P. J. Measures to minimize postoperative recurrences of Crohn's disease. In Bayless, T. M., Hanauer, S. B., eds. *Advanced Therapy of Inflammatory Bowel Disease.* Hamilton, Ontario: B. C. Decker, 2001.

32. Cottone, M., Rosselli, M., Orlando, A. *et al.* Smoking habits and recurrence in Crohn's disease. *Gastroenterology* 1994; **106**: 643–648.

33. Aeberhard, P., Berchtold, W., Riedtmann, H. J., & Stadelmann, G. Surgical recurrence of perforating and nonperforating Crohn's disease. A study of 101 surgically treated patients. *Dis. Colon Rectum* 1996; **39**: 80–87.

34. Post, S., Herfarth, C., Bohm, E. *et al.* The impact of disease pattern, surgical management, and individual surgeons on the risk for relaparotomy for recurrent Crohn's disease. *Ann. Surg.* 1996; **223**: 253–260.

35. Buchman, A. L. The clinical management of short bowel syndrome: steps to avoid parenteral nutrition. *Nutrition* 1997; **13**: 907–913.

36. Bernstein, C. N., Blanchard, J. F., Kliewer, E., & Wajda, A. Cancer risk in patients with inflammatory bowel disease: a population-based study. *Cancer* 2001; **91**: 854–862.

37. Gullberg, K., Stahlberg, D., Liljeqvist, L. *et al.* Neoplastic transformation of the pelvic pouch mucosa in patients with ulcerative colitis. *Gastroenterology* 1997; **112**: 1487–1492.

38. Vieth, M., Grunewald, M., Niemeyer, C., & Stolte, M. Adenocarcinoma in an ileal pouch after prior proctocolectomy for carcinoma in a patient with ulcerative pancolitis. *Virchows Arch.* 1998; **433**: 281–284.

39. Heuschen, U. A., Autschbach, F., Allemeyer, E. H., *et al.* Long-term follow-up after ileoanal pouch procedure: algorithm for diagnosis, classification, and management of pouchitis. *Dis. Colon Rectum* 2001; **44**: 487–499.

40. Stern, H., Walfisch, S., Mullen, B., McLeod, R., & Cohen, Z. Cancer in an ileoanal reservoir: a new late complication? *Gut* 1990; **31**: 473–475.

41. Puthu, D., Rajan, N., Rao, R., Rao, L., & Venugopal, P. Carcinoma of the rectal pouch following restorative proctocolectomy. Report of a case. *Dis. Colon Rectum* 1992; **35**: 257–260.

42. Laureti, S., Ugolini, F., D'Errico, A., Rago, S., & Poggioli, G. Adenocarcinoma below ileoanal anastomosis for ulcerative colitis: report of a case and review of the literature. *Dis. Colon Rectum* 2002; **45**: 418–421.

43. Rotholtz, N. A., Pikarsky, A. J., Singh, J. J., & Wexner, S. D. Adenocarcinoma arising from along the rectal stump after double-stapled ileorectal J-pouch in a patient with ulcerative colitis: the need to perform a distal anastomosis. Report of a case. *Dis. Colon Rectum* 2001; **44**: 1214–1217.

44. Thompson-Fawcett, M. W., Marcus, V., Redston, M., Cohen, Z., & McLeod, R. S. Risk of dysplasia in long-term ileal pouches and pouches with chronic pouchitis. *Gastroenterology* 2001; **121**: 275–281.

45. Hulten, L., Willen, R., Nilsson, O., Safarani, N., & Haboubi, N. Mucosal assessment for dysplasia and cancer in the ileal pouch mucosa in patients operated on for ulcerative colitis – a 30-year follow-up study. *Dis. Colon Rectum* 2002; **45**: 448–452.

15

Postoperative gastrointestinal complications

Brian W. Behm and Neil Stollman

East Bay Center for Digestive Health, Oakland, CA

Gut function is often impacted by surgical interventions, and postoperative GI complications are common. Fortunately, most are minor and self-limited, but a number may be severe, and rarely, life threatening. In this chapter, we will review the causes, diagnostic work-up and treatment options for patients with postoperative gastrointestinal bleeding, nausea and vomiting, and diarrhea (Table 15.1).

Table 15.1. Postoperative GI complications

Gastrointestinal bleeding
Early bleeding
- Stress-related mucosal disease (SRMD)
- Anastamotic breakdown
- Ischemic colitis
- Peptic ulcer disease or other pre-existing lesion
Remote bleeding
- Aortoenteric fistula
- Marginal/recurrent ulcer

Nausea and vomiting
- Ileus/gastric atony
- Vagotomy
- Anastomic obstruction or stricture
- Adhesions
- Afferent/efferent loop syndrome
- Bile-reflux gastritis

Diarrhea
- Medications
- Antibiotic related
- Enteral feeding preparations
- Overflow from fecal impaction
- Bacterial overgrowth
- Vagotomy
- Dumping syndrome
- Short bowel syndrome
- Cholerrheic
- Ischemic colitis

Postoperative gastrointestinal bleeding

Postoperative gastrointestinal (GI) bleeding is an uncommon but potentially serious complication. Clinically significant bleeding (defined as overt or evident bleeding, such as melena or hematemesis, accompanied by signs of hemodynamic compromise or decreased hemoglobin) occurs in 0.5%–1% of patients in the acute postoperative setting.[1,2] Major causes of acute postoperative bleeding include stress ulceration, bleeding from an intestinal anastamosis, ischemic colitis, and bleeding from pre-existing lesions such as gastroduodenal ulcers and diverticular disease. Gastrointestinal hemorrhage temporally remote from surgery may also occur due to aortoenteric fistulae and recurrent or marginal ulcer disease.

Stress-related mucosal disease (SRMD)

Stress-related mucosal disease, or stress-ulceration, is the most common cause of postoperative GI bleeding,[3] although its incidence has decreased over the past decade. Ulcers may be due to disturbances in the mucosal microcirculation, with relative "local" hypoperfusion causing a loss of mucosal integrity, an imbalance between aggressive and protective factors and subsequently, multiple gastric erosions and ulcerations.[4,5] Suppressing or neutralizing gastric acid appears to protect against these mucosal events,[6] and antisecretory agents have been employed successfully for prophylaxis of SRMD in high risk patients.

The two main risk factors for clinically important bleeding from SRMD include prolonged mechanical ventilation and coagulopathy.[7] Other factors include perioperative hypotension, sepsis, spinal cord injuries, and severe burns. SRMD prophylaxis should be considered if one or more of these risk factors are present, with several

Medical Management of the Surgical Patient: A Textbook of Perioperative Medicine, ed. M. F. Lubin, R. B. Smith, T. F. Dobson, N. Spell, H. K. Walker. 4th edn. Published by Cambridge University Press. © Cambridge University 2006.

different medications currently available. Antacid medications have been found to decrease the risk of GI bleeding in ICU patients[8] but are limited by the required frequency of administration and the need to monitor gastric pH. H2 blockers have been demonstrated to be effective in SRMD prevention in several studies[8,9] and appear to be both more efficacious and practical than antacid administration.[10] However, tolerance may develop with continued use of H2 blockers, which may limit their effectiveness.[11] Intravenous cimetidine by continuous infusion has been approved by the Food and Drug Administration (FDA) for the prevention of SRMD.

Sucralfate may be used as an alternative to acid suppressive agents, and has been shown in some studies to be as efficacious at H2 blockers.[12,13] Because it does not alkalinize gastric contents, sucralfate may diminish bacterial colonization of the stomach and respiratory tree, and some earlier studies suggested that sucralfate may lower the risk of nosocomial pneumonia compared with antisecretory agents.[14,15] However, more recent studies have found no difference in the incidence of pneumonia with sucralfate compared with antisecretory agents.[16]

Proton pump inhibitors (PPIs) are increasingly being used as prophylactic agents in critically ill patients. Levy found a significantly decreased risk of GI bleeding with oral omeprazole 40 mg qd compared with H2 blockers.[6] Two other open-label trials found no significant bleeding episodes with the use of omeprazole oral suspension in critically ill patients.[17,18] In addition, a recent study suggests that oral lansoprazole may be more cost-effective than famotidine or cimetidine in preventing SRMD-associated bleeding.[19] While no published trials have compared the clinical efficacy of intravenous vs. oral PPIs in SRMD prophylaxis, gastric dysmotility in postoperative patients may make orally administered agents impractical. Intravenous agents such as pantoprazole may be an option for SRMD prophylaxis when medications cannot be given enterally. PPIs appear to be safe and efficacious in preventing SRMD, and oral PPIs may be more cost-effective than H2 blockers in preventing SRMD-associated GI bleeding. Further studies are needed to determine the cost-effectiveness of intravenous PPIs in this setting. While there is limited evidence available to date to either define the subset(s) of postoperative patients at highest risk for bleeding, or to define the best agent for prophylaxis, it would be appropriate to provide either i.v. H2 blockers or i.v. or p.o. PPIs to postoperative patients who have an anticipated need for prolonged ventilatory support, have multiple organ failure postoperatively, or are coagulopathic.

Ischemic colitis

Several vascular disorders may affect the GI tract in the postoperative period, the most common being ischemic colitis. Colonic ischemia is generally due to hypotension and a 'low-flow' state in the perioperative setting, or may be due to embolic phenomena or IMA ligation associated with vascular surgery. The incidence of ischemic colitis is relatively low but carries a significant mortality rate. It occurs in less than 1% of surgical patients overall,[20–23] but may complicate up to 7%[24–26] of elective aortic surgeries and up to 60% of surgeries for ruptured aortic aneurysms.[24] Mortality rates for ischemic colitis may be as high as 54%.[25] Risk factors for ischemic colitis include older age, peripheral vascular disease, operative trauma to the colon, perioperative hypotension and the need for emergent surgery.[23,26–28] Patients with prior colectomy may also be at higher risk due to disturbed collateral blood supply.

Ischemic colitis typically presents insidiously in the week following a surgical procedure. Depending on the degree of ischemic injury, symptoms may range from mild nausea, diarrhea, heme-positive stool and the absence of abdominal pain, to severe colitis presenting with fever, abdominal pain, hematochezia, and peritoneal signs from transmural necrosis and gangrenous bowel. If the patient recovers, chronic sequelae may occur in up to one-third of patients[29] and may include colonic stricture formation or a persistent segmental colitis that mimics ulcerative colitis. Abdominal CT scanning early in the course may be normal or reveal non-specific colonic thickening, but may be useful to exclude other intra-abdominal processes. Barium studies are used infrequently, but may show characteristic "thumbprinting" due to submucosal hemorrhage. Colonoscopy is the diagnostic procedure of choice. In mild disease, colonoscopy may reveal segments of pale mucosa with areas of petechial hemorrhage. After more severe injury, the mucosa may be blue or black with mucosal sloughing and ulceration. Ischemic colitis may be difficult to distinguish endoscopically from other forms of colitis, but biopsy of the affected areas may be useful in establishing the diagnosis.[30] The rectum is typically spared due to collateral circulation from the hemorrhoidal vessels off the internal iliacs.

Treatment of mild ischemic colitis is supportive, with intravenous hydration, bowel rest, and broad spectrum antibiotics. Follow-up endoscopy may be indicated to document lack of disease progression. Increasing abdominal pain, peritoneal signs, and fever suggests colonic infarction and usually requires exploratory surgery and resection of non-viable colon.

Peptic ulcers

The development of recurrent ulcers after previous peptic ulcer surgery occurs in 2%–10% of patients.[31] With the decline in surgery for peptic ulcer disease, more patients are presently being seen with recurrent or marginal ulcers after other gastric procedures, including bariatric surgery and operations for esophageal reflux, with an incidence of up to 3% in some series.[31] Historically, recurrent ulcers are most frequently due to incomplete vagotomy, but other potential factors include retained antrum, Zollinger–Ellison syndrome, *Helicobacter pylori* infection, salicylate or non-steroidal use, bile reflux, and gastric cancer.

Symptoms due to recurrent ulcer are often atypical, with pain frequently absent or difficult to distinguish from other postgastrectomy syndromes. GI hemorrhage may be the presenting symptom in 40%–60% of patients,[32,33] often without a preceding history of ulcerlike pain. Physicians must have a high index of suspicion for recurrent ulcers due to their often atypical presentation. Endoscopy should be considered in patients after gastric surgery with new or persistent unexplained abdominal symptoms. If ulcers are detected endoscopically, biopsies should be taken to exclude malignancy or *Helicobacter* infection. If ulcers recur or persist despite appropriate therapy, serum gastrin (fasting) and calcium levels should be checked to exclude Zollinger–Ellison syndrome and primary hyperparathyroidism respectively. Salicylate levels may also be helpful if salicylate abuse is suspected.

If patients present with evidence of GI hemorrhage, initial management is the same as with patients without previous surgery. Initial priorities include restoring hemodynamic stability, correcting comorbid conditions such as thrombocytopenia and coagulopathy, following serial laboratory values and vital signs, and intubation for airway protection if significant hematemesis is occurring. Details of the patient's previous surgery may be very useful in planning subsequent endoscopy. Upper endoscopy can identify stigmata such as actively bleeding ulcers and ulcers with a visible vessel or an adherent clot, all of which suggest a higher risk of rebleeding and can guide subsequent therapy.[34] After successful hemostasis, acid suppression with PPIs can significantly decrease the rate of rebleeding and the need for surgery. Several studies indicate that in patients with high-risk ulcers, intravenous PPIs, given as a bolus followed by a continuous infusion for 72 hours, are superior to both H2-blockers[35,36] and PPIs used in intermittent dosing regimens.[37]

Approximately 80% of patients with recurrent ulcers heal with standard medical therapy.[38,39] Both PPIs and H2 blockers have been used successfully as maintenance treatment for recurrent ulcers, although PPIs promote faster healing. Patients have a high rate of recurrence if maintenance agents are discontinued. Ulcers that have not healed after 3 months of high dose antisecretory therapy or those that recur while on maintenance therapy may require reoperation.[31]

Aortoenteric fistula

Aortoenteric fistula (AEF) is a rare but potentially life-threatening cause of remote GI bleeding, occurring in approximately 1% of patients with previous abdominal aortic graft surgery.[40] AEF is usually caused by a direct communication between the proximal aortic anastamosis and the bowel lumen, most typically in the duodenum. Patients typically present months to years after their initial operation with evidence of GI hemorrhage. Patients may be seen initially after a minor episode of bleeding, the so-called "herald bleed," with subsequent massive GI hemorrhage occurring hours to months later. However, approximately 50% of patients with AEF initially present with evidence of chronic GI blood loss, intermittent bleeding, or heme-positive stool.[41] A less frequent presentation occurs when the aortic graft erodes into the bowel lumen. This results in a paraprosthetic–enteric fistula (PEF) as the graft is bathed in enteric contents, and may present with fever, abdominal pain, and sepsis. Patients with PEF may also have melena or guaiac-positive stools, but rarely massive bleeding.[41]

Diagnosis of AEF requires a high index of suspicion. Only one-third of AEFs are demonstrated prior to surgery.[42] If patients are hemodynamically stable, EGD may be performed to identify the source of bleeding. Although endoscopy lacks specificity for AEF[43], graft erosion into the bowel lumen may sometimes be seen and is highly suggestive; endoscopy is also useful to exclude other causes of GI hemorrhage. CT scan may be useful if a patient presents with fever and sepsis, but specificity is low for determining the presence of fistulae.[42] If the suspicion for AEF is high, the patient should undergo urgent exploratory laparotomy.

Postoperative nausea and vomiting

Nausea and vomiting occur frequently in the early postoperative setting. Patient characteristics predisposing to an increased risk include female gender, obesity, history of gastroparesis, prior history of motion sickness or previous postoperative vomiting.[44] Procedure characteristics that increase the risk of nausea and vomiting include abdominal surgery, laparoscopic procedures, and increasing procedure length.[44] Anesthetic agents may also depress GI function to some degree postoperatively, but their role in producing postoperative nausea and vomiting does not appear to be clinically significant. Postoperative risk factors for nausea and vomiting include the use of opiate medications, pain, early ambulation, and early enteral feeding.[44] Postoperative ileus is a common problem especially after abdominal surgery, but typically resolves over 3–5 days. Certain therapies may decrease the duration of postoperative ileus, including the use of less invasive surgical techniques such as laparoscopy, opioid-sparing agents such as nonsteroidal antiinflammatory medications, thoracic epidural anesthetics, and early oral nutrition. Nasogastric tubes have been shown to increase the risk of postoperative pulmonary complications, and their routine use should generally be avoided in the postoperative setting.

Treatment of early postoperative nausea is generally supportive, with intravenous hydration, antiemetic medications, and careful advancement of diet. Patients at higher risk of vomiting due to patient or procedure characteristics may benefit from prophylactic antiemetics postoperatively.[44]

Nausea and vomiting that persists more than a few days after abdominal surgery generally warrants further investigation. In addition, dysphagia may be present in several postoperative scenarios. Dysphagia may occur after vagotomy or reflux surgery but tends to resolve spontaneously within several weeks.[45] Patients undergoing bariatric surgery may also complain of dysphagia or present with vomiting due to stomal obstruction, anastomotic intussusception, or overeating.[46] Endoscopy or upper gastrointestinal barium studies may be useful for diagnosis in severe cases of dysphagia. Severe or persistent dysphagia due to obstruction may respond to endoscopic dilation.

There are also several syndromes associated with gastrectomy that may increase the risk of postoperative nausea and vomiting. The afferent loop syndrome may cause postoperative vomiting after Billroth II gastrectomy due to a blockage of the afferent limb of the gastrojejunostomy. Symptoms include postprandial epigastric pain as pressure builds in the blocked limb, followed by bilious emesis as the obstruction is relieved. The recently ingested food is not found in the emesis. Rarely, patients with chronic high-grade limb-related obstruction may present with pancreatitis and/or obstructive jaundice. Efferent limb syndrome is caused by partial obstruction of the intestinal segment draining the stomach. Symptoms are similar to those of afferent loop syndrome, but with efferent limb syndrome there is typically food present in the emesis. Both afferent

and efferent limb syndromes may be diagnosed via barium studies, and treatment is surgical revision.

Alkaline reflux gastritis is a condition caused by reflux of intestinal contents into the gastric remnant after gastrectomy. Typical symptoms include burning epigastric pain that is not relieved with antacids and may be worse with meals and recumbency. Pain may be associated with bilious emesis. Patients with Billroth II gastrectomy may be at higher risk for alkaline reflux. Diagnostic workup may include endoscopy and upper GI series to exclude other causes of pain; scintigraphy may help confirm the diagnosis. Non-operative therapy has generally been disappointing for this condition, although one study suggests ursodeoxycholic acid may be a potentially useful therapeutic agent.[47] Patients with severe symptoms may benefit from reoperation and construction of a Roux limb,[48] although between 10% and 50% of patients subsequently develop a functional gastric outlet obstruction called the Roux stasis syndrome.[49]

Remote postoperative nausea and vomiting may also be caused by intestinal obstruction, most commonly caused by adhesions after abdominal surgery. In addition, strictures at the site of an intestinal anastamosis may cause postoperative obstruction in approximately 2% of patients.[50] Strictures may be located with endoscopic or barium studies. Video capsule endoscopy may be helpful in evaluating more distal anastomoses, although concern for capsule impaction (non-passage) warrants cautious use in potentially obstructed patients. Anastamotic strictures may sometimes be treated with balloon dilation, although many patients with distal or refractory strictures may need surgical revision.

Postoperative diarrhea

Diarrhea is commonly seen in the early postoperative setting. The majority of such patients have diarrhea due to medication side effects, resolving ileus, or colonization with pathogenic bacterial flora. Initial evaluation of early postoperative diarrhea should include a review of recent medications, with attention to antibiotic use, magnesium-containing antacids, elixers containing sorbitol or mannitol, and other medications including colchicine, lactulose, misoprostil, and anticholinergic agents. Diarrhea associated with *Clostridium difficile* infection may present within the first few weeks of surgery and is usually, although not always, associated with antibiotic use. Enteral feeding has been associated with diarrhea as well.[51] Patients with fecal impaction may also present with "overflow" diarrhea.[52]

Persistent or chronic postoperative diarrhea may sometimes be related to the type of surgical procedure performed. Gastric surgery is frequently associated with diarrhea through a number of mechanisms. Early dumping syndrome is a significant problem in 14%–20% of patients after partial gastrectomy.[53] Dumping is characterized by gastrointestinal and vasomotor symptoms due to rapid emptying of hyperosmolar chyme into the small bowel, as well as abnormal release of gut neuroendocrine factors.[54–56] Symptoms typically begin 10–30 minutes after a meal, with patients complaining of postprandial fullness, pain, and explosive diarrhea soon after eating, often associated with generalized weakness, flushing, and dizziness. The incidence of early dumping is reduced with highly selective vagotomy. Diet modification is the mainstay of therapy, with patients instructed to eat smaller meals low in simple carbohydrates and to avoid liquid intake during a meal. Symptoms refractory to diet changes and antidiarrheal agents may improve with subcutaneous octreotide.[57,58]

Diarrhea may also be seen after vagotomy in 20–30% of patients,[59] and may be due to rapid gastric emptying or impaired gall bladder function leading to bile acid related ("cholerrheic") diarrhea.[60] Patients typically present with frequent watery stools, often with nocturnal symptoms, that are not associated with meals. Treatment includes diet modifications similar to those used for the dumping syndrome, antidiarrheal medications, and cholestyramine in severe cases.[60] Patients with refractory postvagotomy diarrhea may occasionally benefit from surgical procedures such as the construction of an antiperistaltic jejunal segment in an attempt to slow intestinal transit, although clinical results have not been uniformly positive.[61]

Bacterial overgrowth syndrome may be caused by any procedure that interferes with normal intestinal motility, permitting stasis and allowing bacteria to colonize the small bowel and interfere with normal bowel function. The hallmarks of bacterial overgrowth include diarrhea, steatorrhea, and malnutrition. Megaloblastic anemia may be present. Patients develop steatorrhea due to bacterial bile acid deconjugation and subsequent fatty acid malabsorption. In the past, the diagnosis of bacterial overgrowth could be made endoscopically by small bowel aspiration and quantitative culture, with greater than 10^6 organisms/mL suggestive of overgrowth. However, studies such as the 14 c xylose breath test may be performed as well and may be a less invasive diagnostic alternative. In cases where the clinical suspicion for bacterial overgrowth is high, empiric treatment with antibiotics may be done without preceding diagnostic testing. Most regimens include agents with effectiveness against both aerobic and anaerobic bacteria. Several regimens, including tetracycline, amoxicillin-clavulanic acid, cephalexin plus metronidazole, and trimethoprim-sulfamethoxazole have been found to be effective as empiric therapy. A short (7–10-day) course of antibiotics is generally given, but rotating antibiotics may be needed if symptoms quickly return.

The short bowel syndrome is characterized by diarrhea, steatorrhea, and malnutrition in the setting of extensive small bowel resection. Generally, short bowel syndrome that requires prolonged nutritional support may develop when less than 25%, or approximately 120 cm, of functional intestine remains,[62] but the severity of symptoms also depends on the site of resection, the presence of the ileocecal valve and colon, and the functional status and adaptive capacity of the remaining small bowel.[63] Major midgut resection may result in rapid intestinal transit and osmotic diarrhea. Distal ileal resection may result in bile acid diarrhea. Removal of the ileocecal valve may result in reflux of bacteria into the small bowel and subsequent bacterial overgrowth. Chronic complications of short bowel syndrome may include malnutrition, cholelithiasis, nephrolithiasis, bacterial overgrowth, and steatohepatitis if parenteral nutrition is required. Short bowel-associated diarrhea in the early postoperative period is frequently impressive, but usually improves with adaptation of the remaining intestine. Early management goals for short bowel syndrome include supportive care with intravenous fluid, electrolyte repletion, and nutritional support with parenteral nutrition. H2-blockers or PPIs are given to suppress gastric hypersecretion occurring in the early postoperative period. Initial enteral feeding may begin when stool output falls to less than 2.5 l per day.[64] Cholestyramine is often given to patients with distal ileal resection and presumed bile acid related diarrhea. Depending on the extent of resection, patients may require prolonged parenteral nutrition.

Ileostomy-associated diarrhea may be due to underlying intestinal disease, bacterial overgrowth, stomal stenosis causing partial bowel obstruction, or pouchitis. Bacterial overgrowth usually responds to antibiotics. Stomal stenosis may require surgical revision. Pouchitis may occur in either IBD or non-IBD patients, with symptoms that include fever, abdominal pain, and increased ostomy output that may be bloody. Pouchitis may respond to metronidazole, 5-ASA agents, or probiotics such as lactobacillus GG or VSL#3.[65,66]

Patients with ileal resection may have bile salt malabsorption that leads to bile acid diarrhea.[67] Treatment may include antidiarrheal agents and cholestyramine to bind bile acids. Diarrhea may also be seen after cholecystectomy. The pathogenesis is not completely understood, but may be related to abnormal bile acid secretion after cholecystectomy. Symptoms may improve with oral cholestyramine.[68]

REFERENCES

1. Egleston, C. V., Wood, A. E., Gorey, T. F., & McGovern, E. M. Gastrointestinal complications after cardiac surgery. *Ann. R. Coll. Surg. Engl.* 1993; **75**: 52–56.

2. Byhahn, C., Strouhal, U., Martens, S. *et al.* Incidence of gastrointestinal complications in cardiopulmonary bypass patients. *World J. Surg.* 2001; **25**: 1140–1144.

3. Schiessel, R., Feil, W., & Wenzl, E. Mechanisms of stress ulceration and implications for treatment. *Gastroenterol. Clin. N. Am.* 1990; **90**: 101–120.

4. Stremple, J. F., Mori, H., Lev, R. *et al.* The stress ulcer syndrome. *Curr. Prob. Surg.* April 1973; 1–64.

5. Durham, R. M. & Shapiro, M. J. Stress gastritis revisited. *Surg. Crit. Care* **71**: 791–810.

6. Levy, M. J., Seelig, C. B., Robinson, N. J., & Ranney, J. E. Comparison of omeprazole and ranitidine for stress ulcer prophylaxis. *Dig. Dis. Sci.* 1997; **42**: 1255–1259.

7. Cook, D. J., Fuller, H. D., Guyatt, G. H. *et al.* Risk factors for gastrointestinal bleeding in critically ill patients. *N. Engl. J. Med.* 1994; **330**: 377–381.

8. Shuman, R. B., Schuster, D. P., & Zuckerman, G. R. Prophylactic therapy for stress ulcer bleeding: a reappraisal. *Ann. Intern. Med.* 1987; **106**: 562–567.

9. Cook, D. J., Reeve, B. K., Guyatt, G. H. *et al.* Stress ulcer prophylaxis in critically ill patients. *JAMA* 1996; **275**: 308–314.

10. Cook, D. J., Witt, L. G., Cook, R. J., & Guyatt, G. H. Stress ulcer prophylaxis in the critically ill: a meta-analysis. *Am. J. Med.* 1991; **91**: 519–527.

11. Merki, H. S. & Wilder-Smith, C. H. Do continuous infusions of omeprazole and ranitidine retain their effect with prolonged dosing? *Gastroenterology* 1994; **106**: 60–64.

12. Ryan, P., Dawson, J., Teres, D. *et al.* Nosocomial pneumonia during stress ulcer prophylaxis with cimetidine and sucralfate. *Arch. Surg.* 1993; **128**: 1353–1357.

13. Fabian, T. C., Boucher, B. A., Croce, M. A. *et al.* Pneumonia and stress ulceration in severely injured patients. *Arch. Surg.* 1993; **128**: 185–191.

14. Eddelston, J. M., Vohra, A., Scott, P. *et al.* A comparison of the frequency of stress ulceration and secondary pneumonia in sucralfate or ranitidine-treated intensive care unit patients. *Crit. Care Med.* 1991; **19**: 1491–1496.

15. Tryba, M. Prophylaxis of stress ulcer bleeding. A meta-analysis. *J. Clin. Gastroenterol.* 1991; **13** (Suppl. 2): S44–S55.

16. Cook, D. J., Guhyat, G., Marshall, J. *et al.* A comparison of sucralfate and ranitidine for the prevention of upper gastrointestinal bleeding in patients requiring mechanical ventilation. *N. Engl. J. Med.* 1998; **338**: 791–797.

17. Phillips, J. O., Metzler, M. H., Palmieri, T. L. *et al.* A prospective study of simplified omeprazole suspension for the prophylaxis of stress-related mucosal damage. *Crit. Care Med.* 1996; **24**: 1793–1800.

18. Lasky, M. R., Metzler, M. H., & Phillips, J. O. A prospective study of omeprazole suspension to prevent clinically significant gastrointestinal bleeding from stress ulcers in mechanically ventilated trauma patients. *J. Trauma* 1998; **44**: 527–533.

19. Schupp, K. N., Schrand, L. M., & Mutnick, A. H. A cost-effectiveness analysis of stress ulcer prophylaxis. *Ann. Pharmacother.* 2003; **37**: 631–635.

20. Aranha, G. U., Pickleman, J., Piffare, R. *et al.* The reasons for gastrointestinal consultation after cardiac surgery. *Am. Surg.* 1984; **50**: 301–304.

21. Christerson, J. T., Schmuziger, M., Maurice, J. *et al.* Postoperative visceral hypotension, the common cause for gastrointestinal complications after cardiac surgery. *Thorac. Cardiovasc. Surg.* 1994; **42**: 152–157.

22. Huddy, S. P. J., Joyce, W. P., & Pepper, J. R. Gastrointestinal complications in 4473 patients who underwent cardiopulmonary bypass surgery. *Br. J. Surg.* 1991; **78**: 293–296.

23. Ernst, C. B., Hagihara, P. F., Daugherty, M. E. *et al.* Ischemic colitis incidence following abdominal aortic reconstruction: a prospective study. *Surgery* 1976; **80**: 417–421.

24. Hagihara, P. F., Ernst, C. B., & Griffen, W. O. Jr. Incidence of ischemic colitis following abdominal aortic reconstruction. *Surg. Gynecol. Obstet.* 1979; **149**: 571–573.

25. Longo, W. E., Lee, T. C., Barnett, M. G. *et al.* Ischemic colitis complicating abdominal aortic aneurysm surgery in the U.S. veteran. *J. Surg. Res.* 1996; **60**: 351–354.

26. Schiedler, M. G., Cutler, B. S., & Fiddian-Green, R. G. Sigmoid intramural pH for prediction of ischemic colitis during aortic surgery. A comparison with risk factors and inferior mesenteric artery stump pressures. *Arch. Surg.* 1987; **122**: 881–886.

27. Ernst, C. B. Prevention of intestinal ischemia following abdominal aortic reconstruction. *Surgery* 1983; **93**: 102–106.

28. Schroeder, T., Christoffersen, J. K., Andersen, J. *et al.* Ischemic colitis complicating reconstruction of the abdominal aorta. *Surg. Gynecol. Obstet.* 1985; **160**: 299–303.

29. Boley, S. J. Colonic ischemia–25 years later. *Am. J. Gastroenterol.* 1990; **85**: 931–934.

30. Price, A. B. Ischaemic colitis. *Curr. Top. Pathol.* 1990; **81**: 229.

31. Thirlby, R. C. Postoperative recurrent ulcer. *Gastroenterol. Clin. N. Am.* 1994; **23**: 295–311.

32. Schirmer, B. D., Meyers, W. C., Hanks, J. B. *et al.* Marginal ulcer – a difficult surgical problem. *Ann. Surg.* 1982; **195**: 653–661.

33. Wychulis, A. R., Priestley, J. T., & Foulk, W. T. A study of 360 patients with gastrojejunal ulceration. *Surg. Gynecol. Obstet.* 1966; **122**: 89–99.

34. Kankaria, A. G. & Fleischer, D. E. The critical care management of nonvariceal upper gastrointestinal bleeding. *Crit. Care Clin.* 1995; **11**: 347–368.

35. Lin, H. J., Lo, W. C., Lee, F. Y., *et al.* A prospective randomized comparative trial showing that omeprazole prevents rebleeding

in patients with bleeding peptic ulcer after successful endo-scopic therapy. *Arch. Intern. Med.* 1998; **158**: 54–58.

36. Lau, J. Y. W., Sung, J. J. Y., Lee, K. K. C. *et al.* Effect of intravenous omeprazole on recurrent bleeding after endoscopic treatment of bleeding peptic ulcers. *N. Engl. J. Med.* 2000; **343**: 310–316.

37. Bustamante, M. & Stollman, N. The efficacy of proton-pump inhibitors in acute ulcer bleeding. *J. Clin. Gastroenterol.* 2000; **30**: 7–13.

38. Stage, J. G., Friis, J., & Nielsen, O. V. Ranitidine treatment of patients with postoperative recurrent ulcers. *Scand. J. Gastroenterol.* Suppl 1983; **86**: 80.

39. Gugler, R., Lindstaedt, H., Miederer, S. *et al.* Cimetidine for anastomotic ulcers after partial gastrectomy: a randomized controlled trial. *N. Engl. J. Med.* 1979; **301**: 1077–1080.

40. Elliott, J. P., Smith, R. F., & Szilagyi, D. E. Aortoenteric and paraprosthetic-enteric fistulas. *Arch. Surg.* 1974; **108**: 479–490.

41. Pipinos, I. I., Carr, J. A., Haithcock, B. E. *et al.* Secondary aor-toenteric fistula. *Ann. Vasc. Surg.* 2000; **14**: 688–696.

42. Peck, J. J. & Eidemiler, L. R. Aortoenteric fistulas. *Arch. Surg.* 1992; **127**: 1191–1194.

43. Kiernan, P. D., Pairolero, P. C., Hubert, J. P. *et al.* Aortic graft-enteric fistula. *Mayo Clin. Proc.* 1980; **55**: 731–738.

44. Watcha, M. F. & White, P. F. Postoperative nausea and vomiting. *Anesthesiology* 1992; **77**: 162–184.

45. Donahue, P. E. Early postoperative and postgastrectomy syndromes. *Gastroenterol. Clin. N. Am.* 1994; **23**: 215–226.

46. Knol, J. A. Management of the problem patient after bariatric surgery. *Gastroenterol. Clin. N. Am.* 1994; **23**: 345–369.

47. Stefaniwsky, A. B., Tint, G. S., Speck, J. *et al.* Ursodeoxycholic acid treatment of bile reflux gastritis. *Gastroenterology* 1985; **89**: 1000–1004.

48. Ritchie, W. P. Jr. Alkaline reflux gastritis: late results of a con-trolled clinical trial. *Ann. Surg.* 1986; **203**: 537–544.

49. Ritchie, W. P. Jr. Alkaline reflux gastritis. *Gastroenterol. Clin. N. Am.* 1994; **23**: 281–294.

50. Jex, R. K., van Heerden, J. A., Wolff, B. G. *et al.* Gastrointestinal anastomoses: factors affecting early complications. *Ann. Surg.* 1987; **206**: 138–141.

51. Heimburger, D. C. Diarrhea with enteral feeding: will the real cause please stand up? *Am. J. Med.* 1990; **88**: 89–90.

52. Powell, D. W. Approach to the patient with diarrhea. In Yamada, T., ed. *Gastroenterology*, 3rd edn. Philadelphia: Lippincott, Williams & Wilkins, 1999: 858–909.

53. Carvajal, S. H. & Mulvihill, S. J. Postgastrectomy syndromes: dumping and diarrhea. *Gastroenterol. Clin. N. Am.* 1994; **23**: 261–279.

54. Jordan, G. L. J., Overton, R. C., & DeBakey, M. E. The postgas-trectomy syndrome: studies on pathogenesis. *Ann. Surg.* 1957; **145**: 471–478.

55. Miholic, J., Reilmann, L., Meyer, H. J. *et al.* Extracellular space, blood volume, and the early dumping syndrome after total gastrectomy. *Gastroenterology* 1990; **99**: 923–929.

56. Blackburn, A. M., Christofides, N. D., Ghatei, M. A. *et al.* Elevation of plasma neurotensin in the dumping syndrome. *Clin. Sci.* 1980; **59**: 237–243.

57. Mackie, C. R., Jenkins, S. A., & Hartley, M. N. Treatment of severe postvagotomy/postgastrectomy symptoms with the somatostatin analogue octreotide. *Br. J. Surg.* 1991; **78**: 1338–1343.

58. Geer, R. J., Richards, W. O., O'Dorisio, T. M. *et al.* Efficacy of octreotide acetate in treatment of severe postgastrectomy dumping syndrome. *Ann. Surg.* 1990; **212**: 678–687.

59. Dragstedt, L. R., Harper, P. V. J., Tovee, E. B. *et al.* Section of the vagus nerves to the stomach in the treatment of peptic ulcer: complications and end results after four years. *Ann. Surg.* 1947; **126**: 687–699.

60. Allan, J. G. & Russell, R. I. Proceedings: double-blind controlled trial of cholestyramine in the treatment of post-vagotomy diarrhoea. *Gut* 1975; **16**: 830.

61. Sawyers, J. L. & Herrington, J. Jr. Superiority of antiperistaltic jejunal segments in management of severe dumping syn-drome. *Ann. Surg.* 1973; **178**: 311–319.

62. Tilson, D. M. Pathophysiology and treatment of short bowel syndrome. *Surg. Clin. N. Am.* 1980; **60**: 1273–1284.

63. Thompson, J. S. Management of the short bowel syndrome. *Gastroenterol. Clin. N. Am.* 1994; **23**: 403–420.

64. Westergaard, H. Short bowel syndrome. In Sleisenger, M. H., Fordtran, J. S., eds. *Gastrointestinal Disease*, 6th edn. Philadelphia: W. B. Saunders; 1998: 1548–1556.

65. Gionchetti, P., Rizzello, F., Venturi, A. *et al.* Oral bacteriotherapy as maintenance treatment in patients with chronic pouchitis: a double-blind, placebo-controlled trial. *Gastroenterology* 2000; **119**: 305–309.

66. Giochetii, P., Rizzello, F., Helwig, U. *et al.* Prophylaxis of pou-chitis onset with probiotic therapy: a double-blind, placebo-controlled trial. *Gastroenterology* 2003; **124**: 1202–1209.

67. Hardison, W. G. M. & Rosenberg, I. H. Bile-salt deficiency in the steatorrhea following resection of the ileum and proximal colon. *N. Engl. J. Med.* 1967; **277**: 337–342.

68. Arlow, F. L., Dekovich, A. A., Priest, R. J., & Beher, W. T. Bile acid-mediated postcholecystectomy diarrhea. *Arch. Intern. Med.* 1987; **147**: 1327–1329.

Hematology

16

Disorders of red cells

James R. Eckman

Emory University School of Medicine, Atlanta, GA

Introduction

The primary consideration in medical management of red cell disorders during surgery is to optimize hemoglobin concentration to provide for adequate oxygen delivery to tissues. Blood hemoglobin concentration is a primary direct and indirect determinant of tissue oxygenation. Blood oxygen content increases directly as hemoglobin concentration increases. Tissue oxygen delivery is a complex function of hemoglobin level, cardiac output, hemoglobin oxygen affinity, and tissue oxygen content. As hemoglobin level (more correctly red cell number) increases, blood viscosity increases and cardiac output may decrease so there is an optimal range of hemoglobin concentration that maximizes tissue oxygen delivery. The goal of preoperative and postoperative management is to maintain this optimal level at reasonable cost. Unfortunately, this optimal level is poorly defined in most clinical settings, varies between patients and within individual patients over time, and, even if well defined, can not be maintained without unacceptable complication rates or costs. Perioperative management involves considering the optimal hemoglobin level for each clinical setting based on an informal cost/benefit analysis that usually is supported by incomplete outcome data.

An initial assessment should be done to determine if the hemoglobin level is too high or too low for the specific patient or surgical procedure. Alterations in hemoglobin level may also suggest underlying clinical conditions that may compromise surgical outcome if not properly diagnosed and treated. Anemia may require partial correction to prevent cardiovascular complications during surgery and may be a manifestation of nutritional problems that may impair healing, hemoglobinopathies that require specific therapy, or autoimmune diseases that may complicate blood transfusion.

Increased hemoglobin level may also require evaluation and therapy in the preoperative patient. Polycythemia may require correction prior to surgery or could be a sign of acute or chronic volume depletion. Polycythemia may also indicate chronic diseases that are associated with hypoxemia or with increased risk of perioperative thrombosis and bleeding.

Anemia

Anemia is generally defined as a hemoglobin concentration of less than 14 g/dl in males and 12.3 g/dl in females. Corresponding lower limits of normal for hematocrit are 42% in males and 36% in females.

Diagnostic considerations

Evaluation of an anemia caused by decreased production of red cells may reveal nutritional deficiencies that can be treated to maximize hemoglobin level and improve healing. Many microcytic and macrocytic anemias result from specific nutritional deficiencies that cause correctable anemia and may delay healing and predispose to infection. Normocytic anemias may indicate the presence of underlying medical disease or may define patients with marginal marrow reserve. Evaluation of hemolytic anemias must exclude hemoglobinopathies requiring special operative management, immune hemolysis that may complicate blood transfusion, and enzyme deficiencies that may influence selection of medications.

Algorithms of use in evaluating anemias are presented in Figs. 16.1 through 16.3. Blood loss always must be excluded because it is a common cause of anemia in surgical patients. Studies used to initiate diagnostic testing for most common anemias are presented in Fig. 16.1. The reticulocyte count is the initial, and most important, test because it determines if the primary cause of the anemia is

Medical Management of the Surgical Patient: A Textbook of Perioperative Medicine, ed. M. F. Lubin, R. B. Smith, T. F. Dobson, N. Spell, H. K. Walker. 4th edn. Published by Cambridge University Press. © Cambridge University 2006.

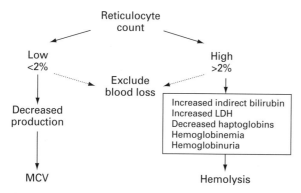

Fig. 16.1. Evaluation of anemia is initiated by obtaining a reticulocyte count to determine if there is decreased production or increased loss of erythrocytes as a primary cause of anemia. Blood loss must always be excluded. The mean corpuscular hemoglobin concentration (MCV) is the next step in determining the cause of anemia when the reticulocyte count is low. Tests are done to establish hemolysis when the reticulocyte count is elevated.

related to decreased production or increased loss of red cells. Anemias caused by decreased red cell production have a low or normal reticulocyte count (corrected percent <2% or <75 000/μl absolute). The mean corpuscular volume (MCV) is the best test to initiate evaluation of anemias caused by decreased red cell production. The diagnostic tests outlined in Fig. 16.2 establish the cause of most common anemias with low reticulocyte counts. Tests indicated by the algorithm should be drawn before surgery or transfusion in all but the most urgent surgical emergencies.

When the reticulocyte count is high (corrected percent >2% or >75 000/μl absolute), the presence of hemolytic anemia is confirmed by excluding blood loss and detecting isolated increase in indirect bilirubin, elevated lactic dehydrogenase, decreased haptoglobin, or free hemoglobin in plasma or urine (see Fig. 16.1). Once hemolysis is confirmed, preoperative diagnosis of the cause of the hemolytic anemia is particularly important because a number of diseases that cause hemolysis require special management of transfusions during surgery. A careful past medical and family history, a direct Coomb's test, and examination of the peripheral blood smear in combination with a few confirmatory tests usually results in a diagnosis (see Fig. 16.3).

Management considerations

Perioperative management of anemia is not difficult because treatment with transfusion of red cells is readily available. Too often, transfusion of red cells is substituted for thoughtful clinical evaluation and optimal medical therapy. Diagnosis and treatment of the cause of the anemia are preferred over transfusion before elective surgery if time permits. If the anemia cannot be corrected or if large blood losses are anticipated, careful planning can allow surgery without transfusion or provide the patient's own blood for transfusion, minimizing the complications. In emergency situations, it is usually best to draw appropriate diagnostic laboratory tests and proceed with transfusion and surgery before the cause of anemia is certain. There are no absolute criteria for management of anemia in the perioperative period, however, a number of useful guidelines have recently been published.

Anemia places increased physiologic demands on patients who are undergoing surgery. There is no evidence showing that mild to moderate anemia slows healing, increases infections, or causes bleeding. The approach to

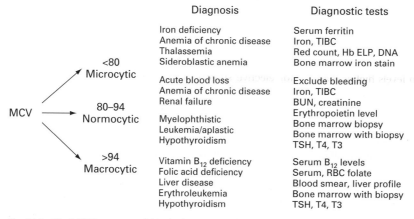

Fig. 16.2. The MCV is most useful in evaluating anemias with decreased red cell production. The most common diagnostic considerations for microcytic, normocytic, and macrocytic anemias are presented with the most useful confirmatory tests.

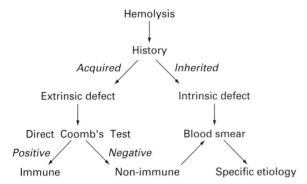

Fig. 16.3. Hemolytic anemias are best evaluated using the patient's history, the direct Coomb's test, and examination of the peripheral blood smear. The history divides hemolysis into acquired disorders where the red cell environment is the cause of increased destruction from inherited disorders where red cell abnormalities shorten survival. The Coomb's test and smear are most useful for acquired disorders, while the smear alone initiates evaluation of inherited disorders.

Table 16.1. Approximate complication rates for homologous red cell transfusion

Immune reaction	
Alloimmunization	1 in 100 to 1 in 150
Acute hemolytic transfusion reaction	1 in 250 000 to 1 in 1×10^6
Delayed transfusion reaction	1 in 100 000
Febrile reaction	1 in 1000
Infection	
HIV	1 in 2×10^6 to 1 in 250 000
Hepatitis B	1 in 30 000 to 1 in 250 000
Hepatitis C (non-A, non-B)	<1 in 30 000 to 1 in 150 000
Other	
Transfusion related acute lung injury	1 in 5000
Bacterial infection	1 in 500 000

preoperative transfusion must be individualized and there is no ideal hemoglobin level required for surgery in all patients. Patients without underlying cardiovascular or respiratory problems have considerable physiologic adaptive capacity and can tolerate significant anemia without increasing surgical morbidity or mortality. Patients with underlying medical problems, those with acute anemia, and those experiencing excessive blood losses, however, may be at risk for increased morbidity and mortality and may require more aggressive treatment of anemia.

Factors in addition to hemoglobin level that affect tissue oxygen delivery include cardiac output, vascular volume, blood viscosity, hemoglobin oxygen affinity, and blood oxygen saturation. With chronic anemia many of these factors are modified to provide optimal oxygen delivery to tissues in spite of the anemia. The "magic" hemoglobin level of 10 gm/dl was challenged in a National Institutes of Health Consensus Conference. Studies show no increased mortality among patients with hemoglobin levels higher than 8 g/dl who lose less than 500 ml of blood during surgery. Because there is no evidence that mild to moderate anemia increases surgical morbidity or mortality, indications for perioperative transfusion must be based on careful assessment of coexisting diseases that may cause reduced tolerance for anemia, patient's physiologic adjustments to the anemia, the stress of the surgical procedure, an estimate of potential operative blood loss based on the nature of the procedure and skill of the surgeon, and the plans for intraoperative procedures to reduce net blood loss such as hemodilution and intraoperative blood salvage.

Informed consent for transfusion, that documents risks of infection, alloimmunization, volume overload, and immediate and delayed transfusion reactions, is required before transfusion in the perioperative period. Patients' religious and cultural beliefs must be recognized and honored. The risks of direct complications from transfusion are not readily quantifiable and are changing because of evolving blood banking techniques. Reasonable estimates are presented in Table 16.1. Alternatives to homologous transfusions should be presented to patients who are undergoing elective surgical procedures that will likely require blood administration. Autologous transfusion of blood without or with administration of erythropoietin is a practical, safe, and under utilized approach to perioperative transfusion. Evidence based literature indicates that these programs not only provide the safest transfusion for the patient, but they also diminish the need for blood donation both by reducing homologous transfusion and by providing unused units for others. Patients must be informed about autologous donation when the decision for elective surgery is made to allow sufficient time to collect the required blood. In patients with concurrent medical problems, medical consultants should supervise blood collection to prevent complications from donation and optimize blood collection. Because liquid blood can be stored up to 42 days, most needs for surgery can be provided as liquid units, reducing cost. Red cells can be frozen for more than ten years to meet greater needs, however, this increases costs significantly.

Intraoperative approaches, such as intraoperative autotransfusion or hemodilution, can be advocated by medical consultants but must be implemented by surgeons and anesthesiologists. Intraoperative blood salvage involves aspirating blood lost in the operative site and centrifuging or washing the cells for reinfusion. Numerous devices make this a practical, but somewhat expensive, approach when loss of large amounts of blood is anticipated. Air embolus is a possible complication and this approach is contraindicated if the operative site is contaminated by microorganisms or tumor cells.

Intraoperative hemodilution involves removal of blood after the induction of anesthesia and replacement with colloid or crystalloid solutions to cause acute normovolemic anemia. This allows the blood to be salvaged for reinfusion, decreases surgical loss of red blood cells, and reduces blood viscosity which may result in increased blood flow. Careful monitoring for volume overload during infusion of salvaged units and accurate identification and labeling of units are critical considerations to ensure safe reinfusion.

In patients with chronic anemia, preoperative transfusion must be planned with the understanding that total blood volume may be increased. Transfusions must be started well in advance of elective surgery and given slowly to prevent acute volume overload and to allow physiologic adaptation to the changes in volume status. Transfusion of packed cells causes minimal volume overload, but does increase the total blood volume by an amount equal to the total volume of the unit and this may persist for 24 hours or longer. In general, volume overload can be kept to a minimum by reducing the amount of cells to 250 ml at one time, reducing the rate to 1 ml/kg body wt/h, and by decreasing right atrial pressure by placing patients in sitting or semiupright position.

Rapid transfusion with diuresis or partial exchange should be reserved for emergent or urgent surgery. Patients with heart failure or renal failure and volume overload, who require rapid transfusion, can be given 20 mg of intravenous furosemide before the transfusion is begun. Additional doses of furosemide can be given by a separate intravenous injection based on urine output and volume of cells infused. Partial exchange transfusion can be used to acutely raise the hemoglobin level in patients with severe anemia and volume overload. One approach is to remove whole blood from one vein as an approximately equal volume of packed red cells is infused through another vein. Severe anemia can be rapidly corrected by infusing a volume of 1000 to 1500 ml of packed red cells as 1200 to 1700 ml of whole blood is removed. The transfused blood should be prewarmed to 37 °C before large volumes are infused rapidly.

In patients with chronic anemia, surgical preparation requires individualized use of transfusion based on the presence of coexisting diseases, chronic hemoglobin levels, and estimates of operative blood losses. If transfusion is required, careful planning may allow use of autologous donation. Preoperative transfusions in patients with chronic anemia should be done well in advance of the surgery to allow physiologic adaptation to the changes in volume and blood viscosity.

Anemias requiring special consideration

Hematologic diseases that require special perioperative management include sickle cell diseases and immune hemolytic anemia. Preoperative screening with a complete blood count, reticulocyte count, and type and cross match will identify most patients with these disorders. The algorithm outlined in Fig. 16.3 should be used to establish a definitive diagnosis before surgery in all but the most emergent situations.

Sickle cell diseases

Patients with sickle cell disease are at significantly increased risk for complications during most operative procedures. Individuals with sickle cell anemia (Hb SS) are at greatest risk. Patients who are compound heterozygotes for Hb S and Hb C (Hb SC disease) or Hb S and β thalassemia (Hb S β thal) may also be at increased risk; however, the perioperative complication rates are not well defined. Carriers of the sickle gene (Hb AS) are not at increased risk for complications unless they experience profound hypoxia or undergo prolonged, complicated cardiovascular surgery. Even in these extreme situations, the risks have not been defined by appropriate controlled studies.

The optimal perioperative management of individuals with sickle cell diseases is not clear. It is generally agreed that the hemoglobin concentration should be corrected by transfusion of packed red cells to a level of 9 to 10 g/dl for all but the simplest procedures. A multicenter collaborative trial found that simple transfusion to a hemoglobin level of 10 g/dl was as effective as exchange transfusion to reduce the hemoglobin S level to less than 30% in reducing complications of surgery and anesthesia and had lower incidence transfusion related complications. Simple transfusion above a hemoglobin level of 10 g/dl should not be done because of the increased viscosity of sickle blood. The level of Hb S can be monitored in the laboratory by using high performance liquid chromatography (HPLC) or by doing standard hemoglobin electrophoresis and estimating the amount of Hb A and Hb S on the membrane using a protein densitometry scanner. This will determine the approximate percentage of erythrocytes with Hb A and Hb S in the patient after transfusion of Hb A-containing erythrocytes. Many advocate transfusion or exchange transfusion to reduce the Hb S level to less than 30% while maintaining the hemoglobin level between 9 and 10 g/dl for cardiovascular bypass surgery, retinal or eye surgery, and major neurosurgery.

There are a number of additional important considerations in planning for transfusion or exchange transfusion in patients with sickle cell disease. The first is the high rate of alloimmunization that accompanies transfusion in these patients. Because up to 20% of patients will develop alloimmunization, some advocate transfusion with red cells that are phenotypically matched for antigens commonly associated with delayed transfusion reactions in this population. Many advocate matching for C, D, E, K antigens in all transfused sickle patients. Patients who have one alloantibody should receive transfusion with blood matched more extensively for antigen phenotype because of the high probability they will develop multiple alloantibodies and may develop autoantibodies. This is especially important with exchange transfusions because of the potential increased severity of a delayed transfusion reaction.

Patients can be prepared with multiple transfusions over the weeks prior to elective surgery. The hemoglobin concentration should be measured before each transfusion to avoid hyperviscosity associated with transfusion to levels greater than 10 g/dl. Repeated HPLC or hemoglobin electrophoresis with densitometry scan can be used to document the percentage of Hb S. If there is insufficient time to achieve desired Hb S percentage by simple transfusion, exchange transfusion is best accomplished by red cell pheresis using an automated cell separator. Manual exchange transfusion using published protocols can achieve the same result; however, these are inefficient and labor intensive in adults and large children.

A multicenter transfusion study in sickle cell indicates that complications will still occur even with extensive exchange transfusion. Transfusion or exchange transfusion cannot be substituted for excellent perioperative management to avoid hypoxia, hypothermia, over-sedation, fluid overload, and acidosis. Acute chest syndrome, acute pain episodes, fever or infection, new alloantibodies, and delayed transfusion reactions appear to be among the most common complications. Predisposing factors for these complications are previous episodes of acute chest syndrome and alloimmunization.

Recommendations for the perioperative management of patients with sickle cell diseases is outlined in Table 16.2.

Table 16.2. Perioperative management of sickle syndromes

- Preoperative transfusion to a hemoglobin level of 10 g/dl using simple transfusion
- Preoperative evaluation to exclude pulmonary, renal, hepatic, or CNS complications.
- Avoidance of hypoxia using careful anesthetic and postoperative respiratory management.
- Hydration with hypotonic intravenous solutions while not taking oral fluids to avoid increased viscosity cellular dehydration, hypoperfusion, or acidosis.
- Careful maintenance of body temperature during and after surgery.
- Early ambulation and intensive respiratory care.
- Postoperative vigilance and aggressive evaluation and treatment of fever or infection.

Data support the need to transfuse to a hemoglobin level of 10 g/dl in all patients. Careful preoperative evaluation and optimization of pulmonary, renal, and hepatic function is important, especially in older patients where end-organ damage may have developed. Intravenous hydration must be adequate to avoid intravascular and intracellular dehydration during the period of restricted oral intake. This is made more important because of the almost universal renal tubular defect that increases obligatory free water loss through the kidneys. Care must also be taken to avoid volume overload in these patients with expanded plasma volumes from chronic anemia. Hypoxia and acidosis should be prevented because of their direct effect of each on the rate of sickling. Decreases in temperature can increase peripheral resistance, reducing local blood flow and predisposing to pain episodes. Early ambulation and intensive respiratory care are important in preventing acute chest syndrome and other pulmonary complications. Incentive spirometry should be used in all patients. Finally, because postoperative complications appear to be more common, diligent assessment of the cause of fevers and the prompt diagnosis and treatment of infection are important in the postoperative period. Close collaboration between surgeons, anesthesiologists, and hematologists helps improve the operative outcome in these patients with high rates of surgical complications.

Autoimmune hemolytic anemia

The perioperative care of patients with immune hemolysis entails several special considerations. Immune hemolytic anemias are mediated by antibodies directed against red cell membrane components or drugs that interact with the red cell membrane. In general, patients should be treated and the immune hemolytic anemia controlled before surgery is undertaken. Immune hemolytic anemias caused by drugs can be managed by stopping the drug and delaying surgery until the anemia is corrected. Autoimmune hemolytic anemias may pose more difficult problems. The diagnosis of hemolysis is made using the studies outlined in Fig. 16.3 and the immune etiology is supported by documenting a positive direct Coomb's test.

Autoimmune hemolytic anemias may be idiopathic but are also commonly associated with autoimmune diseases, lymphomas, chronic lymphocytic leukemia, HIV disease, other infections, and multiple myeloma. Warm antibody hemolytic anemias are caused by IgG antibodies and usually associated with a positive direct Coomb's test for IgG, complement, or both. Initial treatment is prednisone 1 to 1.5 mg/kg per day. Treatment failures are usually treated with splenectomy or immunosuppressive drugs such as cyclophosphamide or azathioprine. Preparation for splenectomy may include the administration of intravenous immunoglobulin, which has been reported to have some activity in controlling immune hemolysis.

Cold reacting autoantibodies are usually IgM antibodies that are associated with positive Coomb's test for complement and high titer cold agglutinin levels. These antibodies are more commonly caused by infections such as mycoplasma pneumoniae, viruses, or lymphoproliferative disease. Management is difficult if the primary disease can not be treated. Steroids and splenectomy are not effective and immunosuppressive drugs are often required for severe, refractory cases. Avoidance of transfusion and supportive care, including hydration, avoidance of cold, and no infusions of fluids with temperatures of less than 37 °C, are the mainstays of therapy.

Autoimmune hemolytic anemias are problematic in patients requiring surgery because anemia may be profound and transfusions of red cells can precipitate a number of serious complications. The autoantibody may cause accelerated destruction of the transfused cells causing renal, coagulation, or pulmonary complications. This is particularly true with cold antibodies because transfusions may increase hemolysis. The autoantibody also causes problems in finding compatible blood for transfusion because typing and cross-matching may be difficult or impossible. Autoantibodies can prevent detection of alloantibodies that may precipitate immediate or delayed transfusion reactions and increase hemolysis caused by the autoimmune process.

Autoantibodies are uncommon, however, and infrequently present preoperative management problems.

When present, they require coordinated management by experienced teams of hematologists, clinical pathologists, and anesthesiologists who understand and will coordinate the special management issues. Elective surgery should be delayed if possible until the autoimmune hemolysis is controlled with therapy. If the autoimmune process is resistant to therapy or if the surgery is emergent, the blood bank should be given sufficient time to use special techniques to detect alloantibodies. In emergent situations, patients often are given the least incompatible blood. Patients with uncontrolled autoimmune hemolytic anemia require careful monitoring and transfusion of the fewest units possible. Treatment with high dose steroids is indicated for warm antibodies. Some advocate increasing steroid doses or administering high dose intravenous immunoglobulin before transfusing patients with poorly controlled autoimmune hemolysis.

Patients with cold antibodies need to be kept warm so the blood temperature exceeds 37 °C throughout the body. All fluids and blood products must be warmed to 37 °C before administration. This may require maintaining the entire operating suite at 37 °C for patients with high titer cold antibodies. Plasmapheresis is effective for the acute removal of these IgM antibodies and may be considered as emergency treatment before surgery in patients with significant, uncontrolled cold antibody immune hemolysis. Plasmapheresis is technically difficult because fluids, blood and the patient must be kept warm.

Polycythemia

Elevated hemoglobin or hematocrit levels require preoperative evaluation to exclude conditions that may increase perioperative complications. The upper limits of normal for hemoglobin and hematocrit are 16.5 g/dl and 55% in males and 15.3 g/dl and 52% in females. Polycythemia or erythrocytosis is defined as an elevation above these levels. The elevation may reflect a true polycythemia (erythrocytosis) with increase in red cell mass or a relative increase in hemoglobin and hematocrit levels caused by a reduction in plasma volume. Relative polycythemia should be diagnosed and corrected because the low plasma volume is usually associated with a reduced total blood volume. This may predispose to hypotension during induction of anesthesia or performance of surgery. True polycythemia may be caused by polycythemia vera, which must be well controlled before surgery to minimize the high incidence of hemorrhagic and thrombotic complications. Secondary polycythemia results from physiologic processes that may predispose to pulmonary and cardiovascular complications in the perioperative period.

Diagnostic considerations

An algorithm for the evaluation of elevated hemoglobin levels in patients undergoing surgery is outlined in Fig. 16.4. The most common cause of elevated hemoglobin is relative polycythemia caused by a reduced plasma volume. This occurs acutely from dehydration or is a chronic state associated with hypertension, adrenergic excess, and increased cardiovascular risk (stress erythrocytosis, Gaisbock's syndrome). If hydration does not return the hemoglobin concentration to normal, a red cell mass should be determined to confirm the presence of true erythrocytosis. Complete blood gas analysis will document chronic hypoxia and detect elevated carbon monoxide in smokers. Exercise-induced hypoxia and sleep apnea should also be considered as a cause of polycythemia because both may increase surgical complications. If there is sufficient time, patients who smoke should stop smoking and be observed to see if the hemoglobin level returns to normal. Determination of carbon monoxide levels may be helpful if the surgery is urgent because the level is usually elevated in smokers with erythrocytosis.

After these more common clinical conditions are excluded, careful evaluation to rule out polycythemia vera is indicated. Splenomegaly is a cardinal feature of polycythemia vera. Spleen scan may be indicated if the spleen is not palpable. If the spleen size is normal, a diagnosis of polycythemia vera is established by the presence of two other indicators of myeloproliferative syndromes such as increased leukocyte or platelet count, elevated white cell mass reflected by an increased B_{12} level, or high leukocyte alkaline phosphatase score. A very low erythropoietin level supports the diagnosis of polycythemia vera. Determination of erythropoietin level and search for occult kidney disease or tumors of a number of organs by intravenous pyelography, sonography, or computerized tomography should be considered if a cause of true polycythemia is not defined by the initial evaluation.

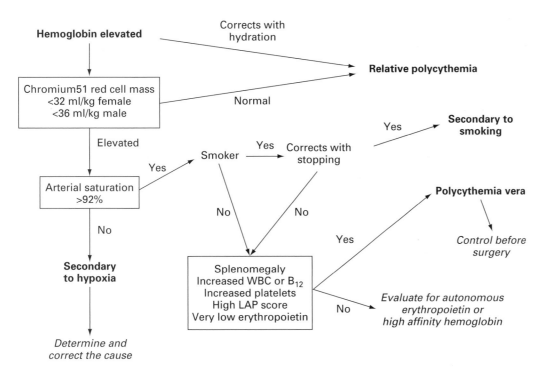

Fig. 16.4. Evaluation of elevated hemoglobin levels is important preoperatively because untreated polycythemia vera is associated with high morbidity and mortality. Evaluation is initiated if hydration does not normalize the hemoglobin level. Determination of red cell mass separates true elevation of the red cell mass from relative elevation caused by low plasma volume. True polycythemia is most commonly secondary to hypoxia or smoking, so blood gases and determining the response to cessation of smoking are important first steps. Splenomegaly or a combination of two of the other manifestations of polycythemia vera establish that diagnosis in true polycythemia without hypoxia. Other less common causes must be sought if these are not present.

Management considerations

Polycythemia rubra vera should be treated to a normal hemoglobin level before surgery because of the high incidence of thrombotic and hemorrhagic perioperative complications in patients with uncontrolled or poorly controlled disease. To assure minimal morbidity and mortality, the general recommendation is that the disease should be well controlled for 4 months before purely elective surgery is undertaken. Before more urgent surgery, the patient should be treated to achieve normal hemoglobin levels. Phlebotomy alone can rapidly control the hemoglobin level in patients with primary elevations. Phlebotomy in combination with hydroxyurea administration should probably be used in patients with elevated hemoglobin levels and platelet counts. The therapeutic goal is a hematocrit level of approximately 45% because of evidence that cerebral blood flow is reduced with higher levels. Phlebotomy can be accomplished rapidly in young individuals by removing 125 to 200 ml every other day. Patients who have acute orthostatic symptoms may benefit from less frequent phlebotomy or concurrent hydration with an equal volume of normal saline. In older patients or those with underlying cardiovascular disease, slower phlebotomy is prudent, removing 100 to 150 ml twice a week. Again, concurrent administration of normal saline may prevent acute orthostatic symptoms.

Reduction of the platelet counts to less than 500 000 is advocated, although there are few data that indicate such treatment reduces thrombotic complications. Drugs that interfere with platelet functioning should be avoided because platelets are often functionally abnormal and bleeding complications are increased.

Patients with polycythemia vera are at higher risk for serious perioperative complications including stroke, myocardial infarction, pulmonary embolus, thrombophlebitis, splenic infarction, and portal or hepatic venous thrombosis. There is also an increased incidence of gastrointestinal and surgical hemorrhage. Alternatives to surgery should be considered. If surgery is necessary, the management plan should be formulated well in advance. Patients require close monitoring for common complications in the perioperative period. For emergency surgery, the hemoglobin level should be returned to normal by removing whole blood and infusion of crystalloid and colloid solutions to maintain blood volume. Anticoagulation is indicated for thrombotic complications but antithrombotic prophylaxis is individualized because of the increased risk of hemorrhage. Recent studies show that treatment with low dose aspirin (80 to 100 mg) reduces the incidence of thrombotic complications without increasing serious bleeding.

Recent publications indicate that patients with relative and secondary polycythemia do not have an increased rate of perioperative complications. It does seem prudent to define the cause of the polycythemia and identify and correct the underlying pathology if possible. Relative polycythemia may indicate acute dehydration that may predispose to hypotension during anesthesia or surgery. Chronic spurious polycythemia is often associated with hypertension and control of blood pressure with antihypertensive agents will often correct the elevated hemoglobin level. Smokers with polycythemia should stop smoking in advance of elective surgery to reduce pulmonary complications. This may also lead to normalization of the hemoglobin concentration.

Although secondary polycythemia probably does not increase the rate of complications, evaluation of this condition may uncover underlying disease requiring special management in the perioperative period. Hypoxia secondary to pulmonary or cardiac disease is a common cause of secondary polycythemia. Certain types of renal disease which cause ischemia in the juxtaglomerular cells increase erythropoietin resulting in secondary polycythemia. Several uncommon tumors, including renal cell carcinoma, hepatoma, cerebellar hemangioblastoma, uterine fibroids, and ovarian carcinoma may cause polycythemia by increasing erythropoietin. Pheochromocytoma and adrenal cortical carcinoma are important rare causes of polycythemia that are important to consider because of the management implications of these tumors during anesthesia and surgery.

If treatment of the underlying condition is impossible or does not correct the polycythemia, phlebotomy to normalize blood viscosity can be considered. Experimental data show that blood flow will be decreased with any true elevation of hemoglobin levels. There is no compelling evidence that phlebotomy is beneficial for either relative or secondary polycythemia with modest elevation of the hemoglobin level. Evidence does suggest that reduction of the hematocrit level may be beneficial if it exceeds 60%, when the elevation is secondary to hypoxia caused by severe pulmonary disease or cyanotic heart disease.

FURTHER READING

Anemia – general

Allen, J. B. & Allen, B. A. The minimum acceptable level of hemoglobin. *Int. Anesth. Clin.* 1982; **20**: 1–22.

Carson, J. L., Poses, R. M., Spence, R. K., & Bonavita, G. Severity of anaemia and operative mortality and morbidity. *Lancet* 1988; **2**: 727–729.

Consensus Conference. Perioperative red blood cell transfusion. *J. Am. Med. Assoc.* 1988; **260**: 2700–2703.

Council on Scientific Affairs. Autologous blood transfusions. *J. Am. Med. Assoc.* 1986; **256**: 2378–2380.

Etchason, J., Petz, L., Keeler, E. *et al.* The cost-effectiveness of preoperative autologous blood donations. *N. Engl. J. Med.* 1995; **332**: 719–724.

Goodnough, L. T. The role of recombinant growth factors in transfusion medicine. *Br. J. Anaesth.* 1993; **70**: 80–86.

Goodnough, L. T., Rudnick, E., Price, T. H. *et al.* Increased preoperative collection of autologous blood with recombinant human erythropoietin therapy. *N. Engl. J. Med.* 1989; **321**: 1163–1168.

Goodnough, L. T., Brecher, M. E., Kanter, M. H., AuBuchon, J. P. Transfusion medicine – blood transfusion. *N. Engl. J. Med.* 1999; **340**: 438–447.

Health and Public Policy Committee, American College of Physicians. Practice strategies for elective red blood cell transfusion. *Ann. Intern. Med.* 1992; **116**: 403–406.

Herbert, P. C., Wells, G., Blajchman, M. A. *et al.* A multicenter, randomized controlled clinical trial of transfusion requirements in critical care. *N. Engl. J. Med.* 1999; **340**: 409–417.

Hillyer, C. D., Silberstein, L. E., Ness, P. M., Anderson, K. C., & Roush, K. S. *Blood Banking and Transfusion Medicine: Basic Principles and Practice.* Philadelphia, PA: Churchill Livingstone, 2003.

Irving, G. A. Continuing medical education. Perioperative blood and blood component therapy. *Can. J. Anaesth.* 1992; **39**: 1105–1115.

Leone, B. J. & Spahn, D. R. Anemia, hemodilution, and oxygen delivery. *Anesth. Analg.* 1992; **75**: 651–653.

McFarland, J. G. Perioperative blood transfusions: indications and options. *Chest* 1999; **115**: 113S–121S.

Toy, P. T. C. Y., Strauss, R. G., Stehling, L. C. *et al.* Predeposited autologous blood for elective surgery. A National Multicenter Study. *N. Engl. J. Med.* 1987; **316**: 517–520.

Vengelen-Tyler, V., ed. *AABB Technical Manual.* 14th edn, Bethesda, MD: American Association of Blood Banks, 2002.

Welch, H. G., Meehan, K. R., & Goodnough, L. T. Prudent strategies for elective red blood cell transfusion. *Ann. Intern. Med.* 1992; **116**: 393–402.

Anemia – sickle syndromes

Adu-Gyamfi, Y., Sankarakutty, M., & Marwa, S. Use of a tourniquet in patients with sickle-cell disease. *Can. J. Anaesth.* 1993; **40**: 24–27.

Bischoff, R. J., Williamson, II, A., Dalali, M. J., Rice, J. C., & Kerstein, M. D. Assessment of the use of transfusion therapy perioperatively in patients with sickle cell hemoglobinopathies. *Ann. Surg.* 1988; **207**: 434–438.

Burrington, J. D. & Smith, M. D. Elective and emergency surgery in children with sickle cell disease. *Surg. Clin. N. Am.* 1976; **56**: 55–71.

Davis, S. C. & Robets-Harewood, M. Blood transfusion in sickle cell disease. *Blood Rev.* 1997; **11**: 57–71.

Esseltine, D. W., Baster, M. R. N., & Bevan, J. C. Sickle cell states and the anaesthetist. *Can. J. Anaesth.* 1988; **35**: 385–403.

Forrester, K. Anesthetic implications in sickle cell anemia. *J. Assoc. Nurs. Anesth.* 1986; **54**: 314–324.

Fullerton, M. W., Philippart, A. I., Sarnaik, S., & Lusher, J. M. Preoperative exchange transfusion in sickle cell anemia. *J. Pediatr. Surg.* 1981; **16**: 297–300.

Gibson, J. R. Anesthesia for the sickle cell diseases and other hemoglobinopathies. *Semin. Anesth.* 1987; **6**: 27–35.

Janik, J. & Seeler, R. A. Perioperative management of children with sickle hemoglobinopathy. *J. Pediatr. Surg.* 1980; **15**: 117–120.

Milner, P. F. & Coker, N. J. Elective surgery in patients with sickle cell anemia. *Arch. Otolaryngol.* 1982; **108**: 547–576.

Morrison, J. C., Whybrew, W. D., & Bucovaz, E. T. Use of partial exchange transfusion preoperatively in patients with sickle cell hemoglobinopathies. *Am. J. Obstet. Gynecol.* 1978; **132**: 59–63.

Oduro, K. A. & Searle, J. R. Anaesthesia in sickle-cell states: a plea for simplicity. *Br. Med. J.* 1972; **4**: 596–598.

Schlanger, M. & Cunningham, A. J. Intraoperative hypoxemia complicating laparoscopic cholecystectomy in a patient with sickle hemoglobinopathy. *Anesth. Analg.* 1992; **75**: 838–843.

Vichinsky, E. P., Earles, A., Johnson, R. A., Hoag, M. S., Williams, A., & Lubin, B. Alloimmunization in sickle cell anemia and transfusion of racially unmatched blood. *N. Engl. J. Med.* 1990; **322**: 1617–1621.

Vishinsky, E. P., Haberkern, C. M., Neumayr, L. *et al.* A comparison of conservative and aggressive transfusion regimens in the perioperative management of sickle cell disease. *N. Engl. J. Med.* 1995; **333**: 206–213.

Vichinsky, E. P. Current issues in blood transfusion in sickle cell disease. *Semin. Hematol.* 2001; **38**: 14–22.

Ware, R., Filston, H. C., Schultz, W. H., & Kinney, T. R. Elective cholecystectomy in children with sickle hemoglobinopathies. *Ann. Surg.* 1988; **208**: 17–22.

Autoimmune hemolytic anemia

Garratty, G. & Petz, L. D. Approaches to selecting blood for transfusion to patients with autoimmune hemolytic anemia. *Transfusion* 2002; **42**: 1390–1392.

Petz, L. D. Transfusing the patient with autoimmune hemolytic anemia. *Clin. Lab. Med.* 1982; **2**: 193–210.

Plapp, F. V. & Beck, M. L. Transfusion support in the management of immune haemolytic disorders. *Clin. Haematol.* 1984; **13**: 167–183.

Sokol, R. J., Hewitt, S., Booker, D. J., & Morris, B. M. Patients with red cell antibodies: selection of blood for transfusion. *Clin. Lab. Haematol.* 1988; **10**: 257–264.

Polycythemia

Berk, P. D., Goldberg, J. D., Donovan, P. B., Fruchtman, S. M., Berlin, N. I., & Wasserman, L. R. Therapeutic recommendations in polycythemia vera based on polycythemia vera study group protocols. *Semin. Hematol.* 1986; **23**: 132–143.

Fitts, W. T., Erde, A., Peskin, G. W., & Frost, J. W. Surgical implications of polycythemia vera. *Ann. Surg.* 1960; **152**: 548–558.

Fruchtman, S. M. & Wasserman, L. R. Therapeutic recommendations for polycythemia vera. In Wasserman, L. R., Berk, P. D., Berlin, N. I., eds. *Polycythemia Vera and the Myeloproliferative Syndromes.* Philadelphia: W. B. Saunders; 1995: 337–350.

Hoffman, R. & Wasserman, L. R. Natural history and management of polycythemia vera. *Adv. Intern. Med.* 1979; **245**: 255–283.

Kaplan, M. E., Mack, K., Goldberg, J. D., Donovan, P. B., Berk, P. D., & Wasserman, L. R. Long-term management of polycythemia vera with hydroxyurea: a progress report. *Semin. Hematol.* 1986; **23**: 167–171.

Lubarsky, D. A., Gallagher, C. J., & Berend, J. L. Secondary polycythemia does not increase the risk of perioperative hemorrhagic or thrombotic complications. *J. Clin. Anesth.* 1991; **3**: 99–103.

Tartaglia, A. P., Goldberg, J. D., Berk, P. D., Wasserman, L. R. Adverse effects of antiaggregating platelet therapy in the treatment of polycythemia vera. *Semin. Hematol.* 1986; **23**: 172–176.

Wallis, P. J. W., Skehan, J. D., Newland, A. C., Wedzicha, J. A., Mills, P. G., & Empey, D. W. Effects of erythrapheresis on pulmonary haemodynamics and oxygen transport in patients with secondary polycythaemia and cor pulmonale. *Clin. Sci.* 1986; **70**: 91–98.

Wasserman, L. R. The treatment of polycythemia vera. *Semin. Hematol.* 1976; **13**: 57–78.

Wasserman, L. R. & Gilbert, H. S. Surgery in polycythemia vera. *N. Engl. J. Med.* 1963; **269**: 1226–1230.

17

Assessment of bleeding risk in the patient with no history of hemostatic problems

Eve Rodler[1] and Ted Wun[2]

[1]Robert Wood Johnson School of Medicine, Camden, NJ
[2]Division of Hematology Oncology, UC Davis SOM VA Northern California Health Care System, Sacramento, CA

"There is perhaps more money wasted and blood unnecessarily shed in this setting than in any other in medicine."

Sabiston's Textbook of Surgery

When patients are evaluated for the potential of abnormal bleeding before surgery, the intensity of screening is determined by the hemostatic challenge of the procedure and the likelihood that the patient has an underlying congenital or acquired disorder that would predispose to bleeding. The risk of bleeding associated with the type of surgical procedure ranges from low risk (lymph node biopsies, dental extractions) to moderate risk (laparotomy, thoracotomy, mastectomy) to high risk (neurosurgical, ophthalmic, plastic, cardiopulmonary bypass, prostatic, surgery to stop bleeding). A screening history should reveal if the patient has experienced any abnormal bleeding or bruising, if there is a history of an acquired medical disorder which could affect hemostasis, if family members have bled abnormally, or if the patient is taking any drugs which could interfere with hemostasis. Physical examination can also provide important information about a patient's surgical bleeding risk. Ecchymoses, petechiae, or purpura may suggest a systemic hemostatic defect. Stigmata of chronic liver disease include hepatomegaly, splenomegaly, jaundice, spider angiomas, palmar erythema, and dilated abdominal veins.

The preoperative hemostatic screening recommendations by Rapaport provide a reasonable basis for selecting laboratories for individual patients.[1] Level 1 are patients with a reassuring history who are undergoing surgeries with only minimal potential blood loss such as excisional biopsies or dental extractions. No screening is required for theses patients as the low predictive value of laboratory screening outweighs the cost of treating minor bleeding episodes in the few individuals who will have mild bleeding disorders undetected by history prior to surgery.

Level 2 are patients with a negative bleeding history who have had prior surgical challenges to hemostasis, and are undergoing surgeries such as bowel resection or orthopedic procedures which have a moderate, but not the highest, risk for bleeding. A partial thromboplastin test (aPTT) and platelet count are recommended as screening tests to assess the risk of bleeding episode in patients who may have an undiagnosed moderate to severe hemostatic defect. Level 3 are patients whose bleeding history suggests a possible defect in hemostasis and who require surgery with a high risk of bleeding. These surgeries include cardiopulmonary bypass in which the pump–oxygenator can damage platelets and coagulation factors, prostatectomies, and all procedures, in which even a small amount of bleeding could be catastrophic, e.g., surgeries of the central nervous system. A more extensive evaluation is recommended for these patients. This includes: the platelet count; aPTT and INR to ensure adequate coagulation. Of note, the classic template bleeding time has not been shown to be predictive of postprocedural bleeding complications and it should not be performed. Group 4 are patients whose history is highly suggestive of a bleeding disorder and should have a thorough evaluation prior to surgery, regardless of the type of procedure. The initial laboratory work-up is the same as that for Group 3 patients, but also includes a von Willebrand panel, platelet function test, and specific coagulation factor assays for factors VIII and IX to detect mild hemophilia (in males). A thrombin time can be checked to detect patients with dysfibrinogenemia.

Common causes of unexpected intraoperative and postoperative bleeding and treatment

Most intraoperative and postoperative bleeding is due to a local lesion at the operative site, with minimal or no

Medical Management of the Surgical Patient: A Textbook of Perioperative Medicine, ed. M. F. Lubin, R. B. Smith, T. F. Dobson, N. Spell, H. K. Walker.
4th edn. Published by Cambridge University Press. © Cambridge University 2006.

abnormalities of the hemostatic system. The treatment generally involves surgical intervention to control bleeding vessels. There are special causes of intra- and postoperative hemostatic failure related to particular types of surgery where the nature of the surgery itself is a risk factor for bleeding. If unexpected bleeding occurs that is not due to a local lesion or to the specific type of surgery being performed, but rather may be due to an undiscovered preexisting hemostatic defect of the patient, then proper evaluation and management must be undertaken expeditiously.

Cardiopulmonary bypass

The high risk for blood loss during cardiopulmonary bypass surgery is multifactorial: the large size of the surgical wound; exposure of blood to artificial surfaces in the extracorporeal oxygenator; injury to platelets and coagulation factors; and activation of fibrinolysis during and after surgery, and heparin. Significant hemorrhage has been reported in 6% to 25% of patients and bleeding requiring re-exploration occurs in approximately 2% to 7%.[2] Of those patients who return to the operating room, only half will have an identifiable surgical bleeding source.

Some experts recommend platelet transfusions following cardiac bypass in patients with normal coagulation values and platelet counts below 100 000/ul if unexplained bleeding occurs.[3] However, the value of this strategy is uncertain. The effect of the vasopressin analogue desmopressin (DDAVP) on reducing postoperative blood loss after cardiac surgery has been studied in several randomized studies, with conflicting results. A recent meta-analysis of 17 randomized, double-blind, placebo-controlled trials showed that DDAVP reduced blood loss by 9%, but had no significant impact on transfusion requirements.[4] Studies have shown that treatment with DDAVP reduced blood loss,[5] or transfusion requirements[6] in patients treated with aspirin up to the time of surgery. DDAVP is administered at a dose of 0.3 µg/kg over 30 minutes.

Several prospective trials have found significant decreases in blood loss as well as transfusion requirements with the use of aprotinin, tranexamic acid, and aminocaproic acid.[2,7–9] Aprotinin, a polypeptide extracted from bovine lung, inhibits the action of several serine proteases, including trypsin, chymotrypsin, plasmin, and tissue and plasma kallikrein through the formation of reversible enzyme inhibitor complexes. Thus, aprotinin inhibits both coagulation and fibrinolysis. Several double-blind studies have demonstrated the effectiveness of aprotinin in reducing blood loss in coronary artery bypass operations.[10] The treatment is most effective when used as prophylaxis. It is recommended for patients who are most likely to require blood transfusions (i.e., patients with hemostatic defects, those taking aspirin, those undergoing repeat sternotomy) or for patients who refuse transfusions. The standard dosing regimen is 2 million kallikrein inactivation units KIU (280 mg) given as a loading dose, followed by continuous infusion of 500 000 KIU/h (70 mg/l), and an addition of 1 to 2 million KIU (140 to 280 mg) to the pump prime intraoperatively.[11]

Aminocaproic acid and tranexamic acid are two synthetic anti-fibrinolytic agents which can reduce blood loss in cardiac surgery by 30 to 40 percent, as demonstrated in clinical trials involving at least 1000 patients.[12] These agents act by forming a reversible complex with plasminogen, preventing its activation to plasmin. Aminocaproic acid can be given as a bolus intravenous dose of 150 mg/kg before the operation, followed by an infusion of 15 mg/kg per h during the operation[13] or a bolus intravenous dose of 80 mg/kg, followed by an infusion of 30 mg/kg per h during the operation, with an additional 80 mg/kg dose to the pump prime.[7] Tranexamic acid has been administered in a 10-mg/kg bolus followed by continuous infusion of 1 to 3 mg/kg per h.[14]

If postoperative hemorrhage occurs, ensure that the patient is not hypothermic and that heparin has been fully reversed with protamine sulfate. A full neutralizing dose is 1 mg of protamine sulfate per 100 units of heparin used intravenously. An antifibrinolytic agent can be used along with transfusions of platelets, red blood cells, and cryoprecipitate or fresh frozen plasma as guided by laboratory evaluation.

Fibrin sealants, also referred to as "fibrin glue" or "fibrin tissue adhesives" are used in cardiovascular procedures as well as a broad range of surgeries to control bleeding during and after surgery and reduce blood loss. Those available commercially (e.g., Tisseel, Hemaseel) consist of human fibrinogen and human or bovine thrombin which are applied to the local tissue site. Some of the commercial products also contain human factor XIII and bovine aprotinin. Although pooled plasma has the theoretical risk of viral transmission, only parvovirus B19 has documented transmission from fibrin sealants.[15] Before the introduction of effective viral inactivation techniques, bovine thrombin was used in fibrin sealants to reduce the risk of viral transmission. The use of bovine thrombin carries the risk of coagulopathies due to the development of thrombin and factor V inhibitors. A recent meta-analysis which reviewed the efficacy of fibrin sealants in reducing perioperative blood loss and allogeneic red blood cell transfusion concluded that the use of fibrin sealant resulted in a mean reduction in blood loss of 150 ml per patient, and a reduction in average transfusion requirements by about 0.6 units, though conclusions are weakened due to lack of blinding in most of the studies.[16]

Prostatectomy

In prostatectomy, enhanced local fibrinolysis related to high concentrations of urokinase likely contributes to bleeding risk. The use of aminocaproic acid or tranexamic acid resulted in significantly decreased postoperative blood loss compared with placebo controls.[12,17] These therapies are contraindicated in patients with bleeding from the upper urinary tract because of the risk of clots causing obstruction. Recombinant activated factor VIIa (rFVIIa), which was originally approved for use in hemophiliacs with factor inhibitors (see below), has recently been approved for other uses including stopping bleeding after radical prostatectomy.[18]

Liver transplantation

Patients undergoing liver transplantation are at high risk for intraoperative blood loss due to coagulopathy and fibrinolysis.[19] Intraoperatively, there is an anhepatic phase during which coagulation factors are not produced and there is excessive fibrinolysis. During the reperfusion phase, t-PA is released from the stored organ and there is proteolytic breakdown of von Willebrand's factor. These patients may need replacement with blood products and antifibrinolytic therapy. rFVIIa has also been approved for liver transplantation.[18] Fibrin sealant has been used successfully in the management of hemorrhage from cut surfaces of parenchymal liver, which is difficult to suture.[20]

Major neurosurgery

After head trauma and in patients with brain tumors, DIC can occur. A recent prospective study demonstrated the association of decreased perioperative factor XIII with an increased risk of postoperative hematoma in neurosurgical patients.[21] Neurological surgery may require a platelet count of $100\,000/\mu l$[22] although this practice has never been validated in a prospective trial.

Damage control surgery

So-called "damage control surgery" is performed for exsanguinating, major trauma patients. It involves rapid restoration of circulating volume, normothermia, maintenance of oxygen delivery, and correction of transfusion related coagulopathy so that expeditious re-operation and completion of definitive surgical management can be attained.[23–25] In an effort to save these patients, a three-component damage control surgery was developed originally for patients with massive abdominal trauma with vascular injury. One component of this process is induced hypothermia, which can lead to platelet dysfunction. Hypothermia also impairs the intrinsic and extrinsic coagulation cascades.[26] In rapidly exsanguinating patients, lab values are not usually helpful because the resuscitation proceeds faster than the ability of the laboratory to return information. Platelets and fresh frozen plasma should be transfused after rapid transfusion of eight or more units of blood in the presence of ongoing bleeding.[24]

Massive transfusion

Massive transfusion is defined as replacement of more than 1 blood volume (apx. 5000 ml in a 70 kg adult) within 4 hours. As many as 51% of all deaths in the first 48 hours of hospitalization are related to lack of hemostasis in patients with trauma. Transfusion of fresh frozen plasma is indicated if a patient's history or clinical course suggests coagulopathy and active bleeding is present, or prior to an invasive procedure in the presence of abnormal coagulation factors.[22] If there is excessive operative bleeding, platelet transfusion to greater than or equal to $100\,000/\mu l$ empirically is indicated.[22] Recombinant factor VIIa has been utilized in severe trauma[18] and appears to be effective despite the presence of a hypothermic and dilutional coagulopathy.[27] Fibrin foams have been used to reduce blood loss by binding to damaged surfaces.[28]

An approach to intraoperative or postoperative bleeding

First, it is crucial to determine if bleeding is related to a hemostatic defect or to a local lesion that requires surgical intervention, e.g., "factor XIV (surgical silk) deficiency". Suspect a problem with local control if bleeding is rapid, if it is confined to the operative site, or if there is excessive blood on dressings, in the operative drains or chest tube. In contrast, bleeding is likely due to a systemic hemostatic abnormality if it is generalized, slower, and "oozing" at multiple sites is found.

There are several congenital or acquired hematological abnormalities, which may not have been detected on preoperative personal or family history or labs, which could account for unanticipated perioperative hemorrhage. Mild deficiencies of factor VIII, factor IX, and factor XI can be present without prolongation of aPTT. Factor XIII deficiency requires a specific test for detection. Mild von Willebrand's disease or a platelet granule disorder may also be discovered after a surgical procedure. Review of the patient's medication record could reveal an acquired platelet dysfunction from aspirin, antibiotics or other medications. If a complete blood count was not checked prior to a simple surgical procedure, the patient could have undetected thrombocytopenia.

If possible, review the patient's past medical history, family history, and recent medications for clues to an underlying hemostatic abnormality. Perform a physical examination to see if it is more consistent with a platelet problem (mucosal bleeding) or coagulation problem (soft tissue bleeding), or both. Additional laboratory tests should be sent, including aPTT, PT, thrombin time, fibrinogen, CBC and peripheral smear. If these laboratory values are all normal, bleeding is unlikely to be due to a systemic bleeding disorder. However, if the clinical suspicion of a hemostatic abnormality is still high, it is reasonable to also test for factor XIII, and von Willebrand's disease, although the results of these tests are likely to be delayed unless there is a full-time special coagulation laboratory available. It is important to draw all laboratories through a peripheral venipuncture and not through a catheter, in order to avoid effects of heparin on coagulation testing.

Patients with known disorders of hemostasis

Hemophilia A and B

There are several inherited disorders of blood clotting, but discussion will focus on the four most common: hemophilia A and B; von Willebrand's disease; and factor XI deficiency. In general, perioperative management of hemophilia A and B, aspirin products, intramuscular and subcutaneous injections should be avoided. It is important to determine if the patient has mild hemophilia (factor VIII or IX level >5%), moderate (factor level 1% to 5%) or severe (factor level <1%).[29] A baseline factor level and mixing study should be done to determine if a circulating alloantibody or autoantibody (inhibitor) is present.

Therapeutic agents used in patients with hemophilia

If no inhibitors are present, pre- and postoperative recombinant or human factor replacement may be used. For major surgery factor VIII and factor IX levels should be 100% of normal. Continuous infusion with high purity products is recommended to avoid level fluctuations and to decrease overall factor utilization. In patients with hemophilia B, high purity products are preferred to avoid the possible thrombotic side effects of the less pure factor IX concentrates in hemophilia B. Treatment should begin a few hours before surgery and continue intraoperatively. Postoperative factor levels should be monitored daily. Infusion of factor replacement should continue at least 10 to 14 days and up to several weeks after major surgery. For moderate risk procedures, such as dental extractions, factor VIII and IX levels should be 50% of normal.

If factor VIII or IX inhibitors are present, there are several approaches to treatment depending on the level of inhibitor and whether bleeding is minor or major.[30,31] Recombinant factor VIIa (Novoseven; rFVIIa) has been used successfully in the perioperative management of patients with inhibitors.[32]

It is hypothesized that factor VIIa activates factor X on the surface of activated platelets without the need for tissue factor.[33,34] Since this is occurring at a localized site of vascular injury, factor VIIa has not been found to cause general activation of coagulation resulting in thrombogenicity, though randomized trials are necessary to test the thrombogenicity of factor VIIa.[32,35] A variety of surgical procedures have been carried out successfully, including amputations, major orthopedic surgeries, and liver biopsies with the use of rFVIIa in hemophiliacs with inhibitors.[36,37] The dosing recommendation is 90 to 110 mcg/kg bolus every 2 hours, followed by the same dose at longer intervals of 3 to 6 hours thereafter.[38] There are reports of giving rFVIIa as a continuous infusion following surgery, but the target maintenance level has varied and there is no consensus on the optimal regimen for continuous infusion.[39] Porcine factor VIII can sometimes be used in patients with inhibitors to human factor VIII. Hemophilia A patients with inhibitors can be tested to see if their inhibitor cross-reacts with porcine factor VIII, as measured in a Bethesda assay. The recommended starting dose of porcine factor VIII is 100–150 units/kg with measurements of factor VIII levels to guide therapy.

Prothrombin complex concentrates (FEIBA, Autoplex) are products with variable amounts of activated factors, including VIIa, IXa, and Xa. It is postulated that the prothrombin complex concentrate "bypasses" inhibitors by enhancing the tissue factor–factor VIIa pathway of coagulation. The presence of factors in an activated form generates a risk of thrombotic complications.[40,41] The risk is increased in patients receiving high or multiple doses of prothrombin complex concentrates or concurrent fibrinolytic therapy or those with significant liver disease. The recommended dose is 75 to 100 units/kg, which can be repeated after 8 to 12 hours.

Desmopressin (DDAVP) may be used in patients with mild or moderate hemophilia A, who have shown a capacity to raise the level of factor VIII to a hemostatic level in response to DDAVP. The dose is 30 μg/kg in saline solution given over 30 minutes. DDAVP has no activity in hemophilia B.

Antifibrinolytic agents can be useful as adjunctive therapy, not for initial hemostasis but to prevent clot lysis after hemostasis. These agents mainly are used in cases of mucous membrane bleeding and after dental extractions.[42,43] Aminocaproic acid can be given as an oral tablet or elixir at a dose of 100 mg/kg (maximum 10 g) initially (if available), then 50 mg/kg (maximum 5 g) every 6 hours. Tranexamic acid can be administered orally at a dose of 25 mg/kg every 6 to 8 hours, or intravenously at 10 mg/kg every 8 hours.

Local control of bleeding can be improved with fibrin glue as an adjunctive therapy to factor replacement in hemophiliac patients after dental procedures and orthopedic procedures or for surgical wounds.[44]

Factor XI deficiency is the least rare of the non-hemophiliac congenital coagulation factor deficiencies. It occurs most often in Ashkenazi Jews but also occurs in non-Jewish populations.[45] Three different point mutations account for most of the cases. Factor XI deficiency is inherited as an autosomal recessive trait. There is no clear correlation between the genotype and the bleeding tendency; very low factor XI levels are not always associated with a bleeding tendency.[46] The phenotype of the family is important. If a patient with factor XI deficiency is to undergo surgery and has never had surgery, dental extractions, or prior trauma, then the bleeding history of the family provides the only clue whether the patient will bleed. Prior to surgery, perform a specific factor XI assay. Most patients whose levels are below 0.15 IU/ml will experience excessive bleeding after surgery, and some patients with factor XI levels as high as 60–70% of normal will have a bleeding tendency.[35]

There is some evidence that desmopressin is effective in patients with partial factor XI deficiency due either to modest increases in factor XI or to larger increases in VIII or von Willebrand factor. DDAVP may also be used for minor bleeding in mildly affected patients.[47] Antifibrinolytics can be used for surface or mucosal bleeding. Patients with severe factor XI deficiency often require plasma replacement. The dose of plasma is a loading dose of 15–20 ml/kg body weight, followed by 3–6 ml/kg every 12 hours until hemostasis is achieved. For major surgery, transfusion of fresh frozen plasma should be given for 10 to 14 days maintaining a trough level of 45% of normal.[48] For minor or moderate risk surgeries fresh frozen plasma can be transfused for 5 to 7 days with a goal to maintain factor XI levels 30% of normal. Factor XI concentrates from plasma can be used, if available. These products allow efficient replacement therapy but they have thrombogenic potential.[49] Peak levels should not be greater than 0.70 IU/ml, and individual doses should not be greater than 30 IU/kg.

von Willebrand's disease is the most common inherited bleeding disorder with a prevalence of 1% of the general population. In general, the treatment of von Willebrand's disease depends on the subtype and the response to desmopressin. Factor VIII:C and ristocetin cofactor activity levels are used to monitor the effect of therapy.

Type I von Willebrand's disease is the most common type accounting for approximately 90% of patients with von Willebrand disease. Most of these patients will respond to DDAVP with a three- to fivefold increase in plasma vWF.[49,50] It may be given by the intravenous or intranasal route. A single daily infusion is frequently sufficient for minor procedures. The response to DDAVP is variable, but consistent within an individual over time. A trial of desmopressin is recommended prior to a major surgery. If the vWF activity (as measured by the ristocetan cofactor assay) increases to >100% (u/dl), the patient can be given DDAVP alone. Perioperatively, daily levels of vWF activity should be measured.

For other types of vWD, or if tachyphalaxis develops with DDAVP, a factor VIII concentrate that contains sufficient vWF multimers, such as Humate P or Koate-HP,[51] is required. Von Willebrand factor/VIII concentrates are now commonly labeled and prescribed in ristocetan cofactor (RCof) units. The recommended dose is 40–80 RCof units/kg depending on the severity of bleeding. For severe hemorrhage or major surgery, repeat doses can be given at 8–12-hour intervals until hemostasis is achieved.[34] The target nadir for major surgery is 50% activity. Adjuvant therapies are the same as used for hemophilia A and B.

Thrombocytopenia

The platelet count needed for adequate surgical hemostasis is not well defined. According to the National Institutes of Health Consensus Development Conference, a minimum platelet count of 50 000 is recommended for surgery.[52] A reasonable approach is the following: low risk surgery, either no platelets or transfuse platelets to 50 000; moderate risk general surgery 50 000 to 100 000; and high-risk surgery transfuse to level of 100 000.[53] An exception is immune thrombocytopenia. In this case lower levels of platelets are tolerated, and transfusions generally are not performed unless life-threatening bleeding occurs.

Platelet dysfunction

Patients with platelet dysfunction may be asymptomatic but normally they have a history of excessive mucocutaneous bleeding and bruising, menorrhagia, petechiae, epistaxis, gingival bleeding, or excessive bleeding following surgery or injury. Hereditary causes of platelet dysfunction include Glanzmann's thrombasthenia, Bernard–Soulier disease, Scott syndrome, and storage pool deficiencies and are less common than acquired causes. Transfusion of platelets to the target levels discussed above should provide adequate platelets for primary hemostasis. There are now reports that factor VIIa can be used to stop hemorrhage in this and other intrinsic platelet defect disorders.[54]

Medications are the most common reason for an acquired platelet functional defect. The Physician's Health Study Research Group examined the clinical importance of aspirin on hemostasis in normal individuals by giving aspirin 325 mg every other day or placebo to 22 071 physicians over 5 years. They found a decrease in risk of myocardial infarction for aspirin treated patients but more patients in the aspirin treated group had easy bruising, hematemesis, melena, and epistaxis than in the control group (RR1.32, $P < 0.00001$) and more people in the aspirin group required a blood transfusion over the 5 years ($P = 0.02$). Thus aspirin does have an impact on normal hemostasis, but it is generally small.[55] For the surgical patient, some, but not all studies have shown that aspirin taken preoperatively increases the amount of blood loss following cardiothoracic surgery.[3] Increased chest tube loss in aspirin treated patients is not associated with worse clinical outcomes.[56] Performing epidural and spinal anesthesia in patients who ingested aspirin was found to be safe in a retrospective study.[57] Aspirin should be avoided in patients with known hemostatic defects. It is reasonable to discontinue aspirin ingestion in patients scheduled for non-emergent invasive procedures or surgery 5 days prior to the procedure, as this is enough time for half of the circulating platelets to be replaced by new platelets.

Other non-steroidal anti-inflammatory drugs also inhibit platelet cyclooxygenase, thus impairing platelet aggregation and secretion. This effect is reversible and of short duration, so the hemostatic risk with these drugs disappears a few hours after the drug is stopped, with the exception of piroxicam, which has a half-life of greater than 2 days.

Ticlopidine and clopidogrel are thienopyridines that are used for secondary prevention of strokes and myocardial infarctions. Thienopyridines have an additive effect with aspirin. The effects of oral ticlopidine and clopidogrel are seen within 24 to 48 hours of the first dose, are maximal in 4 to 6 days, and last for 4 to 10 days after the drugs have been discontinued.[58]

Beta-lactam antibiotics have also been associated with platelet dysfunction. This platelet dysfunction may not subside for several days after the antibiotic is discontinued. It is postulated that these antibiotics inhibit platelet surface receptor functions through a lipophilic association with the plasma membrane.[3] Clinically important bleeding associated with antibiotic induced platelet dysfunction has mainly occurred in patients with multiple hemostatic defects.

Chronic renal disease

The cause of the bleeding tendency in uremia is multifactorial. Platelet dysfunction has been implicated as a major cause of bleeding risk.[3] However, the relationship between platelet dysfunction and clinical bleeding in patients with renal failure is unclear. Anemia, which correlates with the severity of renal failure, plays a role in the platelet adhesion defect and in the prolonged bleeding time.[59] A prolonged bleeding time in uremic patients is common but does not correlate with the risk for perioperative hemorrhage. The frequency of bleeding in uremic patients after biopsies or surgical procedures is not known but based on reports, it is felt to be uncommon.[60] No prospective randomized study has been done to evaluate the effectiveness of therapeutic regimens for improving hemostasis in the uremic patient. Dialysis can often, but not always, correct the bleeding time and reduce the risk of clinical bleeding in patients with uremia.[61,62] DDAVP has been reported to shorten the bleeding time in 50% to 75% of patients with uremia and may be effective in preventing perioperative bleeding in uremic patients.[63] Correction of anemia to a hematocrit >32% can correct the bleeding time and reduce clinical bleeding in uremic patients.[64]

Some uncontrolled studies have found that infusion of cryoprecipitate can correct the bleeding time in uremic patients and decrease bleeding, but other studies have not shown these results. Conjugated estrogens have also been reported to shorten the bleeding time in patients with uremia both in uncontrolled and in double blind randomized studies.[65,66]

Thrombocytosis

Thrombocytosis may be due to a primary myeloproliferative disorder, or to secondary causes such as inflammation, iron deficiency anemia, or the postoperative state.

The risk of thrombosis or hemorrhage is low in patients with secondary thrombocytosis or chronic myelogenous leukemia, and there is no correlation between platelet count and risk in patients with polycythemia rubra vera (PRV) or essential thrombocytosis (ET). In PRV and ET, the risk of complications is greater in older patients and in those patients with a history of bleeding or thrombosis.[67] Empirically, in patients with PRV or ET, the platelet count should be lowered to normal or near normal pre-operatively with plateletpheresis, chemotherapy, or anagrelide. Aspirin should be avoided.[68]

Polycythemia

Patients with uncontrolled polycythemia vera have a high surgical morbidity and mortality mainly due to thromboembolic events resulting from an increase in blood viscosity. In patients with polycythemia vera, the hematocrit should be reduced to less than 45% by phlebotomy prior to elective surgery. In physiologically inappropriate secondary polycythemia, such as polycystic kidney disease and erythropoietin secreting tumors, the hematocrit should be lowered to 45% to 50%. In physiologically appropriate polycythemia, usually from diseases causing significant hypoxia such as COPD, patients may need to maintain a higher hematocrit. Therefore, a preoperative hematocrit between 50% and 60% has been suggested.[67]

Liver disease

Hemostatic defects of liver disease are complex and include coagulopathy from liver synthetic dysfunction, vitamin K deficiency, thrombocytopenia, and platelet defects. A PT (INR) test is a good measure of the severity of liver dysfunction as it evaluates the vitamin K dependent factors and factor V. Although some have suggested that the measurement of individual procoagulant factors is useful in distinguishing between liver synthetic dysfunction, vitamin K deficiency, and concurrent DIC, in practice this is usually not possible.

If patients with liver disease have a PT prolongation less than 3 seconds, serious surgical bleeding is unlikely unless there are other pre-existing hemostatic defects. For patients undergoing high risk surgery or who have a more prolonged PT, prophylactic fresh frozen plasma is recommended. If peri-operative bleeding occurs, aggressive replacement therapy should be undertaken. Prothrombin complex concentrates is not generally recommended in patients with chronic liver disease because activated factors present in the concentrates are not adequately cleared by the liver and can lead to thrombotic complications.[69] Fibrinogen can be maintained with cryoprecipitate, and vitamin K should be empirically given. The effectiveness of platelet transfusions may be limited by splenic sequestration. Checking the platelet count one hour after transfusion will provide information on the degree of splenic sequestration that is occurring. Recombinant factor VIIa has more recently been found to be useful in this setting.

Anemia

Although there are data to suggest the preoperative hemoglobin is predictive of surgical mortality, other studies have shown that the degree of peri-operative blood loss, rather than the degree of anemia is more predictive of postoperative complications. In a study by Spence et al.,[70] 107 patients undergoing elective surgeries were prospectively studied to evaluate the influence of pre-operative hemoglobin level and operative blood loss in patients who refused blood transfusions. They found that mortality was significantly increased with an estimated blood loss of greater than 500 ml, regardless of the preoperative hemoglobin level ($P < 0.025$). Further, there was no mortality if estimated blood loss was less than 500 ml, regardless of the preoperative hemoglobin level.

The appropriate "transfusion trigger" for preoperative transfusion has not been established in prospective trials. Many physicians have used a threshold hemoglobin of 10 g/dl and a hematocrit of 30% (the "10/30" rule) but practices vary widely.[71,72] In a related area, in a recent randomized prospective clinical trial,[73] 838 patients admitted to the intensive care unit with hemoglobin levels less than 9.0 mg/dl were allocated to a liberal transfusion group (hemoglobin 10 to 12 g/dl) or to a restrictive group (hemoglobin levels 7 to 9 g/dl). The study found that the overall in-hospital mortality was significantly lower in the restrictive group, although the 30-day mortality rate was not significantly different. However, in those patients who were less ill (APACHE, 20) or younger (<55 years of age), the 30-day mortality rates were significantly lower for the patients in the restrictive transfusion group. Interestingly, no difference in mortality between the two groups was seen in cardiac patients.

The transfusion trigger concept has shifted in the literature from arbitrary levels to that of a level of hemoglobin required to maintain adequate oxygenation of tissues for a particular patient. While minimum hemoglobin levels may be well tolerated in the clinically stable patient, this range might be suboptimal for the critically ill anemic patients. Volume status in anemic patients appears to influence surgical outcome.

Perioperative erythropoietin

Concern about the risks of allogeneic transfusion is widespread but disproportionate to the risk. Autologous transfusion is misperceived to be safer. In a retrospective analysis, the risk to the donor of a severe reaction requiring hospital admission was 6:100 000 when patients made preoperative autologous blood donations (PABD) and 18:100 000 if it was the donor's first experience, compared to 0.5:100 000 for allogeneic donors. Autologous donors are less likely to receive homologous blood but more likely to be transfused than those who do not donate. The risks of transfusion due to clerical error, bacterial contamination, and blood processing are equally great in both groups. Methods of decreasing allogeneic blood transfusion include lowering the "transfusion trigger" when appropriate as discussed above, autologous blood donation techniques and perioperative erythropoietin therapy.[74]

In the United States rHUEpo has been approved by the FDA for anemic patients scheduled for elective surgery (with the exception of cardiac and vascular surgery). rHUEpo has been used to improve the collection of autologous blood in patients undergoing elective surgery, to correct anemia before surgery, and to hasten the postoperative erythropoietic response.[75]

Preoperative autologous blood donation continues to be used as a blood conserving technique and appears most beneficial for patients at risk for blood transfusion who are undergoing procedures with substantial blood loss.[74] Erythropoietin has been used to augment the number of preoperative autologous units collected. Treatment may also be indicated in patients who reject transfusions because of religious convictions and in bone marrow donors.[75] The optimal treatment schedule is 250 to 300 IU/kg of rHUEpo administered subcutaneously twice weekly over the 3-week period prior to surgery. Intravenous iron supplementation (iron saccharate 200 mg) should be administered at each preoperative autologous donation visit. Alternatively, at least 200 mg of oral elemental iron can be given daily.[75]

Patients who do not accept blood products

Surgical experience with Jehovah's witnesses has demonstrated that people can tolerate very low hemoglobin levels and survive. A review of 16 series published between 1983 and 1990, involving 1404 operations on Jehovah's Witnesses found that anemia was the primary cause of death in only 8 (0.6%) patients and a contributor to death in an additional 12 patients (0.9%).[76] Another large review involving 4722 Jehovah's Witnesses revealed only 23 deaths due to anemia, nearly all of whom had a hemoglobin of less than 5 mg/dl.[77] The general management of

these patients includes maximizing preoperative hemoglobin by eliminating any causes of impaired hematopoiesis. Recombinant erythropoietin has human albumin as a stabilizer, so some Jehovah's Witnesses will decline use of this product. Some patients will permit the use of intraoperative cell savers. If abnormal bleeding occurs, permissible hemostatic agents include DDAVP, antifibrinolytic agents, aprotinin, bovine thrombin and possibly recombinant factor VIIa.

Perioperative DVT prophylaxis

Recent venous thromboembolism greatly increases the risk of postoperative thromboembolism. Recommendations regarding heparin therapy are based on the interval between the thromboembolic event and the operative procedure. Untreated, there is a 50% risk of recurrent thromboembolism in the first month after a deep venous thrombosis (DVT). Warfarin therapy reduces the risk to 5%. Recurrent episodes of thromboembolism have a 6% fatality rate. Similarly, recurrent arterial embolism has a 20% fatality rate and a 40% risk of serious permanent disability. Among patients on anticoagulants the risk of severe postoperative hemorrhage is estimated to be about 3% and, of those, about 3% (0.09% overall) are fatal, making the risk of fatal embolic disease without anticoagulation about 30 times greater than the risk of death from hemorrhage with anticoagulation. However, 50% of major postoperative bleeding events lead to re-operation and 1.5% result in permanent disability. Total knee and hip replacement surgery is especially thrombogenic, as is neurosurgery. In a meta-analysis, total knee replacement, for example, carried a 64% risk of DVT if no prophylaxis was used, a proximal DVT risk of 15% and a DVT-related fatality rate of 0.2% to 0.7%. In one study, DVT rates were reduced to 30% by use of low-molecular-weight heparin (LMWH). It is worth noting that most postoperative DVTs in this setting are asymptomatic. European orthopedists generally begin LMWH therapy 12 h before surgery at half doses, whereas approved usage in the USA calls for 30 mg LMWH every 12 h starting 12–24 h after surgery and continuing for 7–10 days. The bleeding rates are low, 0.9% and 3.5%, respectively. Even so, many American orthopedists are reluctant to use LMWH because of hemorrhagic risk. Prophylactic warfarin therapy in these patients, in contrast, especially if begun just before or immediately after surgery, is less commonly associated with hemorrhage into the replaced knee, but is also less effective in reducing the risk of DVT. A meta-analysis showed that hip surgery is more commonly associated with symptomatic venous thromboembolic events (VTE) than is knee surgery. Another meta-analysis showed that hip replacement under spinal anesthesia is less often followed by VTE than when it is performed under general anesthesia. A variety of new anticoagulant drugs, such as pentassacharide, are under study for use as an alternative to unfractionated heparin (UFH) and LMWH in high-risk patients. The interested reader is referred to a review.[78]

Duration of anticoagulation for surgery-related DVT

Recent data from randomized studies show that indefinite anticoagulation with either moderate intensity vitamin K antagonist (INR 1.5–2.0) or conventional intensity (INR 2.0–3.0) significantly reduces the risk of recurrent VTE in patients with idiopathic DVT (not related to surgery, trauma, or pregnancy). However, the optimal duration of anticoagulation therapy for postoperative VTE without an ongoing risk factor has not been defined in randomized trials. The standard practice is to give secondary prophylaxis with an oral vitamin K antagonist for 3 months.

Asymptomatic coagulopathies

In the course of a preoperative laboratory evaluation or during a hospitalization, it is not unusual to find prolonged aPTT or INR in a patient without a significant bleeding history. In some, a more detailed, focused history may reveal abnormal bleeding. However, for many there will be no such history or a lack of previous hemostatic challenge. The evaluation of these laboratory findings should proceed along the lines of the evaluation of an outpatient with similar findings, with the following points in mind.

1. Minute quantities of heparin in indwelling catheters may prolong coagulation times. Thus, samples for coagulation tests should always be obtained by peripheral venipuncture; even "wasting" the initial blood drawn through a catheter does not ensure lack of contamination.

2. Up to 10% of hospitalized patients will be found to have a slightly prolonged aPTT (up to 40 seconds) without an identifiable cause.

3. A mixing study (1:1 dilution) should always be performed in a patient with a new coagulopathy to determine if there is the presence of an inhibitor. Lupus inhibitors (see appropriate section) are common in hospitalized patients and are associated with increased thrombotic risk in certain populations.

4. Mild hemophilia A and B, and especially von Willebrand disease, may not be diagnosed until adulthood in conjunction with a major hemostatic stress (such as postpartum in the case of von Willebrand disease). Thus, if there is a history of bleeding and/or the

planned procedure is high-risk for hemorrhage, an appropriate diagnostic evaluation should be performed.

REFERENCES

1. Rapaport, S. I. Preoperative hemostatic evaluation–which tests, if any? *Blood* 1983; **61**(2): 229–231.

2. Katsaros, D., Petricevic, M., Snow, N. J. *et al.* Tranexamic acid reduces postbypass blood use: a double-blinded, prospective, randomized study of 210 patients. *Ann. Thorac. Surg.* 1996; **61**(4): 1131–1135.

3. George, J. N. & Shattil, S. J. The clinical importance of acquired abnormalities of platelet function. *N. Engl. J. Med.* 1991; **324**(1): 27–39.

4. Cattaneo, M., Harris, A. S., Stromberg, U., & Mannucci, P. M. The effect of desmopressin on reducing blood loss in cardiac surgery – a meta-analysis of double-blind, placebo-controlled trials. *Thromb. Haemost.* 1995; **74**(4): 1064–1070.

5. Sheridan, D. P., Card, R. T., Pinilla, J. C. *et al.* Use of desmopressin acetate to reduce blood transfusion requirements during cardiac surgery in patients with acetylsalicylic-acid-induced platelet dysfunction. *Can. J. Surg.* 1994; **37**(1): 33–36.

6. Dilthey, G., Dietrich, W., Spannagl, M., & Richter, J. A. Influence of desmopressin acetate on homologous blood requirements in cardiac surgical patients pretreated with aspirin. *J. Cardiothorac. Vasc. Anesth.* 1993; **7**(4): 425–430.

7. Menichetti, A., Tritapepe, L., Ruvolo, G. *et al.* Changes in coagulation patterns, blood loss and blood use after cardiopulmonary bypass: aprotinin vs tranexamic acid vs epsilon aminocaproic acid. *J. Cardiovasc. Surg. (Torino).* 1996; **37**(4): 401–407.

8. Janssens, M., Hartstein, G., & David, J. L. Reduction in requirements for allogeneic blood products: pharmacologic methods. *Ann. Thorac. Surg.* 1996; **62**(6): 1944–1950.

9. Rich, J. B. The efficacy and safety of aprotinin use in cardiac surgery. *Ann. Thorac. Surg.* 1998; **66**(5 Suppl): S6–S11.

10. Mannucci, P. M. Desmopressin: a nontransfusional form of treatment for congenital and acquired bleeding disorders. *Blood* 1988; **72**(5): 1449–1455.

11. Royston, D., Bidstrup, B. P., Taylor, K. M., & Sapsford, R. N. Effect of aprotinin on need for blood transfusion after repeat open-heart surgery. *Lancet* 1987; **2**(8571): 1289–1291.

12. Mannucci, P. M. Hemostatic drugs. *N. Engl. J. Med.* 1998; **339**(4): 245–253.

13. Vander Salm, T. J., Kaur, S., Lancey, R. A. *et al.* Reduction of bleeding after heart operations through the prophylactic use of epsilon-aminocaproic acid. *J. Thorac. Cardiovasc. Surg.* 1996; **112**(4): 1098–1107.

14. Horrow, J. C., Van Riper, D. F., Strong, M. D. *et al.* The dose-response relationship of tranexamic acid. *Anesthesiology* 1995; **82**(2): 383–392.

15. Reece, T. B., Maxey, T. S., & Kron, I. L. A prospectus on tissue adhesives. *Am. J. Surg.* 2001; **182**(2 Suppl.): 40S–44S.

16. Carless, P.A., Anthony, D.M., & Henry, D.A. Systematic review of the use of fibrin sealant to minimize perioperative allogeneic blood transfusion. *Br. J. Surg.* 2002; **89**(6): 695–703.

17. Vinnicombe, J. & Shuttleworth, K. E. Aminocaproic acid in the control of haemorrhage after prostatectomy. Safety of aminocaproic acid – a controlled trial. *Lancet* 1966; **1**(7431): 232–234.

18. Hedner, U. NovoSeven as a universal haemostatic agent. *Blood Coagul. Fibrinol.* 2000; **11** Suppl 1: S107–S111.

19. Porte, R. J. Coagulation and fibrinolysis in orthotopic liver transplantation: current views and insights. *Semin. Thromb. Hemost.* 1993; **19**(3): 191–196.

20. Morikawa, T. Tissue sealing. *Am. J. Surg.* 2001; **182**(2 Suppl): 29S–35S.

21. Gerlach, R., Tolle, F., Raabe, A. et al. Increased risk for postoperative hemorrhage after intracranial surgery in patients with decreased factor XIII activity: implications of a prospective study. *Stroke* 2002; **33**(6): 1618–1623.

22. Lundberg, G. D. Is there a need for routine preoperative laboratory tests? *J. Am. Med. Assoc.* 1985; **253**(24): 3589.

23. Shapiro, M. B., Jenkins, D. H., Schwab, C. W., & Rotondo, M. F. Damage control: collective review. *J. Trauma* 2000; **49**(5): 969–978.

24. Martin, R. R. & Byrne, M. Postoperative care and complications of damage control surgery. *Surg. Clin. N. Am.* 1997; **77**(4): 929–942.

25. Johnson, J. W., Gracias, V. H., Schwab, C. W. et al. Evolution in damage control for exsanguinating penetrating abdominal injury. *J. Trauma* 2001; **51**(2): 261–269.

26. Gubler, K. D., Gentilello, L. M., Hassantash, S. A., & Maier, R. V. The impact of hypothermia on dilutional coagulopathy. *J. Trauma* 1994; **36**(6): 847–851.

27. Martinowitz, U., Kenet, G., Segal, E. et al. Recombinant activated factor VII for adjunctive hemorrhage control in trauma. *J. Trauma* 2001; **51**(3): 431–438.

28. Holcomb, J. B., McClain, J. M., Pusateri, A. E. et al. Fibrin sealant foam sprayed directly on liver injuries decreases blood loss in resuscitated rats. *J. Trauma* 2000; **49**(2): 246–250.

29. Lozier, J. N. & Lessler, C. M. Clinical aspects and therapy of hemophilia. In Hoffman, R., Benz, E. J., Shattil, S. J. et al. eds. *Hematology Basic Principles and Practice*. Philadelphia: Churchill Livingstone; 2000: 1884–1885.

30. White, G. C. & Roberts, H. R. The treatment of factor VIII inhibitors – a general overview. *Vox Sang* 1996; **70** Suppl 1: 19–23.

31. Roberts, H. R. & Hofmann, M. Hemophilia A and hemophilia B. In Beutler, E., Lichtman, M. A., Coller, B. S. et al., eds. *Williams Hematology*. New York: McGraw-Hill, 2001: 1650–1655.

32. Lusher, J. M. Recombinant factor VIIa (NovoSeven) in the treatment of internal bleeding in patients with factor VIII and IX inhibitors. *Haemostasis* 1996; **26**(Suppl 1.): 124–130.

33. Monroe, D. M., Hoffman, M., Oliver, J. A., & Roberts, H. R. A possible mechanism of action of activated factor VII independent of tissue factor. *Blood Coagul. Fibrinol.* 1998; **9**: S15–S20.

34. Kjalke, M., Monroe, D. M., Hoffman, M. et al. Active site-inactivated factors VIIa, Xa, and IXa inhibit individual steps in a cell-based model of tissue factor-initiated coagulation. *Thromb. Haemost.* 1998; **80**(4): 578–584.

35. Aledort, L. M., Green, D., & Teitel, J. M. Unexpected bleeding disorders. *Hematology (Am. Soc. Hematol. Educ. Program).* 2001; 306–321.

36. Kenet, G., Walden, R., Eldad, A., & Martinowitz, U. Treatment of traumatic bleeding with recombinant factor VIIa. *Lancet* 1999; **354**(9193): 1879.

37. Ingerslev, J. Efficacy and safety of recombinant factor VIIa in the prophylaxis of bleeding in various surgical procedures in hemophilic patients with factor VIII and factor IX inhibitors. *Semin. Thromb. Hemost.* 2000; **26**(4): 425–432.

38. Hedner, U. Recombinant factor VIIa (NovoSeven (R)) as a hemostatic agent. *Semin. Hematol.* 2001; **38**(4): 43–47.

39. Schulman, S. Continuous infusion of recombinant factor VIIa in hemophilic patients with inhibitors: safety, monitoring, and cost effectiveness. *Semin. Thromb. Hemost.* 2000; **26**(4): 421–424.

40. Kasper, C. K. Problems with the potency of factor VIII concentrate. *N. Engl. J. Med.* 1981; **305**(1): 50–51.

41. Chavin, S. I., Siegel, D. M., Rocco, T. A., Jr., & Olson, J. P. Acute myocardial infarction during treatment with an activated prothrombin complex concentrate in a patient with factor VIII deficiency and a factor VIII inhibitor. *Am. J. Med.* 1988; **85**(2): 245–249.

42. Walsh, P. N., Rizza, C. R., Matthews, J. M. et al. Epsilon-aminocaproic acid therapy for dental extractions in haemophilia and Christmas disease: a double blind controlled trial. *Br. J. Haematol.* 1971; **20**(5): 463–475.

43. Forbes, C. D., Barr, R. D., Reid, G. et al. Tranexamic acid in control of haemorrhage after dental extraction in haemophilia and Christmas disease. *Br. Med. J.* 1972; **2**(809): 311–313.

44. Martinowitz, U. & Saltz, R. Fibrin sealant. *Curr. Opin. Hematol.* 1996; **3**(5): 395–402.

45. Asakai, R., Chung, D. W., Davie, E. W., & Seligsohn, U. Factor XI deficiency in Ashkenazi Jews in Israel. *N. Engl. J. Med.* 1991; **325**(3): 153–158.

46. Edson, J. R., White, J. G., & Krivit, W. The enigma of severe factor XI deficiency without hemorrhagic symptoms. Distinction from Hageman factor and "Fletcher factor" deficiency; family study; and problems of diagnosis. *Thromb. Diath. Haemorrh.* 1967; **18**(3–4): 342–348.

47. Castaman, G., Ruggeri, M., & Rodeghiero, F. Clinical usefulness of desmopressin for prevention of surgical bleeding in patients with symptomatic heterozygous factor XI deficiency. *Br. J. Haematol.* 1996; **94**(1): 168–170.

48. Seligsohn, U. Factor XI deficiency. *Thromb. Haemost.* 1993; **70**(1): 68–71.

49. Mannucci, P. M., Bauer, K. A., Santagostino, E. et al. Activation of the coagulation cascade after infusion of a factor XI concentrate in congenitally deficient patients. *Blood* 1994; **84**(4): 1314–1319.

50. Mannucci, P. M. Desmopressin (DDAVP) in the treatment of bleeding disorders: the first 20 years. *Blood* 1997; **90**(7): 2515–2521.

51. Mannucci, P. M., Tenconi, P. M., Castaman, G., & Rodeghiero, F. Comparison of four virus-inactivated plasma concentrates for treatment of severe von Willebrand disease: a cross-over randomized trial. *Blood* 1992; **79**(12): 3130–3137.

52. Platelet transfusion therapy. National Institutes of Health Consensus Conference. *Transfus. Med. Rev.* 1987; **1**(3): 195–200.

53. Francis, C. W. & Kaplan, K. L. Hematologic problems in the surgical patient: bleeding and thrombosis. In Hoffman, R., Benz, E. J., Shattil, S. J. *et al.*, eds. *Hematology Basic Principles and Practice*. Philadelphia: Churchill Livingstone, 2000: 2381–2383.

54. Peters, M. & Heijboer, H. Treatment of a patient with Bernard–Soulier syndrome and recurrent nosebleeds with recombinant factor VIIa. *Thromb. Haemost.* 1998; **80**(2): 352.

55. Final report on the aspirin component of the ongoing Physicians' Health Study. Steering Committee of the Physicians' Health Study Research Group. *N. Engl. J. Med.* 1989; **321**(3): 129–135.

56. Despotis, G. J., Filos, K. S., Zoys, T. N. *et al.* Factors associated with excessive postoperative blood loss and hemostatic transfusion requirements: a multivariate analysis in cardiac surgical patients. *Anesth. Analg.* 1996; **82**(1): 13–21.

57. Horlocker, T. T., Wedel, D. J., & Offord, K. P. Does preoperative antiplatelet therapy increase the risk of hemorrhagic complications associated with regional anesthesia? *Anesth. Analg.* 1990; **70**(6): 631–634.

58. McTavish, D., Faulds, D., & Goa, K. L. Ticlopidine. An updated review of its pharmacology and therapeutic use in platelet-dependent disorders. *Drugs* 1990; **40**(2): 238–259.

59. Castillo, R., Lozano, T., Escolar, G. *et al.* Defective platelet adhesion on vessel subendothelium in uremic patients. *Blood* 1986; **68**(2): 337–342.

60. Diaz-Buxo, J. A. & Donadio, J. V., Jr. Complications of percutaneous renal biopsy: an analysis of 1,000 consecutive biopsies. *Clin. Nephrol.* 1975; **4**(6): 223–227.

61. Castaldi, P. A., Rozenberg, M. C., & Stewart, J. H. The bleeding disorder of uraemia. A qualitative platelet defect. *Lancet* 1966; **2**(7454): 66–69.

62. Hutton, R. A. & O'Shea, M. J. Haemostatic mechanism in uraemia. *J. Clin. Pathol.* 1968; **21**(3): 406–411.

63. Bolan, C. D. & Alving, B. M. Pharmacologic agents in the management of bleeding disorders. *Transfusion* 1990; **30**(6): 541–551.

64. Shattil, S. J., Abrams, C. S., & Bennett, J. S. Acquired qualitative platelet disorders due to diseases, drugs, and foods. In Beutler, E., Lichtman, M. A., Coller, B. S. *et al.*, eds. *Williams Hematology*. New York: McGraw-Hill, 2001: 1585.

65. Livio, M., Benigni, A., Vigano, G. *et al.* Moderate doses of aspirin and risk of bleeding in renal failure. *Lancet* 1986; **1**(8478): 414–416.

66. Heistinger, M., Stockenhuber, F., Schneider, B. *et al.* Effect of conjugated estrogens on platelet function and prostacyclin generation in CRF. *Kidney Int.* 1990; **38**(6): 1181–1186.

67. Fellin, F. & Murphy, S. Hematologic problems in the preoperative patient. *Med. Clin. N. Am.* 1987; **71**(3): 477–487.

68. van Genderen, P. J., Mulder, P. G., Waleboer, M. *et al.* Prevention and treatment of thrombotic complications in essential thrombocythaemia: efficacy and safety of aspirin. *Br. J. Haematol.* 1997; **97**(1): 179–184.

69. Marassi, A., Manzullo, V., di C. V., & Mannucci, P. M. Thromboembolism following prothrombin complex concentrates and major surgery in severe liver disease. *Thromb. Haemost.* 1978; **39**(3): 787–788.

70. Spence, R. K., Carson, J. A., Poses, R. *et al.* Elective surgery without transfusion: influence of preoperative hemoglobin level and blood loss on mortality. *Am. J. Surg.* 1990; **159**(3): 320–324.

71. Hebert, P. C., Wells, G., Martin, C. *et al.* A Canadian survey of transfusion practices in critically ill patients. *Crit. Care Med.* 1998; **26**(3): 482–487.

72. Hebert, P. C., Wells, G., Martin, C. *et al.* Variation in red cell transfusion practice in the intensive care unit: a multicentre cohort study. *Crit. Care* 1999; **3**(2): 57–63.

73. Hebert, P. C., Wells, G., Blajchman, M. A. *et al.* A multicenter, randomized, controlled clinical trial of transfusion requirements in critical care. *N. Engl. J. Med.* 1999; **340**(6): 409–417.

74. Goodnough, L. T., Brecher, M. E., Kanter, M. H., & AuBuchon, J. P. Transfusion medicine. Second of two parts – blood conservation. *N. Engl. J. Med.* 1999; **340**(7): 525–533.

75. Cazzola, M., Mercuriali, F., & Brugnara, C. Use of recombinant human erythropoietin outside the setting of uremia. *Blood* 1997; **89**(12): 4248–4267.

76. Kitchens, C. S. Are transfusions overrated? Surgical outcome of Jehovah's Witnesses. *Am. J. Med.* 1993; **94**(2): 117–119.

77. Viele, M. K. & Weiskopf, R. B. What can we learn about the need for transfusion from patients who refuse blood? The experience with Jehovah's Witnesses. *Transfusion* 1994; **34**(5): 396–401.

78. Ansell, J. E., Weitz, J. I., & Comerota, A. J. Advances in therapy and the management of antithrombic drugs for venous thromboembolism, I. New anticoagulant drugs. *Hematology (Am. Soc. Hematol. Educ. Prog.)* 2000: 266–284.

18

Surgical issues affecting patients with hematologic malignancies

Eve Rodler[1] and Ted Wun[2]

[1]Robert Wood Johnson School of Medicine, Camden, NJ
[2]VA Northern California Health Care System, Sacramento, CA

Introduction

Hematologic malignancies are a heterogeneous group of malignant disorders that affect cells originating from bone marrow or lymphatic tissue.[1] Patients with a diagnosis of leukemia, lymphoma, or multiple myeloma are susceptible to life-threatening crises such as leukostasis, disseminated intravascular coagulation, tumor lysis syndrome, infection, respiratory distress due to enlarging masses, and neutropenic enterocolitis (typhlitis). These serious problems may require surgical management or they may have an impact on the perioperative management of patients with hematologic malignancies. Surgery plays a role in the diagnosis of hematologic malignancies, including excisional lymph node biopsies, mediastinoscopy, or laparoscopy, in Hodgkin's and non-Hodgkin's lymphoma. Patients with hematologic malignancies may also present with common surgical problems, such as appendicitis, cholecystitis, bowel obstruction, ureteral obstruction, or bowel perforation due to infiltration of organs by malignant cells. There are also unique problems associated with the different types of hematologic malignancies which may require surgical intervention, such as: osteolytic bone lesions in multiple myeloma causing pathologic fractures; spinal cord compression due to multiple myeloma, lymphoma or solid tumors; hypersplenism in hairy cell leukemia; and neutropenic enterocolitis, perirectal abscesses, and locally invasive fungal infections during acute leukemia.

Indwelling venous access devices are often placed surgically for chronic central venous access to administer chemotherapy, long-term antibiotic therapy, blood and blood products, and total parenteral nutrition. Intraoperative complications related to the placement of central venous catheters are rare but include hemorrhage, pneumothorax, and hemothorax. Postoperative complications such as thrombosis, infection, and catheter shear can occur and require careful management to avoid significant adverse outcomes for patients.[2]

Preoperative considerations in patients with hematologic malignancies include leukocytosis, cytopenias, infection, hemostatic disorders, coagulopathies, and metabolic disturbances. Leukemia, lymphoma, and myeloma patients undergoing surgery who require blood or blood products should receive only leukocyte-depleted, irradiated, CMV-appropriate products to avoid the risk of alloimmunization and graft versus host disease. Patients who have received prior chemotherapy require preoperative evaluation to exclude the possibility of treatment related toxicities to the heart, lungs, kidneys, or liver, which could affect surgical outcome.

Acute leukemias

Brief description

Leukemia is a malignant disease of the hematopoietic system in which a somatic mutation occurs in a bone marrow progenitor cell, followed by unrestrained clonal proliferation of the progeny of that altered cell. The leukemias are broadly divided into acute leukemias, which progress rapidly and, if left untreated, cause death in a few weeks to months, and chronic leukemias, which have a more indolent course, with survival extending from months to years.

Acute myelogenous leukemia (AML) is characterized by a defect in early progenitor cells at some point along the pathway of differentiation into not only myeloid, but also monocytoid, megakaryocytic, and occasionally erythroid cells. AML accounts for 80% of the acute leukemias in adults. AML is usually treated with an anthracycline and

Medical Management of the Surgical Patient: A Textbook of Perioperative Medicine, ed. M. F. Lubin, R. B. Smith, T. F. Dobson, N. Spell, H. K. Walker. 4th edn. Published by Cambridge University Press. © Cambridge University 2006.

cytarabine for induction. High dose chemotherapy with either autologous stem cell infusion or allogeneic stem cell transplantation may be used to treat patients who have relapsed after chemotherapy or who are at high risk for relapse. Although 60% to 70% of adult AML patients can achieve complete response to induction, long-term survival is only approximately 20%.

Acute lymphoblastic leukemia (ALL) originates in a single B- or T-lymphocyte progenitor cell that has undergone somatic genetic mutation leading to arrested maturation and dysregulated growth. ALL accounts for less than 1% of all adult malignancies and approximately 20% of acute leukemias. In addition to presenting with symptoms and signs typical of cytopenias, ALL patients may have hepatosplenomegaly and nodal enlargement. Similar to AML, treatment for ALL involves chemotherapy to try to induce a remission. Unlike AML, central nervous system relapse is common and prophylaxis is routine. Allogeneic peripheral stem cell transplantations can be offered to ALL patients with an HLA-identical sibling donor and other alternatives include unrelated donor or autologous transplants. Long-term survival rates for adult patients with ALL range from 20% to 40% depending on associated risk factors.

Abdominal pain in the neutropenic patient with acute leukemia

Patients with acute leukemias either present with neutropenia (neutrophil count less than $1000/mm^3$) because of their disease or as the result of treatment with chemotherapy. Surgeons may be consulted to evaluate acute leukemia patients with abdominal pain. This discussion will focus on neutropenic enterocolitis, disseminated abdominal infections, and unique causes of abdominal pain in bone marrow transplant patients. However, other causes of abdominal pain common in non-neutropenic patients should also be considered in the evaluation of acute abdominal pain.

Neutropenic enterocolitis

Neutropenic enterocolitis, known also as typhlitis (from the Greek word meaning cecum), is characterized by neutropenia, bowel wall inflammation, and edema that can progress to necrosis. It is the most common cause of abdominal pain in the neutropenic patient.[3] The true incidence of neutropenic enterocolitis is difficult to determine. While it may only occur in 2.6% of all adults with leukemia,[4] the incidence may be as high as 35% to 62%.[5-7] In two studies, neutropenic enterocolitis was the cause of 61% to 100% of acute abdominal problems necessitating surgery in leukemic patients.[8,9]

The pathogenesis of neutropenic enterocolitis appears to be multifactorial and is thought to result from neutropenia, chemotherapy or radiotherapy-induced destruction of normal mucosa, intramural hemorrhage caused by severe thrombocytopenia and change in the normal gastrointestinal flora caused by antibiotics, antifungal agents, and colonization by hospital pathogens.[10,11] The cecum appears to be at increased risk because it is the least vascularized and most distensible region of the colon, and as distension increases, blood flow to the cecum further decreases.[12] Neutropenic enterocolitis occurs most commonly after chemotherapy-induced neutropenia, with a peak incidence 7 to 14 days after the initiation of therapy. The bowel develops transmural edema with patchy areas of ulceration and necrosis, which become portals of entry for microorganisms into the circulation. Organisms include *Pseudomonas aeruginosa*, *Klebsiella pneumoniae*, *Escherichia coli*, Enterobacteriaceae, *Candida* and Clostridia species.[13-15] In particular, *Clostridium septicum* has been identified as a primary pathogen in neutropenic enterocolitis.[16,17] In 40% to 74% of cases of neutropenic enterocolitis, bacteria are isolated from the blood.[6,7,9,17]

Neutropenic enterocolitis most commonly presents with fever and classic peritoneal signs and symptoms.[18] However, the use of steroids may obscure the diagnosis by masking the symptom of abdominal pain. Physical examination may reveal peritoneal signs, decreased bowel sounds, and in some cases, a right lower quadrant mass.[19] Aside from blood and urine cultures, stool for *C. difficile* toxin should be sent to assess for pseudomembranous colitis.

Radiographs usually show nonspecific findings such as mild ileus and focal dilatation of scattered small bowel loops.[20] Computed tomography (CT) scan shows diffuse bowel wall thickening, occasional low attenuation areas consistent with edema or necrosis, thickening of fascial planes, pericolonic fluid, and pneumatosis.[21] CT scan is especially helpful in distinguishing between appendicitis and neutropenic enterocolitis since often the differential diagnosis is between these two conditions.

Treatment for neutropenic enterocolitis is somewhat controversial. Some authors support surgical therapy[4,9,19] while others favor conservative, nonoperative management.[7] Most recommend individualized treatment, which utilizes both medical and surgical management.[5,12,16,18,20] Initial management should be early and aggressive since the mortality rate in neutropenic enterocolitis varies from 50% to 100%.[22] It includes nasogastric decompression, fluid and nutritional support and antibiotics with broad coverage of aerobic and anaerobic pathogens. Surgery is reserved for perforation, hemorrhage, abscess, obstruction, or failure to improve with medical management.

Disseminated abdominal infections

Disseminated fungal infection involving the liver and or the spleen may cause abdominal pain in acute leukemia patients following chemotherapy. Fungal organisms are the second most common cause of infection in neutropenic patients after bacteria. In adult patients with acute lymphoblastic leukemia, *Candida* and *Aspergillus* species are responsible for approximately 90% of fungal infections.[21] When disseminated fungal infection involves the liver or spleen it is called focal hepatic candidiasis, hepatosplenic candidiasis, or hepatic candidiasis. Clinically it is characterized by fever, abdominal pain which can be diffuse or localized to the right upper quadrant, anorexia, nausea, and vomiting.[23,24] Symptoms are caused by abscesses in the liver, spleen, and occasionally the kidneys. CT scan or ultrasound has characteristic "bull's eye lesions" which become evident as the white blood cell count recovers.[23] Surgical intervention has occurred rarely in patients who developed biliary tract candidiasis and involved cholecystectomy.[25] In addition, there are cases of neutropenic patients with acute leukemia who developed splenic abscesses from candidiasis and did not improve on antifungal therapy. Ultimately, they required splenectomy.[26]

Viral infections such as herpes simplex virus (HSV) and cytomegalovirus (CMV) are common in acute leukemic patients and occasionally necessitate surgery. When HSV involves the gastrointestinal tract, surgical intervention may become necessary if complications such as perforation or obstruction occur. CMV is the most common viral infection in the period following bone marrow transplantation. It is also usually due to viral reactivation and can result in abdominal involvement, including gastritis, esophagitis, and enterocolitis. As in the case of severe HSV infection, CMV infection of the abdominal viscera can lead to necrosis, perforation, or obstruction, requiring surgery.[3]

Abdominal pain in the bone marrow transplant patient

Although surgical intervention for abdominal pain in bone marrow transplant (BMT) patients is not common, surgeons are often consulted to evaluate abdominal pain in these patients. In one retrospective study of 45 autologous BMT patients followed for 100 days post-transplantation, abdominal pain was documented in 51% and surgical consultation was obtained in 22% of the cases. Of the patients who had a surgical evaluation, 40% required laparotomy.[27]

Infectious enteritis of bacterial, viral, fungal, or parasitic origin occurs in BMT patients, and occasionally requires surgery for complications in severe disease.

Graft-versus-host disease (GVHD) occurs when transplanted donor-derived T cells recognize and react to histoincompatible recipient antigens and cells, leading to significant morbidity and mortality.[28] Acute GVHD usually develops 25–35 days following transplantation. The major organs involved are the skin, liver, and gastrointestinal tract. Clinical manifestations of acute GVHD of the gut include nausea, vomiting, crampy abdominal pain, distention, ileus, intestinal bleeding and voluminous diarrhea (often bloody).[29] Chronic GVHD develops in 60% to 80% of long-term survivors of allogeneic stem cell transplantation. It occurs 100 or more days post-transplant and is often preceded by acute GVHD.[30] Gastrointestinal involvement is not usually a prominent manifestation of chronic GVHD.

Abdominal pain in the post transplant patient may be caused by infections such as enteritis or disease as mentioned above. In addition, abdominal pain, particularly right upper quadrant pain, can be due to cholecystitis, hepatic veno-occlusive disease (VOD), hepatic GVHD, and gastroduodenal ulcerations or erosions.[3] Hepatic VOD is a common complication of allogeneic BMT, occurring in 20% to 30% of patients within 2 to 3 weeks of transplant. It is caused by the intensive preparative regimen of chemotherapy or combined chemoradiation and is characterized initially by an increase in abdominal girth with weight gain and jaundice which can progress to abdominal pain, ascites, and encephalopathy.[29] Generally, there is no role for surgical therapy in VOD, but surgeons should be aware of this common cause of right upper quadrant pain to avoid unnecessary exploratory laparotomy or laparoscopy.

Anorectal infections in the patient with acute leukemia

Anorectal infection is a severe complication in acute leukemic patients, with an incidence of approximately 3.5% to 8% and a mortality rate of 45% to 78%.[31–33] These patients are often neutropenic, febrile, and complain of rectal pain. Examination may show mild to moderate erythema with induration and tenderness and rarely reveal fluctuance.[31,34] Digital rectal examination should not be performed due to the risk of infection and bleeding, but inspection and gentle palpation of the area should be done. The most common pathogens isolated at surgery or from wound aspirations are the Enterobacteriaceae, anaerobes, group D streptococci, and *Pseudomonas aeuruginosa*.[31,35]

Treatment options for perirectal infections include conservative medical management, and/or surgical drainage or debridement. However, there is hesitation to debride due to the perception these wounds heal very poorly. To date, there are no randomized trials upon which to base therapy. Troiani and DuBois[36] performed a review of the literature, which included five series of case reports, evaluating a total of 128 patients with anorectal infections. They concluded that, if the perirectal infection does not drain spontaneously early in the course with conservative measures including warm compresses, sitz baths, and broad spectrum antibiotics, surgical drainage and debridement should be undertaken, even if the patient is neutropenic. In the largest of these series, 54 leukemic patients with anorectal infections treated at M. D. Anderson over a 40-year period were reviewed.[37] Surgical drainage of abscess was achieved in all eleven cases in which it was attempted. Poor wound healing after either surgical or spontaneous drainage was documented in only one case. In sum, indications for surgery should include progression of local disease or sepsis despite adequate antibiotic coverage, obvious tissue necrosis, or fluctuance.

Invasive fungal infections in the patient with acute leukemia

Aspergillosis

Fungal infections in patients with acute leukemia who undergo induction chemotherapy are caused by *Aspergillus* in 30% of cases.[38] The prognosis of invasive pulmonary aspergillosis may be improved by early recognition of the infection, shortening the neutropenic period with the use of granulocyte colony-stimulating factor (G-CSF) and granulocyte–macrophage colony-stimulating factor (GM–CSF), effective antifungal treatment, and surgical resection of localized invasive pulmonary aspergillosis.[39–43] Therapy for invasive aspergillosis in neutropenic patients and in BMT patients involves high dose conventional amphotericin B (1.0 to 1.5 mg/kg per day) or a lipid formulation of amphotericin B. A third generation triazole, voriconazole may also be effective based on in vitro sensitivity data.[44]

Indications for and timing of thoracic surgery for localized invasive pulmonary aspergillosis are controversial. Early surgical resection can be effective in preventing life-threatening hemoptysis when pulmonary aspergillosis, which lies adjacent to major vessels, is surgically removed.[45] Relapse rates for patients who have recovered from an episode of invasive aspergillosis and receive subsequent chemotherapy for their underlying disease can be very high.[46] This rate can be decreased significantly with

the use of secondary antifungal prophylaxis and should be recommended even after successful surgical resection of a lesion.[47]

Zygomycosis

Zygomycosis (also called mucormycosis) is another invasive fungal infection that can lead to extremely high mortality in the neutropenic patient if left untreated. Zygomycosis can cause rhinocerebral or pulmonary disease after inhalation of spores. Patients may experience fever, facial pain, headache, and show signs of proptosis as the infection spreads through the nasal sinus, penetrates the cribiform plate, and extends into the meninges. The respiratory tract may also become involved. Presenting symptoms include pleuritic chest pain and hemoptysis and radiographic changes include patchy infiltrates, bronchopneumonia, consolidation, and cavitation sometimes with fungus ball formation. Zygomycosis (or any invasive fungal infection) of the sinuses in a neutropenic patient should be considered a surgical emergency requiring prompt and aggressive debridement followed by antifungal therapy.[47] Despite this, mortality rates are high.

Preoperative concerns

Evaluations and management of neutropenic fevers

Acute leukemic patients who have febrile neutropenia due to their underlying illness or to myeloablative therapy should receive adequate antibiotic coverage and await granulocyte cell count recovery prior to surgical procedures, unless a life-threatening problem necessitates early surgical intervention. A neutropenic acute leukemic patient with fever represents a medical urgency.[47]

The initial evaluation of the febrile neutropenic patient may be difficult because symptoms and signs of inflammation may be diminished or absent. Sites that are commonly infected should be inspected and evaluated, including the oropharynx, the periodontium, the paranasal sinuses, the perineum and anus, the fundus of the eye (for evidence of fungal infections), and the skin, particularly vascular catheter access sites. Peripheral blood cultures and samples from central venous access devices should be obtained. If the patient has diarrhea, stool cultures and *Clostridium difficile* toxin may reveal an infectious source. Examination of cerebrospinal fluid is not a routine procedure for neutropenic patients, but this should be undertaken if CNS symptoms are present and/or a CNS infection is suspected.

Empiric antibiotic therapy is an important part of therapy for acute leukemic patients with neutropenia and fevers. Detailed guidelines have been formulated for the treatment of such patients.[48] The following is a brief summary of the recent guidelines by the Infectious Diseases Society of America (IDSA) concerning management of high risk inpatients who have declining neutrophil counts or no indication of marrow recovery in the near term. Note also that afebrile patients who are neutropenic but who have signs or symptoms compatible with an infection should also have empirical antibiotic therapy begun in the same manner as for febrile patients.

Several studies have shown no significant difference in efficacy between monotherapy and multidrug combinations for empirical treatment of uncomplicated episodes of fever in neutropenic patients.[49–59] Any initial antibiotic regimen should include drugs with antipseudomonal activity. A two-drug regimen may be recommended over monotherapy for management of complicated cases such as infections associated with hypotension likely due to sepsis.[48] If there is suspicion of a gram-positive infection, vancomycin may be added to an empiric regimen. Further management should be tailored if an etiologic agent is identified. Persistent fever generally necessitates the empiric addition of an antifungal agent and/or changing the antibiotic coverage. Antibiotics continue until neutrophil recovery and fever lysis.

Transfusion of blood products

In patients with acute leukemia, blood and platelet transfusions are essential. Hemoglobin levels are generally maintained at 8 g/dl or higher in patients with other medical comorbidities. Prophylactic platelet transfusions should be given if platelets fall below 10 000/μl, based on recent randomized studies.[60] Higher levels should be maintained for patients with bleeding or fever. For acute leukemic patients undergoing operations a platelet level of 50 000 cells/mm^3 is felt to be safe based on retrospective data.[61] The use of aspirin and nonsteroidal anti-inflammatory agents should be avoided prior to surgery.

Cellular blood products given to acute leukemic patients should be irradiated to prevent potentially lethal transfusion-associated GVHD (TA-GVHD). Transfusion-associated GVHD occurs when donor immunocompetent T and natural killer cells attack recipient cells. Mortality is approximately 90% and there is no known effective therapy for transfusion-associated GVHD. Irradiating cellular blood products with 2500 cGy inactivates donor lymphocytes and inhibits their proliferation, thus preventing TA-GVHD.[62] Irradiation of blood components is recommended for all patients undergoing autologous or allogeneic bone marrow or peripheral stem cell transplants.

Leukocyte reduction of all blood products is recommended to decrease the incidence of subsequent refractoriness to platelet transfusion caused by HLA alloimmunization in patients requiring long-term platelet support.[63] The combination of irradiation and leukocyte depletion of platelet products can reduce HLA alloimmunization by about 50% by removing antigen-presenting cells.[64] Leukocytes can be removed from red cell and platelet concentrates by bedside leukocyte reduction filters or by pre-storage leukocyte reduction. Current standards by the American Association of Blood Bank require that red cell and platelets labeled as leukoreduced should contain less than 5×10^6 residual white cells. Leukocyte-reduced products are recommended for all autologous and allogeneic bone marrow and peripheral stem cell transplant recipients and candidates for transplant, and for all patients with acute leukemia and lymphoma.

Although the number of patients who will become alloimmunized by repeated transfusion of blood products is significantly reduced by leukocyte reduction and irradiation techniques, some patients can become refractory to platelet transfusions due to alloimmunization from prior pregnancies and transfusions in which leukodepleted products were not used. Platelet refractoriness can be defined as a 1-hour post-transfusion platelet count increment of less than 5000 cells/mm^3 after two sequential transfusions.[64] In these cases, HLA-matched or platelet cross-matched platelets from single donors may be required. Leukocyte reduction will also help prevent febrile non-hemolytic transfusion reactions.[63] Febrile non-hemolytic transfusion reactions are caused by antibodies in the recipient directed against HLA and/or neutrophil specific antigens on donor white blood cells and platelets ("leukoagglutinins").

Finally, leukocyte reduction reduces the risk of CMV transmission.[63] CMV is a leading cause of mortality and morbidity in leukemic patients undergoing allogeneic bone marrow or peripheral stem cell transplantation. While most CMV infections develop as a result of latent reactivation in the recipient, CMV can be transmitted via blood products. CMV-seronegative blood products should be provided to CMV sero-negative bone marrow and peripheral stem cell transplant recipients. Some transfusion experts believe that leukocyte reduction methods yield components that may be equivalent to CMV-seronegative components in terms of reducing the risk of transmission of CMV.[63,65]

Disseminated intravascular coagulation in acute leukemia

Acute leukemia, in particular the subtype acute promyelocytic leukemia (APL), is associated with a coagulopathy that results from disseminated intravascular coagulation (DIC), abnormal fibrinolysis, or both. Up to 90% of APL patients present with hemorrhagic complications.[66] Elective surgical procedures should be postponed until the coagulopathy is fully treated, and emergent procedures should be done with the assistance of a specialist familiar with the management of coagulopathies. Fibrinolysis also plays an important role in the hemorrhagic diathesis of APL.

There are several therapeutic approaches to managing the bleeding complications of acute leukemia in general and acute promyelocytic leukemia, in particular. The most important therapeutic intervention is to initiate treatment for the underlying illness. APL is notable for its response to all-*trans*-retinoic acid (ATRA), which induces differentiation, rather than destruction, of the leukemic promyelocytes. With the use of ATRA in APL patients, there is often early resolution of the bleeding diathesis. The abnormal lab findings indicating DIC and hyperfibrinolysis usually resolve within 2 to 3 days of starting ATRA. Aggressive platelet support should be implemented in the acute leukemic patient with bleeding, maintaining platelets above 50 000 cells/mm^3. Fresh frozen plasma may need to be transfused multiple times daily in order to maintain fibrinogen levels above 120 mg/dl. In severe or persisting DIC or bleeding, empiric low dose heparin (5 to 10 U/kg per h) can be initiated, although this is controversial. The benefit of heparin therapy has never been proven by prospective randomized trials. Patients with continued active bleeding while on heparin may be treated with antifibrinolytic agents such as epsilon aminocaproic acid or tranexamic acid as beneficial effects from these agents has been suggested.[67] These must be used with extreme caution because of the risk of thrombotic complications. For persistent perioperative bleeding local hemostatic products such as fibrin sealant can also be used.

Tumor lysis syndrome

Electrolyte disturbances are common in patients with hematologic malignancies and many of the chemotherapeutic agents used can exacerbate them. Tumor lysis syndrome can be precipitated by chemotherapy for rapidly proliferating malignancies such as acute leukemia and can lead to life threatening electrolyte disturbances and acute renal failure. Correction of electrolyte imbalances and maintenance of adequate hydration and urinary flow are important preoperative concerns.

Acute tumor lysis syndrome (ATLS) is characterized by the rapid development of hyperuricemia, hyperkalemia, hyperphosphatemia, hypocalcemia, and azotemia with acute renal failure.[68–70] It can occur spontaneously or during chemotherapy or radiation of hematologic malignancies. ATLS is caused by increased release of intracellular contents into the circulation during cell lysis.

The goal of management of ATLS is to prevent it. Patients at risk for ATLS should be treated with allopurinol and vigorous hydration for 24 to 48 hours before cytotoxic therapy. A high urine flow should be achieved to decrease the likelihood of uric acid and/or calcium phosphate precipitation in the kidneys. Uric acid nephropathy can also be prevented by alkalinization of the urine by the addition of sodium bicarbonate to intravenous fluids. Over zealous administration of bicarbonate can increase the likelihood of calcium phosphate precipitation, and can induce metabolic alkalosis which may exacerbate symptoms of hypocalcemia. Thus, administration of bicarbonate in the intravenous fluids should be discontinued after the serum uric acid level is normalized.

Urgent leukocyte reduction for acute leukemia

Acute leukemia can present with very high (100 000/mm^3) blast counts, leading to a phenomenon known as hyperleukocytosis. Patients often present in critical condition with respiratory failure, intracranial bleeding and altered mental status, and severe metabolic abnormalities. These complications have been attributed to leukostasis. The incidence of symptomatic hyperleukocytosis is higher in acute myelogenous leukemias than in acute lymphocytic leukemias because leukemic myeloblasts have a larger mean cell volume than leukemic lymphoblasts. Acute leukemic patients with symptomatic leukostasis are not stable for a surgical procedure requiring general anesthesia. Rarely such patients may need emergent surgery. In these cases, immediate cytoreduction with leukapheresis may enable the patient to proceed to surgery in a timely manner.

Leukapheresis has been shown to reduce early mortality in patients with AML with high white cell counts, but it has not been shown conclusively to improve long term survival.[71] The advantages of leukapheresis are its immediate cytoreductive effect and its ability to correct metabolic or coagulation problems rapidly by providing fresh plasma and electrolytes, decreasing the risk of hemorrhage and tumor lysis syndrome. A single leukapheresis can reduce the leukocyte count by 20% to 50%. It is unclear how leukapheresis should be used in patients with hyperleukocytosis but no clinical signs of leukostasis.

Chronic leukemias

Description

Chronic myelogenous leukemia (CML) is a pluripotent stem cell disease characterized by excessive proliferation of marrow granulocytes, a large proportion of mature neutrophils, anemia, basophilia, normal or elevated plate-let counts and often splenomegaly. The molecular basis for CML is a rearrangement between the ableson proto-oncogene and the breakpoint cluster region (bcr–abl) associated with the Philadelphia chromosome. CML accounts for 15% of all cases of leukemia. If they have a severe leukocytosis, patients may present with neurologi-cal symptoms or with respiratory distress (see discussion below). Untreated the disease inevitably progresses from a chronic phase to an accelerated phase that often termi-nates in acute leukemia, at which point therapy is usually unsuccessful and the patient has only a matter of weeks to months of life. Chronic phase CML is generally not asso-ciated with significant immune defects.

Chronic lymphocytic leukemia (CLL) is an indolent B-cell lymphoid malignancy, is the most common form of adult leukemia in the Western hemisphere and accounts for 25% of all leukemias. Complications of CLL include autoimmune hemolytic anemia, immune thrombocytopenic purpura, and pure red cell aplasia, and often hypogammaglobulin-emia with recurrent infections. To date, chemotherapy has not been successful at altering the natural history of CLL, although the use of fludarabine as a single agent has led to a prolonged progression free survival. Median survival for CLL patients is approximately 9 years.

Surgical issues

Splenectomy

Surgical involvement with patients who have chronic leu-kemia primarily relates to splenectomy. In addition, patients with CML and CLL may require other types of surgeries, not directly related to their disease, for which they would need perioperative care.

Splenectomy may be an effective treatment for CLL in specific situations. These include: patients with extensive splenomegaly unresponsive to chemotherapy; significant anemia or thrombocytopenia secondary to hypersplenism; and, those with autoimmune hemolytic anemia or throm-bocytopenia who have an inadequate response. Patients with CLL are predisposed to bacterial infection due to their underlying immunodeficiency. Splenectomy further adds to the risk of infection with encapsulated organisms. Therefore, pneumococcal as well as *Haemophillus* influenza type B, and meningococcal vaccines should be administered to these patients at least ten days prior to splenectomy to provide for optimal develop-ment of protective immunity.[72] When performed by experienced surgeons, the mortality of splenectomy is less than 10%.[73] Splenectomy is rarely performed for patients with CML.[74]

Preoperative concerns

Immunocompromised state of chronic leukemic patients

Chronic lymphocytic leukemia

As stated, perioperative infections are the major cause of morbidity and mortality in patients with CLL.[75] Patients with CLL have an underlying immunodeficient state caused by reduced serum immunoglobulins, a reduced percentage of CD4 + helper T-cells and an increased per-centage of CD8 + suppressor T-cells, and a reduced response to antigens. The pathogenesis of infection in CLL patients is further influenced by the disease stage and subsequent treatment with corticosteroids and che-motherapeutic agents, which are immunosuppressive.

Hypogammaglobulinemia is common in CLL, especially in patients with advanced disease. Patients have an inabil-ity to produce specific antibodies and an abnormal com-plement system making them more susceptible to infection. For CLL patients with repeated bacteria infec-tions due to hypogammaglobulinemia, administration of intravenous gammaglobulin may be considered. It is unclear, however, whether the administration of IVIG has any impact on survival in CLL patients.

In patients treated with conventional chemotherapy agents such as alkylators (e.g., chlorambucil) and/or cor-ticosteroids, the infections that occur are usually of bac-terial origin. With the introduction of purine analogue chemotherapy agents in the treatment of CLL patients such as fludarabine, a different spectrum of infectious complications has been seen. There has been an increase in opportunistic infections such as *Pneumocystis carinii*, Candida, Listeria, Cytomegalovirus, atypical mycobac-terial infections, Nocardia, and Herpesvirus infections. It is common practice to place patients on high-dose ste-roids or fludarabine on pneumocystis prophylaxis; some clinicians also place patients on anti-viral prophylaxis as well.[76]

Leukocytoreduction in chronic leukemia

Leukocytoreduction with a combination of leukapheresis and hydroxyurea therapy may be necessary for patients with CML in the perioperative setting. On the other hand, CLL is less likely to produce symptoms of leukostasis, but it may be treated with leukapheresis in certain situations where there is a rapidly rising white blood cell count.

Transfusion of blood products in chronic leukemia

Blood products for all patients with chronic leukemia should be leukocyte reduced to decrease the risk of alloimmunization. In addition, blood products should be irradiated in chronic leukemic patients who are bone marrow or peripheral blood stem cell transplant recipients to decrease the risk of transfusion related graft versus host disease. Patients with CLL who have been treated with fludarabine or other purine analogues should also only receive irradiated blood products.[77] CMV negative blood products should be provided for CMV seronegative chronic leukemic patients who are transplant recipients or candidates.

Hairy cell leukemia

Description

Hairy cell leukemia is an uncommon type of chronic B-cell leukemia characterized by pancytopenia and splenomegaly, and less commonly, lymphadenopathy. It tends to occur in older patients and makes up about 2% of all adult leukemias. Patients present with symptoms consistent with cytopenias, including infections, fatigue, and bleeding and sometimes with left upper quadrant pain from splenomegaly. The diagnosis is made by identification of lymphocytes with villous cytoplasmic projections in the peripheral blood and bone marrow.[78] The hairy cells exhibit tartrate-resistant acid phosphate (TRAP) activity. The disease can have a prolonged indolent course and approximately 10% of patients never need any therapy. Indications for treatment include massive or progressive splenomegaly, recurrent infections, constitutional symptoms such as fever or night sweats, anemia (Hgb <10 g/dl), thrombocytopenia (platelets $<100\,000$ cells/mm^3), neutropenia (absolute neutrophil count, 1000 cells/mm^3), or bulky lymphadenopathy.

Surgical issues

Splenectomy

In the past, splenectomy was the standard treatment for hairy cell leukemia.[79,80] Since the introduction of purine analogues for the treatment of hairy cell leukemia in the 1980s, splenectomy is no longer front line therapy. The preferred treatment for hairy cell leukemia is now the purine analogues, 2-deoxycoformycin (pentostatin) or 2-chlorodeoxyadenosine (2-CdA) which both produce complete responses in the majority of patients. Complete response rates for pentostatin have ranged from 72% to 76% compared with 50% to 88% with 2-CdA.[81]

Preoperative concerns

Risk of infection

Purine analogues cause immunosuppression due to a reduction in the number of immunocompetent lymphocytes as well as inhibition of lymphocyte activity. Both pentostatin and 2-CdA produce a significant fall in CD4+ and CD8+ cells following treatment. CD8+ cells may recover within 3 months, but CD4+ cells may take longer than 3 years to normalize.[82] Documented infections include bacteremia, herpes simplex reactivation, herpes zoster reactivation, and cytomegalovirus retinitis.[81]

Blood transfusions

Patients with hairy cell leukemia who are undergoing treatment or who have had prior treatment with one of the purine analogues are at increased risk of developing transfusion-associated graft versus host disease. Thus, they should receive only irradiated blood products. Leukocyte reduced blood products are also recommended for all leukemic patients.

Lymphoma

Description

Lymphomas are a heterogenous group of malignancies of the lymphatic system that typically arise in lymph node tissue, but may also occur outside of the lymphatic system. Broadly, lymphomas are categorized by histology into Hodgkin's lymphoma and non-Hodgkin's lymphoma (NHL).

Hodgkin's lymphoma is defined by the presence of the malignant Reed Sternberg and Hodgkin's cells in a background of reactive cells, which include lymphocytes, eosinophils, histiocytes, plasma cells and neutrophils. Clinically, patients often present with painless lymphadenopathy, especially in the cervical lymph nodes. Supradiaphragmatic lymph node involvement is present in about 90% of patients. The extent of disease involvement is strongly prognostic in Hodgkin's lymphoma. Treatment of Hodgkin's lymphoma involves a combination of chemotherapy and radiation therapy for all patients, except for those with Stage I-A with very favorable features (discussed below). With current polychemotherapy regimens, including ABVD (adriamycin, bleomycin, vinblastine, and prednisone) and the Stanford V (mechlorethamine, adriamycin, vinblastine, vincristine, bleomycin, etoposide, prednisone), 5-year survival rates have ranged from 56% (in patients with five or more risk factors)[83] up to 96% for patients with advanced stage (Stage IIB through IV) Hodgkin's lymphoma.[84]

Non-Hodgkins lymphoma refers to a heterogenous group of neoplastic diseases that all arise from somatic mutations in a lymphocyte progenitor cell and the resulting clone of malignant cells can have a B-cell or T-cell phenotype. The site of origin of the disorder can be any primary site in the lymphatic system, lymph nodes, spleen, or mucosa-associated lymphoid tissue; however, any organ in the body can be involved. Patients may present with B symptoms of fevers, weight loss, night sweats or enlarging peripheral nodes. Staging is the same as for Hodgkin's lymphoma, although anatomical stage is less prognostic in lymphomas. The revised European–American classification of lymphoid neoplasm (REAL) distinguishes B-cell and T-cell lymphomas, as does the World Health Organization (WHO) classification. Further subclassification divided each of the B-cell and T-cell lymphomas into: indolent lymphomas (low risk); aggressive lymphomas (intermediate risk); and very aggressive lymphomas (high risk). Low grade lymphomas are treatable but incurable in the majority of patients. Diffuse large B-cell lymphoma is the most common and comprises 40% of all cases. Prognostic factors for patients with aggressive lymphomas, as defined by the International Lymphoma prognostic factor index (IPI), include age greater than 60, elevated serum LDH, poor performance status, stage III or IV disease, and more than one extradnodal site of disease. Combination chemotherapy and radiotherapy is used as well as newer agents such as Rituximab, which is a human mouse chimeric monoclonal antibody that binds to the CD20 antigen. The role of autologous and allogeneic transplantation has been established in intermediate-risk and high-risk lymphomas and is being investigated in low-risk lymphomas.

Surgical issues

Biopsy for diagnosis of lymphoma

Currently, the role of surgery in the management of lymphoma is to establish a tissue diagnosis by performing excisional core biopsy of peripheral nodes or using more invasive techniques including mediastinoscopy and intraabdominal laparoscopy when less invasive methods fail to establish a definitive tissue diagnosis. The accurate histologic diagnosis of lymphoma requires assessment of the total architecture. Whenever possible, it is preferable to excise the entire intact node. Fine needle aspiration of a node does not provide an adequate amount of tissue to make an accurate histologic diagnosis of the subtype of lymphoma so this is not recommended. If multiple nodes are present, biopsy of cervical nodes is preferable to inguinal or axillary nodes because of lower morbidity and less chance of finding only non-diagnostic reactive changes. Each lymph node should be sent in fresh in saline for examination. Use of formalin precludes evaluation by flow cytometry, which is an important diagnostic and prognostic tool in lymphoma.

Staging laparotomy

Patients with lymphoma almost never require intraabdominal staging with laparoscopy or laparotomy as findings will rarely, if ever, affect overall prognosis or treatment decisions. Splenectomy is indicated for cases of isolated splenomegaly when lymphoma is suspected and there is no other tissue to biopsy. It is therapeutic in some indolent lymphomas. From the late 1960s to recent years, laparotomies were performed as the gold standard for staging patients with clinical stage I or II Hodgkin's lymphoma (no or inconclusive disease below the diaphragm) to help guide therapy. With recent changes to a less toxic standard chemotherapy regimen, and the excellent results obtained from giving combined chemoradiotherapy to early stage patients, staging laparotomies are no longer necessary.

Rebiopsy for residual disease

Residual intrathoracic masses are present in about 20% of patients after treatment for NHL or Hodgkin's lymphoma.[85] Such findings may be due to relapsing disease, fibrosis, or new and different pathology. While gallium scan and positron emission tomography (PET) allow for diagnosis in most cases, surgical biopsy is sometimes necessary to achieve an unequivocal diagnosis.

Gallium scan has been found to be more reliable than CT or MRI for evaluating residual disease, with a high specificity of up to 91% and positive predictive value of 81% after treatment for Hodgkin's disease.[86] One important cause of false positive results on gallium scan is "rebound" thymic hyperplasia which can occur after chemotherapy in more than 11% of patients.[85] False-negative findings on gallium scan can be due to partially necrotic or small sized tumors. PET scan is highly sensitive and specific for carcinomas but is still being evaluated for staging of lymphoma. PET has been shown in one study to have a specificity of 96% for evaluating residual masses in patients with Hodgkin's disease and 100% in NHL[87] and a positive predictive value (PPV) of 100% in another study.[88] The PPV in Hodgkin's disease may be less.

Gastrointestinal perforation in the lymphoma patient

When a tumor invades the bowel wall and is treated with effective chemotherapy, cell lysis with perforation can occur, especially with lymphoma. The true incidence of perforation in lymphoma patients is difficult to estimate but in one large review of 104 lymphoma cases, 13% experienced hemorrhage or perforation during therapy.[89] Steroids may mask the typical presenting symptoms, which can make the diagnosis difficult. In addition, pneumoperitoneum can be absent in 51% to 67% of immunocompromised or neutropenic patients.[3] Mortality rates for intestinal perforation in patients receiving steroids have been reported to range from 27% to 100%.[90]

Small bowel perforation is treated by resection and primary anastomosis and colonic perforations are treated with resection and diversion.[3] If a patient presents with a large lymphoma of the colon and is at high risk of perforation, resection of the mass prior to systemic therapy may be a consideration. However, there has never been a randomized study to demonstrate the superiority of resection in this setting, and chemotherapy ± radiation is effective therapy.

Preoperative concerns

Immunocompromised state of lymphoma patients

Patients with Hodgkin's lymphoma have abnormal cellular immunity, which persists after treatment. Patients continue to have suppressed hypersensitivity to neoantigens for several years after they are disease free. Defects in CD4+ and CD8+ T-cells persist for up to 30 years in Hodgkin's patients treated with mediastinal radiation.[91]

Patients with NHL are immunosuppressed from treatment and/or they may have associated inherited or acquired conditions, which contribute to their immunodeficiency. Patients with acquired immunodeficient conditions such as AIDS and following solid organ transplantation are at an increased risk for NHL.

Transfusion of blood products

Patients with Hodgkin's lymphoma are at high risk of developing transfusion-associated GVHD due to their immunodeficient state.[92–94] Patients with NHL appear to be at lesser risk, but cases of transfusion-associated GVHD have been reported.[95,96] Therefore, irradiated blood products should be provided for all patients with a history of or who are undergoing treatment for NHL or Hodgkin's lymphoma. Leukocyte reduced blood products are recommended for all lymphoma patients.

Tumor lysis syndrome

As discussed above, tumor lysis syndrome occurs in the setting of tumors that have high growth fractions. This is typical of acute leukemias as well as high-grade lymphomas, especially Burkitt's lymphoma. Tumor bulk as well as effective chemotherapy plays a role in determining who experiences tumor lysis syndrome. Although most often seen in the setting of chemotherapy, administration of other treatments such as ionizing radiation and steroids, has resulted in tumor lysis syndrome.[68] Careful monitoring and correction of electrolyte imbalances, maintenance of adequate hydration and urinary flow, administration of allopurinal and urinary alkalinization are important means of preventing this potentially lethal consequence for lymphoma patients who may require any type of surgery (see above section for details).

Superior vena cava syndrome

The superior vena cava syndrome is characterized by obstruction of blood flow through the superior vena cava, which is the major vessel for drainage of venous blood from the head, neck, upper extremities, and upper thorax. The major etiology is lung cancer, but NHL has been reported to be the primary pathologic diagnosis of SVC syndrome in 2% to 21% of patients in some series.[97] Although Hodgkin's disease can present with a mediastinal mass, it is rarely associated with SVC syndrome. Patients with SVC syndrome usually present with dyspnea and a sensation of fullness in the head and facial swelling. Other symptoms include cough, arm swelling, chest pain, and dysphagia. Physical examination may reveal venous distension of the neck and chest wall, facial edema, plethora, and cyanosis. Chest radiograph usually shows a chest mass and CT scan of the chest provides more detailed information about the SVC.

If a patient presents with severe dyspnea requiring emergent treatment of the venous obstruction, direct opening of the occlusion may be considered. Endovascular stenting and angioplasty with and without thrombolysis have been performed successfully in such cases.[98] More often, SVC syndrome requires urgent treatment rather than emergent treatment, and there is sufficient time to make an accurate histologic diagnosis to guide treatment. If other clinical features point to lymphoma, biopsy of a peripheral node, if available, can be performed to confirm the diagnosis. Mediastinoscopy has been shown to provide a high diagnostic yield in patients with SVC syndrome, with no perioperative mortality in two studies, and a complication rate of about 5%.[99,100] However, many thoracic surgeons are reluctant to perform mediastinoscopy in the setting of SVC syndrome.

When a diagnosis of lymphoma or Hodgkin's disease is established, chemotherapy is the treatment of choice for SVC syndrome as it provides rapid local control and systemic benefits. Radiation therapy is used following chemotherapy in patients with bulky mediastinal lymphadenopathy or residual masses.

Multiple myeloma

Description

Multiple myeloma is a B cell malignancy of neoplastic differentiated plasma cells, usually slowly proliferating, in which there is an accumulation of clonal plasma cells in the bone marrow, secretion of monoclonal immunoglobulins in the serum and/or urine, and formation of osteolytic bone lesions. It accounts for 1% of all malignant diseases and 10% of hematologic malignancies. It is primarily a disease of older individuals with a median age of 65 years. Clinical manifestations include: infection due to hypogammaglobulinemia resulting from decreased secretion of immunoglobulins by normal plasma cells; anemia due to cytokine production; pain and occasionally spinal cord compression from tumor mass effect; renal failure from protein deposition in the kidneys; hypercalcemia and bone destruction from stimulation of osteoclasts by cytokines; hyperviscosity from excessive serum paraprotein levels; and coagulopathy due to paraprotein interference with platelet function and the coagulation cascade. Current treatments including standard chemotherapy, high dose chemotherapy with autologous stem cell transplantation, and more novel therapies such as thalidomide, have been shown to extend survival and provide significant palliative benefits.

Surgical issues

Pathologic bone fractures

Bone loss in multiple myeloma results from stimulation of osteoclasts by cytokines released from multiple myeloma cells as well as from non-malignant cells of the bone marrow microenvironment, including IL-1-beta, TNF-beta, and IL-6.[101–103] There is generally no increased ostoblast activity in multiple myeloma so routine bone scans are not useful for diagnosing osteolytic lesions. Rather, plain skeletal films are more sensitive for detecting lesions and fractures.

Multiple myeloma patients who have an impending or existing pathologic fracture should receive input from oncologists as well as orthopedic specialists and radiation oncologists to determine an appropriate plan of care that incorporates systemic chemotherapy, radiation, and surgical intervention. It is easier to stabilize the bone while it is still intact and it saves the patient from suffering a painful fracture.

In terms of management of a pathologic fracture, radiographs of the entire length of the affected bone should be obtained first to identify any other lesions that may at a later point develop into a fracture so that these lesions can be stabilized and included in the radiation field as well. The most effective way to relieve pain and restore function in myeloma patients with pathologic fractures is through internal fixation or prosthetic replacement, realizing that most of these fractures will be non-healing, unlike normal traumatic injuries. Resection of the tumor is an important part of the management of pathologic fractures.

Spinal cord compression and vertebral instability

Spinal cord compression can result either from encroachment of an enlarging mass, or from a pathologic fracture with extrusion of bone fragments into the spinal canal, or vertebral collapse. Pain and/or neurologic deficits are the most common presenting complaints/findings. MRI is the study of choice because it can identify lesions throughout the spine, if there is tumor present in the canal, and the degree of spinal cord compression. Cord compression in multiple myeloma has been treated with local radiotherapy and/or surgical spinal decompression and stabilization. In the case of cord compression resulting from fracture or vertebral collapse without an identifiable plasmacytoma, radiation therapy may not be beneficial and decompressive surgery should be the treatment of choice.[104] Patients in whom spinal instability is likely to develop in spite of radiotherapy should undergo surgical stabilization before starting radiotherapy.[105] An alternative to surgery, but one that requires surgical back up, is percutaneous vertebroplasty.

Preoperative concerns

Hemostatic and coagulopathic disorders

Patients with multiple myeloma may acquire coagulation abnormalities related to an increased level of paraproteins interfering with the coagulation cascade and platelet function.[106] Clinically significant bleeding has been described in about 15% of patients with IgG myeloma and 60% of patients with IgA myeloma. The pathogenesis of bleeding is multifactorial.

Myeloma patients may have an acquired von Willebrand's syndrome. The paraprotein can bind the von Willebrand factor and result in clearance of the complex from the circulation. Treatment consists of therapy for the myeloma, plasmapheresis to remove existing paraprotein, and von Willebrand factor replacement with an appropriate purified product.

Bleeding complications are common with amyloidosis and up to 10% of multiple myeloma patients have amyloidosis. Bleeding occurs because of amyloid infiltration that causes fragility of tissues and blood vessels. Factor X can be adsorbed onto amyloid fibrils and renally excreted resulting in an acquired Factor X deficiency. Bleeding due to this condition has been difficult to treat and usually involves supportive measures such as fibrinolytic inhibitors, factor replacement, and even dialysis.

The paraprotein in multiple myeloma can also act as a circulating anticoagulant (interfering with proteins in the coagulation cascade) to cause clinically significant bleeding. Treatment options, aside from treating the underlying malignancy, include plasmapheresis followed by administration of fibrinogen concentrate, or the use of an anti-fibrinolytic agent.

Finally, bleeding complications associated with multiple myeloma relate to impairment of platelet function. This is seen more commonly in patients with IgM Waldenstrom's macroglobulinemia (see below) but may also be seen in patients with IgG myeloma paraproteins. Qualitative platelet defects are due to abnormalities in platelet aggregation and patients may have unexpected post-operative hemorrhage despite normal platelet counts and normal coagulation studies. The abnormality can be diagnosed by doing platelet function studies. Treatment for myeloma patients with bleeding secondary to qualitative platelet defects is to administer normal platelets, with or without plasmapheresis. DDAVP can also be given as a temporizing measure. Use of recombinant factor VIIa (Novo-seven) should also be considered in the case of persisting or life-threatening bleeding episodes.

Paraproteinemia predisposes myeloma patients to hemorrhagic diatheses as described above,[106] but occasionally thrombotic complications can occur as well. A high incidence of deep venous thrombosis was observed in multiple myeloma patients receiving thalidomide in combination with chemotherapy (28%).[107]

A recent prospective randomized trial[108] of 62 newly diagnosed multiple myeloma patients treated with intensive chemotherapy with or without thalidomide showed that, at baseline, a large percentage of the patients (23%) have reduced response to activated protein C (in the absence of factor V Leiden mutation). The risk of DVT was highest (50%) in patients with activate protein C resistance on thalidomide. Further studies are examining whether multiple myeloma patients have an inhibitor of the protein C pathway and whether activated protein C resistance disappears over time with anti-myeloma therapy.

Hypercalcemia

Skeletal complications in multiple myeloma are caused by osteoclastic resorption of bone that is not accompanied by increased bone formation. This can also lead to hypercalcemia with severe symptoms. In acute hypercalcemia, standard treatment involves intravenous fluid hydration, and treatment with antiresorptive drugs.

Bisphosphonates are the most commonly used drug to treat hypercalcemia, both for acute and chronic administration. Pamidronate is the most widely used bisphosphonate and is highly effective at decreasing bone resorption with an onset of action of 24 to 48 hours. Pamidronate is usually given at doses of 60 or 90 mg infused over two hours. Zoldedronate may also be used and can be given over a shorter period of time. Most patients with myeloma will be on monthly bisphosphonate therapy as this has been shown to significantly decrease the incidence of skeletal complications.

Hyperviscosity syndrome

The elevated levels of paraproteins in multiple myeloma can cause abnormalities of blood flow resulting in hyperviscosity. These proteins increase red cell aggregation, manifested on peripheral smear as rouleaux formation of red cells. The hyperviscosity syndrome occurs in less than 5% of myeloma patients but may be fatal if left untreated.[109] It is most common in IgM Waldenstrom's macroglobulinemia, followed by IgA due to the frequent polymerization of the IgA paraprotein, and is least common in IgG myeloma. The degree of hyperviscosity is evaluated by measurements of the serum viscosity, usually using a capillary tube viscometer. Normal serum has a relative viscosity of 1.4 to 1.8, whereas patients symptomatic from elevated paraproteins usually have a serum viscosity which exceeds 4.0.[110]

Patients with hyperviscosity syndrome present with neurological symptoms such as headache, dizziness, visual defects, peripheral neuropathy, and altered mental status, and coma. Fundoscopic exam may reveal retinal hemorrhage and exudates. The syndrome may also cause acute pulmonary distress and renal dysfunction and bleeding. The treatment should be urgent plasmapheresis to relieve acute symptoms and reverse end organ damage prior to any surgical intervention. IgM and IgA are present in the intravascular space and can be removed most effectively by plasma exchange. The frequency of plasmapheresis should be guided by clinical symptoms and serial viscosity measurements. Disease directed therapy should be started as soon as possible to treat the underlying disease.

Renal impairment

The etiology of renal failure in multiple myeloma patients is multifactorial. The most common cause is the presence of urinary light chains that form casts and cause interstitial nephritis.[111] Light chain deposition can also cause renal impairment, often associated with amyloidosis. Factors that can worsen renal function include the use of non-steroidal drugs for analgesia, nephrotoxic antibiotics for infection, intravenous contrast dye in radiologic studies, and hypercalcemia.[104]

Anemia and transfusion of blood products

Malignant myeloma plasma cells replace the normal hematopoietic cells of the bone marrow that usually causes a progressive anemia. Anemia is further exacerbated by a decreased production of erythropoietin.[104] Patients may benefit from administration of erythropoietin to help maintain hemoglobin levels perioperatively. All multiple myeloma patients should receive irradiated and leukocyte reduced, CMV appropriate blood products since they often require frequent transfusions and many will undergo autologous or even allogeneic stem cell transplants.

Infection risk

Multiple myeloma patients have profound cellular and humoral immune dysfunction. These patients often have hypogammaglobulinemia, other than abnormal paraprotein. Thus, they are at greater risk for bacterial infections that normally would be opsonized by specific antibody. As multiple myeloma improves with treatment, there is often recovery of the uninvolved immunoglobulins.

Waldenstrom macroglobulinemia

Waldenstrom's macroglobulinemia is a B-cell lymphoproliferative disorder characterized by secretion of monoclonal IgM protein by malignant plasmacytoid lymphocytes in the bone marrow.[112] Clinical manifestations include hepatomegaly (20%), splenomegaly (15%), and lymphadenopathy (15%). The most common symptoms are fatigue related to anemia, weight loss, and a peripheral neuropathy. Occasionally high levels of the IgM monoclonal protein can produce a hyperviscosity syndrome (see above discussion). In up to 10% of patients with monoclonal IgM, the abnormal protein reacts with the I-antigen on red blood cell, resulting in hemolysis in this temperature range. Therapy for Waldenstrom's macroglobulinemia has included alkylating agents, particularly chlorambucil, purine nucleoside analogues such as fludarabine, and most recently the anti-CD20 antibody, rituxi mab. Patients are treated when they become symptomatic.

Myelodysplastic syndromes

The myelodysplastic syndromes (MDS) are clonal stem cell disorders characterized by ineffective hematopoiesis and dysplastic changes in one or more lineages that result clinically in peripheral blood cytopenias. Patients with MDS can have a chronic indolent course lasting years or they can progress quickly to leukemic transformation. The median age of onset is 70 years. Some patients with prior exposure to marrow toxins or who were treated with chemotherapy or chemotherapy plus radiation develop a secondary MDS that is generally a more aggressive disease. The percentage of myeloblasts in the bone marrow, the degree of derangement of the hematopoietic cell lines, as well as the number and type of cytogenetic abnormalities, predict survival in MDS. Signs and symptoms are the result of cytopenias with infection, bleeding, and fatigue most common. Supportive care is the mainstay of therapy for MDS. All blood products should be leukoreduced to avoid platelet alloimmunization in these patients who require frequent transfusions. Granuloctye colony-stimulating factor (G-CSF) and recombinant human erythropoietin have been used in MDS patients to try to support both leukoctyes and erythrocytes with some success.

Perioperative risks which should be considered in MDS patients who are being evaluated for surgery include: age and comorbidities; the degree of cytopenias and transfusion requirements; a history of recent or recurrent infections; prior treatment of MDS which may indicate a significant level of immunosuppression. Many MDS patients are neutropenic and will be at risk for perioperative infections. The use of G-CSF should be considered, although no prospective studies demonstrate utility in this setting. MDS patients who are transplant recipients or candidates should receive irradiated blood products to minimize the risk of transfusion associated graft-versus host disease.

Central venous catheters

Surgeons are involved in the placement and removal of central venous catheters (CVC) and therefore should understand the indications for each. The need for frequent blood testing and multiple transfusions; the administration of repetitive doses of chemotherapeutic agents, many of which can sclerose peripheral blood vessels; the use of prolonged courses of intravenous antibiotics; and the occasional need for parenteral nutritional support are among the reasons why these catheters are used for patients with hematological malignancies.

For long-term venous access, three types of CVC are used: peripherally inserted central venous catheters (PICC) which are inserted into the basilic, cephalic, or brachial veins; tunneled cuffed central venous catheters which are implanted into the subclavian, internal jugular, or femoral veins; and totally implantable catheters ("ports") which are tunneled beneath the skin and have a subcutaneous port accessed with a needle, placed in the subclavian or internal jugular vein. Implantable catheter ports require minimal care by patients and are often desirable for patients because they are located beneath the skin. Catheters with external ports are preferred for patients with acute leukemia or in the stem cell transplant setting, as they are perceived to be associated with fewer infections, as they do not necessitate insertion of a needle through the skin. Catheter placement should never delay the initiation of urgently needed chemotherapy. Catheters should not be placed during an active untreated infection or while patients are actively bleeding.

Although central venous catheters have become an important component of care for patients with hematologic malignancies, they represent a leading source of nosocomial infection. Catheter-related infections are often difficult to treat because they are caused by organisms that embed themselves in a biofilm layer on the catheter surface and attach to the thrombin sheath on the surface of intravascular devices.[113] Catheter-related infections are generally caused by coagulase-negative staphylococci, coagulase-positive *Staphylococcus aureus*, Enterococcus, aerobic gram-negative bacilli, and *Candida albicans*. Coagulase-negative staphylococci, the most common organism isolated as a cause of CRBSI, has a low mortality rate of 0.7%, in contrast to *S. aureus* which has a high rate of mortality at 8.2%.[114] Catheter infection rates are substantially lower with tunneled catheters than in patients with non-tunneled catheters. Among the possible insertion sites for CVC, the subclavian vein is associated with the lowest risk of infection.[115]

When should a central venous catheter be removed in the setting of an infection? Raad *et al.* have recommended management of catheter-related infections based on the level of risk of CRBSI. A *low-risk* CRBSI is an uncomplicated infection caused by a pathogen of low virulence such as coagulase-negative staphylococci. The majority of these infections can be treated successfully with antibiotics without removal of the CVC.

A *moderate-risk* CRBSI is caused by pathogens of moderate to high virulence in a clinically stable patient, such as *S. aureus* and Candida species. The rapid removal of long-term tunneled catheters is controversial. Some experts might try to salvage the catheter in patients who are clinically stable and who are responding to antimicrobial therapy, by using antimicrobial flush solution with

systemic therapy for at least 14 days.[113] Others recommend rapid catheter removal once positive blood cultures are obtained for either *S. aureus* or *Candida* species.[116,117] Our practice is to remove CVC in the presence of a *Candida* infection. Antibiotic therapy for these types of infections ranges from 10 to 14 days.

A *high-risk* CRBSI is a complicated infection associated with one or more of the following: (a) hypotension or organ hypoperfusion; (b) persistence of fever or positive blood culture results for more than 48 hours after the initiation of appropriate antimicrobial therapy; (c) septic thrombosis of the great vein, septic emboli, or deep seated infections such as endocarditis or osteomyelitis; or (d) a tunnel or pocket (port) infection. In any of these cases, it is necessary to remove the catheter.

In addition to infection, delayed complications of catheter placement can include pneumothorax, hemothorax, thrombosis, tunnel bleeding, incorrect catheter placement, and inadvertent arterial puncture.[118] Suppport with platelet transfusions to achieve a platelet count >50 000/μl prior to the procedure may decrease the incidence of hemorrhagic complications and is generally practiced, but is not evidenced based.

Effects of chemotherapy

In performing a preoperative evaluation of patients with hematologic malignancies who require surgery, it is important to take into account possible side effects from prior chemotherapy treatments, which could affect their perioperative course. Agents commonly used in hematologic malignancies, which have potential complications, include anthracyclines, bleomycin, L-asparaginase, and cytarabine, and methotrexate.

Of the two most widely used anthracyclines, doxorubicin is active against lymphoma and daunorubicin is used primarily in the treatment of acute leukemia. Cardiomyopathy is a major chronic toxicity of the anthracyclines and is related to the total cumulative dose. Cardiotoxicity occurs with significant frequency beginning at approximately 450 to 550 mg per m^2 of doxorubicin and this is similar for daunorubicin. Since the cardiomyopathy can result in a significant decrease in left ventricular ejection fraction and an increased risk for congestive heart failure, patients who have had anthracyclines, especially elderly patients, should undergo a thorough history, physical examination, and, if appropriate, an updated cardiac study to measure left ventricular ejection fraction prior to surgery.

Bleomycin is used to treat Hodgkin's lymphoma. Bleomycin produces a dose-limiting toxicity of pulmonary fibrosis of unknown etiology in approximately 10% of patients. There is also an acute hypersensitivity form of bleomycin toxicity. Progression of pulmonary fibrosis can continue for months after stopping bleomycin. Symptoms include non-productive cough and pleuritic chest pain. Chest radiographs can show nodules and cavitary lesions or interstitial infiltrates. Pulmonary function tests may reveal a decline in diffusing capacity. Even after the drug has been stopped, the fibrosis may be only partially reversible and it may become fatal. Therapy of the disorder includes corticosteroids, bronchodilators, and antioxidants but responses are inconsistent. Patients who have received bleomycin should have careful preoperative evaluation of their pulmonary function status. High oxygen saturations can further damage the lung, presumable via increased reactive oxygen intermediates and should be avoided, if possible.

L-Asparaginase is used in the induction therapy of acute lymphoblastic leukemia in combination with other antileukemic drugs. Toxic effects of L-asparaginase include abnormal liver enzymes and a risk of acute pancreatitis. In addition, L-asparaginase leads to a reduction in clotting factors and fibrinogen levels that can cause bleeding, and a reduction in antithrombin III, protein C and S, which can cause thrombosis and embolism. Therefore, these parameters should be evaluated prior to an operation in a patient receiving L-asparaginase.

Cytarabine (Ara-C) is used in the treatment of acute myelogenous leukemia, acute lymphoblastic leukemia, chronic lymphocytic leukemia, non-Hodgkin's lymphoma, and myelodysplastic syndrome. Ara-C can cause transaminitis, increased levels of bilirubin, and intrahepatic cholestasis. Neurologic side effects can be seen with high-dose regimens in about 10% of patients that manifests predominantly as cerebellar toxicity.

Methotrexate, in combination with other agents, is indicated for the treatment of non-Hodkin's lymphoma (Burkitt's) and acute lymphoblastic lymphoma. Methotrexate can cause nephrotoxicity from precipitation of the drug and its metabolites in the renal tubules and through a direct toxic action on the renal tubules. The incidence of renal failure can be reduced through vigorous fluid hydration and urinary alkalinization. Care must be taken to maintain high urinary flow and avoid acidosis in a patient on methotrexate.

REFERENCES

1. Holleb, A. I., Fink, D. J., & Murphy, G. P. *Textbook of Clinical Oncology*, 1st edn. Atlanta: American Cancer Society, 1991.

2. Eastridge, B. J. & Lefor, A. T. Chronic venous access in the cancer patient. In Lefor, A. T., ed. *Surgical Problems Affecting the Patient with Cancer: Interdisciplinary Management.* Philadelphia: Lippincott-Raven, 1996.

3. Midis, G. P. & Skibber, J. Abdominal pain in the neutropenic cancer patient. In Lefor, A. T., ed. *Surgical Problems Affecting the Patient with Cancer: Interdisciplinary Management.* Philadelphia: Lippincott-Raven, 1996.

4. Mower, W. J., Hawkins, J. A., & Nelson, E. W. Neutropenic enterocolitis in adults with acute leukemia. *Arch. Surg.* 1986; **121**(5): 571–574.

5. Wade, D. S., Douglass, H., Jr., Nava, H. R., & Piedmonte, M. Abdominal pain in neutropenic patients. *Arch. Surg.* 1990; **125**(9): 1119–1127.

6. Villar, H. V., Warneke, J. A., Peck, M. D. *et al.* Role of surgical treatment in the management of complications of the gastrointestinal tract in patients with leukemia. *Surg. Gynecol. Obstet.* 1987; **165**(3): 217–222.

7. Starnes, H. F., Jr., Moore, F. D., Jr., Mentzer, S. *et al.* Abdominal pain in neutropenic cancer patients. *Cancer* 1986; **57**(3): 616–621.

8. Glenn, J., Funkhouser, W. K., & Schneider, P. S. Acute illnesses necessitating urgent abdominal surgery in neutropenic cancer patients: description of 14 cases and review of the literature. *Surgery* 1989; **105**(6): 778–789.

9. Martell, R. W. & Jacobs, P. Surgery for the acute abdomen in adults with leukaemia. *Postgrad. Med. J.* 1986; **62**(732): 915–918.

10. Weinberger, M., Hollingsworth, H., Feuerstein, I. M. *et al.* Successful surgical management of neutropenic enterocolitis in two patients with severe aplastic anemia. Case reports and review of the literature. *Arch. Intern. Med.* 1993; **153**(1): 107–113.

11. Baerg, J., Murphy, J. J., Anderson, R., & Magee, J. F. Neutropenic enteropathy: a 10-year review. *J. Pediatr. Surg.* 1999; **34**(7): 1068–1071.

12. Keidan, R. D., Fanning, J., Gatenby, R. A., & Weese, J. L. Recurrent typhlitis. A disease resulting from aggressive chemotherapy. *Dis. Colon Rectum* 1989; **32**(3): 206–209.

13. Newbold, K. M. Neutropenic enterocolitis. Clinical and pathological review. *Dig. Dis.* 1989; **7**(6): 281–287.

14. Dosik, G. M., Luna, M., Valdivieso, M. *et al.* Necrotizing colitis in patients with cancer. *Am. J. Med.* 1979; **67**(4): 646–656.

15. Coleman, N., Speirs, G., Khan, J. *et al.* Neutropenic enterocolitis associated with *Clostridium tertium. J. Clin. Pathol.* 1993; **46**(2): 180–183.

16. Ettinghausen, S. E. Collagenous colitis, eosinophilic colitis, and neutropenic colitis. *Surg. Clin. North Am.* 1993; **73**(5): 993–1016.

17. Newbold, K. M., Lord, M. G., & Baglin, T. P. Role of clostridial organisms in neutropenic enterocolitis. *J. Clin. Pathol.* 1987; **40**(4): 471.

18. Moir, C. R., Scudamore, C. H., & Benny, W. B. Typhlitis: selective surgical management. *Am. J. Surg.* 1986; **151**(5): 563–566.

19. Alt, B., Glass, N. R., & Sollinger, H. Neutropenic enterocolitis in adults. Review of the literature and assessment of surgical intervention. *Am. J. Surg.* 1985; **149**(3): 405–408.

20. Adams, G. W., Rauch, R. F., Kelvin, F. M. *et al.* CT detection of typhlitis. *J. Comput. Assist. Tomogr.* 1985; **9**(2): 363–365.

21. Frick, M. P., Maile, C. W., Crass, J. R. *et al.* Computed tomography of neutropenic colitis. *Am. J. Roentgenol.* 1984; **143**(4): 763–765.

22. Wade, D. S., Nava, H. R., & Douglass, H. O., Jr. Neutropenic enterocolitis. Clinical diagnosis and treatment. *Cancer* 1992; **69**(1): 17–23.

23. von Eiff, M., Essink, M., Roos, N. *et al.* Hepatosplenic candidiasis, a late manifestation of Candida septicaemia in neutropenic patients with haematologic malignancies. *Blut* 1990; **60**(4): 242–248.

24. Blade, J., Lopez-Guillermo, A., Rozman, C. *et al.* Chronic systemic candidiasis in acute leukemia. *Ann. Hematol.* 1992; **64**(5): 240–244.

25. Morris, A. B., Sands, M. L., Shiraki, M. *et al.* Gallbladder and biliary tract candidiasis: nine cases and review. *Rev. Infect. Dis.* 1990; **12**(3): 483–489.

26. Page, C. P., Coltman, C. A., Robertson, H. D., & Nelson, E. A. Candidal abscess of the spleen in patients with acute leukemia. *Surg. Gynecol. Obstet.* 1980; **151**(5): 604–608.

27. Significance and implications of abdominal pain in autologous bone marrow transplant patients. 89 May 21; 1989.

28. Vogelsang, G. B. Acute and chronic graft-versus-host disease. *Curr. Opin. Oncol.* 1993; **5**(2): 276–281.

29. McDonald, G. B., Shulman, H. M., Sullivan, K. M., & Spencer, G. D. Intestinal and hepatic complications of human bone marrow transplantation. Part I. *Gastroenterology* 1986; **90**(2): 460–477.

30. Goker, H., Haznedaroglu, I. C., & Chao, N. J. Acute graft-vs-host disease: pathobiology and management. *Exp. Hematol.* 2001; **29**(3): 259–277.

31. Barnes, S. G., Sattler, F. R., & Ballard, J. O. Perirectal infections in acute leukemia. Improved survival after incision and debridement. *Ann. Intern. Med.* 1984; **100**(4): 515–518.

32. Birnbaum, W. & Ahlquist, R. Rectal infections and ulcerations associated with blood dyscrasias. *Am. J. Surg.* 1955; **90**(2): 367–372.

33. Blank, W. A. Anorectal complications in leukemia. *Am. J. Surg.* 1955; **90**(5): 738–741.

34. Quadri, T. L. & Brown, A. E. Infectious complications in the critically ill patient with cancer. *Semin. Oncol.* 2000; **27**(3): 335–346.

35. Glenn, J., Cotton, D., Wesley, R., & Pizzo, P. Anorectal infections in patients with malignant diseases. *Rev. Infect. Dis.* 1988; **10**(1): 42–52.

36. Troiani, R. T., Jr., DuBois, J. J., & Boyle, L. Surgical management of anorectal infection in the leukemic patient. *Milit. Med.* 1991; **156**(10): 558–561.

37. Boddie, A. W., Jr. & Bines, S. D. Management of acute rectal problems in leukemic patients. *J. Surg. Oncol.* 1986; **33**(1): 53–56.

38. Bodey, G., Bueltmann, B., Duguid, W. *et al.* Fungal infections in cancer patients: an international autopsy survey. *Eur. J. Clin. Microbiol. Infect. Dis.* 1992; **11**(2): 99–109.

39. Baron, O., Guillaume, B., Moreau, P. *et al.* Aggressive surgical management in localized pulmonary mycotic and nonmycotic infections for neutropenic patients with acute leukemia: report of eighteen cases. *J. Thorac. Cardiovasc. Surg.* 1998; **115**(1): 63–68.

40. Moreau, P., Zahar, J. R., Milpied, N. *et al.* Localized invasive pulmonary aspergillosis in patients with neutropenia. Effectiveness of surgical resection. *Cancer* 1993; **72**(11): 3223–3226.

41. Robinson, L. A., Reed, E. C., Galbraith, T. A. *et al.* Pulmonary resection for invasive Aspergillus infections in immunocompromised patients. *J. Thorac. Cardiovasc. Surg.* 1995; **109**(6): 1182–1196.

42. Wong, K., Waters, C. M., & Walesby, R. K. Surgical management of invasive pulmonary aspergillosis in immunocompromised patients. *Eur. J. Cardiothorac. Surg.* 1992; **6**(3): 138–142.

43. Young, V. K., Maghur, H. A., Luke, D. A., & McGovern, E. M. Operation for cavitating invasive pulmonary aspergillosis in immunocompromised patients. *Ann. Thorac. Surg.* 1992; **53**(4): 621–624.

44. Sutton, D. A., Sanche, S. E., Revankar, S. G. *et al.* In vitro amphotericin B resistance in clinical isolates of *Aspergillus terreus*, with a head-to-head comparison to voriconazole. *J. Clin. Microbiol.* 1999; **37**(7): 2343–2345.

45. Caillot, D., Casasnovas, O., Bernard, A. *et al.* Improved management of invasive pulmonary aspergillosis in neutropenic patients using early thoracic computed tomographic scan and surgery. *J. Clin. Oncol.* 1997; **15**(1): 139–147.

46. Offner, F., Cordonnier, C., Ljungman, P. *et al.* Impact of previous aspergillosis on the outcome of bone marrow transplantation. *Clin. Infect. Dis.* 1998; **26**(5): 1098–1103.

47. Segal, B. H., Walsh, T. J., & Holland, S. M. Infections in the cancer patient. In Devita, V. T. Jr. HSRS, ed. *Cancer Principles and Practice of Oncology.* Philadelphia: Lippincott-Raven, 2001: 2827–2828.

48. Hughes, W. T., Armstrong, D., Bodey, G. P. *et al.* 2002 guidelines for the use of antimicrobial agents in neutropenic patients with cancer. *Clin. Infect. Dis.* 2002; **34**(6): 730–751.

49. Akova, M., Akan, H., Korten, V. *et al.* Meropenem Study Group of Turkey. Comparison of meropenem with amikacin plus ceftazidime in the empirical treatment of febrile neutropenia: a prospective randomised multicentre trial in patients without previous prophylactic antibiotics. *Int. J. Antimicrob. Agents* 1999; **13**(1): 15–19.

50. Cometta, A., Calandra, T., Gaya, H. *et al.* The International Antimicrobial Therapy Cooperative Group of the European Organization for Research and Treatment of Cancer and the Gruppo Italiano Malattie Ematologiche Maligne dell'Adulto Infection Program. Monotherapy with meropenem versus combination therapy with ceftazidime plus amikacin as empiric therapy for fever in granulocytopenic patients with cancer. *Antimicrob. Agents Chemother.* 1996; **40**(5): 1108–1115.

51. de Pauw, B. E., Deresinski, S. C., Feld, R. *et al.* The Intercontinental Antimicrobial Study Group. Ceftazidime compared with piperacillin and tobramycin for the empiric treatment of fever in neutropenic patients with cancer. A multicenter randomized trial. *Ann. Intern. Med.* 1994; **120**(10): 834–844.

52. Feld, R., DePauw, B., Berman, S. *et al.* Meropenem versus ceftazidime in the treatment of cancer patients with febrile neutropenia: a randomized, double-blind trial. *J. Clin. Oncol.* 2000; **18**(21): 3690–3698.

53. Pizzo, P. A., Hathorn, J. W., Hiemenz, J. *et al.* A randomized trial comparing ceftazidime alone with combination antibiotic therapy in cancer patients with fever and neutropenia. *N. Engl. J. Med.* 1986; **315**(9): 552–558.

54. Ramphal, R. Is monotherapy for febrile neutropenia still a viable alternative? *Clin. Infect. Dis.* 1999; **29**(3): 508–514.

55. Wang, F. D., Liu, C. Y., Hsu, H. C. *et al.* A comparative study of cefepime versus ceftazidime as empiric therapy of febrile episodes in neutropenic patients. *Chemotherapy* 1999; **45**(5): 370–379.

56. Malik, I. A., Abbas, Z., & Karim, M. Randomised comparison of oral ofloxacin alone with combination of parenteral antibiotics in neutropenic febrile patients. *Lancet* 1992; **339**(8801): 1092–1096.

57. Del Favero, A., Menichetti, F., Martino, P. *et al.* A multicenter, double-blind, placebo-controlled trial comparing piperacillin-tazobactam with and without amikacin as empiric therapy for febrile neutropenia. *Clin. Infect. Dis.* 2001; **33**(8): 1295–1301.

58. Yamamura, D., Gucalp, R., Carlisle, P. *et al.* Open randomized study of cefepime versus piperacillin-gentamicin for treatment of febrile neutropenic cancer patients. *Antimicrob. Agents Chemother.* 1997; **41**(8): 1704–1708.

59. A randomized trial of cefepime vs. cefaidime as initial therapy for patients with prolonged fever and neutropenia after intensive chemotherapy [abstract].: 1993.

60. Schiffer, C. A., Anderson, K. C., Bennett, C. L. *et al.* Platelet transfusion for patients with cancer: clinical practice guidelines of the American Society of Clinical Oncology. *J. Clin. Oncol.* 2001; **19**(5): 1519–1538.

61. Rebulla, P. Platelet transfusion trigger in difficult patients. *Transfus. Clin. Biol.* 2001; **8**(3): 249–254.

62. Williamson, L. M. & Warwick, R. M. Transfusion-associated graft-versus-host disease and its prevention. *Blood Rev.* 1995; **9**(4): 251–261.

63. Ratko, T. A., Cummings, J. P., Oberman, H. A. *et al.* Evidence-based recommendations for the use of WBC-reduced cellular blood components. *Transfusion* 2001; **41**(10): 1310–1319.

64. Slichter, S. J. Platelet refractoriness and alloimmunization. *Leukemia.* 1998; **12** Suppl 1: S51–S53.

65. British Committee for Standards in Haematology, Blood Transfusion Task Force. Guidelines on the clinical use of leucocyte-depleted blood components. *Transfus. Med.* 1998; **8**(1): 59–71.

66. Kwaan, H. C., Wang, J., & Boggio, L. N. Abnormalities in hemostasis in acute promyelocytic leukemia. *Hematol. Oncol.* 2002; **20**(1): 33–41.

67. Rodeghiero, F., Avvisati, G., Castaman, G. *et al.* Early deaths and anti-hemorrhagic treatments in acute promyelocytic leukemia. A GIMEMA retrospective study in 268 consecutive patients. *Blood* 1990; **75**(11): 2112–2117.

68. Fleming, D. R. & Doukas, M. A. Acute tumor lysis syndrome in hematologic malignancies. *Leuk. Lymphoma.* 1992; **8**(4–5): 315–318.

69. Jeha, S. Tumor lysis syndrome. *Semin. Hematol.* 2001; **38**(4 Suppl 10): 4–8.

70. Flombaum, C. D. Metabolic emergencies in the cancer patient. *Semin. Oncol.* 2000; **27**(3): 322–334.

71. Giles, F. J., Shen, Y., Kantarjian, H. M. *et al.* Leukapheresis reduces early mortality in patients with acute myeloid leukemia with high white cell counts but does not improve long-term survival. *Leuk. Lymphoma* 2001; **42**(1–2): 67–73.

72. Leonard, A. S., Giebink, G. S., Baesl, T. J., & Krivit, W. The overwhelming postsplenectomy sepsis problem. *World J. Surg.* 1980; **4**(4): 423–432.

73. Seymour, J. F., Cusack, J. D., Lerner, S. A. *et al.* Case/control study of the role of splenectomy in chronic lymphocytic leukemia. *J. Clin. Oncol.* 1997; **15**(1): 52–60.

74. Kalhs, P., Schwarzinger, I., Anderson, G. *et al.* A retrospective analysis of the long-term effect of splenectomy on late infections, graft-versus-host disease, relapse, and survival after allogeneic marrow transplantation for chronic myelogenous leukemia. *Blood* 1995; **86**(5): 2028–2032.

75. Morrison, V. A. The infectious complications of chronic lymphocytic leukemia. *Semin. Oncol.* 1998; **25**(1): 98–106.

76. Anaissie, E. J., Kontoyiannis, D. P., O'Brien, S. *et al.* Infections in patients with chronic lymphocytic leukemia treated with fludarabine. *Ann. Intern. Med.* 1998; **129**(7): 559–566.

77. Maung, Z. T., Wood, A. C., Jackson, G. H. *et al.* Transfusion-associated graft-versus-host disease in fludarabine-treated B-chronic lymphocytic leukaemia. *Br. J. Haematol.* 1994; **88**(3): 649–652.

78. Lee, G. R., Foerster, J., Lukens, J., Paraskevas, F., Greer, J. P., & Rodgers, G. M. eds. *Hairy Cell Leukemia.* Baltimore: Lippincott, Williams & Wilkins, 1999.

79. Golde, D. W. Therapy of hairy-cell leukemia. *N. Engl. J. Med.* 1982; **307**(8): 495–496.

80. Magee, M. J., McKenzie, S., Filippa, D. A. *et al.* Hairy cell leukemia. Durability of response to splenectomy in 26 patients and treatment of relapse with androgens in six patients. *Cancer* 1985; **56**(11): 2557–2562.

81. Andrey, J. & Saven, A. Therapeutic advances in the treatment of hairy cell leukemia. *Leuk. Res.* 2001; **25**(5): 361–368.

82. Savoie, L. & Johnston, J. B. Hairy cell leukemia. *Curr. Treatm. Options Oncol.* 2001; **2**(3): 217–224.

83. Hasenclever, D. & Diehl, V. A prognostic score for advanced Hodgkin's disease. International Prognostic Factors Project on Advanced Hodgkin's Disease. *N. Engl. J. Med.* 1998; **339**(21): 1506–1514.

84. Horning, S. J., Rosenberg, S. A., & Hoppe, R. T. Brief chemotherapy (Stanford V) and adjuvant radiotherapy for bulky or advanced Hodgkin's disease: an update. *Ann. Oncol.* 1996; **7**(Suppl. 4): 105–108.

85. Gossot, D., Girard, P., de Kerviler, E. *et al.* Thoracoscopy or CT-guided biopsy for residual intrathoracic masses after treatment of lymphoma. *Chest* 2001; **120**(1): 289–294.

86. Ionescu, I., Brice, P., Simon, D. *et al.* Restaging with gallium scan identifies chemosensitive patients and predicts survival

of poor-prognosis mediastinal Hodgkin's disease patients. *Med. Oncol.* 2000; **17**(2): 127–134.

87. Stumpe, K. D., Urbinelli, M., Steinert, H. C. *et al.* Whole-body positron emission tomography using fluorodeoxyglucose for staging of lymphoma: effectiveness and comparison with computed tomography. *Eur. J. Nucl. Med.* 1998; **25**(7): 721–728.

88. Jerusalem, G., Beguin, Y., Fassotte, M. F. *et al.* Whole-body positron emission tomography using 18F-fluorodeoxyglucose for posttreatment evaluation in Hodgkin's disease and non-Hodgkin's lymphoma has higher diagnostic and prognostic value than classical computed tomography scan imaging. *Blood* 1999; **94**(2): 429–433.

89. Weingrad, D. N., DeCosse, J. J., Sherlock, P. *et al.* Primary gastrointestinal lymphoma: a 30-year review. *Cancer* 1982; **49**(6): 1258–1265.

90. Torosian, M. H. & Turnbull, A. D. Emergency laparotomy for spontaneous intestinal and colonic perforations in cancer patients receiving corticosteroids and chemotherapy. *J. Clin. Oncol.* 1988; **6**(2): 291–296.

91. Horning, S. Hodgkin lymphoma. In Beutler, E., Lichtman, M. A., Coller, B. S., Kipps, T. J., & Seligsohn, U. eds. *Williams Hematology*. 6th edn. New York: McGraw Hill, 2001: 1215–1236.

92. Dinsmore, R. E., Straus, D. J., Pollack, M. S. *et al.* Fatal graft-versus-host disease following blood transfusion in Hodgkin's disease documented by HLA typing. *Blood* 1980; **55**(5): 831–834.

93. von F. V., Higby, D. J., & Kim, U. Graft-versus-host reaction following blood product transfusion. *Am. J. Med.* 1982; **72**(6): 951–961.

94. Decoste, S. D., Boudreaux, C., & Dover, J. S. Transfusion-associated graft-vs-host disease in patients with malignancies. Report of two cases and review of the literature. *Arch. Dermatol.* 1990; **126**(10): 1324–1329.

95. Gelly, K. J., Kerr, R., Rawlinson, S. *et al.* Transfusion-associated graft vs. host disease in a patient with high-grade B-cell lymphoma. Should cellular products for patients with non-Hodgkin's lymphoma be irradiated? *Br. J. Haematol.* 2000; **110**(1): 228–229.

96. Spitzer, T. R., Cahill, R., Cottler-Fox, M. *et al.* Transfusion-induced graft-versus-host disease in patients with malignant lymphoma. A case report and review of the literature. *Cancer* 1990; **66**(11): 2346–2349.

97. Yahalom, J. Oncologic Emergencies. In Devita, V. T., Jr., Hellman, S., & Rosenberg, S. A. eds. *Cancer Principles and Practice of Oncology*. Philadelphia: Lippincott, Williams and Wilkins, 2001: 2609–2616.

98. Schindler, N. & Vogelzang, R. L. Superior vena cava syndrome. Experience with endovascular stents and surgical therapy. *Surg. Clin. North Am.* 1999; **79**(3): 683–694, xi.

99. Jahangiri, M. & Goldstraw, P. The role of mediastinoscopy in superior vena caval obstruction. *Ann. Thorac. Surg.* 1995; **59**(2): 453–455.

100. Mineo, T. C., Ambrogi, V., Nofroni, I., & Pistolese, C. Mediastinoscopy in superior vena cava obstruction: analysis of 80 consecutive patients. *Ann. Thorac. Surg.* 1999; **68**(1): 223–226.

101. Cozzolino, F., Torcia, M., Aldinucci, D. *et al.* Production of interleukin-1 by bone marrow myeloma cells. *Blood* 1989; **74**(1): 380–387.

102. Garrett, I. R., Durie, B. G., Nedwin, G. E. *et al.* Production of lymphotoxin, a bone-resorbing cytokine, by cultured human myeloma cells. *N. Engl. J. Med.* 1987; **317**(9): 526–532.

103. Mundy, G. R., Raisz, L. G., Cooper, R. A. *et al.* Evidence for the secretion of an osteoclast stimulating factor in myeloma. *N. Engl. J. Med.* 1974; **291**(20): 1041–1046.

104. Barlogie, B., Shaughnessy, J., Munshi, N., & Epstein, J. Plasma cell myeloma. In Beutler, E., Lichtman, M. A., Coller, B. S., Kipps, T. J., & Seligsohn, U. eds. *Williams Hematology*. 6th edn. New York: McGraw Hill, 2001: 1279–1304.

105. McLain, R. F. & Bell, G. R. Newer management options in patients with spinal metastasis. *Cleve. Clin. J. Med.* 1998; **65**(7): 359–366.

106. Glaspy, J. A. Hemostatic abnormalities in multiple myeloma and related disorders. *Hematol. Oncol. Clin. North Am.* 1992; **6**(6): 1301–1314.

107. Zangari, M., Anaissie, E., Barlogie, B. *et al.* Increased risk of deep-vein thrombosis in patients with multiple myeloma receiving thalidomide and chemotherapy. *Blood* 2001; **98**(5): 1614–1615.

108. Zangari, M., Saghafifar, F., Anaissie, E. *et al.* Activated protein C resistance in the absence of factor V Leiden mutation is a common finding in multiple myeloma and is associated with an increased risk of thrombotic complications. *Blood Coagul. Fibrinol.* 2002; **13**(3): 187–192.

109. Bloch, K. J. & Maki, D. G. Hyperviscosity syndromes associated with immunoglobulin abnormalities. *Semin. Hematol.* 1973; **10**(2): 113–124.

110. Kwaan, H. C. & Bongu, A. The hyperviscosity syndromes. *Semin. Thromb. Hemost.* 1999; **25**(2): 199–208.

111. Solomon, A., Weiss, D. T., & Kattine, A. A. Nephrotoxic potential of Bence Jones proteins. *N. Engl. J. Med.* 1991; **324**(26): 1845–1851.

112. Gertz, M. A., Fonseca, R., & Rajkumar, S. V. Waldenstrom's macroglobulinemia. *Oncologist* 2000; **5**(1): 63–67.

113. Raad, I. I. & Hanna, H. A. Intravascular catheter-related infections: new horizons and recent advances. *Arch. Intern. Med.* 2002; **162**(8): 871–878.

114. Byers, K., Adal, K., Anglim, A., & Farr, B. Case fatality rate for catheter-related blood stream infections (CRBSI): a meta-analysis. *Infect. Contr. Hosp. Epidemiol.* 1995;16–23.

115. Pearson, M. L. Guideline for prevention of intravascular device-related infections. Part I. Intravascular device-related infections: an overview. The Hospital Infection Control Practices Advisory Committee. *Am. J. Infect. Contr.* 1996; **24**(4): 262–277.

116. Lane, R. K. & Matthay, M. A. Central line infections. *Curr. Opin. Crit. Care.* 2002; **8**(5): 441–448.

117. Nucci, M. & Anaissie, E. Should vascular catheters be removed from all patients with candidemia? An evidence-based review. *Clin. Infect. Dis.* 2002; **34**(5): 591–599.

118. Wagman, L. D., Kirkemo, A., & Johnston, M. R. Venous access: a prospective, randomized study of the Hickman catheter. *Surgery* 1984; **95**(3): 303–308.

19

Prophylaxis for deep venous thrombosis and pulmonary embolism in surgery

Geno J. Merli

Thomas Jefferson University Hospital, Philadelphia, PA

Venous thrombosis is a major cause of disability and death in all patient populations. Autopsy studies of hospitalized patients have demonstrated that massive pulmonary embolism (PE) is the cause of death in 5% to 10% of all hospital deaths and have suggested that two-thirds of all clinically important venous emboli are never recognized during life.[1,2] In a population-based study, Anderson and colleagues estimated that 170 000 patients are treated for a clinically recognized initial episode of venous thromboembolism in US hospitals each year and that 90 000 patients are treated for recurrent disease.[3] In addition, venous thromboembolism has been well documented as a common, serious, and, in some cases, fatal complication in the postoperative period. Despite the plethora of articles, books and courses on the prevention of this complication, physicians continue to underuse prophylactic regimens to prevent thromboembolic disease. Anderson and colleagues showed that 44% of university hospitals use prophylaxis compared to 19% of community hospitals.[4] More striking was the fact that only 32% of the patients in this study who were at high risk for deep venous thrombosis (DVT) or PE received prophylaxis.[4]

Pathophysiology

The pathophysiologic changes of stasis, intimate injury, and hypercoagulability predispose surgical patients to the development of DVT or PE. The supine position on the operating room table, the anatomic position of the extremities for some surgical procedures, and the effect of anesthesia all contribute to stasis during surgery. Venographic contrast studies have shown that the supine position on the operating table decreases venous return.[5,6] In orthopedic, gynecologic, and urologic surgeries, the anatomic position of the extremities that provides the best surgical access to the joint impairs adequate venous drainage during the procedure.[7] For example, in total hip replacement and hip fracture repair, the flexion and adduction of the hip that is required for better anatomic access to the surgical field has been shown to impair venous return.[7] Anesthesia causes peripheral venous vasodilation, which results in increased venous capacitance and decreased venous return during the operative procedure.[8–10]

Intimal injury may be caused by anatomic positioning and the excessive vasodilation that results from anesthesia. Flexion and adduction of the hip during surgery has been shown to compress the femoral vein. Three intraoperative venographic studies provided clear evidence of distortion of the femoral vein during certain phases of total hip replacement.[11–13] The use of a tourniquet on the proximal thigh and flexion of the knee during total knee replacement also compresses the underlying venous structures. These positions for prolonged periods may damage the delicate venous endothelium. Anesthesia also contributes to injury by causing excess vasodilation and endothelial damage.[14–17] Comerota and associates[14] demonstrated in dogs that the endothelial lesions occurred as multiple tears around the junction of small side branches with the major receiving veins (jugular and femoral veins).[14] These tears extended through the endothelium and through the basement membrane, exposing subendothelial collagen, which is highly thrombogenic. On electron microscopic evaluation, the lesions were infiltrated with leukocytes, platelets, and red blood cells.[15] Limited studies have demonstrated the presence of biologically active substances such as histamine, complement fragment C3a, and leukotrienes, which may contribute to venous vasodilation and endothelial damage.[16] These may be the factors that contribute to thrombus formation at sites distant from the surgical procedure.[17] All these mechanisms produce endothelial cell damage, creating a nidus for clot formation.

Medical Management of the Surgical Patient: A Textbook of Perioperative Medicine, ed. M. F. Lubin, R. B. Smith, T. F. Dobson, N. Spell, H. K. Walker. 4th edn. Published by Cambridge University Press. © Cambridge University 2006.

The third factor contributing to the development of postoperative DVT is hypercoagulability. Assessing this state has proved challenging. The current approach focuses on either coagulation cascade modulators or impairment of the fibrinolytic system. Levels of anti-thrombin III (AT) have been shown to be decreased for 3–5 days after total hip and knee surgery.[18] This results in impaired modulation of the clotting cascade at factors Xa and IIa, with an increased propensity toward thrombus formation. The fibrinolytic system also has been evaluated by the measurement of tissue plasminogen activator and plasminogen activator inhibitor-1 levels before and after operation.[19] Several surgical studies have demonstrated a shutdown of the fibrinolytic system as evidenced by reductions in these levels.[20] An increased level of plasminogen activator inhibitor-1 before operation appears to indicate an increased risk for the development of thrombosis in patients undergoing orthopedic surgery.[21] Another marker of an activated fibrinolytic system is the presence of alpha 2-antiplasmin, the primary function of which is to inactivate plasmin. Increased levels of alpha 2-antiplasmin complexes are indicative of active fibrinolysis, which is an indirect measure of active thrombus formation.[21] This radioimmunoassay requires further study as a predictor of postoperative DVT. Coupled with stasis and intimal injury, however, it seems to suggest an increased risk for DVT or PE.

As Virchow postulated in 1856, the three factors (stasis, intimal injury, hypercoagulability) described increase the risk for the development of DVT and PE. Our responsibility as consultants is to ameliorate these risk factors wherever possible.

Risk factor classification

In assessing the risk for DVT or PE before surgery, patient age, length and type of procedure, previous DVT or PE, and secondary risk factors must be documented. Secondary risk factors include prolonged immobilization, paralysis, malignancy, obesity, varicose veins, and estrogen therapy.[1,22] Using these criteria, patients are classified as being at low, moderate, high risk and very high risk for the development of DVT or PE. (Table 19.1)[23]

Patients at low risk are younger than 40 years, have no secondary risk factors, and are undergoing minor, elective abdominal or thoracic surgery under general anesthesia for less than 30 minutes. In this group the risk of DVT/PE is as follows: calf DVT 2%, proximal DVT 0.4%, clinical PE 0.2%, and fatal PE 0.002%. Patients at moderate risk can be divided into three groups: (a) patients having minor surgery with secondary risk factors, (b) non-major surgery in

patients aged 40–60 years with no secondary risk factors, (c) major surgery in patients <40 with no secondary risk factors. The risk of DVT/PE in the moderate risk category are calf DVT 10%–20%, proximal DVT 2%–4%, clinical PE 1%–2%, and fatal PE 0.1%–0.4%. The high-risk group is composed of patients >60 having non-major surgery with secondary risk factors and major surgery in patients >40 with secondary risk factors. The incidence of venous thromboembolic events is 20%–40% calf DVT, 4%–8% proximal DVT, 2%–4% clinical PE, and 0.4%–1% fatal PE. The very high-risk group includes major surgery in patients older than 40 years plus either prior history of DVT/PE, malignancy, hereditary or acquired coagulopathies (e.g., proteins C and S, AT, anticardiolipin antibodies, Factor V Leiden, Prothrombin Gene Mutation 20210), hip or knee arthroplasty, hip fracture, major trauma, or spinal cord injury. This group has a 40% to 80% risk of calf vein thrombosis, a 10% to 20% risk of proximal vein thrombosis, 4%–10% clinical PE, and a 1% to 5% risk of fatal PE if prophylaxis is not used.

Although this classification may appear to be artificial, it does serve as a guide for documenting risk factors in the history and physical examination that affect perioperative prophylactic therapy and identifies high and very high risk patients who must receive DVT/PE prophylaxis.

Techniques of prophylaxis

A number of modalities are used for the prophylaxis of DVT and PE in patients undergoing surgery. Each approach is reviewed with respect to dosage, administration, and length of therapy.

Unfractionated heparin

Unfractionated heparin (UFH) is administered at an initial dose of 5000 U given subcutaneously 2 hours before surgery. After surgery, 5000 U is given subcutaneously every 8 to 12 hours until patients are discharged from the hospital. In double-blind trials, the incidence of major hemorrhagic events using this regimen was 1.8% compared to 0.8% in the control group.[24] This difference is not statistically significant. The incidence of minor bleeding such as injection site and wound hematomas, however, was significant with heparin prophylaxis (6.3% compared to 4.1% in the control group). Rare complications of low-dose UFH therapy include skin necrosis, thrombocytopenia, and hyperkalemia.[25–28]

Adjusted low-dose UFH therapy was devised for use in patients undergoing total hip replacement. This adjusted dose regimen is impractical for the current shortened

Table 19.1. Classification of risk for postoperative deep venous thrombosis (DVT) or pulmonary embolism (PE)

Level of risk	Calf DVT	Proximal DVT	Clinical PE	Fatal PE
Low risk Minor surgery, age <40 yrs No risk factors	2%	0.4%	0.2%	0.002%
Moderate risk Minor surgery with risk factors Non-major surgery 40–60 yrs with no risk factors, major surgery 40 yrs or with risk factor	10–20%	2–4%	1–2%	0.1–0.4%
High risk Non-major surgery >60 yrs or with risk factors, major surgery >40 yrs or with risk factors	20–40%	4–8%	2–4%	0.4–1%
Very High risk Major surgery >40 yrs plus prior VTE, cancer, thrombophilia, THA, TKA, FH, major trauma, ASCI	40–80%	10–20%	4–10%	0.2–5%

Source: From Geerts, W. *et al. Chest* 2001; **119**: 132S–175S.

length of stay for surgical patients. In the original description by Leyvraz and associates,[29] prophylaxis with UFH was begun at a dose of 3500 U given subcutaneously every 8 hours for 2 days before surgery. Adjustments were made on a sliding scale to maintain the partial thromboplastin time at the highest normal value of the laboratory. The practice of admitting patients on the same day of surgery makes this regimen impractical. We administer 3500 U of UFH subcutaneously 2 hours before surgery, followed by 3500 U every 8 hours beginning the evening of the procedure. The UFH dose is adjusted, based on the activated partial thromboplastin time 6 hours after the postoperative afternoon dose. The next adjustment is based on the activated partial thromboplastin time 6 hours after the morning dose on the first postoperative day. Subsequent adjustments are made every other day. The UFH dose is derived from a sliding scale schedule of 4 seconds plus or minus the highest normal activated partial thromboplastin time value of the laboratory. The object is to maintain the activated partial thromboplastin time within 4 seconds of the highest normal value of the laboratory. The dose of UFH is adjusted for 7 to 10 days after surgery, at which point warfarin or the last total daily adjusted dose of UFH is given every 12 hours until discharge. Two studies using this method reported no increase in the risk of bleeding.[29,30]

Low-molecular-weight heparin

Low-molecular-weight heparin (LMWH) preparations have become the primary agents for the prevention of postoperative DVT/PE in orthopedic surgery. LMWH

Table 19.2. Low-molecular-weight heparins

Drug	Molecular weight (daltons)	Xa/IIa	Half-Life (hr)(s)
Ardeparin	5000	2:1	3–3 ½
Dalteparin	5000	2:1	2–2 ½
Enoxaparin	4500	4:1	4–4 ½
Tinzaparin	4500	2:1	2
Fraxiparin	4500	3:1	2–3
Fondaparinux	1728		13–20

have been observed to have a more significant inhibitory effect on factor Xa than on factor IIa, as well as a lower bleeding risk than standard heparin.[31] Three LMWH preparations are approved in the United States, one preparation has been approved for general surgery and three have been approved for orthopedic surgery. Each of these LMWH preparations has a different molecular weight, anti-Xa to anti-IIa activity, rate of plasma clearance, and recommended dosage regimen. (Table 19.2)[32]

LMWH preparations are fragments of commercial-grade standard heparin prepared by either chemical or enzymatic depolymerization. The resulting LMWH contains the pentasaccharide required for specific binding to AT.[32–34] This binding inhibits Xa and IIa without forming the complex that occurs when standard heparin binds with these factors. UFH molecules with fewer than 18 saccharides (molecular weight less than 5400 daltons) are unable to bind thrombin and AT but retain their ability to catalyze the inhibition of factor Xa by AT.[32–34]

LMWH formulations are not bound to plasma proteins (histidine-rich glycoprotein, platelet factor 4, vitronectin, fibronectin, and von Willebrand's factor), endothelial cells, or macrophages as is standard heparin.[32,33] This lower affinity contributes to a longer plasma half-life, more complete plasma recovery at all concentrations, and clearance that is independent of dose and plasma concentration.

In comparing the potential for hemorrhagic complications with standard heparin and LMWH, three factors must be considered. Standard UFH inhibits both collagen-induced and von Willebrand's factor-dependent platelet aggregation and increases vascular permeability.[32] These three qualities result in a higher bleeding potential with standard UFH than with LMWH, which does not have these effects.

In reviewing the literature regarding the safety and efficacy of LMWH preparations for the prevention of postoperative DVT, it must be remembered that these agents are distinct compounds with unique properties and different dosage regimens.

In contrast to UFH, the LMWHs are administered 6 to 12 hours following the surgical procedure. The dose of dalteparin for general surgical and orthopedic surgery is 5000 units, subcutaneous once daily. Enoxaparin is administered at 40 mg, subcutaneous, once daily for general surgery where as the orthopedic dose most commonly used in this country is 30 mg, subcutaneous every 12 hours.

The newest LMWH is fondaparinux. It is a synthetically prepared molecule of the active pentasaccaride sequence of unfractionated heparin.[35] Like unfractionated heparin and LMWHs this drug binds to AT which inhibits Factor Xa. The pharmacokinetics of fondaparinux demonstrates that it occupies only a part of the heparin-binding site on antithrombin and the conformational change induced by the binding differs from UFH.[35] Because fondaparinux is a catalyst, each molecule serves several times in activating AT. The peak plasma level was obtained around 2 hours after subcutaneous injection, and significant levels were reached within 25 minutes.[35] This indicates a rapid onset of antithrombotic activity. The elimination half-life is dose-independent and ranges from 17 to 20 hours. Fondaparinux is renally excreted and therefore precaution is necessary in renal failure. Fondaparinux is administered 2.5 mg, subcutaneous beginning 6 hours after surgery and subsequently once daily.

Warfarin

Three protocols have been devised for the use of warfarin prophylaxis (Table 19.3). The first involves the administration of 10 mg of warfarin the night before surgery, followed

Table 19.3. Warfarin prophylaxis

Method 1

10 mg orally the evening before surgery

5 mg orally the evening of surgery

Adjust dose daily based on a prothrombin time INR of 2–3

Continue for 4 to 6 weeks after discharge at a prothrombin time INR of 2–3

Method 2

Begin warfarin administration at home 14 days before hospital admission

Maintain the prothrombin time at 1.5–3 seconds above the control value

Postoperatively day 1, begin adjusting the dose to maintain a prothrombin time INR 2–3

Continue for 4 to 6 weeks after discharge at a prothrombin time INR of 2–3

Method 3

10 mg orally the evening of surgery

No warfarin postoperative day 1

Postoperative day 2, begin warfarin administration to adjust the prothrombin time INR 2–3

Continue for 4 to 6 weeks after discharge at a prothrombin time INR of 2–3

by 5 mg the evening of surgery.[36] The daily dose is determined by the prothrombin time/INR (INR), which should be kept between 2 and 3. If oral intake is not possible, warfarin can be administered through a nasogastric tube. The second method involves the initiation of warfarin therapy 10 to 14 days before surgery.[37] The dose is adjusted to maintain the PT at 1.5 to 3 seconds longer than the laboratory control value before surgery. On the first postoperative day, the dose of warfarin is regulated to maintain an INR between 2 and 3. This method may not be clinically practical since a high percentage of patients receive spinal or epidural anesthesia and the risk of epidural hematoma could be potentially increased. The third protocol begins with the administration of 10 mg of warfarin on the evening after surgery.[38] No warfarin is given on the first postoperative day. On the second postoperative day, the dose of warfarin is regulated to maintain an INR between 2 and 3. This therapy is continued until discharge. Prophylaxis for DVT after hospital discharge has been recommended as a management strategy for patients who have undergone total hip replacement.[39] Warfarin therapy is continued to maintain the INR between 2 and 3 for a total of 6 weeks.[23] Further studies are necessary to support this clinical approach. The incidence of major postoperative bleeding with warfarin therapy has varied from 5% to 10%. The rare complication of warfarin, skin necrosis, has never been reported in studies using this agent as prophylaxis for DVT or PE.

Antithrombin III

Antithrombin III (AT) has been approved for use in the United States for hereditary AT deficiency but has an off label indication for acquired AT deficiency secondary to surgery. It is derived from purified human plasma. There have not been any reported cases of viral transmission with its use. A postoperative decrease in AT has been reported after orthopedic surgery. This decrease has been cited as one of the factors contributing to the increased incidence of DVT. A DVT prophylaxis trial was undertaken to evaluate the efficacy of the combination of AT plus heparin versus dextran in patients undergoing total hip replacement.[40] Fifteen hundred units of AT and 5000 U of subcutaneous unfractionated heparin were given 2 hours before surgery, followed by 1000 U of intravenous AT each day and 5000 U of subcutaneous unfractionated heparin every 12 hours for 5 days. Two of 41 patients (5%) who received this therapy had documented thrombosis, compared with 12 of 42 patients (40%) who received dextran.

For patients with hereditary AT deficiency the initial dose calculation equals the desired AT level minus the current AT level as a percentage of normal level times the weight (kg) divided by 1.4. The initial target AT level should be 80% to 120% of normal activity. Maintenance dose is given every 24 hours to maintain AT levels greater than 80% of normal. At the present time the use of AT can be combined with either dalteparin, enoxaparin, or fondaparinux for patients undergoing orthopedic procedures. For all other surgeries unfractionated heparin can be maintained with AT for DVT/PE prophylaxis.

Mechanical methods

External pneumatic compression (EPC) sleeves are mechanical methods of improving venous return from the lower extremities.[41] They reduce stasis in the gastrocnemius–soleus pump and may increase fibrinolysis as a concomitant mechanism. These devices are placed on patients in the preoperative preparation room on the morning of surgery. They are worn throughout the surgical procedure and for 3 to 5 days afterwards. When patients resume walking, the sleeves can be removed and warfarin, UFH, LMWH therapy initiated, depending on the surgical procedure performed. In patients who do not resume walking quickly, the sleeves should be kept in place. These patients may not tolerate the sleeves, however, because of increased warmth, sweating, or sleep disturbance. Warfarin, UFH, or LMWH therapy can be initiated and maintained until patients are discharged from the hospital. The sleeves may be removed temporarily from bedridden patients for skin care, bathing, physical therapy, or bedside commode use. Each manufacturer (e.g., Kendall, Venodyne, Jobst, Baxter, Huntleight) provides specifications regarding the operation and cycle time of its device, but no statistically significant difference in the incidence of DVT has been demonstrated. If patients have been bedridden or immobilized for more than 72 hours without any form of prophylaxis, the placement of pneumatic sleeves is not recommended because of the possibility of embolizing newly formed clot. The lower extremity should be evaluated through non-invasive testing.

In 1984, Gardner and colleagues[42] described a previously unrecognized physiologic pump mechanism in the sole of the foot that is activated by the flattening of the plantar arch that occurs with weight bearing. The arteriovenous impulse system foot pump (A–V impulse system) was developed to perform this function. Fordyce and coworkers[43] randomly assigned 84 patients to treatment with either placebo or the A–V impulse system. The incidence of DVT was 40% in the control group and 10% in the treated group. In a nonrandomized study of patients undergoing total knee arthroplasty, Wilson and associates[44] reported the incidence of DVT to be 50% in patients treated with the A-V Impulse System compared to 68.5% in those who received placebo therapy. Although it was not statistically significant, the incidence of proximal vein thrombosis was 17.8% in the treatment group versus 59.4% in the control group. Like the above pneumatic devices, the foot pump modalities should be managed the same as the calf or thigh length intermittent pneumatic devices.

Calf-length gradient elastic stockings are worn during surgery and until discharge from the hospital. The stockings can be removed for skin care and bathing.

Prophylaxis for specific surgery

Table 19.4 outlines the incidence and prophylaxis of DVT in various surgical procedures.

Orthopedic surgery

The number of orthopedic joint replacement procedures performed has increased over the past 10 years

Table 19.4. Incidence and prophylaxis of deep venous thrombosis (DVT) in surgery

Procedure	DVT incidence	Recommended prophylaxis
Orthopedic surgery		
Total hip replacement	40%–60%	LMWH (enoxaparin 30 mg, s.c., Q 12 h, dalteparin 5000 IU, s.c., Q day, fondaparinux 2.5 mg, s.c., Q day)
		Warfarin (INR 2–3)
		Adjusted dose heparin
Fractured hip replacement	40%–50%	LMWH (enoxaparin 30 mg, s.c., Q 12 h, dalteparin 5000 IU, s.c., Q day, fondaparinux 2.5 mg, s.c., Q day)
		Warfarin (INR 2–3)
		Adjusted dose heparin
Total knee replacement	40%–84%	LMWH (enoxaparin 30 mg, s.c., Q 12 h, fondaparinux 2.5 mg, s.c., Q day)
		Warfarin (INR 2–3)
General Surgery	20%–30%	UFH 5000 U, s.c., Q 8 h
		LMWH (enoxaparin 40 mg, s.c., Q day, dalteparin 5000 IU, s.c., Q day)
		EPC sleeves
Neurosurgery		
Craniotomy	19%–40%	EPC sleeves
		UFH 5000 U, s.c., Q 8 h
		LMWH (enoxaparin 40 mg, s.c., Q day)
Spinal surgery	4%–60%	EPC sleeves
		EPC sleeves plus UFH (5000 U, s.c., Q 8 h)
Gynecologic surgery		
Not related to malignancy		
Abdominal hysterectomy	12% – 15%	UFH 5000 U, s.c., Q 12 h,
		LMWH (enoxaparin 40 mg, s.c., Q day, dalteparin 5000 U, s.c., Q day)
		EPC sleeves
Vaginal hysterectomy	6%–7%	UFH 5000 U, s.c., Q 12 h,
		LMWH (enoxaparin 40 mg, s.c., Q day, dalteparin 5000 U, s.c., Q day)
		EPC sleeves
Related to malignancy	35%–38%	UFH 5000 U, s.c., Q 8 h,
		LMWH (enoxaparin 40 mg, s.c., Q day, dalteparin 5000 U, s.c., Q day)
		EPC sleeves plus UFH or LMWH
		EPC sleeves
Urologic surgery		
Transurethral resection of the prostate	7%–10%	EPC sleeves
		Gradient elastic stockings
Open prostatectomy for malignancy	21%–51%	UFH 5000 U, s.c., Q 8 h
		LMWH (enoxaparin 40 mg, s.c., Q day, dalteparin 5000 U, s.c., Q day)
		EPC sleeves plus UFH or LMWH
		EPC sleeves

Notes:

agents selected were those that had FDA approval for these indications.

UFH = unfractionated heparin.

LMWH = low-molecular-weight heparin.

EPC = external pneumatic compression sleeves.

commensurate with the aging of the population. The incidence of DVT has been documented at 40% to 50% in total hip replacement, 45% to 50% in hip fracture, and 72% in total knee replacement. The incidence of fatal PE is about 1% to 5% for all these procedures.[23] The high incidence of thrombotic complications in the absence of prophylaxis is a pressing concern. The prophylactic interventions shown to be effective in reducing the incidence of DVT and PE in this high-risk population are reviewed here (Table 19.4).

Venography is the gold standard for assessing the efficacy of DVT prophylaxis in orthopedic surgery. Thrombosis in this type of surgery can occur in an isolated proximal, proximal and distal, or isolated distal pattern. The non-invasive studies of venous imaging and impedance plethysmography are more sensitive and specific for proximal vein thrombosis and overlook distal vein thrombosis. The studies presented in this section focus on prophylactic techniques that have venographically demonstrated efficacy in reducing postoperative clot formation.

Total hip replacement

The incidence of DVT and fatal PE in total hip replacement surgery varies from 40% to 60% and from 1% to 3%, respectively.[23] In an attempt to reduce these rates, several pharmacologic and mechanical approaches to the prevention of thrombosis have been advocated.

Warfarin is one of the pharmacologic agents of choice for DVT/PE prophylaxis in total hip replacement surgery and may be administered as outlined earlier.[23] The use of warfarin prophylaxis has decreased the incidence of DVT from 40%–60% to 17%–30%, with a marked reduction in proximal vein thrombosis.

The use of fixed-dose unfractionated heparin therapy was not supported by the American College of Chest Physicians Consensus Conference on antithrombotic therapy.[23] In a metaanalysis of the literature, Collins and coworkers[45] reported that fixed-dose unfractionated heparin therapy was associated with a lower incidence of proximal thrombosis and fatal PE in orthopedic surgery but with the same overall number of thrombi. Levine and colleagues[46] demonstrated a 23% incidence of DVT using 7500 U of subcutaneous UFH every 12 hours compared to a 19% incidence of DVT in an experimental group that received LMWH (enoxaparin). In a study by Planes and associates,[47] fixed-dose UFH reduced the incidence of DVT in total hip replacement surgery to 25%.

Leyvraz and colleagues[29] adapted an adjusted low-dose UFH regimen that proved to be effective in reducing the incidence of DVT. This regimen has not been readily accepted, however, because of the necessity of frequent

dose adjustment. Dextran 40 or 70 is another single pharmacologic agent that has been successful in DVT prophylaxis, but its use has been discontinued because of the risk of fluid overload, the occurrence of hypersensitivity reactions, and the availability of more effective techniques.

Finally, the replacement of AT levels depleted by surgery combined with the delivery of low-dose subcutaneous UFH therapy at a dose of 5000 U every 12 hours has been studied by Francis and coworkers.[40] DVT was identified in 5% of the patients who received AT plus low-dose UFH and in 40% of those who received dextran 40. Although it is effective, AT is expensive and exposes patients to the risks inherent in the use of human blood products and is only used for patients with hereditary AT deficiency.

The use of mechanical techniques to prevent DVT has been increasing in orthopedic surgery. Several studies have evaluated the use of calf-length or thigh-length EPC sleeves along, or in combination, with a pharmacologic agent. The overall incidence of DVT was reduced significantly by this approach (from 40% to 60% to 6% to 35%).[48–53] Although these devices have been successful in reducing the incidence of calf vein DVT, they have not been as effective in decreasing proximal vein thrombosis. In these studies, the sleeve on the operated extremity was activated immediately after surgery, whereas the contralateral extremity was compressed through the procedure. The sleeves should be worn for 7 days and removed only for bathroom use and physical therapy. No study has compared different types of sleeves (i.e., calf-length versus thigh-length sleeves or sequential versus single-chamber compression devices).

The largest number of studies evaluating LMWH has been conducted in patients undergoing elective total hip replacement (Table 19.5). Turpie and associates[54] compared placebo with enoxaparin and demonstrated a reduction in the incidence of DVT from 51.3% to 10.8%. Hoek and colleagues[55] evaluated 196 patients who were randomly assigned to receive either lomoparan or placebo. The incidence of DVT was 57% in the placebo group and 10% in the lomoparin group. Planes and coworkers[47] randomly assigned 237 patients to receive either enoxaparin or UFH after hip surgery. The incidence of DVT was reduced from 25% with UFH to 12.5% with LMWH. A fourth study by Levine and associates[46] compared LMWH with heparin (7500 U given subcutaneously every 12 hours). There was no difference in the incidence of DVT in either group but there was a lower incidence of bleeding in the LMWH treated patients.

Lassen and associates[56] completed a randomized prospective trial in total hip replacement surgery comparing enoxaparin (40 mg, s.c., Q day) with fondaparinux

Table 19.5. Prophylaxis of deep venous thrombosis (DVT) with low-molecular-weight heparin in various orthopedic procedures[a]

Study	Number of patients	Prophylaxis	All DVT	Prox DVT	Bleeding
Total hip replacement					
Turpie	50	Placebo	20 (51%)	9 (45%)	2 (4%)
	50	Enoxaparin	4 (11%)	2 (50%)	2 (4%)
Planes	113	UFH	27 (25%)	20 (19%)	2 (2%)
	124	Enoxaparin	15 (12%)	9 (8%)	3 (2%)
Levine	263	UFH	61 (23%)	17 (7%)	31 (9%)
	258	Enoxaparin	50 (19%)	14 (5%)	17 (5%)
Lassen		Enoxaparin Fondaparinux			
Turpie	797	Enoxaparin	66 (8%)	10 (1%)	8 (0.7%)[a]
	787	Fondaparinux	48 (6%)	14 (2%)	18 (2%)[a]
Total knee replacement					
LeClerc	54	Placebo	8 (19%)	11 (20%)	5 (8%)
	41	Enoxaparin	35 (65%)	0 (0%)	4 (6%)
Hull	317	Tinzaparin	116 (37%)	20 (7%)	14 (4%)
	324	Warfarin	154 (48%)	34 (11%)	8 (2%)
Ardeparin	150	Ardeparin	37 (25%)	9 (6%)	10 (6%)
	149	Ardeparin	41 (28%)	7 (5%)	11 (6%)
	147	Warfarin	60 (41%)	15 (10%)	10 (6%)
Bauer	363	Enoxaparin	101 (27.8%)	20 (5.4%)	0
	361	Fondaparinux	45 (12.5%)	9 (2.4%)	9 (1.7%)[a]
Fractured hip repair					
Gerhart	131	Warfarin	28 (21%)	7 (5%)	3 (2%)
	132	Danaparoid	9 (7%)	3 (2%)	5 (4%)
Eriksson	624	Enoxaparin	119 (19.1%)	28 (4.3%)	16 (1.9%)[a]
	626	Fondaparinux	52 (8.3%)	6 (0.9%)	15 (1.8%)[a]

Note:

[a] Bleeding index >2 = The bleeding index was calculated as the number of units of packed red cells or whole blood transfused plus the hemoglobin values before the bleeding episode minus the hemoglobin values after the episode (grams per deciliter).

(2.5 mg, s.c., 6 h postop then Q day). The incidence of DVT was 9% in the enoxaparin group while 4% receiving fondaparinux had thrombotic events. The major bleeding incidence was 3% with enoxaparin and 3% with fondaparinux. Turpie and colleagues[57] evaluated enoxaparin (30 mg, s.c., Q 12 h) vs. fondaparinux (2.5 mg, s.c., 6 h postop then Q day) in elective hip replacement surgery. DVT was documented in 8% of the patients receiving enoxaparin while 6% of those on fondaparinux developed thrombotic events. The major bleeding incidence was 0.7% with enoxaparin vs. 2% with fondaparinux.

These studies in total hip replacement indicate that the possible methods of prophylaxis for this group of patients are varied. Low molecular weight heparins, warfarin (INR 2–3), and adjusted-dose UFH are the primary agents used. Adjuvant prophylaxis with external pneumatic compression may provide additional efficacy. More studies are needed to assess the additive effect of EPC plus a single pharmacologic agent.

Hip fracture

The incidence of DVT in patients who undergo surgery for hip fracture without prophylaxis varies from 40% to 50%.[58,59,60] This increased risk results from the immobilization that is caused by both the fracture and surgical procedure. Several prophylactic regimens have been evaluated in these patients but no consensus has been reached regarding the most effective approach.

An early study by Bergqvist and coworkers[58] evaluated the use of dicumarol and dextran as prophylaxis for DVT in patients with fracture hips. The incidence of DVT was about 30% with both agents. Taberner and associates[60] assessed the effectiveness of heparin as a prophylactic intervention in this population. In a small cohort study, adjusted-dose UFH reduced the incidence of DVT from 14% in patients receiving fixed doses to 7% in those receiving the adjusted regimen. This was a small study of 28 patients but the trend in outcome appears to be real. Powers and colleagues[59] compared three methods of prophylaxis in patients with hip fractures: placebo, warfarin, and aspirin. DVT was documented in 46% of the placebo group, 40.9% of the aspirin group, and 20% of the warfarin group. This was a significant reduction in the incidence of thrombosis.

Eriksson and associates[61] evaluated hip fracture patients in a randomized prospective trial comparing enoxaparin (40 mg, s.c., preop then Q day) with fondaparinux (2.5 mg, s.c., 6 h postop then Q day)(Table 19.5). The incidence of DVT was 19% with enoxaparin versus 8.3% in those receiving fondaparinux. The major bleeding incidence was 2.1% with enoxaparin and 4% in the cohort receiving fondaparinux.

Based on these few studies with venography as their end point, the use of low-molecular-weight heparin, warfarin or adjusted-dose heparin is recommended for prophylaxis.

Total knee replacement

The incidence of DVT in patients undergoing total knee replacement surgery without prophylaxis is 40% to 84% for isolated calf vein thrombosis and 3% to 20% for proximal vein thrombosis.[62–65] The high incidence of proximal thrombosis is significant because PE has been reported in about 1.7% of patients.[65,66] Despite the high incidence, the following methods of prophylaxis have been shown to have an impact on preventing this postoperative complication: adjusted dose warfarin, AT plus unfractionated heparin, external pneumatic compression sleeves, and LMWH.

As part of a larger study of total hip replacement, Francis and colleagues[37] compared dextran 40 with two-step warfarin therapy in a few patients undergoing total knee replacement. All 8 patients who were given dextran 40 developed DVT compared to 3 of the 14 patients who were given warfarin (21%). A much larger, nonrandomized and nonblinded study by Stulberg and associates[66] evaluated 638 patients undergoing unilateral (338 patients), bilateral (121 patients), and unilateral revision (58 patients) knee replacement surgery. The overall incidence of calf thrombosis was 46.1% and the incidence of proximal vein thrombosis was 10.7%. In a small pilot study, Francis and coworkers[40] used AT replacement in two different doses with subcutaneous unfractionated heparin as prophylaxis in patients undergoing total knee replacement. Fifty percent of those who received low dose AT

and 27% of those who received high-dose AT developed DVT. Although the latter was effective the cost of AT is prohibitive for wide spread use.

Three studies have evaluated the use of mechanical methods of prophylaxis either alone or in combination with pharmacologic agents.[49,63,69] Hull and colleagues[48] compared the use of calf-length EPC sleeves plus acetylsalicylic acid to the use of acetylsalicylic acid alone. The incidence of DVT was 6.3% in the former group and 65.5% in the latter group. All the thrombi occurred in the calf vein in patients who received EPC plus acetylsalicylic acid, whereas 36.8% of the thrombi extended from the calf into the popliteal and femoral veins in the control group. The EPC sleeves in this study were worn an average of 12 days. These devices had a 20-second, 50-mmHg compression cycle with a 60-second relaxation phase. Two problems with this study are the fact that different knee surgeries were performed and acetylsalicylic acid use was not randomized. Despite these inadequacies, the data regarding the efficacy of EPC in preventing DVT was significant.

In another study by Stulberg and colleagues, bilateral and unilateral total knee replacement were evaluated using EPC sleeves versus acetylsalicylic acid, the prophylactic regimen outlined earlier.[66] The incidence of DVT in patients who underwent bilateral total knee replacement was 48% in those who were treated with EPC and 68% in those who were treated with acetylsalicylic acid. Among patients who underwent unilateral total knee replacement, 22% of those in the EPC group developed DVT compared to 47% of those in the acetylsalicylic acid group. All the thrombi occurred in the calf vein in patients who underwent unilateral total knee replacement. The thrombi extended into the popliteal veins in 16.6% of patients who underwent bilateral total knee replacement with EPC compared to only 6.6% of those who received acetylsalicylic acid alone. The EPC sleeves were thigh-length, sequential compression devices. They had an 11-second inflation time at a pressure of 35 to 55 mmHg followed by a 60 second venting cycle. The EPC sleeves were worn for 5 to 7 days. An unexpected finding in this study was a higher incidence of high probability lung scans among asymptomatic patients treated with EPC sleeves who had undergone single or bilateral knee replacement. The lung scan results were not confirmed by angiography.

The final mechanical intervention evaluated was continuous passive motion plus acetylsalicylic acid vs. acetylsalicylic acid with active range of motion exercises.[65] (Table 19.5). A Kinetec 3080 provided the continuous range of motion for an average of 10 hours daily for 5 to

7 days. DVT prevalence was not significantly reduced in these two groups, 45.3% in the former and 37.3% in the latter. The rates of proximal extension of thrombosis were 10.7% and 14.7% respectively. This form of mechanical prophylaxis is not as effective as EPC for the reduction of both distal and proximal vein thrombosis.

LeClerc and colleagues[70] performed a randomized study of 111 patients undergoing total knee arthroplasty who were given either placebo or enoxaparin. The incidence of DVT was reduced from 65% in the placebo group to 20% in the enoxaparin group. Two other studies have been performed comparing LMWH to warfarin therapy in patients undergoing total knee replacement surgery.[71,72] Bauer and associates[71] evaluated patients undergoing elective total knee arthroplasty. The patients were randomized to enoxaparin (30 mg, s.c., Q 12 h) or fondaparinux (2.5 mg, s.c., 6 h postop then Q day). In this trial 27.8% of the patients receiving enoxaparin developed DVT while 12.5% of the fondaparinux cohort had thrombotic events. The incidence of major bleeding was 0.2% with enoxaparin and 2% with fondaparinux.

After reviewing these studies, we recommend the use of low molecular weight heparin or warfarin (INR 2 to 3 range) as DVT prophylaxis in patients who undergo total knee replacement. External pneumatic compression sleeves are an alternative modality but because of the shortened length of stay and extended prophylaxis pharmacologic prophylaxis is preferred.

General surgery

The variety of procedures performed in general surgery make it difficult to accurately assess the incidence of DVT in this patient population. When reviewing studies, it is impossible to segregate patients according to procedure. Individual surgical procedures are included in the next sections under their appropriate specialty heading (Table 19.4).

Five trials were reviewed to document the incidence of DVT in general surgery.[72–76] These studies used ^{125}I fibrinogen scanning as the test of therapeutic efficacy. Only one study confirmed the accuracy of all positive ^{125}I fibrinogen from 20% to 30%. A review by Clagett and coworkers[24] reported an incidence of 25%. Calf vein thrombosis has been the predominant type of thrombosis in these studies.

The approach to prophylaxis in general surgery has been directed toward single pharmacologic agents. Five studies used low-dose subcutaneous UFH, 5000 U given 2 hours before surgery and then Q 8 or 12 h until discharged from the hospital. The incidence of postoperative DVT was reduced by 4% to 17% in the general surgery population studied. Clagett and associates[24] performed a metaanalysis of trials that were controlled, uncontrolled, or involved the comparison of heparin and other prophylactic methods. There appeared to be a trend toward a lower incidence of DVT when prophylactic UFH was administered on an 8-hour rather than a 12-hour schedule. Other methods of prophylaxis have been evaluated in general surgery, including dextran and dihydroergotamine plus UFH. Dextran did not prove to be effective in this population but dihydroergotamine plus UFH was beneficial.[72,76] This combination was withdrawn from the American market, however, because of the adverse reports related to dihydroergotamine. EPC sleeves have been adopted as a mechanical means of preventing postoperative DVT. These devices have been studied primarily in orthopedic, urologic, neurologic, and gynecologic surgery, and not in general surgery.

Four studies using ^{125}I fibrinogen scanning as a thrombotic end point for comparing LMWH to low-dose UFH were reviewed (Table 19.6).[77–81] A large multicenter study[81] showed a significant reduction in the incidence of DVT in patients receiving LMWH. The remaining studies did not demonstrate any change. Only one study by Bergqvist and coworkers[78] recorded a lower bleeding risk in patients treated with LMWH. A recent metaanalysis of LMWH studies in Europe did not reveal any advantage with these agents.[80]

For moderate risk general surgery UFH (5000 units, s.c., Q 12 h) is an appropriate prophylaxis. In the high and very high risk general surgery patients UFH (5000 units, s.c., Q 8 h) or LMWHs are effective selections for DVT/PE prophylaxis. The use of EPC sleeves concomitantly with each of the above pharmacologic modalities may provide an additive effect.

Neurosurgery

The risk of pulmonary embolism in neurosurgical patients has been reported to be as high as 5%, with a mortality rate ranging from 9% to 50%.[82] The incidence of clinically overt deep vein thrombosis has been reported to range from 1.6% to 4%.[83] The incidence of objectively proven DVT has been estimated to range from 19% to 43% in case series using ^{125}I fibrinogen scanning to 33% in clinical trials using venographic endpoints.[84] In six studies, patients underwent craniotomy for either tumor or vascular injury (e.g., subdural hematoma, ruptured aneurysm).[85–90] The largest study that separated supratentorial and infratentorial procedures for tumors was conducted by Valladares and colleagues[90] and did not show a difference in DVT.

Table 19.6. Deep venous thrombosis (DVT) prophylaxis in general surgery with low-molecular-weight heparins (LMWH)

Author	Number of patients	LMWH	DVT	Major bleeding
Encke	960	Fraxiparin	27 (2.8%)	47 (4.9%)
	936	UFH (Q 8 h)	42 (4.5%)	42 (4.5%)
Bergqvist	505	Dalteparin	28 (5.5%)	30 (6%)
	497	UFH (Q 12 h)	41 (8.3%)	15 (3%)
Leizorovicz	430	Tinzaparin	16 (3.7%)	13 (3%)
	429	UFH (Q 12 h)	18 (4.2%)	14 (3.3%)
Samama	159	Enoxaparin	6 (3.8%)	4 (2.5%)
	188	UFH (Q 8 h)	12 (7.6%)	4 (2.5%)

Notes:
UFH = unfractionated heparin.
All patients screened with ^{125}I fibrinogen scanning.
Fraxiparin = 7500 IU, s.c., Q day.
Dalteparin = 5000 IU, s.c., 2 hrs prior to surgery, then 5000 IU, s.c., Q day.
Tinzaparin = 3500 IU, s.c., Q day.
Enoxaparin = 40 mg, s.c., Q day.

Constantini and associates[91] did demonstrate a difference in thrombotic events in supratentorial compared to infratentorial surgery, but the study was not included in this assessment because only patients with a suspicion of DVT were evaluated by noninvasive or invasive testing. With significant risk for the development of thrombosis in this very high risk patient population prophylaxis must be applied (Table 19.4).

Turpie and coworkers[85] and Black and associates[89] were the only authors who addressed the issue of duration of risk for DVT in patients undergoing intracranial procedures. In the study by Turpie's group, the intervention portion lasted for 5 days.[85] After that time, patients continued to be monitored for DVT without being given prophylaxis. Seven of 52 patients (13.4%) in the initial treatment group developed thrombosis between postoperative days 6 and 14. Five of the seven patients were not ambulatory and had paralyzed extremities. Black and colleagues[89] maintained prophylaxis until patients became ambulatory, were discharged from the hospital, or died.

The incidence of DVT is not as well defined in spinal surgery as in craniotomy studies. To assess the former group, three studies with mixed neurosurgical procedures were reviewed and the patients undergoing spinal surgery were abstracted for evaluation.[87–90] These patient groups were small and the spinal surgeries were performed for a variety of conditions, including tumors, disk disease, and undefined problems. The reported incidence of DVT varied from 4% to 60%. Rossi and colleagues[92] and Merli and

associates[93] studied patients with spinal cord injuries who were undergoing fusion or stabilization procedures. Venographically confirmed thrombosis developed in 72% of patients in the former study and in 47% of patients in the latter study within the first 14 days after surgery.

In assessing the efficacy of prophylactic interventions, only those studies that used an accurate measure of DVT were chosen. Approaches to preventing DVT in this surgical population have been tempered by the risk of bleeding into such vulnerable tissues as the brain and spinal cord. Despite this potential risk, Cerroto and associates[90] showed that low-dose heparin reduced the incidence of DVT from 34% in control subjects to 6% in the treated group. UFH (5000 U) was administered subcutaneously every 8 hours. A safe prophylactic dose was achieved by evaluating a plasma heparin concentration obtained 3 hours after the initial dose was given. A UFH level of less than 0.18 U/ml was desired. If a level higher than 0.18 U/ml was obtained, the heparin dose was decreased and the level was reassessed. Once the desired level was achieved, heparin was administered at that dose every 8 hours for 7 days. The risk of bleeding was not increased with this regimen.

Three trials have been completed using LMWHs as DVT/PE prophylaxis in neurosurgery patients (Table 19.7 and 19.8). Melon and associates[94] compared enoxaparin (20 mg, s.c., Q day) and placebo. All patients were given prophylaxis for 10 days at which time bilateral venography was performed. DVT/PE was documented in 15.6% (10/64) of patients in the enoxaparin group while 24.1% (14/58) in

Table 19.7. DVT/PE prophylaxis in neurosurgical patients

Author	Group	DVT/PE	RR	Major bleed
Melon *et al.*	Enoxaparin[a]	10/64 (16.9%)	0.65	0%
	Placebo	14/58 (24.1%)		0%
Nurmohamed	Nadroparin + GCS[b]	31/166 (18.7%)	0.71	2.5%
	Placebo + GCS	47/179 (26.3%)		0.8%
Agnelli	Enoxaparin + GCS[c]	22/130 (16.9%)	0.51	2.6%
	Placebo + GCS	43/130 (33.1%)		2.6%

Notes:

[a] Enoxaparin = 20 mg, s.c., Q day.

[b] Nadroparin = 7500 IU, s.c., Q day.

[c] Enoxaparin = 40 mg, s.c., Q day.

Table 19.8. DVT/PE prophylaxis in neurosurgical patients: incidence of proximal DVT

Author	Group	Proximal DVT/PE	Odds ratio	RR
Nurmohamed	Nadroparin + GCS[a]	12/174 (6.9%)	0.58	.60
	Placebo + GCS	21/182 (11.5%)		
Agnelli	Enoxaparin[b] + GCS[c]	7/130 (5.4%)	0.38	.39
	Placebo + GCS	18/130 (13.8%)		

Notes:

[a] Nadroparin = 7500 IU, s.c., Q day.

[b] Enoxaparin = 40 mg, s.c., Q day.

[c] GCS = gradient compression stockings.

the placebo group developed thromboembolic events. Another study by Nurmohamed and associates[95] compared nadroparin (7500 IU, s.c., Q day) plus gradient compression stockings (GCS) and placebo plus GCS. Screening was completed by clinical assessment, venous compression ultrasound, and venography. In the nadroparin group 18.7% (31/166) developed thromboembolic events while 26.3% (47/179) had thrombotic events in the placebo group. In a similar study design, Agnelli and associates[96] evaluated enoxaparin (40 mg, s.c., Q day) plus GCS versus placebo plus GCS. All patients had bilateral venography at the completion of 7 days of prophylaxis. The placebo group had a 33.1% (43/130) incidence of DVT/PE while 16.9% (22/130) had thromboembolic events in the enoxaparin cohort. The incidence of major bleeding was not increased in the Melon and Agnelli papers while the Nurmohamed study demonstrated an increased incidence of major hemorrhagic events.

An alternative approach to the prevention of postoperative DVT in neurosurgical patients is the use of mechanical devices to reduce stasis and hypercoagulability. Two studies using single-chamber, calf-length EPC sleeves demonstrated a decrease in the incidence of DVT from 18% to 19% in the control group to 1.9% to 5.5% in the treated patients.[85,89] The EPC sleeves were used for an extended period by Black and colleagues[89] (until patients resumed ambulation, were discharged from the hospital, or died) but were only applied for 5 days after the surgical procedure by Turpie and associates.[85] The extended treatment period used by Black was related to the longer postoperative recovery period after craniotomy for subarachnoid hemorrhage.[89] Turpie and coworkers[85] used thigh-length sequential compression sleeves. Turpie and coworkers selected a thigh-length, six-chamber sequential compression sleeve with and without gradient elastic stockings.[85] This device reduced the incidence of thrombosis from 19.8% to 9%.

Patients undergoing spinal surgery have not been evaluated with respect to the indication for their procedures. Skillman and coworkers[88] compared calf-length EPC sleeves to placebo in patients undergoing cervical, thoracic, or lumbar laminectomies. No difference in the number of thrombi could be documented. In patients undergoing spinal surgery for traumatic injury with paralysis, both Green and Associates[97] and Merli and colleagues[93,98] demonstrated a significant reduction in the incidence of DVT using EPC and low-dose UFH. Green and associates[97] compared prophylaxis with EPC sleeves to prophylaxis with EPC sleeves plus aspirin and dipyridamole. It was believed that mechanical methods plus antiplatelet therapy would be ideal for this patient population. The results were compared to historical controls and showed a reduction in the incidence of thrombosis. In their initial work, Merli and colleagues demonstrated a significant reduction in DVT using electrical stimulation plus low-dose heparin versus low dose heparin alone. All patients had bilateral lower extremity venography as the end point of the study. In a second study, EPC sleeves were combined with gradient elastic stockings and low-dose unfractionated heparin.[98] Again, a significant reduction in DVT was documented. A recent paper again supported the use of UFH (5000 units, s.c., Q 8 h) plus EPC sleeves or enoxaparin (30 mg, s.c., Q 12 h) as prophylaxis modalities in acute spinal cord injured patients.[99] In all the studies of spinal cord injury, the risk for the development of DVT was highest in the first 2 weeks after injury.

Currently, the recommendations for DVT prophylaxis for patients undergoing neurosurgical procedures include the following as reviewed in the above paragraphs: EPC sleeves with or without gradient elastic stockings, low-dose unfractionated heparin, LMWH, or combinations of either EPC sleeves with low-dose unfractionated heparin or LMWH. Since the risk of intracranial bleeding is always a significant concern of the neurosurgeon, mechanical prophylaxis is the most frequently preferred modality.

Gynecologic surgery

The incidence of DVT in gynecologic surgery varies according to the type of procedure performed and whether the disease process is malignant or benign. Numerous approaches to prophylaxis have been evaluated and have substantially reduced the incidence of DVT (Table 19.4). Studies using ^{125}I fibrinogen scanning, impedance plethysmography, or venography have been selected to define the incidence of DVT and evaluate appropriate prophylactic interventions.

Four studies examined the incidence of DVT demonstrated on ^{125}I fibrinogen scanning in patients undergoing gynecologic surgery for benign indications.[104–107] Both Bonnar and coworkers[100] and Walsh and associates[101] separated their study populations according to abdominal or vaginal hysterectomy and reported the incidence of thrombosis in each group. Thrombosis was documented in 12% to 15% of patients undergoing abdominal hysterectomy and in 6% to 7% of those undergoing vaginal hysterectomy. Taberner and colleagues[102] and Walsh and associates[101] evaluated mixed gynecologic procedures, including both vaginal and abdominal hysterectomy, and documented thrombosis in 20% to 29% of patients. The discrepancy between these results and those of the other studies is most likely related to variation in the procedures included in the populations studied.

Gynecologic surgery for malignancy is associated with a much higher incidence of postoperative thrombotic events. Seven studies were reviewed.[101–108] Walsh,[101] Clarke-Pearson,[105] and Crandon[106] demonstrated a 35% to 38% incidence of DVT in patients undergoing major pelvic procedures for malignancy. In contrast, the remaining four studies documented rates of DVT between 12% and 23%.[102,103,106,107] The surgical procedures performed were similar, as were the methods used to assess thrombosis. The reason for the differences in results is not known.

In assessing the efficacy of prophylactic interventions, the studies reviewed are divided according to whether they used pharmacologic interventions or mechanical devices and whether they involved surgery for malignant or benign conditions. This separation demonstrates the dual clinical approach used throughout the country.

Seven studies were evaluated.[102–104,106,108,109] Bonnar and colleagues[100] compared dextran to a control group in patients undergoing vaginal or abdominal hysterectomy. The dextran was administered during and shortly after the procedure. The incidence of thrombosis was reduced from 15% to 0% in patients undergoing abdominal hysterectomy and from 6% to 1% in those undergoing vaginal hysterectomy. Taberner and coworkers[102] assessed the efficacy of low-dose heparin, warfarin, and placebo. Both low-dose heparin and warfarin reduced the incidence of DVT from 23% in the placebo group to 6% in the treated groups. The prothrombin ratios were maintained between 2 and 2.5 for the study. Ballard and associates[103] compared low-dose heparin with a control group and found that the incidence of DVT was decreased from 29% to 3.6%. Based on the results of these studies, the use of low-dose UFH or dextran alone is recommended as prophylaxis for DVT in patients undergoing gynecologic surgery for benign conditions. Because so few studies have been done on warfarin, I would not use this agent in this patient population unless no other alternative was available. As mentioned previously in this chapter dextran is no longer used as prophylaxis modality in this country.

The efficacy of low-dose UFH for DVT prophylaxis in gynecologic surgery for malignancy has been assessed in three studies. In a study of 185 patients, Clarke-Pearson and colleagues[105] reported no difference in the incidence of DVT between patients who received low-dose UFH (14.8%) and a control group (12.4%). The same authors completed a second study comparing three protocols: the administration of a placebo, the administration of low-dose heparin only after surgery, and the administration of low-dose heparin both 2 or 3 days before surgery and after surgery.[108] The 18.4% incidence of DVT was reduced to 8% with postoperative administration of low-dose UFH. More recently, a third study by Clarke-Pearson[109] comparing the administration of low-dose UFH (5000 U subcutaneously 2 hours before surgery and every 8 hours after surgery) to the use of EPC sleeves demonstrated heparin's effectiveness in reducing the incidence of DVT. Based on these results, we recommend low-dose UFH (5000 units, s.c., Q 8 h) as a single pharmacologic agent of choice.

A large double-blind randomized multi-center trial evaluated enoxaparin (40 mg, s.c., Q day) vs. UFH (5000 units, s.c., Q day) in elective surgery in patients with pelvic and abdominal malignancies.[110] All patients received prophylaxis for 10 ± 2 days at which time bilateral lower extremity venography was performed. In the enoxaparin group 14.7% (46/312) had documented thrombotic events while 18.2% (58/319) of the patients in the UFH cohort had DVT/PE. The two prophylactic interventions were equivalent in efficacy. There was no significant difference in the incidence of major hemorrhagic events.

Prophylaxis may also be accomplished with mechanical devices. Two studies of such techniques have been completed using single-chamber calf compression devices for 5 days after surgery. The first study compared EPC sleeves to a control and documented DVT rates of 12.7% and 34.6%, respectively.[106] The second study compared EPC sleeves to low-dose UFH (5000 U given subcutaneously every 8 hours) and demonstrated no statistical difference in DVT incidence (1.9% vs. 4.6%).[109] The patients who received low-dose UFH in this study required more blood transfusions after surgery and had an increased volume of retroperitoneal drainage. Mechanical methods are an effective alternative to pharmacologic therapy in this high-risk population.

The recommendations for DVT prophylaxis in gynecologic surgery can be broken down into those with benign or malignant disease. For patients having major surgery for benign gynecologic disease the use of either low-dose unfractionated heparin, LMWH, or EPC sleeves are recommended. Those patients having extensive surgery for gynecologic malignancy should receive low-dose unfractionated heparin or LMWH with EPC sleeves. All prophylaxis in either of the above patient groups should maintain DVT prophylaxis until the patient is discharged from the hospital.

Urologic surgery

It is difficult to evaluate the incidence of DVT in patients undergoing urologic surgery because of the lack of uniform study procedures and the variety of surgical procedures evaluated. Urologic studies that had defined cohorts and objective end points for DVT are discussed here (Table 19.4).

Transurethral resection of the prostate is a frequently performed surgical procedure in the United States. Two small studies have shown the incidence of DVT in patients undergoing this procedure to be 7% to 10% using ^{125}I fibrinogen scanning as the thrombosis end point.[111,112] Because of this low incidence, few studies of prophylaxis have been performed in these patients. In an uncontrolled randomized trial, Van Arsdalen and coworkers[113] compared EPC and gradient elastic stockings as prophylactic interventions. They reported DVT rates of 7.6% with EPC and 6.2% with gradient elastic stockings. This difference was not statistically significant. The low incidence of thrombosis in transurethral resection of the prostate requires a large cohort of patients to demonstrate the clinical benefit of a prophylactic intervention. The present

recommendation for DVT prophylaxis in transurethral resection of the prostate is the use of EPC, low-dose UFH, or gradient elastic stockings.

Open prostatectomy is the primary surgical approach for the treatment of patients with prostate cancer. Seven studies using either ^{125}I fibrinogen scanning or venography have documented the incidence of DVT after this procedure to vary between 16% and 51%.[111–117] Two of the studies by Becker and colleagues[114,115] used venography at varying times after surgery. This approach did not provide an accurate natural history of the development of thrombosis after open prostatectomy. Even if these two studies are not included, the incidence of DVT remains high at 21% to 51%.

Preventing this postoperative complication is a major significance in urologic surgery. Six studies using several methods of prophylaxis for thrombosis have been completed.[116–122] The study populations in these protocols underwent a variety of urologic procedures, with open prostatectomy predominating. In four of the studies, EPC sleeves reduced the incidence of DVT significantly to about 6% to 12% compared to the control rate of 25% to 34%. Vandendris and associates[123] reported a reduction in the incidence of DVT from 39% in the control group to 10% in the patients who received low-dose warfarin and reported no case of DVT by duplex scanning in 53 patients studied. No fatal PE occurred in any of these studies.

Patients undergoing radical prostatectomy or major urologic procedures should receive EPC sleeves with either low-dose unfractionated heparin (5000 U, s.c., Q 8 h) or LMWH (enoxaparin 40 mg, s.c., Q day or dalteparin 5000 U, s.c., Q day). All prophylaxis regimens should be maintained until the patient is discharged.

Duration of risk for deep venous thrombosis or pulmorary embolism following surgery

The length of time during which patients are at risk for the development of DVT after surgery has become an important issue because of dramatic reductions in the duration of hospitalization after procedures. The publications reviewed earlier in this chapter focused on DVT/PE during the patient hospital stay and did not assess the risk of thrombosis after discharge from the hospital. All the research subjects underwent evaluation for thrombosis before they were discharged. Importantly, the recommended prophylactic regimens do not eliminate the incidence of thrombosis. In practice, venous imaging or venography cannot be performed before hospital discharge on all patients to detect the small percentage who will develop thrombosis despite prophylaxis. Determining the incidence of clinically significant thromboembolic disease after discharge and the risk-benefit ratio of prophylaxis is of critical importance.

In a study by Scurr,[124,125] 51 patients who underwent major abdominal surgery for benign and malignant disease were followed up for 6 weeks after discharge from the hospital. All patients underwent ^{125}I fibrinogen scanning and plethysmography studies. Thirteen of the 51 patients (25%) developed DVT during the 6-week study period. Only patients with positive results on noninvasive studies underwent venography. The highest incidence of DVT occurred during days 4 through 10 after discharge from the hospital.

In a study by Paiement and coworkers,[126] 268 patients undergoing elective total hip replacement were evaluated. All patients received warfarin prophylaxis during their hospitalization and for 6 months after discharge. No standard non-invasive or invasive testing for DVT or PE was performed. Patients were assessed clinically on an outpatient basis. No fatal PE occurred during the study period and no known PE occurred after the patients were discharged from the hospital.

Lausen and colleagues[127] assessed 89 general surgery patients. All received postoperative prophylaxis with low-molecular-weight heparin (Tinzaparin). At the time of hospital discharge, 45 patients were given no extended prophylaxis and 44 were given LMWH for 3 weeks. The patients were followed up and DVT was assessed by venous imaging. None of the patients in the group that received LMWH developed DVT compared to 15.6% of the group that did not receive prophylaxis. DVT occurred predominantly in the calf between days 15 and 29 after discharge.

Nationally, orthopedic surgeons are the primary group advocating the use of extended prophylaxis after hospital discharge. Bergqvist and associates[128] treated 262 total hip arthroplasty patients with enoxaparin (40 mg, s.c., Q day) for an average of 10 days. At the end of the hospitalization, the patients were randomized to either enoxaparin (40 mg, s.c., Q day) or placebo. Bilateral leg venography was performed within 19 to 23 days. Thrombotic events in the placebo group were 37% (45 of 116 patients) with 24% (28 of 116 patients) proximal thrombi. In the enoxaparin group, the overall incidence of DVT was 18% (21/117) with 7% (8/117) proximal thrombi. Extended prophylaxis with enoxaparin had a lower incidence of thrombotic events ($P = <0.001$).

In a study by Planes and associates[129] 173 patients were treated in the hospital with enoxaparin (40 mg, s.c., Q day) for 13 to 15 days. Bilateral leg venography was performed before discharge, and the patients without thrombosis were randomized to placebo or enoxaparin. After 21 days, all patients had bilateral lower extremity venography. The incidence of total DVT was 19.3% (17/88) in the placebo group and 7.6% (6/85) in the enoxaparin group. Proximal thrombosis was present in 7.9% (7/88) of the placebo patients vs. 5.9% in the enoxaparin group. In this study, the overall incidence of thrombosis was reduced significantly ($P = 0.018$), but there was not a reduction in proximal events.

A study by Lassen et al.[130] evaluated the use of dalteparin (5000 IU, s.c., Q day) for 7 days in patients undergoing primary and revision total hip arthroplasty. After 7 days, patients were randomized to receive dalteparin (5000 IU, s.c., Q day) or placebo for 28 days as outpatients. All patients had bilateral lower extremity venography performed on the 35th day of prophylaxis. In the placebo group 11.8% (12/102) developed DVT vs. 4.4% (5/113) in the enoxaparin group. Proximal vein thrombosis was diagnosed in 5% (5/102) of the placebo group whereas the enoxaparin group had 1% (1/113). This study demonstrated that 35 days of prophylaxis following total hip arthroplasty was more effective than 7 days of in-hospital prophylaxis.

Dahl and associates[131] evaluated 218 total hip arthroplasty patients given prophylaxis with dextran 70, gradient elastic stockings, and dalteparin (5000 IU, s.c., Q day). On the seventh postoperative day, all patients had bilateral leg venography, ventilation-perfusion lung scanning, and a chest radiograph. Patients without thrombosis were randomized to dalteparin (5000 IU, s.c., Q day) or placebo. On day 35, the three studies were repeated, and 31.7% (33/104) of the placebo group developed DVT while only 19.3% (22/114) of the dalteparin group had thrombotic events. The incidence of proximal thrombosis was 9% in the dalteparin group and 13% in the placebo group. This study shows that prolonged thromboprophylaxis with dalteparin for 35 days significantly reduces the frequency of DVT and should be recommended for 5 weeks after total hip arthroplasty.

Hull and associates[132] randomized patients to preoperative and postoperative dalteparin dosing vs. warfarin for 7 to 10 days, at which time patients had bilateral leg venography. The patients without thrombosis continued dalteparin or placebo. Repeat venography was performed on day 35. In the placebo group 37% (69/188) developed DVT vs. 20% (68/345) in the dalteparin cohort. The proximal thrombosis incidence was 9% in the placebo treated patients and 3% in the dalteparin group.

The above studies used venography or lung scanning as endpoints to evaluate the efficacy and safety of prophylactic interventions in this orthopedic population. The incidence of symptomatic DVT/PE was very low in these studies.

The next group of trials will focus on not extending prophylaxis but following patients post orthopedic surgery and evaluating only symptomatic disease. Robinson and associates[133] performed lower extremity ultrasound or sham ultrasound studies on 1000 patients at the completion of 7 to 10 days of warfarin prophylaxis. The patients were followed for 90 days, with all symptomatic patients fully evaluated for thromboembolic disease. In the total hip arthroplasty group, 1.2% (6/506) had symptomatic venous thromboembolic events and 0 incidence of fatal PE. The total knee arthroplasty patients had a 0.6% (3/518) incidence of thromboembolic events and 1 (0.2%) fatal PE. This study concluded that the use of 7 to 10 days of postoperative warfarin prophylaxis resulted in a low rate of symptomatic DVT or PE after hospital discharge.

Leclerc and associates[134] evaluated the incidence of symptomatic thromboembolic disease in patients undergoing total hip arthroplasty or total knee arthroplasty during the 90 days after surgery. All patients had a mean of 9 days of enoxaparin (30 mg, s.c., Q 12 h) during the hospitalization and no prophylaxis during the 90-day follow-up period. Symptomatic patients were evaluated for DVT or PE by appropriate testing. Of 1142 total hip arthroplasty patients, 49 (4.3%) developed thrombotic events while 33 (3.9%) of 842 total knee arthroplasty patients were diagnosed with DVT or PE. Three patients (0.4%) in the total knee arthroplasty sustained fatal PE during the outpatient follow-up. The conclusion of this trial was that 7 to 10 days of postoperative prophylaxis with enoxaparin was associated with a clinically acceptable rate of symptomatic venous thromboembolic events.

Colwell and associates[135] evaluated patients up to 90 days after total hip or knee arthroplasty for which they had received either 7 days of enoxaparin or warfarin prophylaxis. Of the 1516 total hip arthroplasty patients on enoxaparin (30 mg, s.c., Q 12 h), 3.6% (55/1516) developed symptomatic DVT and 0.1% (2/1516) had fatal pulmonary embolism. Of the 1495 total knee arthroplasty patients receiving warfarin, 3.7% (56/1495) had symptomatic DVT and 0.1% (2/1495) had fatal pulmonary emboli. This study had the same conclusion as the Leclerc study.

Heit and associates[136] treated 1195 patients undergoing total hip or total knee arthroplasty with ardeparin (50 IU/kg, s.c., Q 12 h) for an average of 7 days. After discharge, the patients were randomized to placebo or ardeparin (100 IU/kg, s.c., Q day to a maximum of 10 000 IU) and followed for 6 weeks, during which time any symptoms or signs of venous thrombotic events were evaluated. The placebo group had a 2% incidence of symptomatic DVT, PE, or death and the ardeparin group had 1.5% such events. This study also did not support the continued use of extended prophylaxis.

White and associates[137] evaluated 9586 primary total hip arthroplasties and 24 059 primary total knee arthroplasties from the state of California's discharge database. The cumulative incidence of DVT or PE within 3 months of surgery was 556 (2.8%) after total hip arthroplasty and 508 (2.1%) after total knee arthroplasty. This study documented that the diagnosis of DVT or PE occurred after hospital discharge in 76% of total hip arthroplasties and in 47% of total knee arthroplasties. This incidence is similar to the 64% of all thromboembolic complications after total hip athroplasty in patients reported by Warwick and associates. The White study documented the median time of diagnosis of DVT or PE after surgery was 17 days for total hip arthroplasties and 7 days after total knee arthroplasties.

The above data supports the use of LMWH (enoxaparin 40 mg, s.c., Q day) or warfarin (INR 2–3) for 29–35 days as extended DVT/PE prophylaxis in the prevention of clinically significant venous thromboembolic events following orthopedic surgery. The recent College of Chest Physicians guidelines recommended that extended DVT/PE prophylaxis be considered for general surgery patients, who, in the judgment of the clinician, have continued risk for developing DVT/PE following discharge. The recommendation was LMWH (enoxaparin 40 mg s.c. daily or dalteparin 5000 units s.c.) for 30 days.[138]

REFERENCES

1. Carter, C. & Gent, M. The epidemiology of venous thrombosis. In Colman, R., Hirsh, J., Marder, V., & Salzman, E., eds. *Hemostasis and Thrombosis*. Philadelphia: J. B. Lippincott, 1982: 805–819.

2. Dismuke, S. & Wagner, E. Pulmonary embolism as a cause of death: the changing mortality in hospitalized patients. *J. Am. Med. Assoc.* 1986; **255**: 2039–2042.

3. Anderson, F., Wheeler, H., Goldberg, R. *et al.* A population based perspective of the hospital incidence and case fatality rate of deep vein thrombosis and pulmonary embolism: the Worchester DVT study. *Arch. Intern. Med.* 1991; **151**: 933–938.

4. Anderson, F., Wheeler, H., Goldberg, R. *et al.* Physician practice in the prevention of venous thromboembolism. *Ann. Intern. Med.* 1991; **115**: 591–595.

5. Nicolaides, A., Kakkar, V., & Renney, J. Soleal sinuses and stasis. *Br. J. Surg.* 1970; **57**: 307.

6. Nicolaides, A., Kakkar, V., Field, E. *et al.* Venous stasis and deep vein thrombosis. *Br. J. Surg.* 1972; **59**: 713–716.

7. Stamatakis, J., Kakkar, V., Sagar, S. *et al.* Femoral vein thrombosis and total hip replacement. *Br. Med. J.* 1977; **112**: 223–225.

8. Clark, C. & Cotton, L. Blood flow in deep veins of the legs: recording technique and evaluation of method to increase flow during operation. *Br. J. Surg.* 1968; **55**: 211–214.

9. Lindstrom, B., Ahlman, H., Honsson, O. *et al.* Blood flow in the calves during surgery. *Acta Chir. Scand.* 1977; **143**: 335–339.

10. Linstrom, B., Ahlman, H., Jonsson, O. *et al.* Influence of anesthesia on blood flow to the calves during surgery. *Acta Anaesthesiol. Scand.* 1984; **28**: 201–203.

11. Johnson, R., Carmichael, J., Almond, H. *et al.* Deep vein thrombosis following charneley arthroplasty. *Clin. Orthop.* 1978; **132**: 24–30.

12. Planes, A., Vochelle, N., & Fagola, M. Total hip replacement and deep vein thrombosis: a venographic and necropsy study. *J. Bone Joint Surg.* 1990; **72B**: 9–13.

13. Stamatakis, J., Kakkar, V., Sagar, S. *et al.* Femoral vein thrombosis and total hip replacement. *Br. Med. J.* 1977; **2**: 223–225.

14. Comerota, A., Stewart, G., Alburger, P. *et al.* Operative venodilation: a previously unsuspected factor in the cause of postoperative deep vein thrombosis. *Surgery* 1989; **106**: 301–309.

15. Schaub, P., Lynch, P., & Stewart, G. The response of canine veins to three types of abdominal surgery: a scanning and transmission electron microscope study. *Surgery* 1978; **83**: 411–422.

16. Stewart, G., Schaub, R., & Niewiarowske, S. Products of tissue injury: their induction of venous endothelial damage and blood cell adhesion in the dog. *Arch. Pathol. Lab. Med.* 1980; **104**: 409–413.

17. Stewart, G., Alburger, P., Stone, E. *et al.* Total hip replacement induces injury to remote veins in a canine model. *J. Bone Joint Surg.* 1983; **65A**: 97–102.

18. Gitel, S., Salvanti, E., Wessler, S. *et al.* The effect of total hip replacement and general surgery on antithrombin III in relation to venous thrombosis. *J. Bone Joint Surg.* 1979; **61A**: 653–656.

19. Eriksson, B., Eriksson, E., Wessler, S. *et al.* Thrombosis after hip replacement: relationship to the fibrinolytic system. *Acta Orthop. Scand.* 1989; **60**: 159–163.

20. Kluft, C., Verheijen, J., Jie, A. *et al.* The postoperative fibrinolytic shutdown: a rapidly reverting acute phase pattern for the fast acting inhibitor of tissue type plasminogen activator after trauma. *Scand. J. Clin. Lab. Invest.* 1985; **45**: 605–610.

21. D'Angelo, A., Kluft, C., Verheijen, J. *et al.* Fibrinolytic shut down after surgery: impairment of the balance between tissue plasminogen activator and its specific inhibitors. *Eur. J. Clin. Invest.* 1985; **15**: 308–312.

22. Salzman, E. & Hirsh, J. Prevention of venous thromboembolism. In Colman, R., Hirsh, J., Marder, V. *et al.*, eds. *Hemostasis and Thrombosis: Basic Principles of Clinical Practice.* Philadelphia: J. B. Lippincott, 1987: 986–999.

23. Geerts, W., Heit, J., Clagett, G. *et al.* Prevention of venous thromboembolism. *Chest* 2001; **119**: 132S–175S.

24. Clagett, G. & Reisch, J. Prevention of venous thromboembolism in general surgical patients: results of meta-analysis. *Ann. Surg.* 1988; **208**: 277–239.

25. Hall, J., McConahay, D., Gibson, D. *et al.* Heparin necrosis: an anticoagulation syndrome. *J. Am. Med. Assoc.* 1980; **244**: 1831–1832.

26. White, P., Sadd, J., & Nensel, R. Thrombotic complications of heparin therapy. *Ann. Surg.* 1979; **190**: 595–608.

27. Hrushesky, W. Subcutaneous heparin-induced thrombocytopenia. *Arch. Intern. Med.* 1978; **138**: 1489–1491.

28. Edes, T., Edeste, Sunderrajan, E. Heparin induced hyperkalemia. *Arch. Intern. Med.* 1985; **145**: 1070–1072.

29. Leyvraz, P., Richard, J., Bachmann, F. *et al.* Adjusted versus fixed dose subcutaneous heparin in the prevention of DVT after total hip replacement. *N. Engl. J. Med.* 1983; **309**: 954–958.

30. Leyvraz, P., Bachman, F., Vuilleumier, B. *et al.* Adjusted subcutaneous heparin versus heparin plus dihydroergotamine in prevention of deep vein thrombosis after total hip arthroplasty. *J. Arthroplasty* 1988; **3**: 81–86.

31. Nurmohamed, M., Rosendaal, F., Buller, H. *et al.* Low molecular weight heparin versus standard heparin in general and orthopedic surgery: a meta-analysis. *Lancet* 1992; **340**: 152–156.

32. Hirsh, J. & Levine, M. Low molecular weight heparin. *Blood* 1992; **79**: 1–17.

33. Weitz, J. Low molecular weight heparins. *N. Engl. J. Med.* 1997; **337**: 688–698.

34. Young, E., Prins, M., Levine, M., & Hirsh, J. Heparin binding to plasma proteins, an important mechanism for heparin resistance. *Thromb. Haemost.* 1992; **67**: 639–643.

35. Samama, M. Synthetic direct and indirect factor Xa inhibitors. *Thromb. Res.* 2002; **106**: 267–273.

36. Harris, W., Salzman, E., Athanasoulis, C., Waltman, A.C., Baum, S., & DeSanctis, R.W. Comparison of warfarin, low molecular weight dextran, aspirin, and subcutaneous heparin in prevention of venous thromboembolism following total hip replacement. *J. Bone Joint Surg.* 1974; **56A**: 1552–1562.

37. Francis, C., Marder, V., Evart, C. *et al.* Two-step warfarin therapy: prevention of postoperative venous thrombosis without excessive bleeding. *J. Am. Med. Assoc.* 1983; **249**: 374–378.

38. Amstutz, H., Friscia, D., Dorey, F. *et al.* Warfarin prophylaxis to prevent mortality from pulmonary embolism after total hip replacement. *J. Bone. Joint Surg.* 1989; **71A**: 321–326.

39. Goldhaber, S., Morpurgo, M., for the WHO/ISFC Task Force on Pulmonary Embolism. Diagnosis, treatment, and prevention of pulmonary embolism. *J. Am. Med. Assoc.* 1992; **268**: 1727–1733.

40. Francis, C., Pellegrini, V., Marder, V. *et al.* Prevention of venous thrombosis after total hip arthroplasty: antithrombin III and low dose heparin compared with dextran 40. *J. Bone Joint Surg.* 1989; **71A**: 327–335.

41. Caprini, J., Scurr, J., & Hasty, J. Role of compression modalities in a prophylactic program for deep vein thrombosis. *Semin. Thromb. Hemost.* 1988; **14**: 77–87.

42. Gardner, A. & Fox, R. The venous pump of the human foot: a preliminary report. *Bristol Med. Chir. J.* 1983; **98**: 109–114.

43. Fordyce, M. & Ling, R. A venous foot pump reduces thrombosis after total hip replacement. *J. Bone Joint Surg.* 1992; **74B**: 45–49.

44. Wilson, N., Das, S., Kakkar, V. *et al.* Thrombo-embolic prophylaxis in total knee replacement: evaluation of the A-V impulse system. *J. Bone Joint Surg.* 1992; **74B**: 50–52.

45. Collins, R., Scrimogeour, A., Yusuf, S. *et al.* Reduction in fatal pulmonary embolism and venous thrombosis by perioperative administration of subcutaneous heparin: overview of results of randomized trials in general, orthopedic, and urologic surgery. *N. Engl. J. Med.* 1988; **318**: 1162–1173.

46. Levine, M., Hirsh, J., Gent, M. *et al.* Prevention of deep vein thrombosis after elective hip surgery: a randomized trial comparing low molecular weight heparin with standard unfractionated heparin. *Ann. Intern. Med.* 1991; **114**: 545–551.

47. Planes, A., Vochelle, N., Mazas, F. *et al.* Prevention of postoperative venous thrombosis: a randomized trial comparing unfractionated heparin with low molecular weight heparin in patients undergoing total hip replacement. *Thromb. Haemost.* 1988; **60**: 407–410.

48. Hull, R., Delmore, J., Hirsh, M. *et al.* Effectiveness of intermittent pulsatile elastic stockings for the prevention of calf and thigh vein thrombosis in patients undergoing elective knee surgery. *Thromb. Res.* 1979; **16**: 37–45.

49. Hull, R., Raskob, G., McLoughlin, D. *et al.* Effectiveness of intermittent pneumatic leg compression for preventing deep vein thrombosis after total hip replacement. *J. Am. Med. Assoc.* 1990; **263**: 2313–2317.

50. Bailey, J., Kruger, M., Salano, F. *et al.* Prospective randomized trial of sequential compression devices vs low-dose warfarin for deep vein thrombosis prophylaxis in total hip arthroplasty. *J. Arthroplasty* 1991; **6**: S29–S35.

51. Francis, C., Pellegrini, V., Marder, V. *et al.* Comparison of warfarin and external pneumatic compression in prevention of venous thrombosis after total hip replacement. *J. Am. Med. Assoc.* 1992; **267**: 2911–2915.

52. Gallus, A., Raman, K., & Darby, T. Venous thrombosis after elective hip replacement: the influence of preventive intermittent calf compression and of surgical technique. *Br. J. Surg.* 1983; **70**: 17–19.

53. Paiement, G., Wessinger, S., Waltman, A. *et al.* Low dose warfarin versus external pneumatic compression against venous thromboembolism following total hip replacement. *J. Arthroplasty* 1987; **2**: 23–26.

54. Turpie, A., Levine, M., Hirsh, J. *et al.* A randomized controlled trial of a low molecular weight heparin (enoxaparin) to prevent deep vein thrombosis in patients undergoing elective hip surgery. *N. Engl. J. Med.* 1986; **315**: 925.

55. Hoek, J., Nurmohamed, M., ten Cate, H. *et al.* Prevention of deep vein thrombosis following total hip replacement by a low molecular weight heparinoid. *Thromb. Haemost.* 1989; **62**: 1637.

56. Lassen, M., Bauer, K., Erikssson, B. *et al.* European Pentasaccharide Elective Surgery Study (EPHESUS) Steering Committtee: Postoperative fondaparinux versus preoperative enoxaparin for prevention of venous thromboembolism in elective hip replacement surgery: a randomized double blind comparison. *Lancet* 2002; **359**: 1715–1720.

57. Turpie, A., Bauer, K., Eriksson, B., & Lassen, M. The PENTATHLON 2000 Study Steering Committee. Postoperative fondaparinux versus postoperative enoxaparin for prevention of venous thromboembolism after elective hip replacement surgery: a randomized double-blind trial. *Lancet* 2002; **359**: 1721–1726.

58. Bergqvist, E., Berqvist, D., & Bronge, A. An evaluation of early thrombosis prophylaxis following fracture of the femoral neck: a comparison between dextran and dicoumarol. *Acta Chir. Scand.* 1972; **138**: 689.

59. Powers, P., Bent, M., Jay, R. *et al.* A randomized trial of less intense postoperative warfarin or aspirin therapy in the prevention of venous thromboembolism after surgery for fractured hip. *Arch. Intern. Med.* 1989; **149**: 771–774.

60. Taberner, D., Poller, L., Thomson, J. *et al.* Randomized study of adjusted versus fixed low dose heparin prophylaxis of deep vein thrombosis in hip surgery. *Br. J. Surg.* 1989; **76**: 933–935.

61. Eriksson, B. *et al.* for the Steering Committee of the Pentasaccharide in major knee surgery group. Fondaparinux compared with enoxaparin for the prevention of venous thromboembolism after hip fracture surgery. *N. Engl. J. Med.* 2001; **345**: 1298–1304.

62. Cohen, S., Ehrlich, G., Kauffman, M. *et al.* Thrombophlebitis following knee surgery. *J. Bone Joint Surg.* 1973; **55A**: 106–112.

63. Lynch, A., Bourne, R., Rorabeck, C. *et al.* Deep vein thrombosis and continuous passive motion after total knee arthroplasty. *J. Bone Joint Surg.* 1988; **70A**: 11–14.

64. Colwell, C., Spiro, T., Trowbridge, A., *et al.* Efficacy and safety of enoxaparin versus unfractionated heparin for prevention of deep venous thrombosis after elective knee arthroplasty. *Clin. Orthop.* 1995; **321**: 19–27.

65. Stringer, M., Steadman, C., Hedges, A. *et al.* Deep vein thrombosis after elective knee surgery. *J. Bone Joint Surg.* 1989; **71B**: 492–497.

66. Stulberg, B., Insall, J., William, G. *et al.* Deep vein thrombosis following total knee replacement: an analysis of six hundred and thirty-eight arthroplasties. *J. Bone Joint Surg.* 1984; **66A**: 194–201.

67. Haas, S., Insall, J., Scuderi, G. *et al.* Pneumatic sequential compression boots compared with aspirin prophylaxis of deep vein thrombosis after total knee arthroplasty. *J. Bone Joint Surg.* 1990; **72A**: 27–31.

68. Leclerc, J., Geerts, W., Desjardins, L. *et al.* Prevention of deep vein thrombosis after major knee surgery: a randomized, double-blind trial comparing a low molecular weight heparin fragment (enoxaparin) to placebo. *Thromb. Haemost.* 1992; **67**: 417–423.

69. Leclerc, J., Geerts, W., Desjardins, L. *et al.* Prevention of venous thromboembolism after knee arthroplasty: a

randomized, double blind trial comparing enoxaparin with warfarin. *Ann. Intern. Med.* 1996; **124**: 619–626.

70. Heit, J., Berkowitz, S., Bona, R. *et al.* Efficacy and safety of low molecular weight heparin (ardeparin sodium) compared to warfarin for the prevention of venous thromboembolism after total knee replacement surgery: a double blind, dose ranging study. *Thromb. Haemost.* 1997; **77**: 32–38.

71. Bauer, K., Eriksson, B., Lassen, M. *et al.* Fondaparinux compared with enoxaparin for the prevention of venous thromboembolism after elective major knee surgery. *N. Engl. J. Med.* 2001; **345**: 1305–1310.

72. A multi-unit controlled trial. Heparin versus dextran in the prevention of deep vein thrombosis. *Lancet* 1974; **11**: 118.

73. An international multi-center study. Prevention of fatal postoperative pulmonary embolism by low doses of heparin. *Lancet* 1975; **11**: 45.

74. Gallus, A., Hirsh, J., O'Brien, S. *et al.* Prevention of venous thrombosis with small subcutaneous doses of heparin. *J. Am. Med. Assoc.* 1976; **235**: 1980.

75. Groote-Schuur Hospital Thromboembolism Study Group. Failure of low dose heparin to prevent significant thromboembolic complications in high risk surgical patients: interim report of a prospective trial. *Br. Med. J.* 1979; **1**: 1447.

76. Multi-Center Trial Committee. DHE/heparin prophylaxis of postoperative DVT. *J. Am. Med. Assoc.* 1984; **251**: 2960–2966.

77. Nurmohamed, M., Verhaege, R., Haas, S. *et al.* A comparative trial of a low molecular weight heparin (enoxaparin) versus standard heparin for the prophylaxis of postoperative deep vein thrombosis in general surgery. *Am. J. Surg.* 1995; **169**: 567–571.

78. Bergqvist, D., Matzsch, T., Burmark, U. *et al.* Low molecular weight heparin given the evening before surgery compared with conventional low dose heparin in prevention of thrombosis. *Br. J. Surg.* 1988; **75**: 888–891.

79. Leizorowicz, A., Haugh, M., Chapuis, F. *et al.* Low molecular weight heparin in prevention of perioperative thrombosis. *Br. Med. J.* 1992; **305**: 913–920.

80. Kakkar, V., Boeckl, O., Boneu, B. *et al.* Efficacy and safety of a low molecular weight heparin and standard unfractionated heparin for prophylaxis of postoperative venous thromboembolism: European multicenter trial. *World. J. Surg.* 1997; **21**: 2–9.

81. Bergqvist, D. Review of clinical trials of low molecular weight heparins. *Eur. J. Surg.* 1992; **158**: 67–78.

82. Hamilton, M., Hull, R., & Pineo, G. Venous thromboembolism in neurosurgery and neurology patients: a review. *Neurosurgery* 1994; **34**: 280–296.

83. Levi, A., Wallace, M., Bernstein, M., & Walters, B. Venous thromboembolism after brain tumor surgery: a retrospective review. *Neurosurgery* 1991; **28**: 859–863.

84. Agnelli, G. Prevention of venous thromboembolism after neurosurgery. *Thromb. Haemost.* 1999; **82**: 925–930.

85. Turpie, A., Gallus, A., Beatties, W. *et al.* Prevention of venous thrombosis in patients with intracranial disease by intermittent pneumatic compression of the calf. *Neurology* 1977; **27**: 435–438.

86. Cerroto, D., Ariano, C., & Fiacchino, F. Deep vein thrombosis and low-dose heparin prophylaxis in neurosurgical patients. *J. Neurosurg.* 1978; **49**: 378–381.

87. Joffe, S. Incidence of postoperative deep vein thrombosis in neurosurgical patients. *J. Neurosurg.* 1975; **42**: 201–203.

88. Skillman, J., Collins, R., Coe, N. *et al.* Prevention of deep vein thrombosis in neurosurgical patients: a controlled, randomized trial of external pneumatic compression boots. *Surgery* 1978; **83**: 354–358.

89. Black, P., Crowell, R., & Abbott, W. External pneumatic calf compression reduces deep venous thrombosis in patients with ruptured intracranial aneurysms. *Neurosurgery* 1980; **6**: 138–141.

90. Valladares, J. & Hankinson, J. Incidence of lower extremity deep vein thrombosis in neurosurgical patients. *Neurosurgery* 1980; **6**: 138–141.

91. Constantini, S., Kornowski, R., Pomeranz, S. *et al.* Thromboembolic phenomena in neurosurgical patients operated upon for primary and metastatic brain tumors. *Acta Neurochir (Wien)* 1991; **109**: 93–97.

92. Rossi, E., Green, D., Rosen, J. *et al.* Sequential changes in factor VIII and platelets preceding deep vein thrombosis in patients with spinal cord injury. *Br. J. Haematol.* 1980; **45**: 143–151.

93. Merli, G., Herbison, G., Ditunno, J. *et al.* Deep vein thrombosis: prophylaxis in acute spinal cord injured patients. *Arch. Phys. Med. Rehabil.* 1988; **69**: 661–664.

94. Melon, E., Keravel, Y., Gaston, A. *et al.* Deep venous thrombosis prophylaxis by low molecular weight heparin in neurosurgical patients [abstract]. *Anesthesiology* 1987; **75**: A214.

95. Nurmohamed, M., van Riel, A., Henkens, C. *et al.* Low molecular weight heparin and compression stockings in the prevention of venous thromboembolism in neurosurgery. *Thromb. Haemost.* 1996; **75**: 233–238.

96. Agnelli, G., Piovella, F., Buoncristiani, P. *et al.* Enoxaparin plus compression stockings compared with compression stockings alone in the prevention of venous thromboembolism after elective neruosurgery. *N. Engl. J. Med.* 1998; **339**: 80–85.

97. Green, D., Rossi, E., Yao, J. *et al.* Deep vein thrombosis in spinal cord injury: Effect of prophylaxis with calf compression, aspirin, and dipyridoamole. *Paraplegia* 1982; **20**: 227–234.

98. Merli, G., Crabbe, S., Doyle, L. *et al.* Mechanical plus pharmacological prophylaxis for deep vein thrombosis in acute spinal cord injury. *Paraplegia* 1992; **30**: 558–562.

99. Spinal Cord Injury Thromboprophylaxis Group. Prevention of venous thrombosis in the acute phase after acute spinal cord injury: a randomized, multicenter trial comparing low molecular weight heparin plus intermittent pneumatic compression with enoxaparin. *J. Trauma Injury Infect. Crit. Care* 2003; **54**(6): 1116–1124.

100. Bonnar, J. & Walsh, J. Prevention of thrombosis after pelvic surgery by British dextran 70. *Lancet* 1972; **1**: 614.

101. Walsh, J., Bonnar, J., & Wright, F. A study of pulmonary embolism and deep leg vein thrombosis after major gynecologic surgery using labeled fibrinogen-phlebography and lung scanning. *J. Obstet. Gynaecol. Br. Commun.* 1974; **81**: 311.

102. Taberner, D., Poller, L., Burslem, R. *et al.* Oral anticoagulants controlled by the British comparative thromboplastin versus low heparin prophylaxis of DVT. *Br. Med. J.* 1978; **1**: 272.

103. Ballard, R., Bradley-Watson, P., Johnstone, F. *et al.* Low doses of subcutaneous heparin in the prevention of DVT after gynecologic surgery. *J. Obstet. Gynaecol. Br. Commun.* 1973; **80**: 469.

104. Clarke-Pearson, D., Colman, R., Synan, I. *et al.* Venous thromboembolism prophylaxis in gynecologic oncology: a prospective, controlled trial of low dose heparin. *Am. J. Obstet. Gynecol.* 1983; **145**: 606–613.

105. Clarke-Pearson, D., Synan, I., Colman, R. *et al.* The natural history of postoperative venous thromboembolism in gynecologic oncology: a prospective study of 382 patients. *Am. J. Obstet. Gynecol.* 1984; **148**: 1051–1054.

106. Crandon, A. & Koutts, J. Incidence of postoperative deep vein thrombosis in gynecological oncology. *Aust. N Z J. Obstet. Gynaecol.* 1983; **23**: 216–219.

107. Clarke-Pearson, D., Creasman, W., Colman, R. *et al.* Perioperative external pneumatic compression as thromboembolism prophylaxis in gynecologic oncology. *Gynecol. Oncol.* 1984; **18**: 226–232.

108. Clarke-Pearson, D., DeLong, E., Synan, I. *et al.* A controlled trial of two low dose heparin regimens for the prevention of postoperative DVT. *Obstet. Gynecol.* 1990; **75**: 684–689.

109. Clarke-Pearson, D., Synan, I., Dodge, R. *et al.* A randomized trial of low dose heparin and intermittent pneumatic compression for the prevention of deep venous thrombosis after gynecologic oncology surgery. *Am. J. Obstet. Gynecol.* 1913; **168**: 1146–1154.

110. ENOXACAN Study Group. Efficacy and safety of enoxaparin versus unfractionated heparin for prevention of deep vein thrombosis in elective cancer surgery: a double blind randomized multicenter trial with venographic assessment. *Br. J. Surg.* 1997; **84**: 1099–1103.

111. Mayo, M., Hall, T., & Browse, N. The incidence of deep vein thrombosis after prostatectomy. *Br. J. Urol.* 1971; **43**: 739–742.

112. Nicolaides, A., Field, E., Kakkar, V. *et al.* Prostatectomy and deep vein thrombosis. *Br. J. Surg.* 1972; **50**: 487.

113. Van Arsdalen, K., Barnes, R., Clarke, G. *et al.* Deep vein thrombosis and prostatectomy. *Urology* 1983; **21**: 461–463.

114. Becker, J., Borgstrom, S., & Salzman, C. Occurrence and course of thrombosis following prostatectomy: a phlebographic investigation. *Acta Radiol. Diagn.* 1970; **10**: 513.

115. Becker, J. & Borgstrom, S. Incidence of thrombosis associated with epsilon-aminocaproic acid administration and with combined epsilon-aminocaproic acid and subcutaneous heparin therapy. *Acta Chir. Scand.* 1968; **134**: 343.

116. Gordon-Smith, I., Hickman, J., & Masri, S. The effects of the fibrinolytic inhibitors epsilon-aminocaproic acid on the incidence of deep vein thrombosis after prostatectomy. *Br. J. Surg.* 1972; **59**: 522–524.

117. Nicolaides, A., Fernandes, J., & Pollock, A. Intermittent sequential pneumatic compression of the legs in the prevention of venous stasis and postoperative deep vein thrombosis. *Surgery* 1980; **87**: 69–76.

118. Rosenberg, I., Evans, M., & Pollock, A. Prophylaxis of postoperative leg vein thrombosis by low dose subcutaneous heparin or preoperative calf muscle stimulation: a controlled clinical trial. *Br. Med. J.* 1975; **1**: 649.

119. Coe, N., Collins, R., Klein, L. *et al.* Prevention of deep vein thrombosis in urological patients: a controlled, randomized trial of low dose heparin and external pneumatic compression boots. *Surgery* 1978; **83**: 230–234.

120. Salzman, E., Ploetz, J., Bettmann, M. *et al.* Intra-operative external pneumatic calf compression to afford longer term prophylaxis against deep vein thrombosis in urologic surgery. *Surgery* 1980; **87**: 239–242.

121. Hansberry, K., Thompson, I., Bauman, J. *et al.* A prospective comparison of thromboembolic stockings, external sequential pneumatic compression stockings and heparin sodium/dihydroergotamine mesylate for the prevention of thromboembolic complications in urological surgery. *J. Ruol.* 1991; **145**: 1205–1208.

122. Chandhoke, P., Gooding, G., & Narayan, P. Prospective randomized trial of warfarin and intermittent pneumatic leg compressions as prophylaxis for postoperative deep venous thrombosis in major urological surgery. *J. Urol.* 1992; **147**: 1056–1059.

123. Vandendris, M., Kutnowski, M., & Futeral, B. Prevention of postoperative deep vein thrombosis by low-dose heparin in open prostatectomy. *Urol. Res.* 1980; **8**: 219–222.

124. Scurr, J. How long after surgery does the risk of thromboembolism persist? *Acta Chir. Scand.* 1990; **556**: 22–24.

125. Scurr, J., Coleridge-Smith, P., & Hasty, J. Deep vein thrombosis: a continuing problem. *Br. Med. J.* 1988; **297**: 28.

126. Paiement, G., Wessinger, S., Hughes, R. *et al.* Routine use of adjusted low dose warfarin to prevent venous thromboembolism after hip replacement. *J. Bone Joint Surg.* 1993; **75A**: 893–898.

127. Lausen, I., Jorgensen, L., Jorgensen, P. *et al.* Late occurring deep vein thrombosis following general surgery: incidence and prevention. *Thromb. Haemost.* 1993; **69**: 1210.

128. Bergqvist, D., Benoni, G., Bjorgell, O. *et al.* Low molecular weight heparin (enoxaparin) as prophylaxis against venous thromboembolism after total hip replacement. *N. Engl. J. Med.* 1996; **335**: 697–700.

129. Planes, A., Vochelli, N., Darmon, J. *et al.* Risk of deep venous thrombosis after hospital discharge in patients having undergone total hip replacement: double blind randomized comparison of enoxaparin versus placebo. *Lancet* 1996; **348**: 224–228.

130. Lassen, M., Borris, L., Anderson, B. *et al.* Efficacy and safety of prolonged thromboprophylaxis with a low molecular weight heparin (dalteparin) after total hip arthroplasty. The Danish Prolonged Prophylaxis (DaPP) Study. *Thromb. Res.* 1998; **89**: 281–287.

131. Dahl, O., Andreassen, G., Aspelin, T. *et al.* Prolonged thromboprophylaxis following hip replacement surgery: results of a

double-blind, prospective, randomized, placebo controlled study with dalteparin. *Thromb. Haemost.* 1997; **77**: 26–31.

132. Hull, R., Pineo, G., Francis, C. *et al.* Low molecular weight heparin prophylaxis using dalteparin extended out-of-hospital warfarin versus out-of-hospital placebo in hip arthroplasty patients: a double blind, randomized comparison. *Arch. Intern. Med.* 2000; **160**: 2208–2215.

133. Robinson, K., Anderson, D., Gross, M. *et al.* Ultrasonographic screening before hospital discharge for deep venous thrombosis after arthroplasty: The Post-Arthroplasty Screening Study: a randomized controlled trial. *Ann. Intern. Med.* 1997; **127**: 4329–4445.

134. Leclerc, J., Gent, M., Hirsh, J. *et al.* The incidence of symptomatic VTE during and after prophylaxis with enoxaparin: a multi-institutional cohort study in patients who underwent hip or knee arthroplasty. *Arch. Intern. Med.* 1998; **158**: 873–878.

135. Colwell, C., Collis, D., Paulson, R. *et al.* Comparison of enoxaparin and warfarin for the prevention of venous thromboembolic disease after total hip arthroplasty: evaluation during hospitalization and three months after discharge. *J. Bone. Joint Surg.* 1999; **83**: 336–345.

136. Heit, J., Elliott, G., Trowbridge, A. *et al.* Ardeparin sodium for extended out-of-hospital prophylaxis against VTE after total hip or knee replacement: a randomized, double blind, placebo controlled trial. *Ann. Intern. Med.* 2000; **132**: 853–861.

137. White, R., Romano, P., Zhou, H. *et al.* Incidence and time course of thromboembolic outcomes following total hip or knee arthroplasty. *Arch. Intern. Med.* 1998; **158**: 1525–1531.

138. Geerts, W., Pineo, G., Heit, J. *et al.* Prevention of venous thromboembolism. *Chest* 2004; **126**: 338s–400s.

20

Blood transfusion/preoperative considerations and complications

Cassandra D. Josephson, Krista L. Hillyer, and Christopher D. Hillyer

Emory University Transfusion Medicine, Atlanta, GA

Introduction

This chapter is a guide for the physicians who selects, orders, or administers blood components. Blood component descriptions, alternative therapies, and general and specific product indications and contraindications are specifically addressed. Special surgical situations requiring blood components are covered, such as emergency release of blood units and massive transfusion. Technical considerations including pretransfusion evaluation, blood bank component inventory, and general aspects of transfusion are also discussed. Finally, adverse infectious and non-infectious complications are described in detail.

Whole blood and packed red blood cells

Description

Whole blood (WB) is the starting point for the manufacture of most of the components used in transfusion. Whole blood contains red blood cells, plasma, clotting factors, platelets, and approximately 10^9 white blood cells. However, packed red blood cells (pRBCs) are the most commonly transfused blood component. pRBCs are made from whole blood collections by centrifugation or by apheresis techniques. In the USA, over 12 million units of pRBCs are transfused each year. Table 20.1 provides important information on WB and pRBC products including approximate volumes, compositions, and storage periods.

Indications

Historically, WB was used to replace volume and red cell mass, usually during resuscitation of a patient when masssive transfusion was required. Availability of WB is dependent upon each institution and blood center. Its use is discouraged, however, as the use of specific blood components may be best tailored to the individual and unique needs of each patient.

Packed red blood cells are widely available and transfusions should be reserved for use in anemic patients who have compromised oxygen-carrying capacity and are predisposed to an ischemic event. Their use, regardless of additive solution or special processing, is almost always indicated in those patients whose hemoglobin concentration is less than 7 g/dl, and is usually not indicated when hemoglobin concentration is greater than 10 g/dl except as defined below.[1]

The decision to transfuse pRBCs, however, should be based on an evaluation of the patient's vital signs, presence of symptoms of decreased tissue oxygenation, rate and extent of blood loss, increased oxygen consumption, and presence of significant atherosclerosis. Transfusing based on specific "trigger" hemoglobin values (e.g., <10 g/dl, or hematocrits of <30%) have little scientific foundation.[2] The following guidelines, published in the International Anesthesiology Clinics in 2000, stratify patients into three risk groups: (a) "low-risk" patients (<55 years of age, no evidence of heart disease, and APACHE II scores <20), should receive pRBC transfusion only when hemoglobin <6–7 g/dl; (b) "moderate risk" patients ("well compensated" and "stable" cardiac disease) may be transfused when hemoglobin <8 g/dl; (c) "high-risk" patients (those older than 55 years and/or those with postoperative complications who cannot compensate for anemia) should be transfused to keep hemoglobin >10 g/dl. Additionally, some experts still recommend maintaining a hemoglobin of >10 g/dl for perioperative patients thought to be at risk for myocardial ischemia.[3]

Medical Management of the Surgical Patient: A Textbook of Perioperative Medicine, ed. M. F. Lubin, R. B. Smith, T. F. Dobson, N. Spell, H. K. Walker. 4th edn. Published by Cambridge University Press. © Cambridge University 2006.

Table 20.1. Whole blood and packed red blood cell products

Component	Approximate volume (ml)	Composition	Storage period	Hematocrit	Comments
Whole blood	500	250 ml red cells 250 ml plasma 63 ml anticoagulant	35 days (CPDA-1)[a]	35%–40%	• Storage 4 °C • Platelets, granulocytes, labile factors V and VII are not reliable
Packed red blood cells (pRBCs)	250	200 ml red cells 50 ml plasma	35 days (CPDA-1)	50%–80%	• Made from WB • Storage 4 °C • Contains 10^8 WBCs • Can't be infused as rapidly as WB due to increased viscosity
Packed red blood cells (additive solution)	350	200 ml red cells 50 ml plasma 100 ml adenine saline solution[b]	42 days	50%–60%	• Made from WB • Storage 4 °C • Contains 10^8 WBCs • Red cell product most commonly available
Prestorage Leukoreduced (LR-pRBCs)	250–350	Depends on additive solution and anticoagulant	35–42 days	50%–80%	• Made from WB • $< 5 \times 10^6$ WBCs • $\geq 85\%$ of original red cell mass • Does *not* prevent transfusion associated graft vs. host disease (TA-GVHD)
Washed pRBCs	200	180 ml red cells 20 ml isotonic saline (0.9%)	24 hours (after washing)		• Washing removes most plasma and approximately 80% of leukocytes
Irradiated pRBCs	250–350	Depends on additive solution and anticoagulant	28 days post-irradiation, or by original expiration date, whichever comes first		• Reduces storage time due to potassium leak after irradiation • Prevents TA-GVHD
Frozen deglycerolized pRBCs	200	180 ml red cells 20 ml isotonic saline/dextrose solution	24 hours (after deglycerolization)		• Usually reserved for rare blood phenotypes • May be stored frozen for 10 years • Plasma reduced • Approximately 90% leukocyte reduced after deglycerolization and washing

Notes:

[a] Citrate, phosphate buffer, adenine, dextrose.

[b] Adenine, dextrose, saline, mannitol (most plasma removed and replaced with additive solution).

Adverse reactions

This information will be addressed in detail later in the chapter under transfusion complications. Refer to Table 20.5 for details on each type of reaction, diagnosis, laboratory evaluation, and management.

Special processing to prevent complications

Leukoreduction

Most pRBC products are leukoreduced: this means that most of the white blood cells (WBCs) have been removed during a pre-storage procedure at the blood center. Leukoreduction is performed in order to prevent or delay the following complications: febrile non-hemolytic transfusion reactions, human leukocyte antigen (HLA) alloimmunization, transfusion transmitted cytomegalovirus (CMV) and possibly related herpes viruses, and transfusion-related immunomodulation (TRIM). In one study, pRBCs were prestorage filter leukoreduced and stored at 4 °C for 42 days, resulting in a WBC reduction of 3.2 logs, with individual reduction of monocytes, lymphocytes, and neutrophils of 4.1, 3.8 and 2.5 logs, respectively.[4] Because of these WBC-associated complications, Great Britain and Canada have moved to universal prestorage leukoreduction of all blood components. However, in the USA this has not yet been mandated by the American Association of Blood Banks (AABB) or the Food and Drug Administration (FDA). Currently, however, most blood centers do leukoreduce pRBCs and platelet products as standard practice.

Gamma-irradiation

Leukoreduction does not abrogate transfusion-associated-graft-vs.-host-disease (TA-GVHD), which has a 90% mortality rate.[5] Thus, gamma-irradiated, leukoreduced pRBCs are indicated for use in patients who are immunocompromised and at risk for TA-GVHD. The irradiation process (25Gy) covalently cross-links the DNA of the donor T-cells, which inhibits the T-cells ability to replicate and engraft in the host.

The following patients should receive gamma-irradiated products: (a) immunocompromised patients including low-birth weight neonates, intrauterine transfusion recipients, allogeneic stem cell transplant recipients, congenital immunodeficiency syndrome patients, Hodgkin's and non-Hodgkin's lymphoma patients, acute leukemia patients, and (b) patient's receiving HLA matched products including units donated by blood relatives. Patients with other conditions may also be at risk for developing TA-GVHD and may require these specialized products; for these patients, a transfusion medicine physician should be consulted.

Washing

Packed red blood cell washing is performed to remove most plasma and plasma proteins from the product. Washed pRBCs are indicated to reduce the recurrence of severe allergic or anaphylactic transfusion reactions. Washed pRBCs are not adequately leukoreduced to prevent some WBC-associated complications, nor do they protect against the development of TA-GVHD. Also, they are not generally adequate for prevention of reactions in patients with IgA deficiency and subsequent antibodies.

Alternatives to allogeneic pRBC transfusion

Autologous donation

Preoperative whole blood collection can be performed in most stable patients undergoing elective surgical procedures which may require blood transfusion, most often including orthopedic, vascular, cardiac, or thoracic surgeries and radical prostatectomies.[6,7] Autologous donation can significantly reduce patient exposure to allogeneic red cell antigens and infectious elements.[8] A patient's hemoglobin should be at least 11 g/dl in order for him or her to safely donate autologous blood. The following are considered absolute contraindications to autologous donation: infection or risk of bacteremia, aortic stenosis, unstable angina, active seizure disorder, myocardial infarction or cerebrovascular accident during previous 6 months, high-grade left main coronary artery disease, cyanotic heart disease, uncontrolled hypertension, and significant pulmonary or cardiac disease not yet evaluated for surgery by a physician. Donating blood ≥4 weeks in advance of the surgical procedure is recommended to allow time for adequate erythropoiesis to occur; thus, reducing the risk of anemia at the time of surgery. Weekly collection is most common. The latest time that auto-donation can take place is 72 hours before surgery. Dietary supplementation with iron is recommended prior to the start of autologous blood collections. The WB product is stored at 4 °C for up to 35 days, after which it must be frozen or discarded. If the product is not used, it cannot be crossed over for allogeneic use, because autologous donors do not meet the strict criteria required of the general blood donor population.

Intraoperative blood collection ("Cell Saver")

Machines that collect the blood lost during surgery are called "cell savers." The red blood cells are washed with normal saline and concentrated to make an approximate 225 ml unit with a hematocrit of ~55%. The RBC unit can be either directly transfused into the patient or washed again and stored.[9] If the unit is stored, it must be properly labeled and can only be stored for 6 hours at room temperature, or for 24 hours at $1-6\,°C$, if it is chilled within 6 hours of beginning the collection. Patients are excluded from this procedure if they have malignant neoplasms, infections, or contaminated operative fields. The drawback of this procedure is that a lower percentage of RBCs are recovered than in preoperative autologous donation.

Acute normovolemic hemodilution (ANH)

This technique involves the collection of WB from patients immediately prior to a procedure in which blood loss is anticipated. The blood volume removed is quickly replaced with crystalloid or colloid solution prior to surgery. The collected sample is reinfused, typically toward the end of the procedure, or as soon as major bleeding has stopped.[10] The purpose of this technique is to reduce RBC loss during surgery.

Postoperative blood collection

This procedure differs from cell salvage in that the blood is recovered from surgical drains and is usually filtered, but not always washed, prior to reinfusion. The salvaged blood may in fact be hemolyzed and quite dilute. Most surgeons set 1400 ml as the upper limit of volume to be captured that can then be reinfused. The product must be transfused within 6 hours or it must be discarded. Orthopedic and cardiac surgery cases are the primary indications for postoperative blood collection.

Pharmacologic alternatives

DDAVP (vasopressin) induces release of stored von Willebrand Factor (vWF) from Weibel–Palade bodies in endothelial cells. As a result, circulating factor VIII levels are increased, and intraoperative bleeding may be reduced due to improved coagulation.[11] Its side effects include headache, hypertension, tachycardia, and tachyphylaxis. DDAVP is used to treat bleeding patients with mild hemophilia A, certain forms of von Willebrand Disease, and various platelet dysfunction conditions. DDAVP is contraindicated in Type II b vWD.

Aprotinin, a serine protease, inhibits plasmin and kallikrein activity while maintaining platelet activation and aggregation. Administered intraoperatively, aprotinin reduces surgical blood loss, primarily during cardiac surgery or in patients receiving aspirin therapy prior to surgery.[12] Aprotinin has recently been shown to be effective in a randomized, double-blinded, dose-ranging study in major orthopedic surgeries. When compared with placebo, aprotinin was found to reduce the measured and calculated bleeding, which translated to fewer units of pRBCs transfused.[13] Side effects include anaphylaxis to bovine protein and renal toxicity.[14]

Recombinant erythropoietin is a red blood cell growth factor that stimulates the bone marrow to produce new red blood cells. By the seventh day of therapy, the equivalent of 1 unit of blood is produced. Furthermore, by the 28th day, approximately 5 units of new blood are made when iron is also given.[22] Erythropoietin (Epo) has been approved for anemic patients undergoing surgery and recommended for patients prior to surgery to reduce the potential intraoperative or postoperative allogeneic transfusion needs. Epo allows for autologous presurgical donation by increasing hemoglobin concentrations. Additionally, Epo enhances the benefit of ANH (see above). Clinical trials have shown the most benefit in elective surgical patients with initial hemoglobins of 11–13 g/dl and anticipated blood losses of 1000–3000 ml. A wide variety of dosing schedules have been utilized. One possible regimen for a presurgical patient would be 100–600 U/kg SQ weekly × 4 wks; dosing should be individualized based on each patient's clinical needs. Recombinant erythropoietin can cause polycythemia, hypertension, and rarely red cell aplasia and thus is contraindicated in patients at risk of polycythemia or those with uncontrolled hypertension.

Topical agents (fibrin sealants, fibrin glue)

Fibrin glue is made by mixing fibrinogen from cryoprecipitate with thrombin in the operating room and applying the mixture immediately to the surgical site to achieve local hemostasis. This method is not FDA approved. However, there are newly FDA-approved products called fibrin sealants. These contain a protein-concentrate-fibrinolytic inhibitor solution. The concentrate is reconstituted in a bovine fibrinolysis inhibitor solution containing both aprotinin and plasmin. When warmed at $37\,°C$, mixed, and applied to the bleeding site, a solid, adherent sealant is produced. Both fibrin glue and fibrin sealant work by the action of thrombin on fibrinogen, inducing clot formation

Table 20.2. Clinical uses for fibrin glue and fibrin sealant

FDA-approved uses (for fibrin sealant only)
Cardiopulmonary bypass
Heparinized patients undergoing coronary artery bypass
   graft (CABG)
Splenic injury
Colostomy closure

Selected investigational uses
Orthopedic surgery: meniscal tear repair
Urology: establishing patency of vasovasotomy
Neurosurgery: wound closure; securing prosthetic devices;
   nerve anastomoses; dura repair; fascial repair
Pediatric surgery: postoperative neonatal chylothorax repair

Note: Refs. 15–21.

at the bleeding site. Table 20.2 lists the clinical uses for fibrin glue and sealants.

The major adverse reaction caused by fibrin glue and sealants is the occurance of allergic or anaphylactoid reactions to bovine proteins; its use is contraindicated in patients with known bovine allergies. Factor V antibodies have also been reported to develop subsequent to bovine thrombin exposure. If Factor V antibodies are suspected postoperatively, hematologic consultation is recommended.

Blood substitutes

There are a variety of blood substitutes being developed, including human, bovine, and recombinant hemoglobin-based products. However, none of these products are available in the USA at this time. Currently, US clinical studies are still being performed. The only US FDA-approved oxygen-carrying volume expander available is a first-generation perfluocarbon emulsion, which is restricted to use for perfusion of coronary arteries during angioplasty.

Platelets

Description

There are two types of platelet components available to most hospitals: pooled platelet concentrates (also called "random donor platelets") and apheresis platelets (also called "single-donor platelets"). Platelet concentrates contain less platelets ($\sim 7 \times 10^{10}$ platelets/concentrate) compared to apheresis platelets (3–6×10^{11} platelets). Thus, it takes 5–8 pooled platelet concentrates to achieve

the same dose of platelets as a single apheresis platelet unit. As a result, a recipient of pooled platelet concentrates is exposed to 5–8 blood donors per transfusion. Furthermore, a platelet concentrate unit must go through a separate leukofiltration procedure to be rendered leukoreduced ($WBC < 5 \times 10^6$) while an apheresis platelet unit is already "process" leukoreduced ($WBC < 10^4$–10^6), where the machine filters the product. Finally, RBC contamination is often less in the apheresis product than in whole blood-derived platelet concentrates; thus, apheresis platelets may induce less Rh sensitization. Table 20.3 lists the types of platelet products, with their approximate volumes, compositions, and storage periods.

Indications

In a healthy adult or child, the normal peripheral blood platelet count is 150 000–450 000/μl. Most clinically stable, non-bleeding patients tolerate platelet counts as low as 5–10 000/μl without experiencing major bleeding.[23] In tertiary-care hospitals, therapeutic platelet transfusions are often administered to patients who are actively bleeding at higher baseline platelet counts, ranging between 50–100 000/μl. However, prophylactic transfusions to prevent future bleeding are the most common reason for platelet transfusions.[24] Hanson and Slichter *et al.* showed that 7000 platelets/μl per day are required to maintain endothelial integrity in normal individuals.[25]

Two recent prospective clinical trials support that the platelet transfusion trigger should be 10 000/μl instead of 20 000/μl, in stable patients receiving prophylactic transfusions without coexisting conditions.[26,27] Still, a level of 20 000/μl is recommended for use in patients with fever, active bleeding, or coexisting coagulation defects. Of note, platelet usage has been reduced by 20%–40% since adoption of these more restrictive transfusion practices.

Prophylactic transfusion prior to invasive procedures does not have adequate scientific evidence to support or discard its standard clinical practice. Many surgeons will transfuse a patient when the platelet count is <50 to 100 000/μl, prior to minor and major surgeries, respectively. Platelets should also be administered prior to a procedure when a congenital or acquired platelet dysfunction is present and the patient is actively bleeding or likely to bleed.

Contraindications

There are several contraindications to platelet transfusions. (a) Surgical or local measures should first be sought to attain hemostasis when a single anatomic site is

Table 20.3. Platelet products

Component	Approximate volume (ml)	Composition	Storage period	Comments
Platelet, apheresis (single donor)	300	$\geq 3 \times 10^{11}$ platelets; $<10^4$–10^6 WBCs and plasma	4 hours if system opened (i.e., volume reduction or washing) 5 days (closed system)	• Storage 22–26 °C (room temp) with constant horizontal agitation • Equivalent to 5–8 units of platelet concentrates • Decreased number donor exposures to patient • Fewer lymphocytes than equivalent dose of platelet concentrates • HLA-matched products may be provided • Cost equivalent to 6–8 units of concentrate
Platelet concentrate (random donor)	50	$\geq 5.5 \times 10^{10}$ platelets; variable numbers RBC, WBCs, and plasma	4 hours if system opened (i.e., volume reduction or washing) 5 days (closed system)	• Storage 22–26 °C (room temp) with constant horizontal agitation • Average adult dose is 5–8 units which are pooled for infusion

bleeding. Platelet transfusions are indicated in this situation only if the patient is thrombocytopenic. (b) Any hemorrhage of >5 ml WB/kg per hour is considered likely due to an anatomic lesion requiring surgical intervention, rather than platelet transfusion. (c) Patients with thrombotic thrombocytopenic purpura (TTP) and heparin induced thrombocytopenia (HIT) should generally not be transfused with platelets, as the addition of platelets may exacerbate thrombotic complications. Although not absolutely contraindicated, ITP patients are unlikely to benefit from platelet transfusions, due to immune-mediated peripheral platelet destruction. Finally, in uremic patients who are bleeding, platelets alone are not helpful. However, if administered with DDAVP, pRBCs to keep hct >30 g/dl, and/or concurrent dialysis, bleeding uremic patients may respond well to platelet transfusion.

Adverse reactions

There are three main adverse reactions that occur most often with platelet transfusion: (a) hypotension, (b) human leukocyte antigen (HLA) and/or human platelet antigen (HPA) alloimmunization, and (c) post-transfusion purpura. Other transfusion complications will be discussed later in the chapter. The hypotensive reaction to platelets is occasionally accompanied by respiratory distress. It differs from transfusion-related acute lung injury (TRALI) in that no infiltrates are seen on chest X-ray,

fever is not present, and flushing and gastrointestinal discomfort are common symptoms. The reaction ceases rapidly after the transfusion is discontinued.[28] This bradykinin-induced hypotension effect is potentiated in the presence of an ACE inhibitor due to inhibited breakdown of bradykinin. Therefore, patients receiving ACE inhibitor medication and platelet or plasma therapy should be evaluated by a transfusion medicine specialist or hematologist.

The rate of HLA and/or HPA alloimmunization in some studies is found to be as high as 85% in heavily transfused patients.[29] However, the Trial of Reduced Alloimmunization to Platelets (TRAP) study demonstrated that leukoreduction by filtration can significantly decrease the incidence of alloimmunization and platelet refractoriness to less than 4% of transfused patients.[30]

Post-transfusion purpura is an alloimmune mediated thrombocytopenia, caused by the absence of HPA-1 antigen on the patient's platelets. Subsequent to a transfusion with HPA-1 antigen positive platelets, antibodies are produced, resulting in antibody mediated destruction of the donor platelets, as well as destruction of the recipient's platelets. Fortunately, this is a rare complication. If it occurs, washing future products is required.

Platelet refractory state

This situation should be suspected when the post-transfusion platelet count increment is lower than expected after the proper weight adjusted dose of platelets has been administered and other reasons for decreased platelet retention are not present (active bleeding, infection, splenomegaly, etc.). The corrected count increment (CCI) formula can help the physician in this determination:

$$CCI = \frac{\left(\begin{array}{c}\text{1 hour post-}\\\text{transfusion}\\\text{platelet count}\end{array} - \begin{array}{c}\text{Pretransfusion}\\\text{platelet count}\end{array}\right) \times \begin{array}{c}\text{(Body surface}\\\text{area in m}^2)\end{array}}{\text{Number of platelets transfused}}$$

The expected CCI is around $15\,000/\text{ml} \times 10^{11}/\text{ml}$ platelets transfused per m^2 body surface area. If the CCI is less than 5000 to 7500/ml on two successive days, the patient is considered to be refractory. When this situation arises, the blood bank should be notified so they can assist with the next steps in providing either cross-matched platelets or HLA-matched platelets. Both specialized products may require hours to days for the blood center to obtain and prepare.

Crossmatching of platelets is not routinely performed, but can be supplied upon special request. Donor platelets are cross-matched by different methods, using serum from the patient. If no agglutination is detected, then the platelets are considered compatible with the recipient's serum. Alternatively, HLA matching of platelets is indicated in those platelet refractory states where cross-matched platelets have failed and the patient is shown to have an HLA-directed antibody by special testing. This procedure entails testing of the patient's HLA type and the donor's HLA type, and then harvesting platelets from that particular donor. Cross-matched and HLA-matched platelets are labor-intensive and expensive products to collect and supply, and thus they should only be ordered when a patient has been shown to be refractory by CCI and/or has demonstrable HLA antibody.

Pharmacologic alternatives

Thrombopoietin (Tpo) is a platelet growth factor which has a recombinant form, rHuTpo. In clinical trials, it has effectively increased circulating platelet counts in oncology patients who were receiving non-myelosuppressive chemotherapy. However, it was ineffective in those receiving myeloablative therapy.[31] It has not been FDA approved for routine use.

IL-11, another platelet growth factor, also has a recombinant form rHuIL-11. It has been FDA approved for use in patients undergoing myelosuppressive, but not myeloablative, chemotherapy.

Plasma products

Description

Plasma is the aqueous, acellular portion of whole blood, consisting of proteins, colloids, nutrients, crystalloids, hormones, and vitamins. Albumin is the most abundant of the plasma proteins and will be discussed in its own section. Other plasma proteins include immunoglobulins, complement (C3, predominantly), coagulation factors, enzymes, and transport molecules. The coagulation factors in plasma include fibrinogen (2–3 mg/ml), factor XIII (60 µg/ml), von Willebrand factor (5–10 µg/ml), Factor VIII, primarily bound to its carrier protein vWF, at approximately 100 ng/ml, and vitamin K-dependent coagulation factors II, VII, IX, X (1 unit of activity/ml for each factor).

Several types of plasma products can be made from WB or plasmapheresis collections. Single donor plasma or source plasma is made by plasmapheresis and is stored at $-20\,°\text{C}$. The rest of the plasma products are derived from WB, and the time after collection to time of freezing determines its storage time. To be called FFP, the plasma must be frozen within 6–8 hours of collection and stored at $-18\,°\text{C}$ or colder. F24 plasma must be frozen within 24 hours of collection and frozen at $-18\,°\text{C}$ or colder. FFP and F24 are essentially equivalent products, with the exception of Factor VIII levels, which are lower in F24. However, as Factor VIII is an acute phase reactant, its levels are quickly regenerated in recipients without hemophilia A, and specific Factor VIII concentrates and recombinant Factor VIII are available for use in patients with hemophilia A. Thus, FFP and F24 may be used interchangeably in patients without hemophilia A. Finally, cryosupernatant is plasma with its cryoprecipitate fraction depleted; the cryosupernatant is then refrozen at the above temperature. Table 20.4 lists the plasma derived products, appropriate volumes, compositions, and storage periods.

Indications

Frozen plasma products (FFP and F24) are used primarily for the treatment of coagulation factor deficiencies in which specific factor concentrates are not available or when immediate control of bleeding is imperative. Specifically, FFP and F24 are indicated in the following situations: bleeding diathesis associated with acquired coagulation factor deficits, such as end-stage liver disease, massive transfusion, and disseminated intravascular coagulation; the rapid reversal of

Table 20.4. Plasma derived products

Component	Approximate volume (ml)	Composition	Storage period	Comments
Source plasma (single donor plasma)	180–300	• Plasma proteins • Immunoglobulins • Complement • Coagulation factors (II, VII, IX, X, VIII, XIII, vWF, fibrinogen) • Albumin	• 1 year if frozen • 24 hours if maintained at 1–6 °C	• Obtained through single donor plasmapheresis • Stored at –20 °C after collection • Not for volume expansion or fibrinogen replacement
Recovered plasma	180–300	Same as above	• 1 year if frozen • 24 hours if maintained at 1–6 °C	• Plasma obtained from WB of regular donor • Not for volume expansion or fibrinogen replacement
Fresh frozen plasma (FFP)	180–300	Same as above	• 1 year if frozen • 1–5 days after thawing	• Separated from WB within 6–8 hours of collection • Stored frozen at –18 °C • Not for volume expansion or fibrinogen replacement
Plasma frozen within 24 h (F24)	180–300	Same as above	• 1 year if frozen • 1–5 days after thawing	• Separated from WB and frozen within 24 hours of collection • Stored frozen at –18 °C • Not for volume expansion or fibrinogen replacement
Cryosupernatant plasma (Cryopoor plasma)	180–300	• Same as above except depleted levels of Factors VIII, XIII, fibrinogen, and vWF	• 1 year if frozen • 24 hours after thawing	• Depleted of its cryoprecipitate fraction

warfarin effect; plasma infusion or exchange for TTP; congenital coagulation defects (except when specific therapy is available); and C1-esterase inhibitor deficiency.

Contraindications

The use of FFP or F24 is not without risk to the recipient (see adverse effects, below). Due to the availability of better alternative therapies, FFP and F24 should not be used to expand plasma volume, increase plasma albumin concentration, or bolster the nutritional status of malnourished patients. Even when considering the indication for factor replacement in the context of burns, meningococcal sepsis, or acute renal failure, other alternative therapies, such as antithrombin (ATIII) or Activated Protein C concentrates may offer an advantage over FFP or F24 use.[32,33] These alternative therapies should be pursued with guidance from a hematologist or transfusion medicine expert.

Adverse effects

Life-threatening allergic reactions have been attributed to antibodies in the donor's plasma that react with the recipient's WBCs, although this is an uncommon occurrence. In addition, the presence of isohemagglutinins may cause mild hemolytic reactions or result in a positive direct antiglobulin test ("Coomb's" test) if "out-of-group" plasma is administered to the patient. Finally, the IgA-deficient patient who has anti-IgA antibodies must receive IgA-deficient plasma from a national rare donor registry to avoid life-threatening anaphylaxis. However, the presence of absolute IgA deficiency with anti-IgA antibodies is an extremely rare event, and should be confirmed by demonstration of 0% IgA levels and presence of anti-IgA antibodies prior to requesting these rare plasma components.

Alternatives to plasma therapy

Depending on the patient's clinical situation, replacement with specific factor concentrates including Factor VIII, activated prothrombin concentrate (aPCCs), Factor VIIa, Factor IX, Factor XIII, ATIII concentrate, Protein C concentrate, activated Protein C concentrate, C1-esterase inhibitor concentrate, and alpha$_1$-antitrypsin concentrate should be considered when clinically indicated. A hematology consult is recommended when the above factors and concentrates are being considered for use. If fibrinogen is the main substance to be replaced, cryoprecipitate administration is recommended. In vitamin-K deficient states, or in non-emergent situations necessitating warfarin reversal, parenteral Vitamin-K replacement should be considered, rather than frozen plasma infusion.

Cryoprecipitate

Description

Cryoprecipitate contains the highest concentrations of Factor VIII, vWF, Factor XIII, fibrinogen, and fibronectin. It is manufactured by isolating the insoluble precipitate formed after thawing FFP between 1 and 6 °C. The precipitate, which contains the highest molecular weight proteins in FFP, is refrozen in 10–15 ml of plasma within 1 hour of precipitation and stored at ≤ -18 °C for up to 1 year. Prior to the 1980s, cryoprecipitate was primarily used for the treatment of von Willebrand Disease and hemophilia A. However, with the development of recombinant factor products and improved viral inactivation procedures, cryoprecipitate's therapeutic role in treating these diseases has been diminished. Currently, it is primarily used for fibrinogen replacement, due to its high fibrinogen content, 150–250 mg per unit.

Indications

Cryoprecipitate has few indications, due to the development of safer factor concentrates. It is indicated for congenital or acquired fibrinogen deficiencies, factor XIII deficiency, DIC, orthotopic liver transplantation, post-streptokinase therapy (hyperfibrinogenolysis), and renal stone removal as a glue. Other possible investigational uses include uremic bleeding, as a component of fibrin glue/sealant, in hemophilia A (if FVIII concentrate is not available), and as a source of fibronectin for wound healing.

Contraindications

The use of cryoprecipitate is contraindicated in sepsis when the fibrinogen is high and DIC with thrombosis is occurring.

Adverse reactions

Refer to FFP adverse reactions.

Albumin

Description

Albumin is the most abundant of the plasma proteins (3500–5000 mg/dl) and has many functions. Primarily, albumin maintains plasma colloid oncotic pressure and blood pressure. Synthesis of albumin occurs in the liver, and there are small body stores which undergo rapid turnover. Each molecule remains intact for approximately 15–20 days. Albumin for transfusion is separated from human plasma through a cold ethanol fractionation procedure. Commercially available human albumin preparations include a 5% solution, a 25% solution, and a plasma protein fraction 5% solution (PPF). All are prepared from pooled plasma and have a balanced physiological pH, contain 145 meq of sodium and contain less than 2 meq of potassium per liter. The products contain no preservatives or coagulation factors.

Indications

Albumin has a wide variety of uses. Specifically, it is indicated after large-volume paracentesis, for nephrotic syndrome resistant to diuretics, for ovarian hyperstimulation syndrome, and for volume/fluid replacement in plasmapheresis. Relative indications include adult respiratory distress syndrome; cardiopulmonary bypass pump priming; fluid resuscitation in shock, sepsis, and burns; neonatal kernicterus; and enteral feeding intolerance. The use of albumin is investigational for cadaveric renal transplant, cerebral ischemia, and stroke.

Contraindications

Albumin use is contraindicated due to its ineffective result and increased risk to the patient in the following situations: correction of nutritional hypoalbuminemia or hypoproteinemia, nutritional deficiency requiring total parenteral nutrition, preeclampsia and wound healing.

Albumin should not be used for resuspending RBCs or simple volume expansion (i.e., in surgical or burn patients).

Other blood and recombinant products

Granulocytes and intravenous immune globulin (IVIG) are whole blood derivatives and Factor VIIa is produced by recombinant technology. Each has very specific indications that are beyond the scope of this chapter. A hematologic or transfusion medicine consultation should be sought to oversee the proper use of these specialized products.

Special transfusion situations

Massive transfusion effect

Massive transfusion typically occurs under a surgeon's care in those patients experiencing trauma, gastrointestinal bleeding, and undergoing certain surgical procedures. Massive transfusion may be defined in several ways: (a) replacement of a patient's blood volume (70 ml/kg) within 24 hours; (b) replacement of 50% of the patient's circulating blood volume (35 ml/kg) within 3 hours; or (c) transfusion of more than 10 units of whole blood or 20 units of pRBCs in a 24-hour period.[34] Approximately 35% of the patient's original plasma and platelets remain after one blood volume has been replaced with pRBC units.

As dilutional thrombocytopenia and coagulopathy may result from massive transfusion, the physicians managing these patients must regularly monitor critical lab values, including platelets, PT, aPTT, and fibrinogen. Platelet count should be maintained >50 000–60 000/μl to achieve good surgical hemostasis, though some experts recommend platelet counts >80 000–100 000/μl for trauma patients. After a patient receives 10 units of pRBCs, the PT and aPTT may become prolonged. When the plasma coagulation factor levels fall below 30% activity, the PT and aPTT will be prolonged, and hemostasis will be compromised. Furthermore, if fibrinogen levels are below 90–100 mg/dl, the PT or PTT is 1.5 its normal value, then FFP should be administered at 10 ml/kg to raise the plasma levels of clotting factors by 20% to 30%. If the fibrinogen levels are <100 mg/dl, cryoprecipitate should be administered rather than FFP, because cryoprecipitate contains a greater amount of fibrinogen (≥150 mg/dl per unit) in a smaller volume of product.

Metabolic derangements can occur as a result of massive transfusion. Citrate is used in all blood products to chelate calcium for anticoagulant purposes. FFP and platelet products contain more citrate than pRBCs. In patients with normal liver function, citrate is metabolized by the liver into bicarbonate. However, patients with abnormal liver function who receive large, rapid infusions of citrate may become hypocalcemic and hypomagnesemic, resulting in depressed myocardial contractility, ventricular tachyarrhythmias, and neuromuscular irritability. Furthermore, the alkalosis produced from citrate metabolism may worsen the hypocalcemia. Thus, ionized calcium levels should be monitored regularly and calcium gluconate should be administered when hypocalcemia is present.

As hypothermia from refrigerated blood products can also be a problem, blood warmers should be used during massive transfusion. Also, hyperkalemia can occur due to the pRBCs "storage lesion." Older pRBCs leak more potassium into the plasma phase of the product. Thus, when large amounts of blood are infused, hyperkalemia can result. Finally, when a massive transfusion is occuring or is predicted, alerting the blood bank is necessary. To obtain the requested products for the patient as quickly as possible, the surgeons, anesthesiologists, emergency room physicians, nurses, and blood bank staff must work as a team. Thawing of frozen products and obtaining additional products from the blood supplier takes time, and thus advance notice and continued communication with the blood bank is essential for optimal patient care.

Technical considerations

Red blood cell transfusion

ABO and Rh cross-match
Prior to a red blood cell transfusion, ABO and Rh compatibility testing must be done. If the recipient were to receive ABO-incompatible blood, it could cause a severe acute hemolytic transfusion reaction (AHTR). Additionally, if anti-D alloantibodies form in a female recipient of childbearing age due to Rh incompatibility, it could lead to eventual hemolytic disease of the newborn (HDN). Both of these potential reactions can cause fatal consequences.

Ordering pRBCs
A *type and screen* should be ordered when non-urgent transfusion is anticipated. A patient's ABO and Rh antigen types are determined, and an indirect antiglobulin test (IAT) screen is performed on the patient's serum to detect

unexpected alloantibodies to red blood cells. These alloantibodies are typically formed after exposure to foreign red blood cells via prior transfusions or by prior pregnancies (where feto-maternal hemorrhage may have occurred). Type and screen testing requires approximately 30–45 minutes to complete. If no unexpected antibodies are discovered, it should take 15–30 minutes to provide cross-matched pRBC units after an order is submitted (see below). However, if the antibody screen is positive, further tests must be performed to determine if the antibody detected is clinically significant. Once specificity is determined, antigen-negative pRBCs can be provided by the blood bank, though this can significantly delay a transfusion.

A *type and cross-match* order should be submitted if blood is needed within the next 12 hours. Patients are typed for ABO and Rh antigens, and an antibody screen is performed. However, with this order, the appropriate blood product is crossmatched with the patient's serum prior to being issued. All blood banks perform a cross-match procedure prior to issuing any WB or pRBC component, except in an emergency situation.

Emergency transfusions or emergency release

When transfusion of pRBCs is required immediately, there is often not enough time for ABO or Rh typing of the recipient. Group O, Rh negative, uncrossmatched pRBCs may be administered to all recipients in this situation. However, an emergency order requires a signature from a physician to ensure that it is clear the units are **not cross-matched**. Group O, Rh negative pRBCs are a scarce and valuable resource and may be unavailable in the amounts required. As a result, Group O, Rh positive pRBC may be substituted. Transfusion medicine services try to limit this substitution to males and postmenopausal women, in order to avoid the risk of immunizing Rh negative females who may later become pregnant with an Rh positive fetus, predisposing to HDN.

Surgeons and emergency room physicians frequently encounter semi-emergent transfusion needs. In these situations, a limited amount of time is available prior to transfusion, and the blood bank can only provide type-specific blood (A to A, B to B). In this case, screening and cross-matching are not performed prior to the pRBCs leaving the blood bank.

Ideally, if a patient's sample can be obtained quickly and delivered immediately to the blood bank, or if a current, prior sample is available, an emergency cross-match can be performed within 15–20 minutes. However, complete compatibility testing, including ABO/Rh type and antibody screen (assuming negativity) and cross-match,

requires 45–60 minutes. As described earlier, more time must be allotted if the antibody screen is positive, so that antibody specificity can be determined and the appropriate antigen-negative pRBCs can be provided.

Inventory in the blood bank is guided by many factors. Most hospitals have guidelines noting what surgical procedures do not typically require blood products, which require a type and screen order, and which require a type and cross-match order. These maximum surgical blood order schedules (MSBOSs) help set the maximum standard of pRBC units needed and that will be cross-matched for each procedure. The MSBOS aids blood bank staff in preventing unnecessary issue of red cells when cross-matches are ordered for procedures in which pRBCs are not likely to be used.

Component and recipient identification

Labeling of samples is critical in the blood bank. The sample tube must reflect the recipient's name and hospital identification number, which in turn must exactly match the information on the recipient's hospital identification band. Within the blood bank, a technologist labels the donor pRBC units and matches them with the recipient's identification number before the units are issued. The healthcare provider administering the transfusion must check the identity of the recipient and match it with the pRBC unit before transfusing the patient. All of these steps are crucial, since clerical errors remain the leading cause of fatal hemolytic transfusion reactions.[35,36]

Platelets

ABO and Rh compatibility

Platelets should be ABO and Rh matched, when possible, in order to attain the best response from the platelet transfusion and decrease the potential for red blood cell hemolysis. However, ABO and Rh matching are not absolutely necessary, and platelet transfusion should not be denied if type-specific platelets are not available. Rh immunoglobulin should be given (estimate 1 ml of pRBC transfused, per platelet concentrate) if the platelet Rh type is mismatched. When ABO-mismatched platelet transfusions occur, they may contribute to an eventual platelet refractory state.[37] Furthermore, in an attempt to prevent HLA alloimmunization, leukoreduction is recommended.

Hemolysis of red blood cells has been reported when patients have received either large volumes of ABO-incompatible plasma or plasma with high-titer isohemagglutinins.[38] Therefore, it is generally recommended that the volume of mismatched plasma transfused be limited in adults to 1 liter per week. Alternatively, the volume of mismatched plasma transfused in ABO-mismatched platelet transfusions could be limited by volume-reducing platelets prior to transfusion. This method is preferred in neonates receiving ABO-mismatched platelets, but since this practice decreases the number and possibly the function of the platelets (as well as reducing the storage time to 4 hours), volume-reduction is not routinely recommended for older children or adult patients.

Plasma products

ABO and Rh compatibility

No specific compatibility testing is performed prior to infusion of plasma products. As plasma contains isohemagglutinins, it must be compatible with the recipient's blood type, otherwise hemolysis will ensue. However, if the recipient's ABO type is unknown prior to plasma infusion, AB plasma may be administered to all recipients. Rh alloimmunization rarely occurs due to Rh mismatch of plasma products, as there are few red blood cells in the plasma component. Therefore, Rh compatibility is not as critical as is ABO type when transfusing plasma.

Cryoprecipitate

ABO and Rh compatibility

Cryoprecipitate units have a small volume compared with plasma products or pRBCs, thus anti-A and anti-B isohemagglutinins are present only in small amounts. While the AABB standards recommend ABO compatibility for cryoprecipitate transfusions, especially in pediatric patients, compatibility testing is not required. Furthermore, since cryoprecipitate does not contain red cells, Rh matching is unnecessary.

Albumin

Albumin is an acellular product devoid of blood group isohemagglutinins. As a result, neither serologic testing nor ABO or Rh compatibility is necessary prior to administration.

Blood product infusion

Blood products can be warmed prior to infusion to decrease the risk of cardiac arrhythmias, cardiac arrest,

and cold-induced coagulopathy. Warming is indicated for patients receiving multiple transfusions of pRBCs at a fast rate, for example, trauma or plasma exchange patients. It is also recommended for patients with cold agglutinin disease, in order reduce the risk of antibody-mediated hemolysis. However, routine blood warming for all transfusions is not necessary. If it is clincially indicated, the blood should not exceed 42 °C to avoid hemolysis. pRBCs should not be heated in a microwave, under tap water, or in a hot water bath.[39]

Intravenous (IV) solution compatibility with blood product infusions is critical for successful, safe transfusion. Medications and IV fluids should not be added to pRBC products, except for normal saline (0.9%), plasma, 5% albumin, and plasma protein fractions. Dextrose solutions cause hemolysis, and Lactated Ringer's Solution causes clotting in the tubing. If the tubing has been used for other fluids, it should be flushed with normal saline prior to blood product infusion.

pRBCs can be infused as quickly as the patient can tolerate. In the adult, this can be up to 100 ml/minute. One unit of pRBCs may not be infused during more than a 4 hour period, as the risk of bacterial contamination increases as the blood sits at room temperature. If the transfusion is anticipated to require more than 4 hours, the blood bank can split the unit into two separate aliquots in a sterile manner prior to transfusion.

Transfusion complications

Non-infectious hazards of transfusion (NiSHOTs)

Non-infectious hazards of transfusion include: mistransfusion and ABO/Rh incompatibility, TA-GVHD, massive transfusion, and transfusion-related acute lung injury (TRALI).

Hemolytic reactions, both acute and delayed, and non-hemolytic reactions, both febrile and allergic are described in Table 20.5. These reactions, including their symptoms and laboratory findings, as well as cause and management information are listed. Fatal acute hemolytic transfusion reactions occur at a rate of 1–250 000–1 000 000.[43] Delayed hemolytic transfusion reactions have been reported to occur at a rate of 1:1000.[44]

TRALI is a syndrome characterized by dyspnea, hypotension, fever, and bilateral pulmonary infiltrates on X-ray. Onset of TRALI can be at anytime from initiation of the transfusion up to 4 hours post-transfusion. Most patients' symptoms resolve within 3–4 days, but usually require oxygen support and often mechanical ventilation. TRALI is the leading cause of transfusion related mortality

Table 20.5. Transfusion reactions, diagnosis, laboratory evaluation, and management

Transfusion reactions	Signs and symptoms	Laboratory evaluation	Cause/management
Hemolytic transfusion reactions			
Acute hemolytic transfusion reactions (AHTR)	Fever, chills, anxiety, shock, DIC, dyspnea, chest pain, flank pain, hemoglobinemia, hemoglobinuria	• Complete blood count • Coagulation panel • Urine analysis • Direct Coombs (DAT) • Free plasma hemoglobin in post-transfusion specimen	1. ABO incompatibility #1 cause 2. Stop transfusion 3. Hydrate with normal saline to maintain renal blood flow 4. Diuretics can be used 5. Support BP with vasopressors 6. Corticosteriods may be administered 7. Treat DIC 8. Monitor renal status – may need dialysis
Delayed hemolytic transfusion reactions (DHTR)	Occurs 3–14 days post-transfusion, unexplained fever	• Anemia • Indirect hyperbilirubinemia • Increase in LDH • Direct Coombs ±(DAT)	1. Sensitization 2. Monitor hemoglobin and renal function 3. Coagulation panel 4. No acute transfusion usually required
Non-hemolytic transfusion reactions			
Febrile non-hemolytic transfusion reactions (FNHTR)	Fever, chills, rarely hypotension	• Blood culture of recipient • Blood product gram stain and culture to rule out bacterial contamination	1. Antibodies to leukocytes or cytokine infusion 2. Stop transfusion 3. Give antipyretic (acetominophen) 4. Next transfusion: order leukocyte-reduced product
Allergic transfusion reactions	Urticaria, hives, rash, rarely hypotension or anaphylaxis	• None	1. Antibodies to plasma proteins usual cause 2. Stop transfusion 3. Give diphenhydramine i.v. or p.o. 4. Give epinephrine/steroids if reaction is severe 5. May restart transfusion if patient responds to antihistamine and vital signs are stable after 15 minutes 6. If severe and repetitive reactions occur, may need to wash products – consult transfusion medicine service

Table 20.6. Estimated risk of collecting blood during the infectious window period (repeat donors)

Agent	Window period (days)	Risk (rate of infectious donations)
HBV, no correction	59	1:488 000
HCV, antibody test only	70	1:276 000
HCV, plus NAT	10	1:1 935 000
HIV, antibody plus p24 antigen	16	1:1 468 000
HIV, plus NAT	11	1:2 135 000
HTLV, 1998–1999	51	1:514 000
HTLV, 2000–2001	51	1:2 993 000

reported to the FDA. Granulocyte antibodies, HLA class I antibodies, and HLA class II antibodies in donor plasma have been implicated in TRALI reactions. Recognition of TRALI remains underdiagnosed, since it occurs most often in extremely ill patients. Surgeons should be aware and alert to the potential consequences of this transfusion-associated complication. Swift recognition is critical to provide appropriate supportive therapy, as TRALI is often misdiagnosed as volume overload, and the use of diuretics in a TRALI patient can significantly worsen outcome.[40]

A less commonly encountered hazard is transfusion-related immuno-modulation (TRIM). Surgeons have observed an increased rate of postoperative infections in transfused patients. Leukocytes are thought to modulate the immunosuppression. The TRIM phenomenon was demonstrated in a study in which surgical patients were randomized to receive non-leukoreduced vs. leukoreduced pRBCs. The results showed significantly fewer post-operative infections in the leukoreduced group.[41] Furthermore, reactivation of latent viruses has also been reported in patients who have received non-leukoreduced products.[42]

Infectious complications of transfusion

Transfusion-transmitted infectious diseases are another less common complication of transfusion. Viral, bacterial, fungal, and parasitic organisms all pose risks. Only the viral and bacterial risks will be emphasized in this chapter, as they are the most common. All volunteer-donated blood is tested for the following: syphilis, hepatitis B surface antigen (HbsAg), antibodies to HIV-1/ HIV-2, p24 antigen, Human T-cell lymphotrophic virus (HTLV I and II), Hepatitis B core antibody (HbcAb), and hepatitis C

(HCV). HIV and HCV testing now includes FDA-approved nucleic acid testing (NAT) in order to shorten both viruses' infectious window period. Table 20.6 was adapted from Dodd *et al.*, published in August of 2002, which depicts the estimated risk of collecting blood during the infectious window period for HBV, HCV, HIV, and HTLV.[45]

Bacterial contamination of blood products has been estimated as pRBC risk at 1:65 000–500 000[46,47] and platelet risk at 1:12 000.[46] However, the spectrum of symptoms and outcomes following infusion of a bacterially contaminated blood product is wide ranging. Mild bacterial contamination may cause fever only, whereas heavy contamination may cause sepsis, shock, and death. If this type of reaction is suspected, the transfusion needs to be stopped. The patient must have a blood culture drawn prior to initiation of antibiotics, and the blood product unit must be gram stained and cultured. The blood bank and microbiology lab should be notified immediately. *Yersinia enterocolitica* has been implicated most often in pRBCs, as it has been found in asymptomatic bacteremic donors. When *Pseudomonas* and *Serratia* species are cultured, from blood product units, breakdowns in aseptic technique during collection is the suspected etiology.[48]

REFERENCES

1. Anonymous. Practice guidelines for blood component therapy: a report from the American Society of Anesthesiologists Task Force on Blood Component Therapy. *Anesthesiology* 1996; **84**: 732–747.

2. Carson, J. L., Hill, S., Carless, P. *et al.* Transfusion triggers: a systematic review of the literature. *Transfus. Med. Rev.* 2002; **16**(3): 187–199.

3. Wall, M. H. & Prielipp, R. Transfusion in the operating room and the intensive care unit: current practice and future directions. *Int. Anesth. Clin.* 2000; **38**(4): 149–169.

4. Roback, J. D., Bray, R. A., & Hillyer, C. D. Longitudinal monitoring of WBC subsets in packed RBC units after filtration: implications for transfusion transmission of infections. *Transfusion* 2000; **40**: 500–506.

5. Akahoshi, M., Takanashi, M., & Masuda, M. A case of transfusion-associated graft-versus host disease not prevented by leukocyte depletion filters. *Transfusion* 1992; **32**: 169–172.

6. Goodnough, L. T. & Brecher, M. E. Autologous blood transfusion. *Intern. Med.* 1998; **37**: 238–245.

7. Brecher, M. (ed.) *Technical Manual*, 14th edn. American Association of Blood Banks, 2002: Bethesda, MD: 106.

8. Henry, D. A., Carless, P. A., Moxey, A. J. *et al.* Pre-operative autologous donation for minimising perioperative allogeneic blood transfusion [Review]. *Cochrane Database Syst. Rev.* 2002; **3**.

9. Goodnough, L. T., Monk, T. G., Sicard, G. *et al.* Intraoperative salvage in patients undergoing elective abdominal aortic

aneurysm repair: an analysis of cost and benefit. *J. Vasc. Surg.* 1996; **24**: 213–218.

10. Goodnough, L. T., Brecher, M. E., & Monk, T. G. Acute normovolemic hemodilution in surgery. *Hematology* 1992; **2**: 413–420.

11. Manucci, P. M. Drug therapy: hemostatic drugs. *N. Engl. J. Med.* 1998; **339**: 245–253.

12. Henry, D. A., Moxey, A. J., Carless, P. A. *et al.* Anti-fibrinolytic use for minimising perioperative allogeneic blood transfusion [Review]. *Cochrane Database Syst. Rev.* 2002; **3**.

13. Samama, C. M., Langeron, O., Rosencher, N. *et al.* Aprotinin versus placebo in major orthopedic surgery: a randomized, double-blinded, dose-ranging study. *Anesth. Analg.* 2002; **95**: 287–93.

14. Peters, D. C. & Noble, S. Aprotinin: An update of its pharmacology and therapeutic use in open heart surgery and coronary artery bypass surgery. *Drugs* 1999; **57**: 233–260.

15. Donovan, J. F. Microscopic vasovasotomy: current practice and future trends. *Microsurgery* 1995; **16**: 325–332.

16. Kollias, S. L. & Fox, J. M. Meniscal repair. Where do we go from here? *Clin. Sports Med.* 1996; **15**: 621–630.

17. Martinowitz, U., Schulman, S., Horoszowski, H. *et al.* Role of fibrin sealants in surgical procedures on patients with hemostatic disorders. *Clin. Orthop. Related Res.* 1996; **328**: 65–75.

18. Mccarthy, P. M. Fibrin glue in cardiothoracic surgery. *Transfus. Med. Rev.* 1993; **7**: 173–229.

19. Rousou, J., Levitsky, S., Gonzalez-Lavin, L. *et al.* Randomized clinical trials of fibrin sealant in patients undergoing resternotomy or reoperation after cardiac operations. A multicenter study. *J. Thorac. Cardiovasc. Surg.* 1989; **97**: 194–203.

20. Schlag, G. Immuno's fibrin sealant: The European experience. Abstract from Symposium on Fibrin Sealant: Characteristics and Clinical Uses. Uniformed Services University of the Health Sciences, Bethesda, MD, 1994. Dec. 8–9.

21. Bucur, S. Z. & Hillyer, C. D. Cryoprecipitate and related products. In Hillyer, C. D., Hillyer, K. L., Strobel, F. J. *et al. Handbook of Transfusion Medicine*, 1/e. California: Academic Press, 2001: 50.

22. Goodnough, L. T., Monk, T. G., & Andriole, G. L. Current concepts: erythropoietin therapy. *N. Engl. J. Med.* 1997; **336**: 933–938.

23. Gmur, J., Burger, J., Schanz, U. *et al.* Safety of stringent prophylactic platelet transfusion policy for patients with acute leukemia. *Lancet* 1991; **338**: 1223–1226.

24. Pisciotto, P. T., Benson, K., Hume, H. *et al.* Prophylactic versus therapeutic platelet transfusion practices in hematology and/or oncology patients. *Transfusion* 1995; **35**: 498–502.

25. Hanson, S. R. & Slichter, S. J. Platelet kinetics in patients with bone marrow hypoplasia: evidence for a fixed platelet requirement. *Blood* 1985; **66**: 1105–1109.

26. Rebulla, P., Finazzi, G., Marangoni, F. *et al.* The threshold for prophylactic platelet transfusions in adults with acute myeloid leukemia. Gruppo Italiano Malattie Ematologiche Maligne dell'Adulto. *N. Engl. J. Med.* 1997; **337**: 1870–1875.

27. Wandt, H., Frank, M., Ehninger, G. *et al.* Safety and cost effectiveness of a $10 \times 10(9)/$L trigger for prophylactic platelet transfusions compared with the traditional $20 \times 10(9)/$L

trigger: a prospective comparative trial of 105 patients with acute myeloid leukemia. *Blood* 1998; **91**: 3601–3606.

28. Takahashi, T., Abe, H., Nakai, K., & Sekiguchi, S. Bradykinin generation during filtration of platelet concentration with a white cell-reduction filter [letter]. *Transfusion* 1995; **35**; 967.

29. Friedman, D. F., Lukas, M. B., Jawad, A. *et al.* Alloimmunization to platelets in heavily transfused patients with sickle cell disease. *Blood* 1996; **88**: 3216–3222.

30. TRAP. Leukocyte reduction and ultraviolet B irradiation of platelets to prevent alloimmunization and refractoriness to platelet transfusions. The Trial to Reduce Alloimmunization to Platelets Study Group. *N. Engl. J. Med.* 1997; **337**: 1861–1869.

31. Kutar, D. J., Cebon, J., Harker, L. A. *et al.* Platelet growth factors: potential impact on transfusion medicine. *Transfusion* 1999; **39**: 321–332.

32. Churchwell, K. B., McManus, M. L., Kent, P. *et al.* Intensive blood and plasma exchange for treatment of coagulopathy in Meningococcemia. *J. Clin. Apher.* 1995; **10**: 171–177.

33. Cohen, H. Avoiding misuse of fresh frozen plasma. *Br. Med. J.* 1993; **307**: 395–396.

34. Crosson, J. T. Massive transfusion. *Clin. Lab. Med.* 1996; **16**: 873–882.

35. Linden, J. V., Wagner, K., Voytovich, A. E., & Sheehan J. Transfusion errors in New York State: an analysis of 10 years' experience. *Transfusion* 2000; **40**: 1207–1213.

36. Myhre, B. A. & McRuer D. Human error – a significant cause of transfusion mortality. *Transfusion* 2000; **40**: 879–885.

37. Carr, R., Hutton, J. L., Jenkins, J. A. *et al.* Transfusion of ABO mismatched platelets leads to early platelet refractoriness. *Br. J. Haematol.* 1990; **75**: 408–413.

38. Pierce, R. N., Reich, L. M., & Mayer, K. Hemolysis following platelet transfusions from ABO-incompatible donors. *Transfusion* 1985; **25**: 60–62.

39. Iserson, K. V. & Huestis, D. W. Blood warming: current applications and techniques. *Transfusion* 1991; **31**: 558–571.

40. Kopko, P. M., Marshall, C. S., MacKenzie, M. R. *et al.* Transfusion-related acute lung injury – report of a clinical look-back investigation. *J. Am. Med. Assoc.* 2002; **287**(15): 1968–1961.

41. Vamvakas, E. C. & Carven, J. H. Allogeneic blood transfusion, hospital charges, and length of hospitalization: a study of 487 consecutive patients undergoing colorectal cancer resection. *Arch. Pathol. Lab. Med.* 1998; **122**: 145–151.

42. Hillyer, C. D., Lankford, K. V., Roback, J. D. *et al.* Transfusion of the HIV seropositive patient: immunomodulation, viral reactivation, and limiting exposure to EBV (HHV-4), CMV (HHV-5), and HHV – 6, 7, and 8. *Transfus. Med. Rev.* 1999; **13**: 1–17.

43. Linden, J. V., Tourault, M. A., & Scribner, C. L. Decrease in frequency of transfusion fatalities. *Tranfusion* 1997; **37**: 243–244.

44. Ness, P. M., Shirley, R. S., Thoman, S. K., & Buck, S. A. The differentiation of delayed serologic and delayed hemolytic transfusion reactions: incidence, long-term serologic findings, and clinical significance. *Transfusion* 1990; **30**: 688–693.

45. Dodd, R. Y., Notari, E. P., & Stramer, S. L. Current prevalence and incidence of infectious disease markers and estimated window-period risk in the American Red Cross blood donor population. *Transfusion* 2002; **42**: 975–979.

46. Goodnough, L. T., Brecher, M. E., Kanter, M. H., & AuBuchon, J. P. Transfusion Medicine. First of two parts. *Blood Transfus. N. Engl. J. Med.* 1999; **340**: 438–447.

47. Blajchman, M. A. Bacterial contamination and proliferation during the storage of cellular blood products. *Vox Sang.* 1998; **74**: 155–159.

48. Goldman, M. & Blajchman, M. A. Blood product-associated bacterial sepsis. *Transfus. Med. Rev.* 1991; **5**: 73–83.

Infectious disease

21

Prevention of surgical site infections

Hien H. Nguyen and Stuart H. Cohen

Division of Infectious Diseases, University of California, Davis School of Medicine, Sacramento, CA

Introduction

Prevention of surgical infections has helped to revolutionize surgery from a practice that had been plagued by frequent infection and death into the discipline it is today. As the development of antimicrobial prophylaxis and the prevention of postoperative infection have progressed, the development of more invasive, technical procedures has also evolved.

However, infections related to surgery continue to remain a problem. Over 27 million surgeries are performed in US hospitals each year with average infection rates over the past decade ranging from 0.14% for clean uncomplicated eye surgery to well over 17% for high-risk cardiothoracic surgeries, with an overall infection rate of approximately 2.6% from 1986–1996.[1,2] Data from the Centers for Disease Control and Prevention (CDC), through the National Nosocomial Infections Surveillance (NNIS) System, indicate surgical site infections (SSIs)[3] are the third most common infection reported, accounting for 14%–16% of all nosocomial infections.[4] SSIs are the most common nosocomial infection in surgical patients.[2] In turn, these complications result in longer and costlier hospital stays. In 1995, it was estimated that nosocomial infections accounted for approximately $4.5 billion of the healthcare budget, with surgical wound infections the most costly.[5] In fact, when readmissions are accounted, Kirkland and colleagues estimated in 1999 that the total excess hospitalization and direct costs attributable to one surgical site infection were 12 additional hospital days and $5038, respectively.[6]

For some procedures, SSIs not only impact cost but also quality of life. Whitehouse and colleagues published their findings in 2002 that SSIs following orthopedic procedures not only increased hospitalization by 14 days and cost by approximately $18 000, but also negatively impacted quality of life significantly using the Medical Outcome Study Short Form.[7] In addition, patients who develop surgical site infections carry an overall twofold higher mortality rate, which is independent of their initial surgical risk and other survival predictors.[6,8,9] Thus, the prevention of this surgical complication represents a significant impact not only on cost and quality of life but also on mortality.

While the benefits of preventing surgical infections are apparent, we must also keep in mind the disadvantages of excess antimicrobial use. It is overly simplistic to believe we can prevent all infections from occurring. Humans are not sterile beings; surgery is not performed in a vacuum; and each patient has a unique set of immune defenses and risks for infection. The goal of surgical prophylaxis is not to sterilize a patient but rather to decrease the bacterial burden at the surgical site. Prophylaxis augments the host's natural immune defense mechanisms by increasing the magnitude of a bacterial inoculum needed to cause an infection.[10]

Use of broad-spectrum antibiotics contributes to the development of multidrug-resistant organisms.[11] The past decade has seen a rise in the incidence of methicillin resistant *S. aureus* (MRSA) as well as *Candida* spp. in SSIs.[12,13] For each individual patient, infections due to resistant organisms are associated with a worse clinical outcome.[14] In addition, the impact on hospital ecology may be detrimental to other patients as well.[15] Therefore, there must be a balance in the use of antimicrobial agents to prevent infection and the overuse of antimicrobial agents resulting in excess cost and the development of multidrug-resistant organisms.

Fortunately, studies done over the past 50 years have helped to provide the foundation for guidelines for appropriate antimicrobial prophylaxis. This section provides general guidelines in the use of antibiotic prophylaxis, other considerations to decrease the rate of postsurgical

Medical Management of the Surgical Patient: A Textbook of Perioperative Medicine, ed. M. F. Lubin, R. B. Smith, T. F. Dobson, N. Spell, H. K. Walker. 4th edn. Published by Cambridge University Press. © Cambridge University 2006.

Table 21.1. Classification of surgical wounds and risk of subsequent infection

Wound classification	Definition	Infection rate (%)	
		Without preoperative antibiotics	With preoperative antibiotics
Clean wound	A non-traumatic wound in which no inflammation was encountered, no break in surgical technique occurred, and the respiratory, gastrointestinal, and genitourinary tracts were not entered	5.1	0.8
Clean-contaminated wound	A non-traumatic wound in which a break in surgical technique occurred or the respiratory, gastrointestinal, or genitourinary tracts were entered without significant spillage	10.1	1.3
Contaminated wound	A fresh, traumatic wound from a relatively clean source or an operative wound with a major break in technique such as gross spillage from the gastrointestinal tract or entrance into infected urinary or biliary tract. This includes incisions encountering acute non-purulent inflammation	21.9	10.2
Dirty wound	Traumatic wounds from a dirty source or with delayed treatment, fecal contamination, foreign bodies, a devitalized viscus, or pus from any source that is encountered	40	10

infections, and evidence based antimicrobial prophylaxis for specific procedures.

General guidelines of surgical prophylaxis

Surgical prophylaxis is defined as the administration of antibiotics at the time of surgery to patients without evidence of established infection in order to prevent infection. Therefore, patients with a pre-existing infection such as pneumonia, a ruptured appendix, or an infected heart valve, where the use of antibiotics is considered therapeutic, are excluded from this discussion, since the choice of an antimicrobial agent, dosing and duration may differ dramatically. General principles to consider in surgical prophylaxis include (a) assessing a patient's underlying risk of surgical site infection, (b) weighing the risks and benefits of surgical prophylaxis prior to initiating prophylaxis, (c) understanding the microbiology of the surgical site and resultant infections, and (d) choosing the dose and timing of the antimicrobic.

Assessing patient risk

In the prevention of surgical infections, it is first important to understand the limitations of antimicrobial prophylaxis

and the inherent infection risk. Historically, a patient's risk of developing a postoperative infection correlated with the type of surgical procedure being performed and the bacterial load already present within the surgical field. Surgeries are divided into one of four different categories (Table 21.1), each intrinsically carrying different potential for infection.[16] They cover the range of possibilities from clean procedures where reservoirs of endogenous patient flora are not encountered to clean-contaminated procedures where these reservoirs of bacteria are entered under controlled conditions; contaminated procedures include everything short of a dirty-infected procedure, where there may be evidence of clinical infection or a perforated viscus.

While this classification has served to crudely estimate infection risk, it does not take into account individual patient or procedural risk factors for infection. Epidemiologic studies have identified a number of patient-centered risk factors associated with SSIs, including extremes of age, diabetes, use of steroids, prior site irradiation, hypoxemia, nicotine use, a low preoperative serum albumin level, skin test allergy, a long preoperative hospitalization, severe malnutrition or obesity, and the presence of a remote infection at the time of surgery.[17,18] In order to assess the independent importance of each underlying risk of infection, the Study on the Efficacy of

Nosocomial Infection Control (SENIC) was conducted in 1985. Using a multivariate analysis, Haley *et al.* found and confirmed that operations involving the abdomen, procedures lasting longer than 2 hours, and the presence of three or more discharge diagnoses (as a surrogate for identifying the complicated patient) were independent risk factors for infection. While the addition of other risk factors did not improve the predictive capability of the model, they are useful in targeted populations where specific measures can be used in an attempt to reduce SSIs. A model that stratified patients within each of the four wound categories further into low, medium, and high risk of infection was developed. As a result, the ability to identify risk of infection for individual patients improved by twofold when compared to the traditional classification of wound contamination.[19]

Finally, in 1991, the CDC modified the ASA risk index into what is used today to assist in predicting a patient's risk of developing a surgical site infection.[20] Instead of using the number of discharge diagnoses as a measure of a patient's underlying health status, the American Society of Anesthesia (ASA) Score, which has the advantage of being available at the time of surgery, was substituted. In addition, instead of using a standard time of two hours as a risk factor for infection, a customized time representative of the 75th percentile of the average time for each surgical procedure was used to account for procedures that traditionally take a longer or shorter time to complete. Each additional risk factor increased the rate of infection significantly. These data demonstrated the limitations of wound classification system as the sole predictor of infection risk. By assessing a patient's risk for infection, we can determine how aggressive we may need to be in preventing a surgical site infection.

Cost (risk)/benefit assessment

The financial aspects of prophylactic therapy can be staggering especially with the institution of prospective payment systems for hospitals. In Belgium, antimicrobials account for 30% of hospital pharmacy budgets with prophylactic antibiotics estimated to represent one-third of all antimicrobials administered in hospitals.[21] As detailed above, all surgical procedures do not carry the same risk of infection. The administration of antibiotics routinely in all surgical settings is not cost effective. The potential benefit of preventing infection in each individual circumstance must be balanced against the risk and cost of surgical prophylaxis.

In addition to the tremendous financial cost of antimicrobial prophylaxis, there are costs that are more difficult to calculate. With each dose of antibiotic, there is an ecological cost in the development of antimicrobial resistance.[22] There have been attempts to assign a value to the ecologic cost of antimicrobial resistance. However, it is difficult to weigh the risk of future antimicrobial resistance, however great, against the immediate benefit of preventing a surgical site infection, however small. Other considerations of the risk of prophylaxis must include toxic or allergic reactions that increase as larger numbers of patients receive these medications. *Clostridium difficile*-associated diarrhea can be associated with any antibiotic agent and has certainly been associated with antibiotic prophylaxis.[23,24] In weighing all of these factors, the answer to the cost-benefit question lies in the specifics for each surgical procedure and the results of rigorous clinical trials.[25]

For clean surgical procedures, the risk of infection is approximately five percent. The risks of antibiotic prophylaxis for these patients appear to out weigh the benefit of their use. Except in a few defined circumstances discussed below, prophylaxis is generally not indicated in clean surgical procedures. Knight *et al.* retrospectively reviewed clean general surgery patients from a private hospital comparing cases that received antibiotic prophylaxis with cases that did not.[26] Although there may be some bias related to patient selection, infection rates did not differ significantly whether the patients received prophylactic antibiotics or not.

Conversely, studies indicate that, for a select number of clean procedures, antimicrobial prophylaxis is beneficial. Two general indications include the placement of intravascular prosthetic material and procedures in which a SSI would result in a grave risk for the patient. Elek and Conen[27] clarified the role of prosthetic material in the pathogenesis of wound infection. They showed that the inoculum of bacteria needed to cause an infection was reduced 10 000 fold with the addition of foreign material. They also suggested that devitalized tissue or burns represent a similar circumstance that could allow a small inoculum to cause infection. Studies conducted in the late 1970s and early 1980s suggest that peripheral (non-cardiac) vascular surgery with graft implantation benefits from prophylaxis with an antistaphylococcal agent.[28] Examples of infections that pose a catastrophic risk to patients include all types of cardiac surgery, including cardiac pacemaker placement.[29] Breast surgery and herniorrhaphy also seem to benefit from surgical prophylaxis;[30] however, in general, the infection rates for these procedures are low thus having little impact on overall patient care.

Table 21.2. Likely pathogens for specific operations

Operation	Likely pathogens
Clean surgeries	
Orthopedic	*S. aureus*; coagulase-negative staphylococci; gram-negative bacilli
Total joint replacement	
Closed fractures/use of nails, bone plates	
Functional repair without implant	
Neurosurgical	*S. aureus*; coagulase-negative staphylococci
Cardiothoracic	*S. aureus*; coagulase-negative staphylococci
Vascular	*S. aureus*; coagulase-negative staphylococci
Clean-contaminated surgeries	
Head and neck	*S. aureus*; streptococci; oropharyngeal anaerobes (e.g., peptostreptococci)
Incisions through the oropharyngeal mucosa	
Gastrointestinal	Gram-negative bacilli; enterococci; group B streptococci; anaerobes
Biliary	Gram-negative bacilli; anaerobes
Colorectal	Gram-negative bacilli; anaerobes
Genitourinary	Gram-negative bacilli
May not have pathogens if urine is sterile	
Gynecologic and obstetric	Gram-negative bacilli; enterococci; group B streptococci; anaerobes
Trauma	*S. aureus*; coagulase-negative staphylococci; gram-negative bacilli
Burn	First week: group A streptococci; S. *aureus*
	Afterwards: Gram-negative bacilli; anaerobes; *Candida sp.*

Microbiology of prophylaxis (Table 21.2)

Integral to the choice of antimicrobial agents must be the understanding of the microorganisms that commonly cause surgical site infections. For clean surgical procedures, wound infections are, by definition, caused by skin or exogenous airborne microorganisms since other reservoirs of bacteria, such as the gastrointestinal tract are not entered. The elimination of reservoirs of *S. aureus* by the use of intranasal mupirocin ointment may decrease SSIs by this organism.[31] For other procedures, endogenous polymicrobial flora are potential pathogens, depending on the location. When oropharyngeal mucous membranes are excised, staphylococci, streptococci, and oropharyngeal anaerobes (e.g., peptostreptococci) are usually isolated. For procedures involving the gastrointestinal tract, gram-negative organisms (e.g., *E. coli*), gram-positive organisms (e.g., enterococci), and occasionally anaerobes (e.g., *Bacillus fragilis*) are typically implicated. Procedures in the perineum or groin involve fecal flora. Table 21.2 lists the likely pathogens associated with individual procedures. Seeding of the surgical site from a distant focus is less commonly implicated. This route of infection may be important in the setting of insertion of prosthetic material, which provides a nidus for attachment for microorganisms.[32–36] Additionally, fungi causing infection may arise either from exogenous or endogenous sources, although the pathogenesis is not well understood.[37]

While the patient's endogenous flora is a largely held accountable for SSIs, surgical team personnel and the operating room environment also deserve discussion. Members of the surgical team who have direct contact with the sterile operating field have been linked with unusual outbreaks. Use of artificial nails has been shown to increase carriage of gram-negative organisms and fungi.[38,39] An outbreak of *Serratia marcescens* SSIs in cardiovascular surgery patients has been associated with the use of artificial nails.[40] Anesthesia personnel also may play a role in postsurgical infections. Although not directly involved in the surgical field during the time of the surgery, they perform a variety of procedures leading up to surgery. Outbreaks of bloodstream and surgical site infections have been linked to the re-use of propofol vials and other breaks in aseptic technique by anesthesiologists.[41]

Choosing an antibiotic

While specific antibiotic choices will be discussed later, it is not uncommon for internists or surgeons to have to make *ad hoc* choices in surgical prophylaxis due to extenuating circumstances like drug allergies, drug interactions, or other contraindications to the usual prophylactic regimens. The initial factor in the choice of an antibiotic for prophylaxis is the spectrum of activity of the drug. The chosen antibiotic may not be active against the entire gamut of organisms encountered, but it must be effective against the bacteria that most commonly cause infections. Other factors to consider include the pharmacokinetics and pharmacodynamics of the drug. Specifically, the agent must have a half-life that covers the decisive interval (the first 3 hours after incision or contamination) with therapeutic tissue concentrations from the time of incision to the time of closure. Failure to maintain adequate tissue concentrations of the drug above the minimum inhibitory concentration (MIC) increases the risk of wound infection.[42,43] Redosing of antibiotics may be necessary if the procedure is long, multiple transfusions are needed, or if the antibiotic is cleared rapidly.

In addition, the drug chosen for prophylaxis should take into account the resistance patterns of the hospital. The routine use of vancomycin prophylactically is not recommended for any procedure.[3] However, if the prevalence of methicillin-resistant S. aureus exceeds 20% for a hospital, the use of vancomycin may be indicated prophylactically for major vascular, orthopedic, or neurosurgical procedures involving prostheses.[44,45] When used appropriately, this targeted approach can lead to a significant decrease in the incidence of SSIs.[46]

Ideally, the drug chosen for prophylaxis should not be the same one used routinely as the treatment of choice for therapy should an infection occur. Infections with organisms resistant to antibiotics chosen for prophylaxis can occur by two different mechanisms. Selective pressure from the antibiotic may allow for small populations of antibiotic resistant bacteria to flourish in an individual patient and cause infection.[22] Also, resistant organisms endemic within an institution may cause a nosocomial infection via exogenous contamination.[47] In addition, due to the concerns of resistance, use of an antibiotic for prophylaxis having a broad spectrum of activity may limit its utility as a therapeutic agent. Therefore, another characteristic of an optimal prophylactic agent chosen is relative specificity for the organisms likely to be encountered as pathogens.

Cost should be the final consideration. Cost should include drug monitoring, administration, redosing, adverse effects, and failure of prophylaxis (i.e., SSI).[18] Given all of these factors, the most thoroughly studied class of antibiotics for prophylaxis has been the cephalosporins. Specifically, cefazolin, a first-generation cephalosporin, has been the recommended choice for prophylaxis for most surgical procedures due to its acceptable safety profile, relatively long half-life, good tissue penetration, sufficiently specific spectrum of action, and reasonable cost per dose.[18,48]

Timing of administration of prophylaxis

One of the most important determinants of successful use of perioperative antibiotics is the timing of administration. Burke first demonstrated this observation in a guinea pig model of subcutaneous S. aureus infection.[49] Administration of antibiotics before or shortly after inoculation with S. aureus helped to significantly reduce the extent of infection. A delay in administration of an hour resulted in a greater infection and the greater the delay, the greater the extent of infection. Delays up to 4 hours resulted in infections that were similar to guinea pig controls that did not receive antibiotics. Classen and colleagues demonstrated this phenomenon in a clinical setting. The administration of antibiotics too late, after the start of a procedure, resulted in a greater number of postsurgical infections. In addition, they showed that the administration of antibiotics too far ahead of time resulted in an infection rate five times greater than if the antibiotics were administered within 2 hours of the procedure.[50] Thus, the old practice of administrating antibiotics "on call" to the operating room has been revised to ensure appropriate timing. Antibiotics should optimally be administered within 30 minutes of the skin incision.[18]

Duration of prophylaxis

In general, the duration of antibiotics should not be longer than 24 hours after the procedure, and ideally should last only to the end of the procedure. One of the most difficult areas for physician adherence to published guidelines has been the continuation of antibiotic prophylaxis after a procedure.[51] The general misconception is that if antibiotics are useful in preventing infection at the time of incision, the continuation of antibiotics would further benefit a freshly inoculated, surgical wound. There is a growing body of evidence suggesting that postoperative doses of antibiotics are unnecessary. Burke's seminal paper sheds some light on the utility of antibiotics after the inoculation of bacteria into a wound. He clearly showed that antibiotics administered more than 3 hours after inoculation of S. aureus did not prevent infection.[49] Similarly, one should not expect the continuation of antibiotics for 24 to 48 hours after surgical manipulation to have much effect on the prevention of surgical site infection either. In addition, clinical studies, summarized by Dipiro in 1986, have shown that, for most surgical procedures, the use of single dose antibiotic prophylaxis is as effective in the prevention of surgical site infections as multiple doses for up to 24 to 48 hours after the procedure.[52] This excludes procedures where redosing of an antibiotic may be necessary due to the length

Table 21.3. Modifying risk of surgical site infection with interventions other than antibiotics

Modifying factor	Risk modification
Patient-centered factors	
Glucose control	Aggressive control of perioperative glucose levels below 200 mg/dl with an insulin drip reduced the incidence of deep sternal wound infections from 2% to 0.8% ($P = 0.01$) in patients undergoing cardiothoracic surgery
Intranasal mupirocin	For patients who are colonized with *S. aureus*, the rate of nosocomial *S. aureus* infections decreased from 7.7% to 4% (OR = 0.49, $P = 0.02$), but did not show a decrease in surgical site infections with *S. aureus*
Environmental factors	
Temperature	In patients undergoing colorectal surgery, normothermia (mean operative core body temperature of $36.6 \pm 0.5\,^{\circ}C$) reduced the surgical site infection rate from 19% to 6% ($P = 0.009$) compared to hypothermia (mean temperature of $34.7 \pm 0.6\,^{\circ}C$)
Supplemental oxygen	In patients undergoing colorectal surgery, 80% inspired oxygen reduced the surgical site infection rate from 11.2% to 5.2% ($P = 0.01$) compared to 30% inspired oxygen

of time of the surgery or blood loss and the need for transfusion. There is no value in administering antibiotics after the operation has been completed to prevent an SSI.

However, controversy continues to exist. Studies in three different types of surgical procedures support a longer duration of prophylaxis. While these studies do not definitively justify a longer duration of antibiotics, they do call for additional data and larger trials to help reach a consensus regarding the optimal duration of antibiotic prophylaxis for these areas. First, for cesarean sections, 3 days of antimicrobial prophylaxis with ampicillin had a lower incidence of endometritis than a shorter course of 18 hours.[53] Next, in major joint repairs, one study suggests that five doses of cefamandole were more effective in preventing infections than one dose.[54] Finally, debate continues over the duration of antibiotic therapy after vascular procedures where patients require the use of invasive monitoring. The concern is possible hematogenous seeding of the operative wound. Hall and colleagues found infection rates were two times higher in patients who received short courses of prophylaxis versus patients who continued prophylaxis until lines and drains were removed (not exceeding 5 days).[55]

Additional measures to help prevent infection (Table 21.3)

While the emphasis of this chapter is on the perioperative use of antibiotics, the prevention of infection certainly does not start or end with antibiotics. Just as the cause of infection can be multifactorial, the prevention efforts must be multifactorial as well. One of the most important determinants of infection risk is the surgeon's skill.

Surgeons who perform more procedures have lower infection rates for many reasons.[56] Surgeons must have the ability to clear the surgical field of devitalized tissue, prevent hematomas, and perform these tasks in a manner that is timely and devoid of intraoperative complications. In fact, while a surgeon's volume and expertise may play a role, a hospital's volume of a procedure may have an even greater impact not only on morbidity but on mortality, stressing the importance of a multidisciplinary approach to optimizing good outcomes.[57]

Authoritative guidelines have served to disseminate appropriate use of antimicrobials based on rigorous clinical trials. However, the application of this intervention has not been universal. While studies attempting to define the reasons for inappropriate use (overuse when not indicated and lack of use despite evidence for use) of antibiotics have not been conclusive, overwhelming evidence exists showing that there is room for improvement.[51] One adjunctive measure to insure optimal antimicrobial prophylaxis has been the use of computer-assisted systems. At LDS Hospital in Salt Lake City, the percentage of patients receiving prophylactic antibiotics within two hours of a procedure increased from 58% in 1986 to 72% in 1988 to 97–99% in 1998 with the implementation of computerization. Additionally, from 1988 to 1998, the percentage of patients receiving antibiotics for more than 24 hours decreased from 29.8% to 5.8%.[58]

Topical prophylaxis

Theoretically, the combination of topical and systemic antibiotics should decrease the chance of wound infection. The presumption is that infections occur with the inoculation of bacteria; thus topical irrigation of the wound with antibiotics could help reduce the amount of infecting bacteria, since high concentrations of the drug would be present at the site of bacterial entry, acting as an additional barrier to infection. A number of prospective trials studying the use of "non-absorbable" antibiotics during surgery has proven its benefit in colorectal surgery.[59] Moreover, the use of topical, luminal decontamination of the bowel seems to enhance the systemic use of antibiotics.[64] Other strategies involving topical antimicrobials, such as the use of antibiotic cement as prophylaxis in joint replacement surgery, are still controversial.[60] Early retrospective studies of antimicrobial cement seemed to show a significant decrease in the rate of surgical infections; however, more recent data with larger numbers of patients showed similar infection rates with longer periods of follow-up.[60,61] The use of antibiotic laden prosthetic material is less controversial; the use of antibiotic beads and spacers in the setting of osteomyelitis with two-stage revisions seem to show higher success rates.[62] Use of antimicrobials as an irrigation solution has not provided benefit when compared to saline irrigation.[64]

Glucose control

Of the multiple host immune defense mechanisms involved in overcoming a bacterial challenge, neutrophils play the most important role in killing the most common wound pathogens. In diabetics, poor glucose control can impair neutrophil and monocyte function;[65] thus, controlling a patient's glucose should theoretically assist in preventing infections. In a retrospective analysis, Golden and colleagues found that diabetics with progressively higher perioperative glucose levels had higher rates of infectious complications including SSIs, pneumonia, and urinary tract infections.[66] They recommended that glucose values be kept under 200 mg/dl. Furnary and colleagues not only confirmed this observation in diabetics undergoing cardiac procedures involving a median sternotomy, but also found that the use of continuous intravenous insulin infusion further reduced the rate of sternal wound infection versus intermittent subcutaneous insulin injection.[67]

The surgical environment

The operating room (OR) environment has been the focus of a number of studies to define its role in the development of SSIs. Measures to insure a sterile environment have been shown to directly impact the rate of postoperative infections. These include the use of hand/forearm antisepsis, OR ventilation, including laminar airflow, and the use of sterile instruments.[3] More recent studies have shown other factors in the OR environment may also have an impact on SSIs. Kurtz and colleagues studied the rates of postoperative wound infections in patients undergoing colorectal surgery. In a prospective, blinded protocol, they randomized patients to receive measures to insure normothermia versus standard intraoperative management that allowed patients to become mildly hypothermic to 34.5 °C. They found a threefold increased rate of postoperative wound infection and longer hospital stays in the group assigned to mild hypothermia versus normothermia.[68] There was no change in mortality. This evidence confirms animal data that perioperative hypothermia may impair host immune functions, such as chemotaxis and phagocytosis of granulocytes. In addition, hypothermia leads to vasoconstriction as the body tries to regulate temperature. In turn, vasoconstriction decreases the partial pressure of oxygen in tissues, which decreases bacterial killing, partly because the production of oxygen free radicals is dependent on the partial pressure of oxygen in wounds.[68]

Along the same line of reasoning, supplemental oxygen during surgery also seems to impact the rate of postoperative wound infections. Patients undergoing colorectal surgery were assigned to receive 80% inspired oxygen vs. 30% inspired oxygen. Those who received supplemental oxygen presumably had higher partial pressures of oxygen in tissue allowing for improved oxidative killing of bacteria by neutrophils. As a result, surgical wound infection rates decreased by half (11.2% vs. 5.2%, $P = 0.01$). However the duration of hospitalization was similar in the two groups.[69]

Other factors prior to surgery may impact the rate of surgical wound infections. However, many of these associations have confounders clouding their true impact on surgical site infections. These include a short preoperative stay in the hospital, careful hair removal at the surgical site, preoperative cleansing, and preoperative treatment of remote infections.

For most elective procedures, patients are admitted on the morning of surgery or the day before surgery. In addition, a number of procedures are being done on an outpatient basis, which serves to decrease the impact of hospital stay on surgical site infections. While some authors have documented exponential increases in the rates of infection for each week of hospitalization prior to surgery,[70] longer preoperative hospitalization, usually for medical problems, may be a surrogate for comorbidities and severity of illness rather than an independent predictor of SSIs.[3] Nonetheless, some authors have recommended that patients should not undergo elective

Table 21.4. Prophylaxis for endocarditis

Procedure	Recommended regimen	Comments
Dental, upper respiratory tract, esophageal or minor GI/GU procedures	Amoxicillin 2 g p.o. 1 hour before the procedure	For penicillin allergic patients, use clindamycin 600 mg p.o. 1 hour before the procedure. Alternatively, may use azithromycin or clarithromycin 500 mg p.o. 1 hour before the procedure For patients unable to take orals, Ampicillin 2 g i.m. or i.v. within 30 minutes of the procedure. For penicillin allergic and unable to take orals, clindamycin 600 mg i.v. within 30 minutes of procedure
Major GI/GU procedures	Ampicillin 2 g i.m. or i.v. plus Gentamicin 1.5 mg/kg (not to exceed 120 mg) within 30 minutes of procedure	For penicillin allergic patients, Vancomycin 1 gm IV over 1–2 hours plus Gentamicin 1.5 mg/kg, complete infusion within 30 minutes of procedure

operations during the same hospital stay due to the risk of infection with nosocomial organisms.[71]

Increased SSIs due to perioperative shaving have been attributed to microscopic breaks in the skin which serve as portals of entry for bacteria, causing infection. Shaving with a razor greater than 24 hours before surgery is associated with the highest rates of SSIs, followed by hair clipping the night before, shaving within 24 hours, shaving immediately before surgery, and hair clipping immediately before surgery. Use of a depilatory agent or no hair removal at all was associated with the lowest rates of SSIs.[3]

Use of preoperative cleansing with an antibacterial solution, like chlorhexidine or other antiseptics, has been shown to decrease the bacterial burden of normal skin flora. However, this has not definitively been shown to translate into decreased rates of SSIs.[3]

Remote infections of the urinary tract, skin, or respiratory tract have been shown to be associated with an increase in the development of SSIs.[72] Valentine and colleagues retrospectively studied the impact of remote infections on SSIs in clean surgeries. They conclude that the use of antibiotics therapeutically, defined as treatment for a remote infection initiated greater than 24 hours before surgery, decreased the rate of SSIs to levels similar to patients without remote infections.[73]

Surgical prophylaxis for specific procedures

This section will first review prophylaxis for patient groups who may require additional considerations to prevent infections when undergoing procedures. Then, recommendations for specific procedures will be discussed with regards to the pathogenesis, key microbiological organisms, and prophylactic regimens.

Prophylaxis of patients with valvular heart disease

In 1997, the American Heart Association revised guidelines for the prevention of bacterial endocarditis.[74] Similar to the use of antibiotics to prevent surgical wound infections, the use of antibiotics to prevent bacterial endocarditis involves assessing a procedure's likelihood of causing transient bacteremia within the context of the patient's underlying risk for the development of endocarditis. In addition, when taking into account the potential adverse events associated with the use of antibiotics and the cost–benefit analysis, they recommend the administration of prophylaxis to patients with underlying structural heart disease placing them at high or moderate risk of endocarditis for surgical procedures, which are likely to cause bacteremia. In contradistinction to the previous guidelines, the new guidelines limit the duration of prophylactic antibiotics and eliminate the use of erythromycin in prophylaxis (Table 21.4).

Prophylaxis for patients at risk for distant site infections

An area of continued debate is the use of antibiotic prophylaxis for dental or urological procedures in patients who may have a predisposition to infections at distant sites other than structural heart disease. These include patients with hip or knee replacements, dialysis catheters or shunts, vascular grafts, pacemakers, or ventriculoperitoneal shunts. In addition, should patients with immune dysfunction such as those with systemic lupus erythematosus, poorly controlled diabetes, or neutropenia secondary to cancer chemotherapy be managed differently to prevent distant site infections? In a joint statement, the American Dental Association and the American Academy of Orthopedic Surgeons recommend against routine administration of antibiotics for patients with orthopedic implants.[76] A survey of infectious disease consultants largely showed that they do not routinely use antibiotic prophylaxis for the patient populations noted above. However, 25%–40% of infectious disease physicians recommended prophylaxis for neutropenic patients and those with prosthetic joints or vascular grafts, mainly citing medicolegal issues for this practice.[77]

Prophylaxis for HIV-positive patients

With improved therapy for human immunodeficiency virus, more individuals are surviving with this infection. As this population increases and lives longer, more surgeries will be done on this patient group. Retrospective studies indicate that wound healing is delayed when CD4+ T-cell lymphocyte count is less than 50 cells/ml.[78] In addition, rates of postoperative infection appear to be increased as well. Grubert and associates reviewed the rates of postoperative morbidity in HIV-positive women undergoing obstetric and gynecological procedures.[79] In a case-control design they found that HIV-positive women had a significantly higher rate of postoperative infection compared to matched HIV-negative controls, which was especially significant for patients undergoing abdominal surgeries. Paiement and colleagues found similar results looking at asymptomatic HIV-positive orthopedic trauma patients undergoing surgery.[80] Increased rates of postoperative infection were most pronounced in HIV patients with open fractures, 55.6% infection rate vs. 11.3% in HIV-negative patients (Fisher's exact test, $P = 0.004$). Overall, while very low CD4+ T-lymphocyte seems to play a role in wound healing, it does not appear to be a reliable predictor of postoperative infection.[79,81] HIV seropositivity alone predisposes to infectious complications. Measures to prevent surgical site infections in this patient population need further study.

Clean surgical procedures (Table 21.5)

Orthopedic surgery

Although most clean procedures do not require the use of prophylactic antibiotics, the placement of a foreign body during most orthopedic procedures predisposes to surgical infections. Moreover, because of the severe consequences of infection after joint replacement, prophylaxis is recommended. By definition, the environment plays an important role in the pathogenesis of the SSI. Microorganisms seeded during the operation cause most postoperative infections of joint replacements. While most

infections will manifest themselves within the first month after the procedure, many infections will take years to manifest clinically. Infections occurring over 2 years after the procedure are thought to be a result of hematogenous seeding of the joint rather than direct inoculation of bacteria at the time of surgery, although controversy exists. *Staphylococcus aureus* and coagulase-negative staphylococci are the two most common pathogens accounting for up to 90% of cases that occur within the first 2 years. Cefazolin is usually chosen for prophylaxis due to its efficacy against gram-positive pathogens, reasonable cost, and favorable safety profile.[82] However, in some centers where the prevalence of methicillin resistance is high, the use of vancomycin for prophylaxis is warranted.

Additionally, since environmental contamination may account for early infection, investigators have studied the use of ultraclean-air technology, enclosed operating rooms with laminar airflow and surgeons wearing body-exhaust systems. In conjunction with systemic antibiotics, they find a further reduction in the rates of infection although the data are not overwhelming.[83,84]

As discussed earlier, the use of antibiotic cements alone for the prevention of postoperative infection does not seem to alter the infection rate or the rate of revisions of joint replacement. However, the use of antibiotic cements in addition to systemic antimicrobial prophylaxis is better than the use of systemic antibiotics alone. Espenhaug's observational study showed that the rates of infection or revision were lower if patients had received a combined regimen as compared to systemic antibiotics alone. The positive results were seen in early infection, and the difference was even greater with 8 years of follow-up.[61]

The use of mupirocin ointment to eradicate *S. aureus* colonization of the nares has been studied for orthopedic procedures. While the use of mupirocin twice a day from the time of admission to the hospital to surgery was able to eradicate *S. aureus* colonization in some patients, when studied in a placebo-controlled fashion, no statistically significant effect on the rates of postoperative infections could be found.[85,86]

Neurosurgery

The infection rate associated with clean neurosurgical procedures is very low. When prosthetic materials are inserted, antibiotic prophylaxis is commonly used. Prospective randomized, clinical trials have not shown a clear benefit for the use of prophylaxis. However, these trials included all kinds of neurosurgical procedures, which carry different baseline infection rates. Meta-analyses by Barker indicate that when data are analyzed

Table 21.5. Prophylaxis for clean surgical procedures

Orthopedic surgery	Recommended regimen	Comments
Arthroplasty of joints including joint replacements	Cefazolin 1 g preoperatively and every 6 hours for 3 doses for patients with normal renal function	When using a tourniquet for knee replacement surgery a higher cefazolin dose should be considered (2 g)
Open reduction of fracture	Cefazolin 1 g preoperatively and every 6 hours for 3 doses for patients with normal renal function	Complex (open) fractures would not be considered a clean procedure and would require treatment as a contaminated procedure with a course of antimicrobials
Lower limb amputation	Cefoxitin 2 g preop and every 6 hours for 4 doses for patients with normal renal function	Cefotetan or cefmetazole may be substituted. Other combinations of 3rd gen. Cephalosporin and Metronidazole would also be acceptable

Laminectomy, spinal fusion without prosthesis placement do not require prophylaxis in non-compromised patients

Neurosurgery	Recommended regimen	Comments
Craniotomy	Clindamycin 300 mg preop and at 4 hours	Vancomycin 10 mg/kg (up to 500 mg) and gentamicin 2 mg/kg (up to 120 mg) with an aminoglycoside irrigating solution
Spinal fusion	See above	

Cardiothoracic surgery	Recommended regimen	Comments
Median sternotomy, coronary artery bypass surgery, or repair of a valve	Cefazolin 1 g preop and every 4 hours intraoperatively or if massive hemorrhage occurs	Vancomycin could be considered in hospitals with rates of MRSA > 20% or allergy to cefazolin; give vancomycin 15 mg/kg slowly in a dilute solution over 1 hour preop; duration is often continued postop, although no data indicate efficacy in adults
Pacemaker insertion	Cefazolin 1 g preop	With cefazolin allergy, due to low incidence of infection, may be reasonable to give no prophylaxis
Thoracic surgery, including lobectomy and pneumonectomy	Cefazolin 1 g preop and every 4–6 hours intraoperatively	Vancomycin or clindamycin for cefazolin allergy

Vascular surgery	Recommended regimen	Comments
Aortic and femoral vascular procedures, including bypass and reconstruction	Cefazolin 1 g preop and every 4–6 hours intraoperatively	Vein stripping and carotid endarterectomy do not require prophylaxis unless baseline infection rates are high.

Laparoscopic surgery – no data to indicate benefit of prophylaxis

for individual neurosurgical procedures, a benefit for surgical prophylaxis is significant for those involving a craniotomy or spinal surgery.[87,88] No difference could be found between single and multiple doses of antibiotics or between different antibiotic regimens. While benefits can be demonstrated, caution must be used in the interpretation of data and larger randomized trials must be conducted in order to draw definite conclusions about clean neurosurgical procedures that do not involve placement of a foreign body.

While normothermia may be helpful in the prevention of surgical infections, the benefit of hypothermia may be greater for neurosurgery. Hypothermia may prevent cerebral ischemia during neurosurgical procedures. Thus, hypothermia should continue to be recommended for patients undergoing craniotomy who are at risk for cerebral ischemia despite the potential negative impact on infection.[87]

Cardiothoracic surgery

Although regarded as a clean procedure, the risks of infection associated with open-heart surgery, such as mediastinitis or pericarditis, are life threatening and justify the use of prophylactic antibiotics. In addition, while initial studies of prophylaxis in cardiac surgery did not show a statistical benefit of antibiotic prophylaxis, a subsequent study by Fong and colleagues, applying more stringent experimental methods, showed a significant benefit of a short course of antistaphylococcal antibiotics over placebo.[88,89] While cefazolin remains the recommended choice of antimicrobial, the use of vancomycin may be indicated in specific clinical situations. See section "Choosing an antibiotic" for further discussion.

The duration of antibiotic prophylaxis in cardiac surgery is controversial. Not only is the duration of antibiotics postoperatively debated, but also the redosing of antibiotics during the procedure is debated. Zanetti and colleagues retrospectively studied the effect of redosing of cefazolin in cardiac surgery. They found that redosing in procedures lasting >400 minutes significantly reduced the SSI rate by 16%. This supports the theoretical pharmacokinetic guidelines recommended for redosing of cefazolin every 3–4 hours to maintain adequate tissue levels of antibiotics during a procedure to prevent infection.[3,90]

Antimicrobial prophylaxis is continued for 48 hours after the procedure in most studies and shorter regimens have not been well studied. Owing to the concern of postoperative infection and potential hematogenous seeding of a surgical prosthesis, some cardiac surgeons prefer to continue prophylactic antibiotics until all "tubes" are removed. No data support this practice in adults. One non-randomized, retrospective study in pediatric cardiac surgery patients showed that this practice was potentially beneficial, however, the authors note that this population differs greatly from the adult cardiac patient.[91]

Vascular surgery

Considered a "clean" surgery, the rates of wound infection after vascular surgery differ greatly depending on the site of surgery. Surgeries involving an incision in the groin area carry a higher infection rate than carotid or upper extremity procedures.[92,93] Thus, prophylaxis is recommended for procedures involving aortic or femoral reconstructions. The risk of infection in upper extremity procedures does not outweigh the risks of drug administration.

Data for the use of antibiotics prophylactically in aortic or femoral vascular procedures come mainly from the work of Hasselgren and colleagues. In a prospective, randomized, double-blind study of patients undergoing lower extremity vascular reconstructive surgery, they demonstrated that the use of cefuroxime for 24 hours decreased the wound infection rate from 16.7% to 3.8% ($P < 0.05$).

Extension of antibiotics to 72 hours showed no difference when compared to 24 hours.[94]

Placement of a prosthesis should include prophylaxis. Bennion and colleagues showed that the use of antibiotics perioperatively reduced the overall infection rate in patients undergoing placement of vascular access hemodialysis grafts.[95]

Lower extremity amputation for ischemia should also receive prophylaxis. Sonne-Holm and colleagues studied 152 patients undergoing lower extremity amputation for ischemia. Postoperative wound infection rates decreased from 38.7% in the placebo arm to 16.9% in the antibiotic group ($P < 0.005$). Clostridial infections occurred in the placebo arm that were not seen with the cefoxitin arm. Prophylaxis should include coverage of anaerobic flora.[96]

Laparoscopic surgery

The use of laparoscopic surgery has dramatically decreased the infection rate associated with elective cholecystectomy. McGuckin and colleagues note that the rate of SSIs in this surgery is 0.4%. Randomized prospective trials have not been able to show a benefit for the use of perioperative antibiotics in uncomplicated, elective laparoscopic cholecystectomy. Although data are needed to make firm conclusions, antibiotic prophylaxis does not appear to be beneficial in other kinds of laparoscopic surgeries.

Clean–contaminated surgical procedures (Table 21.6)

Head and neck surgery

Clean head and neck surgeries, such as thyroidectomy, parotidectomy, or submandibular gland resection have very low postoperative infection rates and do not require antimicrobial prophylaxis. In reviewing 438 cases, Johnson and Wagner demonstrated that, with an infection rate of 0.7%, the addition of antibiotics is unnecessary.[97] However, prophylactic antibiotics in clean neck dissections may be useful. Carrau and colleagues retrospectively reviewed the use of antibiotics in neck dissections that were not contaminated by endogenous bacterial flora. They found that the use of antibiotics decreased the infection rate from 10% to 3.3% ($P = 0.09$).[98] Subsequent studies have clearly demonstrated that there is no benefit to continuing antibiotics longer than 24 hours.[99]

Clean-contaminated head and neck surgeries, where contamination of the surgical wound occurs by

Table 21.6. Prophylaxis for clean contaminated surgical procedures

Head and neck surgery	Recommended regimen	Comments
Major procedures involving contamination with oropharyngeal secretions	Cefazolin 1 g preop and every 4–6 hours intraoperatively and metronidazole 0.5 g preop and every 8 h intraoperatively	Clindamycin as a single agent could be used as an alternative 300 mg preop and every 8 h intraop
Tonsillectomy, with or without, adenoidectomy, or rhinoplasty and repair of the nose – no data to indicate benefit of prophylaxis		
Gastroduodenal surgery	**Recommended regimen**	**Comments**
Procedures involving the esophagus or stomach, with risk factors for decreased acid production	Cefazolin 1 g preop and every 4–6 hours intraoperatively	Risk factors for decreased acid production include elderly, tumor, use of antacids, or disease states with decreased acid production (i.e. pernicious anemia or atrophic gastritis)
As above without risk factors for decreased acid production	None recommended	Adequate acid production and motility in the stomach acts as bacteriostatic agents, with few remaining bacteria, therefore procedures do not require prophylaxis
General/colorectal surgery	**Recommended regimen**	**Comments**
Biliary tract surgery	Cefazolin 2 g i.v. preop and every 6 hours intraoperatively	1st gen ceph as effective as others studied. Required for high risk patients. Acute cholecystitis or ascending cholangitis need treatment. With beta-lactam allergy, can use gentamicin 80 mg i.v. preop and every 8 hours intraoperatively
Colorectal surgery	Gastrointestinal lavage followed by neomycin and erythromycin base 1 g of each p.o. at 1, 2, 11 pm the day prior to surgery	For more emergent procedures or cases where preop oral prophylaxis is not possible, use ceftizoxime or gentamicin plus metronidazole; or cefoxitan, cefotetan, or cefmetazole 2 g i.v. preop and every 3 hours during surgery or if massive hemorrhage
Appendectomy, non-perforated	Gentamicin 5 mg/kg i.v. preop plus Metronidazole 0.5 mg preop or Ceftizoxime 1 g preop plus Metronidazole 0.5 g preop	Alternative is cefoxitin 2 g i.v. preop and every 6 h intraop. For gangrenous or perforated appendix, would treat as a contaminated procedure or infection
Genitourinary surgery	**Recommended regimen**	**Comments**
Data are lacking in the use of perioperative antibiotics for urologic procedures in which the urine is sterile prior to the procedure, no foreign body is inserted and no colonic contamination is expected.		
Urinary diversion surgery	Mechanical bowel prep as per colonic procedure and Gentamicin 5 mg/kg preop plus Metronidazole 0.5 g preop	Transrectal procedures may not need bowel preparation; data are inconclusive

oropharyngeal secretions, carry infection rates up to 87% and require the use of prophylactic antibiotics.[100] Additional risks factors for SSI include bilateral neck dissection, stage IV cancer, total laryngectomy, and prior tracheostomy. Prior irradiation and diabetes were not risk factors for postoperative infection.[101,102] The authors hypothesize that more extensive surgery increases the risk of infection due to the inability to achieve a watertight closure, closure of the mucosal suture lines under tension, or application of complex reconstructions. Prior tracheostomy may simply increase the burden and inoculum of bacteria existing in the upper airway, leading to increased rates of infection despite prophylactic antibiotics.

The choice of antibiotics should address the most common causes of postoperative infection, including *Staphylococcus aureus*, streptococcal species, and anaerobes. To further characterize the bacteria that cause postoperative infections, Rubin and colleagues reviewed the cases of SSI at their institution. In 96% of cases, infections were polymicrobial, involving aerobes and, in 74% of cases, anaerobes. Prophylaxis therefore should include adequate anaerobic coverage.[103] When cefazolin was compared to the combination of cefazolin and metronidazole, the latter regimen, with adequate anaerobic coverage, demonstrated a lower rate of SSI 11.9% vs. 23.9% ($P < 0.05$).[104] The role of gram-negative organisms in the development of SSI in head and neck surgery is controversial. Studies comparing the use of clindamycin, which has no gram-negative coverage, showed equal efficacy to the regimen of clindamycin plus an agent with gram-negative activity, suggesting that a broader agent with gram-negative coverage is not necessary in prophylaxis.[105,106]

The duration of prophylaxis has been studied with a number of regimens. Extending the duration of prophylactic antibiotics beyond 24 hours was not beneficial.[102,107] The potential infection of myocutaneous reconstructive flaps has led to the prolonged use of antibiotic prophylaxis. However, the only prospective, multi-center trial, comparing 1 day to 5 days of antibiotic prophylaxis for this type of surgery did not show any benefit for prolonged antibiotic use (18.9% vs. 25%; $P > 0.05$).[108]

Gastroduodenal surgery

Surgical infections involving the stomach and duodenum can be predicted, based upon the presence and function of gastric acid within the stomach prior to surgery. Patients with normal gastric acid output and gastric motility harbor few bacteria in the stomach and proximal intestine due to the bacteriostatic action of acid and the mechanical cleansing action of normal motility.[109] However, in patients with obstructing ulcers, tumors or decreased or lessened acidity of the stomach (for example: upper gastrointestinal bleeding, being elderly, use of antacid medications) infections due to endogenous bacterial overgrowth are common. Antibiotic prophylaxis is beneficial for these high-risk individuals.[110,111] Prophylaxis with an agent that has activity against oral flora and coliforms, such as a first- or second-generation cephalosporin perioperatively is efficacious.[111]

Biliary surgery

Surgery involving the biliary system without the presence of infection is limited mainly to elective cholecystectomy. In this situation, prophylaxis is not always beneficial. The work of Keighley and colleagues has defined a group of patients who will benefit from the use of perioperative antibiotics. In a multivariate analysis of patients undergoing surgery of the biliary tract without prophylactic antibiotics, they defined a high-risk group for postoperative

infectious complications as patients with one or more of the following clinical risk factors: age greater than 70 years, history or presence of jaundice, previous biliary tract surgery, chills or fevers within 1 week of surgery, common duct disease, operations done within 1 month of an acute attack of cholecystitis or diabetes mellitus.[112]

Use of an antimicrobial agent with high concentrations within the biliary tract has not been shown to be more efficacious than systemic agents in the prevention of surgical wound infections after biliary tract surgery.[113] The use of a short course of a first-generation cephalosporin is the recommended regimen as it has been as effective as other antibiotics studied.[114]

Colorectal surgery

Of the clean–contaminated surgeries discussed, colorectal surgery encounters the largest amount of bacteria and is thus the most formidable task in the prevention of surgical infections. The use of mechanical cleansing has been employed to reduce the bacterial load of the colon prior to surgery. However, it is clear from clinical trials that mechanical cleansing alone is not sufficient.[115] Placebo-controlled studies have established the role of antibiotics, shown by a reduction in SSIs from 40.2% to 12.9%.[116] While it is clear that antibiotics should be used, the ideal regimen and route of administration are debated. The decision to use oral versus parenteral antibiotics depends on whether one believes in the importance of reducing the number of microorganisms in the bowel lumen (oral) or in the importance of adequate tissue concentrations of an antimicrobic prior to opening the colon (parenteral). For surgeries lasting less than 3 hours, there does not appear to be a difference between use of an oral regimen or an intravenous regimen with activity against facultative aerobes and anaerobes. However, in surgeries lasting longer than 4 hours, or procedures involving rectal resection lasting longer than 215 minutes, the combination of an oral and parenteral prophylactic regimen was superior to use of a parenteral regimen alone.[117,118] It is unclear if redosing of the parenteral antibiotic would change the rate of wound infections in longer procedures.

The most widely studied oral preparation is neomycin–erythromycin base. When used, the first of three doses should be given starting 19 hours prior to surgery.[119] Owing to the critical timing of this regimen and the need for a functional bowel, use of an oral antibiotic preparation during emergency procedures is not recommended. Numerous parenteral regimens have been studied, all of which have similar rates of efficacy to the combination of mechanical preparation and oral antibiotics, as long as there is adequate activity against both facultative aerobes and anaerobes. Effective regimens used in clinical trials have included a second-generation cephalosporin with anaerobic activity like cefoxitin or cefotetan, doxycycline, or the combination of an agent with facultative aerobic activity like cefotaxime, ceftriaxone, cefepime, cefuroxime, gentamicin, or amikacin, plus an agent with anaerobic activity like metronidazole or clindamycin.[71] First-generation cephalosporins are not effective in prophylaxis of infections for colorectal surgeries.[120]

Genitourinary surgery

Clinical studies examining surgical prophylaxis for urologic surgery have been criticized for a lack of uniformity.[121] Unlike surgical wound infections associated with other procedures, complications of urologic surgery may include bacteriuria, pyelonephritis, bacteremia, and sepsis. One of the main problems revolves around the importance of post procedure bacteriuria. Some authors believe that even small numbers of bacteria may be significant since it may lead to other complications, while others suggest that clinical symptoms should be the end point. Thus, without convincing data, there is a lack of consensus among recommendations. Surgeries involving the genitourinary tract can be divided into clean procedures and clean–contaminated procedures. However, when there is clinically significant bacteriuria prior to a procedure, use of antibiotics can be considered therapeutic not prophylactic. Most authorities agree that the use of antibiotics in this scenario improves the rate of postoperative infectious complications.[122] Elective procedures should ideally be delayed until after therapy and repeat urine culture confirm sterilization of the urine.

Clean urologic procedures, in which the preoperative urine culture is sterile, do not require prophylactic antibiotics. These include ureterolithotomy, pyelolithotomy, nephrectomy, and cystotomy.[123] Cystoscopy and urodynamic evaluation also carry a low rate of infection. For these procedures, Kraklau and Wolf conclude that, in low-risk patients, with sterile urine, and no history of UTI, voiding dysfunction, foreign body, or immunosuppression, antibiotic prophylaxis is not necessary.[124] Clean procedures that may benefit from surgical prophylaxis include surgeries with placement of a prosthesis or foreign body.[122,125]

Clean–contaminated urologic procedures include urinary diversion surgery and transrectal urologic procedures. Prophylaxis for the latter should include mechanical and antibiotic bowel preparations.[126] Intravenous prophylaxis should include coverage of both gram-negative and anaerobic organisms. Clinical studies evaluating the role of enemas in transrectal procedures, such as ultrasound guided transrectal prostate biopsy, have conflicting conclusions. However, there is no role in prolonging the duration of antibiotics past 24 hours in low-risk patients.[127]

Gynecologic surgery

Normal vaginal flora consists of many aerobic and anaerobic organisms, dominated by lactobacilli. A transvaginal approach has been associated with a higher risk of infection compared to an abdominal approach. The use of a short course of perioperative antibiotics has been shown to reduce net health care costs for procedures like transvaginal hysterectomy or cervical cone procedures.[128] The value of prophylaxis in uncomplicated abdominal hysterectomy is debated due to low baseline infection rates, however, a benefit probably exists, and both the American College of Obstetricians and Gynecologists and the American Society of Health-System Pharmacists recommend a single dose of prophylactic antibiotics. Cefazolin appears to be more effective than ampicillin for elective abdominal hysterectomy.[129]

Obstetric surgery

Cesarean section carries a 5–20-fold greater risk of infectious complications than vaginal delivery. Killian and colleagues conducted a prospective cohort study to determine the risk factors for SSIs following C-section. Multiple logistic regression analysis found that infections were associated with absence of antibiotic prophylaxis, having less than seven pre-natal visits, hours of ruptured membranes, and surgical time.[130] Smaill and Hofmeyr, in a Cochrane review, determined that prophylaxis is beneficial for C-sections.[131] The rates of endometritis in both elective and non-elective C-sections are significantly reduced with a relative risk of 0.39 (95% CI 0.22–0.64, and 0.31–0.46, respectively). In addition, wound infection rates were also reduced for elective procedures (RR 0.73, 95% CI 0.53–0.99) and non-elective procedures (RR 0.36, 95% CI 0.26–0.51).

Trauma surgery

Ten to fifteen percent of trauma victims with penetrating abdominal injury acquire infections, with an attributable mortality rate of 30% in those who develop severe abdominal infections.[132] The use of antibiotics in the setting of trauma has been traditionally considered therapeutic rather than prophylactic. Unlike the controlled operative setting where antibiotics are ideally administered 30 minutes prior to the incision, antibiotics cannot be given prior to injury. Additionally, the wounds sustained from trauma are commonly grossly contaminated. While intuition would support the use of antibiotics, the duration of therapy may not be as intuitive. Kirton and colleagues conducted a randomized, double-blind, placebo-controlled study to compare 1 vs. 5 days of perioperative antibiotics on the risk of surgical site or non-surgical site infections in patients with high-risk penetrating hollow viscus injury.[133] They found that antibiotic duration of 5 days vs. 24 hours did not result in a difference in SSIs (10% vs. 8%, $P = 0.74$) or non-surgical-site infections (11% vs. 20%, $P = 0.16$). However, a multivariate analysis showed that the total number of red cell transfusions and the penetrating abdominal trauma index (PATI) score greater than 25 were associated with infections. Although the study excluded patients who required more than 15 units of packed red cells, patients at risk for imminent death, and patients with soft tissue or orthopedic injuries requiring antibiotics greater than 24 hours, it suggests that surgical technique is as important as the use of perioperative antibiotics in the prevention of infectious complications in these patients.

For abdominal trauma, the spectrum of activity of the antibiotic(s) chosen should be broad. Coverage should include skin as well as bowel flora. Studies using one day perioperative antibiotics have included beta-lactam/beta-lactamase inhibitors and cephamycins, such as cefotetan or cefoxitin.[134,135] Other combinations studied have used an aminoglycoside combined with an antianaerobic agent such as metronidazole.[136]

For chest trauma, prophylaxis is suggested for esophageal injuries, especially when repair is delayed for longer than 12 hours.[20] One day of cefazolin is recommended for patients with little or no contamination, and depending on the extent of mediastinal spillage, a longer course is usually given although not evidence based. Similarly, patients with cardiac trauma are frequently given prophylaxis with cefazolin for 24 hours, due to the risk of sternal wound infection.[20]

Burn surgery

Infection remains the leading cause of morbidity and mortality in patients with burns.[137] However, the prevention of systemic infection from a burn wound remains difficult despite antibiotics due to the underlying disease process. Burn wounds typically have avascular, or necrotic areas where systemic antibiotics cannot be delivered in adequate concentrations. In addition, depressed humoral and cellular immune functions make prevention of infection more challenging.

Risk factors associated with a higher risk of infection include larger surface area burns, full vs. partial thickness burns, and the age of the patient (children > elderly > others). Thus, the utility of antibiotics in the prevention of infection increases as the risk of infection increases. The use of topical antimicrobials, such as silver nitrate, mafenide acetate, chlorhexidine, and silver sulfadiazine, have been shown to delay colonization of moderate burns (under 50% of total body surface area); however, in large burns (over 50% total body surface area), neither topical nor systemic antibiotics will prevent colonization.[138]

The use of systemic antibiotics has focused on the initial days of hospitalization as well as on perioperative antibiotics at the time of skin grafting or wound debridement. Traditionally, penicillin or penicillin-like drugs are given during the first 3–5 hospital days to prevent group A streptococcal infection, which was the most common cause of infectious morbidity and mortality in the preantibiotic era. However, with improved surgical and ICU management, Durtschi and colleagues did not find a reduction in cellulitis or burn sepsis with the use of penicillin for the first 5 days vs. placebo.[139] The use of perioperative antibiotics in adults undergoing wound debridement appears to be beneficial in burns greater than 60% body surface area.[140] In contrast, cefazolin prophylaxis in children undergoing debridement did not show a benefit.[141]

Transplant surgery

In the early postoperative period up to 2 months, 33–68% of liver transplants, 54% of lung transplants, 47% of kidney transplants, 35% of pancreas transplants, and 21%–30% of heart transplants develop bacterial infections.[142–144] These infections include SSIs, pneumonias, UTIs, and line infections. Despite the frequency of infections, controlled trials to evaluate the effect of antimicrobial prophylaxis during transplant surgery have only been done in kidney transplants.[145,146] The confounding effects of immunosuppressive therapy as well as other immunomodulatory therapies makes it difficult to measure the benefits of antimicrobial prophylaxis. Nonetheless, the demonstrable benefit in kidney transplants has led to the standard practice of using prophylaxis for other organs as well.

The choice of antibiotics should be dictated by the bacterial flora of the transplanted site and the antibiotic susceptibilities of the institution. Kidney transplants should receive prophylaxis for uropathogens and staphylococci; pancreas transplants should receive gram-negative, enterococci, and staphylococci coverage; liver transplants should receive prophylaxis for any biliary tract manipulation, cholangiogram or liver biopsy. The use of selective bowel decontamination for liver transplants has been shown to be effective in randomized trials.[147] For patients with cystic fibrosis undergoing lung transplants, therapy should be tailored to sputum cultures. In some centers, prophylactic sinus surgery is also considered.

The duration of therapy should be <24 hours for kidney transplants and <3 days for other solid organs. Typically, for thoracotomies, antibiotics are continued until drains are pulled, but data do not demonstrate benefit of this practice. Finally, the duration of prophylaxis in cystic fibrosis should continue for 14 days after transplantation or until purulent secretions are no longer seen.[147]

Owing to the net state of immunosuppression, the prevention of infection in these patients goes beyond the use of perioperative antibiotics. The risks of infection can be anticipated by the patient's epidemiologic exposures. Potential hospital exposures that can be preventable include water and air-conditioning systems with *Legionella* sp. and construction zones with *Aspergillus* spores.

Conclusions

As the surgical scalpel evolves, we must continue to balance the double-edged sword of antimicrobial prophylaxis. While the benefit of prophylaxis is evident in many surgical procedures, the detrimental ecologic effects can be seen with the overutilization of antibiotics. Further data will elucidate some of the areas of controversy.

REFERENCES

1. Centers for Disease Control and Prevention, National Center for Health Statistics. *Vital and Health Statistics, Detailed Diagnoses and Procedures, National Hospital Discharge Survey, 1994.* Vol 207. Hyattsville, Maryland: DHHS Publication; 1997.
2. Centers for Disease Control and Prevention. National nosocomial infections surveillance (NNIS) report, data summary from October 1986–April 1998, issued June 1998. *Am. J. Infect. Control* 1998; **26**: 522–533.
3. Mangram, A. J., Horan, T. C., Pearson, M. L., Silver, L. C., & Jarvis, W. R. The Hospital Infection Control Practices Advisory Committee. Guideline for Prevention and Surgical Site Infection, 1999. *Infect. Cont. Hosp. Epidemiol.* 1999; **20**: 247–278.
4. Emori, T. G. & Gaynes, R. P. An overview of nosocomial infections, including the role of the microbiology laboratory. *Clin. Microbiol. Rev.* 1993; **6**: 428–442.
5. Akalin, H. E. Surgical prophylaxis: the evolution of guidelines in a era of cost containment. *J. Hosp. Infect.* 2002; **50**(Suppl A): S3–S7.
6. Kirkland, K. B., Briggs, J. P., Trivette, S. L., Wilkinson, W. E., & Sexton, D. J. The impact of surgical-site infections in the 1990s: attributable mortality, excess length of hospitalization, and extra costs. *Infect. Cont. Hosp. Epidemiol.* 1999; **20**: 725–730.
7. Whitehouse, J. D., Friedman, N. D., Kirkland, K. B., Richardson, W. J., & Sexton, D. J. The impact of surgical-site infections following orthopedic surgery at a community hospital and a university hospital: adverse quality of life, excess length of stay, and extra cost. *Infect. Cont. Hosp. Epidemiol.* 2002; **23**: 183–189.
8. Poulsen, K. B., Wachmann, C. H., Bremmelgaard, A. *et al.* Survival of patients with surgical wound infection: A case-control study of common surgical interventions. *Br. J. Surg.* 1995; **82**: 208–209.
9. Astagneau, P., Rioux, C., Golliot, F., Brucker, G., for the INCISO Network Study Group. Morbidity and mortality associated with surgical site infections: results from the 1997–1999 INCISO surveillance. *J. Hosp. Infect.* 2001; **48**: 267–274.
10. Houang, E. T. & Ahmet, Z. Intraoperative wound contamination during abdominal hysterectomy. *J. Hosp. Infect.* 1991; **19**: 181–189.
11. McGowan, J. E. Jr. Antimicrobial resistance in hospital organisms and its relation to antibiotic use. *Rev. Infect. Dis.* 1983; **5**: 1033–1048.
12. Schaberg, D. R., Culver, D. H., & Gaynes, R. P. Major trends in the microbial etiology of nosocomial infection. *Am. J. Med.* 1991; **91**(3B): 72S–75S.
13. Jarvis, W. R. Epidemiology of nosocomial fungal infections, with emphasis of *Candida* species. *Clin. Infect. Dis.* 1995; **20**: 1526–1530.
14. Bhavnani, S. M., Drake, J. A., Forrest, A. *et al. Diagn. Microbiol. Infect. Dis.* 2000; **36**: 145–158.
15. Bonten, M. J., Slaughter, S., Ambergen, A. W. *et al.* The role of colonization pressure in the spread of vancomycin-resistant entercocci: an important infection control variable. *Arch. Intern. Med.* 1998; **158**: 1127–1132.
16. Garner, J. S. CDC guidelines for the prevention and control of nosocomial infections: guideline for prevention of surgical wound infections, 1985. *Am. J. Infect. Control.* 1986; **14**: 71.
17. Ad Hoc Committee of the Committee on Trauma, National Research Council Division of Medical Sciences. Postoperative wound infections: the influence of ultraviolet irradiation of the operating room and of various other factors. *Ann. Surg.* 1964; **160**(Suppl. 2): 1–132.
18. Page, C. P., Bohnen, J. M. A., Fletcher, J. R. *et al.* Antimicrobial prophylaxis for surgical wounds: guidelines for clinical care. *Arch. Surg.* 1993; **128**: 79–88.
19. Haley, R. W., Culver, D. H., Morgan, W. M., White, J. W., Emori, T. G., & Hooton, T. M. Identifying patients at high risk of surgical wound infection. *Am. J. Epidemiol.* 1985; **121**: 206–215.

20. Culver, D. H., Horan, T. C., Gaynes, R. P. and the National Nosocomial Infections Surveillance Systems (NNIS): Surgical wound infection rates by wound class, operation and risk index in U.S. Hospitals. *Am. J. Med.* 1991; **91**(Suppl 3B): 152S–157S.

21. Sasse, A., Mertens, R., Sion, J. P. *et al.* Surgical prophylaxis in Belgian hospitals: estimate of costs and potential savings. *J. Antimicrob. Chemother.* 1998; **41**: 267–272.

22. Kernodle, D. S., Barg, N. L., & Kaiser, A. B. Low-level colonization of hospitalized patients with methicillin-resistant coagulase-negative staphylococci and emergence of the organisms during surgical antimicrobial prophylaxis. *Antimicrob. Agents Chemother.* 1988; **32**: 202–208.

23. Kreisel, D., Savel, T. G., Silver, A. L. *et al.* Surgical antibiotic prophylaxis and *Clostridium difficile* toxin positivity. *Arch. Surg.* 1995; **130**: 989–993.

24. Yee, J., Dixon, C. M., McLean, P. H. *et al. Clostridium difficile* disease in a department of surgery: The significance of prophylactic antibiotics. *Arch. Surg.* 1991; **126**: 241–246.

25. McGowan, J. E. Jr. Cost and benefit of perioperative antimicrobial prophylaxis: methods for economic analysis. *Rev. Infect. Dis.* 1991; **13**(Suppl 10): S879–S889.

26. Knight, R., Charbonneau, P., Ratzer, E., Zeren, F., Haun, W., & Clark, J. Prophylactic antibiotics are not indicated in clean general surgery cases. *Am. J. Surg.* 2001; **182**: 682–686.

27. Finland, M. Antibacterial agents: uses and abuses in treatment and prophylaxis. *Rhode Island Med. J.* 1960; **43**: 499–520.

28. Hopkins, C. C. Antibiotic prophylaxis in clean surgery: peripheral vascular surgery, noncardiovascular thoracic surgery, herniorrhaphy, and mastectomy. *Rev. Infect. Dis.* 1991; **13**(Suppl. 10): S869–S873.

29. Da Costa, A., Kirkorian, G., Cucherat, M. *et al.* Antibiotic prophylaxis for permanent pacemaker implantation: a meta-analysis. *Circulation* 1998; **97**: 1796–1801.

30. Platt, R., Zucker, J. R., Zaleznik, D. F. *et al.* Prophylaxis against wound infection following herniorrhaphy or breast surgery. *J. Infect. Dis.* 1992; **166**: 556–560.

31. Perl, T. M., Cullen, J. J., Wenzel, R. P. *et al.* Intranasal mupirocin to prevent postoperative *Staphylococcus aureus* infections. *N. Engl. J. Med.* 2002; **346**: 1871–1877.

32. Cioffi, G. A., Terezhalmy, G. T., & Taybos, G. M. Total joint replacement: a consideration for antimicrobial prophylaxis. *Oral Surg. Oral Med. Oral Pathol.* 1988; **66**: 124–129.

33. Heggeness, M. H., Esses, S. I., Errico, T., & Yuan, H. A. Late infection of spinal instrumentation by hematogenous seeding. *Spine* 1993; **18**: 492–496.

34. Mont, M. A., Waldman, B., Banerjee, C., Pacheco, I. H., & Hunderford, D. S. Multiple irrigation, debridement, and retention of components in infected total knee arthroplasty. *J. Arthroplasty.* 1997; **12**: 426–433.

35. Ozuna, R. M. & Delamarter, R. B. Pyogenic vertebral osteomyelitis and post-surgical disc space infections. *Orthop. Clin. North Am.* 1996; **27**: 87–94.

36. Schmalzried, T. P., Amstutz, H. C., Au, M. K., & Dorey, F. J. Etiology of deep sepsis in total hip arthroplasty. The significance of hematogenous and recurrent infections. *Clin. Orthop.* 1992; **280**: 200–207.

37. Giamarellou, H. & Antoniadou, A. Epidemiology, diagnosis and therapy of fungal infections in surgery. *Infect. Cont. Hosp. Epidemiol.* 1996; **17**: 558–564.

38. Pottinger, J., Burns, S., & Manske, C. Bacterial carriage by artificial versus natural nails. *Am. J. Infect. Control.* 1989; **17**: 340–344.

39. McNeil, S. A., Foster, C. L., Hedderwick, S. A., & Kauffman, C. A. Effect of hand cleansing with antimicrobial soap or alcohol-based gel on microbial colonization of artificial fingernails worn by health care workers. *Clin. Infect. Dis.* 2001; **32**: 367–372.

40. Passaro, D. J., Waring, L., Armstron, R. *et al.* Postoperative *Serratia marcescens* wound infections traced to an out-of-hospital source. *J. Infect. Dis.* 1997; **175**: 992–995.

41. Bennett, S. N., McNeil, M. M., Bland, L. A. *et al.* Postoperative infections traced to contamination of an intravenous anesthetic, propofol. *N. Engl. J. Med.* 1995; **333**: 147–154.

42. Polk, H. C. Jr., Trachtenberg, L., & Finn, M. P. Antibiotic activity in surgical incisions: The basis for prophylaxis in selected operations. *J. Am. Med. Assoc.* 1980; **244**: 1353–1354.

43. Scher, K. S. Studies on the duration of antibiotic administration for surgical prophylaxis. *Am. Surg.* 1997; **63**: 59–62.

44. Fraise, A. P. Guidelines for the control of methicillin-resistant *Staphylococcus aureus. J. Antimicrob. Chemother.* 1998; **42**: 287–289.

45. De Lalla, F. Surgical prophylaxis in practice. *J. Hosp. Infect.* 2002; **50**(Suppl A): S9–S12.

46. Spelman, D., Harrington, G., Russo, P., & Wesselingh, S. Clinical, microbiological and economic benefit of a change in antibiotic prophylaxis for cardiac surgery. *Infect. Cont. Hosp. Epidemiol.* 2002; **23**: 402–404.

47. Archer, G. L. & Armstrong, B. C. Alteration of staphylococcal flora in cardiac patients receiving antibiotic prophylaxis. *J. Infect. Dis.* 1983; **147**: 642–649.

48. Anonymous. Antimicrobial prophylaxis in surgery. *Med. Letter Drugs Ther.* 1999; **39**(1012): 97–102.

49. Burke, J. F. The effective period of preventive antibiotic action in experimental incisions and dermal lesions. *Surgery* 1961; **50**: 161–168.

50. Classen, D. C., Evans, R. S., Pestotnik, S. L. *et al.* The timing of prophylactic administration of antibiotics and the risk of surgical-wound infection. *N. Engl. J. Med.* 1992; **326**: 281–286.

51. Burnett, K. M., Scott, M. G., Kearney, P. M., Humphreys, W. G., & McMillen, R. M. The identification of barriers preventing the successful implementation of a surgical prophylaxis protocol. *Pharm. World Sci.* 2002; **24**: 182–187.

52. Dipiro, J. T., Cheung, R. P., Bowden, T. A., & Mansberger, J. A. Single dose systemic antibiotic prophylaxis of surgical wound infections. *Am. J. Surg.* 1986; **152**: 552–559.

53. Elliott, J. P., Reeman, R. K., & Dorchester, W. Short versus long course of prophylactic antibiotics in cesarean section. *Am. J. Obstet. Gynecol.* 1982; **143**: 740–744.

54. Gatell, J. M., Garcia, S., Lozano, L. *et al.* Perioperative cefamandole prophylaxis against infections. *J. Bone Joint Surg.* 1987; **8**: 1189–1193.

55. Hall, J. C., Christiansen, K. J., Goodman, M. *et al.* Duration of antimicrobial prophylaxis in vascular surgery. *Am. J. Surg.* 1998; **175**: 87–90.

56. Farber, B. F., Kaiser, D. L., & Wenzel, R. P. Relation between surgical volume and incidence of postoperative wound infections. *N. Engl. J. Med.* 1981; **305**: 200–204.

57. Birkmeyer, J. D., Siewers, A. E., Finlayson, E. *et al.* Hospital volume and surgical mortality in the United States. *N. Engl. J. Med.* 2002; **346**: 1128–1137.

58. Burke, J. P. Maximizing appropriate antibiotic prophylaxis for surgical patients: an update from LDS Hospital, Salt Lake City. *Clin. Infect. Dis.* 2001; **33**(Suppl 2): S78–S83.

59. Halasz, N. A. Wound infection and topical antibiotics: the surgeon's dilemma. *Arch. Surg.* 1977; **112**: 1240–1244.

60. Van de Belt, H., Neut, D., Schenk, W. *et al.* Infection of orthopedic implants and the use of antibiotic-loaded bone cements. *Acta Orthop. Scand.* 2001; **72**: 557–571.

61. Espenhaug, B., Engesaeter, L. B., Vollset, S. E. *et al.* Antibiotic prophylactics in total hip arthroplasty. *J. Bone Joint Surg. (Br.)* 1997; **79**: 590–595.

62. Nelson, C. L., Evans, R. P., Blaha, J. D. *et al.* A comparison of gentamicin-impregnated polymethylmethcrylate bead implantation to conventional parenteral antibiotic therapy in infected total hip and knee arthroplasty. *Clin. Orthop.* 1993; **295**: 96–101.

63. Dirschl, D. R. & Wilson, F. C. Topical antibiotic irrigation in the prophylaxis of operative wound infections in orthopedic surgery. *Orthop. Clin. North Am.* 1991; **22**: 419–426.

64. Lewis, R. T. Oral versus systemic antibiotic prophylaxis in elective colon surgery: a randomized study and meta-analysis send a message from the 1990s. *Can. J. Surg.* 2002; **45**: 173–180.

65. Calvet, H. M. & Yoshikawa, T. T. Infections in diabetics. *Infect. Dis. Clin North Am.* 2001; **15**: 407–421.

66. Golden, S. H., Pert-Vigilance, C., Kao, W. H., & Brancati, F. L. Perioperative glycemic control and the risk of infectious complications in a cohort of adults with diabetes. *Diabetes Care* 1999; **22**: 1408–1414.

67. Furnary, A. P., Zerr, K. J., Grunkemeier, G. L., & Starr, A. Continuous intravenous insulin infusion reduces the incidence of deep sternal wound infection in diabetic patients after cardiac surgical procedures. *Ann. Thorac. Surg.* 1999; **67**: 352–362.

68. Kurz, A., Sessler, D. L., & Lenhardt, R. Perioperative normothermia to reduce the incidence of surgical-wound infection and shorten hospitalization. *N. Engl. J. Med.* 1996; **334**: 1209–1215.

69. Grief, R., Akca, O., Horn, E. P., Kurz, A., & Sessler, D. I. Supplemental perioperative oxygen to reduce the incidence of surgical-wound infection. *N. Engl. J. Med.* 2000; **342**: 161–167.

70. Cruse, P. J. & Foord, R. The epidemiology of wound infection: a 10 year prospective study of 62,939 wounds. *Surg. Clin. North Am.* 1980; **60**: 27–40.

71. Nichols, R. L. Prophylaxis for surgical infections. In Gorbach, S. L., Barlett, J. G., & Blacklow, N. R. Infectious Diseases. Chapter 44. 2nd edn. 1998; 471.

72. Edwards, L. D. The epidemiology of 2056 remote site infections and 1966 surgical wound infections occurring in 1865 patients: A four year study of 40,923 operations at Rush-Presbyterian-St. Luke's Hospital, Chicago. *Ann. Surg.* 1976; **184**: 758–766.

73. Valentive, R. J., Weigelt, J. A., Dryer, D., & Rodgers, C. Effect of remote infections on clean wound infection rates. *Am. J. Infect. Control* 1986; **14**: 64–67.

74. Dajani, A. S., Taubert, K. A., Wilson, W. *et al.* Prevention of bacterial endocarditis. recommendations by the American Heart Association. *J. Am. Med. Assoc.* 1997; **277**: 1794–1801.

75. Strom, B. L., Abrutyn, E., Berlin, J. A. *et al.* Dental and cardiac risk factors for infective endocarditis. *Ann. Int. Med.* 1998; **129**: 761–769.

76. American Dental Association, American Academy of Orthopedic Surgeons. Antibiotic prophylaxis for dental patients with total joint replacements. *J. Am. Dent. Assoc.* 1997; **128**: 1004–1007.

77. Lockhart, P. B., Brennan, T., Fox, P. C. *et al.* Decision-making on the use of antimicrobial prophylaxis for dental procedures: a survey of infectious disease consultants and review. *Clin. Infect. Dis.* 2002; **34**: 1621–1626.

78. Lord, R. V. N. Anorectal surgery in patients infected with human immunodeficiency virus. *Ann. Surg.* 1997; **226**: 92–99.

79. Grubert, T. A., Reindell, D., Kastner, R. *et al.* Rates of postoperative complications among human immunodeficiency virus – infected women who have undergone obstetric and gynecologic surgical procedures. *Clin. Infect. Dis.* 2002; **34**: 822–830.

80. Paiement, G. D., Hymes, R. A., LaDouceur, M. S., Gosselin, R. A., & Green, H. D. Postoperative infections in asymptomatic HIV-seropositive orthopedic trauma patients. *J. Trauma* 1994; **37**: 545–550.

81. Emparan, C., Iturburu, I. M., Portugal, V. *et al.* Infective complications after minor operations in patients infected with HIV: role of CD4 lymphocytes in prognosis. *Eur. J. Surg.* 1995; **161**: 721–730.

82. Hill, C., Mazas, F., Flamant, R., & Evrard, J. Prophylactic cefazolin versus placebo in total hip replacement. *Lancet* 1981; **1**: 795–796.

83. Lidwell, O. M., Lowbury, E. J. L., Whyte, W. *et al.* Infection and sepsis after operations for total hip or knee-joint replacement: influence of ultraclean air, prophylactic antibiotics and other factors. *J. Hyg. (Lond.)*. 1984; **93**: 505–529.

84. Hanssen, A. D. & Osmon, D. R. Prevention of deep wound infection after total hip arthroplasty: the role of prophylactic antibiotics and clean air technology. *Semin. Arthroplasty* 1994; **5**: 114–121.

85. Gernaat-van der Sluis, A. J., Hoogenboom-Verdegall, A. M. M., Edixhoven, P. J. *et al.* Prophylactic mupirocin could reduce orthopedic wound infections. *Acta Orthop. Scand.* 1998; **69**: 412–414.

86. Kalmeijer, M. D., Coertjens, H., van Nieuwland-Bollen, P. M. *et al.* Surgical site infections in orthopedic surgery: the effect of mupirocin nasal ointment in a double-blind, randomized, placebo-controlled study. *Clin. Infect. Dis.* 2002; **35**: 353–358.

87. Winfree, C. H., Baker, K. Z., & Connolly, E. S. Perioperative normothermia and surgical-wound infection. *N. Engl. J. Med.* 1996; **335**: 749–750.

88. Fekety, F. R., Cluff, L. E., Sabiston, D. C. *et al.* A study of antibiotic prophylaxis in cardiac surgery. *J. Thorac. Cardiovasc. Surg.* 1969; **57**: 757–763.

89. Fong, I. W., Baker, C. B., & McKee, D. C. The value of prophylactic antibiotics in aortacoronary bypass operations. *J. Thorac. Cardiovasc. Surg.* 1979; **78**: 908–913.

90. Zanetti, G., Giardina, R., & Platt, R. Intraoperative redosing of cefazolin and risk for surgical site infection in cardiac surgery. *Emerg. Infect. Dis.* 2001; **7**: 828–831.

91. Maher, K. O., VanDerElzen, K., Bove, E. L. *et al.* A retrospective review of three antibiotic prophylaxis regimens for pediatric cardiac surgical patients. *Ann. Thorac. Surg.* 2002; **74**: 1195–1200.

92. Szilagyi, D. E., Smith, R. F., Elliott, J. P., & Vrandecic, M. P. Infection in arterial reconstruction with synthetic grafts. *Ann. Surg.* 1972; **176**: 321–333.

93. Kaiser, A. B., Clayson, K. R., Mulherin, J. L. *et al.* Antibiotic prophylaxis in vascular surgery. *Ann. Surg.* 1978; **188**: 283–289.

94. Hasselgren, P., Ivarsson, L., Risberg, B., & Seeman, T. Effects of prophylactic antibiotics in vascular surgery. *Ann. Surg.* 1984; **200**: 86–92.

95. Bennion, R. S., Hiatt, J. R., Williams, R. A., & Wilson, S. E. A randomized, prospective study of perioperative antimicrobial prophylaxis for vascular access surgery. *J. Cardiovasc. Surg.* 1985; **26**: 270–274.

96. Sonne-Holm, S., Boeckstyns, M., Menck, H. *et al.* Prophylactic antibiotics in amputation of the lower extremity for ischemia. *J. Bone Joint Surg.* 1985; **67A**: 800–803.

97. Johnson, J. T., & Wagner, R. L. Infection following uncontaminated head and neck surgery. *Arch. Otolaryngol. Head Neck Surg.* 1987; **113**: 368–369.

98. Carrau, R. L., Byzakis, J., Wagner, R. L., & Johnson, J. T. Role of prophylactic antibiotics in uncontaminated neck dissections. *Arch. Otolaryngol. Head Neck Surg.* 1991; **117**: 194–195.

99. Slattery, W. H., Stringer, S. P., & Cassisi, N. J. Prophylactic antibiotic use in clean, uncontaminated neck dissection. *Laryngoscope* 1995; **105**: 244–246.

100. Becker, G. D. & Parell, G. J. Cefazolin prophylaxis in head and neck cancer surgery. *Ann. Otol. Rhinol. Laryngol.* 1979; **88**: 183–186.

101. Coskun, H., Erisen, L., & Basut, O. Factors affecting wound infection rates in head and neck surgery. *Otolaryngol. Head Neck Surg.* 2000; **123**: 328–333.

102. Tabet, J.-C. & Johnson, J. T. Wound infection in head and neck surgery: prophylaxis, etiology, and management. *J. Otolaryngol.* 1990; **19**: 197–200.

103. Rubin, J., Johnson, J. T., Wagner, R. L., & Yu, V. L. Bacteriologic analysis of wound infection following major head and neck surgery. *Arch. Otolaryngol. Head Neck Surg.* 1988; **114**: 969–972.

104. Robbins, K. T., Byers, R. M., Cole, R. *et al.* Wound prophylaxis with metronidazole in head and neck surgical oncology. *Layrngoscope* 1988; **98**: 803–806.

105. Piccart, M., Dor, P., & Klastersky, J. Antimicrobial prophylaxis of infections in head and neck cancer surgery. *Scand. J. Infect. Dis. Suppl.* 1983; **39**: 92–96.

106. Johnson, J. T., Yu, V. L., Myers, E. N., & Wagner, R. L. An assessment of the need for gram-negative coverage in antibiotic prophylaxis for oncological head and neck surgery. *J. Infect. Dis.* 1987; **155**: 331–333.

107. Righi, M., Manfredi, R., & Farneti, G. Short-term versus long-term antimicrobial prophylaxis in oncologic head and neck surgery. *Head Neck.* 1996; **18**: 399–404.

108. Johnson, J. T., Schuller, D. E., Silver, F. *et al.* Antibiotic prophylaxis in high-risk head and neck surgery: one day vs. five day therapy. *Otolaryngol. Head Neck Surg.* 1986; **95**: 554–557.

109. LoCicero, J. & Nichols, R. J. Sepsis after gastroduodenal operations: relationship to gastric acid, motility, and endogenous microflora. *South Med. J.* 1980; **73**: 878–880.

110. Lewis, R. T., Allan, C. M., Goodall, R. G. *et al.* Discriminate use of antibiotic prophylaxis in gastroduodenal surgery. *Am. J. Surg.* 1979; **138**: 640–643.

111. Nichols, R. L., Webb, W. R., Jones, J. W. *et al.* Efficacy of antibiotic prophylaxis in high risk gastroduodenal operations. *Am. J. Surg.* 1982; **143**: 94–98.

112. Keighley, M. R. B., Flinn, R., & Alexander-Williams, J. Multivariate analysis of clinical and operative findings associated with biliary sepsis. *Br. J. Surg.* 1976; **63**: 528–531.

113. Keighley, M. R. B., Baddeley, R. M., Burdon, D. W. *et al.* A controlled trial of parenteral prophylactic gentamicin therapy in biliary surgery. *Br. J. Surg.* 1975; **62**: 275–279.

114. Ulualp, K. & Condon, R. E. Antibiotic prophylaxis for scheduled operative procedures. *Infect. Dis. Clin. North Am.* 1992; **6**: 613–625.

115. Clarke, J. S., Condon, R. E., Barlett, J. G. *et al.* Preoperative oral antibiotics reduce septic complications of colon operations: results of prospective, randomized, double-blind clinical study. *Ann. Surg.* 1977; **186**: 251–259.

116. Song, F. & Glenny, A. M. Antimicrobial prophylaxis in colorectal surgery: a systematic review of randomized controlled trials. *Health Technol. Assessm.* 1998; **2**: 1–110.

117. Kaiser, A. B., Herrington, J. L. Jr., Jacobs, J. K. *et al.* Cefoxitin versus erythromycin, neomycin, and cefazolin in colorectal operations. Importance of the duration of the surgical procedure. *Ann. Surg.* 1983; **198**: 525–530.

118. Coppa, G. F. & Eng, K. Factors involved in antibiotic selection in elective colon and rectal surgery. *Surgery* 1988; **104**: 853–858.

119. Nichols, R. L. Surgical antibiotic prophylaxis. *Med. Clin. North Am.* 1995; **79**: 509–522.

120. Antonelli, W., Borgani, A., Machella, C. *et al.* Comparison of two systemic antibiotics for the prevention of complications

in elective colorectal surgery. *Ital. J. Surg. Sci.* 1985; **15**: 255–258.

121. Chodak, G. W. & Plaut, M. E. Systemic antibiotics for prophylaxis in urologic surgery: a critical review. *J. Urol.* 1979; **121**: 695–699.

122. Grabe, M. Perioperative antibiotic prophylaxis in urology. *Curr. Opin. Urol.* 2001; **11**: 81–85.

123. Childs, S. J. Genitourinary surgical prophylaxis. *Infect. Surg.* 1983; **2**: 701–710.

124. Kraklau, D. M. & Wolf, J. S. Jr. Review of antibiotic prophylaxis recommendations for office-based urologic procedures. *Tech. Urol.* 1999; **5**: 123–128.

125. Scherz, H. C. & Parsons, C. L. Prophylactic antibiotics in urology. *Urol. Clin. North Am.* 1987; **14**: 265–271.

126. Ferguson, K. H., McNeil, J. J., & Morey, A. F. Mechanical and antibiotic bowel preparation for urinary diversion surgery. *J. Urol.* 2002; **167**: 2352–2356.

127. Webb, N. R. & Woo, H. H. Antibiotic prophylaxis for prostate biopsy. *B. J. U. International* 2002; **89**: 824–828.

128. Shapiro, M., Schoenbaum, S. C., Tager, I. B. *et al.* Benefit–cost analysis of antimicrobial prophylaxis in abdominal and vaginal hysterectomy. *J. Am. Med. Assoc.* 1983; **249**: 1290–94.

129. Chongsomchai, C., Lumbiganon, P., Thinkhamrop, J. *et al.* Placebo-controlled, double-blind, randomized study of prophylactic antibiotics in elective abdominal hysterectomy. *J. Hosp. Infect.* 2002; **52**: 302–306.

130. Killian, C. A., Graffunder, E. M., Vinciguerra, T. J., & Venezia, R. A. Risk factors for surgical-site infections following cesarean section. *Infect. Control Hosp. Epidemiol.* 2001; **22**: 613–617.

131. Smaill, F. & Hofmeyr, G. J. Antibiotic prophylaxis for cesarean section (Cochrane Review). In *The Cochrane Library.* 2002; Issue 4.

132. Fabian, T. C. Infection in penetrating abdominal trauma: risk factors and preventive antibiotics. *Am. Surg.* 2002; **68**: 29–35.

133. Kirton, O. C., O'Neill, P. A., Kestner, M., & Tortella, B. J. Perioperative antibiotic use in high-risk penetrating hollow viscus injury: a prospective randomized, double-blind, placebo-control trial of 24 hours vesus 5 days. *J. Trauma* 2000; **49**: 822–832.

134. Fabian, T. C., Croce, M. A., Payne, L. W. *et al.* Duration of antibiotic therapy for penetrating abdominal trauma; a prospective trial. *Surgery* 1992; **112**: 788–795.

135. Nichols, R. L., Smith, J. W., Klein, D. B. *et al.* Risk of infection after penetrating abdominal trauma. *N. Engl. J. Med.* 1984; **311**: 1065–1070.

136. Dellinger, E. P. Antibiotic prophylaxis in trauma. *Rev. Infect. Dis.* 1991; **13**(Suppl 10): S847–S857.

137. Nguyen, T. T., Gilpin, D. A., Meyer, N. A., & Herndon, D. N. Current treatment of severely burned patients. *Ann. Surg.* 1996; **223**: 14–25.

138. American College of Surgeons, Committee on Surgical Infections. *Manual on Control of Infection in Surgical Patients*, 2nd edn. Philadelphia: J. B. Lippincott, 1984.

139. Durtschi, M. B., Orgain, C., Counts, G. W., & Heimbach, D. M. A prospective study of prophylactic penicillin in acutely burned hospitalized patients. *J. Trauma.* 1982; **22**: 11–14.

140. Mousa, H. A. Aerobic, anaerobic, and fungal burn wound infections. *J. Hosp. Infect.* 1997; **37**: 317–323.

141. Edwards-Jones, V. & Shawcross, S. G. Toxic shock syndrome in the burned patient. *Br. J. Biomed. Sci.* 1997; **54**: 110–117.

142. Patel, R. & Paya, C. V. Infections in solid organ transplant recipients. *Clin. Microbiol. Rev.* 1997; **10**: 86–124.

143. Rubin, R. H. & Tolkoff-Rubin, N. E. Antimicrobial strategies in the care of organ transplant recipients. *Antimicrob. Agents Chemother.* 1993; **37**: 619–624.

144. Wagener, M. M. & Yu, V. L. Bacteremia in transplant recipients: a prospective study of demographics, etiologic agents, risk factors and outcomes. *Am. J. Infect. Control.* 1992; **20**: 239–247.

145. Tillegard, A. Renal transplant and wound infection: the value of prophylactic antibiotic treatment. *Scand. J. Urol. Nephrol.* 1984; **18**: 215–221.

146. Townsend, T. R., Rudolf, L. E., & Westervelt, F. B. Jr. Prophylactic antibiotic therapy with cefamandole and tobramycin for patients undergoing renal transplantation. *Infect. Control* 1980; **1**: 93–96.

147. Soave, R. Prophylaxis strategies for solid-organ transplantation. *Clin. Infect. Dis.* 2001; **33**(Suppl 1): S26–31.

22

Medical care of the HIV-infected surgical patient

Jeffrey L. Lennox

Emory University School of Medicine, Atlanta, GA

The epidemic of HIV infection that began in the late twentieth century has become one of the dominant health issues worldwide for the early twenty-first century. In the developed world, advances in the treatment of HIV infection have dramatically extended the lifespan of infected patients. As a result of these therapeutic advances, deaths from HIV infection in the USA fell by over 50% between 1995 and 2000. In developing areas of the world, HIV continues to spread among sexually active adults and their offspring. In some areas of Africa as much as 20% of the adult population is infected. HIV infection rates are also accelerating in the developed nations of Asia, and in areas of the former Soviet Union. The combined effects of increased longevity and accelerated worldwide dissemination are likely to result in increasing opportunities for internists and surgeons to collaborate in the management of HIV-infected patients.

The clinical course of HIV infection has been well described and should be familiar to most general internists. HIV infection is associated with abnormalities in the number and function of CD4 positive T-lymphocytes. Because the CD4 positive lymphocytes are essential to the regulation of the human immune system, progressive immune dysfunction is a natural consequence of HIV infection in most patients. This progressive immune dysregulation is associated with decreased cell-mediated immune function, alterations in the humoral immune response, chronic inflammation and depressed mucosal immunity. The late stages of HIV infection are associated with pathologic processes in many organ systems and eventual death due to opportunistic infections or tumors. This natural history of the disease has been dramatically altered by the widespread use in the developed world of highly active antiretroviral therapy (HAART). HAART is an acronym that refers to combinations of antiretroviral agents that have been shown in clinical trials to result in undetectable plasma HIV RNA levels in the majority of patients. These combinations may include two to three nucleoside analogs plus either a protease inhibitor or a non-nucleoside reverse transcriptase inhibitor. Guidelines for the use of these agents in HIV-infected adults and children have been developed, are frequently updated, and are available through the worldwide web.[1]

The use of HAART is associated with significant increases in the levels of CD4 positive T-lymphocytes, decreases in levels of inflammatory markers, decreases in lymphocyte activation and apoptosis, improvement in antibody mediated immune responses and reductions in infections and tumors. In HAART-treated patients it may be expected that CD4 positive T-lymphocytes will increase by approximately 100–150 cells/mm^3 over the first year of therapy. Patients who in an earlier era would have died of AIDS-related complications may present for surgical care with conditions which are related to the normal aging process, or to other underlying risk factors such as smoking. There is also evidence that survival on HAART is associated with an increased risk for diabetes, cardiovascular disease, and osteoporosis.[2,3] The extent and magnitude of the risk is best established for cardiovascular disorders. The adjusted relative rate of myocardial infarction increases each of the first 4 years of protease inhibitor use.[4] However, it is likely that surgeons and internists will be called upon to care for an increasing number of patients undergoing typical surgical interventions which have been used in their HIV-uninfected brethren.

The immune improvements experienced as a result of HAART may also give rise to certain conditions which can necessitate surgical intervention. It is important to recognize these conditions in order to help guide proper surgical intervention. In those individuals who begin HAART at a time when their T-helper cell count is <200 cells/mm^3 there may occur a syndrome of

Medical Management of the Surgical Patient: A Textbook of Perioperative Medicine, ed. M. F. Lubin, R. B. Smith, T. F. Dobson, N. Spell, H. K. Walker. 4th edn. Published by Cambridge University Press. © Cambridge University 2006.

immune response to occult infections. This syndrome, sometimes referred to as "Immune reconstitution inflammatory syndrome," or IRIS is most likely to occur in the first 16 weeks following HAART initiation.[5] In most treated patients CD4 positive T-cell counts in peripheral blood rise acutely following the initiation of HAART. It is during this T-cell rise that the manifestations of immune reconstitution are most likely to occur. The most frequently described manifestations are painful inflammatory lymphadenitis due to mycobacterial infection, retinitis due to cytomegalovirus (CMV), meningitis due to cryptococcus, hepatitis due to chronic hepatitis C or B. After 16 weeks, late manifestations include thyroiditis and sarcoidosis. Optimal management of these conditions has not been elucidated, but in general the severity of the disorder dictates the approach. In patients with mild symptoms, simple observation or anti-inflammatory medication may suffice. In patients with severe inflammatory manifestations, corticosteroids are sometimes prescribed to reduce the inflammation. Surgery may be indicated to drain large abscesses, to place lumbar–peritoneal shunts to relieve intracranial hypertension, or to do a biopsy to aid in diagnosis. Whether to stop the HAART during a severe episode of the immune reconstitution syndrome is a question the answer to which is currently driven mostly by opinion.

Perioperative evaluation and care

Surgical risk

The risk of surgical procedures in HIV-infected patients is influenced by many of the same factors that determine risk for uninfected patients. Age, operative procedure, other underlying diseases and the experience of the surgical team are but a few of these factors. In addition, the immunodeficiency caused by HIV may pose an increased risk for infected patients. Most of the data regarding operative risk in patients with HIV infection was collected in the pre-HAART era. Considering the profound effect of HAART on immune function in HIV-infected patients, it is likely that any assessment of surgical risk that relies on these data is an overestimate. In general, studies from the pre-HAART era indicated that HIV-infected patients are at a somewhat increased risk for postoperative morbidity and mortality.[6–8] However, the absolute degree and clinical significance of this risk is controversial. The majority of the studies were retrospective, case-control reports that included small numbers of patients. In addition, staging of the degree of immunosuppression was not routinely reported in all series.

An estimation of the maximal likely risk due to AIDS may be made by determining the mortality associated with urgent abdominal surgery. In four studies reported between 1994 and 1999, 205 patients underwent urgent abdominal surgery.[9–12] The majority of these patients had an AIDS defining illness prior to the operation. The most common reasons for abdominal operation were appendicitis (93 patients) and cholecystitis/cholangitis (66 patients). In these 159 patients, the operative mortality was 3%. The remaining 46 patients had undergone surgery for intestinal bleeding (10 patients), intestinal obstruction (12 patients), perforation (8 patients), trauma (6 patients) and other causes (10 patients). In many of these patients the underlying reason for the operation was either an obstructive tumor or an infectious complication of HIV infection. Of these 46 patients, 17 (37%) died in the 30-day postoperative period.

Based on these studies, most of the risk associated with urgent surgery is likely to be observed in patients who have an active opportunistic infection or a tumor causing obstruction or bleeding. As detailed in a recent review, those who only have HIV-associated immunosuppression are at a lower risk for death than those who have other active AIDS diagnoses.[13] In addition to active infections and tumors, hypoalbuminemia and leukopenia have been associated in some series with an increased operative mortality.[9,10]

Given the dysregulation of the immune function associated with HIV infection, it has been suggested that HIV-infected patients may have an increased risk for postoperative wound infections. The literature on this subject suffers again from its retrospective nature, poor controls and limited sample sizes. The results of analyses reported in the literature are conflicting, with some papers indicating a marked increased risk of wound infection and others indicating no increased risk.

Buehrer et al. reported on 169 invasive procedures performed in patients with hemophilia or other clotting disorders between 1979 and 1988.[14] The wound infection rate in the HIV-infected patients was 1.4%, which was not statistically significant from that reported in the HIV-uninfected patients. French et al. reported on 99 HIV-infected patients who underwent coloproctostomy.[15] The 2% wound infection rate in this group was the same as that seen for non-HIV-infected patients. In contrast are the recent results from Emparan et al. who described an increased infection rate in patients who had less than 200 CD4 cells/mm^3.[16] However, this study included a total of only 24 patients, and the validity of its findings must therefore be considered unproven. Based on the available literature, patients with HIV infection appear to have little increased risk for surgical wound infections.

If there is an increased risk, it may be mostly found in those with an AIDS-defining condition. Patients with AIDS have been shown to have an increased carriage rate of *Staphylococcus aureus* compared to HIV-uninfected controls.[17] This may account for some of the possible increased risk. A recent study indicates that preoperative reduction in staphylococcus colonization rates may reduce postoperative wound infection rates and bacteremia.[18] However, the results of another study show less benefit, and whether this strategy will be beneficial in HIV-infected patients has not been determined.[19]

Given the contradictory data regarding wound infection rates, and the paucity of data regarding the efficacy of colonization eradication in this patient population, no formal recommendations can be made regarding this strategy.

Other operative complications besides mortality and wound infection have also been the subject of concern. Albaran *et al.* studied all operative complications in 43 patients who underwent abdominal surgery.[20] In the 11 patients who had greater than 200 CD4 positive lymphocytes/mm^3 there were only two postoperative complications. In the 32 patients who had less than 200 cells/mm^3, there were a total of 31 major complications in 19 patients. The most common complication was pneumonia, which sometimes resulted in respiratory failure. Other complications included pancreatitis, intravenous line infections, and pseudomembranous colitis.

Comparing patients who developed postoperative complications to those who did not, complications were more frequently observed in those who had lower levels of CD4 positive T-helper cells and lower platelet counts. The two groups did not differ in regards to the white blood cell count, hematocrit, or serum albumin level. These findings are somewhat contradicted by a meta-analysis published by Rose *et al.*[21] In their analysis of 22 studies that compared outcomes in HIV-infected and uninfected patients, no difference in postoperative complications was found in 15 of the 22 studies.

Taken together, the available data indicate that the presence of HIV infection itself is not a contraindication to surgical intervention. It is likely, however, that patients in advanced stages of HIV infection are at increased risk for postoperative complications. The primary care provider and the surgeon must therefore evaluate the degree of immunosuppression, concurrent disease processes and the inherent risk of the surgical procedure in order to adequately inform the patient of the anticipated likelihood of major complications. For patients who have advanced immunosuppression, in whom elective surgery is being considered, it seems prudent to recommend that HAART be instituted in anticipation of the immunologic benefits

that have been noted in the majority of treated patients. It must be recognized, however, that this recommendation is not founded on peer-reviewed publications. For patients requiring immediate surgery, additional attention should be given to *Pneumocystis* pneumonia prophylaxis, airway management, and antibiotic utilization.

General assessment

A thorough medical history should be performed prior to elective surgery in any HIV-infected patient. It is essential that the degree of the patient's current immune function be determined. The most reliable determinant of this function is the total CD4 positive T-lymphocyte count. For patients who are on HAART, an existing CD4 count and viral load may be used if the results have been obtained within the last 2 to 3 months prior to operation. In patients who are on a stable antiretroviral regimen, which has fully suppressed the viral load to less than 50 copies of HIV RNA/ml, it is unlikely that the CD4 lymphocyte count will vary significantly over this period of time. In patients who are not on therapy, a CD4 cell count should be performed in the 2–4 weeks prior to surgery in order to determine if the patient is at an increased risk for postoperative complications and to assess for the need for prophylactic therapy to prevent opportunistic infections. In addition, patients should be questioned closely to determine whether they have received immunization against pneumococcal and influenza associated disease, and for the need for prophylactic therapy to prevent *Pneumocystis* pneumonia as recommended by the Public Health Service.[22]

Given the widespread use of antivirals and antibiotic therapy, a thorough medication history should be documented for each patient. Certain medications have important drug interactions and the interactions must be anticipated prior to the operative intervention. Table 22.1 lists the antiretroviral medications and potential drug interactions that should be anticipated in the operative setting. In general, the antiretroviral drugs that are of the greatest concern are those that primarily act as inhibitors of the cytochrome P450 enzyme system. These drugs include the class of antiretroviral protease inhibitors, and also certain members of the azole family of antifungal agents. Medications which fall into these two categories may be anticipated to prolong the effects of any other medications which are metabolized by CYP450 3A enzymes in the liver. General classes of medications affected include: anxiolytics, certain analgesics, certain calcium channel blockers and certain antiarrhythmics.

Table 22.1. Selected interactions between antiretrovirals and medications potentially used in the operative setting[a]

Drug A	Drug B					
	Analgesics	Cardiovascular		GI	Psychotropic	
	Codones Fentanyl Meperidine Propoxyphene	Amiodarone Encainide Flecainide Propafenone Quinadine	Diltiazem Felodipine Nifedipine Nicardipine Warfarin Lidocaine	Cisapride (PPI)	Midazolam Triazolam	Alprazolam Clorazepate Diazepam Flurazepam
Amprenavir	B Increased	B Increased	B Increased	Do not use	Do not use	B Increased
Atazanavir	B Increased	B Increased (Use β-blockers and Digoxin with caution, monitor PR interval)	B Increased	Do not use (Do not use proton pump inhibitors)	Do not use	
Delavirdine	B Increased	B Increased	B Increased	Do not use (Do not use proton pump inhibitors)	Do not use	B Increased
Efavirenz	B Increased		Warfarin effect varies	Do not use	Do not use	
Indinavir	B Increased	B Increased	B Increased	Do not use	Do not use	B Increased
Lopinavir/ Ritonavir	B Increased	Do not use	B Increased	Do not use	Do not use	B Increased
Nelfinavir	B Increased	B Increased	B Increased	Do not use	Do not use	B Increased
Nevirapine	B Increased		B Decreased	Avoid	Avoid	
Ritonavir	B Increased (Do not use Mepiridine or Propoxyphene)	Do not use	B Increased	Do not use	Do not use	B Increased
Saquinavir	B Increased	B Increased	B Increased	Do not use	Do not use	B Increased
Tiprinavir	Effect varies	Do not use	Effect varies	Do not use	Do not use	

Note:

[a] Based on pharmacokinetics, and the package inserts for each drug. Interactions with other medications exist, see reference 1 for more details.

In general, the strongest inhibitors of this system include the protease inhibitors Ritonavir and Nelfinavir, the non-nucleoside reverse transcriptase inhibitor Delavirdine and the azole antifungal drugs Ketoconazole and Itraconazole. These medications may prolong the effects of the analgesics Meperidine and Fentanyl, and may have variable effects on Methadone and Codone derivatives. In general, Propofol, Methohexital and Morphine sulfate levels should not be affected since their metabolism is not via the CYP450 system. Certain anxiolytics such as Midazolam, Diazepam, Alprazolam and others may also be affected. If anxiolytics must be used in the operative setting, an alternative is Lorazepam, which is also not metabolized by the CYP450 system.

In addition to the interactions noted above, certain patients will require anticoagulation in the postoperative setting. Warfarin, which is metabolized by the cytochrome isoenzymes, will have its activity increased by the protease inhibitors and the azoles mentioned above. Careful monitoring of the international normalized ratio (INR) or the prothrombin time (PT) should be undertaken in patients who are receiving coumadin in the postoperative setting.

In contrast to the inhibition of liver cytochromes as outlined above, some medications are primarily inducers of the cytochrome system. These medications include the non-nucleoside reverse transcriptase inhibitors Efavirenz and Nevirapine, and both Rifampin and Rifabutin. These medications would be expected to decrease the activities

Table 22.2. Adverse effects of medications commonly used to treat HIV infection or its complications[a]

Acidosis, hepatic steatosis	All nucleoside reverse transcriptase inhibitors
Bleeding	Protease inhibitors (in hemophiliacs)
Bone marrow suppression	Cidofovir, dapsone, flucytosine, ganciclovir, hydroxyurea, interferon, lamivudine (rare), linazolid, primaquine, pyrimethamine, ribavirin, rifabutin, stavudine, sulfadiazine, TMP-SMX, trimetrexate, valganciclovir, zidovudine
Bronchospasm	Pentamidine
Cardiovascular	PR interval prolongation (atazanavir)
Dermatologic – rash	Abacavir, amprenavir, atovaquone, dapsone, delavirdine, efavirenz, nevirapine, pyrimethamine, ribavirin, rifabutin, rifampin, sulfadiazine, TMP-SMX, zalcitabine
Dermatologic – other	Fluconazole (hair loss at high dose), emtricitabine (hyperpigmentation), foscarnet (genital ulcers), indinavir (hair loss, ingrown toenails), zalcitabine (oral and genital ulcers), zidovudine (hyperpigmentation)
Diabetes/glucose intolerance	Didanosine, growth hormone, pentamidine, protease inhibitors
Diarrhea	Atovaquone, clindamycin, protease inhibitors, tenofovir
Hepatotoxicity	All antiretrovirals, all azole antifungals, azithromycin, clarithromycin, isoniazid, pyrazinamide, rifabutin, rifampin, TMP-SMX
Hyperlipidemia	Delavirdine, efavirenz, nevirapine, protease inhibitors except atazanavir, stavudine
Hypersensitivity – fever, rash, nausea, vomiting, cough, multiorgan failure	Abacavir
Lipodystrophy	Protease inhibitors, stavudine, zidovudine
Myopathy	All nucleoside analog antiretrovirals
Nephrotoxicity	Acyclovir (high-dose), adefovir, aminoglycosides, amphotericin B, cidofovir, foscarnet, ganciclovir, indinavir (nephrolithiasis), pentamidine, tenofovir, TMP-SXT, valganciclovir
Neurotoxicity – central	Acyclovir (high-dose), azithromycin, clarithromycin, efavirenz, interferon, quinolones
Neurotoxicity – peripheral	Didanosine, hydroxyurea (with didanosine), growth hormone (carpal tunnel syndrome), isoniazid, metronidazole, ritonavir (paresthesias), stavudine, zalcitabine
Ocular toxicity	Cidofovir (hypotony), didanosine, ethambutol (color blindness), interferon (retinal lesions), rifabutin (uveitis), voriconazole
Ototoxicity	Azithromycin, clarithromycin
Pancreatitis	Didanosine, lamivudine (rare), pentamidine, ritonavir, stavudine, TMP-SMX, zalcitabine

Note:

[a] This table does not include common upper gastrointestinal, electrolyte or psychiatric disorders.

of many of the same medications listed above. In addition to these important drug interactions, many of the medications used in the setting of HIV infection have toxicities that may become apparent during the perioperative and postoperative setting. Table 22.2 gives a listing of some of the commonly used medications and their associated toxicities. For simplicity's sake the common side effects of nausea, headache and malaise are not included in this table.

Hematopoietic disorders

Patients with advanced HIV infection frequently have leukopenia, anemia, and thrombocytopenia. These hematological abnormalities may increase the likelihood of postoperative complications. Such conditions may also be worsened by certain antivirals and prophylactic antibiotics (See Table 22.2). The antibiotic Dapsone can also

cause methemoglobinemia, which at high levels may result in cyanosis. In general, any medication that is being used to prevent or to suppress an opportunistic infection may be safely withheld for a brief period of time (i.e., 2 to 3 days) if necessary. Longer periods of interruption should prompt the selection of alternative regimens that have fewer hematological side effects.

In addition to the above abnormalities, some HIV-infected patients may have an increased propensity for thrombosis. Conditions associated with thrombosis include acquired deficiencies of Protein S and Protein C, anticardiolipin antibodies, and nephrotic syndrome.[23] The efficacy of screening for these conditions prior to surgery has not been studied. Thrombotic complications have primarily been described in patients who are not being treated with antiretroviral therapy. Patients with untreated HIV infection should therefore be considered at increased risk for thrombosis, and appropriate preventive measures instituted.

Respiratory disorders

It is important to assess for upper airway disease prior to the intubation of an HIV-infected patient. The physician should examine for oral candidiasis and treat it appropriately if possible prior to the procedure. In addition, patients with advanced immunosuppression are at an increased risk for aphthous ulceration. This painful condition impairs the ability of the patient to tolerate food and oral medications. Aphthous ulceration may be treated with either systemic corticosteroids or with thalidomide.[24]

Patients with HIV infection are also at an increased risk for pulmonary complications in the postoperative setting.[20] All patients who have a CD4 positive T-lymphocyte count less than 200 cells/mm^3, or who have a history of oral candidiasis, should receive prophylaxis to prevent pneumocystis pneumonia. For patients who have not received prophylaxis, a high degree of suspicion must be maintained for pneumocystosis if pulmonary complications are noted in the postoperative setting.

Since pneumonia is the most commonly reported postoperative complication, physicians should be familiar with the spectrum of HIV-associated pathogens. Common bacterial etiologies of pneumonia in HIV-infected patients include *Streptococcus pneumoniae, Hemophilus influenzae, Legionella pneumophila,* and *Pseudomonas aeruginosa.* Common opportunistic infections include *Mycobacterium tuberculosis, Mycobacterium kansasii,* Cytomegalovirus, *Aspergillus* species, *Cryptococcus neoformans, Coccidioides immitis* and *Histoplasma capsulatum.* Patients who have suffered recurrent episodes of opportunistic pulmonary infections may develop chronic obstructive pulmonary disease. It should also be noted that women with HIV infection appear to have an increased risk for primary pulmonary hypertension, although this complication remains rare.[25]

Cardiovascular disorders

The spectrum of cardiac disease associated with HIV infection is broad. HIV-1 infection itself and many opportunistic infections have been reported to cause either cardiac dysfunction or pericardial effusion. These include tuberculosis, toxoplasmosis, Cytomegalovirus, cryptococcosis, and others.

In addition to these infectious complications, nucleoside reverse transcriptase inhibitors may be associated with cardiac dysfunction. This cardiomyopathy is felt to be due to mitochondrial dysfunction.[26] Tissues that have an increased need for mitochondrial activity, particularly muscle and liver, are more likely to be adversely affected by long-term nucleoside analogue use. Such patients may present with isolated signs of cardiac failure, or may present with signs or symptoms of more extensive mitochondrial dysfunction (see Hepatobiliary disorders).

Untreated HIV infection is known to be associated with elevated triglyceride levels. Certain antiretrovirals can cause additional elevations in LDL cholesterol and triglycerides (Table 22.2). Protease inhibitors may also be associated with reduced arterial endovascular function, glucose intolerance and diabetes. Given the presence of these factors, it is likely that HIV-infected patients who are receiving antiretroviral therapy may be at an increased risk for cardiovascular disease.[2,4,27] Given the lipid abnormalities observed with certain HAART regimens, a cardiac risk assessment should be performed prior to elective surgery. In general, such assessment should follow the guidelines for operative risk as outlined elsewhere in this textbook.

Hepatobiliary disorders

Patients with HIV infection utilize a variety of medications which are potentially hepatotoxic, as outlined in Table 22.2. Nevirapine, in particular, may cause severe hepatitis, especially in women with CD4 and T-cell counts >250 cells/mm^3 and men with CD4 counts >400 cells/mm^3. This affliction is usually observed in the first few months of therapy. Careful follow-up and weekly or every other week monitoring of liver transaminases for the first 16 weeks should be routine. There is also an increased prevalence of hepatitis B and hepatitis C virus infection in patients with HIV infection. In patients who are seropositive for hepatitis B surface antigen or for hepatitis C virus antibodies, a history and physical assessment to determine the likelihood of liver disease should be performed.

Physicians should also be aware of the signs and symptoms of hepatic steatosis due to nucleoside-induced mitochondrial dysfunction.[28] Symptoms of this disorder include fatigue, malaise, weakness, and abdominal pain. On physical examination patients may be noted to have hepatomegaly. In the late stages of mitochondrial dysfunction patients present with lactic acidosis, hepatic steatosis, myopathy, and at times with pancreatitis. Patients who have symptoms or signs of mitochondrial dysfunction should have a resting serum lactate level determined and an ultrasound or CAT scan of the liver. Appropriate management should be instituted prior to surgery if at all possible. Such management should include the withholding of antiretroviral therapy if the lactate level is greater than two to five times the upper limit of normal, the patient is symptomatic, and no other cause of lactic acidemia is present.[29] Depending on the degree of dysfunction, certain B vitamins and other mitochondrial nutrients may be indicated, although the evidence for the efficacy of these agents is anecdotal.[30,31] Recovery of full mitochondrial function may take several weeks, and as such may delay elective surgery.

Late stage, HIV-infected patients are also at an increased risk for biliary tract disease. This typically presents in patients who have less than 100 CD4 positive T-lymphocytes/mm^3. Common complaints include right upper quadrant pain (88%), nausea (83%), diarrhea (59%), and weight loss (41%).[32] Biliary tract disease may be due to cholelithiasis (33%), opportunistic infection (34%), or idiopathic (acalculous) (33%). The opportunistic infections most commonly associated with biliary tract disease include CMV, *Cryptosporidium* and Microsporidiosis. In patients with an opportunistic infection the alkaline phosphatase level tends to be elevated to a greater degree than that observed in patients with acalculous cholecystitis.[33] Patients with acalculous cholecystitis are more likely to have a normal right upper quadrant ultrasound and a normal HIDA scan than patients who have an opportunistic infection. In contrast, patients with opportunistic infections are more likely to have a thickened gall bladder wall or sludge noted by ultrasound.[33] Our anecdotal experience at Grady Memorial Hospital indicates that patients with an opportunistic infection of the biliary tree may present with worsening of this condition in the setting of the immune reconstitution syndrome. Operative intervention in late stage patients with an opportunistic infection of the biliary system is prone to complications. However, laparoscopic cholecystectomy is a safe procedure in HIV-infected patients and should be considered for any patient in which there are operative indications.[34]

Gastrointestinal disorders

Candidiasis, aphthous ulceration, and CMV are common causes of esophageal disease in HIV-infected patients who are immunosuppressed. In a patient who complains of odynophagia or dysphagia, a course of oral azole antifungal therapy should be given, whether or not oral candidiasis is present. If there is no improvement after 48–72 hours, an esophagoscopy should then be performed.

Kaposi's sarcoma and many opportunistic infections may be associated with diarrhea. These infections include bacterial pathogens (Shigella, Salmonella, Campylobacter, *Clostridium difficile*), viruses (CMV, HSV), parasites (Giardia, Microsporidiosis, Isospora), and mycobacteria (Tuberculosis, disseminated *Mycobacterium avium–intracellulare* complex (DMAC)). Protease inhibitors are also noted for their propensity to cause diarrhea. Patients who complain of diarrhea should have an evaluation for infectious causes prior to elective surgery. In residents of the developed world in whom symptoms of proctitis are absent, it is reasonable to perform stool cultures and a stool smear for Giardia. A stool smear for Microsporidiosis and other intestinal parasites should be done for those in whom these initial results are negative. A stool test for *C. difficile* toxin should be performed if the patient is febrile or has a peripheral blood leukocytosis. Patients with symptoms of proctitis should initially be tested for HSV, gonorrhea and Chlamydia by collecting rectal swab specimens. If these are negative, then further testing as outlined above, and a proctoscopy or flexible sigmoidoscopy, may be performed.

Patients with DMAC or CMV frequently complain of abdominal pain. For DMAC a blood mycobacterial culture should be performed. For CMV a computer-assisted tomography scan of the abdomen may reveal thickening of the colonic wall. A colonoscopy with biopsy is the typical diagnostic procedure. However, for patients who refuse this procedure and who have active ophthalmic CMV, a presumptive diagnosis may be made if there is a symptomatic response to therapy. Preliminary evidence indicates that a positive blood CMV antigen assay or DNA PCR assay correlates with the development of active CMV disease, although the clinical utility of these tests for diagnosing CMV colitis is not well established.[35]

Renal disorders

African-American patients with HIV infection are at an increased risk for renal dysfunction due to HIV-associated nephropathy (HIVAN).[36] This condition is rare in Caucasians and other racial groups. HIVAN is characterized by focal and segmental glomerulosclerosis, glomerular collapse, and progressive azotemia. In the early stages, HIVAN may be detected by increased protein excretion in the urine. In the later stages nephrotic range proteinuria and renal dysfunction become evident. Ultrasound examination of the kidneys will frequently reveal enlarged kidneys with increased echogenicity. There is no known effective treatment, although anecdotal reports have indicated possible benefit from HAART in delaying the onset and progression. Patients who have asymptomatic proteinuria may be at an increased risk for medication induced renal toxicity. A screening urinalysis should be performed in HIV-infected, African-American patients in order to assess for this potential complication. Table 22.2 includes a listing of commonly used medications that are potentially nephrotoxic.

Miscellaneous disorders

Since HIV infection can affect every organ system of the body, the internist should perform a thorough assessment for miscellaneous conditions. These include adrenal insufficiency, pancreatic disease, central nervous system disease, peripheral nervous system disease and musculoskeletal disease. All of these general conditions are noted to be more prevalent in HIV-infected patients either due to the disease process or due to medications. For those who desire to learn more about the myriad clinical manifestations of HIV infection, the *Textbook of AIDS Medicine* is a useful resource.[37]

Occupational transmission of HIV

HIV can be transmitted from infected patients to healthcare workers. However, the risk of acquiring infection in the surgical setting is small. For example, in the first 19 years of the HIV-epidemic only 56 US healthcare personnel were documented to have occupationally acquired HIV infection.[38] In addition, another 138 healthcare workers had a possible work-related infection. However, the majority of the healthcare workers infected as a result of an occupational exposure were not physicians or operating room personnel.

The risk of developing HIV infection in the healthcare setting includes several elements. Among these are the prevalence of HIV infection in the patient population, the size of the blood inoculum, the depth of penetration and the duration of contact with the inoculum. Another important factor is the stage of illness of the patient. Patients with advanced stages of HIV infection typically have higher plasma viral loads than patients with earlier stages. High risk needle sticks are caused by hollow bore needles that have been in the vein of an HIV-infected patient, and which cause a deep penetrating injury to the healthcare worker. Factors which potentially reduce the infectious inoculum include injury from a solid needle or instruments, the use of antiretroviral therapy in the source patient and the wearing of gloves. Laboratory studies have suggested that double gloving has the potential to additionally reduce HIV transmission.

The Centers for Disease Control and Prevention estimates that the average rate of transmission of HIV after a percutaneous exposure is approximately 0.32%.[39] This estimate is derived from data collected during an era when HAART therapy was not available for either patients or healthcare workers. The risk should be much lower if the source patient and the health care worker are appropriately treated. Concern about the potential transmission of HIV should therefore not be a significant consideration of whether to perform an operative procedure. However, since even one high-risk exposure can result in infection, appropriate measures to reduce the risk to operating room personnel should be utilized. These universal precautions, which should be used for all patients, involve the use of fluid-resistant gowns, gloves, masks and eyewear that reduce contact with infectious fluids.

The risk of infection for healthcare workers can be reduced further by the appropriate administration of postexposure prophylaxis. Based on available data, postexposure prophylaxis reduces the risk of transmission by approximately 80%.[40] In general, the efficacy of postexposure prophylaxis is dependent upon rapid evaluation and appropriate medical treatment. The Public Health Service recommendations indicate that all healthcare workers who sustain percutaneous injuries from HIV-infected patients should be considered for post exposure prophylaxis.[40] For small volume percutaneous injuries, such as solid needle and a superficial injury, two to three drugs are recommended depending on the stage of illness of the patient. For patients with >500 CD4+ T-cells, or for those known to have a low viral load, a regimen of two nucleoside analogues is considered acceptable. For advanced stage patients, or for more severe injuries, an expanded three-drug regimen is recommended. The guidelines recommend that three-drug regimens include two nucleoside analogue inhibitors and either a protease inhibitor or Efavirenz. However, it is also recommended that the regimen be tailored to the virus harbored by the individual source patient. There are documented cases where postexposure prophylaxis was administered, but failed due to resistant virus present in the source patient's blood. Healthcare workers should receive postexposure medications to which the source patient's virus is likely to be sensitive. A useful resource for those involved in the management of occupational exposures is the National Needlestick Hotline. This hotline is available 24 hours a day and may be reached at 001-800-969-4152.

The optimal duration of prophylaxis is unknown. Based on the available data, the Public Health Service recommends that healthcare workers who receive prophylaxis be treated for 4 weeks. Cohort studies have indicated that approximately 50% of healthcare workers will experience drug-associated adverse events. The majority of these are gastrointestinal upset, although more severe toxicities have also been reported. In general, Nevirapine should be avoided for prophylaxis due to the potential for hepatitis and Stevens–Johnson syndrome. Unusual or severe toxicity should be reported to the Food and Drug Administration at 001-800-332-1088. Occupationally acquired HIV infection or failure of postexposure prophylaxis should be reported to the CDC at 001-800-893-0485.

REFERENCES

1. Guidelines for the use of antiretroviral agents among HIV-infected adults and adolescents: recommendations of the panel on clinical practices for treatment of HIV. http://AIDSinfo.nil.gov.

2. Beherns, G., Schmidt, H., Meyer, D. *et al.* Vascular complications associated with use of HIV protease inhibitors. *Lancet* 1998; **351**: 1958.

3. Allison, G. T., Bostrom, M. P., & Glesby, M. J. Osteonecrosis in HIV disease: epidemiology, etiologies, and clinical management. *AIDS* 2003; **17**(1): 1–9.

4. The data collection on adverse events of anti-HIV drugs Study Group. Combination antiretroviral therapy and the risk of myocardial infarction. *N. Engl. J. Med.* 2003; **349**: 1993–2003.

5. Sempowski, G. D. & Haynes, B. F. Immune reconstitution in patients with HIV infection. *Ann. Rev. Med.* 2002; **53**: 269–284.

6. Ferguson, C. M. Surgical complications of human immunodeficiency virus infection. *Am. Surg.* 1988; **54**(1): 4–9.

7. Wexner, S. D., Smithy, W. B., Trillo, C. *et al.* Emergency colectomy for cytomegalovirus ileocolitis in patients with the acquired immune deficiency syndrome. *Dis. Colon Rectum* 1988; **31**(10): 755–761.

8. Robinson, G., Wilson, S. E., & Williams, R. A. Surgery in patients with acquired immunodeficiency syndrome. *Arch. Surg.* 1987; **122**(2): 170–175.

9. Whitney, T. M., Brunel, W., Russell, T. R. *et al.* Emergent abdominal surgery in AIDS: experience in San Francisco. *Am. J. Surg.* 1994; **168**: 239–243.

10. Bizer, L. S., Pettorino, R., & Ashikari, A. Emergency abdominal operations in the patient with acquired immunodeficiency syndrome. *J. Am. Coll. Surg.* 1995; **180**: 205–209.

11. Flum, D. R., Steinberg, S. D., Sarkis, A. Y. *et al.* Appendicitis in patients with acquired immunodeficiency syndrome. *J. Am. Coll. Surg.* 1997; **184**: 481–486.

12. Ricci, M., Puente, A. O., Rothenberg, R. E. *et al.* Open and laparoscopic cholecystectomy in acquired immunodeficiency syndrome: indications and results in fifty-three patients. *Surgery* 1999; **125**(2): 172–177.

13. Harris, H. W. & Schecter, W. P. Emergency abdominal surgery. In Flum, D. R. & Wallack, M. K., eds. *The Role of Surgery in*

AIDS: an Outcomes-based Approach. Baltimore: Lippincott, Williams & Wilkins, 1999.

14. Buehrer, J. L., Weber, D. J., Meyer, A. A. *et al.* Wound infection rates after invasive procedures in HIV-1 seropositive versus HIV-1 seronegative hemophiliacs. *Ann. Surg.* 1990; **211**: 492–498.

15. Emparan, C., Iturburu, I. M., Oritz, J. *et al.* Infective complications after abdominal surgery in patients infected with human immunodeficiency virus: role of CD4+ lymphocytes in prognosis. *World J. Surg.* 1998; **22**: 778–782.

16. Ganesh, R., Castle, D., McGibbon, D. *et al.* Staphylococcal carriage and HIV infection. *Lancet* 1989; **2**: 558.

17. Kalmeijer, M. D., Coertjens, H., van Nieuwland-Bollen, P. M. *et al.* Surgical site infections in orthopedic surgery: the effect of mupirocin nasal ointment in a double-blind, randomized, placebo-controlled study. *Clin. Infect. Dis.* 2002; **35**(4): 353–358.

18. VandenBergh, M. F., Kluytmans, J. A., van Hout, B. A. *et al.* Cost-effectiveness of perioperative mupirocin nasal ointment in cardiothoracic surgery. *Infect. Control Hosp. Epidemiol.* 1996; **17**(12): 786–792.

19. Perl, T. M., Cullen, J. J., Wenzel, R. P. *et al* and the mupirocin and the risk of *Staphylococcus aureus* study team. Intranasal mupirocin to prevent postoperative *Staphylococcus aureus* infections. *N. Engl. J. Med.* 2002; **346**(24): 1871–1877.

20. Albaran, R. G., Webber, J., & Steffes, C. P. CD4 cell counts as a prognostic factor of major abdominal surgery in patients infected with the human immunodeficiency virus. *Arch. Surg.* 1998; **133**: 626–631.

21. Rose, D. N., Collins, M., & Kleban, R. Complications of surgery in HIV-infected patients. *AIDS* 1998; **12**: 2243–2251.

22. Centers for Disease Control and Prevention. Guidelines for preventing opportunistic infections among HIV-infected persons – 2002 recommendations of the U.S. Public Health Service and the Infectious Diseases Society of America. *Morb. Mortal. Wkly Rep.* 2002; **51**(No. RR-8): 1–51.

23. Saif, M. W., Bona, R., & Greenberg, B. AIDS and thrombosis: retrospective study of 131 HIV-infected patients. *AIDS Patient Care Stds* 2001; **15**(6): 311–320.

24. Patton, L. L. & van der Horst, C. Oral infections and other manifestations of HIV disease. *Infect. Dis. Clin. North Am.* 1999; **13**(4): 879–900.

25. Seoane, L., Shellito, J., Welsh, D. *et al.* Pulmonary hypertension associated with HIV infection. *South. Med. J.* 2001; **94**(6): 635–639.

26. Lewis, W. & Dalakas, M. C. Mitochondrial toxicity of antiviral drugs. *Nature Med.* 1995; **1**(5): 417–422.

27. Henrey, K., Melroe, H., Huebsch, J. *et al.* Severe premature coronary artery disease with protease inhibitors. *Lancet* 1998; **351**: 1328.

28. Fortgang, I. S., Belitsos, P. C., Chaisson, R. E. *et al.* Hepatomegaly and steatosis in HIV-infected patients receiving nucleoside analog antiretroviral therapy. *Am. J. Gastroenterol.* 1995; **90**: 1433–1436.

29. Carr, A. Lactic acidemia in Human Immunodeficiency Virus. *Clin. Infect. Dis.* 2003; **36**(Suppl 2): S96–S100.

30. Luzzati, R., del Bravo, P., Di Perri, G. *et al.* Riboflavin and severe lactic acidosis. *Lancet* 1999; **353**: 901–902.

31. Patrick, L. Nutrients and HIV: Part three: N-acetylcysteine, alpha-lipoic acid, L-glutamine, and L-carnitine. *Alt. Med. Rev.* 2000; **5**(4): 290–305.

32. Nash, J. A. & Cohen, S. A. Gallbladder and biliary tract disease in AIDS. *Gastroenterol. Clin. North Am.* 1997; **26**(2): 323–335.

33. French, A. L., Beaudet, L. M., Benator, D. A. *et al.* Cholecystectomy in patients with AIDS: clinicopathologic correlations in 107 cases. *Clin. Infect. Dis.* 1995; **21**: 852–858.

34. Ricci, M., Puente, A. O., Rothenberg, R. E. *et al.* Open and laparoscopic cholecystectomy in acquired immunodeficiency syndrome: indications and results in fifty-three patients. *Surgery* 1999; **125**(2): 172–177.

35. Rasmussen, L., Zipeto, D., Wolitz, R. A. *et al.* Risk for retinitis in patients with AIDS can be assessed by quantitation of threshold levels of cytomegalovirus DNA burden in blood. *J. Infect. Dis.* 1997; **176**(5): 1146–1155.

36. Szczech, L. A. Renal diseases associated with human immunodeficiency virus infection: epidemiology, clinical course, and management. *Clin. Infect. Dis.* 2001; **33**(1): 115–119.

37. Merigan, T. C., Bartlett, J. G., & Bolognesi, D. eds. *Textbook of AIDS Medicine*, 2nd edn. Baltimore: Lippincott Williams & Wilkins, 1999.

38. Centers for Disease Control and Prevention. Surveillance of health care workers with HIV/AIDS. http://www.cdc.gov/hiv/pubs/facts/hcwsurv.htm.

39. Cardo, D. M., Culver, D. H., Ciesielski, C. A. *et al.* A case-control study of HIV seroconversion in health care workers after percutaneous exposure. *N. Engl. J. Med.* 1997; **337**: 1485–1490.

40. Centers for Disease Control and Prevention. Updated U.S. Public Health Service guidelines for the management of occupational exposures to HBV, HCV, and HIV and recommendations for postexposure prophylaxis. *Morb. Mortal. Wkly Rep.* 2001; **50**(No. RR-11): 1–52.

23

Fever and infection in the postoperative setting

James P. Steinberg[1] and Shanta M. Zimmer[2]

[1]Emory University School of Medicine, and Crawford Long Hospital of Emory University, Atlanta, GA
[2]Emory University School of Medicine, Atlanta, GA

Fever is common in the postoperative period, and its causes are diverse (Table 23.1). Fever may result from a benign process such as the release of pyrogens from traumatized tissue and have no bearing on the clinical outcome. Alternatively, fever may be an early sign of a potentially life-threatening infection. The clinician's challenge is to distinguish those fevers from the large pool of "routine" fevers, while avoiding the excessive use of diagnostic resources and therapeutic interventions such as antibiotics.

Evaluation of a febrile surgical patient begins with a careful history and review of the medical record. The presence of symptoms or signs of infection before the operative procedure or underlying medical problems that increase the likelihood of postoperative complications are valuable clues. The type of surgical procedure performed, operative findings, and the temporal relationship between the operation and the onset of fever are also important. Although prolonged endotracheal intubation, indwelling bladder catheters, and intravascular catheters may be important components of patient care, they violate normal host defenses and increase the likelihood of postoperative infection. When a patient has a significant infection, symptoms and signs in addition to fever usually are present. Thus, a careful physical examination is essential. Laboratory and radiographic studies should be directed by the relevant clinical data and not obtained by an undirected "shotgun" approach.

The incidence of postoperative fever varies widely depending on the surgical procedure performed and the definition of fever. There is no consensus regarding what constitutes fever in the postoperative setting. Investigators have used temperatures ranging from 37.5 °C to 38.5 °C to define fever with 38 °C as the most common cut-off point. In addition, some investigators require that the temperature be elevated on consecutive measurements to meet their

Table 23.1. Causes of postoperative fever

Non-infectious	Infectious
Adrenal insufficiency	Abscess
Alcohol withdrawal	Bloodstream infections
Atelectasis	Cholecystitis
Blood (hematoma/CSF)	*Clostridium difficile* colitis
Dehydration	Endocarditis
Drug fever (including	Infusion-related infections
anesthetics)	Intravascular device infections
Factitious	Parotitis
Malignant hyperthermia	Peritonitis
Myocardial infarction	Pneumonia
Neoplasms	Prostatitis
Pancreatitis	Surgical site infections
Pheochromocytoma	superficial incisional
Pericarditis/Dressler's	deep incisional
syndrome	organ/space
Pulmonary embolism	Transfusion related (CMV,
Thrombophlebitis	hepatitis)
Thyrotoxicosis	Urinary tract infection
Tissue trauma	
Transfusion reaction	

definition of fever, whereas others require that the temperature be elevated for two consecutive days. Thus, it is not surprising that the reported incidence of postoperative fever ranges from 13.7% after general surgery to nearly 100% following cardiac surgery.[1,2] Even among studies that involve only abdominal operations, there still is a considerable variation in the reported incidence of fever (Table 23.2).[3–6]

Postoperative fever can be divided into two broad categories – infectious and non-infectious. The reported proportion of febrile episodes attributed to bacterial infection also varies widely. In general, high fevers are more likely caused by infection, but considerable overlap exists.

Medical Management of the Surgical Patient: A Textbook of Perioperative Medicine, ed. M. F. Lubin, R. B. Smith, T. F. Dobson, N. Spell, H. K. Walker. 4th edn. Published by Cambridge University Press. © Cambridge University 2006.

Table 23.2. Incidence of fever and infection causing fever following abdominal surgery

Procedure	Definition of fever	N	% with fever	% of those febrile with infection
Major abdominal[3]	≥38.5 °C (rectally) on 2 consecutive measurements during first 6 postoperative days	464	15	27[c]
Cholecystectomy[4]	≥38.4 °C or ≥38.0 °C (orally) on consecutive measurements 4 hours apart	176	16	7[a,b]
Abdominal[5]	≥38.1 °C during first 7 postoperative days	434	38	16[c]
Intra-abdominal, duration >1 hour[6]	≥38.0 °C (rectally) on 2 measurements >1 hour apart	608	43	36
	Group A – 38°–38.4 °C		A–5	A–19
	Group B – ≥38.5 °C		B–27	B–45

Notes:

[a] 8 other patients had infection but were afebrile.

[b] Uses CDC definition of infection.

[c] Required culture confirmation.

Temporal aspects of postoperative fever

The time of onset of postoperative fever is a helpful clue that can suggest a particular cause. Fever that develops within 24 hours after surgery usually is not caused by infection (Fig. 23.1). The time-honored dogma that atelectasis causes most early postoperative fever[7,8] may be inaccurate.[2,9] Garibaldi and colleagues[9] found that unexplained (and presumed non-infectious) early post-operative fever did not occur more frequently after thoracic and upper abdominal surgeries, procedures that predispose to atelectasis and pneumonia. In addition, Roberts and associates did not find a strong correlation between early fever (48 hours or less) following abdominal surgery and radiographic evidence of atelectasis.[10] Cytokine release during surgery appears to be the major cause of early postoperative fevers. A shift in the core temperature curve has been observed in all postoperative patients (Fig. 23.2).[11] In this study, the highest temperature occurred 11.5 ± 5.8 hours after surgery. Tissue trauma during surgery causes a release of proinflammatory cytokines, the levels of which correlate with increases in core temperature.[11] Duration and perhaps extent of surgical intervention appear to impact the degree of temperature elevation. Other non-infectious causes of early postoperative fever include drug hypersensitivity reactions (including anesthetic agents) and transfusion reactions, which may cause hemolysis. Malignant hyperthermia usually manifests with high fever (39 °C to 44 °C) beginning within 30 minutes of the administration of an anesthetic agent. Rarely, the fever associated with malignant hyperthermia is delayed and develops several hours after operation.

On occasion, infection does occur within one to two days after surgery. *Streptococcus pyogenes* and *Clostridium perfringens* infections, although rare, are the classic causes of early postoperative wound infections and can produce high fever within 24 hours of surgery. With streptococcal infections, erythema around the surgical site develops early and spreads rapidly. Clostridial wound infections typically occur after biliary tract or intestinal surgery. Severe pain is present and tense edema develops at the surgical site. A bronze or violaceous hue may develop followed by hemorrhagic bullae and the formation of tissue gas.

Toxic shock syndrome also produces high fever early in the postoperative period. Hypotension, diffuse erythematous rash, confusion, and other signs of toxemia often are present. In contrast to other wound infections, signs of local inflammation are absent, even though the surgical site harbors the toxigenic *Staphylococcus aureus*. If significant aspiration of oropharyngeal or gastric contents occurred during induction of anesthesia, a postoperative pneumonia may manifest within 1 or 2 days of surgery. If the surgery is prompted by infection (such as peritonitis following a ruptured viscus), fever can antedate or occur shortly after the procedure. On occasion, an unrelated infection is incubating at the time of surgery and produces early fever. Accurate diagnosis can be difficult, especially when patients are intubated or sedated after operation and are unable to relate their histories.

Fever that develops 72 hours or more after operation suggests the presence of infection. Rates of infection vary considerably with the type of operation performed, ranging from 2% after herniorrhaphy to 20.8% after gastric

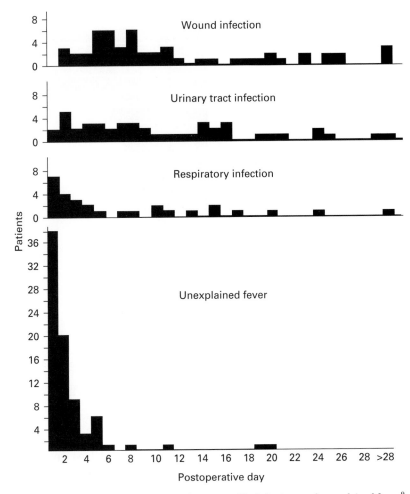

Fig. 23.1. Day of onset of postoperative fever caused by infections and unexplained fever.[9]

surgery (Fig. 23.3).[12] Although the causes of postoperative infection are numerous (Table 23.1), surgical site infections, bloodstream infections, pneumonia, and urinary tract infections (UTIs) account for 80% to 90% of all cases. Surgical site infections are most common overall but the distribution of infections depends on the type of operation performed (Table 23.3). Surgical site infections typically manifest themselves 5 to 10 days after operation, although deep organ space abscesses may appear later. Bacterial pneumonias are often precipitated by perioperative aspiration or early postoperative atelectasis and, consequently, tend to occur within the first week after surgery. UTIs can appear at any time; the major risk factors for UTI development are instrumentation of the urinary tract and indwelling urinary catheter placement. The probability of bacterial colonization in the bladder increases with duration of catheterization. Bloodstream infections may result from any of these infections but are most commonly

caused by intravascular devices. The risk of bloodstream infection increases with the duration of intravascular access.

Fever may accompany postoperative myocardial infarction, which occurs most commonly within 72 hours. Clinical clues may be difficult to assess in the intubated and sedated patient but include tachycardia, arrhythmia, congestive heart failure, and diaphoresis. Postpericardiotomy syndrome, including Dressler's syndrome, may be another non-infectious cause of postoperative fever, and careful auscultation for a pericardial friction rub aids in this diagnosis.

Thrombophlebitis, pulmonary embolism, and pulmonary infarction are important causes of postoperative fever that can occur early or late in the postoperative period, depending on the clinical situation. Diagnosis can be difficult and a high index of suspicion is necessary. Hematomas can produce occult fevers or mimic an

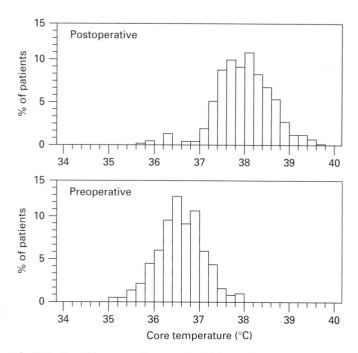

Fig. 23.2. These histograms illustrate the shift in maximum postoperative core temperatures in the first 24 hours following surgery patients compared with preoperative core temperatures (N=271).[11]

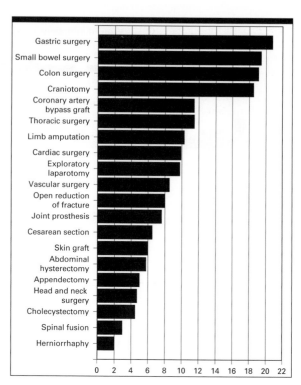

Fig. 23.3. Overall infection rate by type of operation (number of nosocomial infections at all sites per 100 operations). Data from National Nosocomial Infection Surveillance System.[12]

intra-abdominal abscess. The possibility of a hematoma should be considered when the hematocrit continues to decline after the operation in the absence of other explanations such as gastrointestinal blood loss. Resorption of blood can produce hyperbilirubinemia and an elevated lactate dehydrogenase level. Hematomas also can become secondarily infected, further complicating the clinical picture.

Medications are an important cause of postoperative fever. Drug fever caused by antibacterial agents classically develops 7 to 10 days after administration of the agent is begun.[13] Misconceptions abound regarding drug fever; rash, eosinophilia, and other signs of drug allergy are frequently absent. In addition, drug fever can produce a hectic fever curve.

Late fever, developing more than 2 weeks after surgery, usually occurs in patients with underlying medical problems or complicated hospital courses. Prolonged intravenous access, bladder catheterization, or endotracheal intubation presents ongoing risks for infection. Transient bacteremias can lead to metastatic foci of infection that declare themselves in the late postoperative period. Drug fevers can occur several weeks or longer after a new medication is introduced. Transfusion-related infections, particularly cytomegalovirus infection, can produce fever

weeks to months after the receipt of blood products. Screening of blood products for human immunodeficiency virus, hepatitis B and C has reduced transfusion associated infection to extremely low levels. *Clostridium difficile* diarrhea occurs days to several weeks after antibiotics are administered. Single dose antibiotic prophylaxis before surgery rarely induces this infection.

Surgical site infections

The term *surgical site infection* is preferred to *surgical wound infection* because it allows for a more precise categorization of infections. According to the CDC definitions, surgical site infections are divided into incisional or organ/space infections.[14] Superficial incisional infections involve the skin and subcutaneous tissues whereas deep incisional infections involved the fascia and muscle. Organ/space surgical site infections involve any anatomic part other than the incised body wall layers opened or manipulated during the procedure. The term surgical "wound" in standard parlance extends from the skin to the deep soft tissues and not to the organ space. Thus, the

Table 23.3. Distribution of nosocomial infections in surgical patients by site for operations

Operation	Number of infections	Incisional surgical site infection (%)	Organ/space surgical site infection	Urinary tract infection (%)	Pneumonia (%)	Primary bloodstream infection (%)
Coronary artery bypass graft	4,559	25	8	19	21	8
Thoracic surgery	1,418	11	6	18	34	11
Open reduction of fracture	3,507	18	4	48	14	4
Joint prosthesis	2,742	21	7	52	9	2
Cesarean section	4,908	19	55	12	3	2
Abdominal hysterectomy	2,491	22	24	37	6	2
Colon surgery	5,312	26	12	26	15	8
Cholecystectomy	2,245	24	9	26	19	7
Vascular surgery	4,057	29	4	23	20	8
Exploratory laparotomy	4,024	25	8	23	18	10
Appendectomy	817	51	24	6	8	2
Herniorrhaphy	787	46	4	21	15	4

Source: Adapted from reference 12.

term *deep wound infection*, referring to infections at or deep to the fascial layers, is ambiguous. The distinction between incisional and organ/space infections has relevance because certain procedures (e.g., cesarean section) are more likely to lead to organ/space infection, whereas other procedures (e.g., herniorrhaphy, appendectomy, exploratory laparotomy) are complicated more often by incisional infections (Table 23.3).

The standard classification of surgical wound infections has four categories – clean, clean–contaminated, contaminated, and infected – based on the degree of bacterial contamination at the time of the procedure. Although it is helpful, this system has limited capability to stratify the risk of surgical site infections.[15] Host factors that contribute to the development of postoperative infections include diabetes, advanced age, obesity, tobacco use, malnutrition, other immunosuppression, and infection or colonization at other body sites.[16] Prolonged duration of the operation independently predicts risk of infection. For some operations including cholecystectomy and colon resection, the laproscopic approach is associated with lower infection rates compared to open surgery.[17] Prolonged hospital stay prior to surgery or prolonged stay in intensive care following surgery also increases the likelihood of surgical site infection.[18]

Superficial incisional infections are heralded by pain at the surgical site disproportionate to usual postoperative pain. Edema, tenderness, erythema, and purulent drainage are frequently evident on inspection of the wound. The wound should be examined closely for areas of fluctuance. Occasionally, crepitus is present and suggests the involvement of anaerobic organisms. Deep incisional infections may not show the typical local signs and diagnosis may be delayed. Fever and leukocytosis are usually present but are not invariable.

Effective wound drainage, which usually includes suture removal, is the cornerstone of therapy for incisional infections. Purulent drainage should be sent to the microbiology laboratory for Gram stain and culture. If cellulitis and systemic signs of infection are absent, drainage is usually curative and the use of systemic antibiotics can be avoided. Antibiotic selection should be based on Gram stain results, if these are available. Staphylococci and streptococci are the major causes of superficial incisional infections. The emergence of methicillin-resistant *S. aureus* (MRSA) as a significant nosocomial pathogen complicates empiric antibiotic coverage. The need to consider vancomycin as part of empiric therapy depends on the prevalence of methicillin-resistant *S. aureus* at the particular institution, the severity of the infection, the duration of hospitalization, and previous antibiotic administration.

Organ/space infections involving the peritoneal cavity or the pelvis are frequently polymicrobial, and empiric antibiotics should have activity against gram-negative and anaerobic pathogens. Peritonitis typically occurs following procedures that enter contaminated areas such as the bowel or the biliary tract. Procedures that include anastomoses of the gastrointestinal tract pose an increased risk of peritonitis. Anastomotic leaks usually occur between the third and fifth postoperative days, when edema of the suture line begins to resolve. The diagnosis of peritonitis in the postoperative period is usually straightforward. Signs of peritoneal irritation are often heralded by fever, tachycardia, and abdominal pain.

Intraabdominal or pelvic abscesses occurring after gastrointestinal or gynecologic surgery can have a subtle presentation. Abdominal pain and other localizing signs may or may not be present. Persistent or recurrent fever and leukocytosis may be early clues. Computed tomography is invaluable, both for diagnosis and percutaneous drainage of abscesses. On average, computed tomographic scans are obtained 1 week after the initial surgery if abscess is suspected. During this interval, some of the expected inflammatory changes in the operative area should resolve, whereas any infection that is present may evolve into a discrete abscess.

Infection after median sternotomy may be superficial, involve the sternum, or result in mediastinitis. After the procedure, the sternum is contiguous with the deeper mediastinal structures and the pericardium. Thus, differentiating superficial from deep infection may be difficult. When mediastinitis is present, patients are often critically ill with accompanying bacteremia. On occasion, fever and systemic signs of infection develop before other clinical signs of wound infection such as purulent drainage. *S. aureus* and coagulase-negative staphylococci are common causes of sternal wound infections. Therapy involves prolonged administration of intravenous antibiotics and aggressive surgical debridement. Prolonged surgery, reoperation, underlying diseases such as diabetes mellitus, cigarette smoking, obesity, and use of internal mammary arteries are risk factors for the development of sternal wound infections. Postoperative stays in the intensive care unit of more than 72 hours have also been associated with an increased risk of sternal wound infection.[18]

Bloodstream infections

Bloodstream infections in the postoperative setting can result from localized processes such as surgical site infections, pneumonias, or UTIs. The rate of secondary bloodstream infection varies considerably depending on the operative procedure performed. Rates of bacteremia accompanying incisional and organ/space infections are the highest (13.2% and 39.7%, respectively) after cardiac surgery.[12] Postoperative pneumonia is more likely to lead to secondary bacteremia in patients who are mechanically ventilated than in those who are not.

Primary bloodstream infections, usually a consequence of intravascular access devices, are more common than

secondary bloodstream infections and account for 7% of nosocomial infections in surgical patients.[12] Although any device can serve as the source for a bacteremia or fungemia, most device-related bloodstream infections in the postoperative setting are caused by central venous catheters. Several studies of percutaneously inserted subclavian or internal jugular (IJ) vein catheters have found a septicemia rate of 3% to 5%.[19] Cutaneous colonization of the insertion site by bacteria, increased duration of placement, frequent manipulation, and poor line care are risk factors for central venous catheter-related infection. The risk of infection with internal jugular vein catheters is higher than with subclavian catheters, probably because the former are more difficult to secure and are located close to oropharyngeal secretions. Femoral venous catheters are also associated with higher rate of infection and a higher rate of non-infectious complications, primarily thrombosis, compared to subclavian catheters.[20] Swan-Ganz catheters inserted with maximal barrier precautions (e.g., surgical gowns, masks, sterile gloves, and large sterile sheet drape) are less prone to infection than catheters inserted in the operating room under less stringent conditions.[21] With short-term catheters (vs. cuffed tunneled lines such as Hickman catheters), most bloodstream infections are caused by bacteria that colonize the skin site and then gain access to the bloodstream from the insertion wound (i.e., outside the lumen). With increased manipulation of the catheter, the hub may become colonized and serve as the source of bacteremia. Contaminated infusates are uncommon but can be the source of epidemic nosocomial bacteremias. The insertion site may show erythema or purulence, although these findings are often absent with catheter-associated bacteremia, especially if the catheter hub or infusate is the source of infection.

Peripheral catheters can be the source of phlebitis and bloodstream infection. Phlebitis manifests with pain, erythema, tenderness, and an indurated thrombosed vein. Phlebitis is a reaction to the catheter material or the infusate and does not imply that infection is present. However, phlebitis predisposes to the development of catheter-related infection and should prompt catheter removal. The inflammation associated with phlebitis can produce fever. The absence of phlebitis does not exclude a catheter-related bloodstream infection. With routine replacement every 72–96 hours, peripheral venous catheters rarely cause bloodstream infection. An erythematous or indurated catheter site should be assessed for signs of suppurative phlebitis which include fluctuance over the course of the vein and purulence that can be expressed from the insertion site by milking the vein. Suppurative phlebitis is the cause of a sustained bacteremia; patients frequently appear septic with high spiking fevers. Excision of the involved vein is often necessary.

In the assessment of febrile postoperative patients, any intravascular catheter should be considered a potential source of infection, especially if no other site of infection is apparent. If catheter-associated infection is suspected, the device should be removed and the tip sent for semi-quantitative cultures. Two sets of blood cultures should be obtained, at least one by peripheral venopuncture. A negative line-drawn blood culture is evidence against an intravascular catheter-related infection. However, blood cultures obtained through the device have a higher contamination rate, emphasizing the importance of clinical interpretation of a positive line culture.[22]

If intravascular catheter-related bacteremia is suspected, empiric antibiotic therapy is warranted. Coagulase-negative staphylococci and *S. aureus* are the most common pathogens but many types of bacteria and fungi have been associated with catheter-related infections. Prolonged antibiotic therapy, hyperalimentation, acute renal failure, underlying medical problems such as diabetes mellitus, central venous access, and previous surgery are risk factors for catheter-related fungemia.[23] If patients with central venous catheter-related bacteremia remain febrile despite the administration of appropriate antibiotics and if follow-up blood cultures show a sustained bacteremia, an infected thrombus or endocarditis should be suspected. Unlike septic phlebitis of peripheral veins, there are few clues on the physical examination to suggest septic thrombosis of a central vein.

Pneumonia

Pneumonia and other pulmonary sources of postoperative fever are discussed in Chapter 9.

Urinary tract infections

According to CDC data, UTIs account for 27% of post-operative infections.[12] Although they are the second most common infection in surgical patients, UTIs cause less morbidity and mortality than do pneumonias, bloodstream infections, or surgical site infections. UTIs occur almost exclusively in patients with bladder catheterization or previous urinary tract manipulation. The risk of bacteriuria increases with duration of catheterization. The microbiology of nosocomial UTIs is much broader than that of community acquired UTIs, with *Escherichia coli* accounting for only about 30%. The intensive use of broad-spectrum antibiotics, including third-generation cephalosporins, in the postoperative setting has contributed to the increase in the number of UTIs caused by enterococci, resistant gram-negative bacilli, and yeast. Removal of the bladder catheter as soon as feasible is the best means of minimizing the risk of UTI.

Seventy to 80% of patients with catheter-associated bacteriuria are asymptomatic. The presence of the bladder catheter obscures the symptoms of lower tract infection. Pyuria is common even when symptoms are absent. Signs of upper tract infection, including fever and flank pain, are rare; secondary bacteremia occurs in about 1% of patients with bacteriuria. Because bacteriuria is common and the course usually benign, other sources of infection should be considered in febrile postoperative patients who have positive results on urine cultures. After the removal of short-term urinary catheters, symptomatic lower UTIs developed in 7 of 42 patients (17%) with catheter-associated bacteriuria.[24] Consequently, it is prudent to treat patients with asymptomatic bacteriuria after catheter removal.

Candida species have surpassed bacteria as the most common organisms isolated from the urine of surgical intensive care unit patients. Distinguishing between fungal colonization, contamination and infection can be very difficult if not impossible. Consequently, determining the clinical significance of funguria in the febrile postoperative patient is problematic. In addition, the role of antifungal therapy is not straightforward. In one prospective study, funguria resolved in most patients without antifungal therapy. In half of the patients who received antifungal therapy, the funguria recurred.[25] These data suggest that routine antifungal treatment of funguria is not warranted. In general, treatment should be reserved for those patients with documented infection (pyuria and funguria on more than one urine specimen) who are symptomatic or have unexplained fever. Candida can seed the urinary tract through hematogenous dissemination. Thus, in the patient at risk for disseminated fungal infection, the presence of funguria may be a clue to bloodstream infection and disseminated candidiasis. This increasing prevalence of funguria underscores the importance of minimizing risk factors such as inappropriate antibiotic use and indwelling urinary catheters.

Other infections

Ten to 20% of infections in the surgical patient are from other sources. The diagnosis may be cryptic, especially in critically ill patients in the intensive care units. Physical examination, although difficult to perform, is nonetheless essential. Careful inspection of the skin, including the sacrum, for evidence of decubitus ulcers, phlebitis, or rashes is important. Maxillary sinusitis, often staphylococcal, occurs in patients with nasotracheal intubation or nasogastric tubes. Sinus tenderness may be present, even in obtunded patients. A boggy, tender, and enlarged parotid gland suggests parotitis, an uncommon complication seen in sick patients with volume depletion. A careful funduscopic examination should be performed to search for evidence of fungal endophthalmitis, especially in patients with risk factors for candidemia. Acute cholecystitis can occur following surgery remote to the gall bladder. Right upper quadrant pain is usually present but recognition can be delayed in the sedated and paralyzed patients. Calculi may be absent on imaging studies. Without prompt diagnosis and surgical intervention, perforation, peritonitis and sepsis can develop. Diarrhea is sometimes absent or mild with *C. difficile* colitis; this diagnosis should be considered in any postoperative patient with fever and abdominal tenderness.

Antibiotic usage in the perioperative and postoperative setting

Perioperative prophylactic antibiotics effectively reduce the postoperative infection rates following a variety of operative procedures.[26,27] Timing of the preoperative dose is critical; infection rates are higher if the antibiotic is administered more than 2 hours before surgery or after the incision is made.[28] One preincisional dose is usually sufficient, although a second dose administered during procedures that last more than 3 to 4 hours is advised. Current guidelines recommend that the pre-incision antibiotic should be administered within 60 minutes of incision (120 minutes) for antibiotics requiring prolonged infusion (including vancomycin) and that antibiotics should be discontinued within 24 hours of completion of the operation.[27] Antibiotics given beyond this time should be considered therapeutic and not prophylactic. Prolonging therapy longer than 48 hours in the absence of established infection should be avoided because of the increased cost and the increased likelihood of colonization and infection with antibiotic resistant bacteria. The use of broad-spectrum agents also exerts selective pressure on the microbiologic flora. These agents, especially third-generation cephalosporins, have no role in perioperative prophylaxis. There is temptation to continue the administration of perioperative antibiotics because of early postoperative fever. This temptation should be balanced by the realization that

fever on the first postoperative day is rarely due to infection and by knowledge of the hazards of prolonged antibiotic coverage. Data from the CDC show an increase in surgical site and other nosocomial infections caused by antibiotic resistant pathogens including methicillin-resistant *S. aureus*, enterococci, coagulase negative staphylococci, *Enterobacter* sp., and *Candida albicans*.[29,30] The intensive use of antibiotics has played a major role in the selection of these and other resistant organisms. In choosing an antibiotic regimen for a postoperative infection, the clinician must be cognizant not only of the likely pathogens but also of the previous antibiotics administered to the patients and resistance trends in the hospital.

REFERENCES

1. Galicier, C. & Richet, H. A prospective study of postoperative fever in a general surgery department. *Infect. Control* 1985; **6**: 487.

2. Livelli, F. D. Jr., Johnson, R. A., McEnany, M. T. *et al.* Unexplained in-hospital fever following cardiac surgery. *Circulation* 1978; **57**: 968.

3. Freischlag, J. & Busuttil, R. W. The value of postoperative fever evaluation. *Surgery* 1983; **94**: 358.

4. Giangobbe, M. J., Rappaport, W. D., & Stein, B. The significance of fever following cholecystectomy. *J. Fam. Pract.* 1992; **34**: 437.

5. Mellors, J. W., Kelly, J. J., Gusberg, R. J., Horwitz, S. M., & Horwitz, R. I. A simple index to estimate the likelihood of bacterial infection in patients developing fever after abdominal surgery. *Am. Surg.* 1988; **54**: 558.

6. Jorgensen, F. S., Sorensen, C. G., & Kjaergaard, J. Postoperative fever after major abdominal surgery. *Ann. Chir. Gynaecol.* 1988; **77**: 47.

7. Hiyama, D. T. & Zinner, M. J. Surgical complications. In Schwartz, S. I., ed. *Principles of Surgery*. 6th edn. New York: McGraw-Hill, 1994: 455.

8. Fry, D. E. Postoperative fever. In Mackowiak, P. A., ed. *Fever: Basic Mechanisms and Management*. New York: Raven Press, 1991: 243.

9. Garibaldi, R. A., Brodine, S., Matsumiya, S., & Coleman, M. Evidence for the non-infectious etiology of early postoperative fever. *Infect. Control* 1985; **6**: 273.

10. Roberts, J., Barnes, W., Pennock, M., & Browne, G. Diagnostic accuracy of fever as a measure of postoperative pulmonary complications. *Heart Lung* 1988; **17**: 166.

11. Frank, S. M., Kluger, M. J., & Kunkel, S. L. Elevated thermostatic setpoint in post-operative patients. *Anesthesiology* 2000; **93**(6): 1426.

12. Horan, T. C., Culver, D. H., Gaynes, R. P., Jarvis, W. R., Edwards, J. R., & Reid, C. R. Nosocomial infections in surgical patients in the United States, January 1986–June 1992. National Nosocomial Infections Surveillance (NNIS) System. *Infect. Control Hosp. Epidemiol.* 1993; **14**: 73.

13. Mackowiak, P. A. Drug fever. In Mackowiak, P. A., ed. *Fever: Basic Mechanisms and Management*. New York: Raven Press, 1991: 255.

14. Horan, T. C., Gaynes, R. P., Martone, W. J., Jarvis, W. R., & Emori, T. G. CDC definitions of nosocomial surgical site infections, 1992: a modification of CDC definitions of surgical wound infections. *Infect. Control Hosp. Epidemiol.* 1992; **13**: 606.

15. Culver, D. H., Horan, T. C., Gaynes, R. P. *et al.* Surgical wound infection rates by wound class, operative procedure, and patient risk index. National Nosocomial Infections Surveillance System. *Am. J. Med.* 1991; **91**: 152S.

16. Consensus paper on the surveillance of surgical wound infections. The Society for Hospital Epidemiology of America; The Association for Practitioners in Infection Control; The Centers for Disease Control; The Surgical Infection Society. *Infect. Control Hosp. Epidemiol.* 1992; **13**: 599.

17. Gaynes, R. P., Culver, D. H., Horan, T. C., Edwards, J. R., Richards, S., & Tolson, J. S. Surgical site infection rates in the United States, 1992–1998: The National Nosocomial Infections Surveillance System basic SSI risk index. *Clin. Infect. Dis.* 2001; **33**(Suppl 2): S69.

18. Kohli, M., Yuan, L., Escobar, M. *et al.* A risk index for sternal surgical wound infection after cardiovascular surgery. *Infect. Control Hosp. Epidemiol.* 2003; **24**: 17.

19. Maki, D. G. Infections due to infusion therapy. In Bennett, J. V., Brachman, P. S., eds. *Hospital Infections*. 3rd edn. Boston/Toronto/London: Little, Brown, 1992: 849.

20. Merrer, J., DeJonghe, B., Golliot, F. *et al.* Complications of femoral and subclavian venous catheterization in critically ill patients. *J. Am. Med. Assoc.* 2001; **286**(6): 700

21. Mermel, L. A., McCormick, R. D., Springman, S. R., & Maki, D. G. The pathogenesis and epidemiology of catheter-related infection with pulmonary artery Swan–Ganz catheters: a prospective study utilizing molecular subtyping. *Am. J. Med.* 1991; **91**(Suppl. 3B): 197S.

22. Mermel, L. A., Farr, B. M., Sherertz, R. J. *et al.* Guidelines for the management of catheter-related intravascular infections. *Clin. Infect. Dis.* 2001; **32**: 1249.

23. Blumberg, H. M., Jarvis, W. R., Soucie, J. M. *et al.* and the NEMIS Study Group. Risk factors for candidal bloodstream infections in surgical intensive care unit patients: the NEMIS Prospective Multicenter Study. *Clin. Infect. Dis.* 2001; **33**: 177.

24. Harding, G. K. M., Nicolle, L. E., Ronald, A. R. *et al.* How long should catheter-acquired urinary tract infections in women be treated? *Ann. Intern. Med.* 1991; **114**: 713.

25. Kauffman, C. A., Vazquez, J. A., Sobel, J. D. *et al.* and the National Institute for Allergy and Infectious Diseases (NIAID) Mycoses Study Group. Prospective multicenter surveillance study of funguria in hospitalized patients. *Clin. Infect. Dis.* 2000; **30**: 14.

26. Page, C. P., Bohnen, J. M. A., Fletcher, J. R., McManus, A. T., Solomkin, J. S., & Wittmann, D. H. Antimicrobial prophylaxis for surgical wounds. *Arch. Surg.* 1993; **128**: 79.

27. Bratzler, D. W., Houck, P. M. for the Surgical Infection Prevention Guidelines Writers Group, Antimicrobial Prophylaxis for Surgery: an advisory statement from the National Surgical Infection Prevention Project. *Clin. Infect. Dis.* 2004; **38**: 1706–1715.

28. Classen, D. C., Evans, R. S., Pestotnik, S. L., Horn, S. D., Menlove, R. L., & Burke, J. P. The timing of prophylactic administration of antibiotics and the risk of surgical-wound infection. *N. Engl. J. Med.* 1992; **326**: 281.

29. Schaberg, D. R., Culver, D. H., & Gaynes, R. P. Major trends in the microbial etiology of nosocomial infection. *Am. J. Med.* 1991; **91**: 3B–73S.

30. NNIS System. National Nosocomial Infections Surveillance (NNIS) System Report, data summary from January 1992–June 2001, issued August 2001. *Am. J. Infect. Control* 2001; **29**: 404.

Renal disease

24

Surgery in the patient with renal disease

Jane Y. Yeun[1] and Burl R. Don[2]

[1]Department of Veterans Affairs Northern California Health Care System, Mather, CA and University of California Davis, Sacramento, CA
[2]University of California Davis, Sacramento, CA

Introduction

Kidney disease encompasses a wide spectrum of diseases: nephrotic syndrome or nephritic syndrome, mild chronic kidney disease (CKD) (Stage 1 and 2 $C_{Cr} \geq 0$ ml/min), moderate CKD (Stage 3 C_{Cr} 30–59 ml/min), severe CKD (Stage 4 C_{Cr} 15–29 ml/min), end-stage renal disease (ESRD) or CKD (Stage 5 $C_{Cr} < 15$ ml/min) on some form of renal replacement therapy, and acute renal failure (ARF). Since CKD, ESRD, and ARF are more common and have more associated perioperative complications, this discussion will focus on patients with renal failure.

In general, patients with CKD, ESRD, and ARF are subject to the same potential complications perioperatively. In the patients with ESRD, there are the added considerations of the dialysis modalities or kidney allograft. Where appropriate, these also will be addressed. However, a thorough discussion of the perioperative management of patients with functioning kidney allografts is beyond the scope of this chapter. Therefore, we will focus on general principles in managing transplant patients.

End-stage renal disease (ESRD) develops in about 3.3 in 10 000 Americans each year and has a four times higher incidence in blacks than in whites.[1] Diabetes mellitus and hypertension are the major causes of CKD and ESRD. More than 275 000 patients are now on dialysis, and the incidence is increasing by 3%–5% a year.[1] Patients with CKD and ESRD are becoming increasingly common as the patient population ages, concomitant with a potential need for more surgical interventions for coronary artery disease, peripheral vascular disease, and vascular access for dialysis. Despite the increase in this patient population, most of the literature is anecdotal and based on opinions and clinical practice.

Perioperative morbidity and mortality

The perioperative mortality is 4% for ESRD patients undergoing general surgery and 10% for cardiac surgery.[2] Not much is known about mortality in patients with CKD undergoing surgical procedures. However, morbidity is extremely high at >54% for general surgery in ESRD patients and >46% for cardiac surgery.[2] The goal of this review is to help reduce this unacceptably high morbidity.

Surgery in patients with kidney disease may be complicated by hyperkalemia, infections, hypotension or hypertension, bleeding, arrhythmias, or clotted fistulas. The complications result in part from an impaired ability of diseased kidneys to concentrate and dilute the urine; to regulate volume and sodium balance; to excrete acid, potassium, and medications; to synthesize erythropoietin; and to eliminate waste products that interfere with platelet and white blood cell function. Mortality usually results from a cardiovascular complication, hyperkalemia induced arrhythmia, or sepsis with associated multiorgan failure.[2–4]

Preoperative evaluation

The incidence of heart disease is high in patients with CKD, ESRD, and kidney transplant. Cardiac-related deaths account for over 50% of all deaths in the United States dialysis patient population.[5] Even patients with CKD not yet on dialysis[6–8] and successful kidney transplant[9] have a high incidence of cardiovascular complications. Concentric left ventricular hypertrophy is also highly prevalent in CKD and ESRD patients, up to 90% in some studies.[6,8,10] Therefore, a careful search for heart disease must be undertaken preoperatively and measures taken to

Table 24.1. Sensitivity and specificity of various cardiac screening tests in patients with kidney disease

Cardiac screening	"Gold standard"	Sensitivity	Specificity	NPV
Exercise thallium	Coronary angiogram[26]	50%	67%	
	Cardiovascular events[25]	88%	70%	86%
Persantine thallium	Coronary angiogram[16,26,31,35]	37–92%	37–89%	61–98%
	Cardiovascular events[27,31]	67–100%	81–88%	91–100%
Dobutamine stress echocardiography	Coronary angiogram[32,34,37]	75–95%	60–86%	57–97%
	Cardiovascular events[34,36]	52–82%	74%	80–94%
Persantine and exercise stress echocardiography	Coronary angiogram[17]	83%	84%	93%
	Cardiovascular events[17]	86%	94%	96%

Note:
NPV – negative predictive value.

ensure optimal cardiac function before any surgical procedure is performed.

The sections on "Preoperative testing" and "Cardiology in perioperative care of the surgical patient" (Part 1) of this textbook address many of these issues in detail for the general population undergoing surgery. However, important differences exist between patients with kidney disease and the general population. First, traditional cardiac risk factors such as hypertension, smoking, and hyperlipidemia poorly predict the presence of coronary artery disease in patients with kidney disease.[11] Second, 25% to 30% of dialysis patients with angina[12] and 25% to 50% of renal failure patients with an abnormal functional study[13–16] do not have significant coronary artery disease on angiogram, likely reflecting small vessel disease from severe left ventricular hypertrophy or diabetes. Third, about 20% of asymptomatic dialysis patients have evidence for coronary artery disease on cardiac catheterization.[17,18]

Although several studies have addressed the issue of cardiac evaluation in patients with kidney disease,[13–17,19–39] all have significant confounding variables. Many studies were small and retrospective in nature. Most studies included only patients already on dialysis, and dealt only with diabetic patients undergoing evaluation for kidney transplantation or combined kidney and pancreas transplantation, not for vascular access creation or other types of surgery. The "gold standard" employed in the studies differed significantly, ranging from subsequent clinical cardiac events to significant coronary artery stenosis by angiography or a combination of both. Given the high prevalence of demand ischemia from left ventricular hypertrophy and diabetic microvascular disease, angiography may not be the appropriate gold standard. Even if angiography is an appropriate gold standard, the studies that chose to use this modality did not perform an angiogram in all of their subjects. These study design flaws make interpretation of what little data are available even more difficult.

Cardiac screening tests in patients with kidney disease include exercise stress testing with thallium administration,[14,15,19,23–26] the dipyridamole thallium stress test,[13,15,16,20,26–31,33,35,39] the dobutamine stress echocardiography,[32,34,36,37] and more recently a combined dipyridamole and stress echocardiography.[17] Studies reporting the sensitivity, specificity, and negative predictive values or containing sufficient detail to allow their calculation are summarized in Table 24.1. None of the screening modalities offers absolute confidence in predicting the absence of significant coronary artery disease (defined as stenosis of >50%–75%). However, a negative screening test offers some reassurance (negative predictive value of 80%–100%) that the patient will not have an adverse cardiovascular event in the near future (variably defined as in the postoperative period up to several years). Many dialysis patients are unable to exercise sufficiently to achieve target heart rate and blood pressure, excluding the use of exercise stress testing. Dipyridamole radionuclide stress testing requires the use of isotopes and specialized imaging equipment that may not be widely available. Therefore, dobutamine stress echocardiography and exercise stress echocardiography, when appropriate, are gaining popularity.

Given the high prevalence of cardiovascular disease in patients with kidney disease and the low sensitivity of various screening tests in some studies, should all patients with kidney disease undergo cardiovascular risk stratification before elective surgery (Table 24.2)? Unfortunately, there are insufficient data to support or refute this approach. The cost obviously is very high. West *et al.*[37] only screened high-risk patients, defined as those patients having diabetes mellitus, prior myocardial infarction, age ≥50 years, cerebral and/or peripheral vascular disease,

Table 24.2. Potential criteria for selecting patients at high risk for cardiac events to improve cost-effectiveness for further cardiac screening

West[37]	Le[20]	UC Davis
Age ≥50 years	Age ≥50 years	Age ≥65 years
Diabetes mellitus	Diabetes mellitus I	Diabetes mellitus and peripheral vascular disease
Class I or II angina	Angina	Functional class III or IV angina
Myocardial infarction	Congestive heart failure	Congestive heart failure from systolic dysfunction
Peripheral vascular disease	Abnormal EKG (other than left ventricular hypertrophy)	
Cerebral vascular disease		
Congestive heart failure		
Dialysis >5 years		

congestive heart failure, class I or II angina, or on dialysis >5 years, with dobutamine stress echocardiography prior to kidney transplantation. Unfortunately, the authors do not report on the cardiovascular outcome of the 91 out of 133 dialysis patients who did not undergo non-invasive studies to assess for coronary artery disease. Le et al.[20] defined kidney transplant candidates as being at high risk for a cardiac event if they have any of the following characteristics: age ≥50 years, history of angina, insulin-dependent diabetes, congestive heart failure, or an abnormal electrocardiogram (other than left ventricular hypertrophy). After 4 years of follow-up, patients in the low-risk group (e.g., none of the above characteristics) had a 1% cardiac mortality, compared with 17% in the high-risk group.

At our center, in collaboration with cardiology and transplant surgery, we recently established new guidelines to screen for patients at high risk of cardiovascular complications in preparation for vascular access surgery: age >65 years, history of angina, history of congestive heart failure due to systolic dysfunction, class III or IV symptoms of angina (symptoms of chest discomfort or dyspnea with daily activity or at rest, respectively), and a combination of diabetes and peripheral vascular disease. Patients meeting any of these criteria undergo further work-up with a dobutamine stress echocardiogram prior to surgery. The new guidelines were prompted by an overwhelming demand for preoperative dobutamine stress echocardiogram, resulting in unacceptable delays in surgery. No data are yet available as to the efficacy of these guidelines.

In summary, given the high risk for cardiovascular complications in patients with kidney disease, they must be screened to identify those at high risk of having an adverse cardiovascular event perioperatively. Patients at low risk (Table 24.2) need no further cardiac evaluation prior to surgery. Patients at high risk should be further risk stratified using dobutamine stress echocardiography, exercise radionuclide stress testing, or dipyridamole radionuclide stress testing, depending on their ability to exercise and the availability of the test. A subgroup of patients at very high risk of an adverse cardiac event (symptoms of unstable angina) should be considered for coronary angiography without non-invasive testing. It is unclear at this time whether patients with renal disease should undergo such screening even for minor surgical procedures such as vascular access surgery.

In patients with moderate to high risk of having a perioperative cardiac event, beta blockade therapy prior to high risk surgery (intraperitoneal, intrathoracic, or suprainginal vascular procedures) reduces the cardiac risk.[39a] Although patients with kidney disease were not studied specifically, creatinine ≥2 mg/dl has been identified as a risk factor for perioperative cardiac event.[39a] Therefore, beta blocker therapy should be considered in CKD patients at moderate to high risk for a cardiac event who are undergoing major surgery.

Perioperative considerations

Management of volume status

Perioperatively, it is important to ensure that the patient is euvolemic. Volume overload may lead to poorly controlled hypertension and hypoxia either during surgery or afterwards. Typically, dependent edema in the lower extremities or the sacral area is present, and may be accompanied by hypertension, pulmonary rales, and distended jugular veins. If pulmonary edema is present, congestive heart failure must be ruled out since congestive heart failure will require therapy in addition to diuretics.

In the CKD or ARF patients not requiring dialysis, volume overload is managed with salt and fluid restriction (2 g sodium diet, 1 l fluid) and diuretics, administered either orally or intravenously. Loop diuretics are the most potent and are the diuretic of choice. Since diuretics must be filtered by the glomeruli and/or secreted by the tubular cells into the tubular lumen to be effective, the dose of diuretic given must be appropriate for the degree of kidney failure. The worse the kidney function, the higher the dose of diuretics needed for the desired effect.[40] When C_{Cr} is less than 25 ml/min, furosemide dose in excess of 120 mg and bumetanide dose in excess of 3 mg may be required. Occasionally, metolazone (5–10 mg orally) or chlorothiazide (250–500 mg intravenously) is given 30 minutes before the loop diuretic to augment the diuretic response. Although loop diuretics, particularly in high doses, are associated with ototoxicity, toxicity is generally in the setting of concomitant administration of other ototoxic drugs or bolus injection of the loop diuretic.[40,41] The high peak serum level after intravenous bolus is thought to be the most important factor. Doses in excess of 80 mg should be infused over 30 minutes in a small amount of fluid. When high doses of loop diuretics are necessary to maintain diuresis, a continuous infusion may be preferable because it decreases the total daily dose required to achieve the same diuretic response. After a bolus of 40–80 mg to help achieve steady state blood levels, furosemide is administered continuously at a rate of 10–20 mg/h. If the desired diuresis is not achieved after 2 hours, a repeat bolus should be given and the infusion rate increased by 10–20 mg/h. If excessive diuresis ensues, the infusion rate can be decreased.

Based on clinical experience, patients with ESRD should undergo dialysis within 24 hours of surgery to optimize volume status. Concomitant dietary sodium (2 g) and fluid (1 l) restrictions are very important adjuncts to dialysis. Patients on peritoneal dialysis should have their peritoneal dialysate drained shortly before going to the operating room. Prolonged dwelling time of dialysate in the peritoneum will dissipate the glucose gradient and result in absorption of the peritoneal fluid, contributing to volume overload. In addition, the presence of a large amount of fluid in the abdomen may compromise lung function during surgery.

Excessive fluid removal with diuretics or dialysis before surgery may lead to hypotension perioperatively. Anesthetics administered during surgery may cause vasodilation, which will aggravate hypotension. Fluid sequestration after surgery will further deplete the intravascular volume and also exacerbate hypotension.

Maintenance intravenous fluids should be no more than 0.5 l a day to replace insensible fluid losses. If the patient has large amounts of fluid loss through nasogastric suctioning, high fevers, abdominal drainage, significant urine output, diarrhea, or other additional sources of fluid loss, these also should be replaced. Otherwise, the frequently used 75–125 ml/h of maintenance fluid will lead to pulmonary edema and hypertension in patients on dialysis or with oliguric ARF. The type of fluid used is also important. If the patient has hypotonic losses, then replacement fluid should be with a hypotonic solution such as 0.45% sodium chloride. If only the minimal maintenance fluid (0.5 l a day) is required, 0.9% NaCl solution may be more appropriate to prevent development of hyponatremia (see below).

Control of hypertension

In general, hypertension in patients with kidney disease may be managed in the same manner as for patients without kidney disease (see Chapter 8). However, there are a number of points that bear special emphasis.

Given the high incidence of cardiovascular disease in patients with renal disease, patients on β-blockers preoperatively should be kept on them intraoperatively and postoperatively. If the patient cannot take medications orally, metoprolol and esmolol are available as intravenous preparations. Esmolol is usually given as a continuous intravenous infusion because of its very short half-life.

Postoperative hypertension may be difficult to control in patients with renal disease.[42] Pain, anxiety, and volume overload may be significant contributing factors to hypertension.[42] Adequate pain control and judicious use of anxiolytics and loop diuretics may help to control blood pressure in the immediate postoperative period. For patients on dialysis, dialysis is indicated for control of hypertension if there is significant volume overload.

In patients on clonidine preoperatively, severe rebound hypertension may occur if clonidine is stopped abruptly. Rebound hypertension is especially a concern at a dose of ≥ 0.6 mg a day. Such patients should have a clonidine patch substituted for the oral medication at least 1 day before the surgery, to allow the patch to achieve therapeutic blood levels of clonidine prior to surgery.

Frequently used intravenous medications for treating hypertension postoperatively include β-blockers (metoprolol, esmolol, and labetolol), enalaprilat, hydralazine, and nitroprusside.[42] Beta-blockers are first line agents in patients with tachycardia or ischemia postoperatively, or a history of coronary artery disease and angina. Patients with a history of systolic dysfunction should be treated with enalaprilat for blood pressure control if intravenous medications are needed, unless there is intervening ARF. If possible, hydralazine should be avoided in patients with renal disease because it may cause significant reflex tachycardia and aggravate cardiac ischemia. Lastly, nitroprusside should be reserved for severe hypertension that cannot be controlled by other means, because of the increased risk of thiocyanate and cyanide toxicity in patients with impaired kidney function.[43] In general, nitroprusside should not be administered continuously for more than 48 hours in patients with renal failure. If longer administration is required, close monitoring of thiocyanate level is mandatory. If and when nitroprusside is initiated, simultaneous initiation or dose escalation of oral or other intravenous antihypertensive medications is mandatory to allow titration off of nitroprusside as soon as possible.

Electrolyte, mineral, and acid–base status

Sodium and water disorders

Patients with kidney disease generally do not have problems handling water until creatinine clearance (C_{Cr}) is below 10–15 ml/min, by which time they are generally on dialysis. However, patients with severe renal failure (creatinine clearance ($C_{Cr} < 25$ ml/min)) have little renal reserve and may not be able to excrete an acute water load rapidly,[42] leading to hyponatremia. Factors commonly seen in the postoperative setting such as pain, stress, and nausea may lower serum sodium further by increasing the release of antidiuretic hormone. Because of an intact thirst mechanism in ambulatory patients, hypernatremia is usually not a problem in patients with renal failure. In a postoperative patient in the intensive care unit, hypernatremia may ensue, especially in the setting of significant free water losses from diarrhea, continuous nasogastric suctioning, diuresis with loop diuretics, insensible fluid losses (fever, open wound), osmotic diuresis from hyperglycemia or other osmotic agents (mannitol, contrast). Factors such as intubation and altered mental status may further contribute to the problem by blunting thirst.

Postoperative patients with impaired kidney function should receive sufficient intravenous fluids for (a) insensible fluid losses, approximately 0.5 l of 0.45% NaCl solution, and (b) replacement of fluids lost from other sources, such as urine, wound drainage, fistula drainage, and gastrointestinal tract.[44] Close monitoring of serum chemistries and volume status will allow adjustment of the rate of intravenous infusion as well as type of fluid administered. Dialysis patients without urine output should receive no more than 1 l of fluid a day, unless there are significant fluid losses from other sources. If more than 0.5 l of intravenous fluid is necessary in a dialysis patient, it should be administered as an isotonic solution such as 0.9% NaCl unless there is significant hypotonic fluid losses. The anuric patient is unable to excrete the excess free water present in 0.45% NaCl beyond the 0.5 l or so of insensible fluid loss and will develop hyponatremia. When the patient resumes oral intake, intravenous fluids should be discontinued and the patient placed on a 1 l/day fluid restriction to avoid volume overload or water balance disorders. The daily fluid restriction encompasses both the patient's oral intake as well as any intravenous fluids accompanying administration of heparin, antibiotics, parenteral nutrition, or other medication.

Patients with renal failure and volume overload and/or congestive heart failure being treated with loop diuretics should be monitored closely with serum electrolytes, because loop diuretics tend to generate a hypotonic urine.[42] If hypernatremia ensues, the patient should receive an infusion of at least 0.5 ml of 5% dextrose in water for each milliliter of urine to prevent worsening hypernatremia. Additional free water must be administered to correct the hypernatremia. Often, there is concern that administration of 5% dextrose in water will worsen the congestive heart failure, but only 83 ml of one liter of water remains in the intravascular space. The remainder distributes to the interstitial and intracellular fluid compartments.

Potassium disorders

Perioperatively, hyperkalemia is more common than hypokalemia in patients with kidney disease. Unless the patient is diabetic and has a Type IV renal tubular acidosis, hyperkalemia generally does not occur until C_{Cr} is below 20 ml/min.[45] As with water handling, renal reserve is decreased and the diseased kidneys may not be able to excrete an acute potassium load. In addition, patients with CKD and ESRD may have a defect in non-renal potassium homeostasis (impaired response to insulin, catecholamines, and/or aldosterone), such that potassium shifts less readily from the intravascular into the intracellular compartment.[46] These two impaired limbs of potassium homeostasis may act in concert to cause life-threatening hyperkalemia in the postoperative period.

Sources of potassium in perioperative patients include (a) administration in intravenous fluid, total parenteral nutrition, or enteral nutrition, (b) increased catabolism, (c) red blood cell transfusion, (d) reabsorption of hematoma, (e) tissue breakdown, and (f) red blood cell salvage and re-infusion intraoperatively (Table 24.3). If hypokalemia is not present, routine supplementation of intravenous fluids and total parenteral nutrition with potassium should be avoided. With advanced CKD and ESRD, enteral nutrition preparations containing the least amount of potassium is preferred. Dialysis patients should receive the freshest blood available to minimize the amount of potassium infused. If possible, blood should be transfused during dialysis to allow simultaneous removal of the

Table 24.3. Causes of perioperative hyperkalemia

Mechanism	Cause
Increased potassium load	Increased catabolism
	Blood transfusion
	Reabsorption of hematoma
	Tissue breakdown
	Red blood cell salvage
	Potassium administration
Impaired transcellular potassium shift	Fasting state (insulinopenia)
	β-blockers
Decreased potassium excretion	Volume depletion
	Constipation
	Medications
	Trimethoprim-sulfamethoxazole
	Potassium sparing diuretics
	Angiotensin converting
	enzyme inhibitors
	Angiotensin receptor blockers

excess volume and potassium. However, blood transfusion during heparin-free dialysis can increase the risk of dialyzer thrombosis because of the high viscosity of packed red blood cells.

Potassium elimination may be reduced perioperatively through volume depletion in patients with CKD (Table 24.3). Volume depletion limits renal potassium excretion because distal sodium delivery is required to allow exchange of potassium for sodium.[42] Constipation is another important cause of hyperkalemia in patients with severe CKD and ESRD.[42,47] Unlike subjects with normal kidney function who eliminate 10% of their daily potassium load through the gastrointestinal tract, patients with advancing renal failure secrete 30%–40% of their daily potassium load in the colon. Constipation limits potassium secretion into the gastrointestinal tract. Medications that limit renal potassium secretion, such as trimethoprim/sulfamethoxazole, potassium sparing diuretics, angiotensin converting enzyme inhibitors, and angiotensin receptor blockers, will worsen hyperkalemia. Medications that antagonize aldosterone action also will exacerbate hyperkalemia through inhibition of colonic secretion of potassium.

Basal levels of insulin is vital to the cellular uptake of potassium (Table 24.3).[46,48] When patients with CKD and ESRD fast, insulin release is suppressed, leading to hyperkalemia.[49] Administering a glucose containing solution to fasting patients will prevent this occurrence.

Previously, metabolic acidosis was thought to cause hyperkalemia through shift of potassium from the intracellular to the extracellular compartment. It is now clear that organic metabolic acidosis (lactic acidosis, ketoacidosis alone, and acidosis from renal failure) does not cause such a potassium shift.[45,50] This has obvious implications for the treatment of hyperkalemia.

Treatment of hyperkalemia in the postoperative period is identical to that in other situations.[42,50] Intravenous calcium gluconate is administered acutely to stabilize the myocardial cell membrane should there be electrocardiographic changes. Insulin and 50% dextrose is administered intravenously to shift the potassium intracellularly. Inhaled β-agonists will shift potassium intracellularly as well. Intravenous bicarbonate may not lower the potassium level and should be used only as an adjunct to other treatment for hyperkalemia.[46,50,51] Cation exchange resins such as polystyrene (Kayexalate) to remove potassium can be given either orally or as a retention enema if oral therapy is not possible. When given orally, sorbitol must accompany the polystyrene. Additional doses of sorbitol should be given if the patient does not have a bowel movement within 1–2 hours. Transplant patients requiring a retention enema must receive only the cation exchange resin without the sorbitol because of reported cases of colonic perforation when the two are given concomitantly.[52] In cases of severe hyperkalemia (>7 meq/l) or contraindication to the use of cation exchange resin, dialysis should be instituted.

Hypokalemia usually results from aggressive diuresis or diarrhea in the perioperative period. Frequent use of inhaled β-agonists also may cause hypokalemia. Given the high incidence of cardiovascular disease in patients with renal disease, hypokalemia, even in dialysis patients, should be treated with cautious potassium repletion. The impaired transcellular shift of potassium makes it imperative that only small doses of potassium be given at a time, not to exceed 40 meq orally or 10 meq intravenously, with sufficient elapsed time between doses. Rapid administration of potassium will result in iatrogenic hyperkalemia.

Magnesium disorders

Patients with severe CKD and ESRD are unable to excrete magnesium. Therefore, medications such as milk of magnesia, magnesium citrate, and magnesium-containing antacids should not be used. Constipation may be treated with sorbitol, lactulose, and polyethylene glycol solutions (Colyte, Miralax), or with enemas that do not contain phosphorus. Aluminum containing antacids may be used in the short term instead of magnesium-containing antacids, but will result in aluminum toxicity with prolonged use (more than 3–6 months). If stronger anti-acid treatment is needed, proton pump inhibitors and H_2-blockers may be used, keeping in mind that cimetidine and raniti-dine are cleared by the kidney and may cause altered mental status.

Phosphorus disorders

Impaired phosphorus excretion occurs at a $C_{Cr} < 40$ ml/min, but hyperphosphatemia is not seen clinically until a $C_{Cr} < 25$ ml/min. The main concern of acute hyper-phosphatemia is symptomatic hypocalcemia, sufficient to cause cardiac arrhythmias.[53] Chronic hyperphosphatemia causes secondary hyperparathyroidism, increased bone turnover, and metastatic calcification in tissues.[54] Calcium phosphate may deposit in the skin causing pruritus, in the eye giving conjunctivitis, in the heart leading to conduction system disease, in the joint causing a crystal-line arthropathy, and in blood vessels leading to peripheral ischemia.

As soon as patients with severe renal function impairment begin eating, phosphate binders should be restarted. The binders must be given with meals to precipitate with the phosphorus in food and prevent its absorption.[55] Many different types of binders are available: calcium carbonate, calcium acetate, aluminum hydroxide, and sevelamer. Because calcium carbonate is not very effective at phosphate binding[56] compared with calcium acetate or aluminum hydroxide, more of the calcium is available for absorption and may give rise to hypercalcemia. This is obviously undesirable if the phosphorus levels are ele-vated and/or the calcium × phosphorus product exceeds 60, as metastatic calcification may occur. Aluminum hydroxide is the most effective phosphate binder, but longterm use (>3–6 months) may result in aluminum toxicity.[57] Aluminum toxicity can occur acutely if a citrate-containing medication (sodium, potassium, or cal-cium citrate) is given concomitantly with the aluminum.[58] Citrate chelates calcium in the gastrointestinal tract, thereby opening up tight junctions in the mucosa and allowing rapid absorption of aluminum. Sevelamer is a non-calcium and non-aluminum containing resin that selectively binds phosphate, avoiding the problems of excessive calcium and aluminum administration. Unlike aluminum hydroxide solutions or calcium tablets or solu-tions, sevelamer cannot be administered via a nasogastric tube and would be of no use as a phosphate binder in postoperative patients receiving nasogastric feeding. Like all resins, sevelamer quickly becomes a gelatinous mass when exposed to water. In general, if phosphate is <6 mg/dl and the product <60, any of the above binders may be used. If either is high, then aluminum hydroxide or seve-lamer is the initial choice, keeping in mind that sevelamer is not as effective as aluminum at phosphate binding.

Once the phosphate and the product is lower, another binder should be substituted for aluminum hydroxide.

Dietary phosphorus intake must be restricted to less than 700 mg a day. Common sources of phosphorus include cola drinks, milk products, and protein sources including beans and legumes. In addition, some of the enemas such as Fleet's enema or Phosphosoda contain large amounts of phosphorus and must be avoided in patients with renal failure. In severe cases of hyperphos-phatemia, continuous dialysis or extended daily dialysis (see below) will effectively correct the phosphate within two to three days.[59,60]

Rarely, hypophosphatemia occurs. Refeeding hypophos-phatmia is the likely cause if the patient is nutritionally depleted and begins feeding.[61] Another common cause is the use of continuous or extended hemodialysis treat-ments since these modalities may remove large amounts of phosphorus.[59] Lastly, sucrafate, used in the intensive care unit as gastrointestinal bleeding prophylaxis, is an excellent phosphate binder and can cause hypophosphatemia.[62]

Calcium disorders

New onset hypercalcemia is unusual in the perioperative patient with acute or chronic renal failure, since patients with renal failure tend to be hypocalcemic. Hypercalcemia noted preoperatively is likely due to (a) continued use of calcium containing phosphate binders despite poor oral intake, allowing the calcium to be absorbed, (b) excessive calcitriol administration which responds quickly to with-holding the calcitriol, and (c) severe secondary or tertiary hyperparathyroidism, as in the ESRD patient awaiting para-thyroidectomy. De novo hypercalcemia rarely may be seen in the setting of prolonged immobilization.[63] Treatment consists of removing calcium containing drugs, vitamin D analogues, and dialysis against a low calcium dialysate in severe cases. The hypercalcemia from prolonged immobi-lization may respond to bisphosphonate therapy,[64] such as pamidronate or alendronate. Renal dose adjustment for alendronate is 5 mg orally daily. It is unknown whether weekly administration of alendronate is safe.

Hypocalcemia most commonly occurs as a result of hyperphosphatemia, and should not be treated with intra-venous calcium because of the risk of precipitating meta-static calcification, unless life-threatening arrhythmias are present. Instead, efforts should be directed at correcting the hyperphosphatemia. Use of regional citrate antico-agulation (see below) may also lead to symptomatic and/ or life-threatening hypocalcemia and should be corrected by raising the calcium infusion rate. Finally, patients who undergo parathyroidectomy to treat severe secondary or tertiary hyperparathyroidism can develop severe hypocalcemia from the "hungry bone syndrome."[65] They require large amounts of elemental calcium and calcitriol. Initially, the calcium may need to be administered as an infusion, until the patient stabilizes on oral doses of calcium administered apart from meals and calcitriol. Hemodialysis against a higher dialysate calcium concentration will correct severe hypocalcemia quickly.

Acid–base status

Patients with renal failure usually have a mild metabolic acidosis because of the accumulation of non-volatile acids resulting from the metabolism of food (about 1 mmol/kg per day). In most cases, the acidosis can be corrected easily by oral base supplementation (e.g., sodium bicarbonate) or by dialysis. If stable patients with renal failure develop progressive acidosis, other causes should be vigorously investigated. These include lactic acidosis, ketoacidosis, intoxications (e.g., ethylene glycol), and severe diarrhea.

A fall in arterial pH to less than 7.10 can precipitate potentially fatal ventricular arrhythmias and reduce both cardiac contractility and inotropic response to catecholamines.[66–68] Neurologic symptoms ranging from lethargy to coma have been described in patients with metabolic acidosis, which appear to be related to a decrease in cerebrospinal fluid pH.[69] The initial goal in the management of severe metabolic acidosis (blood pH less than 7.2) is to treat the underlying cause. The next important step in managing profound metabolic acidosis in a ventilated patient is vigorous use of the ventilator to augment carbon dioxide excretion by the lungs. Increasing ventilation to lower the pCO_2 is a very powerful treatment in ameliorating the severity of the metabolic acidosis and is frequently underutilized in the surgical intensive care unit for the management of metabolic acidosis. For example, a patient with a pCO_2 of 38 mm Hg and bicarbonate level of 10 mmol/l will have a pH of 7.04. Simply increasing the ventilation to lower the pCO_2 to 25 mm Hg will increase the pH to 7.23 and quickly attenuates the severity of the profound metabolic acidosis.

Metabolic acidosis in the perioperative patient with either acute or chronic renal failure can be effectively treated with acute hemodialysis or hemofiltration with bicarbonate-containing replacement fluids, which is the treatment of choice. If the patient has a profound metabolic acidosis (pH < 7.10) and dialysis treatment has not been initiated, administering intravenous sodium bicarbonate may help raise the pH to a safer level (>7.20) at which abnormalities in cardiovascular function become less likely. Another indication for sodium bicarbonate therapy is in patients with metabolic acidosis due to massive gastrointestinal bicarbonate loss from severe diarrhea.

However, rapid intravenous administration of bicarbonate can lead to fluid overload, worsening tissue oxygenation, hypokalemia, and worsening cerebrospinal fluid acidosis (because the blood–brain barrier is more permeable to CO_2 than to bicarbonate).[67] To minimize these complications, intravenous bicarbonate therapy either should be stopped or infused at a much slower rate once the blood pH has reached 7.2. Other complications of treatment with sodium bicarbonate include hypernatremia (if hypertonic bicarbonate solutions are used), hyponatremia (if hypotonic solutions are used), and metabolic alkalosis (if excessive bicarbonate is given). In addition, there is ongoing controversy concerning the use of sodium bicarbonate therapy in patients with lactic acidosis. Based on a number of experimental and clinical studies, bicarbonate therapy in the setting of lactic acidosis only transiently increases serum bicarbonate levels but worsens intracellular acidosis.[70] However, if the lactic acidosis is profound (pH < 7.10), bicarbonate should be administered judiciously to attenuate the severity of the acidosis and its untoward effects on cardiovascular function.[71,72]

Although equations exist to allow calculations of the bicarbonate deficit,[72] serial measurements of the blood pH and serum bicarbonate are mandatory to monitor the rate and extent of correction of the metabolic acidosis.

Another option for the treatment of metabolic acidosis is the use of tromethamine (THAM). THAM is an inert amino alcohol that buffers both acids and CO_2 by accepting a proton forming $THAM\text{-}NH_3^+$.[73] The drug has been used to treat severe acidosis but its clinical efficacy compared to the use of sodium bicarbonate is unproven. In addition, serious side effects include hyperkalemia, hypoglycemia, and respiratory depression.

Metabolic alkalosis in patients with renal failure is usually caused by acid losses from vomiting, nasogastric suction, or diuretic use (in those with predialysis disease). The administration of excessive alkali (e.g., sodium bicarbonate, citrate-anticoagulated blood transfusion) also causes metabolic alkalosis because excretion of bicarbonate is markedly reduced in patients with renal failure. Treatment must be directed at the underlying cause. If patients are volume depleted or hypokalemic, then careful volume expansion with isotonic saline or supplementation with potassium chloride is indicated. Hemodialysis or hydrochloric acid administration can be used to treat symptomatic or severe alkalosis.[74]

Management of nutrition in the perioperative patient

Malnutrition is a common problem in patients with either acute or chronic renal failure. Approximately one-third of chronic dialysis patients are malnourished, due to a combination of factors including poor nutritional intake, protein losses during dialysis, and increased catabolism.[75] Decreased serum albumin levels are strong predictors of mortality and hospitalization in chronic dialysis patients. The risk of mortality increases as serum albumin decreases below 4.0 g/dl, doubles in patients with a serum albumin between 3.5 and 4.0 g/dl, and is 15-fold higher when albumin falls below 3.0 g/dl range.[76] Recently, it has been recognized that a substantial number of ESRD patients appear to have serologic evidence of an augmented inflammatory state with activation of the systemic inflammatory response. Moreover, it appears that inflammation may be as or more important than protein intake in causing hypoalbuminemia.[77]

Patients with ESRD undergoing surgical procedures need to receive adequate protein and calorie intake. One problem with dietary intake recommendations for malnourished dialysis patients is choosing the appropriate weight to compute protein and caloric needs, since the actual body weight reflects the effects of malnutrition. Protein and caloric intake estimates should be based on average body weight for healthy subjects of the same sex, height, age, and body frame.[78] The dialysis outcomes quality initiative (DOQI)[79] recommends that stable hemodialysis patients should ingest 1.2 g of protein per kilogram of average body weight per day (g/kg per day), and peritoneal dialysis patients 1.5 g/kg per day because of increased protein losses in the dialysate. At least 50% of the protein should be of high biologic value. Caloric intake should be 35 kcal/kg per day in dialysis patients less than 60 years of age and 30–35 kcal/kg per day in those over 60 years,[79] because this level of caloric intake is necessary to maintain neutral nitrogen balance and prevent protein breakdown in dialysis patients. At least half of the calorie intake should be from carbohydrates.

For the surgical patient with acute renal failure or ESRD, both the caloric and protein requirements are much greater because of increased catabolism, protein losses, and higher energy demands. Rocco and Blumenkrantz[78] have adapted adjustment factors from the literature for determining energy requirements (non-protein calories) in patients with renal failure (Table 24.4). The amino acid or protein requirements for these patients should be in the range of 1.2 to 2.0 g/kg per day. For patients with acute renal failure, augmenting protein intake beyond these levels does not improve nitrogen balance or survival[80] and serves only to increase nitrogenous waste products and hence the uremic environment.

Perioperative patients with either acute or chronic renal failure who are unable to ingest sufficient calories and

Table 24.4. Adjustment factors for determining energy requirements

Clinical condition	Adjustment factor
Mechanical ventilation	
Without sepsis	1.10–1.20
With sepsis	1.25–1.35
Peritonitis	1.15
Infection	
Mild	1.00–1.10
Moderate	1.10–1.20
Sepsis	1.20–1.30
Soft-tissue trauma	1.10
Bone fractures	1.15
Burns (% of body surface area)	
0%–20%	1.15
20%–40%	1.50
40%–100%	1.70

Source: From ref. 78, p. 437.

protein may require nasogastric or parenteral nutritional support. When initiating nutritional support, special attention should be given to the potassium, sodium, phosphorus, and free water content of the solution to avoid precipitating electrolyte disturbances (see above).

Management of anemia in the perioperative patient

Anemia in renal disease is due mainly to insufficient production of erythropoietin by the diseased kidney. Other factors may contribute to the anemia including folate and vitamin B_{12} deficiency, chronic gastrointestinal bleeding, shortened red blood cell survival, and uremic inhibition of red cell synthesis.[81] The development of recombinant erythropoietin (EPO) was one the greatest advances in the care of this population since the advent of chronic dialysis.[82] Patients with ESRD or advanced CKD admitted for surgical procedures should be maintained on their outpatient EPO regimen, generally administered two to three times a week either subcutaneously or intravenously and titrated to achieve a target hematocrit of 33%–36%.[83] The stimulation of erythropoiesis usually depletes iron stores and periodic parenteral iron administration may be required. The rate of rise in hematocrit is dose dependent but should not exceed 1%–3% per week, since higher rates of rise may result in severe hypertension and seizures. If the perioperative patient with renal disease is profoundly anemic (hematocrit <25%), treatment with EPO may not raise the hematocrit fast enough to prevent perioperative complications from the anemia, especially in patients with underlying cardiac disease or where significant surgical blood loss is anticipated. Blood transfusions are usually required for these patients to raise the hematocrit quickly to a safer level (>30%).

Erythropoietin can be used in patients with ARF although there is a paucity of studies evaluating its use in this setting. Perioperative patients with either acute or chronic renal failure may be resistant to EPO if infection or surgery-induced inflammation is present. Higher doses of EPO may overcome such resistance. Percent iron saturation and ferritin levels should be obtained to evaluate iron stores since relative or absolute iron deficiency is another major cause of EPO resistance. Criteria and treatment protocols for management of iron deficiency are discussed in the DOQI guidelines.[83]

Bleeding diathesis

Patient with either acute or chronic renal failure can manifest derangement in hemostasis with impairment in clot formation in response to vascular injury.[84] Many factors contribute to impairment in clot formation, which largely revolve around defects in platelet function. Platelet aggregation is abnormal in patients with renal failure and may be due to reduced intraplatelet adenosine diphosphate (ADP) and serotonin levels, and defective thromboxane A_2 production. An adhesion receptor, the glycoprotein IIb-IIIa complex, is a key component in controlling the formation of platelet thrombi. For patients with either acute or chronic renal failure, activation of this receptor complex is impaired leading to prolonged bleeding time.[11,85,86] In addition, abnormalities in von Willebrand factor and increased production of nitric oxide have been implicated and contribute to the bleeding diathesis of uremia.[87] Finally, anemia, especially when the hematocrit is less than 30%, appears to impair platelet aggregation leading to prolonged bleeding time.[84]

The perioperative evaluation of any potential coagulopathy in the patient with either acute or chronic renal failure should entail measurement of the platelet count, prothrombin time and partial thromboplastin time. These values should be within the normal range even for patients with renal failure unless there is an additional pathologic process such as liver disease or disseminated intravascular clotting. An important point is that patients with renal failure have a qualitative disorder and platelet counts are normal in this population unless another disease process is present. This bleeding diathesis can be assessed by measuring skin bleeding time.[88] The risk for hemorrhage is increased when the bleeding time exceeds 10 minutes.

Practically, bleeding times are not commonly performed perioperatively, because of the general assumption that there is a bleeding diathesis and that active bleeding should be treated promptly and not delayed by tests. Moreover, bleeding times do not necessarily correlate with clinical bleed events.

Preoperatively, the bleeding diathesis can be mitigated to some extent by performing hemodialysis prior to surgery. Patients who are markedly uremic with very high blood urea nitrogen levels (>100 mg/dl) may benefit from more than one dialysis treatment prior to a major surgical procedure, if time permits, to minimize whatever component the uremic milieu may be contributing to the bleeding diathesis. Postoperatively, if bleeding is still an active issue, intensive dialysis support should be continued to help improve platelet function.[89]

Severely anemic patients with renal failure should receive blood transfusions prior to surgery to achieve a hematocrit of >30%. The increase in hematocrit forces the platelets to flow along the periphery of the blood vessel, making the platelets readily available should the blood vessel become disrupted. This hematocrit should be maintained during the perioperative period to help minimize bleeding.

For the perioperative patient with renal failure who is either actively bleeding or at high risk for bleeding during a major surgical procedure, the administration of either cryoprecipitate or desamino-8-D-arginine vasopressin (DDAVP) can be effective in improving the qualitative platelet defect of uremia.[84,85,90] Cryoprecipitate is a pooled plasma fraction enriched with factor VIII and von Willebrand factor and has been demonstrated to improve bleeding times. The effect is apparent 1 hour after infusion of ten units with a peak effect between 4 and 12 hours. DDAVP induces the release of endogenous von Willebrand factor. When given intravenously in a dose of 0.3 µg/kg, the bleeding time begins to decrease by 1 hour with a duration of 6–8 hours. A similar effect can be achieved with subcutaneous administration, but the onset of action is delayed by 2 hours. Repeated administration of DDAVP more often than every 48 hours results in decreased efficacy, probably due to depletion of endogenous stores of von Willebrand factor.

Conjugated estrogens also improve bleeding times in patients with renal failure. Although the onset of action is much slower with estrogens compared with DDAVP or cryoprecipitate, the duration of action is much longer (7–10 days). The use of conjugated estrogens may be helpful in improving the bleeding diathesis in renal failure patients undergoing elective procedures with a high risk for bleeding, since the drug can be started 1 week prior to the planned surgery. It may also be beneficial in improving the bleed diathesis in renal failure patients with prolonged postoperative bleeding and is given as conjugated estrogen 0.6 mg/kg intravenously daily for 5 days.[85,91]

The use of anticoagulation during hemodialysis for the perioperative patient with either acute or chronic renal failure may contribute to the bleeding diathesis. For a full discussion, see the section below.

Medical imaging in the perioperative patient with renal disease

Risk of acute renal failure with medical imaging

Medical imaging in the perioperative patients with renal disease may result in worsening renal function because of the use of iodinated radiocontrast agents. The mechanism is not well understood but is probably due to intense renal vasoconstriction and/or direct tubular toxicity. The renal vasoconstriction may result from contrast-induced release of endothelin and adenosine, although there is controversy as to the role of endothelin in ARF.

Risk factors for developing ARF following iodinated radiocontrast agents include: (a) underlying CKD (plasma creatinine >1.5 mg/dl), (b) diabetic nephropathy with renal insufficiency, (c) hypovolemia or impaired renal perfusion, (d) volume of contrast administered, and (e) presence of multiple myeloma.[92,93] Since perioperative patients may be intravascularly volume depleted, especially in the setting of trauma, they are at increased risk for contrast-induced ARF. The risk increases further if the patient has concomitant preexisting CKD and/or diabetic nephropathy.

Worsening of renal function from radiocontrast agents usually begins soon after the infusion of the contrast (<24 hours), peaks in 2–3 days, and resolves over the next 3 to 5 days. Complete recovery with renal function returning to baseline levels is the norm. Patients are usually non-oliguric and the majority does not require dialysis. However, if the patient has advanced renal failure (creatinine >4 mg/dl) at baseline, there may be insufficient renal reserve to avoid dialysis.

The use of iodinated contrast agents is not contraindicated in dialysis patients since they are committed already to long-term renal replacement therapy. However, contrast may reduce further any residual renal function of the native kidneys. It is important for the non-nephrologist to appreciate that residual renal function does help in the overall solute clearance and volume removal and may be critical in peritoneal dialysis patients. Despite this caveat, the benefits of a radiocontrast-requiring imaging study probably outweigh any theoretical concern for loss of residual renal function. In addition, the belief that

dialysis should be performed immediately following contrast administration is unfounded.[94] By the time dialysis begins (at least 30 minutes after contrast administration), the contrast has circulated already through the kidneys innumerable times. The effectiveness of hemodialysis in removing contrast media depends on many factors, including the protein binding, hydrophilicity, and electrical charge of the contrast medium, and several sessions are required to remove the contrast completely.

Prevention and treatment of contrast-induced acute renal failure

As discussed above, the use of iodinated radiocontrast agents mainly impacts patients with CKD and/or diabetic nephropathy, exacerbated in the perioperative patient by the potential for intravascular volume depletion. When one or more risk factors are present in a perioperative patient, use of an alternative medical imaging test such as ultrasound or magnetic resonance imaging should be considered. Paramagnetic contrast agents such as the gadolinium used in magnetic resonance angiography do not have any significant nephrotoxicity.[95]

If medical imaging requiring iodinated radiocontrast is deemed essential in the evaluation of a high-risk perioperative patient, some measures can be undertaken to help prevent or attenuate the severity of the ARF. First, a number of studies have demonstrated that adequate hydration with either 0.45% or 0.9% saline prior to administering a radiocontrast agent attenuates or prevents ARF in high-risk patients.[92,93,96] Most studies infused saline starting 12 hours before the contrast administration and continuing for 12 hours afterwards, at a rate of 75–125 ml/h. Despite potential theoretical benefits, recent studies have failed to show any benefit in the use of mannitol or furosemide to prevent contrast-induced ARF.[96] In fact, furosemide was associated with a worse outcome compared with saline alone. Using lower volumes of contrast may be beneficial. In addition, the newer non-ionic iso-osmolar agents may be associated with less nephrotoxicity.[97]

Two new and very popular agents for the prevention of contrast-induced ARF in high risk patients is the use of oral *N*-acetylcysteine (600 mg po BID) given the day prior to and the day of the radiocontrast study. Although some studies suggest that acetylcysteine prophylaxis reduce and NaHCO$_3$ the incidence of acute deterioration of renal function in high-risk patients,[98,99] other studies did not.[100–102] Since acetylcysteine and sodium bicarbonate (NaHCO$_3$ 154 meq/l) given intravenously at 3 ml/kg for 1 hour before and 1 ml/kg/hour during and for 6 hours after contrast exposure[102a] have little or no toxicity, it seems reasonable to continue using them for prophylaxis against contrast nephropathy despite the negative studies. However, adequate hydration must be administered concomitantly.

A number of other measures have been tried to prevent contrast-induced acute renal failure with no clear-cut benefits, including dopamine, fenoldopam, atrial natriuretic peptide, and endothelin antagonists. In addition, it has been proposed that acute hemodialysis after the contrast study may help prevent ARF through removing the radiocontrast agent. Despite this potential theoretical benefit, no definitive study has shown any value for prophylactic hemodialysis after a radiocontrast study.

In summary, it appears that the most beneficial measures to help prevent acute renal failure in high risk patients are: (a) intravenous hydration with saline, (b) use of a low osmolality and non-ionic agent, (c) use of acetylcysteine and/or $NaHCO_3$, and (d) reduced amount of contrast.

Dialytic management of the surgery patient with renal disease

For patients with ESRD

Patients with ESRD on chronic hemodialysis usually will receive dialysis the day prior to elective surgery to minimize the risks for volume overload and hypertension, hyperkalemia, and metabolic acidosis. The dialysis treatment preceding surgery also will optimize control of the uremic environment, which in turn mitigates platelet dysfunction (as noted above), impaired immune function, malnutrition, and possibly impaired wound healing. The goals of dialysis therapy for these patients are to achieve euvolemia or "dry weight," normalize serum potassium level, and increase serum bicarbonate levels to attenuate metabolic or respiratory acidosis. As discussed above, maintaining euvolemia will improve blood pressure control and reduce congestive heart failure.

Patients who are chronically underdialyzed (blood urea nitrogen >100 mg/dl) and hypervolemic may benefit from daily dialysis for a few days preceding elective surgery. Reducing nitrogenous waste products may improve immune function, malnutrition and wound healing. Whether intensive dialysis actually improves these parameters has not been proven rigorously, but most nephrologists agree that the degree of azotemia should be minimized prior to surgery. Underdialyzed patients are at increased risk of developing pericarditis, which obviously should be avoided perioperatively.

Approximately 10% of the ESRD population in the USA are on peritoneal dialysis. Patients can continue on peritoneal dialysis perioperatively to manage volume overload and electrolyte and acid–base abnormalities. Before surgery, all of the peritoneal dialysis fluid is drained from the abdominal cavity, to allow ease of surgery for abdominal procedures and to prevent respiratory compromise intraoperatively from increased abdominal pressure. For simple abdominal procedures, the peritoneal dialysis catheter can be left in place and the patient should receive hemodialysis via a temporary venous catheter until the abdominal incision has healed sufficiently to permit resumption of peritoneal dialysis. For abdominal procedures in which the catheter may be contaminated, such as perforated bowel cases, it is probably prudent to remove the peritoneal dialysis catheter and switch the patient to hemodialysis temporarily. Other situations when a peritoneal dialysis patient will require surgical removal of the catheter are recurrent bacterial peritonitis, a peritoneal catheter tunnel infection, and fungal peritonitis. When the patient has completely healed from the abdominal surgery and/or peritonitis and there is no issue of continued intra-abdominal infection, a new peritoneal dialysis catheter can be placed and peritoneal dialysis resumed.

For patients with ARF

Acute renal failure can develop during the preoperative, intraoperative, or the postoperative period in high-risk patients, especially in the setting of trauma and major vascular procedures during which renal blood flow is compromised. The ARF is usually due to the development of acute tubular necrosis (see above). Important questions are: (a) what are the indications for dialysis therapy in patients with ARF, and (b) which renal replacement modality should be used to treat such patients?

The indications for dialysis in a perioperative patient with ARF are the same as for any patient with ARF. The most common indication is the presence of the signs and symptoms of uremia (Table 24.5), such as pericarditis and an otherwise unexplained worsening of mental status. Hyperkalemia, severe acidosis, and volume overload that cannot be managed with drugs are common indications for acute dialysis. Patients with perioperative ARF are generally quite catabolic and are receiving large volumes of fluid in the form of total parenteral nutrition and various medications. Thus, dialysis support, and more specifically hemofiltration, is crucial in preventing or attenuating volume overload and congestive heart failure. The goal of therapy is to maintain adequate oxygenation while

Table 24.5. Indications for acute dialysis

Symptoms and signs associated with uremia in patients with creatinine clearance <20–25 ml/min per 1.73 m²:

- Nausea, vomiting, anorexia
- Other gastrointestinal symptoms (gastritis with hemorrhage, colitis with or without hemorrhage)
- Altered mental status (lethargy, somnolence, malaise, stupor, coma, or delirium)
- Signs of uremic encephalopathy (asterixis, multifocal clonus, or seizures)
- Pericariditis
- Bleeding diathesis from uremic platelet dysfunction

Refractory or progressive fluid overload
Uncontrolled hyperkalemia
Severe metabolic acidosis, especially in an oliguric patient
Acute and progressive worsening of renal function with

- Blood urea nitrogen levels >70–100 mg/dl
- Measured creatinine clearance <15–20 ml/min

keeping the inspired oxygen concentration below 50% to minimize pulmonary oxygen toxicity.

Many nephrologists will initiate hemodialysis in patients with ARF when the blood urea nitrogen level reaches 70–100 mg/dl or when the creatinine clearance is below 15 ml/min, even if the patient has no overt clinical indications for dialysis. This practice is common and has been the practice at our center, especially in catabolic and oliguric patients with a rapid rise in blood urea nitrogen (>20 mg/dl per day) and serum creatinine (>2 mg/dl per day). There are conflicting studies in the literature as to whether prophylactic dialysis will alter the course or outcome of patients with ARF.[103,104] Moreover, early dialysis may be detrimental to renal function because of hypotension[105] or use of bio-incompatible dialysis membranes (see below).[106] Hypotension is seen commonly during hemodialysis in the critically ill patient, and repeated episodes of hypotension may lead to recurrent ischemic tubular injury in a patient who already has acute tubular necrosis.

There is general consensus among nephrologists that the synthetic and more biocompatible hemodialysis membranes should be used in treating patients with ARF, and not the older bioincompatible cuprophane membranes. The cuprophane membranes are associated with complement activation and upregulation of adhesion molecules,[106] and clinically with a delay in recovery from ARF and worse survival when compared with biocompatible membranes.[107,108] Our practice is to use biocompatible dialysis membranes also when treating perioperative patients with ESRD.

Continuous renal replacement therapy in catabolic patients

There are three general therapeutic modalities that can be used for treatment of renal failure (either acute or chronic) in the perioperative patient: peritoneal dialysis, intermittent hemodialysis, and continuous renal replacement therapy. Most patients with ARF in the perioperative period are catabolic, resulting in high urea, potassium, and phosphate levels. They are also frequently volume overloaded because of the administration of total parenteral nutrition, antibiotics, blood products, and pressor agents. The discussion that follows focuses on dialytic management of catabolic patients with ARF, but the discussion applies equally to ESRD patients who are catabolic in the perioperative period.

Although peritoneal dialysis is rarely used in the USA to treat ARF, there are some advantages to its use in such patients. Since solute and volume removal is much slower with peritoneal dialysis, it may be more desirable in hemodyamically unstable patients. Moreover, systemic anticoagulation is not required. However, there are also major disadvantages. Acute peritoneal dialysis is contraindicated after major abdominal surgery because of the need for abdominal wound healing, the presence of drains, and the increased risk for infection. There may be pleuro-peritoneal communications after thoracic surgery, leading to large pleural effusions with peritoneal dialysis. Moreover, instillation of fluid in the peritoneal cavity may increase intra-abdominal pressure and compromise respiratory effort, a major issue in the perioperative patient with ARF who frequently has concomitant respiratory failure and adult respiratory distress syndrome. Finally, the slow nature of peritoneal dialysis renders it inefficient in treating the catabolic and hyperkalemic perioperative patient with ARF and pulmonary edema. For these reasons, it is not our practice to use peritoneal dialysis in the treatment of ARF.

The major modalities used to treat ARF are either intermittent hemodialysis or some form of continuous renal replacement therapy. Perioperative patients with ARF are often hypercatabolic and volume overloaded, and require more frequent dialysis treatments to achieve acceptable or target solute, acid–base, potassium, and volume levels. Recent studies suggest that more intensive dialysis in patients with ARF may improve survival.[109,110] One hundred and sixty patients with ARF were randomized to either daily dialysis or every other day dialysis. The patients in the daily dialysis arm of the study had a significant reduction in mortality (28 vs. 46%), fewer hypotensive episodes, and more rapid recovery from ARF. This and other studies support the notion that increased or daily dialysis may be beneficial in patients with ARF and moderate to high APACHE scores.[109]

A major difficulty in performing dialysis in patients with perioperative ARF is hypotension because of underlying sepsis, respiratory failure, and other organ-system problems. Use of continuous renal replacement therapy (CRRT) can mitigate worsening hypotension during dialysis. There are various forms of CRRT, including continuous venous-venous hemofiltration, continuous venous-venous hemodiafiltration, continuous hemodialysis, extended daily dialysis, and sustained low efficiency dialysis.[111] A discussion of the technical aspects of these modalities is beyond the scope of this chapter. The basic concept is that a slower and prolonged form of hemodialysis or hemofiltration may be better tolerated than intermittent hemodialysis in critically ill patients with ARF and tenuous hemodynamic status. Moreover, in patients with increased catabolism and profound metabolic acidosis, CRRT is very effective in correcting azotemia and metabolic acidosis.[112] Clinical trials are in progress to determine which modality of CRRT is superior in treating ARF.

Anticoagulation during hemodialysis

Heparin is used routinely during hemodialysis to prevent clotting of blood through the dialysis circuit. Postoperatively, hemodialysis can be performed without heparin to help minimize bleeding, using periodic saline flushes during the procedure to help prevent clotting of the circuit.

In perioperative patients with active bleeding requiring daily dialysis or CRRT (see above) yet frequent clotting of the dialysis circuit, an alternative to systemic heparin is regional citrate anticoagulation. This procedure involves administering citrate into the blood in the extracorporeal circuit and using a calcium-free dialysate. By chelating all available calcium, coagulation is prevented in the extracorporeal circuit. When the blood is returned to the patient, the process is reversed by infusing calcium to prevent hypocalcemia and systemic anticoagulation. Approximately one-third of the citrate is dialyzed off, and the remaining two-thirds is metabolized quickly by the patient to form bicarbonate. Although regional citrate anticoagulation is very effective in preventing clotting of the extracorporeal circuit, the major disadvantages are symptomatic and possibly life-threatening hypocalcemia and metabolic alkalosis. Serum calcium levels must be monitored very closely and the calcium infusion must be adjusted to maintain normal calcium levels.[113]

Since perioperative patients with acute or chronic renal failure and multi-organ failure tend to have higher risks for bleeding, the use of periodic saline flushes or regional citrate anticoagulation may be preferable to heparin.

Care of the dialysis access

Peritoneal dialysis catheters must receive daily care to the exit site, consisting of washing the area with soap and water, thoroughly drying it, and then applying a new dressing over the exit site. Such exit site care is best provided by someone with expertise. Each time the peritoneal dialysis catheter is manipulated to start or complete an exchange, everyone in the room should wear a mask. In addition, thorough handwashing should precede handling of the peritoneal dialysis catheter.

A common complication in hemodialysis patients postoperatively is thrombosis of the vascular access, either due to hypotension or applying a torniquet or blood pressure cuff above the arteriovenous fistula or graft. Preventing hypotension and conspicuous labeling of the access arm may help to avoid access thrombosis and delay in subsequent dialysis. If the vascular access for dialysis is a tunneled catheter, then the catheter should be labeled clearly that it is for dialysis use only. Frequent accessing of the dialysis catheter increases the risk of catheter-related infection and catheter thrombosis, because non-dialysis personnel are unfamiliar with the degree of heparinization required and the need for strict sterile technique. In addition, non-dialysis personnel may flush all or part of the heparin-lock in the catheter ($\geq$5000 u/port) into the venous circulation, causing systemic anticoagulation.

Perioperative acute renal failure

Prevention of renal injury is the perioperative goal in the management of patients with functioning kidneys. Acute renal failure that develops after anesthesia and surgery is associated with increased mortality. Mortality rates for acute postoperative ARF requiring dialysis has ranged from 47% to 81% in a number of clinical series.[114] Risk factors for increased mortality for patients with ARF include male gender, presence of oliguria, mechanical ventilation, acute myocardial infarction, acute stroke or seizure, and chronic immunosuppression.[115] Despite advances in intensive care and dialysis technology, the outcome in perioperative patients with ARF has not improved.

A number of risk factors have been identified as contributing to perioperative ARF, most often due to acute tubular necrosis (Table 24.6). These can be broadly divided into two categories: decreased renal perfusion

Table 24.6. Causes of perioperative renal failure

Decreased renal perfusion
- Intravascular volume depletion
- Congestive heart failure
- Sepsis
- Cardiopulmonary bypass
- Anesthetic effects on renal blood flow
- Aortic cross-clamping
- Use of non-steroidal anti-inflammatory drugs or cycloxygenase inhibitors
- Use of angiotensin converting enzyme inhibitors/angiotensin receptor blockers

Nephrotoxin exposure
- Aminoglycosides
- Radiocontrast agents
- Anesthetic agents
- Myoglobin/rhabdomyolysis

and exposure to nephrotoxins. Postoperative patients are at increased risk for acute tubular necrosis because preoperative fluid depletion, anesthesia, and intraoperative fluid losses can lead to volume depletion and reduction in renal blood flow and glomerular filtration rate. Most patients can tolerate these procedures, but the likelihood of tubular injury is increased if the patient has pre-existing CKD. In addition, the presence of hypotension and hemolysis exacerbates tubular injury.

Surgical risk factors

Three surgical procedures are associated with the highest risk for developing acute tubular necrosis: abdominal aortic aneursym repair, cardiac surgery with cardiopulmonary bypass, and surgery to correct obstructive jaundice.[116] In abdominal aortic aneursym repair, the kidneys may receive no blood flow for prolonged periods if the aorta is clamped above the renal arteries during surgery. In the setting of cardiac surgery, underlying heart disease with impaired left ventricular function plus hypotension contributes to the increased risk for ARF from acute tubular necrosis. Furthermore, prolonged cardiopulmonary bypass and hemolysis during bypass may contribute further to acute tubular necrosis. Finally, surgery to correct obstructive jaundice is associated with greater decreases in glomerular filtration rate than other types of abdominal surgery, perhaps due to higher rates of sepsis and increased gut absorption of endotoxin.

Sepsis with and without hypotension is an important cause of acute tubular necrosis in the perioperative patient. Multiple organ dysfunction and probable endotoxemia frequently accompany the sepsis syndrome in this population.[117] The mechanism by which sepsis causes acute tubular necrosis is not well understood, but may involve systemic hypotension with tubular ischemia, direct renal vasoconstriction, the release of a number of cytokines such as tumor necrosis factor, and activation of neutrophils which leads to direct renal injury.

Use of drugs that affect renal hemodynamics

Many anesthetic agents have been associated with decreases in renal blood flow, glomerular filtration rate, and urine output. It is not clear if these decreases in renal function reflect direct effects of the anesthetic or indirect effects of sympathetic and neurohumoral activation and anesthetic-induced hypotension. Although the role of anesthetics in causing ARF is not well understood, surgical anesthesia combined with hypotension appear to increase the risk for acute tubular necrosis.

A number of pharmacologic agents such as non-steroidal anti-inflammatory drugs (NSAIDs), cyclooxygenase-2 (COX-2) inhibitors, angiotensin converting enzyme (ACE) inhibitors, and angiotensin receptor blockers (ARBs) can impair renal perfusion. NSAIDs and COX-2 inhibitors block the production of important vasodilatory prostaglandins such as prostaglandin E_2. In the setting of impaired renal perfusion as seen in the perioperative patient, the kidney augments the production of these locally produced autacoids to enhance renal blood flow and maintain glomerular filtration rate. NSAIDs and COX-2 inhibitors prevent this adaptive vasodilatory response leading to relative renal vasoconstriction and decrease in renal blood flow and glomerular filtration rate.[118,119] These drugs should not be used in the perioperative patient, especially in the setting of major surgery where decreased renal perfusion or elevated serum creatinine concentration is present.

ACE inhibitors and ARBs are commonly used antihypertensive agents, especially in patients with left ventricular dysfunction and/or diabetes mellitus. As noted in an earlier section, perioperative patients with ESRD taking these drugs should continue on them for their antihypertensive and cardiac benefits. However, for patients with CKD not yet on dialysis, these drugs may worsen renal function, especially if the patient is volume depleted or develops postoperative ARF. During intravascular volume depletion and/or impaired renal perfusion, the renin–angiotensin system is stimulated and angiotensin II production increased. By selectively increasing efferent arteriolar vasoconstriction, angiotensin II maintains intraglomerular capillary pressure and glomerular filtration rate despite reduced renal blood flow. ACE inhibitors or ARBs block, respectively, the production and action of angiotensin II.[120,121] Therefore, if volume depletion or acute renal failure develops, ACE inhibitors and ARBs should be avoided or discontinued, and alternative antihypertensives such as beta-blockers or calcium channel blockers used to control hypertension.

Nephrotoxins

The perioperative patient is frequently exposed to a number of nephrotoxins that can cause acute tubular necrosis. Aminoglycoside antibiotics are used perioperatively, especially in the setting of trauma and abdominal surgery. Volume depletion, hypotension, sepsis, and pre-existing renal disease appear to act synergistically with aminoglycosides to cause acute tubular necrosis.[122–124] Additional risk factors for aminoglycoside nephrotoxicity include dose and plasma levels, concomitant use of penicillins or cephalosporins, and duration of therapy. Acute renal failure generally develops after at least 5 to 7 days of treatment. However, in the setting of hypotension or volume depletion, the combined insults may lead to earlier development of acute tubular necrosis. Close monitoring of peak and trough plasma levels and adjustment of the dose are key components of aminoglycoside therapy. Recently, there has been evidence that once-daily dosing of aminoglycosides may be less nephrotoxic than the traditional divided dose regimens. However, in the setting of pre-existing CKD, the divided dose regimens with appropriate dose reduction or interval lengthening should be used to avoid toxic peak and trough levels. Most patients with aminoglycoside-induced acute tubular necrosis are non-oliguric and generally do not require dialysis support unless they have prior renal failure and marginal renal reserve or are oliguric because of multiple nephrotoxic insults.

Radiocontrast agent is another nephrotoxin that can cause ARF and has been discussed fully above.

Rhabdomyolysis and myoglobinuria

Surgery services frequently manage patients who have sustained major trauma and accompanying severe muscle injury (rhabdomyolysis). The resulting myoglobinuria causes acute tubular necrosis, because the heme moiety separates from the globin in an acid urine (pH 5–5.5) and releases free iron. In addition, the filtered myoglobin may precipitate in the renal tubules causing intrarenal obstruction. Finally, volume depletion with third space sequestration of fluid leads to impaired renal blood flow and renal ischemia.[125–127]

Early and vigorous intravenous fluid therapy to correct hypovolemia and renal ischemia is important in attenuating renal injury.[128] Since myoglobin is more nephrotoxic in acid urine, most groups advocate the addition of sodium bicarbonate to the intravenous fluids to alkalinize the urine,[125,126,129] which also may ameliorate the hyperkalemia. Mannitol is used in combination with fluid/alkaline therapy to prevent renal injury in rhabdomyolysis.[129] Potential benefits of mannitol include: (a) increase in urine flow and prevention of obstructing cast formation, (b) reduction in renal tubular epithelial swelling and injury, and (c) scavenging of oxygen free radicals.[130]

Although there are no controlled trials to show a direct benefit of forced alkaline-mannitol diuresis in preventing ARF in rhabdomyolysis, there are many case reports suggesting such therapy was instrumental in averting renal injury. We recommend the infusion of both mannitol and sodium bicarbonate solutions if the patient remains oliguric after adequate volume resuscitation with isotonic crystalloid solutions, usually normal saline. The mannitol-bicarbonate solution, made by adding 25 g mannitol (12.5 g/50 ml) and 100 meq $NaHCO_3$ (50 meq/50 ml) to 800 ml of 5% dextrose in water, is infused at 250 ml/h. If urine flow rate increases after 4 hours, the infusion rate should be adjusted to equal urine output and to achieve a urine pH > 6.5 until azotemia improves and all evidence of myoglobinuria disappear. If urine flow does not increase after 4 hours, the patient has established oliguric ARF. The mannitol-bicarbonate solution should be discontinued and the patient treated conservatively until dialysis is required.[127] This approach corrects oliguria, hastens the clearing of azotemia, and avoids the need for dialysis in roughly half of the patients with myoglobinuric ARF. Patients who responded have less muscle damage and better preservation of renal function than those that did not respond.[131] Whether this reflects earlier intervention, a less severe degree of muscle injury, or just vigorous volume expansion is not known.

Once ARF is established, dialysis is required. Early and intensive hemodialysis may be associated with significantly lower morbidity and mortality. Daily hemodialysis or some form of CRRT is often required for the first several days, because these patients tend to be quite catabolic and develop metabolic acidosis, hyperkalemia, hyperphosphatemia, and concomitant hypocalcemia. Full recovery of renal function is the rule, provided other coexisting organ-system dysfunction resolves.

Treatment

The best treatment for ARF is its prevention. As discussed above, the patient with underlying kidney disease is at increased risk of developing further renal injury from a variety of drugs and renal ischemia. Avoidance of NSAIDs, aminoglycosides, and radiocontrast where possible, and optimization of hemodynamic and volume status will prevent much of the ARF.

Surgery in the patient with a stable kidney transplant

A full discussion of perioperative care in the kidney transplant recipient in the immediate post-transplant period is beyond the scope of this chapter, as is a full discussion of perioperative care in the patient with a stable kidney transplant. Nephrology or transplant nephrology consultation must be obtained. However, a few points deserve emphasis.

Immunosuppressive medications must be continued in the perioperative period, according to the outpatient schedule. Usually, prednisone is taken early in the morning, along with the morning dose of a calcineurin inhibitor (either cyclosporin or tacrolimus) and antimetabolite (usually azathioprine or mycophenolate mofetil). The evening dose of the calcineurin inhibitor and antimetabolite must be given 12 hours later. If the patient cannot take medications orally, the steroid must be given intravenously at an equivalent dose (e.g., convert prednisone orally to solumedrol intravenously). Cyclosporin and tacrolimus may be administered intravenously as an infusion, but the dose is one-third of the oral dose because of increased bioavailability. Stress dose steroids must be given in most patients to prevent adrenal insufficiency, since chronic suppression of the adrenal glands renders them less capable of mounting a stress response. Finally, an indwelling urinary catheter should be avoided if at all possible or removed as soon as possible, due to the increased risk of and susceptibility to urinary tract infection and pyelonephritis.

Drugs

The kidneys eliminate many drugs either primarily or secondarily. Secondary clearance occurs in drugs that require hepatic metabolism to render the drug water soluble; the kidney then clears this metabolite. Therefore, these drugs or their metabolites accumulate in renal failure and can cause significant side effects. Furthermore, the volume of distribution of some drugs may be affected by renal disease because of alteration in protein binding, increasing the free drug level and its effect. We will discuss briefly some of the frequently encountered problems in the perioperative period.

General principles of drug therapy in kidney disease

Drug toxicity is an important cause of morbidity in patients with kidney disease, and there are several responsible mechanisms. First, drugs that are renally cleared will accumulate in kidney failure. The dose and/or frequency of administration of such medications must be adjusted. While some medications, such as some of the penicillins and cephalosporins, require dose adjustment only when kidney function is severely impaired ($C_{Cr} < 25$ ml/min), others require dose adjustment even at higher levels of kidney function.

Second, medications that are cleared by the liver may be metabolized into conjugated moieties that then require renal clearance. If these metabolites have activity or serious side effects, such effects will be prolonged because of the delay in clearance. Examples of such medications are procainamide and morphine (see below). Procainamide is metabolized in the liver to N-acetylprocainamide, which accumulates in renal failure and can induce torsade de pointe.[132,133]

A third mechanism is decreased absorption via the gastrointestinal tract because of concomitant use of phosphate binders, which may also bind medications.[134,135] Coumadin, immunosuppressive medications used in kidney transplant, and ferrous sulfate are some examples that exhibit this interaction.

The volume of distribution of some drugs is altered in kidney failure because of altered protein binding. Classic examples include digoxin[136] and phenytoin.[137] Both are protein-bound to significant degrees in health, and free levels of both drugs are increased in patients with renal failure. Therefore, the loading dose of such medications must be reduced, since the volume of distribution effectively has decreased. In addition, maintenance levels should be lower than the target for the general population to avoid toxicity, especially when the drug has a narrow therapeutic index.

Finally, appropriate dosing of medications in kidney failure requires an estimated creatinine clearance. Serum creatinine is a poor indicator of kidney function, especially in elderly patients and chronically ill patients who have significant loss of lean muscle mass. A reasonable estimate of creatinine clearance (C_{Cr}) that does not require a

24-hour urine collection is the Cockcroft–Gault equation that is based on age, body weight in kilograms (BW – preferably ideal body weight as opposed to actual body weight), and serum creatinine (S_{Cr}):

$$C_{Cr} = \frac{(140 - age)(BW)}{S_{Cr}}$$

or the MDRD equation using serum creatinine, age, ethnicity, and gender.[138] A recent study in geriatric patients receiving medical care at a tertiary care institution show that medications are frequently inappropriately adjusted in elderly patients with even mild degrees of renal failure.[139]

In addition to non-renal side effects, certain classes of drugs can cause acute deterioration of kidney function in patients with pre-existing CKD (see above). In postoperative patients already experiencing renal perfusion problems, aminoglycosides, radiographic contrast, NSAIDs, ACE inhibitors, and ARBs can reduce further perfusion to the kidneys and cause either pre-renal azotemia or acute tubular necrosis if ischemia is prolonged. Certain antibiotics (penicillins and sulfamethoxazole) and NSAIDs also can induce acute interstitial nephritis. Lastly, overdiuresis can lead to volume depletion and acute tubular necrosis.

Some of the medications commonly used in the perioperative situation are listed in Table 24.7. A good reference source for medication dose adjustment in renal failure is the *ACP Drug Handbook*.[140]

Anesthesia

In general, regional anesthesia is preferred in patients with renal failure because of the increased risk of general anesthesia and the difficulty in selecting the right combination of general anesthetics.[141] These are particularly useful for insertion of arteriovenous shunts and fistula for dialysis access. Spinal and epidural anesthesia, however, are less desirable because of the potential for severe hypotension in patients with autonomic neuropathy, and the risk for spinal hematoma from platelet dysfunction.[141,142]

Many of the agents used in inducing general anesthesia have altered protein binding in renal failure (thiopental, methohexital, diazepam, etomidate, midazolam) (Table 24.7).[141,142] Therefore, the dose of such drugs should be reduced when renal failure is present.

Many muscle relaxants are partially or completely renally cleared, leading to a prolonged half-life in patients with renal failure (Table 24.7).[141,142] Some have active metabolites, further prolonging the drug action (vecuronium and pancuronium). In addition, succinylcholine

may result in significant hyperkalemia and is contraindicated in renal failure. Atracurium and cistracurium do not rely on renal elimination,[141,142] and the metabolite of atracurium has no activity.[142] These are the drugs of choice for muscle relaxants in patients with renal failure.

Some volatile anesthetic agents (enflurane and sevoflurane) are contraindicated in renal failure because of the production of fluoride and the potential for developing fluoride-induced acute renal failure,[141] although there is some controversy.[143,144] Isoflurane, desflurane, and halothane are better tolerated and preferred in renal failure.[141,145]

Propofol appears to be safe in patients with renal failure. Hepatic clearance is unaffected in renal failure, and its metabolite lacks activity. However, ESRD patients may require higher induction doses of propofol.[68] The negative correlation of propofol dose with preoperative hemoglobin concentration suggested that the increased requirement may be a consequence of anemia-induced hyperdynamic circulation.

Fentanyl and sufentanil are commonly used as adjuncts but elimination appears to be impaired in renal failure.[141] Remifentanil is preferred because it is rapidly inactivated by non-specific esterases in blood and does not depend on either renal or hepatic elimination.[141]

Finally, the half-life of drugs that are used to reverse anesthesia, anticholinergic agents and anticholinesterases, are prolonged in patients with renal disease.[141,142] After reversal, patients may develop excessive muscarinic effects to include bradyarrhythmias, respiratory secretions, and bronchospasm, because the half-life of the anticholinesterases is more prolonged than that of the anticholinergic agents.

Pain management/analgesia

Pain control is obviously an important issue in the postoperative patient. However, many pain medications are contraindicated in the patient with renal disease. Nonsteroidal anti-inflammatory drugs should not be administered in the patient with advanced CKD because of the risk of ARF (see above) from renal ischemia. Toradol, in particular, appears to be a common offending agent in the perioperative period, because it is the only NSAIDs that can be given parenterally. Despite the theoretical concern about reducing residual renal function (see above discussion with aminoglycosides), NSAIDs may be used in ESRD patients if there is no gastrointestinal contraindication.

Although narcotics are the mainstay of pain management in the postoperative period, all narcotic drugs may

Table 24.7. Commonly used drugs and/or their metabolites that are cleared by the kidney

Drug class	Drug	Route of elimination	Toxic metabolite	Altered protein binding[a]	Dose adjustment
Anesthetics	Enflurane	Respiratory	Fluoride		Avoid
	Sevoflurane	Respiratory	Fluoride		Avoid
	Etomidate	Hepatic		Yes	Reduced dose
Muscle relaxants	Gallamine	Renal			Avoid
	Demethyl tubocurarine	Renal			Avoid
	Pancuronium	Partial renal	3-Hydroxy-pancuronium		Avoid
	Pipecuronium	Partial renal			Avoid
	D-Tubocurarine	Partial renal			Avoid
	Vecuronium	Partial renal	Desacetyl-vecuronium		Avoid
	Doxacurium	Partial renal			Avoid
	Succinylcholine	Hepatic	Hyperkalemia		Avoid
Barbiturates	Thiopental	Hepatic		Yes	Reduce dose
	Methohexital	Hepatic		Yes	Reduce dose
	Phenobarbital	Partial renal			Reduce dose
Anticholinergic	Atropine	Partial renal			Reduce dose
	Glycopyrrolate	Partial renal			Reduce dose
Cholinergic	Neostigmine	Partial renal			Reduce dose
	Pyridostigmine	Partial renal			Reduce dose
	Edrophonium	Partial renal			Reduce dose
Antibiotics	Vancomycin	Renal			Reduce dose/interval
	Aminoglycosides[b]	Renal			Reduce dose/interval[b]
	Cephalosporins[c]	Renal			Variable[c]
	Penicillins[c]	Renal			Variable[c]
	Imipenem[d]	Renal			Reduce dose/interval[d]
	Fluconazole	Renal			Reduce dose/interval
	Acyclovir	Renal			Reduce dose/interval
	Ganciclovir	Renal			Reduce dose/interval
Cardiovascular	Digoxin	Renal		Yes	Reduce dose/interval
	Procainamide	Renal/Hepatic	NAPA		Avoid
	Quinidine	Partial renal			Reduced dose
	Nitroprusside	Hepatic	Thiocyanate		Avoid after 24–48 hours
	ACE inhibitor	Variable renal			
	ARB	Variable renal			
	Atenolol	Renal			Avoid
Diuretics	Hydrochlorothiazide	Renal			Avoid (ineffective)
	Furosemide	Renal			Increase dose
Psychoactive	Diazepam	Hepatic	Oxazepam	Yes	Reduce dose/interval
	Midazolam	Hepatic	1-Hydroxy-midazolam		Reduce dose/interval
Analgesics	Morphine	Hepatic	Morphine-6-glucuronide		Avoid
	Meperidine	Hepatic	Normeperidine		Avoid
	Other narcotics	Hepatic			Reduce dose/caution
Anti-seizure	Phenytoin	Hepatic		Yes	Reduce dose
H₂ blockers	Cimetidine	Renal			Reduce dose
	Ranitidine	Renal			Reduce dose
	Famotidine	Renal			Reduce dose
Hypoglycemics	Glyburide	Renal			Avoid
	Insulin	Renal			Reduce dose
Others	Allopurinol	Partial renal			Reduce dose

Notes:

[a] Loading dose should be reduced for drugs that exhibit altered protein binding.

[b] The practice of dosing aminoglycosides daily at 3–5 mg/kg does not apply to patients with renal failure. Aminoglycosides should be dosed at 1–2 mg/kg loading, then dose reduced and/or interval lengthened depending on the creatinine clearance.

[c] Renal dose adjustment for cephalosporins and penicillins vary widely, ranging from no dose adjustment to dose adjustment only with creatinine clearance <25 ml/min.

[d] Disagreement exists concerning whether imipenem is absolutely versus relatively contraindicated in the setting of renal failure.

have a prolonged half-life to one degree or another when renal failure is present. However, two drugs are well known for their central nervous system effects in patients with renal failure. Morphine is metabolized in the liver to morphine-6-glucuronide, a metabolite with 40 times the activity of morphine, which then requires renal elimination.[141] Meperidine is also hepatically metabolized to normeperidine, which has neuroexcitatory effects and requires renal excretion.[141] Both morphine and meperidine are contraindicated in patients with ESRD and advanced renal failure. If they are used, patients must be monitored carefully and the drug discontinued at the first sign of undesirable neurologic effects. Other narcotics also must be administered with caution because disposition may vary from individual to individual.

REFERENCES

1. United States Renal Data System. United States Renal Data System 2002 Annual Data Report: Incidence and prevalence. *Am. J. Kidney Dis.* 2003; **41**(4 Suppl. 2): S41–S56.

2. Kellerman, P. S. Perioperative care of the renal patient. *Arch. Intern. Med.* 1994; **154**: 1674–1688.

3. Brenowitz, J. B., Williams, C. D., & Edwards, W. S. Major surgery in patients with chronic renal failure. *Am. J. Surg.* 1977; **134**: 765–769.

4. Pinson, C. W., Schuman, E. S., Gross, G. F. *et al.* Surgery in long-term dialysis patients. Experience with more than 300 cases. *Am. J. Surg.* 1986; **151**: 567–571.

5. United States Renal Data System. United States Renal Data System 2002 Annual Data Report: Survival, mortality, and causes of death. *Am. J. Kidney Dis.* 2003; **41**(4 Suppl. 2): S151–S164.

6. Foley, R. N., Parfrey, P. S., & Sarnak, M. J. Epidemiology of cardiovascular disease in chronic renal disease. *J. Am. Soc. Nephrol.* 1998; **9**: S16–S23.

7. Foley, R. N., Parfrey, P. S., & Sarnak, M. J. Clinical epidemiology of cardiovascular disease in chronic renal disease. *Am. J. Kidney Dis.* 1998; **32**: S112–S119.

8. Foley, R. N., Parfrey, P. S., Harnett, J. D. *et al.* Clinical and echocardiographic disease in patients starting end-stage renal disease therapy. *Kidney Int.* 1995; **47**: 186–192.

9. Kasiske, B. L., Guijarro, C., Massy, Z. A. *et al.* Cardiovascular disease after renal transplantation. *J. Am. Soc. Nephrol.* 1996; **7**: 158–165.

10. Nally, J. V. Jr. Cardiac disease in chronic uremia: investigation. *Adv. Renal Replacem. Ther.* 1997; **4**: 225–233.

11. Koch, M., Gradaus, F., Schoebel, F. C. *et al.* Relevance of conventional cardiovascular risk factors for the prediction of coronary artery disease in diabetic patients on renal replacement therapy. *Nephrol. Dialysis Transpl.* 1997; **12**: 1187–1191.

12. Rostand, S. G., Brunzell, J. D., Cannon, R. O., III, *et al.* Cardiovascular complications in renal failure. *J. Am. Soc. Nephrol.* 1991; **2**: 1053–1062.

13. Mistry, B. M., Bastani, B., Solomon, H. *et al.* Prognostic value of dipyridamole thallium-201 screening to minimize perioperative cardiac complications in diabetics undergoing kidney or kidney-pancreas transplantation. *Clin. Transpl.* 1998; **12**: 130–135.

14. Holley, J. L., Fenton, R. A., & Arthur, R. S. Thallium stress testing does not predict cardiovascular risk in diabetic patients with end-stage renal disease undergoing cadaveric renal transplantation. *Am. J. Med.* 1991; **90**: 563–570.

15. Iqbal, A., Gibbons, R. J., McGoon, M. D. *et al.* Noninvasive assessment of cardiac risk in insulin-dependent diabetic patients being evaluated for pancreas transplantation using thallium-201 myocardial perfusion scintigraphy. *Clin. Transpl.* 1991; **5**: 13–19.

16. Marwick, T. H., Steinmuller, D. R., Underwood, D. A. *et al.* Ineffectiveness of dipyridamole SPECT thallium imaging as a screening technique for coronary artery disease in patients with end-stage renal failure. *Transplantation* 1990; **49**: 100–103.

17. Dahan, M., Viron, B. M., Poiseau, E. *et al.* Combined dipyridamole-exercise stress echocardiography for detection of myocardial ischemia in hemodialysis patients: an alternative to stress nuclear imaging. *Am. J. Kidney Dis.* 2002; **40**: 737–744.

18. Rostand, S. G., Kirk, K. A., & Rutsky, E. A. Dialysis-associated ischemic heart disease: insights from coronary angiography. *Kidney Int.* 1984; **25**: 653–659.

19. Cottier, C., Pfisterer, M., Muller-Brand, J. *et al.* Cardiac evaluation of candidates for kidney transplantation: value of exercise radionuclide angiocardiography. *Eur. Heart J.* 1990; **11**: 832–838.

20. Le, A., Wilson, R., Douek, K. *et al.* Prospective risk stratification in renal transplant candidates for cardiac death. *Am. J. Kidney Dis.* 1994; **24**: 65–71.

21. Kasiske, B. L., Ramos, E. L., Gaston, R. S. *et al.* The evaluation of renal transplant candidates: clinical practice guidelines. Patient Care and Education Committee of the American Society of Transplant Physicians. *J. Am. Soc. Nephrol.* 1995; **6**: 1–34.

22. Verani, M. S. Myocardial perfusion imaging versus two-dimensional echocardiography: comparative value in the diagnosis of coronary artery disease. *J. Nucl. Cardiol.* 1994; **1**: 399–414.

23. Philipson, J. D., Carpenter, B. J., Itzkoff, J. *et al.* Evaluation of cardiovascular risk for renal transplantation in diabetic patients. *Am. J. Med.* 1986; **81**: 630–634.

24. Morrow, C. E., Schwartz, J. S., Sutherland, D. E. *et al.* Predictive value of thallium stress testing for coronary and cardiovascular events in uremic diabetic patients before renal transplantation. *Am. J. Surg.* 1983; **146**: 331–335.

25. Brown, J. H., Vites, N. P., Testa, H. J. *et al.* Value of thallium myocardial imaging in the prediction of future cardiovascular events in patients with end-stage renal failure. *Nephrol. Dialysis Transpl.* 1993; **8**: 433–437.

26. Vandenberg, B. F., Rossen, J. D., Grover-McKay, M. *et al.* Evaluation of diabetic patients for renal and pancreas transplantation: noninvasive screening for coronary artery disease using radionuclide methods. *Transplantation* 1996; **62**: 1230–1235.

27. Camp, A. D., Garvin, P. J., Hoff, J. *et al.* Prognostic value of intravenous dipyridamole thallium imaging in patients with diabetes mellitus considered for renal transplantation. *Am. J. Cardiol.* 1990; **65**: 1459–1463.

28. Derfler, K., Kletter, K., Balcke, P. *et al.* Predictive value of thallium-201-dipyridamole myocardial stress scintigraphy in chronic hemodialysis patients and transplant recipients. *Clin. Nephrol.* 1991; **36**: 192–202.

29. Brown, K. A., Rimmer, J., & Haisch, C. Noninvasive cardiac risk stratification of diabetic and nondiabetic uremic renal allograft candidates using dipyridamole-thallium-201 imaging and radionuclide ventriculography. *Am. J. Cardiol.* 1989; **64**: 1017–1021.

30. Lewis, M. S., Wilson, R. A., Walker, K. W. *et al.* Validation of an algorithm for predicting cardiac events in renal transplant candidates. *Am. J. Cardiol.* 2002; **89**: 847–850.

31. Dahan, M., Viron, B. M., Faraggi, M. *et al.* Diagnostic accuracy and prognostic value of combined dipyridamole-exercise thallium imaging in hemodialysis patients. *Kidney Int.* 1998; **54**: 255–262.

32. Reis, G., Marcovitz, P. A., Leichtman, A. B. *et al.* Usefulness of dobutamine stress echocardiography in detecting coronary artery disease in end-stage renal disease. *Am. J. Cardiol.* 1995; **75**: 707–710.

33. Schmidt, A., Stefenelli, T., Schuster, E. *et al.* Informational contribution of noninvasive screening tests for coronary artery disease in patients on chronic renal replacement therapy. *Am. J. Kidney Dis.* 2001; **37**: 56–63.

34. Herzog, C. A., Marwick, T. H., Pheley, A. M. *et al.* Dobutamine stress echocardiography for the detection of significant coronary artery disease in renal transplant candidates. *Am. J. Kidney Dis.* 1999; **33**: 1080–1090.

35. Boudreau, R. J., Strony, J. T., duCret, R. P. *et al.* Perfusion thallium imaging of type I diabetes patients with end stage renal disease: comparison of oral and intravenous dipyridamole administration. *Radiology* 1990; **175**: 103–105.

36. Bates, J. R., Sawada, S. G., Segar, D. S. *et al.* Evaluation using dobutamine stress echocardiography in patients with insulin-dependent diabetes mellitus before kidney and/or pancreas transplantation. *Am. J. Cardiol.* 1996; **77**: 175–179.

37. West, J. C., Napoliello, D. A., Costello, J. M. *et al.* Preoperative dobutamine stress echocardiography versus cardiac arteriography for risk assessment prior to renal transplantation. *Transpl. Int.* 2000; **13** Suppl. 1: S27–S30.

38. Manske, C. L., Thomas, W., Wang, Y. *et al.* Screening diabetic transplant candidates for coronary artery disease: identification of a low risk subgroup. *Kidney Int.* 1993; **44**: 617–621.

39. Trochu, J. N., Cantarovich, D., Renaudeau, J. *et al.* Assessment of coronary artery disease by thallium scan in type-1 diabetic uremic patients awaiting combined pancreas and renal transplantation. *Angiology* 1991; **42**: 302–307.

39a. Auerbach, A. D., Goldman, L. β-blockers and reduction of cardiac events in noncardiac surgery. *J. Am. Med. Assoc.* 2002; **287**: 1435–1444.

40. Suki, W. N. Use of diuretics in chronic renal failure. *Kidney Int. Suppl* 1997; **59**: S33–S35.

41. Greenberg, A. Diuretic complications. *Am. J. Med. Sci.* 2000; **319**: 10–24.

42. Yee, J., Parasuraman, R., & Narins, R. G. Selective review of key perioperative renal–electrolyte disturbances in chronic renal failure patients. *Chest* 1999; **115**: 149S–157S.

43. Rindone, J. P. & Sloane, E. P. Cyanide toxicity from sodium nitroprusside: risks and management. *Ann. Pharmacother.* 1992; **26**: 515–519.

44. Burke, J. F. Jr. & Francos, G. C. Surgery in the patient with acute or chronic renal failure. *Med. Clin. North Am.* 1987; **71**: 489–497.

45. Bia, M. J. & DeFronzo, R. A. Extrarenal potassium homeostasis. *Am. J. Physiol.* 1981; **240**: F257–F268.

46. Salem, M. M., Rosa, R. M., & Batlle, D. C. Extrarenal potassium tolerance in chronic renal failure: implications for the treatment of acute hyperkalemia. *Am. J. Kidney Dis.* 1991; **18**: 421–440.

47. Martin, R. S., Panese, S., Virginillo, M. *et al.* Increased secretion of potassium in the rectum of humans with chronic renal failure. *Am. J. Kidney Dis.* 1986; **8**: 105–110.

48. Ferrannini, E., Taddei, S., Santoro, D. *et al.* Independent stimulation of glucose metabolism and Na^+–K^+ exchange by insulin in the human forearm. *Am. J. Physiol.* 1988; **255**: E953–E958.

49. Allon, M., Takeshian, A., & Shanklin, N. Effect of insulin-plus-glucose infusion with or without epinephrine on fasting hyperkalemia. *Kidney Int.* 1993; **43**: 212–217.

50. Blumberg, A., Weidmann, P., Shaw, S. *et al.* Effect of various therapeutic approaches on plasma potassium and major regulating factors in terminal renal failure. *Am. J. Med.* 1988; **85**: 507–512.

51. Allon, M. & Shanklin, N. Effect of bicarbonate administration on plasma potassium in dialysis patients: interactions with insulin and albuterol. *Am. J. Kidney Dis.* 1996; **28**: 508–514.

52. Pirenne, J., Lledo-Garcia, E., Benedetti, E. *et al.* Colon perforation after renal transplantation: a single-institution review. *Clin. Transpl.* 1997; **11**: 88–93.

53. Van Der Klooster, J. M., Van Der Wiel, H. E., Van Saase, J. L. *et al.* Asystole during combination chemotherapy for non-Hodgkin's lymphoma: the acute tumor lysis syndrome. *Neth. J. Med.* 2000; **56**: 147–152.

54. Levin, N. W. & Hoenich, N. A. Consequences of hyperphosphatemia and elevated levels of the calcium–phosphorus product in dialysis patients. *Curr. Opin. Nephrol. Hypertens.* 2001; **10**: 563–568.

55. Schiller, L. R., Santa Ana, C. A., Sheikh, M. S. *et al.* Effect of the time of administration of calcium acetate on phosphorus binding. *N. Engl. J. Med.* 1989; **320**: 1110–1113.

56. Sheikh, M. S., Maguire, J. A., Emmett, M. *et al.* Reduction of dietary phosphorus absorption by phosphorus binders. A

theoretical, in vitro, and in vivo study. *J. Clin. Invest.* 1989; **83**: 66–73.

57. Cannata-Andia J. B., Fernandez-Martin J. L. The clinical impact of aluminium overload in renal failure. *Nephrol. Dial. Transpl.* 2002; **17** Suppl. 2: 9–12.

58. Molitoris, B. A., Froment, D. H., Mackenzie, T. A. *et al*. Citrate: a major factor in the toxicity of orally administered aluminum compounds. *Kidney Int.* 1989; **36**: 949–953.

59. Kumar, V. A., Yeun, J. Y., Vu, J. T. *et al*. Extended daily dialysis (EDD) rapidly reduces serum phosphate levels in intensive care unit (ICU) patients with acute renal failure (ARF). *ASAIO J.* 2001; **47**(2): 150.

60. Tan, H. K., Bellomo, R., M'Pis, D. A. *et al*. Phosphatemic control during acute renal failure: intermittent hemodialysis versus continuous hemodiafiltration. *Int. J. Artif. Organs* 2001; **24**: 186–191.

61. Crook, M. A., Hally, V., & Panteli, J. V. The importance of the refeeding syndrome. *Nutrition* 2001; **17**: 632–637.

62. Hemstreet, B. A. Use of sucralfate in renal failure. *Ann. Pharmacother.* 2001; **35**: 360–364.

63. Mechanick, J. I. & Brett, E. M. Endocrine and metabolic issues in the management of the chronically critically ill patient. *Crit. Care Clin.* 2002; **18**: 619–641.

64. Gallacher, S. J., Ralston, S. H., Dryburgh, F. J. *et al*. Immobilization-related hypercalcaemia – a possible novel mechanism and response to pamidronate. *Postgrad. Med. J.* 1990; **66**: 918–922.

65. Cruz, D. N. & Perazella, M. A. Biochemical aberrations in a dialysis patient following parathyroidectomy. *Am. J. Kidney Dis.* 1997; **29**: 759–762.

66. Mitchell, J. H., Wildenthal, K., & Johnson, R. L. The effects of acid–base disturbances on cardiovascular and pulmonary function. *Kidney Int.* 1972; **1**: 375–389.

67. Orchard, C. H. & Ketnish, J. C. Effects of changes of pH on the contractile function of cardiac muscle. *Am. J. Physiol.* 1990; **258**: C967–C981.

68. Goyal, P., Puri, G. D., Pandey, C. K. *et al*. Evaluation of induction doses of propofol: comparison between endstage renal disease and normal renal function patients. *Anaesth. Intens. Care* 2002; **30**: 584–587.

69. Posner, J. B. & Plum, F. Spinal-fluid pH and neurologic symptoms in systemic acidosis. *N. Engl. J. Med.* 1967; **277**: 605–613.

70. Adrogue, H. J. & Madias, N. E. Management of life-threatening acid–base disorders. *N. Engl. J. Med.* 1998; **338**: 26–34.

71. Narins, R. G. & Cohen, J. J. Bicarbonate therapy for organic acidosis: the case for its continued use. *Ann. Intern. Med.* 1987; **106**: 615–618.

72. Rose, B. D. & Post, T. W. Metabolic acidosis. In Rose, B. D. & Post, T. W., eds. *Clinical Physiology of Acid–Base and Electrolyte Disorders*, 5th edn. New York: McGraw Hill, 2001: 578–646.

73. Holmdahl, M. H., Wiklund, L., Wetterberg, T. *et al*. The place of THAM in the management of acidemia in clinical practice. *Acta Anaesthesiol. Scand.* 2000; **44**: 524–527.

74. Swartz, R. D., Rubin, J. E., Brown, R. S. *et al*. Correction of postoperative metabolic alkalosis and renal failure by hemodialysis. *Ann. Intern. Med.* 1977; **86**: 52–55.

75. Hakim, R. M. & Levin, N. Malnutrition in hemodialysis patients. *Am. J. Kidney Dis.* 1993; **21**: 125–137.

76. Lowrie, E. G. & Lew, N. L. Death risk in hemodialysis patients: the predictive value of commonly measured variables and an evaluation of death rate differences between facilities. *Am. J. Kidney Dis.* 1990; **15**: 458–482.

77. Don, B. R. & Kaysen, G. A. Assessment of inflammation and nutrition in patients with end-stage renal disease. *J. Nephrol.* 2000; **13**: 249–259.

78. Rocco, R. V. & Blumenkrantz, M. J. Nutrition. In Daugirdas, J. T., Blake, P. G., & Ing, T. S., eds. *Handbook of Dialysis*, 3rd edn. Philadelphia: Lippincott, Williams & Wilkins, 2001: 420–445.

79. Anonymous. National Kidney Foundation Dialysis Outcomes Quality Initiative: Clinical practice guidelines for nutrition in chronic renal failure. *Am. J. Kidney Dis.* 2000; **35**(6 Suppl. 2): S1–S140.

80. Feinstein, E. I., Kopple, J. D., Silberman, H. *et al*. Total parenteral nutrition with high and low nitrogen intakes in patients with acute renal failure. *Kidney Int.* 1983; **24**: S319–S323.

81. Eschbach, J. W. & Adamson, J. W. Anemia of end-stage renal disease. *Kidney Int.* 1985; **28**: 1–5.

82. Eschbach, J. W., Egrie, J. C., Downing, M. R. *et al*. Correction of the anemia of end-stage renal disease with recombinant human erthyropoietin: results of combined phase I and II clinical trial. *N. Engl. J. Med.* 1987; **316**: 73–78.

83. Anonymous. National Kidney Foundation Dialysis Outcomes Quality Initiative: Clinical practice guidelines for anemia of chronic kidney disease: update 2000. *Am. J. Kidney Dis.* 2001; **37**(1 Suppl. 1): S182–238.

84. Eberst, M. E. & Berkowitz, L. R. Hemostasis in renal disease. *Am. J. Med.* 1994; **96**: 168–179.

85. Rabelink, R. W., Zwaginga, J. J., Koomans, H. A. *et al*. Thrombosis and hemostasis in renal disease. *Kidney Int.* 1994; **46**: 287–296.

86. Escolar, G., Cases, A., Bastida, E. *et al*. Uremic platelets have a functional defect affecting the interaction of von Willebrand factor with glycoprotein IIb–IIIa. *Blood* 1990; **76**: 1336–1340.

87. Noris, M. & Remuzzi, G. Uremic bleeding: Closing the circle after 30 years of controversies. *Blood* 1999; **94**: 2569–2574.

88. Steiner, R. W., Coggins, C., & Carvalho, A. C. A. Bleeding time in uremia: a useful test to assess clinical bleeding. *Am. J. Hematol.* 1979; **7**: 107–117.

89. Lindsay, R. M., Friesen, M., Aronstam, A. *et al*. Improvement in platelet function by increased frequency of hemodialysis. *Clin. Nephrol.* 1978; **10**: 67–70.

90. Mannucci, P. M. Hemostatic drugs. *N. Engl. J. Med.* 1998; **339**: 245–253.

91. Vigano, G., Gaspari, F., Locatelli, M. *et al*. Dose–effect and pharmacokinetics of estrogens given to correct bleeding time in uremia. *Kidney Int.* 1988; **34**: 853–858.

92. Barrett, B. J. Contrast nephrotoxicity. *J. Am. Soc. Nephrol.* 1994; **5**: 125–137.

93. Solomon, R. Contrast-medium-induced acute renal failure. *Kidney Int.* 1998; **53**: 230–242.

94. Morcos, S. K., Thomsen, H. S., & Webb, J. A. Contrast Media Safety Committee of the European Society of Urogenital Radiology. Dialysis and contrast media. *Eur. Radiol.* 2002; **12**: 3026–3030.

95. Tombach, B., Bremer, C., Reimer, P. *et al.* Renal tolerance of a neutral gadolinium chelate (gadoburtol) in patients with chronic renal failure: results of a randomized study. *Radiology* 2001; **218**: 651–657.

96. Solomon, R., Werner, C., Mann, D. *et al.* Effects of saline, mannitol, and furosemide on acute decreases in renal function induced by radiocontrast agents. *N. Engl. J. Med.* 2003; **331**: 1416–1420.

97. Aspelin, P., Aubry, P., Frannson, S. G. *et al.* Nephrotoxic effects in high-risk patients undergoing angiography. *N. Engl. J. Med.* 2003; **348**: 491–499.

98. Tepel, M., Van Der Giet, M., Schwartfeld, C. *et al.* Prevention of radiographic-contrast-agent-induced reduction in renal function by acetylcysteine. *N. Engl. J. Med.* 2003; **343**: 180–184.

99. Diaz-Sandoval, L. J., Kosowsky, B. D., Losordo, D. W. Acetylcysteine to prevent angiography-related renal tissue injury (The APART trial). *Am. J. Cardiol.* 2002; **89**: 356–358.

100. Boccalandro, F., Amhad, M., Smalling, R. W. *et al.* Oral acetylcysteine does not protect renal function from moderate to high doses of intravenous radiographic contrast. *Catheter Cardiovasc. Interv.* 2003; **58**: 336–341.

101. Durham, J. D., Caputo, C., Dokko, J. *et al.* A randomized controlled trial of *N*-acetylcysteine to prevent contrast nephropathy in cardiac angiography. *Kidney Int.* 2002; **62**: 2202–2207.

102. Briguori, C., Manganelli, F., Scarpato, P. *et al.* Acetylcysteine and contrast agent-associated nephrotoxicity. *J. Am. Coll. Cardiol.* 2002; **40**: 298–303.

102a. Merten, G. J., Burgess, W. P., Gray, L. V. *et al.* Prevention of contrast-induced nephropathy with sodium bicarbonate. *J. Am. Med. Assoc.* 2004; **291**: 2328–2334.

103. Conger, J. D. Interventions in clinical acute renal failure: what are the data. *Am. J. Kidney Dis.* 1995; **26**: 565–576.

104. Star, R. A. Treatment of acute renal failure. *Kidney Int.* 1998; **42**: 1817–1831.

105. Myers, B. D. & Morelli, S. M. Hemodynamically mediated acute renal failure. *N. Engl. J. Med.* 1986; **314**: 97–105.

106. Schulman, G., Fogo, A., Gung, A. *et al.* Complement activation retards resolution of acute ischemic renal failure. *Kidney Int.* 1991; **40**: 1069–1074.

107. Hakim, R. A., Wingard, R. L., & Parker, R. A. Effect of the dialysis membrane in the treatment of patients with acute renal failure. *N. Engl. J. Med.* 1994; **331**: 1338–1342.

108. Schiffl, H., Lang, S. M., & Konig, A. Biocompatible membranes in acute renal failure. *Lancet* 1994; **344**: 570–572.

109. Schiffl, H., Lang, S. M., & Fischer, R. Daily hemodialysis and the outcome of acute renal failure. *N. Engl. J. Med.* 2002; **346**: 305–310.

110. Paganini, E. P., Tapolyai, M., Goormastic, M. *et al.* Establishing a dialysis therapy/patient outcome link in intensive care acute dialysis for patients with acute renal failure. *Am. J. Kidney Dis.* 1996; **28**: S81.

111. Kumar, V. A., Yeun, J. Y., Craig, M. *et al.* A new approach to renal replacement therapy for acute renal failure in the intensive care unit. *Am. J. Kidney Dis.* 2000; **36**: 294–300.

112. Golper, T. A. Continuous renal replacement therapy in acute renal failure. In Rose, B. D. *Up To Date* (10.3). 2003. Wellesley, MA.

113. Hertel, J., Keep, D. M., & Caruana, R. J. Anticoagulation. In Daugirdas, J. T., Blake, P. G., & Ing, T. S., eds. *Handbook of Dialysis*, 3rd edn. Philadelphia: Lippincott, Williams & Wilkins, 2001: 182–198.

114. Miller, C. F. Renal Failure. In Breslow, M. J., Miller, C. F., & Rogers, M., eds. *Perioperative Management.* St. Louis: C.V. Mosby Co., 1990: 327–342.

115. Chertow, G. M., Lazarus, J. M., Paganini, E. P. *et al.* Predictors of mortality and the provision of dialysis in patients with acute tubular necrosis. *J. Am. Soc. Nephrol.* 1998; **9**: 692–698.

116. Rose, B. D. Postischemic and postoperative acute tubular necrosis. In Rose, B. D. *Up To Date.* (10.3). 2002. Wellesley, MA.

117. Wardle, E. N. Acute renal failure and multiorgan failure. *Nephron* 1994; **66**: 380–385.

118. Perazella, M. A. & Eras, L. Are COX-2 selective inhibitors nephrotoxic? *Am. J. Kidney Dis.* 2000; **35**: 937–940.

119. Patrono, C. & Dunn, M. J. The clinical significance of inhibition of renal prostaglandin synthesis. *Kidney Int.* 1987; **32**: 1–12.

120. Bakris, G. L. & Weir, M. R. Angiotensin-converting enzyme inhibitor-associated elevations in serum creatinine: is this a cause for concern? *Arch. Intern. Med.* 2000; **160**: 685–693.

121. Oster, J. R. & Materson, B. J. Renal and electrolyte complications of congestive heart failure and effects with angiotensin-converting enzyme inhibitors. *Ann. Intern. Med.* 1992; **152**: 704–710.

122. Humes, H. D. Aminoglycoside nephrotoxicity. *Kidney Int.* 1988; **33**: 900–911.

123. Moore, R. D., Smith, C. R., & Lipsky, J. J. Risk factors for nephrotoxicity in patients treated with aminoglycosides. *Ann. Intern. Med.* 1984; **100**: 352–357.

124. Meyer, R. D. Risk factors and comparisons of clinical nephrotoxicity of aminoglycosides. *Am. J. Med.* 1986; **80**: 119–125.

125. Zager, R. A. Studies of mechanisms and protective maneuvers in myoglobinuric acute renal injury. *Lab. Invest.* 1989; **60**: 619–629.

126. Zager, R. A. Rhabdomyolysis and myohemoglobinuric acute renal failure [editorial]. *Kidney Int.* 1996; **49**: 314–326.

127. Don, B. R., Rodriguez, R. A., & Humphreys, M. H. Acute renal failure associated with pigmenturia or crystal deposits. In Schrier, R. W., ed. *Diseases of the Kidney and Urinary Tract*, 7th edn. Philadelphia: Lippincott, Williams & Wilkins, 2001: 1299–1326.

128. Bywaters, E. G. & Beall, D. Crush injuries with impairment of renal function. *J. Am. Soc. Nephrol.* 1998; **9**: 322–332.

129. Better, O. S. & Stein, J. H. Early management of shock and prophylaxis of acute renal failure in traumatic rhabdomyolysis. *N. Engl. J. Med.* 1990; **322**: 825–829.

130. Zager, R. A. Combined mannitol and deferoxamine therapy for myohemoglobinuric renal injury and oxidant tubular stress. Mechanistic and therapeutic implications. *J. Clin. Invest.* 1992; **90**: 711–719.

131. Eneas, J. F., Schoenfeld, P. Y., & Humphreys, M. H. The effect of infusion of mannitol-sodium bicarbonate on the clinical course of myoglobinuria. *Arch. Intern. Med.* 1979; **139**: 801–805.

132. Connolly, S. J. & Kates, R. E. Clinical pharmacokinetics of *N*-acetylprocainamide. *Clin. Pharmacokinet.* 1982; **7**: 206–220.

133. Vlasses, P. H., Ferguson, R. K., Rocci, M. L. Jr. *et al.* Lethal accumulation of procainamide metabolite in severe renal insufficiency. *Am. J. Nephrol.* 1986; **6**: 112–116.

134. Pruchnicki, M. C., Coyle, J. D., Hoshaw-Woodard, S. *et al.* Effect of phosphate binders on supplemental iron absorption in healthy subjects. *J. Clin. Pharmacol.* 2002; **42**: 1171–1176.

135. Maton, P. N. & Burton, M. E. Antacids revisited: a review of their clinical pharmacology and recommended therapeutic use. *Drugs* 1999; **57**: 855–870.

136. Cheng, J. W., Charland, S. L., Shaw, L. M. *et al.* Is the volume of distribution of digoxin reduced in patients with renal dysfunction? Determining digoxin pharmacokinetics by fluorescence polarization immunoassay. *Pharmacotherapy* 1997; **17**: 584–590.

137. Borga, O., Hoppel, C., Odar-Cederlof, I. *et al.* Plasma levels and renal excretion of phenytoin and its metabolites in patients with renal failure. *Clin. Pharmacol. Ther.* 1979; **26**: 306–314.

138. Levey, A. S., Bosch, J. P., Lewis, J. B. *et al.* A more accurate method to estimate glomerular filtration rate from serum creatinine: a new prediction equation. Modification of Diet in Renal Disease Study Group. *Ann. Intern. Med.* 1999; **130**: 461–470.

139. Hu, K. T., Matayoshi, A., & Stevenson, F. T. Calculation of the estimated creatinine clearance in avoiding drug dosing errors in the older patient. *Am. J. Med. Sci.* 2001; **322**: 133–136.

140. Aronoff, G. R., Berns, J. S., Brier, M. E. *et al. Drug Prescribing in Renal Failure: Dosing Guidelines for Adults*, 4th edn. Philadelphia, 1999.

141. Sladen, R. N. Anesthetic considerations for the patient with renal failure. *Anesthesiol. Clin. North Am.* 2000; **18**: 863–882.

142. Cranshaw, J. & Holland, D. Anaesthesia for patients with renal impairment. *Br. J. Hosp. Med.* 1996; **55**: 171–175.

143. Nishimori, A., Tanaka, K., Ueno, K. *et al.* Effects of sevoflurane anaesthesia on renal function. *J. Int. Med. Res.* 1997; **25**: 87–91.

144. Conzen, P. F., Nuscheler, M., Melotte, A. *et al.* Renal function and serum fluoride concentrations in patients with stable renal insufficiency after anesthesia with sevoflurane or enflurane. *Anesth. Analg.* 1995; **81**: 569–575.

145. Litz, R. J., Hubler, M., Lorenz, W. *et al.* Renal responses to desflurane and isoflurane in patients with renal insufficiency. *Anesthesiology* 2002; **97**: 1133–1136.

25

Postoperative electrolyte disorders

Juliet Kottak Mavromatis

Emory University School of Medicine, Atlanta, GA

A variety of electrolyte disorders are common postoperatively. These result from fluid losses, intravenous fluid administration, and intrinsic regulatory mechanisms that come into play at this time. During surgery, large volumes of isotonic fluids as well as blood products may be given to compensate for the blood loss and third spacing that occurs with the surgical procedure. In the postoperative period patients must remain fasting until bowel function has returned. Frequently, nasogastric, chest, or biliary tubes are present and drain fluids and maintenance intravenous fluids are continued. Parenteral nutrition often complicates fluid balance. There may be shifts in acid–base status such as metabolic acidosis from lactic acidosis secondary to tissue ischemia, or respiratory alkalosis from hyperventilation as a result of pain or mechanical ventilation. Anesthetics, diuretics, steroids, insulin, cardiac medications, and non-steroidal anti-inflammatory drugs administered during this time period may alter plasma electrolytes and further complicate the picture.

Sodium disorders

Abnormalities of serum sodium are generally disorders of water balance. Hyponatremia occurs when there is too much free water, which may be retained appropriately or inappropriately. Hypernatremia occurs in patients who have an impaired thirst mechanism or have limited access to water and are not repleted appropriately. Of the two, hyponatremia is generally more common as a postoperative problem.

Hyponatremia

In order to understand sodium and water disorders one must understand the relationship between plasma sodium concentration and serum osmolality. Plasma osmolality is defined by the equation:

$$P_{osm} = 2 \times [Na^+] + glucose/18 + BUN/2.8 \qquad (25.1)$$

Under normal circumstances plasma urea and glucose contribute minimally to the total, leaving plasma sodium as the main determinant of serum osmolality. Consequently, hyponatremic patients are most often hypoosmolar. Normal serum osmolality ranges from 274 to 290 mosmol/kg. The plasma, or extracellular osmolality, is in balance with the total body osmolality, which is determined by both intracellular solutes and extracellular solutes. Potassium salts make up the primary intracellular solute. Plasma sodium concentration is equal to exchangeable sodium plus exchangeable potassium divided by total body water:

$$Plasma[Na^+] = Na_e^+ + K_e^+ / TBW \qquad (25.2)$$

Thus changes in potassium balance may also affect sodium homeostasis.

Plasma osmolality is carefully regulated by osmoreceptors in the hypothalamus that detect minute changes in osmolality and accordingly affect thirst and output of ADH (anti diuretic hormone) from the posterior lobe of the pituitary. ADH acts in the kidney on the collecting tubules causing resorption of water resulting in an increase in urinary osmolality. In addition, however, extracellular volume status with volume contraction can override the effect of hypoosmolality, stimulating secretion of ADH on its own.

When confronted with a hyponatremic patient, it is first important to determine the patient's serum tonicity. Most often in hyponatremic patients the plasma is hypoosmolar. However, as seen in eq 25.1, patients with an elevation of plasma glucose may be hyperosmolar but hyponatremic. The sodium concentration may fall by 1.7 meq/l

Medical Management of the Surgical Patient: A Textbook of Perioperative Medicine, ed. M. F. Lubin, R. B. Smith, T. F. Dobson, N. Spell, H. K. Walker. 4th edn. Published by Cambridge University Press. © Cambridge University 2006.

for every 100 mg/dl rise in plasma glucose.[1] "Hidden" osmoles may cause an "osmolal gap," which is seen as a difference between the measured and the calculated plasma osmolality. Substances that cause this gap include mannitol, methanol and ethylene glycol, among others. Hyponatremia may be seen in situations where irrigant solutions (mannitol, sorbitol, or glycine) used during surgery are absorbed systemically. The absorption of such solutions most commonly occurs in prostate surgery, and results in "post-TURP syndrome." Irrigant solutions may be either hypo- or isotonic and the resultant hyponatremia may be hypo-, iso- or hyperosmolar, depending on the solution used, its ability to diffuse across the cell membrane, and the extent to which it may induce an osmotic diuresis. The hyponatremia that results may produce severe symptoms and its treatment remains controversial.[1,2] It has been suggested that, if the resulting hyponatremia is near iso-osmolar, observation may be the best therapy. However, if hypoosmolar hyponatremia results, it should be treated the same as for euvolemic hyponatremia – hypertonic saline if symptoms of hyponatremia are present.[3]

Pseudohyponatremia was a problem diagnosed in the past, caused by elevated levels of plasma proteins or high serum triglycerides causing a reduction in plasma water. The newer means of measuring serum sodium with an ion-sensitive electrode, rather than a flame photometer, enables an accurate sodium measurement within the aqueous phase of the plasma.

Hyponatremia is categorized based on extracellular volume status – hypovolemic, normovolemic, or hypervolemic hyponatremia. History and clinical examination with orthostatic blood pressure and pulse measurement, assessment of jugular venous distention and peripheral edema are of primary importance. Determining the urine sodium concentration is often helpful unless the patient has been on diuretics. A urine sodium of less than 25 meq/l indicates a reduction in effective circulating volume, including loss of volume through the gastrointestinal tract, lungs, skin, third spacing of fluids, or loss of effective volume from congestive heart failure and cirrhosis. A urine sodium of greater than 40 meq/l is seen with SIADH (syndrome of inappropriate ADH secretion), renal insufficiency, diuretics, hypothyroidism and adrenal insufficiency. The urine osmolality should also be ordered. A urine osmolality of less than 100 reflects maximally dilute urine. However, most patients with hyponatremia have a defect in water excretion and are not able to achieve this level.[4]

Water intoxication may be iatrogenic, or self-induced by drinking water, as in psychogenic polydipsia. It occurs commonly in the postoperative state and is probably related both to the administration of excessive amounts of hypotonic intravenous fluids along with increased secretion of ADH related to postoperative pain, anesthesia, analgesic use, and third spacing of fluid. In one prospective study postoperative hyponatremia occurred in 4.4% of operations. It was particularly common following cardiovascular and gastrointestinal or biliary surgeries, where it occurred approximately 20% of the time. Of the hyponatremic patients studied, 21% were found to have hyponatremia related to hyperglycemia, 21% were volume overloaded, and 42% were euvolemic. The remaining patients were hypovolemic or had renal failure.[5] Almost all the hyponatremic patients had been given hypotonic fluids in the perioperative period. However, severe postoperative hyponatremia may also arise with the administration of isotonic fluid. In these cases elevated plasma ADH levels may lead to resorption of excretion of hypertonic urine.[3,6] While hyponatremia probably occurs at equal rates in men and women postoperatively, young menstruating women may be at increased risk of permanent brain injury or death related to the hyponatremia.[7,8]

The symptoms of hyponatremia are primarily of central nervous system dysfunction including delirium, nausea, vomiting, and seizures. Patients are generally asymptomatic if serum sodium is greater than 125 meq/l. Symptoms that do occur relate to cerebral edema. The degree of severity of these symptoms depends on the rapidity of change in serum sodium. In chronic hyponatremia protective mechanisms exist, causing a loss of organic osmolytes from the brain, thereby decreasing osmotic pressure and edema. This loss of osmolytes is what makes the rapid correction of hyponatremia particularly dangerous. Patients who have developed hyponatremia on a chronic basis are at higher risk of developing complications relating to the rapid correction of serum sodium than patients who have developed acute hyponatremia. The syndrome of brain demyelination of pontine and extrapontine neurons, known as central pontine myelinolysis, may occur with rapid correction of serum sodium. This results in rapidly deteriorating mental status several days after correction of serum sodium and at times quadriparesis, pseudobulbar palsy and rarely death.[9]

The goal of management of hyponatremia should be to ameliorate the symptoms that it produces; which is generally possible by elevating serum sodium to greater than 125 meq/l. Myelinolysis does not appear to occur provided that the serum sodium is corrected no faster than 12 meq/l per day.[10] For patients who are hypovolemic, normal saline should be administered to restore volume. Serum sodium should be monitored frequently. For patients who are euvolemic resulting from inappropriate ADH secretion, free water restriction is the mainstay of therapy. If symptoms of hyponatremia are present, hypertonic saline may be carefully administered (usually in the form of 3% sodium chloride in water. Five percent solution is also available). Loop diuretics may be used in either situation to increase the excretion of dilute urine. A useful calculation suggested by Androgue in a recent review is the change in serum sodium produced by administering one liter of an infusate.[1] It may be estimated as:

$$\Delta \text{ in serum sodium after one liter of infusate}$$
$$= \frac{(\text{Infusate Na}^+ + \text{infusate K}^+) - \text{serum Na}}{(\text{Total body water} + 1)} \quad (25.3)$$

The infusate sodium in 3% NaCl is 513 mmol per liter. A conservative approach is to target the increase in serum sodium to be no more than 8–10 mmol/l per day or to stop when the serum sodium concentration is greater than 125 mmol/l, or when the symptoms of hyponatremia subside. Initially, the rate of correction may be 1–2 mmol/l per hour. After these goals have been achieved, longer-term measures may be initiated. If SIADH is present demeclocycline, a tetracycline derivative, may be used in a dose of 600 to 1200 mg per day to decrease renal sensitivity to ADH, producing a nephrogenic diabetes insipidus.[4] Water restriction should be continued and loop diuretics may be continued to promote the diuresis of dilute urine.

In the case of hypervolemic patients with hyponatremia, loop diuretics along with free water restriction to less than 1 liter per day are standard treatments.

Hypernatremia

Hypernatremia most often occurs as a postoperative complication in patients who are unable to drink adequately to meet their free water needs. Patients who are on ventilators or elderly patients who have delirium or dementia are common candidates. In one study of patients with hospital acquired hypernatremia, half were intubated; and of those remaining, two thirds had altered mental status.[11] Patients with an intact thirst mechanism and access to water virtually never develop this disorder, even in the case of dramatic wasting of free water.

Causes of hypernatremia include loss of water via insensible losses from skin and lung (e.g., the febrile patient), renal losses through diuretics or diabetes insipidus, and gastrointestinal losses (e.g., osmotic diarrhea). Rarely sodium gain through ingestion of excessive sodium or administration of hypertonic NaCl, sodium bicarbonate, or through primary hyperaldosteronism may occur. Common hospital situations include the initiation of tube feeds without free water supplementation, over-diuresis with loop diuretics, hyperglycemia causing an osmotic diuresis or overzealous administration of lactulose.[4] Neurogenic diabetes insipidous may be seen in patients following transsphenoidal pituitary surgery or as a result of trauma to the hypothalamus. Hypothalamic or pituitary destruction by neoplasms such as craniopharyngioma or infiltration of this area by sardoidosis may also be the culprit.[12] Nephrogenic diabetes insipidus occurs when the collecting tubules are resistant to the effects of ADH. This may be caused by drugs – most commonly lithium, or by hypercalcemia.[13] However, even in this disorder the patient may be able to keep up with free water losses provided he or she has an intact sensorium and access to water. Symptoms of hypernatremia result from cellular dehydration as a result of the hyperosmotic state. As in hyponatremia symptoms are primarily neurological – weakness, coma and seizures – and depend on the acuity of the change in serum sodium concentration. Generally patients are asymptomatic until the serum sodium is greater than 160 mmol/l.[13] With severe cases cerebral bleeding may occur.

The management of hypernatremia involves correcting a volume deficit, if present, in order to restore normal vital signs, followed by correction of the free water deficit. It has been suggested that the maximum rate of lowering serum sodium should not exceed 12 meq/l per day or 0.5 meq/l per hour.[4,13] The water deficit may be estimated as:

$$\text{Water deficit} = 0.6 \times \text{total body weight}$$
$$\times \frac{[(\text{plasma Na}) - 140]}{140} \quad (25.4)$$

One must also take into account insensible losses (30 to 50 ml/h) and any ongoing high levels of urinary or gastrointestinal losses. The primary risks of correcting hypernatremia too fast are cerebral edema and cerebral hemorrhage.

In central, or "neurogenic" diabetes insipidus, desmopressin (dDAVP) may be administered. It comes in nasal and oral forms with a nasal dose ranging from 5 to 20 µg once or twice a day, or an oral dose of 0.1 to 0.8 mg divided in two or three doses daily. Nephrogenic diabetes insipidus may be treated with thiazide diuretics and a low protein, low sodium diet.[14]

Potassium disorders

Potassium disorders are common in the hospitalized patient. Potassium is the major intracellular osmole, and 98% of total body potassium is located in the intracellular compartment. The sodium potassium ATPase pump helps maintain the appropriate balance of sodium and potassium within the extracellular and intracellular spaces. The potassium gradient is important for maintenance of the cell membrane resting potential. When the plasma concentration of potassium is too low, the cell membrane becomes hyperpolarized and easily excitable and when the plasma concentration of potassium is elevated, the cell membrane is depolarized and less excitable. This accounts for the signs and symptoms of hypo- and hyperkalemia, which cause changes in neuromuscular function.

Disorders of potassium balance occur when there are abnormal gains and losses of potassium from the extracellular space or from transcellular shift of potassium between the extracellular and intracellular compartments. Changes in acid–base status affect the transport of potassium. Metabolic acidosis causes a shift of potassium to the extracellular space that is coupled with the intracellular movement of hydrogen ions. Metabolic alkalosis causes movement of potassium into the intracellular space. Increased beta-adrenergic activity and insulin also cause activation of the sodium potassium ATPase pump and movement of potassium to the intracellular space. Losses of potassium may occur from the kidney or the gastrointestinal tract. Diarrhea, vomiting and gastric tube drainage may deplete potassium through the loss of gastrointestinal fluids containing potassium. Potassium depletion is increased by the elevation in aldosterone that results from volume contraction and hypoosmolarity. Renal wasting of potassium commonly occurs as a result of loop and thiazide diuretics, or in states of mineralocorticoid or cortisol excess such as primary hyperaldosteronism or Cushing's syndrome. Aldosterone causes the resorption of sodium and excretion of potassium and hydrogen ion leading to metabolic alkalosis. Treatment with other medications, such as penicillins, may lead to potassium ion secretion by the distal tubule as a result of the production of large concentrations of metabolites that are nonresorbable anions within the distal tubule. Another condition leading to hypokalemia in the hospitalized patient is treatment with amphotericin B, which leads to enhanced secretion of K^+ from the distal tubule and causes a type I renal tubular acidosis. Syndromes that less commonly present in the hospitalized patient include Bartter and Gitelman syndromes.

The most important clinical manifestations of hypo- and hyperkalemia are cardiac, although both disorders may also lead to generalized muscle weakness. Because of its effect on the resting potential of the myocardium, potassium disorders cause cardiac arrythmias. Hypokalemia results in delayed ventricular depolarization. Initial EKG changes include ST segment depression,

decreased amplitude of the T wave and increased amplitude of the U wave in the precordial leads. More severe potassium depletion leads to PR prolongation and QRS widening. Atrioventricular heart block, junctional tachycardia, paroxysmal atrial tachycardia, or ventricular arrythmias may ensue.[4,15,27] Hypokalemia can augment the effect of digitalis, resulting in toxicity at lower than expected levels.

The EKG changes of hyperkalemia include the initial appearance of narrow and peaked T waves and QT interval shortening, followed by PR prolongation and QRS widening. A sine wave may occur as the widened QRS merges with the T wave with life-threatening hyperkalemia. These changes in cardiac conduction may lead to ventricular fibrillation or asystole.[15] A low plasma calcium concentration and metabolic acidosis may make a patient more susceptible to this.

Hyperkalemia results from either increased potassium intake, decreased excretion through urine or transcellular shift. In the hospitalized patient there may be excessive intravenous infusion or oral supplementation of potassium, particularly in a patient with impaired renal function. One often sees transcellular shift causing hyperkalemia in the patient with hyperglycemia, insulin deficiency, and metabolic acidosis. In such patients, although plasma potassium levels are high, total body potassium is usually low as a result of increased renal excretion of potassium. This leads to hypokalemia with correction. Hyperkalemia also may result from tissue breakdown in rhabdomyolysis, tissue necrosis, or during treatment of hematologic malignancies – tumor lysis syndrome. In cardiopulmonary bypass surgeries reperfusion of ischemic areas as well as rewarming of hypothermic tissues can result in significant hyperkalemia.

Drugs such as potassium-sparing diuretics, beta-blockers and succinylcholine may contribute to hyperkalemia. Beta-blockers decrease cellular uptake of potassium, whereas succinylcholine used in general anesthesia may cause hyperkalemia by altering the cell membrane action potential, favoring movement of potassium to the extracellular space. Other drugs may result in hyperkalemia by causing hypoaldosteronism by different mechanisms; these include nonsteroidal anti-inflammatory drugs (NSAIDS) and ACE inhibitors.[16] One review found that in 60% of adult inpatients with potassium levels greater than 5.9 meq/l, a drug was a probable contributing factor. The most common causative drugs were potassium chloride, captopril, NSAIDs, and potassium-sparing diuretics. In these hyperkalemic patients most also had impaired potassium homeostasis secondary to renal insufficiency, diabetes or metabolic acidosis.[17]

Management

The management of hypokalemia involves the oral supplementation or intravenous infusion of potassium, along with addressing the underlying problem that caused the potassium deficiency. The normal daily requirement of potassium is 60 to 100 meq. Oral supplementation of 60 to 80 meq per day plus normal dietary intake is generally sufficient for the patient who is able to eat.[4] If symptoms are more severe or if a patient is unable to eat, intravenous treatment is necessary. The recommended rate of correction is 10 to 20 meq per hour. However, in dire circumstances, up to 40 meq per hour may be administered. Monitoring on telemetry is essential, as the intravenous infusion of potassium can result in heart block. If the rate of infusion exceeds 10 meq per hour, hourly checks on serum potassium are recommended. One must remember to simultaneously correct hypomagnesemia. The peripheral intravenous administration of potassium frequently causes phlebitis; nonetheless, peripheral administration is preferred as central administration may increase the likelihood of cardiac arrythmias.

The initial management of life threatening hyperkalemia includes the administration of calcium, which acts to stabilize the myocardium, improves cardiac conduction, and reduces the likelihood of cardiac arrythmia. Calcium may be administered in a dose of 10 ml of 10% calcium gluconate over 2 to 3 minutes. The effect is immediate, though short-lived, and is recommended in cases where serum potassium concentration exceeds 7.5 meq/l, or where cardiac arrythmias are already present. Next, sodium bicarbonate may be used. This is more helpful in cases of concomitant metabolic acidosis, and less helpful in cases of advanced renal failure. The bicarbonate shifts the potassium to the intracellular space. Onset of action is typically 30 to 60 minutes. A dose of 44 to 50 meq of sodium bicarbonate may be given intravenously over five minutes. Finally, insulin may be administered, typically along with glucose, except in hyperglycemic patients, who require insulin alone. An intravenous dose of 10 units of regular insulin, along with 25 to 50 g of glucose, is typical. Again, potassium is shifted to the intracellular space, the effect of which is somewhat delayed, seen minutes to an hour after its administration. The effect of Kayexalate, sodium polystyrenesulfonate, is even more delayed although it removes potassium from the body. This agent is a cation exchange resin, which causes increased potassium uptake in the gut in exchange for the release of sodium. It is typically given orally in a dose of 40 to 50 g mixed with 100 ml of 20% sorbital every 4 to 6 hours. An enema form is also available – 50 g in 50 ml of 70% sorbital

plus 100 to 150 ml of tap water. It is recommended that this be followed by the administration of a non-sodium irrigant solution because of the possibility of colonic toxicity.[4,27]

In cases of renal insufficiency dialysis may be necessary to treat hyperkalemia. With chronic mild hyperkalemia, drugs such as ace inhibitors and potassium-sparing diuretics should be avoided. If mineralocorticoid deficiency is present, fludrocortisone in a dose of 0.2 to 1 mg per day may be given. If hypertension, congestive heart failure, and/or mild renal insufficiency are present, loop or thiazide diuretics may be the treatment of choice.

Postoperative acid–base disorders

While a comprehensive discussion of acid–base disorders is beyond the scope of this chapter, there are particular acid–base disorders that occur frequently in the postsurgical setting. Metabolic alkalosis is the most common acid–base disturbance to occur in the hospital setting.[18] It occurs when plasma bicarbonate is increased and may be acute, with an elevated plasma pH, or chronic, with a relatively normal plasma pH. In chronic metabolic alkalosis a compensatory respiratory acidosis occurs with an elevation in serum pCO_2 of 0.7 mmHg per 1 meq/l increase in plasma bicarbonate.

The most common etiologies are gastrointestinal or renal losses of hydrogen ion. Gastrointestinal fluids may be lost through postoperative vomiting or nasogastric suction. The concomitant loss of potassium and volume helps to perpetuate the alkalosis. Increased aldosterone secretion leads to depletion of hydrogen ion through the kidney, through the activation of the Na^+-H^+-ATPase. This mechanism does not come into play unless there is adequate delivery of sodium to the distal tubule. This is common in the setting of diuretic use, when distal delivery of sodium is enhanced and hyperaldosteronism may lead to metabolic alkalosis.[4,16] Concurrent hypokalemia plays a role in maintaining the extracellular alkalosis by causing transcellular shift with potassium moving extracellular in exchange for hydrogen ion moving into the cell.

Metabolic alkalosis has been linked with increased morbidity and mortality in critically ill patients, especially those being treated with mechanical ventilation.[19] Through compensatory mechanisms respiratory drive is decreased and hypoxemia and hypercapnia can result. This may make weaning from mechanical ventilation more difficult. In addition, metabolic alkalosis results in peripheral and coronary vasoconstriction and decreased oxygen delivery to tissues. The result may be cardiac arrythmias or neurological changes.[18] The appropriate treatment of metabolic alkalosis most often includes the administration of sodium chloride to correct the volume and chloride deficits, as well as correction of hypokalemia. In cases of mineralocorticoid excess administration of sodium chloride is ineffective. These patients generally are hypertensive, volume expanded and hypokalemic. The alkalosis is generally mild.

Metabolic acidosis is also common postoperatively – particularly in the case of cardiovascular surgeries or trauma. In these situations tissue ischemia or rhabdomyolysis may result in lactic acidosis and hyperkalemia related to transcellular shift. Metabolic acidosis may be classified based on the presence of a normal or an elevated anion gap, which is calculated by the difference between the plasma Na^+ and the measured anions, Cl^- and HCO_3. The anion gap is normally 5 to 11 meq/l.[4]

The most common causes of an elevated anion gap metabolic acidosis in the postoperative setting are lactic acidosis, ketoacidosis and uremia. Hyperchloremic metabolic acidosis may occur after surgical procedures resulting in the loss of biliary fluids that are rich in sodium bicarbonate through ongoing biliary drainage or pancreaticenteric fistulae. Urinary diversion procedures such as ureterosigmoidostomy and ureteroileostomy may result in the resorption of urinary chloride in the ureteral conduit in exchange for increased excretion of bicarbonate into stool.[20] Diarrhea, renal tubular acidosis and drugs (amphotericin, carbonic anhydrase inhibitors and spironolactone, among others) account for other cases of normal anion gap metabolic acidosis. The urinary anion gap (urine sodium plus potassium minus chloride) may be useful in diagnosing the cause of hyperchloremic metabolic acidosis. A negative anion gap generally occurs with gastrointestinal bicarbonate loss whereas a positive gap occurs with disorders of urinary acidification – renal tubular acidosis.[21]

Therapy of metabolic acidosis involves correcting the underlying problems leading to this condition – improving tissue perfusion and oxygenation, treating infection, administering insulin, fluids, or removing an inciting medication. In lactic acidosis and diabetic ketoacidosis the administration of sodium bicarbonate is generally recommended in cases where the plasma pH falls below 7.1, at which point cardiac contractility is decreased, there is peripheral vasodilation, decreased renal and hepatic blood flow, and increased pulmonary vascular resistance.[4,22,23] However, the use of sodium bicarbonate remains controversial; it may be associated with complications, and does not appear to improve survival in these critically ill patients.[25,26]

Respiratory acid–base disturbances may occur following surgery. Respiratory alkalosis frequently results from postoperative pain or anxiety causing hyperventilation. Drugs or hormonal causes of respiratory alkalosis include salicylates, cathecholamines, progesterone, and pregnancy. More serious disorders that increase the respiratory rate include central nervous system events such as stroke or subarachnoid hemorrhage, and fever. Hypoxemia and/or direct stimulation of chest receptors may cause hyperventilation. One must consider pneumonia, pulmonary embolus, pulmonary edema, pneumothorax, and sepsis as potential causes of respiratory alkalosis. Finally, hepatic failure and mechanical hyperventilation are common etiologies in the hospitalized patient. Respiratory alkalosis causes reduced cerebral blood flow and may cause cerebral hypoxia. However, by reducing cerebral blood flow it may be used as a therapeutic measure in neurosurgical patients to reduce cerebral edema and intracranial pressure.[12]

Respiratory acidosis is a result of alveolar hypoventilation. In the postoperative setting there may be neurological, muscular or pulmonary causes. Respiratory acidosis may occur because of overdosing with sedative or anesthetic agents, postoperative delirium, or acute neurological events – though, as mentioned above, strokes and bleeds commonly lead to respiratory alkalosis. Pain may limit motion of the chest wall or diaphragm after transthoracic or intraabdominal procedures. Primary lung problems with severe upper or lower airway obstruction, such as laryngospasm or bronchospasm, pulmonary infection or edema, inadequate intubation or mechanical ventilation frequently result in hypercarbia. The danger of respiratory acidosis lies in the accompanying hypoxemia. Ensuring an adequate airway and treatment with oxygen, either through mechanical or nonmechanical means, is of paramount importance. This is followed by correction of the underlying disorder. In patients with chronic respiratory acidosis (usually from chronic lung disease) with a compensatory metabolic alkalosis, worsening respiratory acidosis should be treated more cautiously, as overzealous oxygen therapy may diminish respiratory drive. In addition, the generation of metabolic alkalosis should be avoided as it leads to suppression of respiratory drive and worsening hypercapnia. When mechanical ventilation is initiated, care must be taken not to overly reduce the plasma carbon dioxide level as this will cause an acute metabolic alkalosis that may worsen neurological function and make patients susceptible to cardiac arrhythmias and reduced cardiovascular output.

In summary, electrolyte and acid–base disorders are common in the postoperative setting. The patient's past medical history, including a history of congestive heart failure, cirrhosis, renal insufficiency, chronic obstructive pulmonary disease, diabetes or dementia, may give clues about a patient's susceptibility to particular disorders of fluid and sodium balance, potassium homeostasis or acid-base disturbances. A review of historical factors, laboratory data, and scrutiny of the patient's operative and postoperative records, with attention to fluids and medications administered in the perioperative period, is necessary for appropriate diagnosis and treatment of these disturbances.

REFERENCES

1. Androgue, H. J. & Madias, N. E. Primary care: hyponatremia. *N. Engl. J. Med.* 2000; **342**: 1581–1589.

2. Agarwal, R. & Emmett, M. The post-transurethral resection of prostate syndrome: therapeutic proposals. *Am. J. Kidney Dis.* 1994; **24**: 108–111.

3. Gowrishankar, M., Lin, S.-H., Oh, M. S., & Halperin, M. L. Acute hyponatremia in the perioperative period: insights into its pathophysiology and recommendations for management. *Clin. Nephrol.* 1998; **50**: 352–360.

4. Rose, B. D. & Post, T. W. *Clinical Physiology of Acid–Base and Electrolyte Disorders.* New York: McGraw-Hill, 2001.

5. Chung, H.-M., Kluge, R., Schrier, R. W., & Anderson, R. J. Postoperative hyponatremia: a prospective study. *Arch. Int. Med.* 1986; **146**: 333–336.

6. Steele, A., Gowrishankar, M., Abrahamson, S., Mazer, C. D. *et al.* Postoperative hyponatremia despite near-isotonic saline infusion: a phenomenon of desalination. *Ann. Int. Med.* 1997; **126**: 20–25.

7. Arieff, A. I. Hyponatremia, convulsions, respiratory arrest, and permanent brain damage after elective surgery in healthy women. *N. Engl. J. Med.* 1986; **314**: 1529–1534.

8. Ayus, C., Wheeler, J. M., & Arieff, A. I. Postoperative hyponatremic encephalopathy in menstruant women. *Ann. Int. Med.* 1992; **117**: 891–897.

9. Laureno, R. & Karp, B. I. Myelinolysis after correction of hyponatremia. *Ann. Int. Med.* 1997; **126**: 57–62.

10. Sterns, R. H., Riggs, J. E., & Schochet, S. S. Osmotic demyelination syndrome following correction of hyponatremia. *N. Engl. J. Med.* 1986; **314**: 1535–1541.

11. Palevsky, P. M., Bhargrath, R., & Greenberg, A. Hypernatremia in hospitalized patients. *Ann. Int. Med.* 1996; **124**: 197–203.

12. Andrews, B. T. Fluid and electrolyte disorders in neurosurgical intensive care. *Neurosurg. Clin. North Am.* 1994; **5**: 707–721.

13. Androgue, H. J. & Madias, N. E. Primary care: hypernatremia. *N. Engl. J. Med.* 2000; **342**: 1493–1499.

14. Sterns, T. H., Spital, A., & Clark, E. C. Disorders of water balance. In Kokko, J. P. & Tannen, R. L., eds. *Fluids and Electrolytes.* Philadelphia: W. B. Saunders, 1996.

15. Lutarewych, M. A. & Battle, D. C. Disorders of potassium balance. In Androgue, H. J., ed. *Contemporary Management in Critical Care: Acid–Base and Electrolyte Disorders.* New York: Churchill Livingstone, 1991.

16. Tannen, R. L. Potassium disorders. In Kokko, J. P. & Tannen, R. L., eds. *Fluids and Electrolytes.* Philadelphia: W. B. Saunders, 1996.

17. Rimmer, J. M., Horn, J. F., & Gennari, J. Hyperkalemia as a complication of drug therapy. *Arch. Int. Med.* 1987; **147**: 867–869.

18. Toto, R. D. & Alpern, R. J. Metabolic alkalosis. In Androgue, H. J., ed. *Contemporary Management in Critical Care: Acid–Base and Electrolyte Disorders.* New York: Churchill Livingstone, 1991.

19. Wilson, R. F., Bibson, D., Percinel, A. K. *et al.* Severe alkalosis in critically ill surgical patients. *Arch. Surg.* 1972; **105**: 197.

20. McDougal, W. S. Metablic complications of urinary intestinal diversion. *J. Urol.* 1992; **147**: 1199–1208.

21. Batlle *et al.* Urinary anion gap and metabolic acidosis. *N. Engl. J. Med.* 1988; **318**: 594–599.

22. Toto, R. D. & Alpern, R. J. Metabolic acid–base disorders. In Kokko, J. P. & Tannen, R. L., eds. *Fluids and Electrolytes.* Philadelphia: W. B. Saunders, 1996.

23. Hood, V. L. & Tannen, R. L. Lactic acidosis. In Androgue, H. J., ed. *Contemporary Management in Critical Care: Acid–Base and Electrolyte Disorders.* New York: Churchill Livingstone, 1991.

24. Androgue, H. J. & Maliha, G. Diabetic ketoacidosis. In Androgue, H. J., ed. *Contemporary Management in Critical Care: Acid–Base and Electrolyte Disorders.* New York: Churchill Livingstone, 1991.

25. Cooper, D. J., Walley, K. R., Wiggs, B. R., & Russell, J. A. Bicarbonate does not improve hemodynamics in critically ill patients who have lactic acidosis. A prospective, controlled clinical study. *Ann. Intern. Med.* 1990; **112**: 492–498.

26. Lever, E. & Jaspan, J. B. Sodium bicarbonate therapy in severe diabetic ketoacidosis. *Am. J. Med.* 1983; **75**: 263–268.

27. Singer, G. G. & Brenner, B. M. Fluid and electrolyte disturbances. In Braunwald, E., Fauci, A. S., Kasper, D. L., Hauser, S. L., Longo, D. L., & Jameson, J. L., eds. *Harrison's Principles of Internal Medicine,* 15th edn. New York: McGraw-Hill, 2001.

Endocrinology

26

Diabetes mellitus

Pamela T. Prescott

University of California at Davis, Division of Endocrinology, Sacramento, CA

Surgery has major effects on carbohydrate metabolism and thus presents special risks for patients with diabetes. Surgical mortality rates for patients with diabetes have declined but the successful perioperative care of these patients requires close cooperation between surgeons, anesthesiologists, and primary physicians to prevent complications. More than 20 million people in the USA have diabetes and at least half of them will require surgery at some point in their lives. In addition to surgical conditions typical of the general population, patients with diabetes experience increased intervention for occlusive vascular disease; cholelithiasis; ophthalmic disease (i.e., cataract extraction, vitrectomy); renal disease; and infection. Three of four patients with diabetes are older than 40 years and are approaching a time of life when surgical indications increase. The presence of diabetes typically is known before operation, although a new diagnosis of diabetes is made in the perioperative period in as many as 20% of cases.

Pathophysiology

The endocrine pancreas, which consists of the islets of Langerhans, accounts for less than 3% of the total pancreatic mass in adults. The islets are unevenly distributed through the pancreas and contain four cell types: A (α) cells, which secrete glucagons; B (β) cells, which secrete insulin; D (δ) cells, which secrete somatostatin; and F cells, which secrete pancreatic polypeptide. Insulin, the major secretory product, is synthesized as a precursor molecule, preproinsulin, in the endoplasmic reticulum and is cleaved by microsomal enzymes to proinsulin. Proinsulin is then converted by proteolysis to insulin and an amino acid residue, c-peptide. After secretion into the portal venous system, insulin passes through the liver and the

Table 26.1. Major biologic effects of insulin

Organ or system	Effect
Liver	Promotes glycogen synthesis and storage, inhibits glycogenolysis
	Promotes triglyceride, very low-density lipo-protein, and cholesterol synthesis
	Inhibits ketogenesis
	Promotes glycolysis, inhibits gluconeogenesis
Fat	Promotes triglyceride storage, inhibits lipolysis
Muscle	Promotes protein synthesis
	Promotes glycogen synthesis and storage
Vascular	Promotes lipoprotein lipase activity

portion that is not extracted enters the peripheral circulation. There, it binds to specific cell-surface receptors, initiating multiple phosphorylations of receptor and intracellular proteins and the internalization of the insulin–receptor complex.

The normal basal production of insulin is about 1 U/h, with an additional 3 to 5 U produced after meals. The usual fasting serum insulin concentration is 10 μU/ml; peak postprandial values rarely exceed 100 μU/ml. Endogenous insulin, which has a half-life of less than 5 minutes in plasma, is metabolized by hepatic and renal insulinases. Its major function is to promote the storage of ingested nutrients in many tissues, especially the liver, muscle, and fat. The major biologic effects are outlined in Table 26.1. Deficiency or reduced effectiveness of insulin has profound consequences on metabolism.

Diabetes mellitus is a metabolic condition characterized by elevated glucose levels resulting from defects in insulin secretion, insulin action, or both. Diabetes mellitus is classified as type 1 diabetes (caused by an absolute deficiency of insulin secretion), and type 2 diabetes (caused

Medical Management of the Surgical Patient: A Textbook of Perioperative Medicine, ed. M. F. Lubin, R. B. Smith, T. F. Dobson, N. Spell, H. K. Walker. 4th edn. Published by Cambridge University Press. © Cambridge University 2006.

by a combination of insulin resistance to insulin action and inadequate insulin secretory response). Occasionally, hyperglycemia can occur in individuals who have other conditions and who have a predisposition for diabetes mellitus. These conditions include sepsis, pancreatitis, corticosteroid use, Cushing's syndrome, pregnancy (gestational diabetes), thyrotoxicosis, acromegaly, glucagonoma, pheochromocytoma, cirrhosis, and obesity.[1] Diabetes mellitus is diagnosed when a fasting glucose level is >126 mg/dl, or a random glucose is >200 mg/dl with classic symptoms (polyuria, polydipsia, unexplained weight loss), or 2 hour glucose tolerance test glucose of >200 mg/dl (glucose load 75 g).[1]

Patients with type 1 diabetes (10% to 20% of all patients with diabetes in the USA) typically have circulating antibodies to islet cells and insulin that precedes the clinical manifestations of the disease and persist for a few years after the onset of illness. Patients with type 1 diabetes secrete little insulin, are prone to ketosis, and require insulin for treatment. Patients with type 2 diabetes commonly are obese (85%), are not prone to ketosis, and demonstrate insulin resistance that precedes impaired insulin secretion.

Effects of diabetes on surgery

Surgical mortality rates for patients with diabetes have declined substantially over the years with improved perioperative care. Uncomplicated diabetes is no longer associated with an increased mortality rate after cholecystectomy or peripheral vascular surgery and is associated with only a slightly increased risk after coronary artery bypass grafting. Nonetheless, multiple anatomic and functional complications of the disease do introduce specific problems during surgery.

Infection and poor wound healing are the most common postoperative complications in patients with diabetes. Diabetic patients who undergo major surgery are at increased risk for postoperative infections compared with non-diabetic patients. Several factors may contribute to the increased incidence of infection in diabetic patients, including impairment of the immune response, especially the response of neutrophils. Neutrophils isolated from diabetic patients demonstrate impaired activity in chemotaxis, oxidative burst, and phagocytosis.[2] Perioperative stress also can worsen hyperglycemia. Counter-regulatory hormone, tumor necrosis factors, and cytokines can impair the function of insulin and cause hyperglycemia.[3] Stress-induced hyperglycemia can worsen ischemic events following

myocardial infarction and cerebral stroke. The mechanisms causing the increased incidence may include impairment of cardiac contractility, increase in the frequency of arrhythmias, impairment of the endothelium-dependent vasorelaxation and increased thrombosis. Controlling or normalizing the glucose levels before, during, and after surgery significantly decreases mortality, decreases myocardial infarction and reinfarction rates, decreases incidence of CHF, and cerebral vascular events.[4,5,6] Controlling glucose levels also shortens hospital stay.[7]

The chronic complications of diabetes may also complicate surgery. The presence of neuropathy, particularly autonomic neuropathy, places patients at increased risk for perioperative cardiac arrest. Resting tachycardia or little change in the pulse with deep inspiration or exercise are warning signs and should encourage close postoperative cardiac and respiratory monitoring. The presence of gastroparesis increases the risk of aspiration, and appropriate perioperative therapy with metoclopramide and H_2 blockers is indicated. Ileus and urinary retention are additional complications of autonomic neuropathy. Renal disease can complicate fluid and electrolyte management. Of critical importance is macrovascular disease affecting coronary, cerebral, and peripheral vessels. Cardiac morbidity and death are also predicted by pre-existing congestive heart failure and valvular disease. Non-cardiac vascular complications are best predicted by the presence of retinopathy, neuropathy, nephropathy, congestive heart failure, and peripheral vascular disease. Control of diabetes has not been shown to be predictive.

Effects of surgery (stress) on diabetes

It has been known for more than 50 years that patients who do not have diabetes can develop hyperglycemia during the stress of surgery. Marked elevations are reached in intraoperative and postoperative levels of the counter-regulatory hormones (glucagons, catecholamines, cortisol, and growth hormone). Experimental data indicate that the effects of these hormones are synergistic. In diabetes, the effects of stress are magnified by limited insulin availability or effectiveness. Furthermore, insulin release is significantly depressed during surgery. The hormonal milieu fosters hyperglycemia, and the markedly increased ratio of glucagon to insulin can result in ketoacidosis. Hormonal effects induced specifically by the newer inhalational anesthetic agents or by spinal anesthesia are not of great significance.

Care of surgical patients with diabetes

A careful history, physical examination, and selected laboratory tests (e.g., blood count, urinalysis, fasting blood glucose level, electrolyte levels, creatinine level, hemoglobin A_{1c}, electrocardiogram, home glucose monitoring records) provide information regarding specific risk factors and assist in the care of surgical patients with diabetes. When possible, optimal control of diabetes should be achieved before surgery, although early admission to the hospital for this purpose often is not possible because of diagnosis-related group regulations.

Surgery should be performed early in the day to limit the time that patients are without food and are not receiving their usual treatment regimens. The goal of diabetes management in the perioperative period is to prevent marked hyperglycemia, ketosis, postoperative infections, and impaired wound healing, while also preventing unrecognized and potentially fatal hypoglycemia. This requires an intense coordinated effort between the internist or endocrinologist, surgeon, anesthesiologist, and nursing staff. Frequent and precise monitoring of the perioperative glucose level is the most important factor in achieving optimal control.

Intensive insulin therapy titrated to maintain blood glucose level between 80 and 120 mg/dl during time of critical illness and surgical recovery can decrease mortality, and septic morbidity, and sepsis-related organ failure. Additional effects of insulin, unrelated to the control of glycemia have also been reported.[4,5]

Patients with type I diabetes

Patients with type 1 diabetes always require insulin before, during, and after surgery. Insulin cannot be withheld, even if the patient is not eating and is NPO. Insulin can be administered subcutaneously (by injection or via an insulin pump), intramuscularly or intravenously. Several approaches exist for preoperative insulin management. If the patient is using an insulin pump, the insulin pump can be left to infuse the patient's usual basal rate preoperatively. If the patients take intermediate acting insulin in the morning, one-third to one-half the usual dose could be given. If the patient takes short-acting insulin before each meal and intermediate acting insulin at night, the intermediate acting insulin should be given the night before the surgical procedure, and half the usual short-acting insulin dose should be given on the morning of the procedure. An infusion including 5% dextrose should be started while the patient is NPO to prevent catabolism. The blood glucose should be monitored every 1 to 2 hours and supplemental insulin should be given to maintain normal glycemia.

Treatment with a regular insulin intravenous infusion can be started at any time. Guidelines for adjusting the insulin infusion include the following.[1,8]

Increased insulin needs to be expected with the stress of surgery, sepsis, surgical procedures, glucose containing intravenous solutions, and hypothermia. Until patients can resume their usual diets, intravenous insulin therapy remains the optimal mode of therapy. Insulin half-life is about 5 to 10 minutes and the biological half-life is 20 to 30 minutes. Total discontinuation of the insulin drip is promptly associated with catabolism leading to hyperglycemia and subsequent ketosis. Thus, a dose or subcutaneous regular insulin should be given 30 minutes before the insulin infusion is stopped.

Patients with type II diabetes

For minor surgery, most patients with diet-controlled type 2 diabetes do not require insulin treatment. Patients who are taking the shorter-acting sulfonylureas (glipizide, tolbutamide, tolazimide), glinides (repaglinide, nateglinide), alpha-glucocidase inhibitors (acarbose) and biguanides (metformin) should hold the doses the day of surgery. Patients who are taking the longer-acting agents (glimepiride, glyburide) should hold the doses the day before and the day of surgery. Blood glucose levels should be checked every 6 hours. When perioperative insulin is required, it should be giving using a sliding scale with intravenous dextrose running at 100 ml/h. Patients with type 2 diabetes who normally use insulin can be treated in the perioperative period either by the traditional method using sliding-scale regular insulin (Table 26.2) or by (Table 26.3). Patients with type 2 diabetes who are undergoing major surgery are best treated with continuous intravenous insulin infusion if adequate glucose monitoring is available.

Postoperative care

In the postoperative period, all patients with diabetes must be closely monitored to prevent both hyperglycemia and hypoglycemia. As soon as possible, patients should resume their usual diets and regimens of insulin or oral

Table 26.2. Traditional method of insulin administration for insulin-requiring type 2 diabetes

On morning of surgery, give one-half to one-third the usual dose of intermediate-acting insulin.

Infuse dextrose 5% in water with 10–20 meq of potassium chloride per liter at 100–150 ml/h.

Monitor blood glucose every 6 hours. Supplement with regular insulin. A representative scale follows:

Blood glucose (mg/dl)	Regular insulin (U) subcutaneously q 6 h
<140	0
141–180	4
181–240	6
241–300	8
>300	10

Table 26.3. Insulin infusion method

Start the insulin infusion at 0.02 U/kg/hr.

Check fingerstick glucose levels every 1 hour.

The goal glucose level is 80–120 mg/dl.

Change the infusion rate according to the fingerstick glucose level.

If glucose level is <80, decrease the infusion rate by 1–2 units per hour.

If the glucose level is >120 but <199, increase the infusion rate by 1–2 units per hour.

If the glucose level is >200 but <300, increase the infusion rate by 2–3 units per hour.

If the glucose level is >300, increase the infusion rate by 3–4 units per hour.

hypoglycemic agents. Because of the increased risk of postoperative infection, wound care must be assiduous and devices such as Foley and vascular catheters should be removed as soon as possible. In patients at high risk for coronary events, postoperative electrocardiographic monitoring can be helpful to monitor for new changes. With careful glucose monitoring and insulin infusions as needed, patients with diabetes can safely undergo major surgical procedures.

REFERENCES

1. ADA Clinical Practice Guidelines 2004. Hyperglycemic crises in patients with diabetes mellitus. *Diabetes Care* 2004; **27**: S5–10.
2. Rassias, A. J., Givan, A. L., Marrin, C. A., Whalen, K., Pahl, J., & Yeager, M. P. Insulin increases neutrophil count and phagocytic capacity after cardiac surgery. *Anesth. Analg.* 2002, **94**: 1113–1119.
3. McCowen, K. C., Malhotra, A., & Bistrian, B. R. Stress-induced hyperglycemia. *Crit. Care Clin.* 2001; **17**: 107–124.
4. Preiser, J. C., Devos, P., & Van den Berghe, G. Tight control of glycaemia in critically ill patients. *Curr. Opin. Clin. Nutr. Metab. Care* 2002; **5**: 533–537.
5. Van den Berghe, G., Wouters, P., Weekers, F. *et al.* Intensive insulin therapy in the critically ill patient. *N. Engl. J. Med.* 2001; **345**: 1359–1367.
6. Golden, S. H., Peat-Vigilance, C., Kao, W. H., & Brancati, F. L. Perioperative glycemic control and the risk of infectious complications in a cohort of adults with diabetes. *Diabetes Care* 1999; **22**: 1408–1414.
7. Medhi, M., Marshall, M. C. Jr., Burke, H. B. *et al.* HbA1c predicts length of stay in patients admitted for coronary artery bypass surgery. *Heart Dis.* 2001; **3**: 77–79.
8. Levetan, C. S. & Magee, M. F. Hospital management of diabetes. *Endocrinol. Metab. Clin. North Am.* 2000; **29**: 745–770.

27

Disorders of the thyroid

Pamela T. Prescott

University of California at Davis, Division of Endocrinology, Sacramento, CA

Because thyroid hormones exert regulatory effects on multiple organ systems, thyroid function should be aggressively evaluated and abnormal function treated in patients who require surgery. Thyroid hormones also significantly affect the metabolism of many drugs, and dose adjustments may be required when function is abnormal. Medical consultants performing preoperative evaluations should include clinical assessments of thyroid function and perform confirmatory tests when indicated.

The adult thyroid gland weighs 15 to 20 g, typically consists of two lobes connected by an isthmus, and is located just below the cricoid cartilage. A remnant of the thyroglossal duct, the pyramidal lobe may be noted arising superiorly from the isthmus or medial side of a lobe. Enlargement of the pyramidal lobe indicates a diffuse thyroidal abnormality. The thyroid gland consists of follicles, which are spheres lined by a single layer of cuboidal cells and are filled with a colloid that is composed primarily of thyroglobulin. A rich capillary network surrounds the follicles, explaining why a bruit is sometimes heard over hyperactive, enlarged thyroid glands. Scattered throughout the thyroid are calcitonin-secreting perifollicular cells. Hyperplasic or malignant transformation of these cells does not result in abnormalities of thyroid function.

Inorganic iodide is actively transported from the blood into the follicular cells, immediately oxidized by peroxidase, and is rapidly incorporated into the tyrosine residues of thyroglobulin. These monoiodotyrosine and diiodotyrosine residues couple to form the iodothyronines thyroxine (T_4) and triiodothyronine (T_3), which are stored in the follicles. In response to thyroid-stimulating hormone (TSH), follicular cells extend pseudopods into the colloid and take it up by endocytosis. Subsequent hydrolysis of thyroglobulin in cellular lysosomes yields T_4 and, to a lesser extent, T_3, which are then secreted into the blood. Thyroid function is closely regulated by the hypothalamic-pituitary-thyroidal axis. Hypothalamic thyrotropin-releasing hormone (TRH) stimulates the synthesis and release of TSH. TSH secretion is modulated by negative feedback from T_3 produced in the pituitary by monodeiodination of T_4. The thyroid gland also exhibits autoregulation in response to iodine availability.

Only 0.03% of T_4 and 0.3% of T_3 circulates as free hormones. The remainder is bound to thyroid-binding globulin, T_4 binding prealbumin, and albumin. Virtually all circulating T_4 is secreted from the thyroid gland, whereas 85% of T_3 is derived from peripheral deiodination of T_4. Deiodination at the 5' and 5 positions on T_4 yields T_3 and the biologically inactive reverse T_3 (rT_3), respectively.

A wide variation of tests are available to evaluate thyroid function and effect in individuals with known or suspected thyroid disease. Tests may be classified as those that measure the concentration and binding of the thyroid products, directly test thyroid function or anatomy, assess the hypothalamic pituitary access.[1-3]

Measuring thyroid products

The first thyroid test of choice is the highly sensitive TSH assay with a lower detection limit of $<0.01\,\mu U/ml$. The TSH measurement can be combined with a single measurement of a free T_4 to improve the detection of thyroid abnormalities. If total T_4 is measured, a T_3 uptake assay is done at the same time to measure the effect of or changes in thyroid-binding proteins. A free thyroid index (FTI) is then calculated. The FTI is an estimation of free T_4. If the TSH is low, but the free T_4 is normal, then a free T_3 assay should be obtained. Thyroid antibody assays (antithyroid peroxidase antibodies, antityroglobulin antibodies, and thyroid stimulating antibodies) can be done to help

Medical Management of the Surgical Patient: A Textbook of Perioperative Medicine, ed. M. F. Lubin, R. B. Smith, T. F. Dobson, N. Spell, H. K. Walker. 4th edn. Published by Cambridge University Press. © Cambridge University 2006.

Table 27.1

Low TSH, raised free T_3 or T_4	Primary hyperthyroidism (Graves' multinodular goiter, toxic nodule)
	Subacute, painful thyroiditis (postviral or de Quervain's)
	Subacute, painless thyroiditis (postpartum)
	Drug-induced (amiodarone, lithium)
	Therapeutic (thyroxine ingestion)
	Factitious
	Ectopic (Struma ovarii, molar pregnancy, Choriocarcinoma, gestational hyperthyroidism)
	Excess iodine ingestion (Jodbasedow)
Low TSH, normal free T_3 or T_4	Therapeutic (thyroxine ingestion, high dose glucocorticoids, dopamine and dobutamine infusions)
	Subclinical hyperthyroidism
	Non-thyroidal illness (euthyroid sick syndrome)
Low or normal TSH, low free T_3 or T_4	Non-thyroidal illness (euthyroid sick syndrome)
	Pituitary disease (secondary hypothyroidism)
	Treated hyperthyroidism[a]
Raised TSH, low free T_3 or T_4	Primary hypothyroidism (autoimmune, postsurgical, postablative)
	Excess iodine ingestion (Wolff–Chaikoff effect)
	Drug induced (amiodarone, lithium)
	Reidel's thyroiditis
	Pendred's syndrome
Raised TSH, normal free T_3 or T_4	Subclinical hypothyroidism
	Antimouse immunoglobulin[b]
	Malabsorption of thyroxine
	Amiodarone
	Pendred's syndrome
	TSH resistance
Normal or raised TSH, raised free T_3 or T_4	Ingestion of high dose thyroxine just before tests
	Antibodies to T_4 or T_3
	Familial dysalbuminemic hyperthyroxinemia
	Amiodarone
	Acute psychiatric disorders
	Methamphetamines (acute response)
	TSH secreting pituitary tumors
	Thyroid hormone resistance
	Recovery from non-thyroidal illness

Notes:

[a] As hyperthyroidism is treated, TSH levels may remain suppressed despite low levels of free T_3 or T_4. The pituitary response may be delayed and the TSH remains suppressed even if the hyperthyroid treatment causes low levels of free T_3 or T_4 During this 2- to 3 month period, the treatment is adjusted according to the free T_3 or T_4 levels.

[b] When TSH does not return to normal after treatment, but T_4 is normal, there may be an anti-mouse immunoglobulin interfering with the TSH assay. Need to repeat the TSH with a different assay.

determine the cause of a thyroid abnormality exists. If the TSH free T_4 and free T_3 are normal, and thyroid antibodies are negative, thyroid disease can be excluded. Measurement of rT3 is usually not necessary but can help to differentiate severe non-thyroidal illness from hypothyroidism because levels are normal to elevated in the former and decreased in the latter. Thyroglobulin is detectable in the serum and usually elevated in hyperthyroidism and subacute thyroiditis, and decreased in hypothyroidism and excessive use of thyroxine. It is used after thyroid cancer surgery and Iodine 131 ablation to detect residual or recurrent disease.[1,2]

Dayan describes six patterns of thyroid function tests and the associated thyroid diseases (Table 27.1).[2]

In addition, there are other conditions not mentioned above that can have varying effects on thyroid function tests, they are pregnancy, psychiatric decompensation, chronic failure, aging, and non-thyroid illness.

Pregnancy can have significant, but reversible changes in thyroid function tests. Both normal pregnancy, and pregnancy complicated by conditions such as hyperemesis gravidarium, can be associated with thyroid function study changes that are strongly suggestive of hyperthyroidism, in the absence of thyroid disease. The earliest and most marked change is an elevation in the serum concentrations of T_4 and T_3. The free T_4 and free T_3 are generally in the normal range, although they may be slightly elevated in the first trimester and slightly reduced in the third trimester. TSH is low in the first trimester, when HCG levels are the highest, and gradually returns to normal after the second trimester. Persistently suppressed TSH into the second trimester can be seen with molar pregnancies and with hyperemisis gravidarium. Serum thyroglobulin levels gradually elevate throughout the pregnancy and are generally proportional to thyroid mass. Anti-thyroid antibody levels fall through the last trimester of pregnancy, but they can rise during the postpartum period.[3]

Acute psychiatric decompensation (schizophrenia, major depression, bipolar disorder) causes transient elevation in serum-free T_4 with a suppressed or normal TSH.[2] Individuals with a rapidly cycling bipolar disorder may have slightly low total T_4 and high TSH.[4]

Chronic renal failure can affect thyroid tests. Both plasma T_3 and T_4 are reduced. The low T_3 is due to impaired extrathyroidal T4 to T3 conversion, and the reduction in T_4 is due to circulating inhibitors that impair binding of T_4 to TBG. Despite decreased T_4 and T_3, TSH levels are normal. The hypothalamo-pituitary axis remains normal. When renal failure patients become hypothyroid the TSH is elevated and when hyperthyroid, the TSH is suppressed. Thyroid hormone is minimally lost during hemodialysis and peritoneal dialysis, but does not require replacement.[5]

Elderly individuals have decreased T_3 levels and lower mean TSH concentrations. Autoimmune thyroid disease is particularly prevalent because frequency of thyroid antibodies increases with age.[6]

Non-thyroidal illness (euthyroid sick syndrome) causes change in hormone production so interpretation of thyroid function studies can be difficult.[4] The changes can be seen in any severe illness, there is a drop in both serum T_3 and T_4 as well as an increase in rT_3. TSH values at the onset of the illness are usually normal, but with progression and increasing severity, the TSH can become suppressed.[4,7] With recovery, the TSH and free T_4 rise and return to normal.[7]

Evaluating thyroid anatomy and function

Although the radioactive iodine uptake test is typically increased in hyperthyroidism and decreased in hypothyroidism, it is not commonly used for differentiation. A low radioactive iodine uptake test result accompanying hyperthyroidism suggests subacute thyroiditis, exogenous thyroid administration, resolving hyperthyroidism, struma ovarii, iodine-induced thyrotoxicosis, or functional thyroid cancer metastases after thyroidectomy. Radionuclide scanning with iodine or technetium isotopes provides information regarding the functional status of nodules and thyroid size but is not helpful with respect to metabolic status. Thyroid ultrasound does not give functional information but does define nodules to help determine whether they are cystic, mixed, or solid. Fine-needle aspiration of thyroid nodules has decreased the need for ultrasound and radionuclide scanning and is typically the first test performed in the elevation of a thyroid nodule.

Assessing the hypothalamic–pituitary thyroidal axis

The measurement of TSH by radioimmunoassay is of great utility in evaluating thyroid function. The new "supersensitive" assays distinguish hyperthyroidism as well as hypothyroidism from normal thyroid activity. A normal or low TSH accompanying hypothyroidism is evidence for hypothalamic or pituitary disease.

Reasons for surgery

The most common reasons for recommending surgery are marked thyroid enlargement, rapidly growing goiter, substernal extension of a goiter, compressive symptoms, an abnormal finding on a fine needle aspiration, failure of medical therapy for the treatment of hyperthyroidism, and patient preference. Patients presenting with well-controlled hypo- and hyperthyroidism do not usually have increased risk of complications during and after surgery. However, patients with uncontrolled hyper- and hypothyroidism are at considerable risk.[9,10]

Preparation for surgery

The history and physical examination of patients scheduled for thyroidectomy should include identification of abnormalities of thyroid function. Besides symptoms and signs of hypo- and hyperthyroidism, evidence for other medical conditions should be sought, including cardio-respiratory disease and associated endocrine disorders. For example, patients who require thyroidectomy for medullary cancer may have an associated pheochromocytoma.[9]

Routine laboratory tests include thyroid function tests, hemoglobin, white cell and platelet count, urea and electrolytes, and serum calcium. If liver abnormalities or clotting disorders are suspected, activated partial thromboplastin time (PTT) and prothrombin time (PT) should be included in the initial laboratory evaluation. Patients may have a fine needle aspiration as a diagnostic test prior to surgery. A chest X-ray may be needed to show evidence of tracheal compression or deviation, and extension of the thyroid tissue into the mediastinum. An EKG should be done in the elderly, those with a history of hypertension, cardiac disease, diabetes mellitus and those with hyperthyroidism.[9,10]

Complications of surgery[1,8–13]

Postoperative complications of surgery include extubation problems, hemorrhage, laryngeal or pharyngeal edema, nerve damage (recurrent laryngeal, superior laryngeal, or phrenic nerve), tracheal collapse, pneumothorax, hypocalcemia, vomiting, wound infection, pain, and thyroid storm in hyperthyroid patients. During extubation, care should be taken to decrease coughing because of the risk of bleeding. Injury to the recurrent and superior laryngeal nerves can be temporary or permanent. Temporary recurrent laryngeal nerve damage occurs in 3%–4% and can cause minor voice hoarseness. Patients usually require only observation. Permanent unilateral vocal cord paralysis occurs in <1% and can lead to hoarseness, aspiration, breathlessness, and stridor. It is usually treated with silicon injections, or vocal cord fixation. Bilateral vocal cord paralysis is extremely rare, and usually requires tracheotomy. Tracheal collapse is rare, but usually occurs from prolonged compression from a large goiter. Once the goiter is removed, the trachea collapses and the patient will develop stridor, and respiratory compromise. Patients may require reintubation and a tracheotomy. Pneumothorax usually results if the lower neck dissection is required.

Hypocalcium from parathyroid stunning or unintentional parathyroidectomy can cause temporary or permanent hypocalcemia. Patients may develop perioral numbness, carpopedal spasms, and anxiety. Symptoms usually appear with 1 to 7 days after surgery. Severe hypocalcemia is treated with intravenous calcium gluconate, and mild hypocalcemia is treated with oral calcium carbonate (starting at 1 gm two to three times a day). Permanent hypocalcemia will require chronic treatment with calcium and vitamin D (see Chapter 29).

Patients undergoing thyroidectomy have a high rate of nausea and vomiting following thyroidectomy (as high as 71% in some studies). Patients typically only have mild to moderate pain, so the nausea and vomiting is their main source of discomfort. Nausea or vomiting with retching can lead to postoperative bleeding with development of a hematoma or hemorrhage leading to need for another surgical procedure or airway obstruction. Control of nausea and vomiting is essential.

Hyperthyroidism

Hyperthyroidism results from Graves' disease (the most common cause), toxic adenoma, toxic multinodular goiter, subacute thyroiditis, the hyperthyroid phase of Hashimoto's thyroiditis (reflecting overlap with Graves' disease), thyrotoxicosis factitia from exogenous hormone, and iodine-induced thyrotoxicosis. Rare causes include ovarian struma, hydatidiform mole, metastatic follicular carcinoma, and a TSH-producing adenoma. Measurement in serum of free T_4 or of the free T_4 index (total T_4 with T_3 resin uptake) plus a sensitive TSH should confirm the diagnosis. Serum T_3 is increased in hyperthyroidism but may be normal after iodine ingestion or when severe non-thyroidal illness is present. A flat TSH response to TRH is confirmatory when the TSH level is equivocal or sensitive measurements are not available. An increased serum thyroid-stimulating immunoglobulin level is seen with Graves' disease. In younger patients, the clinical presentation of hyperthyroidism is typically dramatic, with obvious signs of increased sympathetic activity. The diagnosis is often more subtle in elderly patients, who may be markedly apathetic, with weight loss, weakness, poor appetite, and congestive heart failure without tachyarrhythmias or goiter.

Multiple organs are influenced by hyperthyroidism. The most common alterations with hyperthyroidism include those listed in Table 27.2.

Surgery in patients with hyperthyroidism

The preoperative diagnosis and treatment of hyperthyroidism is of great importance to prevent tachyarrhythmias and life-threatening thyroid storm. If surgery is not emergent, patients should be rendered euthyroid.

Table 27.2. Symptoms and signs of hyperthyroidism

Eye	Upper lid retraction
Cardiovascular	Decreased peripheral vascular resistance
	Tachycardia
	Atrial fibrillation
	Congestive heart failure
	Cardiomyopathy
	Thromboembolic events
Respiratory	Respiratory muscle weakness
Gastrointestinal	Hyperdefecation
	Elevated alanine amniotransferase (ALT)
	Elevated alkaline phosphatase
	Hepatomegaly
	Depletion of hepatic glycogen stores
Nervous system	Nervousness
	Emotional lability
	Hyperkinesia
	Fatigue
Muscle	Muscle weakness
Skeletal	Bone Loss
Metabolic	Hypercalcemia
	Hyperglycemia
	Relative or true adrenal insufficiency
Hematopoietic	Neutropenia
	Thrombocytopenia
Reproductive	Menstrual irregularity
	Infertility
	Increased incidence of miscarriages

β-Adrenergic blockade provides prompt symptomatic relief but does not significantly affect thyroid hormone levels. Some β-blockers (e.g., propranolol, atenolol) block the peripheral conversion of T_4 to T_3 but the therapeutic importance of this is questionable and β-blockers without this action are equally effective. The risks and benefits of β-blockade must be weighed in patients with congestive heart failure or bronchospasm. Both propylthiouracil, 300 to 600 mg in three divided doses daily, and methimazole, 30 to 40 mg in two divided doses daily, are effective inhibitors of thyroid hormone synthesis. Propylthiouracil blocks peripheral conversion of T_4 to T_3 and is favored by some endocrinologists for this reason, but then again, this effect may be of little clinical consequence. The decreased frequency of dosing required with methimazole may improve compliance. Propylthiouracil is preferred during pregnancy and nursing because it crosses the placenta one fourth as well as methimazole and enters breast milk one tenth as well. With adequate doses of antithyroid drugs, patients may be nearly euthyroid within 3 weeks. The clearance of β-blockers is increased in hyperthyroidism. Thus, dose reductions are needed as the euthyroid state is approached.

Emergent surgery in hyperthyroid patients requires a different approach. The antithyroid drugs that only block organification and thyroid hormone synthesis are ineffective because of their slow onset of action. β-Adrenergic blockade alone has been used successfully. If propranolol is selected, it should be given at the rate of 40 to 80 mg orally every 6 hours and continued after operation because fever, tachycardia, and thyroid storm can occur with inadequate dosing or too rapid discontinuation. Propranolol, 1 to 5 mg, can be given slowly by the intravenous route if time does not permit oral administration, and this should be continued every 6 hours as needed through the perioperative period.

Iodide should be used in conjunction with β-blockade in emergency preparation for surgery. Iodide acutely blocks the release of thyroid hormone from the gland as well as inhibits organification. A decline of T_4 levels to normal may be reached in a week using 10 drops of an oral saturated solution of potassium iodide or 1 g of intravenous sodium iodide daily. Occasionally, other agents are needed to quickly prepare patients for surgery when conventional agents like PTU and methimazole cannot be used or have failed. Iopanoic acid, which is an oral iodinated cholecystographic agent that inhibits 5'-deiodinase and causes a reduction in the peripheral conversion of T_4 to T_3, has been used in a small number of patients. There are reports of its use to successfully prepare patients with amiodarone-induced thyrotoxicosis for surgery when they were unresponsive to PTU, methimazole or steroids. Mean dose was 1 g per day for 13 days.[14,15] Very rarely, lithium is used for intractable hyperthyroidism, including amiodarone induced hyperthyroidism, that is resistant to usual therapies. Usual clinical response is seen with 900–1500 mg/day.[16,17]

Although they are not immediately effective, therapy with antithyroid drugs should be initiated in patients who are undergoing emergent surgery. The rectal route has been shown to provide adequate serum levels when oral administration is precluded. If patients develop signs of thyroid storm (e.g., hyperthermia, vomiting, hypertension, tachycardia, altered mental state, impending vascular collapse), prompt treatment with β-blockers, iodide, antithyroid drugs, and glucocorticoids (hydrocortisone, 75 to 100 mg intravenously every 8 hours) is required. Glucocorticoids cover potential inadequate adrenal reserve as well as inhibit 5'-monodeiodinase, thereby lowering T_3 levels. Salicylates should not be used because they displace thyroid hormone from binding proteins, resulting in increased free levels. The diagnosis of thyroid storm is a clinical one. Thyroid hormone levels are not higher than those in hyperthyroidism without storm. Presumably, concomitant stress increases catecholamine levels, with a profound effect on the already increased β-adrenergic receptor activity characteristic of the hyperthyroid state.

Hypothyroidism

The clinical presentation of hypothyroidism ranges from mild symptoms of fatigue to myxedema coma. A higher index of suspicion of the disease is required in the elderly because many mild symptoms and signs of hypothyroidism may be attributed to the aging process *per se*. The diagnosis of hypothyroidism is made by measuring free T_4 and TSH. An increase in TSH preceded the decline in circulating thyroid hormone levels; a low TSH suggests a hypothalamic–pituitary cause. The most common cause of hypothyroidism, Hashimoto's thyroiditis, is associated with high levels of antimicrosomal and antithyroglobulin antibodies.

The results of thyroid hormone deficiency are varied and affect surgery. Cardiovascular manifestations include bradycardia, decreased cardiac output, atrioventricular conduction defects, and pericardial effusions. Respiratory effects include decreased alveolar ventilation because of blunted responsiveness to anoxia and hypercarbia, and pleural effusions. Delayed gastric emptying and intestinal mobility can lead to abdominal distention and ileus. Women may have menorrhagia or amenorrhea. Decreased metabolism of administered drugs may lead to toxicity and trigger respiratory failure.

Surgery in patients with hypothyroidism

When possible, surgery should be postponed until hypothyroidism can be corrected. Studies have shown a small increase in intraoperative hypotension and postoperative congestive heart failure, ileus, and confusion when patients were moderately hypothyroid. These studies support the need for close monitoring of respiratory status, attention to fluid balance, and cautious use of narcotics and sedatives. If surgical patients demonstrate signs of myxedema coma (e.g., stupor, hypothermia, hypoventilation, hypoglycemia, hyponatremia, hypotension), emergency treatment is required. L-Thyroxine is given intravenously at a dosage of 400 µg. Glucocorticoids (hydrocortisone, 75 to 100 mg intravenously every 8 hours) are administered because relative adrenal insufficiency may

be present (e.g., hypopituitarism, coincident autoimmune Addison's disease). Because most patients with hypothyroidism do well in surgery, this vigorous treatment should not be routine. In young patients without evidence of cardiac disease, full replacement with L-thyroxine, 100 to 125 µg intravenously or orally per day, may be initiated and continued through the perioperative period. A 20% reduction in dose is appropriate when long-term parenteral administration is needed. When coronary artery disease is present, a starting dose of 25 µg/d is more appropriate; if angina or arrhythmias occur, the dose should be reduced. For patients undergoing coronary revascularization surgery, thyroid replacement is best not initiated. These patients do well with surgery and the replacement of thyroid hormone often increases angina and induces arrhythmias. If thyroid function tests are inconclusive or not available, and hypothyroidism is clinically suspected, it is prudent to treat patients with replacement doses of L-thyroxine and reevaluate when they are stable.

Patients who are euthyroid while receiving replacement therapy can be maintained on parenteral therapy through the perioperative period. Alternatively, interruption of thyroid replacement for as long as 1 week is not detrimental.

Effect of surgery on thyroid function

Non-thyroidal surgery is associated with several changes in circulating thyroid hormone levels. Most profoundly, an abrupt decline in T_3 levels occurs within 24 hours as a result of inhibition of 5′-monodeiodinase. Reverse T_3 levels rise for the same reason. The effect on T_4 levels is less predictable but a decline is usually noted when the procedure is prolonged and associated with greater stress and extended fasting. Free T_4 and TSH levels are typically normal. These patients are considered to be euthyroid (the "euthyroid sick" syndrome) and should not be treated with thyroid hormone.

REFERENCES

1. Larsen, P. R., Davies, T. F., & Hay, I. D. Thyroid gland. In Wilson, J. D., Foster, D. W., Kronenberg, H. M. *et al.* (eds). *Williams Textbook of Endocrinology*, 9th edn. Philadelphia: W. B. Saunders, 1998: 389–515.
2. Dayan, C. M. Interpretation of thyroid function tests. *Lancet* 2001; **357**: 619–624.
3. Brent, G. A. Maternal thyroid function: Interpretation of thyroid function tests in pregnancy. *Clin. Obstet. Gynecol.* 1997; **40**: 3–15.

4. Langton, J. E. & Brent, G. A. Nonthyroidal illness syndrome: evaluation of thyroid function in sick patients. *Endocrinol. Metab. Clin. North Am.* 2002; **31**: 159–172.

5. Lim, V. S. Thyroid function in patients with chronic renal failure. *Am. J. Kidney Dis.* 2001; **38**: S80–S84.

6. Chiovato, L., Mariotti, S., & Pincera, A. Thyroid diseases in the elderly. *Baillieres Clin. Endocrinol. Metab.* 1997; **11**: 251–270.

7. De Groot, L. J. Dangerous dogmas in medicine: the nonthyroidal illness syndrome. *JCEM* 1999; **84**: 151–164.

8. Mittendorf, E. A. & McHenry, C. R. Thyroidectomy for selected patients with thyrotoxicosis. *Arch. Otolaryngol. Head Neck Surg.* 2001; **127**: 61–65.

9. Farling, P. A. Thyroid disease. *Br. J. Anaesth.* 2000; **85**: 15–28.

10. Graham, G. W., Unger, B. P., & Coursin, D. B. Perioperative management of selected endocrine disorders. *Int. Anesthesiol. Clin.* 2000; **38**: 31–67.

11. McHenry, C. R. Patient volumes and complications in thyroid surgery. *Br. J. Surg.* 2002; **89**: 821.

12. Pulli, R. S. & Coniglio, J. U. Surgical management of the substernal thyroid gland. *Laryngoscope* 1998; **108**: 358–361.

13. Sonner, J. M., Hynson, J. M., Clark, O., & Katz, J. A. Nausea and vomiting following thyroid and parathyroid surgery. *J. Clin. Anesth.* 1997; **9**: 398–402.

14. Bogazzi, F., Miccoli, P., Berti, P. *et al.* Preparation with iopanoic acid rapidly controls thyroxicosis in patients with amiodarone-induced thyrotoxicosis before thyroidectomy. *Surgery* 2002; **132**: 1114–1117.

15. Osman, F., Franklyn, J. A., Sheppard, M. C., & Gammage, M. D. Successful treatment of amiodarone-induced thyrotoxicosis. *Circulation* 2002; **105**: 1275–1277.

16. Dickstein, G., Shechner, C., Adawi, F., Kaplan, J., Baron, E., & Ish-Shalom, S. Lithium treatment in amiodarone-induced thyrotoxicosis. *Am. J. Med.* 1997; **102**: 454–458.

17. Kauschansky, A. & Genel, M. Preoperative treatment of intractable hyperthyroidism with acute lithium administration. *Eur. J. Pediatr. Surg.* 1996; **6**: 301–302.

28

Disorders of the adrenal cortex

Pamela T. Prescott

University of California at Davis, Division of Endocrinology, Sacramento, CA

Serum cortisol levels rise within 30 minutes of the induction of anesthesia and remain elevated for hours to days in the face of postoperative stress. Because of cortisol's critical role in the successful handling of stress, a careful clinical assessment of adrenal function is necessary before surgery. Either deficiency or excess of cortisol can adversely affect surgical outcome. The physiology and metabolism of the adrenal cortex are briefly reviewed in this chapter to help clarify the appropriate selection of tests to verify a clinical diagnosis of adrenal cortex disorder. The adrenal medulla is discussed in Chapter 30.

Human adult adrenal glands weigh 4 to 5 g each and reside in the retroperitoneal space supermedial to the kidneys. The cortex, of mesodermal origin, occupies the outer 90% of the gland. It consists of three concentric histologic zones, two of which have apparently identical function. The outermost zona glomerulosa produces aldosterone but, because it lacks 17 α-hydroxylase activity, is unable to synthesize cortisol or androgens. The middle zona fasciculate is the largest area of the adrenal cortex, and the small innermost zona reticularis encircles the medulla. These two zonae produce cortisol, androgens, and small amounts of estrogen but lack the 18-hydroxysteriod dehydrogenase required for aldosterone synthesis. Histologic evidence suggests that the zona fasciculata responds to acute adrenocorticotropic hormone (ACTH) stimulation, whereas the zona reticularis responds to prolonged stimulation.

Adrenal steroid synthesis is controlled by the hypothalamic–pituitary–adrenal (HPA) axis. Hypothalamic corticotrophin-releasing hormone (CRH) and arginine vasopressin (AVP), also known as antidiuretic hormone (ADH), are the most important regulators of ACTH. ACTH controls cortisol secretion. ACTH is released in quick, pulsatile bursts, followed by a slower, more sustained rise in cortisol and metabolites. Free cortisol is the active hormone and acts directly on tissues.[1] Normal ACTH release and production of cortisol follows a circadian rhythm and is connected to light. It is the highest on awakening in the morning (peaking about 8 hours after the onset of sleep), declines over the day, and is lowest in the middle of the night. The cortisol secretory pattern is usually resistant to acute change. Prolonged bed rest, continuous feeding, or 5 days of fasting, do not alter the rhythm.[1] Occasionally, abrupt time changes of the sleep-awake cycle, as during shift work rotations and jet lag, may have some effect on the 24-hour cortisol patterns.[2] Critical illness, chronic inflammatory conditions, chronic insomnia, coronary artery disease and severe stress often alter the daily rhythm.[3–5] These conditions exert their effect by cytokines, interleukins and tumor necrosis factors. Circulating interleukin-6 is a potent activator of the HPA axis. By stimulating pituitary ACTH, and therefore cortisol, response to inflammation can enhance resistance to inflammatory disease, while a decreased or defective response can increase susceptibility.[3–5]

Glucocorticoids have multiple actions and affect every system of the body. In broadest terms, glucocorticoids affect the metabolism of glucose, protein and lipids, and the function of the immune, renal[6] and circulatory systems. Glucocorticoids increase blood glucose levels by increasing hepatic glucose production, decreasing insulin action, and increasing glucagon secretion. Glucocorticoids increase the availability and release of amino acids, and lipids that are used as substrate for glucose production.[7] During fasting, these processes protect against hypoglycemia. With endogenous or exogenous glucocorticoid excess, hyperglycemia can occur; with glucocorticoid deficiency, hypoglycemia can occur.

Glucocorticoids can cause redistribution of immune cells. They increase intravascular polymorphonuclear cell release from the bone marrow, but cause temporary

Medical Management of the Surgical Patient: A Textbook of Perioperative Medicine, ed. M. F. Lubin, R. B. Smith, T. F. Dobson, N. Spell, H. K. Walker. 4th edn. Published by Cambridge University Press. © Cambridge University 2006.

sequestration of lymphocytes and monocytes into the spleen, lymph nodes and bone marrow.[7] Glucocorticoids increase glomerular filtration by direct effect, and in conjunction with mineralocorticoid activity effect electrolyte and water balance.[8] When in excess, glucocorticoids with mineralocorticoid activity, i.e., cortisol, can cause sodium retention, hypokalemia, and hypertension. Glucocorticoids in conjunction with catecholamines maintain vascular tone, vascular permeability and the vascular distribution of water.[9] Deficiency can result in refractory shock in the stressed state, and excess can cause hypertension. Excess glucocorticoids inhibit connective tissue and bone formation, decrease gastrointestinal absorption of calcium and increase calciuria. Both excess and deficiency of glucocorticoids have major effects on the central nervous system.[1]

Cortisol is the most important glucocorticoid. Cortisol synthesis proceeds through several steps, the final being the hydroxylation in mitochondria of 11-deoxycortisol to cortisol. Adrenal androgen synthesis in adults is stimulated by ACTH. The physiological effects of adrenal androgens in adult men are inconsequential. In women, however, in whom the adrenal androgen supply is roughly 50%, in premenopausal, and in all postmenopausal, excess adrenal production results in acne, hirsutism, and virilization.

The production of aldosterone by the adrenal cortex is controlled primarily by the renin-angiotensin system and secondarily by ACTH. Acute increases in serum potassium, depletion of body sodium, and renin production by the kidneys are also potent stimulators of aldosterone production. Excess production is manifested by hypertension, hypokalemia, suppression of the renin system, and normal to low cortisol secretion.

Adrenal response to stress

Glucocorticoid levels increase immediately with surgery, severe injury or burns, pain, fever, hypothermia, emotional distress, hemorrhage and hypotension or hypovolemia.[8–12] Surgery is a potent activator of the HPA axis. ACTH rises with the incision and during surgery. The highest rise in ACTH is with extubation and the immediate postoperative period.[10] During surgical procedures, such as laparotomy, glucocorticoid levels rise immediately, peaking in the immediate postoperative period and decline to baseline over 24–48 hours.[8,9] After surgery and with severe illness, there is no circadian variation. Glucocorticoid levels tend to be higher than baseline. The normal cortisol response to stress is usually considered to be a level >18 to 20 μg/dl. In patients with traumatic injuries, cortisol levels can peak between 30–45 μg/dl.[9]

In patients with severe illness and in those shortly before death, the cortisol levels can be as high as 30–260 μg/dl.[9] The level of the cortisol response is related to the severity of the illness. There is no known level that distinguishes an adequate from an inadequate adrenal response, but many believe that a random cortisol level in a stressed patient should achieve a threshold of at least 25 μg/dl.[10]

Adrenal insufficiency

Because a patient's response to the stress in associated with surgery requires adequate adrenal reserves, it is critical that adrenal insufficiency be diagnosed and treated before operation. Medical consultants should always inquire about any use of glucocorticoids in patients who are about to undergo surgery. Although the inhaled steroids used to treat obstructive pulmonary disease are usually not associated with adrenal suppression, high doses of these drugs can result in suppression that is sufficient to require the perioperative administration of systemic glucocorticoids.

In the USA, 80% of primary adrenocortical insufficiency (Addison's disease) is a result of autoimmune adrenalitis. This is often associated with other autoimmune disorders, including Hashimoto's thyroiditis, Graves' disease, type I diabetes mellitus, premature ovarian failure, hypoparathyroidism, and, rarely, testicular failure. Associated non-endocrine conditions include mucocutaneous candidiasis, vitiligo, alopecia, pernicious anemia, and chronic active hepatitis. Worldwide, tuberculosis remains the most common cause of Addison's disease; it is the second most common cause in the USA. Rare causes include hemorrhage (a risk of anticoagulant therapy), fungal infections, tumor metastases, surgical adrenalectomy, radiation, amyloidosis, sarcoidosis, hemochromatosis, congenital enzyme defects, and medications (e.g., metyrapone, ketoconazole, aminoglutethimide, etopamide, mitotane).[1,11]

The most common cause of secondary adrenal insufficiency is ACTH deficiency resulting from exogenous glucocorticoid therapy. The administration of replacement doses of glucocorticoids (i.e., 5 mg of prednisone or 20 mg of hydrocortisone daily) for more than 2 weeks is sufficient to suppress the hypothalamic–pituitary–adrenal axis. Subnormal cortisol responses to stimuli can persist for as long as 1 year after the discontinuation of glucocorticoid therapy. Pituitary recovery preceded adrenal recovery by months. Endogenous secondary adrenal insufficiency is most commonly caused by pituitary or hypothalamic tumors.[1,11]

Patients with primary adrenal insufficiency are weak and fatigued. Appetite is decreased despite increased taste and smell sensation; nausea, vomiting, and weight loss are common. Hyperpigmentation, hyponatremia, and fasting hypoglycemia (especially in children) can occur. Because of the associated mineralocorticoid deficiency, volume depletion with orthostatic hypotension, hyperkalemia, and acidosis occur. Acute adrenal crisis is characterized by fever, volume depletion with refractory hypotension, nausea, weakness, depressed mentation, and hypoglycemia. Patients with secondary adrenocortical insufficiency have most of the same symptoms but are not hyperpigmented because the production of ACTH and β-lipotropin is reduced. Because their aldosterone production is typically intact, they do not have volume depletion, hyperkalemia, or acidosis. Hyponatremia from impaired excretion of water does occur, and there is the potential for hypotension with a stress-induced crisis.[11]

Primary adrenal insufficiency is best diagnosed with the ACTH stimulation test. A normal serum cortisol response (at least 20 µg/dl, 30 to 60 minutes after a 250 µg dose of intravenous or intramuscular synthetic ACTH (cosyntropin)) excludes the diagnosis. To rule out the diagnosis of Addison's disease in patients who have been receiving glucocorticoids, several daily doses of synthetic ACTH or an 8-hour infusion of ACTH may be needed to achieve a normal cortisol response because of superimposed secondary adrenal insufficiency.[12] In secondary adrenal insufficiency, the serum cortisol response to ACTH is frequently blunted but can be normal.

Hypothalamic–pituitary–adrenal axis function can be evaluated by the overnight metyrapone test. After bedtime administration of 30 mg/kg of oral metyrapone, an agent that blocks the conversion of 11-deoxycortisol are measured at 8:00 am the next day. A cortisol level of less than 5 µg/dl indicates that the level of blockade was adequate, and a marked increase (80-fold) in 11-deoxycortisol confirms that the adrenal response was normal.

Alternatively, the hypothalamic–pituitary–adrenal axis can be tested with insulin-induced hypoglycemia. After the intravenous injection of 0.1 U/kg of regular insulin, a serum glucose nadir occurs in 20 to 30 minutes. The serum cortisol should increase to more than 20 µg/dl, 30 to 60 minutes after the glucose nadir. Because of the potential morbidity of hypoglycemia, this test requires the presence of a physician and should not be performed in the elderly or in patients with significant cardiovascular or cerebrovascular disease. Measurement of plasma ACTH and serum cortisol after CRH administration has been disappointing in distinguishing between hypothalamic and pituitary disease. Predictably, the ACTH response to CRH is exaggerated in primary adrenal insufficiency.

Adrenal insufficiency is treated with steroid replacement. For primary adrenal insufficiency, maintenance doses are 20 to 30 mg/d of hydrocortisone in at least two divided doses or 5 to 7.5 mg/d of prednisone in a single or divided dose. Patients who are also receiving drugs such as rifampin, barbiturates, and phenytoin, which induce hepatic metabolism of glucocorticoids, may require modest increases in the glucocorticoid dosage. The necessity for mineralocorticoid replacement with Florinef (9α-fluorocortisol) at a dosage of 0.05 to 0.2 mg/d is determined by assessment of the blood pressure and serum potassium level. Patients are instructed to increase their dosages of glucocorticoids two- to fourfold when they are experiencing stress and to notify their physicians if symptoms persist.

Surgery is a major form of stress and traditionally patients are given the maximal stress dose (ten times the maintenance dose or 300 mg of hydrocortisone per day) starting in the perioperative period. Hydrocortisone 100 mg is given intravenously with induction of anesthesia, and 100 mg every 8 hours for at least 24 hours.[15] The patient's status is determined and, if stable, the hydrocortisone is tapered over 4 to 5 days, (i.e., 50 mg every 8 hours for 1 day, 25 mg every 8 hours for 1 day, 25 mg BID for 1 day, then down to maintenance 10–20 mg in the am and 5–10 mg in the pm).[15] There is some evidence that smaller doses of hydrocortisone can be given, thus avoiding some of the adverse effects of high dose steroids.[13,14] The dosing of the hydrocortisone depends on the stress produced by the surgery. For low stress procedures (like an inguinal hernia repair) 25 mg on the day of the procedure, for moderate stress (open cholecystectomy or colon resection) 50–75 mg on the day of surgery and for 1–2 days after, and for major surgery (cardiothoracic surgery or esophagectomy) 100–150 mg on day of surgery and for 1–2 days after.[13,14] The authors stated that abovementioned alterations to the traditional hydrocortisone dosing were clearly only guidelines and the patient's condition, and the level of stress dictate the amount of hydrocortisone given. Daily doses of hydrocortisone exceeding 50 mg supply adequate mineralocorticoid replacement, but comparable doses of methylprednisolone and dexamethasone do not have the same degree of mineralocorticoid activity. Blood pressure, electrolyte, and glucose measurements, as well as fluid status, must be carefully monitored. If patients develop any signs suggestive of acute adrenal crisis, intravenous hydrocortisone at a dosage of 300 mg/d (100 mg every 8 hours) plus glucose and saline infusions must be given emergently. Once the acute stress has

Table 28.1. Perioperative management of adrenal insufficiency

---

Inquire about any preoperative use of glucocorticoids (systemic or inhaled) and symptoms suggestive of adrenal insufficiency.

Administer hydrocortisone 100 mg intravenously q 8 h. Give first dose at least 1 h before induction of anesthesia.

Once the patient is stable after operation, taper the hydrocortisone dose over 3–4 days to maintenance levels (30 mg/d in at least two divided doses) or to the patient's preoperative dose of glucocorticoid.

Prevent volume depletion and hypoglycemia with the use of intravenous saline and glucose.

---

passed, patients can be weaned over several days to maintenance doses. Table 28.1 outlines the perioperative management of adrenal insufficiency.

If the adrenal status is not known, but adrenal insufficiency is suspected in a patient with severe stress, a random serum cortisol should be drawn, and hydrocortisone 100 mg every 8 hours started. If the serum cortisol level subsequently is found to be <25 μg/dl, the hydrocortisone is continued and tapered as the condition warrants.[9]

Cushing's syndrome

The most common cause of Cushing's syndrome (the term for any state characterized by increased glucocorticoid effect) is exogenous glucocorticoid administration, which results in pituitary adrenal suppression. Cushing's disease, adrenal hyperplasia resulting from excess pituitary production of ACTH, is the cause of 70% of all cases of endogenous Cushing's syndrome. A pituitary adenoma is identified in most cases. Autonomous adrenal hyperfunction resulting from an adrenal adenoma or carcinoma, and ectopic production of ACTH by tumors (especially small cell carcinomas of the lung), each account for about 15% of all cases of endogenous Cushing's syndrome. Common signs and symptoms include obesity, facial plethora, hirsutism, menstrual irregularities, hypertension, proximal muscle weakness, back pain, and skin stria. Psychologic symptoms (e.g., euphoria, mania, psychosis) are probably under-reported. Patients with ectopic ACTH production have fewer chronic signs of glucocorticoid excess but demonstrate more mineralocorticoid effect with hypertension and hypokalemia associated with weight loss. Adrenal carcinomas often are accompanied by signs of marked androgenicity as well as glucocorticoid effect.

The two screening tests for Cushing's syndrome are the 1 mg overnight dexamethasone suppression of serum cortisol and measurement of the 24-hour urinary-free cortisol. Suppression of the morning serum cortisol level to less than 5 μg/dl after the administration of 1 mg of oral dexamethasone and the presence of normal secretion of urine cortisol are both strong evidence against abnormal cortisol secretion. High-dose dexamethasone (2 mg orally every 6 hours for 48 hours) suppresses serum cortisol in the face of Cushing's disease but not adrenal tumors. Serum ACTH levels are low with adrenal tumors, normal to slightly elevated in Cushing's disease, and often markedly elevated with ectopic production. Metyrapone and CRH administration each induce exaggerated ACTH responses in Cushing's disease but have little effect in other causes of Cushing's syndrome.

Therapy for Cushing's syndrome involves surgical removal of the pituitary tumor, adrenal tumor, or ectopic source (if possible). Cure rates for pituitary microadenomas are very good and the transsphenoidal surgery itself has low morbidity and mortality. Transient postoperative diabetes insipidus can occur. Complications after the resection of cortisol-producing adrenal tumors are more frequent and include wound infection, bleeding, pulmonary embolism, and respiratory infections. After surgery, a period of secondary adrenal insufficiency ensues. Unfortunately, adrenal carcinoma is often widely metastatic at the time of presentation, and the prognosis is poor. When surgical resection is not possible, medical therapy with ketoconazole, metyrapone, aminoglutethimide, or mitotane may be useful to decrease cortisol levels.

Patients with Cushing's syndrome have an increased incidence of hypertension, cardiovascular disease, diabetes mellitus, thromboembolism, delayed wound healing, and increased susceptibility to infection. Despite this increased risk of operative complications, emergent surgery can usually be safely performed in the face of hypercortisolism. If surgery can be postponed, the carefully monitored use of one or more of the agents mentioned above to control hypercortisolism may be of benefit in reducing surgical complications. After operation, patients must be observed for evidence of steroid withdrawal symptoms, which may require replacement steroids that are then slowly tapered.

Primary aldosteronism

Primary aldosteronism is manifested by hypertension, increased aldosterone levels, low plasma renin levels, metabolic alkalosis, and hypokalemia. In about two-thirds of patients, it results from a unilateral adrenal adenoma; in the remainder, idiopathic hyperplasia is the usual cause. Adrenal carcinoma is an extremely rare cause. Adenomas are treated with adrenalectomy of the affected side, which cures about three-fourths of patients. Before operation, sodium restriction and potassium-sparing diuretic such as spironolactone are used to correct the electrolyte abnormalities and hypertension. It is preferable to treat medically for 1 to 2 months before surgery to reduce the incidence of postoperative complications. After surgery, electrolyte concentrations and blood pressure must be monitored. Recovery of the renin–aldosterone system may take many months but normal function is the usual outcome.

Hypoaldosteronism

Aldosterone deficiency without concomitant glucocorticoid deficiency is usually hyporeninemic hypoaldosteronism and rarely results from a primary abnormality of the adrenal cortex. Diabetes mellitus and tubulointerstitial renal disease are disorders that can be associated with decreased renin secretion, leading to subsequent hypoangiotensinemia and low aldosterone levels. The mineralocorticoid deficiency is manifested by hyperkalemia, hyperchloremic metabolic acidosis, and occasional sodium depletion. Most patients with hyporeninemic hypoaldosteronism are asymptomatic but hyperkalemia and metabolic acidosis can lead to arrhythmias. Treatment with furosemide, 40 to 120 mg/d, helps relieve hyperkalemia and metabolic acidosis, although hypotension may be induced. This is typically combined with Florinef, which increases renal potassium and hydrogen ion excretion and causes salt retention. Correction of hyporeninemic hypoaldosteronism is desirable before surgery to prevent potential complications.

REFERENCES

1. Orth, D. & Kovacs, W. The adrenal cortex. In Wilson, J. D., Foster, D. W., Kronenberg, H. M. *et al.*, eds. *Williams Textbook of Endocrinology*, 9th edn. Philadelphia: W. B. Saunders, 1998: 532, 537, 544–547.

2. Caufriez, A., Moreno-Reyes, R., Leproult, R., Vertongen, F., Van Cauter, E., & Copinschi, G. Immediate effects of an 8-H advance shift of the rest-activity cycle on 24-h profiles of cortisol. *Am. J. Physiol. Endocrinol. Metab.* 2002; **282**: E1147–E1153.

3. Zoli, A., Lizzo, M. M., Ferlisi, E. M. *et al.* ACTH, cortisol and prolactin in active rheumatoid arthritis. *Clin. Rheumatol.*, 2002; **21**: 289–293.

4. Vgontzas, A. N., Zoumakis, M., Papanicolaou, D. A. *et al.* Chronic insomnia is associated with a shift of interleukin-6 and tumor necrosis factor secretion from nighttime to daytime. *Metabolism* 2002; **51**: 887–892.

5. Fantidis, P., Perez De Prada, T., Fernandez-Ortiz, A. *et al.* Morning cortisol production in coronary heart disease patients. *Eur. J. Clin. Invest.* 2002; **32**: 304–330.

6. Baylis, C., Handa, R. K., & Sorkin, M. Glucocorticoids and control of glomerular filtration rate. *Semin. Nephrol.* 1990; **10**: 320–329.

7. Riad, M., Mogos, M., Thangathurai, D., & Lumb, P. D. Steroids. *Curr. Opin. Crit. Care* 2002; **8**: 281–284.

8. Offner, P. J., Moore, E. E., & Ciesla, D. The adrenal response after severe trauma. *Am. J. Surg.* 2002; **184**: 649–653.

9. Marik, P. E. & Zaloga, G. P. Adrenal insufficiency in the critically ill: a new look at an old problem. *Chest* 2002; **122**: 1784–1796.

10. Lamberts, S. W. J., Briuning, H. A., & De Jong, F. H. Corticosteroid therapy in severe illness. *N. Engl. J. Med.* 1997; **337**: 1285–1292.

11. Oelkers, W. Adrenal insufficiency. *N. Engl. J. Med.* 1996; **335**: 1206–1212.

12. Nye, E. J., Grice, J. E., Hockings, G. I. *et al.* Comparison of adrenocorticotropin (ACTH) stimulation tests and insulin hypoglycemia in normal humans: low dose, standard high dose, and 8-hour ACTH- (1–24) infusion tests. *J. Clin. Endocrinol. Metab.* 1999; **84**(10): 3648–3655.

13. Graham, G. W., Unger, B. P., & Coursin, D. B. Perioperative management of selected endocrine disorders. *Int. Anesthesiol. Clin.* 2000; **38**: 31–67.

14. Salem, M., Tainsh, R. E., Bromberg, J., Loriaux, D. L., & Chernow, B. Perioperative glucocorticoid coverage; a reassessment 42 years after emergence of a problem. *Ann. Surg.* 1994; **219**: 416–425.

15. Jabbour, S. A. Steroids and the surgical patient. *Med. Clin. North Am.* 2001; **85**: 1311–1317.

29

Disorders of calcium metabolism

Pamela T. Prescott

University of California at Davis, Division of Endocrinology, Sacramento, CA

Both hypercalcemia and hypocalcemia may be associated with life-threatening cardiac arrhythmias as well as morbidity affecting other organ systems. Effective treatment is available and clinicians should be alert to abnormalities in serum calcium, which are present in more than 2% of hospitalized patients. Furthermore, both hypercalcemia and hypocalcemia suggest significant underlying pathology, and efforts to diagnose and treat these conditions should be instituted.

Adult humans contain more than 1 kg of calcium, of which over 99% is skeletal and dental and only 0.1% is in extracellular fluids. About half the calcium in serum is bound to protein, primarily albumin. Decreases in serum albumin are accompanied by decreases in calcium (a drop of 1 g/dl of albumin lowers the calcium by about 0.8 mg/dl). Several calcium determinations and measurement of ionized (physiologically active) calcium levels may be needed to accurately assess calcium status.[1]

Serum ionized calcium levels are tightly controlled by the interplay of parathyroid hormone, calcitonin, and 1,25-dihydroxycholecalciferol (1,25-$[OH]_2D_3$). Parathyroid hormone is synthesized in the parathyroid glands and, after cleavage of precursor molecules, is released into the circulation as an 84-amino-acid polypeptide and small fragments.[1]

The amino-terminal 1–34 amino acids compose the biologically active portion of the molecule. Highly specific immunoradiometric assays are available that measure the intact hormone, permitting accurate diagnosis. Parathyroid hormone release is primarily controlled by serum calcium levels, although modest hypomagnesemia also evokes a parathyroid hormone response, whereas severe hypomagnesemia impairs release. Parathyroid hormone increases serum calcium by increasing bone resorption, decreasing calciuria, and indirectly increasing gastrointestinal absorption of calcium by its effects on the production of 1,25-(OH_2D_3) and stimulation of the vitamin D-dependent calcium pump. Calcitonin is synthesized in the thyroidal perifollicular cells in response to hypercalcemia. Calcitonin directly inhibits bone resorption and may indirectly increase calciuria. The physiologic importance of calcitonin in humans is questioned. The renal synthesis of 1,25-($OH)_2D_3$ is regulated directly by serum levels of parathyroid hormone and phosphate and, at least indirectly, by serum calcium. This sterol hormone increases intestinal absorption of calcium and phosphorus and is critical for normal mineralization of osteoid.[1]

Hypercalcemia

Hypercalcemia affects the function of many organs. When it is severe, hypercalcemia can cause arrhythmias and heart block. Effects of digitalis are exaggerated. Gastrointestinal symptoms include anorexia, nausea, vomiting, constipation, and ileus. Prolonged hypercalcemia may be associated with peptic ulcer disease and pancreatitis. Affected patients may exhibit polyuria and polydipsia resulting from reversible nephrogenic diabetes insipidus. Acute and chronic renal failure with nephrolithiasis and nephrocalcinosis may occur. Neuropsychiatric symptoms include poor concentration and memory, weakness, lethargy, depression, coma, and, rarely, psychosis.

Causes of hypercalcemia are listed in Table 29.1. The three most common causes of hypercalcemia are primary hyperparathyroidism, malignancy and granulomatous diseases. Hypercalcemia may be discovered when serum calcium is measured as a screening test or as part of the evaluation for fatigue, unexplained weakness, neuromuscular disability, renal stones, or osteopenia.[1–3]

Medical Management of the Surgical Patient: A Textbook of Perioperative Medicine, ed. M. F. Lubin, R. B. Smith, T. F. Dobson, N. Spell, H. K. Walker. 4th edn. Published by Cambridge University Press. © Cambridge University 2006.

Table 29.1. Causes of hypercalcemia

Primary hyperparathyroidism
Familial hypocalciuric hypercalcemia
Malignancy (PTHrP, cytokines, prostaglandin E, 1,25-[OH]$_2$D$_3$)
Granulomatous disease (1,25-[OH]$_2$D$_3$)
   Sarcoid
   Tuberculosis
   Fungal infections
   Leprosy
   Silicone
   Lymphoma
Hyperthyroidism
Hypothyrodism (rare)
Acromegaly (rare)
Calcium ingestion
Vitamin D intoxication
Vitamin A intoxication
Thiazides
Lithium
Immobilization in association with:
   Adolescence
   Paget's disease
   Any state with increased bone resorption
Renal disease
   Diuretic phase of acute renal failure
   Renal transplantation
   Tertiary hyperparathyroidism

Hyperparathyroidism is diagnosed when there is hypercalcemia and inappropriately normal or elevated levels of parathyroid hormone (PTH). Not all patients have elevated serum or ionized calcium levels at every laboratory draw for calcium. In those with mild hyperparathyroidism, the serum calcium may be at the upper limit of normal, and the ionized calcium normal or slightly elevated.[4] Hyperparathyroidism may present as part of a multiple endocrine neoplasia syndrome. With prolonged hyperparathyroidism, hypophosphatemia and a hyperchloremic acidosis may occur. Immunoradiometric assays for intact PTH (IRMA, PTH-intact) are usually used to confirm the elevation in PTH.

The next most common cause is hypercalcemia associated with malignancy. This is believed to virtually always have a systemic or local osseous humoral cause. The most common cause of solid tumor hypercalcemia is excessive elaboration of parathyroid hormone-related protein. This protein, which is a product of many normal tissues, has substantial homology with the amino-terminal end of the parathyroid hormone and binds to the same receptor. It can be measured by specific assays that do not measure parathyroid hormone, permitting laboratory distinction

between these two common causes of hypercalcemia. The hypercalcemia of malignancy may also be mediated by various cytokines, including lymphotoxin, interleukin-1, and tumor necrosis factor, and by tumorous production of 1,25-(OH)$_2$D$_3$ or prostaglandins.

Familial hypocalciuric hypercalcemia may be difficult to discern from hyperparathyroidism. Parathyroid hormone levels are typically not elevated yet are not appropriately suppressed. Lack of tissue damage, onset in childhood, family history, and low urinary calcium levels should help with the diagnosis. Although parathyroidectomy is the usual therapy for primary hyperparathyroidism, it is neither required nor recommended for familial hypocalciuric hypercalcemia.

Granulomatous disease causes hypercalcemia in a few patients and this is typically mediated by 1,25-(OH)$_2$D$_3$ hydroxylated in the granuloma. Vitamin D and vitamin A cause bone resorption. Thiazide diuretics, by decreasing calciuria, can cause a transient hypercalcemia; if this persists, a workup to exclude another cause is appropriate. Lithium alters the set-point for calcium feedback of parathyroid hormone release, resulting in mild hypercalcemia without appropriate suppression of parathyroid hormone. Immobilization leads to hypercalcemia in states of increased bone turnover (adolescence, Paget's disease, hyperthyroidism) and aggravates hypercalcemia resulting from other causes. Other, less common, causes are listed.

Therapy for hypercalcemia

Therapy for asymptomatic hyperparathyroidism may include estrogen for selected postmenopausal women, or bisphosphonates to provide skeletal protection, even though hypercalcemia may persist. For patients with symptoms or severe side effects of the hyperparathyroidism, surgery is suggested. Granulomatous diseases can be treated with corticosteroids. A therapeutic response may take days or weeks to achieve and high doses (5 to 8 times maintenance doses) are typically required. Chloroquine, hydroxychloroquine, and ketoconazole can be used if the patient fails to respond to, or develops, dangerous side effects from corticosteroid therapy.[3] Malignancy-associated hypercalcemia is usually severe and usually requires several modalities to lower the calcium and limit the hypercalcemic effects. Patients with hypercalcemia and thyrotoxicosis may show hypocalcemic responses to beta-blockers. Selected patients with renal failure and hypercalcemia require dialysis.

For severe hypercalcemia, rehydration with intravenous saline and early mobilization are important. Forced saline diuresis with large amounts of normal saline

(150–250 ml/hour) together with furosemide may be needed. Cardiovascular and electrolyte status will need to be monitored. If further treatment is necessary, salmon calcitonin (4 to 12 MRC U/kg every 6 to 12 hours subcutaneously) exhibits a hypocalcemic effect in 2 hours and can be used safely in the presence of hepatic and renal disease. Bisphosphonates, like pamidronate, have become the standard. Pamidronate 60 to 90 mg is infused intravenously over 4 to 24 hours. Slightly less effective are infusions of another bisphosphonate, etidronate disodium, which is given at a rate of 7.5 mg/kg daily for 3 days. Pamidronate is a potent inhibitor of bone resorption but may not affect tubular calcium reabsorption, as seen with some malignancies. In these patients, gallium nitrate is infused at a rate of 200 mg/m² over 5 days. Gallium nitrate has the potential for nephrotoxicity. Plicamycin is currently not used because of its considerable toxicity.[2,3,5]

For patients with hypercalcemia who need surgery, careful evaluation is needed. During anesthesia, several factors may alter the serum ionized calcium level, thus potentiating the adverse effects of hypercalcemia. The duration of non-depolarizing relaxants is likely to be prolonged, especially if muscle weakness coexists. A reduction in the duration of action of atracurium has been reported in a patient whose serum calcium was elevated secondary to hyperparathyroidism.[6]

Hypocalcemia

Modest hypocalcemia commonly occurs in critically ill patients but is not clinically significant. When symptoms do occur, they involve multiple organs. Neuropsychiatric symptoms include tetany, muscle spasms, hyperreflexia, paresthesias (circumoral, extremities), weakness, irritability, depression, dementia, and, rarely, psychosis. The Chvostek's sign is mildly positive in as many as 20% of normocalcemic research subjects but Trousseau's sign is more specific. Cardiovascular manifestations include hypotension, bradycardia, arrhythmias, and digitalis and catecholamine insensitivity. Electrocardiograhic QT intervals are prolonged. Laryngospasm and bronchospasm may occur as well.

Causes of hypocalcemia are listed in Table 29.2. Hypocalcemia results from a deficiency of parathyroid hormone, impaired parathyroid action, a deficiency of vitamin D, impaired vitamin D action, complexing or precipitation of calcium, increased osteoblastic activity, or drugs that inhibit bone resorption. Patients with hypoparathyroidism typically have hyperphosphatemia, whereas those with vitamin D deficiency have low serum

Table 29.2. Causes of hypocalcemia

Hypoparathyroidism (subnormal parathyroid hormone release)
   Idiopathic (autoimmune)
   Postsurgical
   Infiltrative (metastatic cancer, hemochromatosis, amyloidosis, Granulomatous disease, Wilson's disease)
   Irradiation
   Severe hypomagnesemia
Pseudohypoparathyroidism
Vitamin D deficiency
   Decreased absorption
   Decreased 25-(OH)D$_3$ (severe liver disease)
   Decreased 1,25-(OH)$_2$D$_3$ (renal failure, vitamin D-dependent rickets)
Hyperphosphatemia
   Tumor lysis
   Rhabdomyolysis
   Iatrogenic
Massive blood transfusion (citrate)
Osteoblastic metastases
Parathyroidectomy (hungry bones)
Drugs
   Anticalcemic agents (discussed in text)
   Asparaginase
   Cisplatin
   Cytosine arabinoside
   Foscarnet
   Ketoconazole

phosphorus levels. Measurement of serum parathyroid hormone levels distinguishes hypoparathyroidism from pseudohypoparathyroidism because levels are increased in the latter. Levels of 25-(OH)D$_3$ assess renal hydroxylation. Severe hypomagnesemia (less than 1 mg/dl) impairs both parathyroid hormone release and activity.

Surgical patients with hypocalcemia require treatment to prevent the cardiorespiratory and neurologic manifestations of this metabolic derangement. Ionized calcium determinations should be performed in patients with hypoalbuminemia, although the reliability of this measurement is variable. Patients with hyperphosphatemia should be treated with dietary restrictions and phosphate binders (aluminum hydroxide or aluminum carbonate) to lower their serum phosphate levels because vigorous administration of calcium may result in enhanced soft tissue precipitation. Patients with hypomagnesemia require normalization of their serum magnesium levels to achieve normal calcium levels.

Symptomatic hypocalcemia should be treated emergently with intravenous calcium. A 100 to 200 mg bolus of elemental calcium, diluted to minimize venous irritation, should be given over a 10-min period. Several preparations are available. The advantage of calcium gluconate (90 mg elemental calcium per 10 ml ampule) is that it is less irritating to the veins than calcium chloride (272 mg of elemental calcium per 10 ml ampule). Intravenous calcium therapy only raises the calcium level for 1 to 2 hours; if the hypocalcemia is severe, an infusion of 15 mg/kg elemental calcium (about 100 to 200 mg of elemental calcium in 500 ml) over 4 to 6 hours can be given. This will raise the serum calcium by 2 to 3 mg/dl.[6,7] Serum calcium levels should be monitored every few hours during treatment because hypercalcemia, nausea, arrhythmias, bradycardia, and toxicity from digitalis, when used, may occur. When the patient is stable, oral calcium should be started, at a dose of 1 to 4 g elemental calcium per day. If the patient was hypercalcemic prior to neck surgery, subsequent hypocalcemia could be from temporary or permanent damage to the parathyroid glands, or hungry bone syndrome. These patients may require both oral and intravenous calcium therapy, Vitamin D, in the form of $1,25(OH)_2D_3$.

For patients with hypocalcemia who need surgery, several surgical factors alter the serum calcium and ionized calcium levels, and may potentiate the adverse effects of the hypocalcemia. These include abnormal acid–base status and electrolytes; transfusion of large volumes of citrated blood; and the use of cardiopulmonary bypass.[6] Acidosis decreases calcium binding to albumin thus increasing ionized calcium, while alkalosis increases calcium binding resulting in lower ionized calcium levels. Massive blood transfusions and cardiopulmonary bypass (which requires massive blood transfusions) expose the patient to a high amount of citrate that can temporarily lower calcium levels. Calcium levels should be monitored closely, so treatment, if needed, can be started immediately. Symptomatic hypocalcemia should be treated emergently with intravenous calcium. A 100 to 200 mg bolus of elemental calcium, diluted to minimize venous irritation, should be given over a 10 min period. Calcium chloride provides more elemental calcium per gram than does either calcium gluconate or calcium gluceptate but all are acceptable for therapy. Subsequent treatment varies according to the cause of the hypocalcemia. A continuous calcium infusion (100 to 200 mg of elemental calcium in 500 ml over 6 hours) may be adequate in the acute perioperative setting but oral calcium or the addition of vitamin D may be indicated for future long-term therapy with calcium and, if needed, with a short-acting vitamin D preparation such as $1,25(OH)_2D_3$, but should be maintained at mildly hypocalcemic levels to stimulate the remaining parathyroid tissue to recover. Serum calcium levels should be monitored every few hours during treatment because hypercalcemia, nausea, arrhythmias, bradycardia, and toxicity from digitalis, when this is used, may occur.

REFERENCES

1. Bringhurst, F. R., Demay, M. B., & Kroenberg, H. M. Hormones and disorders of mineral metabolism. In Wilson, J. D., Foster, D. W., Kronenberg, H. M., & Larsen, P. R., eds. *Williams Textbook of Endocrinology*, 9th edn. Philadelphia: W. B. Saunders, 1998: 1155–1209.
2. Marcus, R. Diagnosis and treatment of hyperparathyroidism. *Rev. Endocr. Metab. Disord.* 2000; **1**: 247–252.
3. Sharma, O. P. Hypercalcemia in granulomatous disorders: a clinical review. *Curr. Opin. Pulm. Med.* 2000; **6**: 442–447.
4. Bilezkian, J. P., Potts, J. T. Jr., Fuleihan Gel, -H. *et al.* Summary statement from a workshop on asymptomatic primary hyperparathyroidism: a perspective for the 21st century. *J. Clin. Endocrinol. Metab.* 2002; **87**: 5353–5361.
5. Esbrit, P. & Hurtado, J. Treatment of malignant hypercalcaemia. *Expt. Opin. Pharmacother.* 2002; **3**: 521–527.
6. Aguilera, I. M. & Vaughan, R. X. Calcium and the anaesthetist. *Anaesthesia* 2000; **55**: 770–790.
7. Vasa, F. R. Endocrine problems in the chronically critically ill patient. *Clin. Chest Med.* 2001; **22**: 193–208.

30

Pheochromocytoma

Pamela T. Prescott

University of California at Davis, Division of Epidemiology, Sacramento, CA

Although pheochromocytomas are not a common medical/surgical problem (they are estimated to cause only 0.1% to 0.5% of all cases of hypertension, and are operated on only once or twice per year in most centers), medical consultants are likely to be asked to evaluate and prepare for surgery patients with suspected pheochromocytomas at some time during their careers. Because catecholamines have major regulatory effects on many different body systems, it is vital that these be anticipated and properly managed in the perioperative period. Pheochromocytomas are associated with an increased risk of adverse reactions to many commonly prescribed drugs and clinicians must also be aware of this potential hazard. The surgical removal of a pheochromocytoma has great potential for intra- and postoperative complications because of the release of catecholamines during manipulation or stimulation of the tumor.

Pathophysiology

Pheochromocytomas arise from chromaffin cells of the neural crest that migrate to form the adult adrenal medulla and sympathetic ganglia. These cells synthesize catecholamines through a series of enzymatically controlled steps, starting with the conversion of tyrosine to dihydroxyphenylalanine (dopa) by tyrosine hydroxylase. This is the rate-limiting step in catecholamine synthesis. Dopa is then converted to dopamine, which is subsequently decarboxylated to norepinephrine. The methylation of norepinephrine to epinephrine is accomplished through the action of phenylethanilamine-N-methyl transferase, an enzyme that is induced by glucocorticoids that reach the adrenal medulla in high concentrations through the corticomedullary venous sinuses from the adrenal cortex. Norepinephrine and epinephrine are the major products of most pheochromocytomas. Epinephrine is produced mainly in the adrenal medulla; thus, a pheochromocytoma that produces epinephrine is nearly always located in the adrenal. Norepinephrine is produced and secreted in the central nervous system and the sympathetic postganglionic nerve endings as well as in the adrenal medulla. Dopamine is also produced and secreted by some pheochromocytomas. Once catecholamines reach the plasma, they have a half-life of only 1 to 2 minutes before they are taken up by cells or enzymatically degraded. Metanephrine, normetanephrine, and vanillylmandelic acid are the major metabolites.

Catecholamines bind to adrenergic and dopaminergic cell-surface receptors, which in turn induce second messengers. Norepinephrine is primarily an alpha-adrenergic agonist that causes vasoconstriction and hypertension with little metabolic activity. Epinephrine, an alpha- and beta-adrenergic agonist, has positive inotropic and chronotropic effects on the heart and causes vasodilation. Its metabolic effects include inhibition of insulin secretion and stimulation of glycogenolysis in the liver. Hypersecretion of catecholamines has many dramatic physiologic effects. In contrast, adrenal medullary hypo function is not clinically significant because norepinephrine is available from other sources.

Presentation

Pheochromocytoma is a rare endocrine disorder. It is highly treatable, but fatal if misdiagnosed or improperly treated.[1] Nearly 90% of pheochromocytomas in adults occur in the adrenal medulla. Of those that occur outside the adrenal 1% are found in the abdomen, 1% in the chest and 1% in the urinary bladder. As a general rule, pheochromocytomas are approximately 10% familial,

Medical Management of the Surgical Patient: A Textbook of Perioperative Medicine, ed. M. F. Lubin, R. B. Smith, T. F. Dobson, N. Spell, H. K. Walker. 4th edn. Published by Cambridge University Press. © Cambridge University 2006.

10% bilateral, and 10% malignant, and 10% are found outside of the adrenal glands.[1–3] The incidence of pheochromocytomas is increased in familial conditions such as tuberous sclerosis, Sturge–Weber syndrome, von Recklinghousen's disease, VonHippel–Lindau disease, neurofibromatosis, familial pheochromocytoma, and multiple endocrine neoplasia (MEN) syndromes. MEN 1 consists of hyperparathyroidism, pituitary adenomas, pancreatic islet cell tumors, and very rarely pheochromocytoma. MEN 2 A consists of pheochromocytoma, medullary carcinoma of the thyroid, and mucosal neuroma syndromes.[1] In the familial conditions, the incidence of bilateral adrenal tumors increases.

Although the presence of pheochromocytoma in pregnancy is extremely rare, the tumor constitutes a very high risk for both mother and fetus. Pheochromocytoma should be considered in any pregnant woman with hypertension, especially if paroxysmal or labile, or with unexplained "spells." Maternal and fetal survival depends on an early diagnosis, correct medical therapy and correct timing of delivery and surgery.

Clinical features

Because nearly all pheochromocytomas are functional and produce high levels of catecholamines, a wide variety of symptoms and signs can occur. Hypertension is the most common feature and, despite the emphasis usually placed on the intermittent nature of pheochromocytoma symptoms, is more likely to be sustained that intermittent. Only about half of all patients have the classic paroxysmal symptoms of headache, pallor, palpitations, and sweating associated with hypertension. Orthostasis is frequent. The sudden onset of hypertension in a previously normotensive person, especially occurring during the induction of anesthesia, should suggest the possibility of pheochromocytoma. Other reported symptoms include a sense of doom or apprehension, anxiety, trembling, mild abdominal pain, and constipation. Less common presentations include intestinal pseudoobstruction and ileus, cardiomyopathy, Prinzmetal's coronary spasm, and peripheral vascular spasm. In elderly patients, symptoms may be less marked because of the decline in sensitivity to catecholamines that occurs with advanced age. A serious complication of pheochromocytoma is myocarditis and subsequent congestive heart failure. Infiltrates of histiocytes, plasma cells, and other inflammatory cells are seen in the myocardium on postmortem studies.

Few physical findings suggest pheochromocytoma other than hypertension. In the associated endocrine neoplasias and neuroectodermal disorders, thyroid enlargement, neurofibromas, or café au lait spots may be present.

Diagnosis

It is essential to establish the diagnosis of pheochromocytoma preoperatively because intraoperative diagnosis of pheochromocytoma has a mortality approaching 50%.[3] The diagnosis of pheochromocytoma is made by documenting the excess secretion of catecholamines. Biochemical diagnosis can be difficult because of inadequate specificity of biochemical tests, and false-positive and false-negative results are common.[4] Biochemical tests include measurements of plasma and urinary catecholamines, urinary fractionated metanephrines, urinary total metanephrines, and urinary vanillylmandelic acid (VMA). Among all patients with pheochromocytoma, sensitivities for testing are the highest for measurements of plasma free metanephrines at 99%, followed by urinary fractionated metanephrines at 97%. Sensitivities of the other tests are lower with urinary catecholamines at 86%, plasma catecholamines at 84%–93%, urinary total metanephrines at 77%, and urinary VMA at 64%. Plasma free metanephrines and urinary fractionated metanephrines offer the highest sensitivities[4,5] but, no one method can absolutely diagnose or exclude the presence of pheochromocytoma.

Plasma levels of catecholamines and free metanephrines must be obtained under carefully controlled conditions with patients in the supine position, with placement of an indwelling catheter, and after an overnight fast. The laboratory draw for the plasma catecholamines and free metanephrines must be as stress free as possible, the venipuncture itself can cause levels to be falsely elevated. Interfering substances for plasma catecholamines and free metanephrines include coffee, tricyclic antidepressants, nicotine, and phenoxybenzamine.[4] Urinary collections are also prone to false-positive and false-negative results from numerous interfering substances, including decongestants; several antibiotics (choramphenicol, nalidixic acid, tetracycline, erythromycin); antihypertensives (reserpine, guanethindine, labetolol, phentolamine and methyldopa); amphetamines; benzodiazepines; diuretics in doses sufficient to produce sodium depletion; nitrates; bromocriptine; MAO inhibitors; phenothiazines; caffeine; ethanol, and marijuana.[6] Certain clinical situations may increase both plasma catecholamine and urine catecholamine metabolites to levels usually seen in pheochromocytoma. These situations include acute clonidine withdrawal, acute alcohol withdrawal, vasodilator therapy with hydralazine or minoxidil, acute myocardial ischemia or infarction, acute cerebral vascular accident, cocaine abuse, severe congestive heart failure, and hypoglycemia.[7]

The oral clonidine test, which supresses plasma catecholamine secretion in patients with essential hypertension but not in those with pheochromocytomas, may be useful. The failure of 0.3 mg of oral clonidine to reduce plasma levels of norepinephrine in patients with hypertension is suggestive of pheochromocytoma. Provocative tests for catecholamine release such as glucagon, have high rates of morbidity and mortality, and should be used cautiously. A calcium antagonist can be used to blunt the hypertensive response and without interfering with plasma catecholamine determination. A positive glucagon stimulation test requires a twofold to 2.5-fold increase in plasma catecholamine concentration 60 to 120 seconds after a bolus iv administration of 2.0 mg glucagon.[7]

REFERENCES

1. Young, J. B. & Landsberg, L. Pheochromocytoma. In Wilson, J. D., Foster, D. W., Kronenberg, H. M., & Larsen, P. R., eds., *Williams Textbook of Endocrinology*, 9th edn., Philadelphia: W. B. Saunders; 1998: 705–716.

2. Kinney, M. A. O., Narr, B. J., & Warner, M. A. Perioperative management of pheochromocytoma. *J. Cardiothoracic. Vasc. Anesth.* 2002; **16**: 359–369.

3. Graham, G. W., Unger, B. P., & Coursin, D. B. Perioperative management of selected endocrine disorders. *Int. Anesthesiol. Clin.* 2000; **38**: 31–67.

4. Lenders, J. W. M., Pacak, K., Walther, M. M. *et al.* Biochemical diagnosis of pheochromocytoma. Which is best? *J. Am. Med. Assoc.* 2002; **287**: 1427–1434.

5. Van Der Harst, E., De Herder, W. W., Dekrijger, R. R. *et al.* The value of plasma markers for the clinical behavior of pheochromocytomas. *Eur. J. Endocrinol.* 2002; **147**: 85–94.

6. Henry, J. B. (ed.) Adrenal gland. In *Clinical Diagnosis and Management by Laboratory Methods*, 20th edn, Philadelphia: W. B. Saunders; 2001: 313.

7. Bravo, E. L. Pheochromocytoma. *Cardiol. Rev.* 2002; **10**: 44–50.

Rheumatology

31

Rheumatologic diseases

Joe T. Kelley, III[1] and Doyt L. Conn[2]

[1]Sarasota, FL
[2]Rheumatology Division, Emory University School of Medicine, Atlanta, GA

The perioperative evaluation of the patient with rheumatologic disease should include the usual medical evaluation as outlined elsewhere in the text, with special attention to medications and assessing disease activity (Tables 31.1, 31.2). Three important classes of medications are non-steroidal anti-inflammatory drugs (NSAIDs), glucocorticoids, and disease-modifying antirheumatic drugs (DMARDs). Patients should be carefully questioned regarding their use of over the counter NSAIDs as many patients fail to mention these to their physicians. It is vital to continue glucocorticoid therapy during the entire perioperative period. Discontinuing even low doses of glucocorticoids may cause a significant flare of disease activity with profound consequences. As will be discussed later in this chapter, recommendations for glucocorticoid supplementation in the perioperative period have changed during the past few years.

We will discuss two other important issues, fractures in potentially osteoporotic patients and acute arthritis in the postoperative period (Table 31.2).

Medications

Non-steroidal anti-inflammatory drugs (NSAIDs)

Patients with rheumatic diseases commonly use aspirin and non-aspirin NSAIDs. NSAIDs inhibit platelet cyclo-oxygenase-1 (COX-1) thus blocking the formation of thromboxane A_2. The result is impairment of thromboxane-dependent platelet aggregation and prolongation of the bleeding time.[1] Aspirin irreversibly blocks COX; therefore, its actions persist for the circulating lifetime of the platelet, which is about 10 days. Non-aspirin

Table 31.1. Medications in the perioperative period

Aspirin	Discontinue at least 10 days prior to surgery
Non-aspirin NSAIDs	Discontinue in time for complete elimination (5 half-lives)
	Ibuprofen 1 day prior to surgery
	Naproxen 4 days prior to surgery
Glucocorticoids	Always continue glucocorticoid therapy in perioperative period
	See text for details regarding supplementation
Methotrexate	Continue without interruption unless elderly, renal insufficiency, uncontrolled diabetes mellitus, significant lung or liver disease, ethanol abuse, moderate to high dose glucocorticoid therapy (>10 mg/day prednisone), poor functional status if one or more present, hold two weekly doses, one during week before surgery one during week of surgery
Hydroxychloroquine	Continue without interruption
Sulfasalazine Azathioprine	Discontinue 1 day prior to surgery and resume 3 days after surgery
Cyclophosphamide	Discontinue 1 day prior to surgery
Etanercept Infliximab	Discontinue at least 1 week prior to surgery and resume 2 weeks after surgery

Medical Management of the Surgical Patient: A Textbook of Perioperative Medicine, ed. M. F. Lubin, R. B. Smith, T. F. Dobson, N. Spell, H. K. Walker. 4th edn. Published by Cambridge University Press. © Cambridge University 2006.

Table 31.2. Special issues in the perioperative period

Fractures	Always consider osteoporosis in patients with fracture, especially after minor trauma
	Early diagnosis and treatment important
Acute arthritis	Crystal-induced arthritis is common. Always consider infection
	Must perform joint aspiration and synovial fluid examination for WBC, crystals, gram stain and culture
Rheumatoid arthritis	Assess disease activity including cervical spine involvement
	Appropriate medication changes
	Early range of motion exercises/early ambulation to prevent joint contractures

NSAIDs inhibit COX reversibly so the duration of their action depends on the specific drug dose, serum level, and half-life.[2] The selective COX-2 inhibitors, celecoxib and rofecoxib, do not inhibit COX-1, therefore platelet aggregation is not inhibited.

Since NSAIDs can prolong the bleeding time, physicians are often asked about the potential for clinically significant bleeding in the perioperative period. Perioperative bleeding time, however, has not been shown to correlate strongly with surgical bleeding.[1,3,4] A literature review in 1991 found no evidence that a prolonged preoperative bleeding time predicts surgical bleeding.[3] In 1996 a retrospective study examining the clinical utilization and predictive value of the bleeding time failed to show an association between abnormal bleeding time and clinically significant perioperative bleeding.[4] Although preoperative bleeding time does not seem to predict surgical bleeding, several studies have suggested that the use of NSAIDs in the preoperative period does lead to significantly increased perioperative blood loss.[5–8]

Given the available data, we suggest discontinuing aspirin at least 10 days prior to surgery since the lifespan of platelets is 10 days. Non-aspirin NSAIDs should be discontinued in time for complete elimination of the drug to occur which is about 5 half-lives. Ibuprofen has a half-life of about 2.5 hours so it should be stopped 1 day prior to surgery. The half-life of naproxen is about 15 hours, so discontinuation should occur 4 days prior to surgery.

Glucocorticoids

Glucocorticoids were first used to treat rheumatoid arthritis in 1948 at the Mayo Clinic in Rochester, Minnesota, and the dramatic results led to the awarding of the Nobel Prize in Medicine to Kendall, Hench, and Reichstein.[9] Glucocorticoids continue to play an important role in the management of rheumatologic diseases.

Glucocorticoids are produced in the adrenal cortex under negative feedback control of both the hypothalamus and pituitary gland (hypothalamic–pituitary–adrenal [HPA] axis). The hypothalamus produces corticotropin-releasing hormone (CRH), stimulating the pituitary gland to synthesize adrenocorticotrophic hormone (ACTH) which leads to production of corticosteroids, mainly cortisol, by the adrenal gland. The rate of secretion is approximately $5\,mg/m^2$ per day to $10\,mg/m^2$ per day of cortisol, which is the equivalent of about 20–30 mg per day of hydrocortisone or 5–7 mg per day of prednisone.[10,11] This basal rate may increase five- to tenfold under conditions of severe stress and is essential for the maintenance of homeostasis.[12,13,14]

When patients on chronic glucocorticoids undergo episodes of significant stress as in the perioperative period, physicians are frequently concerned about their ability to produce endogenous steroids. This concern originates from case reports, published in the 1950s, which describe two young patients who received chronic glucocorticoids and died unexpectedly after routine surgery, presumably from adrenal insufficiency.[1,15,16] In 1952 Fraser described a patient who developed adrenal insufficiency due to preoperative withdrawal of glucocorticoid therapy.[15] The next year, Lewis described a patient who died after surgery had been performed to correct a flexion contracture of the knee.[16] The patient had been on daily cortisone for 5 months and this therapy was discontinued 1 day prior to surgery. Postmortem examinations revealed diffuse atrophy and hemorrhage in the adrenal glands. This paper suggested increasing perioperative glucocorticoids by about fourfold. Since that time, patients on chronic glucocorticoids are frequently given "stress dose" steroids despite little evidence to support this practice.[1]

The duration of glucocorticoid therapy, the highest dose, and the total cumulative dose have been considered important predictors of HPA axis suppression since the 1960s.[17,19] It is now known, however, that it is difficult to predict, on the basis of the history of glucocorticoid therapy, which patient will have HPA axis suppression.[13,19–22] Even if HPA axis suppression does occur, the time to recovery is highly variable, ranging from 2.5 days up to 1 year.[17,18,22] One recent study suggested that patients who receive 5 mg per day or less of prednisone continue to have an intact HPA axis.[23]

Three recent reviews have addressed the topic of glucocorticoid supplementation and these expert recommendations call for lower doses and shorter duration of therapy than textbooks traditionally suggest.[10,13,24] One supplemental glucocorticoid dose does not accommodate all patients or procedures and excessive doses may lead to hyperglycemia, immunosuppression, accelerated protein catabolism leading to altered wound healing, hypertension, volume overload, and acute psychosis.[10,13,24] The recommendations from these reviews will be summarized below.

All patients on chronic glucocorticoids who undergo any type of procedure or have a medical illness require their normal daily glucocorticoid therapy. It is especially important to continue glucocorticoid therapy in patients with rheumatic diseases, as discontinuing even low doses of glucocorticoids may cause a significant flare of disease activity. Patients who receive 5 mg per day or less of prednisone do not require additional supplementation, regardless of the procedure or illness.[10,25] Patients who undergo a superficial procedure of less than one hour under local anesthesia, such as routine dental work, skin biopsy or minor orthopedic surgery, require their normal daily dose without additional supplementation.[10,13,24]

Minor surgical procedures, such as inguinal hernia repair, and colonoscopy, require hydrocortisone 25 mg or methylprednisolone 5 mg intravenous on the day of procedure only.[10]

Moderately stressful procedures, such open cholecystectomy, and hemicolectomy, require hydrocortisone 50–75 mg or methylprednisolone 10–15 mg intravenous on the day of procedure with a rapid taper over 1–2 days to patient's usual dose.[10]

Severe surgical stress, such as experienced major cardiothoracic surgery, Whipple procedure, and liver resection, require hydrocortisone 100–150 mg or methylprednisolone 20–30 mg intravenous on the day of procedure with a taper over 1–2 days to patient's usual dose.[10]

Critically ill patients, such as with shock or sepsis-induced hypotension, require hydrocortisone 50–100 mg intravenous every 6–8 hours or 0.18 mg/kg per hour as continuous infusion plus 50 µg/day of fludrocortisone until shock resolves. The taper may take several days to a week and should be gradual with attention paid to maintaining blood pressure and good renal function.[10]

If patients on high doses of glucocorticoids present with lethargy, feeling poorly and with vague abdominal distress and distension, they must be evaluated further. Because the higher doses of glucocorticoids have suppressed the normal signs of inflammation or infection such as fever and pain, such a patient should be evaluated for septicemia from such causes as a perforated peptic ulcer, bowel or gall bladder.

Patients on glucocorticoids should also be on calcium, vitamin D and depending on dose, duration of treatment, age and sex. If history of fracture or low bone density, the patient should also be on bisphosphonates.

Methotrexate

Weekly methotrexate therapy became popular among rheumatologists in the 1980s and continues to be one of the most commonly used disease-modifying antirheumatic drugs (DMARDs).[26] The relationship between methotrexate and postoperative complications, such as local infections and poor wound healing, has been a controversial topic over the past decade due to the lack of definitive studies.[27] Most of the studies have involved rheumatoid arthritis patients undergoing elective orthopedic surgery.

A small retrospective study published in 1991 suggested that methotrexate increases the risk of postoperative complications.[28] The authors were unable to draw any definite conclusions however, due to the small number of patients and the non-randomized selection of therapy. Other small studies around the same time failed to show a significant increase in complications in patients taking methotrexate perioperatively.[29–31]

Alarcon et al. planned a randomized, placebo-controlled, multicenter trial to address this issue but they were unable to enroll an adequate number of patients.[32] The major reason cited for failure to enroll enough patients was that many potential investigators declined to participate because of their strong opinions that methotrexate did, or did not, contribute to postoperative complications.[27,32]

In 2001 Grennan et al. published a prospective randomized study of postoperative infection or surgical complications in patients with rheumatoid arthritis who underwent elective orthopedic surgery.[33] Three hundred and eighty-eight patients with rheumatoid arthritis, who were to undergo elective orthopedic surgery, were divided into two groups. One group continued methotrexate and the other group discontinued methotrexate from 2 weeks before surgery until 2 weeks after surgery. Their complication rates were compared with complications occurring in 228 rheumatoid arthritis patients not receiving methotrexate who also underwent elective orthopedic surgery. Methotrexate use was not associated with an increased incidence of complications and, in fact, those patients continuing methotrexate had significantly less complications or infections than either of the other two groups ($P < 0.003$). Additionally, discontinuation of methotrexate led more commonly to disease flares within 6 weeks following surgery.[33]

For the rheumatoid arthritis patient undergoing orthopedic surgery, it has been recommended that two weekly doses of methotrexate be withheld, one during the week before surgery and one during the week of surgery, then resuming methotrexate in the week following surgery.[27] Regardless of the type of surgical procedure, this recommendation seems prudent in the elderly methotrexate-treated patient and those patients with renal insufficiency, uncontrolled diabetes mellitus, significant lung or liver disease, ethanol abuse, moderate to high dose glucocorticoid therapy (>10 mg per day prednisone), or poor functional status. The elderly and those with renal insufficiency are at increased risk of methotrexate related pancytopenia[34–36] and it has been suggested that the perioperative period is an especially hazardous time for methotrexate-treated patients with renal impairment and sepsis.[37] In the absence of the above factors, we believe methotrexate should be continued. If methotrexate therapy is interrupted it is imperative to begin therapy as soon as possible given the risk of having a disease flare.[33]

Other medications

Other medications frequently used in patients with rheumatologic conditions include hydroxychloroquine, sulfasalazine, azathioprine, and cyclophosphamide. Although little data exist on the use of these agents in the perioperative period, it is reasonable to withhold medications that are excreted renally, such as cyclophosphamide.[1] We suggest discontinuing sulfasalazine and azathioprine until a few days postoperatively but hydroxychloroquine can probably be continued without interruption.

The tumor necrosis factor (TNF) inhibitors, etanercept and infliximab, are being used more widely and no data exist regarding their safety in the perioperative period. We believe it is prudent to discontinue these agents at least one week prior to surgery and resume therapy two weeks after surgery.

Special issues

Fractures in potentially osteoporotic patients

Osteoporosis is defined as a disease characterized by low bone mass and microarchitectural deterioration of bone tissue, leading to enhanced bone fragility and a consequent increase in fracture risk.[38] Significant morbidity, excess mortality, and enormous economic costs are associated with osteoporotic fractures with an estimated annual cost of $10 billion in the USA.[39] Patients with

osteoporosis are usually asymptomatic and are likely to come to the attention of the medical profession with fractures as a result of minor trauma.[40] These patients are at increased risk of sustaining another fracture as compared with patients who have not sustained an osteoporotic fracture.[41] This is not a problem only in women as wrist fractures in men have been shown to be powerful predictors of subsequent hip fracture risk.[42,43]

Recent studies have shown that physicians frequently overlook osteoporosis in these patients and do not offer information, diagnostic testing, or treatment.[40,44–46] Smith et al. reported on 218 patients at least 40 years of age who suffered either a hip or wrist fracture.[40] Only 32% had bone mineral density (BMD) measured and 39% were offered treatment for osteoporosis. Freedman et al. presented a large cohort of women at least 55 years of age who sustained a wrist fracture and found that only 3% had a subsequent BMD and only 17% were started on treatment.[45]

Physicians should always consider osteoporosis in patients presenting with a fracture, especially after minor trauma. In those patients with risk factors for osteoporosis, appropriate diagnostic testing should be performed and patient education and treatment should be initiated while the patient is hospitalized or very shortly thereafter.

Acute arthritis in the postoperative period

Although infection should always be considered in the patient with acute arthritis, crystal-induced arthritis commonly occurs in the postoperative period[1]. Both gout and pseudogout (due to monosodium urate (MSU) and calcium pyrophosphate dihydrate (CPPD) crystal deposition, respectively) can occur during periods of stress, such as medical illness or surgery, and they are frequently overlooked as a cause of arthritis in hospitalized patients.[47–49] Institution or withdrawal of medications, such as allopurinol or diuretics[1] can also precipitate crystal-induced arthritis. Fever can be a prominent feature in hospitalized patients with crystal-induced arthritis.[49–51] The swollen joint(s) can easily be overlooked in the delirious or intubated patient unless a careful joint examination is performed.[1] Patients with gout flares in the postoperative period usually have a history of prior attacks. The clinician should remember that flares of crystalline arthritis commonly look like joint infections with significant swelling and erythema of the soft tissue surrounding the joint (pseudocellulitis). Joint aspiration should always be performed and the synovial fluid should be examined for white blood cell count (WBC) and differential, crystal examination, and gram stain and culture.

The three common treatments for acute gout are colchicine, NSAIDs, and glucocorticoids. Colchicine is traditionally administered orally in a dose of 1 mg, followed by 0.5 mg every two hours until abdominal discomfort or diarrhea develops or a total dose of 4 mg has been given. Colchicine should be used cautiously in those with renal or hepatic insufficiency,[52] and some physicians avoid colchicine in the high doses necessary to abort an acute attack given the efficacy of NSAIDs and glucocorticoids. NSAIDs are usually effective in relieving pain and inflammation in patients with acute gout. NSAIDs should not be used to treat acute gout in elderly patients, those with renal dysfunction, and patients with a history of peptic ulcer disease with bleeding. Intraarticular injections of a glucocorticoid are usually effective in acute monoarticular gout. The appropriate dose of glucocorticoid is related to the size of the joint; the dose of methylprednisolone acetate may vary from 5 to 10 mg for a small joint to 20 to 60 mg for a large joint.[53] Systemic glucocorticoid therapy is also effective with oral prednisone (30 to 50 mg per day initially, with a taper over 7 to 10 days), intramuscular corticotropin (40 units), or triamcinolone acetonide IM (60 mg), or Depo Medrol IM (40 to 60 mg).[53,54]

Rheumatoid arthritis (RA)

Perioperative management of the patient with RA involves assessing disease activity including cervical spine involvement and making appropriate medication changes, if necessary. Important postoperative issues include early range of motion (ROM) exercises and early ambulation in order to prevent joint contractures. The importance of continuing glucocorticoid therapy cannot be stressed enough. As stated previously in the chapter, all patients on chronic glucocorticoids who undergo any type of procedure or have a medical illness require at least their normal daily glucocorticoid therapy. Supplemental doses, if necessary can be given as outlined earlier in the chapter. Discontinuing glucocorticoids preoperatively, which is inappropriate, can lead to postoperative flares of disease and these patients have difficulty with postoperative rehabilitation and therefore may be at higher risk for complications.

Rheumatoid arthritis can manifest with both articular and systemic symptoms. Systemic symptoms include low-grade fever, fatigue, weight loss, and significant morning stiffness. Joint examination may reveal tender, swollen joints and the temperature over the involved joints may be elevated. Laboratory evaluation may reveal evidence of systemic inflammation with mild leukocytosis, thrombocytosis, normochromic anemia, elevated erythrocyte sedimentation rate, and elevated C-reactive protein. In the perioperative period, active disease can be treated by a short-term increase in the glucocorticoid dose with

prednisone 10 mg/day or 5 mg b.i.d. being sufficient.[55,56] If DMARDs, such as methotrexate, or TNF inhibitors, such as etanercept or infliximab, are discontinued in the perioperative period, glucocorticoids can be adjusted to control disease. Restarting DMARDs and TNF inhibitors, as outlined earlier in the chapter, and tapering glucocorticoids to the previous dose is important since the side effects of glucocorticoids are dependent on cumulative dose.[57]

Although RA rarely involves the thoracic, lumbar, or sacral spine, cervical spine involvement is common. Natural history studies in patients with RA suggest that clinically significant cervical spine disease occurs in up to 78% of patients.[58–63] Radiographic cervical spine subluxation in one form or another is estimated to affect 43% to 80% of RA patients and atlantoaxial (C1–2) subluxation is the most common type.[58–62] Anterior subluxation is the most prevalent form and is best demonstrated on lateral cervical spine X-ray with the neck in the flexed position.[64,65] The most common symptom of cervical subluxation is neck pain radiating into the occiput and patients may report a clicking in the neck on flexion and sometimes perceive an anterior movement of the head on the neck.[65,66] Less commonly, patients develop slowly progressive spastic quadriparesis, frequently with painless sensory loss in the hands or transient episodes of medullary dysfunction sometimes with paresthesias in the shoulders or arms during movement of the head.[66]

Rheumatoid arthritis patients at high risk for cervical spine involvement are those with neck symptoms, long-standing disease, erosive disease, subcutaneous nodules, and the elderly.[65]

Importantly, in routine clinical practice it is unnecessary to image the cervical spine unless suggestive symptoms are present. Rheumatoid arthritis patients undergoing surgery with the potential for endotracheal intubation should have preoperative routine anteroposterior, lateral, and open-mouth cervical spine radiographs since the presence of even subtle degrees of atlantoaxial instability may be an indication for fiberoptic intubation.[58]

In the postoperative period it is important, especially in the patient with RA, to continue ROM exercises and encourage early ambulation to prevent joint contractures.

Systemic lupus erythematosus (SLE)

Preoperative assessment of the patient with SLE is directed at determining disease activity and making decisions regarding medications. If the patient is coming in for elective surgery unrelated to lupus, the lupus should be controlled and inactive prior to elective surgery.

Clinical features that suggest active lupus include fever, diffuse skin eruption, polyarthritis, pleurisy, pericarditis, seizures, red blood cells and red blood cells casts on microscopic exam of the urine, and proteinuria, diminished complement components, C_3 and C_4, and elevated levels of anti-DNA.

Active lupus may mimic potential surgical situations in the following circumstances. A patient has a febrile illness, chest pain, and shortness of breath. Chest X-ray shows a large heart indicative of a pericardial effusion. After documentation of the pericardial effusion, aspirations may be indicated for analysis (WBC count), and removal of the fluid. Pericarditis is rapidly responsive to prednisone in doses of 60–80 mg per day in divided doses. Consequently, pericardiectomy is not necessary. An acute abdomen may occur in a setting of active lupus. Although one must rule out cholecystitis, and a perforated bowel, a likely cause is inflammatory peritonitis in the setting of active lupus.

Medications were discussed earlier in this chapter but it should be stressed once again that patients should receive at least their normal daily glucocorticoid therapy, with supplemental doses, if necessary, given as outlined. If necessary, glucocorticoids can be used to control disease activity prior to surgery.

Once the activity and the organ systems involved are known, the treatment can be selected: For constitutional features, polyarthritis and mild skin eruptions, prednisone 10 mg/day or 5 mg b.i.d. may be required.

For severe generalized skin eruptions, pleuritis, pericarditis, peritonitis, hemolytic anemia, significant thrombocytopenia, WHO class 3 and 4 glomerulonephritis, seizures, diffuse brain syndrome, prednisone in doses of 60 mg per day, divided bid or tid, will control the acute manifestations, then the dose can be tapered to the lowest dose that will control the features of disease. Depending on the manifestation, other agents may be added. Hydroxy-chloroquine in most cases, cyclophosphamide IV pulse monthly for Class 4 glomerulonephritis and azathiaprine for steroid sparing in other situations.

Scleroderma

Patients with scleroderma may have limited skin involvement or diffuse skin involvement. All patients with scleroderma have Raynaud's phenomenon and esophageal dysfunction. Some may have interstitial lung disease with varying degrees of lung functional impairment. A small percentage of patients may have renal vascular involvement with hypertension and may be at risk for developing renal scleroderma crisis with accelerated hypertension and renal failure.

Most patients with scleroderma will be on a peripheral acting calcium channel blocker (nifedipine), a proton pump inhibitor, and aspirin, 81 mg per day. Those with more recent interstitial lung disease may be on prednisone and perhaps a cytotoxic agent, cyclophosphamide. In these cases, the duration of higher doses of prednisone should be limited to 1 to 2 months and then tapered to a dose of prednisone 10 mg or less.

If the patient is on prednisone, that dose should be maintained through and after surgery. If the patient is going to have major surgery, the dosage of glucocorticoids should be managed as described in the glucocorticoids section of this chapter.

Occasionally a patient with scleroderma and severe Raynaud's may develop ischemia and dry gangrene of a fingertip that may be very painful. Generally, it can be managed medically by protecting the extremity, stopping smoking, using peripheral acting calcium channel blockers, antiplatelet drugs and pain control. X-rays of the digit will usually show dissolution of the distal phalanx, but this is due to ischemia, not to infection. Osteomyelitis is rare. Surgery is only necessary if pain cannot be managed. The ischemic digital tip will often autoamputate over time. Patients with scleroderma should continue their medications through the surgical procedure. Blood pressure must be monitored and managed.

Polymyositis – dermatomyositis

These diseases are characterized by proximal muscle weakness and sometimes dysphagia. Those with dermatomyositis will have diffuse erythematosus skin involvement. Generally active disease is indicated by an active skin eruption, proximal muscle weakness and an elevated serum creatine phosphokinase (CPK). The disease activity should be controlled before any elective surgery. This is done by using higher doses of prednisone, 60 mg per day for several months until the CPK is near normal, then tapering the prednisone to the lowest dose that will control the disease. Usually the patient will also be on a steroid sparing agent, azathiaprine or methotrexate. The patient should be continued on the same drugs and the same dosages through surgery.

Vasculitis

The most common type of vasculitis is giant cell arteritis (GCA). It occurs in individuals over age 60 and is manifest by constitutional features, fever, weight loss, fatigue, polymyalgia rheumatica, and evidence of cranial artery involvement. This may include headaches, jaw claudication, or visual disturbances. There will also be evidence of systemic inflammation with manifestation such as elevated erythrocyte sedimentation rate, C-reactive protein, anemia, thrombcytosis and a diminished serum albumin. Patients with active disease are treated with higher doses of prednisone, 40–60 mg/day. As the inflammation is controlled, the prednisone dose is tapered to the lowest dose that controls the inflammatory features.

Patients with GCA being considered for surgery should be maintained on their current dose of prednisone and modify the dose depending on the type and duration of surgery according to the algorithm described in the glucocorticoid section in this chapter.

There are also other types of vasculitis which are less common. These include polyarteritis nodosa, microscopic polyarteritis, Wegener's granulomatosus and Takayasus arteritis. There are even less common types of disease with arterial inflamation.[67] In each situation it is important to maintain the drugs that the patient has been taking for their disease through the surgical periods according to the recommendations discussed in the section on drugs in this chapter.

REFERENCES

1. Shaw, M. & Mandell, B. F. Perioperative management of selected problems in patients with rheumatic diseases. *Rheum. Dis. Clin. North Am.* 1999; **25**: 623–638.

2. Schafer, A. I. Effects of nonsteroidal antiinflammatory drugs on platelet function and systemic hemostasis. *J. Clin. Pharmacol.* 1995; **35**: 209–219.

3. Lind, S. E. The bleeding time does not predict surgical bleeding. *Blood* 1991; **77**: 2547–2551.

4. Gewirtz, A. S., Miller, M. L., & Keys, T. F. The clinical usefulness of the preoperative bleeding time. *Arch. Pathol. Lab. Med.* 1996; **120**: 353–356.

5. Connelly, C. S. & Panush, R. S. Should nonsteroidal antiinflammatory drugs be stopped before elective surgery? *Arch. Intern. Med.* 1991; **151**: 1963–1966.

6. Bashein, G., Nessly, M. L., Rice, A. L. *et al.* Preoperative aspirin therapy and reoperation for bleeding after coronary artery bypass surgery. *Arch. Intern. Med.* 1991; **151**: 89–93.

7. An, H. S., Mikhail, W. E., Jackson, W. T. *et al.* Effects of hypotensive anesthesia, nonsteroidal antiinflammatory drugs, and polymethylmethacrylate on bleeding in total hip arthroplasty patients. *J. Arthroplasty* 1991; **6**: 245–250.

8. Robinson, C. M., Christie, J., & Malcolm-Smith, N. Nonsteroidal antiinflammatory drugs, perioperative blood loss, and transfusion requirements in elective hip arthroplasty. *J. Arthroplasty* 1993; **8**: 607–610.

9. Hench, P. S., Kendall, E. C., Slocumb, C. H. *et al.* The effect of a hormone of the adrenal cortex (17-hydroxy-11-dehydrocorticosterone; compound E) and of the pituitary adrenocorticotrophic hormone on rheumatoid arthritis. *Proc. Staff. Meet. Mayo Clin.* 1949; **24**: 181.

10. Coursin, D. B. & Wood, K. E. Corticosteroid supplementation for adrenal insufficiency. *J. Am. Med. Assoc.* 2002; **287**: 236–240.

11. Esteban, N. V., Loughlin, T., Yergey, A. *et al.* Daily cortisol production in man determined by stable isotope dilution/mass spectrometry. *J. Clin. Endocrinol. Metab.* 1991; **72**: 39–45.

12. Krasner, A. S. Glucocorticoid-induced adrenal insufficiency. *J. Am. Med. Assoc.* 1999; **282**: 671–676.

13. Lamberts, S. W. J., Bruining, H. A., & DeJong, F. H. Corticosteroid therapy in severe illness. *N. Engl. J. Med.* 1997; **337**: 1285–1292.

14. Munck, A., Guyre, P. M., & Holbrook, N. J. Physiological fractures of glucocorticoids in stress and their relation to pharmacological actions. *Endocr. Rev.* 1984; **5**: 25–44.

15. Fraser, C. G., Preuss, F. S., & Bigford, W. D. Adrenal atrophy and irreversible shock associated with cortisone therapy. *J. Am. Med. Assoc.* 1952; **149**: 1542–1543.

16. Lewis, L., Robinson, R. F., Yee, J. *et al.* Fatal adrenal cortical insufficiency precipitated by surgery during prolonged continuous cortisone infusion. *Ann. Intern. Med.* 1953; **39**: 116–125.

17. Graber, A. L., Ney, R. L., Nicholson, W. E. *et al.* Natural history of pituitary–adrenal recovery following long-term suppression with corticosteroids. *J. Clin. Endocrinol. Metab.* 1965; **25**: 11–16.

18. Axelrod, L. Corticosteroid therapy. *Medicine* 1976; **55**: 39–65.

19. Treadwell, B. L. J., Savage, O., Sever, E. D. *et al.* Pituitary–adrenal function during corticosteroid therapy. *Lancet* 1963; **1**: 355–358.

20. Jasani, M. K., Boyle, J. A., Greig, W. R. *et al.* Corticosteroid-induced suppression of the hypothalamo-pituitary-adrenal axis: observations on patients given oral corticosteroids for rheumatoid arthritis. *Quast. J. Med.* 1967; **143**: 261–276.

21. Meakin, J. W., Tantongco, M. S., Crabbe, J. *et al.* Pituitary–adrenal function following long-term steroid therapy. *Am. J. Med.* 1960; **29**: 459–464.

22. Streck, W. F. & Lockwood, D. H. Pituitary adrenal recovery following short-term suppression with corticosteroids. *Am. J. Med.* 1979; **66**: 910–914.

23. LaRochelle, G. E., LaRochelle, A. G., Ratner, R. E. *et al.* Recovery of the hypothalamic–pituitary–adrenal axis in patients with rheumatic diseases receiving low-dose prednisone. *Am. J. Med.* 1993; **326**: 258–264.

24. Salem, M., Tainsh, R. E., Bromberg, J. *et al.* Perioperative glucocorticoid coverage: a reassessment 42 years after emergence of a problem. *Ann. Surg.* 1994; **219**: 416–425.

25. Streck, W. F. & Lockwood, D. W. Pituitary adrenal recovery following short-term suppression with corticosteroids. *Am. J. Med.* 1979; **66**: 910–914.

26. Kremer, J. M. Rational use of new and existing disease-modifying agents in rheumatoid arthritis. *Ann. Intern. Med.* 2001; **134**: 695–706.

27. Bridges, S. L. Jr. & Moreland, L. W. Perioperative use of methotrexate in patients with rheumatoid arthritis undergoing orthopedic surgery. *Rheum. Dis. Clin. North Am.* 1997; **23**: 981–993.

28. Bridges, S. L., Jr., Lopez-Mendez, A., Han, K. H. *et al.* Should methotrexate be discontinued before elective orthopedic

surgery in patients with rheumatoid arthritis? *J. Rheumatol.* 1991; **18**: 984.

29. Perhala, R. S., Wilke, W. S., Clough, J. D. *et al.* Local infectious complications following knee joint replacement in rheumatoid arthritis patients treated with methotrexate versus those not treated with methotrexate. *Arthritis Rheum.* 1991; **34**: 146.

30. Kasdan, M. L. & June, L. Postoperative results of rheumatoid arthritis patients on methotrexate at the time of reconstructive surgery of the hand. *Orthopedics* 1993; **16**: 1233.

31. Sany, J., Anaya, J. M., Canovas, F. *et al.* Influence of methotrexate on the frequency of postoperative infectious complications in patients with rheumatoid arthritis. *J. Rheumatol.* 1993; **20**: 1129.

32. Alarcon, G. S., Moreland, L. W., Jaffe, K. *et al.* The use of methotrexate perioperatively in patients with rheumatoid arthritis undergoing major joint replacement surgery: Will we ever have a consensus about its use? *J. Clin. Rheumatol.* 1996; **2**: 86.

33. Grennan, D. M., Gray, J., Loudon, J. *et al.* Methotrexate and early postoperative complications in patients with rheumatoid arthritis undergoing elective orthopedic surgery. *Ann. Rheum. Dis.* 2001; **60**: 214–217.

34. Howland, W. L. Methotrexate-associated bone marrow suppression following surgery. *Arthritis Rheum.* 1988; **31**: 1586–1587.

35. Buchbinder, R., Hall, S., Harkness, A. *et al.* Severe bone marrow failure due to low dose methotrexate. *J. Rheumatol.* 1988; **15**: 1586–1588.

36. Gutierrez-Urena, S., Molina, J. F., Garcia, C. O. *et al.* Pancytopenia secondary to methotrexate therapy in rheumatoid arthritis. *Arthritis Rheum.* 1996; **39**: 272–276.

37. Wluka, A. E., Buchbinder, R., Mylvaganam, A. *et al.* Long-term community based methotrexate use in rheumatoid arthritis: 12 year follow up of 460 patients. *J. Rheumatol.* 2000; **27**: 1864–1871.

38. Consensus Development Conference: Prophylaxis and treatment of osteoporosis. *Osteoporos Int.* 1991; **1**: 114–117.

39. Hawker, G. A. The epidemiology of osteoporosis. *J. Rheumatol.* 1996; **23** Suppl. 45: 2–5.

40. Smith, M. D., Ross, W., & Ahern, M. J. Missing a therapeutic window of opportunity: an audit of patients attending a tertiary teaching hospital with potentially osteoporotic hip and wrist fractures. *J. Rheumatol.* 2001; **28**: 2504–2508.

41. Ross, P. D., Davis, J. W., Epstein, R. S. *et al.* Pre-existing fractures and bone mass predict fracture incidence in women. *N. Engl. J. Med.* 1995; **332**: 767–773.

42. Owen, R. A., Melton, L. J., III, Ilstrup, D. M. *et al.* Colles' fracture and subsequent hip fracture risk. *Clin. Orthop. Relat. Res.* 1982; **171**: 37–43.

43. Mallmin, H., Ljunghall, S., Persson, I. *et al.* Fracture of the distal forearm as a forecaster of subsequent hip fracture: a population-based cohort study with 24 years of follow-up. *Calcif. Tissue Int.* 1993; **52**: 269–272.

44. Khan, S. A., deGeus, C., Holroyd, B. *et al.* Osteoporosis follow-up after wrist fractures following minor trauma. *Arch. Intern. Med.* 2001; **161**: 1309–1312.

45. Freedman, K. B., Kaplan, F. S., Bilder, W. B. *et al.* Treatment of osteoporosis: are physicians missing an opportunity? *J. Bone Joint Surg.* 2000; **82-A**: 1063–1070.

46. Broy, S. B., Bohren, A., Harrington, T. *et al.* Are physicians treating osteoporosis after hip fracture? *Arthritis Rheum.* 2000; **43**: S203.

47. Wortmann, R. L. & Kelley, W. N. Gout and hyperuricemia. In Ruddy, S., Harris, E. D. Jr., & Sledge, C. B., eds. *Kelley's Textbook of Rheumatology*, 6th edn. Philadelphia: W. B. Saunders, 2001: 1339–1376.

48. Reginato, A. J. & Reginato, A. M. Diseases associated with deposition of calcium pyrophosphate or hydroxyapatite. In Ruddy, S., Harris, E. D., Jr., & Sledge, C. B. eds. *Kelley's Textbook of Rheumatology*, 6th edn. Philadelphia: W. B. Saunders, 2001: 1377–1390.

49. Ho, G. Jr. Gout and pseudogout in hospitalized patients. *Arch. Intern. Med.* 1993; **153**: 2787–2790.

50. Berger, R. G. Febrile presentation of calcium pyrophosphate dihydrate deposition disease. *J. Rheumatol.* 1988; **15**: 642–643.

51. Mavrikakis, M. E. CPPD crystal deposition disease as a cause of unrecognized pyrexia. *Clin. Exp. Rheumatol.* 1994; **12**: 419–422.

52. Roberts W. N., Liang M. H., Stern S. H. Colchicine in acute gout: reassessment of risk and benefits. *J. Am. Med. Assoc.* 1987; **257**: 1920–1922.

53. Emmerson, B. T. The management of gout. *N. Engl. J. Med.* 1996; **334**: 445–451.

54. Axelrod, D. & Preston, S. Comparison of parenteral adrenocorticotrophic hormone with oral indomethacin in the treatment of acute gout. *Arthritis Rheum.* 1988; **31**: 803–805.

55. Van Everdingen, A. A., Jacobs, J. W. G., van Reesema, D. R. S. *et al.* Low dose prednisone therapy for patients with early active rheumatoid arthritis: clinical efficacy, disease-modifying properties, and side effects. *Ann. Intern. Med.* 2002; **136**: 1012.

56. Conn, D. L. Resolved: Low-dose prednisone is indicated as standard treatment in patients with rheumatoid arthritis. *Arthritis Rheum. (Arthritis Care Res.)* 2001; **45**: 462–467.

57. Zonana-Nacach, A., Barr, S. G., Magder, L. S. *et al.* Damage in systemic lupus erythematosus and its association with corticosteroids. *Arthritis Rheum.* 2000; **43**: 1801–1808.

58. Gurley, J. P. & Bell, G. R. The surgical management of patients with rheumatoid cervical spine disease. *Rheum. Dis. Clin. North Am.* 1997; **23**: 317–332.

59. Conlon, P. W., Isdale, I. C. & Rose, B. S. Rheumatoid arthritis of the cervical spine. An analysis of 333 cases. *Ann. Rheum. Dis.* 1966; **25**: 120–126.

60. Eulderink, F. & Meijers, K. A. E. Pathology of the cervical spine in rheumatoid arthritis. A controlled study of 44 spines. *J. Pathol.* 1976; **120**: 91–108.

61. Pellicci, D. M., Ranawat, C. S., Tsairis, P. *et al.* A prospective study of the progression of rheumatoid arthritis of the cervical spine. *J. Bone Joint Surg. Am.* 1981; **63**: 342–350.

62. Rana, N. A. Natural history of atlantoaxial subluxation in rheumatoid arthritis. *Spine* 1989; **14**: 1054–1056.

63. Smith, P. H., Benn, R. & Sharp, J. Natural history of rheumatoid cervical subluxations. *Ann. Rheum. Dis.* 1972; **31**: 431–439.

64. Komusi, T., Munro, T. & Harth, M. Radiologic review: the rheumatoid cervical spine. *Semin. Arthritis Rheum.* 1985; **14**: 187–195.

65. Crosby, E. T. The adult cervical spine: implications for airway management. *Can. J. Anaesth.* 1990; **37**: 77–93.

66. Harris, E. D. Jr. Clinical features of rheumatoid arthritis. In Ruddy, S., Harris, E. D. Jr., & Sledge, C. B., eds. *Kelley's Textbook of Rheumatology*, 6th edn. Philadelphia: W. B. Saunders, 2001: 967–1000.

67. Vasculitis. In Klippel, J. H. & Dieppe, P. A., eds. *Rheumatology*, 2nd edn. Volume 2. London: Mosby, 1998, Section 7: Chapters 17–31.

Neurology

32

Cerebrovascular disease

Michael R. Frankel[1] and Duncan Borland[2]

[1]Emory University School of Medicine, Atlanta, GA
[2]Portland, OR

Stroke affects about 750 000 people each year in the USA and is a leading cause of long-term adult disability. Over the past decade there have been considerable advances in treatment and prevention. This chapter will review many of these advances with emphasis on issues relevant to surgical patients.

There are two types of stroke: ischemic and hemorrhagic. Ischemic events account for about 80% of all strokes.[2] Most of these are related to atherothromboembolic events.

Atherosclerosis is a systemic disease that most prominently affects the aorta, the coronary arteries, the extracranial carotid and vertebral arteries, and the arteries to the extremities.[3] Atherosclerosis causes stroke by producing progressive stenosis, local thrombosis with occlusion, or distal embolization. Any one of these mechanisms can be the primary cause. For example, progressive atherosclerotic occlusion can cause distal hypoperfusion severe enough to result in tissue ischemia and infarction. Mild or moderate atherosclerotic stenosis that does not cause distal hypoperfusion can be the site of thrombosis and cause intra-arterial embolization leading to occlusion of an intracerebral artery downstream.

The relative significance of local thrombosis versus intra-arterial embolization varies according to the site of atherosclerosis. Most strokes resulting from stenosis of the proximal internal carotid artery are caused by distal embolic occlusion of the middle cerebral artery or its branches. Cerebral infarction in the basilar artery territory usually results from occlusion of the small perforating vessels by local thrombosis.

Ischemic strokes are divided into several categories including cardioembolic, lacunar, and atherosclerotic etiologies. Each of these subtypes accounts for about 25% of ischemic stroke, with the remaining 25% being of undetermined cause. Unusual causes (e.g., arterial disection, hypercoagulability, septic emboli, venous infarction) comprise about 5% of cases. Hemorrhagic causes include intracerebral hemorrhage or hematoma (ICH) and aneurysmal subarachnoid hemorrhage (SAH), the former occurring about twice as often as the latter. Hemorrhagic infarction is a term reserved for cerebral infarcts which become hemorrhagic when perfusion to the ischemic area is restored. The hemorrhage is usually petechial and asymptomatic.

Transient symptoms often precede an ischemic stroke. Patients with a stroke due to atherosclerotic disease will have a history of a TIA 50% of the time, whereas those with lacunar stroke or cardioembolism have a neurological warning only 25% and 5% of the time, respectively. The vast majority of TIAs last less than 15 minutes although they can last for hours.[1] Urgent evaluation of patients with TIAs is essential to identify the cause and institute stroke preventive therapy (e.g., carotid endarterectomy, anticoagulation, or antiplatelet therapy).

Recognition of the warning leak (also called the sentinel hemorrhage) of aneurysmal SAH is extremely important. It is estimated that this occurs 25% to 50% of the time in the few days or weeks preceding a fulminant bleed.[2] The warning leak causes a sudden severe headache, unlike previous headaches, often without neurologic signs. Because symptoms usually resolve spontaneously or with simple analgesic medication they may not be evaluated for the presence of SAH. Once again, prompt recognition and urgent evaluation are essential. Unlike SAH and ischemic stroke, ICH almost always occurs without warning. However, the majority of patients with ICH have a history of hypertension and many have severely elevated blood pressure on presentation suggesting the precipitous cause.

Stroke symptoms

Stroke symptoms are usually sudden and vary based on the location of damage. Common symptoms include weakness (hemiparesis), numbness (hemi-sensory loss), difficulty speaking (dysarthria or aphasia), change in vision (monocular, hemianopia or diplopia), problems with balance (difficulty walking or vertigo), and headache. Other important findings on examination include neglect (lack of awareness of weakness) and gaze preference. Common syndromes occur as a result of specific sites of arterial occlusion. For example, middle cerebral occlusion produces contralateral hemiplegia and gaze preference towards the side of the brain lesion. In right-handed patients (and even most left-handers), left-sided brain injury is often accompanied by aphasia while right sided strokes produce neglect. Signs of basilar artery occlusion include quadriparesis, paralysis of horizontal gaze, and pupilary abnormalities.

Diagnostic tests

The most important part of the evaluation of the patient with suspected stroke is the history and physical exam. Family members, nursing staff, and eyewitness accounts of the onset of symptoms and baseline cognitive and physical function are critical. The examination should focus on recognizable patterns of cerebral dysfunction to aid in localization of the suspected pathology. Causes of ischemic stroke in the anterior circulation (internal carotid artery distribution) differ from those in the posterior circulation (vertebral artery or basilar artery distribution). Vascular imaging studies are much more relevant when the exact location of cerebral infarction is known. Cerebral imaging is necessary to confirm clinical findings. Non-contrast computed tomography (CT) remains the test of choice in the acute setting. It is very sensitive to the presence of hemorrhage. However, patients with ischemic stroke may have normal CT imaging in the first few hours. Magnetic resonance imaging (MRI), and especially the sequence called diffusion weighted imaging (DWI), is more sensitive to focal ischemia. Vascular imaging can help guide therapeutic plans. MR or CT angiography and ultrasound are reliable and relatively non-invasive methods for assessing the cerebral circulation. These studies may reveal sites of occlusive disease or even provide reasonable evidence of the pathophysiology, e.g., atherosclerotic stenosis vs. arterial dissection. Conventional cerebral angiography may be needed to further define the underlying abnormality. Echocardiography is appropriate when cardiac or aortic arch evaluation is necessary. When subarachnoid hemorrhage is suspected (for example, a patient with sudden severe headache), CT imaging will not show blood in about 5%–10% of patients. Lumbar puncture is needed in these patients to evaluate for xanthochromia.

Mechanisms specific to surgical intervention

Surgery and anesthesia may contribute to stroke by several mechanisms. Hypotension resulting from hemorrhage, fluid loss, or anesthetic agents may cause cerebral ischemia. Patients who do not have hypertension or cerebrovascular disease maintain cerebral blood flow at a constant level until cerebral perfusion pressure reaches a mean of 60 mm Hg.[4] This perfusion pressure is the lower level of autoregulation. Chronic hypertension raises this lower limit so that decreases in cerebral blood flow occur at higher mean arterial blood pressures. Arterial occlusive disease also affects tolerance to hypotension. This effect is highly variable and depends on the adequacy of the collateral supply distal to the site of occlusion.[4] Flow across a region of stenosis varies directly with the pressure difference. Therefore, a decrease in pressure proximal to the stenosis requires a decrease in pressure distally to maintain the same perfusion pressure. This is accomplished by decreasing the resistance to flow distally by dilating resistance vessels. If resistance vessels are already maximally dilated, there is no means of decreasing resistance further and the pressure difference decreases, as does the flow.[5] This concept is called hemodynamic reserve. Although this can be evaluated before surgery by several methods, including xenon cerebral blood flow, transcranial Doppler, and EEG the usefulness of such data remains unclear.[6,7] In summary, hypotension increases the risk of brain injury in all patients but particularly in those with atherosclerosis and a history of hypertension.

Dislodged thrombus, fragments of plaque or cholesterol crystals may result in distal embolization and occlusion. This can occur during angiography or intraoperatively with manipulation of vascular structures (i.e., during clamping of the carotid artery or aorta). Intraoperative ultrasound and transesophageal echocardiography can demonstrate extensive atherosclerosis and thrombus in the aortic arch, which likely serves as a source of embolism.[8–11] Aortic manipulation and cross clamping are probably a common cause of perioperative stroke.[12] Marshall and colleagues have suggested that intraoperative ultrasound of the aorta allows the surgeon to modify cannulation and operative techniques, and thereby reduce the risk of perioperative stroke.[13]

Cardiopulmonary bypass plays a definite role in the postoperative encephalopathy that may be seen after coronary artery bypass grafting (CABG), although the mechanism is not well understood.[14] This encephalopathy is a state of general mental slowing, particularly in the frontal lobe functions of planning, concentration, shifting set, and choice reaction time. Microemboli consisting of gas bubbles and particulate matter generated from aortic cannulation appear to have a significant role in causing this disorder.[15] In a study involving 312 CABG patients, 24% of patients experienced moderate to severe intellectual impairment following surgery.[14] A matched control group undergoing comparable vascular surgeries without bypass had no intellectual dysfunction. Some of this decrement is long lasting. Advanced age also increases the risk for loss of cognitive function. The number of microemboli detected by transcranial Doppler during surgery appears to correlate with the neuropsychologic outcome.[16] Increasing age, history of stroke, hypertension, diabetes, and the presence of a carotid bruit predict the development of encephalopathy.[17]

Perioperative stroke risk

Physicians are often asked to assess risk in patients awaiting surgery. Guidelines[1] have been published to assist in cardiac evaluation but a similar source for cerebrovascular risk assessment is lacking. This section addresses some of the important issues in surgical patients at risk for stroke due to atherosclerosis.

Several studies have examined the risk of stroke in patients undergoing major vascular[9,18-22] and minor nonvascular surgical procedures.[3] Surgery and anesthesia may contribute to stroke by several mechanisms. Hypotension resulting from hemorrhage, fluid loss, or anesthetic agents may cause cerebral ischemia. Dislodged thrombus, fragments of plaque or cholesterol crystals may result in distal embolization and occlusion. This can occur during angiography or intraoperatively with manipulation of vascular structures (i.e., during clamping of the carotid artery or aorta).

Specific risk factors that contribute to perioperative stroke include female gender,[32] hypertension,[17,23] smoking,[23] prior stroke,[17,26,29,31,32] abnormal cardiac rhythm,[23] peripheral vascular disease,[26,31] aortic atherosclerosis,[29] chronic obstructive pulmonary disease,[26,32] age,[17,29,31] unstable angina,[31] elevated creatinine,[31] diminished ejection fraction,[32] diabetes,[34] perioperative hypotension,[29,30] and protracted cardiopulmonary bypass time.[29,23]

Although some studies have shown an association between perioperative stroke and the presence of carotid disease,[19,32] many have not. In a prospective study, Ropper and colleagues identified carotid bruits preoperatively in 104 of 735 (14%) patients scheduled for elective surgery.[24] The overall stroke rate was 0.7% (all in CABG patients) and no correlation with the presence of carotid bruits was

identified. A search of ultrasound records for a ten year period at the Mayo Clinic found 284 patients who subsequently underwent general surgery within the year.[27] In this cohort there were 224 patients with a carotid stenosis of 50% or more and 8 (3.6%) suffered a perioperative stroke. Furlan and Cracium found that asymptomatic unilateral internal carotid artery stenosis less than 90%, or internal carotid artery occlusion, did not increase the risk of stroke during CABG.[21] Von Reutern and colleagues monitored middle cerebral artery velocities with transcranial Doppler during CABG in patients with severe carotid stenosis or occlusion and found no change in velocities compared with patients without carotid stenosis.[18] Hise and colleagues reviewed computed tomographic scans and angiographic results in patients who had strokes related to CABG and concluded that "the main mechanism of injury was cerebral embolization rather than cerebral hypoperfusion."[28] A significant number of these patients had evidence of multiple emboli, suggesting a cardiac or aortic source. Moody and colleagues looked at neuropathologic material and found focal arteriolar and capillary dilation as well as evidence of birefringence suggesting the previous presence of air or fat emboli in four of five patients after CABG.[15] Based on this evidence, there does not appear to be an indication for carotid endarterectomy in asymptomatic patients with carotid stenosis before cardiac surgery.

As mentioned, previous stroke has been linked to perioperative risk. A retrospective review of patients with histories of recent or remote strokes receiving open heart surgery compared the incidence of perioperative stroke in these two groups.[30] A recent stroke was defined as one that occurred less than three months before open heart surgery. There was no significant difference in new stroke rates between patients with recent and remote strokes. There was a suggestion that patients with recent strokes were more susceptible to perioperative hypotension.

Data were collected prospectively on 2711 patients undergoing CABG by McKhann and colleagues.[17] All postoperative patients suspected of having suffered a stroke were examined by a neurologist and most underwent CT or MRI. Strokes occurred in 72 patients (2.7%). Prior stroke (OR = 2.11; 95% CI, 1.05–4.23; $P = 0.04$), hypertension (OR = 1.97; 95% CI, 1.05–3.69; $P = 0.04$), and age were identified by logistic regression analysis as significant predictors of stroke during CABG. The authors constructed useful flowcharts that provide probabilities for the development of stroke and encephalopathy in CABG candidates. For example, a patient over the age of 75 with a history of hypertension has a 7% chance of having a stroke related to CABG whereas a similar patient with a history of stroke has almost double this risk (13%).[17]

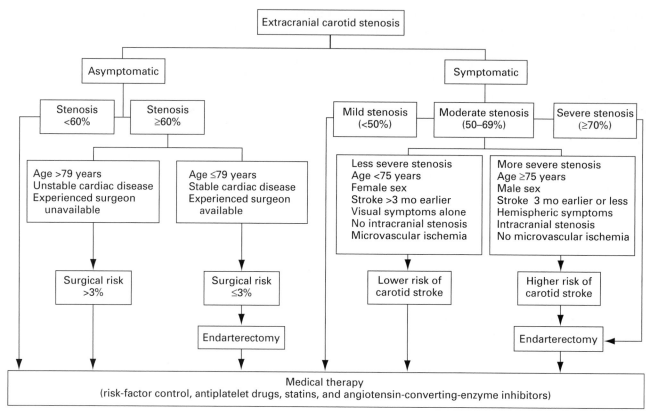

Fig. 32.1. From ref 48.

Carotid endarterectomy

The North American Symptomatic Carotid Endarterectomy Trial (NASCET) was a landmark study establishing the benefit of surgery for symptomatic patients with carotid stenosis greater than 70%.[37] Similar findings were found in the European Carotid Surgery Trial.[38] The Asymptomatic Carotid Atherosclerosis Study (ACAS), demonstrated that selected patients with asymptomatic carotid stenosis of 60% or more would benefit from surgery if the incidence of any stroke and death resulting from angiography and surgery was kept below 3%.[40] This caveat is not so easily achieved as mortality and morbidity vary from 1.8% to 4.7% (or more) depending on patient selection,[41] the surgeon[41,42] and the institution.[43] In ACAS, with a perioperative adverse event rate of 2.3%, the relative risk reduction obtained from surgery over a 5-year period was 53% and the absolute risk reduction was 5.5% when compared with medical treatment alone.

Since the publication of the AHA "Guidelines for Carotid Endarterectomy" the second phase of NASCET has been completed.[44] This study examined the relative merits of medical versus surgical treatment of patients with symptomatic moderate carotid stenoses of 50% to 69%. The five year risk of any ipsilateral stroke was 22.2% in the medical group and 15.7% in the surgical group. An absolute risk reduction of 6.5% ($P = 0.045$) translates into a number needed to treat of 15. The 5-year risk of any stroke or death was 43.3% in the medical group and 33.2% in the surgical group reflecting a significant benefit in those receiving endarterectomy. Gorelick[47] and Sacco[48] have provided detailed reviews of the data surrounding treatment of carotid disease. An algorithm for the management of extracranial carotid stenosis is provided by Sacco (Fig. 32.1). Initial data appears promising for carotid angioplasty and stenting as an alternative to endarterectomy. However, before this new approach can be routinely recommended, the relative risk and long-term benefit need to be defined in ongoing clinical trials.

Prevention and management of perioperative stroke

Patients should be screened before surgery for history of stroke and stroke risk factors such as hypertension, peripheral vascular disease, and coronary artery disease. Because atherosclerosis is a systemic disease, carotid atherosclerosis and coronary artery disease frequently coexist.[3] Myocardial infarction is a major cause of mortality in patients with stroke. All patients with histories of TIA or stroke should be screened before surgery with a thorough history and electrocardiogram looking for cardiac disease. The indications for carotid endarterectomy were outlined earlier.

Perioperative medical therapy does not differ substantially from good routine care except for extra care to prevent hypotension. However, in patients undergoing endarterectomy, careful control of hypertension intraoperatively and post-operatively is necessary to prevent reperfusion injury. In patients with high grade carotid stenosis and especially those with recent cerebral infarction, hypertension after endarterectomy can induce cerebral hemorrhage. Controlling hypertension in this setting may reduce the chance of this complication.

Despite early evidence from small studies, patients with acute ischemic stroke do not appear to benefit from immediate anticoagulation.[84] Two large studies have shown that anticoagulation after acute ischemic stroke does not provide significant benefit.[85,86] Furthermore, even in the high-risk condition of atrial fibrillation, there is no clear benefit of immediate anticoagulation in patients with acute ischemic stroke.[87] Yet controversy remains as proponents continue to emphasize that anticoagulation may be beneficial in certain subsets of patients such as those with cardiac embolism, unstable cerebral ischemia or extracranial carotid or vertebral dissection. National guidelines from the American College of Chest Physicians have indicated that anticoagulation is an acceptable treatment in these high-risk patients but that evidence of benefit is lacking.[49] More recent consensus guidelines on anticoagulation state that early anticoagulation after acute ischemic stroke cannot be recommended for any subgroup because data is insufficient.[87]

The benefit of intravenous administration of recombinant tissue plasminogen activator (rt-PA) in carefully selected patients with acute ischemic infarction was demonstrated in an NIH sponsored study leading to the FDA approval for this indication in 1996.[57] The benefit of intra-arterial thrombolysis was seen in the PROACT II study[58] and is supported by consensus opinion for selected patients although not approved by the FDA.[49] Because of the potential for serious bleeding, recent major surgery is a contraindication to intravenous rt-PA. However, intra-arterial thrombolysis may be an option for some patients with cerebral embolism in the perioperative period.[59] In a recent report, intra-arterial thrombolysis

was given to 6 patients with acute ischemic stroke within as few as 2 days of cardiac surgery. No clinically significant bleeding complications occurred.[59]

Communication, swallowing and mobility concerns need to be addressed in all patients. Range of motion exercises, splints, communication devices, and extra care to prevent bedsores all must be taken into consideration in patients with stroke and limited mobility.

The prevention of deep venous thrombosis and pulmonary embolus is an important concern after almost any major surgery. When patients are hemiplegic, the risk of embolic complications is even greater. Prophylaxis for deep venous thrombosis should be initiated in all patients with stroke who are not ambulatory. This usually consists of the administration of 5000 U of subcutaneous heparin every 12 hours, the application of compression stockings, and the institution of early mobilization for gait training.[52]

Bowel and bladder continence play a major role in quality of life for patients with strokes. These concerns must be addressed during postoperative care. Timed voiding and elimination are the main tools for retraining. Medications should be chosen with their autonomic side effects in mind.

Seizures may occur in patients after stroke.[60] In general, prophylaxis with antiepileptic medication is not used in patients with stroke. These drugs are given only to patients who have had at least one seizure. Patients with histories of seizures who are receiving antiepileptic medications must maintain adequate blood levels in the postoperative setting, when seizures could have serious consequences. Changes in kidney, liver, and heart function can affect the metabolism, protein binding, and volume of distribution of anticonvulsants. The use of various concomitant medications can also have an effect on the efficacy and toxicity of anticonvulsants during the perioperative period.

Medical therapy for stroke prevention

Patients with ischemic stroke are at risk for vascular events (myocardial infarction, stroke, vascular death). Patients with a history of stroke should be identified and appropriate long-term control of risk factors to prevent vascular events should be initiated or considered prior to discharge. The most important aspects include smoking cessation counseling, treatment of hypertension, treatment of hyperlipidemia, diabetic control, and antithrombotic therapy. Several of these will be addressed.

Antiplatelet therapy reduces the risk of recurrent vascular events in patients with recent ischemic stroke or TIA.

Currently available oral preparations that have been shown to be effective in clinical trials of patients with ischemic stroke and/or TIA include aspirin, clopidogrel, extended release dipyramidole with aspirin, and ticlopidine. All are effective in preventing recurrent vascular events in patients who have had an ischemic stroke.

Aspirin is a cost-effective method of stroke prevention for most patients, although the optimal effective dose remains unclear. In 1998, the FDA provided a statement recommending doses between 50 mg and 325 mg to prevent recurrent stroke.[49] After endarterectomy, doses between 81 mg and 325 mg have been shown to be more effective than higher doses.[75]

Are the newer antiplatelet medications better than aspirin? To answer this question, each clinical trial must be reviewed with close attention to the entry criteria and predefined primary endpoint. Although the benefit of ticlopidine over 1300 mg of aspirin for reducing stroke risk in patients with recent ischemic stroke or TIA was reported, there was no effect on stroke-free survival.[76] In the CAPRIE trial, approximately 20 000 patients with recent ischemic stroke, myocardial infarction, or peripheral arterial disease were randomized to receive clopidogrel or 325 mg of aspirin.[77] For the primary endpoint of MI, stroke or vascular death, clopidogrel was more effective than aspirin but the relative benefit (9%) and absolute benefit (0.5%) was small. In the ESPS-2 trial, patients with recent ischemic stroke or TIA were studied using combination therapy with extended-release dipyramidole and 50 mg of Aspirin.[78] The combination therapy was shown to be more effective in preventing stroke than low dose aspirin. However, the combination therapy was not more effective in preventing the primary endpoint of stroke or death. Although combining aspirin with clopidogrel is effective after acute non-Q wave myocardial infarction,[79] there are no data in patients with recent stroke. Ongoing clinical trials are examining this issue. Since all of the above studies had different entry criteria, primary endpoints and doses of aspirin, it is difficult to clearly determine which regimen is the most effective. Therefore, cost, tolerability, and once daily dosing make aspirin a logical choice for initial therapy. For patients who have recurrent events on aspirin, combination antiplatelet therapy is a consideration.

The risk of serious bleeding is low with all of the antiplatelet preparations. The more common but minor side effects may limit compliance. Aspirin containing preparations can cause dyspepsia, especially at the higher doses. Aspirin can also cause gastrointestinal (GI) bleeding.[49] Dipyramidole containing preparations cause headache in some patients.[78] Clopidogrel appears to have fewer side effects compared with ticlopidine and is preferred over ticlopidine for this reason.[77] Ticlopidine causes neutropenia in about 2% of patients and requires blood monitoring every 2 weeks during the first 3 months of therapy.[49] Combining clopidogrel with aspirin increases the risk of serious GI bleeding by about 1%.[79]

The relative benefit of warfarin vs. aspirin differs depending on stroke subtype. Warfarin is clearly more effective in patients with certain cardiac conditions like atrial fibrillation (INR 2.0–3.0); however, it is no better than aspirin in patients without a cardiac source of embolism.[49] The Warfarin Aspirin Recurrent Stroke Study (WARSS) showed that aspirin (325 mg) and warfarin (INR 1.4–2.8) have equivalent effects in patients with ischemic stroke or TIA without a cardioembolic source.[80] Further, predefined substudies of patients within WARSS did not show benefit. For example, patients with a patent foramen ovale or those with anti-phospholipid antibodies did not benefit from warfarin over aspirin therapy.[81,82] Still, there may be higher-risk conditions that have not been adequately studied that may benefit from warfarin such as low ejection fraction, symptomatic intracranial stenosis, or severe proximal aortic arch disease. Each of these is currently being studied in separate clinical trials.

There has been some uncertainty expressed about the results of WARSS due to the lower range of INR values used in the study. Critics have argued that the design of the trial did not test the range most commonly used (INR 2.0–3.0). But if the lower anticoagulation intensity limited the effectiveness of warfarin, there should have been a relationship between the INR value and the risk of recurrent stroke. No such relationship was found, suggesting that the reason for the lack of benefit of warfarin was not due to the range of INR values chosen. Thus, this landmark trial shows that indiscriminate use of warfarin for all patients with ischemic stroke or TIA should be avoided. Careful consideration of the underlying etiology is required.

Transient interruption of anticoagulants is often necessary perioperatively. Recent recommendations have been published for the perioperative management of patients who are currently taking oral anticoagulants.[68] For patients with conditions that require lifelong therapy with oral anticoagulants to prevent cerebral embolism (e.g., atrial fibrillation), transient interruption in therapy may be necessary when surgery is indicated. The risk of embolism during this period is relatively low (0.3%–3.0%) and dependent on the duration of withholding anticoagulation and associated risk factors.[69] For patients with vascular risk factors, early postprocedure anticoagulation with heparin or low molecular weight heparin may be warranted when deemed safe from the surgical perspective.[68]

Statin medications were designed to limit atherosclerosis but also appear to have additional beneficial effects by promoting plaque stabilization, providing an anti-inflammatory effect (decreased CRP) and reducing the risk of thrombosis.[73] The Heart Prevention Study recently published the results of approximately 20 000 high-risk patients.[74] The subset of patients with prior cerebrovascular disease and no coronary heart disease benefited from therapy with simvastatin. Based on the results of this study and other studies of statin medications in patients at risk for vascular events, statins should be considered in all ischemic stroke and TIA patients who have LDL levels higher than 130 and possibly those higher than 100. Targeting an LDL level of less than 100 would be an acceptable but unproven approach in patients who have had an ischemic stroke or TIA.

A number of large multicenter, randomized, prospective studies have provided evidence of reduced long term risk of cardiovascular morbidity and mortality including stroke in patients receiving antihypertensive and lipid lowering agents.[61–63] A review of randomized trials of antihypertensive medications by the Blood Pressure Lowering Treatment Trialists' Collaboration published in 2000 found no strong evidence to suggest that any particular drug or class of drugs was more beneficial in preventing stroke.[64] In a review appearing in *J. Am. Med. Assoc.* in 2002 a similar conclusion was reached. In one of the few trials comparing medications head to head, losartan, a selective angiotensin-II type 1-receptor antagonist, produced a greater reduction in stroke incidence than atenolol.[63]

Patients with prior MI and cholesterol levels <240 mg/dl treated with pravastatin experienced a 31% risk reduction in stroke compared with placebo.[65] The Long-Term Intervention with Pravastatin in Ischemic Disease study (LIPID) compared pravastatin to placebo in 9014 patients with a history of MI or unstable angina and a total cholesterol level of 155 to 271. Over 6 years, the incidence of stroke in those treated with pravastatin was 4.5% vs. 3.7% in placebo-treated patients.[66] Recommendations for the treatment of hyperlipidemia in patients with cerebrovascular disease can be found in the National Cholesterol Education Program guidelines and are no different than for those with cardiovascular disease.[67]

Angiotensin-converting enzyme inhibitor medications (ACE-I) were designed to treat hypertension. However, they appear to have beneficial effects beyond blood pressure control. These effects include antiatherogenesis, endothelial cell modulation, and platelet inhibition.[70] Two studies of Angiotensin-Converting Enzyme inhibitors (ACE-I) show a reduction in stroke risk (HOPE, PROGRESS).[71,72] The HOPE trial studied the effects of ramipril in patients at high risk for ischemic events and found a beneficial effect. The combined endpoint of MI, stroke or vascular death was significantly reduced. Furthermore, the endpoint of stroke was also reduced. PROGRESS tested the effects of combining perindopril with a diuretic, indapamide, in patients with ischemic stroke, TIA or intracerebral hemorrhage and found that the combination therapy dramatically reduced the risk of recurrent stroke. No benefit for perindopril therapy alone was found although the study was not designed to test this. Much of the benefit was related to tighter control of BP. This suggests that the current upper limit of normal for BP is set too high for patients with stroke. Thus, more aggressive long-term control of BP by targeting a lower BP (e.g., <130/80) may be warranted. Recent recommendations offer some guidance.[83] Whether this kind of control will precipitate recurrent stroke or cognitive decline in patients with advanced or extensive intracranial arterial disease is not known and requires further study. Also, further study of ACE-I and statin medications in patients with stroke are needed to determine if patients without hypertension or hyperlipidemia might benefit from treatment.

REFERENCES

1. Guidelines for Perioperative Cardiovascular Evaluation for Noncardiac Surgery: Report of the American College of Cardiology/American Heart Association Task Force on Practice Guidelines (Committee on Perioperative Cardiovascular Evaluation for Noncardiac Surgery). *Circulation* 1996; **93**(6): 1278–1317.

2. Caplan, L. R. Diagnosis and the clinical encounter. In *Caplan's Stroke: A Clinical Approach*. Boston: Butterworth-Heinemann, 2000: 51–71.

3. Caplan, L. R. Strokes, cerebrovascular disease, and surgery. In *Caplan's Stroke: A Clinical Approach*. Boston: Butterworth-Heinemann, 2000: 445–462.

4. Heiss, W. Experimental evidence of ischemic thresholds and functional recovery. *Stroke* 1992; **23**: 1666–1672.

5. Bullock, R., Mendelow, A. D., Bone, T., Patterson, J., Macleod, W. N., & Allardice, G. Cerebral blood flow and CO_2 responsiveness as an indicator of collateral reserve capacity in patients with carotid arterial diseases. *Br. J. Surg.* 1985; **72**: 348–351.

6. Jansen, C., Ramos, L. M., van Heesewijk, J. P., Moll, F. L., van Gijn, J., & Ackerstaff, R. G. Impact of microembolism and hemodynamic changes in the brain during carotid endarterectomy. *Stroke* 1994; **25**: 992–997.

7. Henricksen, L., Hjaims, E., & Lindeburgh, T. Brain hyperperfusion during cardiac operations: cerebral blood flow measured in man by intra-arterial injection of xenon 133 – evidence suggestive of intra operative microembolism. *J. Thorac. Cardiovasc. Surg.* 1983; **86**: 202–208.

8. Karalis, D. G., Chandrasekaran, K., Victor, M. F., Ross, J. J., Jr., & Mintz, G. S. Recognition and embolic potential of intra-aortic atherosclerotic debris. *J. Thorac. Cardiovasc. Surg.* 1991; **17**: 73–78.

9. Kartchner, M. M. & McRae, L. P. Carotid occlusive disease as a risk factor in major cardiovascular surgery. *Arch. Surg.* 1982; **117**(8): 1086–1088.

10. Rakowski, H. & Pearlman, A. Preventing perioperative stroke: look, but don't touch! *Am. Heart. J.* 1999; **138**(4): 609–611.

11. Stern, A., Tunick, P. A., Culliford, A. T. *et al.* Protruding aortic arch atheromas: risk of stroke during heart surgery with and without aortic arch endarterectomy. *Am. Heart J.* 1999; **138** (4 Pt 1): 746–752.

12. Barbut, D. & Caplan, L. R. Brain complications of cardiac surgery. *Curr. Probl. Cardiol.* 1997; **22**(9): 449–480.

13. Marshall, W. G., Jr., Barzilai, B., Kouchoukos, N. T., & Saffitz, J. Intraoperative ultrasonic imaging of the ascending aorta. *Ann. Thorac. Cardiovasc. Surg.* 1989; **48**: 339–344.

14. Shaw, P. J., Bates, D., Cartlidge, N. E. *et al.* Neurologic and neuropsychologic morbidity following major surgery: bypass and peripheral vascular surgery. *Stroke* 1987; **18**: 700–707.

15. Moody, D. M., Bell, M. A., Challa, V. R., Johnston, W. E., & Prough, D. S. *et al.* Brain microemboli during cardiac surgery or aortography. *Ann. Neurol.* 1990; **28**: 477–486.

16. Pugsley, W., Klinger, L., Paschalis, C. *et al.* Microemboli and cerebral impairment during cardiac surgery. *Vasc. Surg.* 1990; **24**: 34–43.

17. McKhann, G. M., Grega, M. A., Borowicz, L. M., Jr. *et al.* Encephalopathy and stroke after coronary artery bypass grafting: incidence, consequences, and prediction. *Arch. Neurol.* 2002; **59**(9): 1422–1428.

18. von Reutern, G. M., Hetzel, A., Birrbaum, D., & Schlosser, V. Transcranial Doppler ultrasonography during cardiopulmonary bypass in patients with severe carotid stenosis or occlusion. *Stroke* 1988; **19**(6): 674–680.

19. Reed, G. L., 3rd, Singer, D. E., Picard, E. H., & DeSanctis, R. W. Stroke following coronary-artery bypass surgery. A case-control estimate of the risk from carotid bruits. *N. Engl. J. Med.* 1988; **319**(19): 1246–1450.

20. Kamik, R., Valentin, A., Bonner, G., Ziegler, B., & Slany, J. Transcranial Doppler monitoring during percutaneous transluminal aortic valvuloplasty. *Angiology* 1990; **41**: 106–111.

21. Furlan, A. J. & Cracium, A. R. Risk of stroke during coronary artery bypass graft surgery in patients with internal carotid artery disease documented by angiography. *Stroke* 1985; **16**(5): 797–799.

22. Breuer, A. C., Furlan, A. J., Hanson, M. R. *et al.* Central nervous system complications of coronary artery bypass graft surgery: prospective analysis of 421 patients. *Stroke* 1983; **14**(5): 682–687.

23. Parikh, S. & Cohen, J. R. Perioperative stroke after general surgical procedures. *N Y State J. Med.* 1993; **93**(3): 162–165.

24. Ropper, A. H., Wechsler, L. R., & Wilson, L. S. Carotid bruit and the risk of stroke in elective surgery. *N. Engl. J. Med.* 1982; **307**(22): 1388–1390.

25. Landercasper, J., Merz, B. J., Cogbill, T. H. *et al.* Perioperative stroke risk in 173 consecutive patients with a past history of stroke. *Arch. Surg.* 1990; **125**(8): 986–989.

26. Limburg, M., Wijdicks, E. F., & Li, H. Ischemic stroke after surgical procedures: clinical features, neuroimaging, and risk factors. *Neurology* 1998; **50**(4): 895–901.

27. Evans, B. A. & Wijdicks, E. F. High-grade carotid stenosis detected before general surgery: is endarterectomy indicated? *Neurology* 2001; **57**(7): 1328–1330.

28. Hise, J. H., Nipper, M. N., & Schnitker, J. C. Stroke associated with CABG. *Am. J. Neuroradiol.* 1991; **12**: 811–814.

29. Gardner, T. J., Horrieffer, P. J., Manolio, T. A. *et al.* Stroke following CABG: a 10 year study. *Ann. Thorac. Surg.* 1985; **12**: 574–581.

30. Rorick, M. B. & Furlan, A. J. Risk of cardiac surgery in patients with prior stroke. *Neurology* 1990; **40**(5): 835–837.

31. Ascione, R., Reeves, B. C., Chamberlain, M. H., Ghosh, A. K., Lim, K. H., & Angelini, G. D. Predictors of stroke in the modern era of coronary artery bypass grafting: a case control study. *Ann. Thorac. Surg.* 2002; **74**: 474–480.

32. Stamou, S. C., Jablonski, K. A., Pfister, A. J. *et al.* Stroke after conventional versus minimally invasive coronary artery bypass. *Ann. Thorac. Surg.* 2002; **74**: 394–399.

33. Bendszus, M., Reents, W., Franke, D. *et al.* Brain damage after coronary artery bypass grafting. *Arch. Neurol.* 2002; **59**(7): 1090–1095.

34. Szabo, Z., Hakanson, E., & Svedjeholm, R. Early postoperative outcome and medium-term survival in 540 diabetic and 2239 nondiabetic patients undergoing coronary artery bypass grafting. *Ann. Thorac. Surg.* 2002; **74**(3): 712–719.

35. American Heart Association. "Guidelines for Carotid Endarterectomy" A Multidisciplinary Consensus Statement From the Ad Hoc Committee. *Stroke* 1995; **26**(1): 188–201.

36. The CASANOVA Study Group. Carotid surgery versus medical therapy in asymptomatic carotid stenosis. *Stroke* 1991; **22**(10): 1229–1235.

37. North American Symptomatic Carotid Endarterectomy Trial Collaborators. Beneficial effect of carotid endarterectomy in symptomatic patients with high-grade carotid stenosis. *N. Engl. J. Med.* 1991; **325**(7): 445–453.

38. European Carotid Surgery Trialists' Collaborative Group. MRC European Carotid Surgery Trial: interim results for symptomatic patients with severe (70–99%) or with mild (0–29%) carotid stenosis. *Lancet* 1991; **337**(8752): 1235–1243.

39. Hobson, R. W., 2nd., Weiss, D. G., Fields, W. S. *et al.* The Veterans Affairs Cooperative Study Group. Efficacy of carotid endarterectomy for asymptomatic carotid stenosis. *N. Engl. J. Med.* 1993; **328**(4): 221–227.

40. National Institute of Neurological Disorders and Stroke. Carotid endarterectomy for patients with asymptomatic internal carotid artery stenosis. *J. Neurol. Sci.* 1995; **129**(1): 76–77.

41. Marcinczyk, M. J., Nicholas, G. G., Read, J. F., 3rd., & Nastasee, S. A. Asymptomatic carotid endarterectomy: patient and surgeon selection. *Stroke* 1997; **82**(2): 291–296.

42. Hannan, E. L., Popp, A. J., Feustel, P. *et al.* Association of surgical specialty and processes of care with patient outcomes for carotid endarterectomy. *Stroke* 2001; **32**(12): 2890–2897.

43. Hannan, E. L., Popp, A. J., Tranmer, B., Feustel, P., Waldman, J., & Shah, D. Relationship between provider volume and mortality for carotid endarterectomies in New York State. *Stroke* 1998; **29**(11): 2292–2297.

44. Barnett, H. J., Taylor, D. W., Eliasziw, M. *et al.* North American Symptomatic Carotid Endarterectomy Trial Collaborators. Benefit of carotid endarterectomy in patients with symptomatic moderate or severe stenosis. *N. Engl. J. Med.* 1998; **339**(20): 1415–1425.

45. Paciaroni, M., Eliasziw, M., Kappelle, L. J., Finan, J. W., Ferguson, G. G., & Barnett, H. J. Medical complications associated with carotid endarterectomy. *Stroke* 1999; **30**: 1759–1763.

46. Streifler, J. Y., Eliasziw, M., Benavente, O. R. *et al.* Prognostic importance of leukoaraiosis in patients with symptomatic internal carotid artery stenosis. *Stroke* 2002; **33**(6): 1651–1655.

47. Gorelick, P. B. Carotid endarterectomy; where do we draw the line? *Stroke* 1999; **30**: 1745–1750.

48. Sacco, R. L. Extracranial carotid stenosis. *N. Engl. J. Med.* 2001; **345**(15): 1113–1118.

49. Albers, G. W., Amarenco, P., Easton, J. D., Sacco, R. L., & Teal, P. Antithrombotic and thrombolytic therapy for ischemic stroke. *Chest* 2001; **119**: 300S–320S.

50. Wolf, P. A., Clagett, G. P., Easton, J. D. *et al.* Preventing ischemic stroke in patients with prior stroke and transient ischemic attack. A statement for healthcare professionals from the Stroke Council of the American Heart Association. *Stroke* 1999; **30**: 1991–1994.

51. Hirsch, J., Anand, S. S., Halperin, J. L., & Fuster, V. Guide to anticoagulant therapy: heparin: a statement for healthcare professionals from the American Heart Association.

52. Hirsh, J. *et al.* Guide to anticoagulant therapy: heparin. A Statement From the American Heart Association. *Circulation* 2001; **103**: 2994–3018.

53. International Stroke Trial Collaborative Group: The International Stroke Trial: a randomized trial of aspirin, subcutaneous heparin, both or neither among 19,435 patients with acute ischemic stroke. *Lancet* 1997; **349**: 1569–1581.

54. The Publication Committee for the Trial of Org 10172 in Acute Stroke Treatment (TOAST) Investigators: Low molecular weight heparinoid, ORG 10172 (danaperoid) an outcome after acute ischemic stroke: a randomized controlled trial. *J. Am. Med. Assoc.* 1998; **279**: 1265–1272.

55. Chimowitz, M. I., Kokkinos, J., Strong, J. *et al.* The warfarin–aspirin symptomatic intracranial disease study. *Neurology* 1995; **45**: 1488–1493.

56. Caplan, L. R. Treatment. In *Caplan's Stroke: A Clinical Approach*. Boston: Butterworth-Heinemann, 2000: 115–161.

57. The National Institute of Neurological Disorders and Stroke rt-PA Stroke Study Group. Tissue plasminogen activator for acute ischemic stroke. *N. Engl. J. Med.* 1995; **333**: 1581–1587.

58. Furlan, A., Higashida, R., Wechsler, L. *et al.* Intra-arterial pro-urokinase for acute ischemic stroke: The PROACT II Study: a randomized controlled trial. *J. Am. Med. Assoc.* 1999; **282**: 2003–2011.

59. Katzan, I. L., Masaryk, T. J., Furlan, A. J. *et al.* Intra-arterial thrombolysis for perioperative stroke after open heart surgery. *Neurology* 1999; **52**(5): 1081–1084.

60. Bladin, C. F. *et al.* What causes seizures after stroke? *Stroke* 1994; **25**: 245.

61. Bosch, J., Yusuf, S., Pogue, J. *et al.* Use of ramipril in preventing stroke: double blind randomised trial. *Br. Med. J.* 2002; **324**: 1–5.

62. MacMahon, S., Neal, B., Tzourio, C. *et al.* Randomised trial of a perindopril-based blood-pressure-lowering regimen among 6105 individuals with previous stroke or transient ischemic attack. Progress Collaborative Group. *Lancet* 2001; **358**: 1033–1041.

63. Dahlof, B., Devereinx, R. B., Kjeldsen, S. E. *et al.* Cardiovascular morbidity and mortality in the Losartan Intervention For Endpoint reduction in hypertension study (LIFE): a randomised trial against atenolol. *Lancet* 2002; **359**: 995–1003.

64. Neal, B., MacMahon, S., & Chapman, N. Blood Pressure Lowering Treatment Trialists' Collaboration. Effects of ACE inhibitors, calcium antagonists, and other blood-pressure-lowering drugs: results of prospectively designed overviews of randomised trials. *Lancet* 2000; **355**: 1955–1964.

65. Sacks, F. M., Pfeffer, M. A., Move, L. A. *et al.* Cholesterol and Recurrent Events Trial investigators. The effect of pravastatin on coronary events after myocardial infarction in patients with average cholesterol levels. *N. Engl. J. Med.* 1996; **335**(14): 1001–1009.

66. White, H. D., Simes, R. J., Anderson, N. E. *et al.* Pravastatin therapy and the risk of stroke. *N. Engl. J. Med.* 2000; **343**(5): 317–326.

67. Executive summary of the third report of the National Cholesterol Education program (NCEP) Expert Panel on Detection, Evaluation and Treatment of High Blood Cholesterol in Adults (Adult Treatment Panel III). *J. Am. Med. Assoc.* 2001; **285**: 2486–2497.

68. Blacker, D. J., Flemming, K. D., Link, M. J. *et al.* The preoperative cerebrovascular consultation: common cerebrovascular questions before general or cardiac surgery. *Mayo Clin. Proc.* 2004; **79**: 223–229.

69. Blacker, D. J., Wijdicks, E. F., & McClelland, R. L. Stroke risk in anticoagulated patients with atrial fibrillation undergoing endoscopy. *Neurology* 2003; **61**: 964–968.

70. Gorelick, P. B. New horizons for stroke prevention: PROGRESS and HOPE. *Lancet Neurology* 2002; **1**: 149–156.

71. The Heart Outcome Prevention Evaluation Study Investigators (HOPE). Effects of an angiotensin-converting enzyme inhibitor, ramipril, on cardiovascular events in high-risk patients. *N. Engl. J. Med.* 2000; **342**: 145–153.

72. PROGRESS Collaborative Group. Randomised trial of a perindopril-based blood-pressure-lowering regimen among 6105 individuals with previous stroke or transient ischaemic attack. *Lancet* 2001; **358**: 1033–1041.

73. Gorelick, P. Stroke prevention therapy beyond antithrombotics. *Stroke* 2002; **33**: 862.

74. MRC/BHF Heart Protection Study of cholesterol lowering with simvastatin in 20,536 high-risk individuals: a randomised placebo controlled trial. *Lancet* 2002; **360**: 7–22.

75. Taylor, D. W., Barnett, H. J., Haynes, R. B. *et al.* ASA and Carotid Endarterectomy (ACE) Trial Collaborators. Low-dose and high-dose acetylsalicylic acid for patients undergoing carotid endarterectomy: a randomised controlled trial. *Lancet* 1999; **353**: 2179–2184.

76. Hass, W. K., Easton, J. D., Adams, H. P. Jr. *et al.* A randomized trial comparing ticlopidine hydrochloride with aspirin for the prevention of stroke in high-risk patients. *N. Engl. J. Med.* 1989; **321**: 501–507.

77. CAPRIE Steering Committee. A randomized, blinded, trial of clopidogrel versus aspirin in patients at risk of ischemic events (CAPRIE). *Lancet* 1996; **348**: 1329–1339.

78. Diener, H. C., Cunha, L., Forbes, C. *et al.* European Stroke Prevention Study 2 (ESPS-2). Dipyridamole and acetylsalicylic acid in the secondary prevention of stroke. *J. Neurol. Sci.* 1996; **143**: 1–13.

79. The Clopidogrel in Unstable Angina to Prevent Recurrent Events (CURE) Trial Investigators. *N. Engl. J. Med.* 2001; **345**: 494–502.

80. Mohr, J. P., Thompson, J. L. P., Lazar, R. M. *et al.* A comparison of warfarin and aspirin for the prevention of recurrent ischemic stroke (WARSS). *N. Engl. J. Med.* 2001; **345**: 1444–1451.

81. Homma, S., Sacco, R. L., Di Tullio, M. R. *et al.* Effect of medical treatment in stroke patients with patent foramen ovale: patent foramen ovale in cryptogenic stroke study. *Circulation* 2002; **105**: 2625–2631.

82. The APASS Investigators. Antiphospholipid antibodies and subsequent thrombo-occlusive events in patients with ischemic stroke. *J. Am. Med. Assoc.* 2004; **291**: 576–584.

83. Chobanian, A. V., Bakris, G. L., Black, H. R. *et al.* The Seventh Report of the Joint National Committee on Prevention, Detection, Evaluation, and Treatment of High Blood Pressure: The JNC 7 Report. *J. Am. Med. Assoc.* 2003; **289**: 2560–2571.

84. Coull, B., Williams, L. S., Goldstein, L. B. *et al.* Anticoagulants and antiplatelets in acute ischemic stroke. *Stroke* 2002; **33**: 1934–1942.

85. Publications Committee for the Trial of ORG 10172 in Acute Stroke Treatment (TOAST) Investigators. Low molecular weight heparinoid, ORG 10172 (danaparoid), and outcome after acute ischemic stroke: a randomized controlled trial. *J. Am. Med. Assoc.* 1998; **279**: 1265–1272.

86. Bath, P. M. W., Lindenstrom, E., Boysen, G. *et al.* Tinzaparin in acute ischaemic stroke (TAIST): a randomized aspirin-controlled trial. *Lancet* 2001; **358**: 702–710.

87. HAEST Study Group. Heparin in Acute Embolic Stroke Trial. *Lancet* 2000; **355**: 1205–1210.

33

Management of the surgical patient with dementia

Madhav Thambisetty[1], James J. Lah[2], and Allan I. Levey[3]

[1]MRC Centre for Neurodegenerative Research, Institute of Psychiatry at the Maudsley, King's College, London, UK
[2]Wesley Woods Center, Atlanta, GA
[3]Emory University School of Medicine, Atlanta, GA

Introduction

Aging and dementia: magnitude of the problem

Health problems affecting an aging population constitute a major public health concern. Management of the elderly in the hospital, particularly those with cognitive impairment in need of surgery, represents a major challenge. These individuals often have multiple medical problems, and are susceptible to superimposed complications such as delirium that increase hospital stay and further increase risk. In the year 2000, the US census recorded 35.0 million people over the age of 65 years in this country. The proportion of the population aged 65 years and older is estimated to be more than 12% of the population. It is also estimated that the group aged 85 years and older is the fastest growing segment of the US population.[1] Moreover, there is a dramatic increase in the incidence of dementia with increasing age. Early studies using review of medical records in the study population reported an incidence of dementia per 1000 person–years to be about 1.6 in the age group 65–69 years, increasing dramatically to 41.4 in the 85–89-year age group.[2,3] More recent cohort-based studies

have reported incidence of dementia from 4.3–7.0 per 1000 person–years in the 65–69-year age group, increasing substantially to 54–118 in the 85–89-year age group.[4–6] A significant number of persons with dementia are often unrecognized by physicians in a primary care setting.[2,7–10] Moreover, the prevalence of dementia in hospitalized patients is considerably higher and has been estimated at 12% to 20%.[11] This chapter discusses some of the challenges posed by elderly individuals with dementia who are in hospital for surgical procedures, and outlines strategies for their management (Table 33.1).

The elderly surgical patient with dementia

The number of older patients presenting with operable disease is on the increase. There is also a growing body of evidence suggesting that a variety of major surgical procedures can be performed safely in the elderly patient with acceptable rates of mortality and morbidity.[12,13] This has in turn, resulted in patients with both previously diagnosed and unrecognized dementia undergoing surgery. The detection of dementia and the management of related conditions such as delirium in the surgical patient,

Table 33.1. Suggested approach to the elderly patient with suspected dementia

1. Administer Informant Questionnaire on Cognitive Decline in the Elderly (IQCODE)[27] to caregiver during initial interview.
2. Ask specific questions about vegetative signs of depression while obtaining history from the patient.
3. Further screen for depression by administering a formal instrument such as Geriatric Depression Scale (GDS) or the Center for Epidemiological Studies Depression Scale CES-D.
4. Formal mental assessment by either a clock-drawing task[41] or the Folstein Mini-Mental State Examination (MMSE).[43] If MMSE is used, further sensitivity in screening for dementia may be achieved by combining IQCODE and MMSE scores.[31]
5. Thorough physical examination to detect comorbid conditions and focused neurological examination for clues to etiology of cognitive decline.
6. If dementia is suspected, consider further laboratory evaluation and CT/MRI scan of the brain according to Practice Parameters of American Academy of Neurology (AAN).[58]

Medical Management of the Surgical Patient: A Textbook of Perioperative Medicine, ed. M. F. Lubin, R. B. Smith, T. F. Dobson, N. Spell, H. K. Walker. 4th edn. Published by Cambridge University Press. © Cambridge University 2006.

together with diagnosis and management of comorbid medical conditions, are of considerable importance in ensuring favorable outcomes after surgery. For instance, the development of delirium in the elderly hospitalized patient is a complication that is associated with increased mortality, duration of hospitalization, and greater rates of nursing home placement.[14] One estimate of healthcare expenditure related to the development of delirium during hospitalization suggests an annual cost of more than four billion dollars.[15] The medical management of the older, demented, surgical patient is thus an important consideration. In this chapter we examine the key issues that must be considered in the medical management of the surgical patient with known or suspected dementia. A brief overview is also presented of the ethical and legal issues surrounding the decision to operate on such patients.

For routine clinical use, the American Academy of Neurology (AAN) recommends the definition of dementia listed in the *Diagnostic and Statistical Manual of Mental Disorders*, Revised Third Edition (DSM-III-R)[16]: Impairment in short- and long-term memory, associated with impairment in abstract thinking, impaired judgment, other disturbances of higher cortical function, or personality change. The disturbance is severe enough to interfere significantly with work or usual social activities or relationships with others. The diagnosis of dementia is not made if these symptoms occur in delirium.

Preoperative considerations

Approach to the demented patient

In the patient with cognitive impairment, careful consideration of the cause of dementia is an important factor before the decision to operate is made. In the United States and Europe, Alzheimer's disease (AD) is the leading cause of progressive and irreversible dementia (50%–60% of cases) is followed by vascular dementia (10%–20% of cases).[17] However, Lewy body dementia and frontotemporal dementia are also now recognized as common causes of dementia that approximate vascular dementia in some populations.[18–21] Dementia may either be the presenting feature or an important manifestation of a wide variety of medical, neurological and psychiatric causes.[22] The recognition of treatable causes of dementia is of considerable practical significance. Studies on the prevalence of dementias that may be amenable to treatment report a wide range (0%–30%)[23] and are dependent on various factors such as clinical setting, diagnostic

criteria and extent of reversibility of cognitive symptoms.[24,25] The prevalence of treatable dementias has decreased considerably in recent years, excepting perhaps, the most common causes of reversible cognitive impairment: iatrogenic drug intoxication and depression.[24,25] Metabolic causes such as vitamin B_{12}/thiamine deficiency and thyroid disorders are less common. Other diagnostic considerations include normal pressure hydrocephalus (NPH), subdural hematoma, neoplasms of the brain, and neurosyphilis.

The initial patient interview should be oriented towards asking whether or not the patient has symptoms suggestive of dementia, delirium and/or depression. In the elderly patient, screening should begin with a detailed history obtained from the family or caregiver(s) about the patient's cognitive status.[26] This should focus on obtaining information about activities of daily living such as cooking, shopping, driving, and managing personal finances. A history suggestive of increasing dependence on others for activities that could previously be accomplished independently may be suggestive of cognitive impairment.[27] The Informant Questionnaire on Cognitive Decline in the Elderly (IQCODE) is an example of a simple, standardized questionnaire that can be administered to the patient's caregiver in the physician's office.[27] It provides information on changes in the patient's cognitive status over the previous 10 years. Therefore, it has the advantage of measuring change rather than current functioning. Moreover, it is not influenced by the patient's educational level and premorbid ability. Several studies have validated the utility of the IQCODE as a screening test for dementia.[28–30] Moreover, the combination of an informant-report tool such as the IQCODE with an easily administered and brief psychometric test such as the Mini Mental State Examination (MMSE) can further increase the accuracy of screening for dementia in the elderly patient.[31]

Depression may masquerade as dementia

Screening for depression must constitute an important component of the evaluation of the demented patient. As demonstrated by prospective studies, individuals with depression and co-existing cognitive impairment are especially likely to have an underlying dementia on longitudinal follow-up.[32–34] An important component of history-taking should focus on vegetative signs suggestive of depression such as loss of appetite, loss of libido and sleep disturbance. Several self-report scales of depression are currently in use and can be easily administered at this stage of the patient interview. The most commonly used scales in the elderly patient are the Center for Epidemiological Studies Depression Scale CES-D and the Geriatric Depression Scale (GDS). Both instruments have been shown to be excellent screening tools for major depression in elderly primary care patients.[35] One advantage of the GDS may be its ease of administration due to its yes or no format.

Assessment of mental status

A formal neuropsychological examination of the patient for confirmation and further evaluation of dementia is often time consuming. In the primary care setting or during a presurgical evaluation, however, a reasonable assessment of the patient's mental status can easily be performed, by administering one or two standardized tests. These can often confirm the clinical diagnosis of dementia, suggested earlier by the history and, in some cases, also suggest the etiology of the cognitive impairment. It is especially important to obtain an objective measure of the degree of cognitive impairment, if present, before surgery. Recent studies indicate that a significant number of patients undergoing coronary artery bypass grafting (CABG) and other major surgery, develop long-term cognitive dysfunction.[36,37] An objective evaluation of cognitive functioning before the surgical procedure may hence be useful in generating a baseline against which later impairment may be compared.

One popular test of cognitive function is the clock-drawing task, which has recently been suggested to be a sensitive measure for discriminating between individuals with dementia and normal subjects. This test is easily and quickly administered in an office setting and only requires a piece of paper and pencil.[38–41] Several studies have shown that individuals with dementia score significantly lower than controls.[38] Moreover, clock scores have been shown to correlate with other measures of dementia.[39] The utility of clock-drawing tasks in the diagnosis of Alzheimer's disease has also been reported by numerous studies.[40,41] Although several scoring systems have been developed for the clock-drawing task, a simple, practical means of assessing performance may include evaluation of the placement and sequence of numbers within a pre-drawn circle and the ability to set the minute and hour hands to a specified time.

Another example of a useful measure of the mental status is a delayed word recall task. Although commonly used, there is considerable disagreement on its utility as a good screening test for dementia and its ability to discriminate Alzheimer's disease from other conditions.[42] The Mini Mental State Examination (MMSE) takes about 10 minutes to administer and has reasonable sensitivity and specificity for detecting moderate dementia.[43] It is one of the most widely used instruments of screening for dementia in older persons. It is, however, significantly dependent on the patient's level of education and may not detect patients with mild cognitive symptoms.[44,45] Other popular brief assessment instruments include the Short Portable Mental Status Questionnaire,[46] Cognitive Capacity Screening Examination[47] and Dementia Rating Scale.[48]

Importance of the physical and neurological examination

The preoperative physical examination is particularly important, as coexisting medical conditions are likely to have an important effect on operative risk. Moreover, they can both cause and exacerbate cognitive impairment. For instance, congestive heart failure, particularly left ventricular failure, cardiac arrhythmias and orthostatic hypotension have all been associated with cognitive impairment in the elderly.[49] Optimization of medical regimens prior to surgery is therefore of great importance and can be appropriately directed by a careful physical examination.

In addition to examination of the mental status, a good neurological examination may also provide clues to the etiology of observed cognitive deficits. While the neurological examination is relatively normal in most primary degenerative dementias, extrapyramidal abnormalities have been reported in some patient series.[50,51] Visual hallucinations, parkinsonian features, fluctuating cognition, and gait disturbance are important signs suggestive of Lewy body dementia.[52,53] Generalized seizures may be a common feature in patients with AD and have been reported to have a prevalence of 10%–20%.[54,55] Dementia occurs frequently in advanced Parkinson's disease (PD)[56] and the presence of tremor, rigidity, bradykinesia, and postural abnormalities accompanying cognitive impairment must raise suspicion of undiagnosed PD. The presence of markedly impaired vertical eye movements, unsteady gait, and dysarthria accompanying dementia must raise suspicion of progressive supranuclear palsy.

As previously mentioned, vascular causes account for 10%–20% of all cases of dementia. Physical signs suggesting vascular dementia include focal neurological deficits that are determined by the vascular territory involved. While hemiparesis, hemianopia, or hemisensory abnormalities may be easily detected, other deficits may accompany the dementia. Examples of such deficits include aphasia (left middle cerebral artery), acute confusional state (right middle cerebral artery), apathy, abulia (anterior cerebral artery), visual field defects, alexia, disturbances of color vision, and cortical blindness (posterior cerebral artery). The commonest type of vascular dementia is called multi-infarct dementia and is the result of multiple, bilateral supratentorial infarcts. These are most commonly seen in the clinical setting of vascular or cardiac valvular disease and patients often have a history of hypertension, diabetes, angina, congestive heart failure, intermittent claudication, and vascular surgery.[57] While patients with cortical infarcts may present with some of the features mentioned previously, those with deep subcortical infarcts may present with motor signs, gait instability and pseudobulbar features such as emotional lability and choking.

Communicating hydrocephalus, commonly referred to as normal pressure hydrocephalus (NPH), classically presents with the triad of gait impairment, urinary incontinence and psychomotor slowing. While this may be difficult to distinguish from a primary degenerative dementia, a shorter course of progression of symptoms makes NPH a more likely diagnosis.

Laboratory evaluation of the demented patient

Further evaluation of the patient may include neuroimaging and laboratory testing. Based on an extensive review of previously published studies, the Quality Standards Subcommittee of the American Academy of Neurology (AAN) recently published an evidence-based review of diagnostic tests in the evaluation of dementia.[58] Based on this review, the AAN has recommended practice parameters for diagnostic testing in dementia. These guidelines suggest that structural neuroimaging with either non-contrasted computed tomography (CT) or magnetic resonance (MR) may be appropriate in the routine initial evaluation of patients with dementia. The importance of CT/MR in such patients is in the detection of brain neoplasms, subdural hematoma or NPH. Earlier guidelines published by the AAN recommended a number of laboratory tests (complete blood count, serum electrolytes, glucose, urea/creatinine, folate, B_{12}, thyroid function, and syphilis serology) in the routine assessment of dementia. The current practice parameter recommends routine estimation of serum B_{12} levels because its deficiency is common in the elderly. Screening for hypothyroidism is also recommended in the elderly patient. Screening for syphilis is not recommended unless the patient has a risk factor, evidence of prior infection or resides in an area with a relatively high number of syphilis cases.

Table 33.2. Important issues to address with patient and family prior to surgery

1. Increased likelihood of confusion and agitation in the immediate postoperative period.
2. Increased risk of long-term cognitive decline.
3. Ascertain and document patient's wishes regarding life-sustaining procedures.
4. Provide information to patient and family on advance directives.

Importance of communication with family and ethical/legal considerations

The demented patient is particularly prone to delirium in the postoperative period and this is an issue that must be addressed early in the preoperative stage (Table 33.2). Educating the family about the increased risk of postoperative agitation, its recognition and management is likely to make its occurrence less stressful. Identification of the patient's principal caregivers and providing them with additional information on the recognition of signs of delirium may aid in its early diagnosis and management.

The issue of obtaining informed consent from a patient with dementia often poses ethical and legal dilemmas. As all but the most emergent surgical procedures require informed consent, the physician is often the judge of the patient's competence to make rational decisions concerning treatment choices and attendant risks. While, in many cases, competence may be easily judged, the physician may face particular problems in others. For instance, the patient with mild dementia may report a reasonably well-preserved ability to perform most activities of daily living, have a non-focal neurological examination and yet show striking abnormalities in discrete cognitive domains such as executive functioning. The assessment of competence to give informed consent may prove considerably more complicated in such cases. In all such scenarios, a formal assessment of mental competence should be carried out by a psychiatrist or neurologist. In such cases, neuropsychological testing may reveal abnormalities in specific cognitive domains that may, in turn, predict competence to provide informed consent to treatment by the demented patient.[59]

A closely related issue is the question of decision making concerning treatment options, life-sustaining measures, withdrawal/withholding of treatment and end-of-life issues in the demented patient. Widely publicized court cases in an increasingly litigious environment have meant that the practicing physician must develop familiarity with common instruments by which incapacitated patients may convey their wishes concerning medical interventions. This is of particular importance in the care of the demented patient. In a landmark judgment in 1990, the Supreme Court ruled in *Cruzan v Director, Missouri Department of Health*, that the state could require "clear and convincing" evidence regarding patients' wishes for life-sustaining procedures.[60] Moreover, the Court noted that affidavits produced by family members specifying the patient's premorbid verbal directives were considered supportive, but not definitive evidence. The Patient's Self-Determination Act passed by Congress in 1990 requires that healthcare providers educate the patient about issues concerning advance directives. This federal law requires all facilities certified by Medicare and Medicaid to furnish timely information enabling patients to express their wishes regarding the use or refusal of medical care. The living will is among the oldest of mechanisms used to communicate a patient's wishes concerning medical interventions. It details those interventions desired by the patient and, more commonly, those not wanted in specific clinical situations. The living will, because of its specific nature regarding interventions, is considered the least useful of the advance directives, although it can be used to guide the actions of a surrogate decision maker.[61]

Durable power of attorney for healthcare is a legal document that names surrogates to make decisions on medical care when the patient is unable to do so. This is the most flexible of advance directives and allows surrogates to receive and process information in a manner identical to the patient. Moreover, it allows them to make decisions on behalf of the patient, even in the event of unexpected or unusual events in the clinical course.[62] The prehospital advance directive (PHAD) is a legal document on a standardized form that is uniform within a state or emergency medical services (EMS) region. It is meant to prevent EMS providers such as paramedics from beginning resuscitative efforts. A common modification of this document is the prehospital do not resuscitate (DNR) form. Unlike the PHAD, these forms are usually initiated, and their provisions agreed to, by the patient's physician. They are particularly relevant in the care of patients in nursing homes or hospices.[61]

Nutritional assessment

The inclusion of formal assessment of nutritional status in the preoperative evaluation is important because of the large number of elderly hospitalized patients at risk for malnutrition. It is estimated that about 60% of elderly patients in hospitals and nursing homes have evidence of malnutrition.[63] While few studies have examined the risk of malnutrition in the hospitalized, demented patient, it is likely that this subgroup of the elderly population would benefit from early detection of risk and prevention of malnutrition. The mini nutritional assessment (MNA) is an example of a screening tool that is easy to administer and patient friendly. It has been found to be useful in the screening of elderly hospitalized patients for malnutrition.[64] If such screening reveals inadequate nutritional intake, a complete assessment of nutritional status and appropriate intervention can be formulated by a clinical dietitian.[65]

Postoperative issues

Cognitive decline in the postoperative patient

With an increasing number of elderly patients undergoing major surgical procedures, postoperative decline in cognitive function is being recognized as a common problem. In a large, multicenter study, the incidence of postoperative cognitive decline was reported to be about 10% at 3 months following major, non-cardiac surgery.[36] Coronary artery bypass grafting (CABG) is a major surgery that has been particularly well studied in relation to the risk of postoperative dementia. It is one of the most commonly performed major operations in the developed world. Detailed cognitive testing reveals that up to 80% of patients may experience significant cognitive impairment at the time of discharge.[66] Moreover, cognitive impairment at discharge has been reported to be a strong predictor of late decline. Two large studies have reported the incidence of cognitive decline after CABG. In a systematic review, the incidence of post-operative cognitive decline was reported to be 22% 2 months after CABG.[67] Newman and colleagues reported an incidence of 53% at discharge, 36% at 6 weeks, 24% at 6 months and 42% at 5 years.[37] Although the etiology of postoperative dementia following cardiac surgery remains controversial, some recent studies have shown that "off-pump" techniques, where cardiopulmonary bypass is avoided by the use of cardiac stabilizing devices, may reduce its incidence.[66] Larger clinical trials, however, will be needed to further substantiate the role of such newer surgical techniques in the prevention of postoperative dementia.

A closely related and contentious issue concerns the role of anesthesia in the causation of postoperative cognitive decline. Concerns about the role of general anesthesia in cognitive decline after surgery were raised nearly 50 years ago.[68] Several studies have compared general and regional anesthesia with regard to the incidence of postoperative cognitive dysfunction. These have reported varying results on the role of general anesthesia as a risk factor for cognitive impairment following surgery.[69]

Depression in elderly patients with dementia may often be overlooked and is an important cause of postoperative cognitive decline.[70] Elderly patients may often deny affective symptoms or manifest atypical depression without prominent emotional features that are more easily recognized in younger patients.[71] Postsurgical patients with depression can be effectively treated by pharmacological and psychotherapeutic interventions.

Delirium is common in the postoperative patient

Delirium is the most common neurological impairment in the immediate postoperative period in the elderly patient. It affects both the demented and normal elderly patient and is characterized by restlessness, confusion and agitation. Distinguishing features include acute onset, altered sleep–wake cycle, fluctuating levels of consciousness and altered psychomotor activity. The incidence of postoperative delirium in the elderly patient ranges from 10%–60%.[72] Moreover, the elderly patient with dementia is at increased risk for development of delirium.[73] The wide range in incidence of delirium in the postoperative period can be attributed to differences in the patient populations studied, the specific surgical procedure performed and techniques used to determine the presence of delirium. For example, while the incidence of delirium in the elderly patient after orthopedic surgery is reported to be 28%–60%, it is only 1%–3% in patients undergoing cataract surgery.[72] Common causes of delirium in the postoperative setting include both intoxication and withdrawal from medications, (Table 33.3) infection, conditions predisposing to hypoxia such as chronic obstructive pulmonary disease and congestive heart failure, and toxic/metabolic causes such as hepatic encephalopathy and electrolyte abnormalities. Other factors that may contribute to the development of delirium include loss of ambient sensory input, sleep deprivation, and transfer to an unfamiliar environment.[74]

Approach to the delirious patient (Table 33.4)

The occurrence of delirium in the hospitalized patient is associated with increases in length of hospital stay, admission to a long-term care facility, disability as well as mortality.[75,76] Although early recognition of this clinical syndrome allows for prompt treatment, delirium in the elderly, hospitalized patient is often undiagnosed.[76] The hyperactive variant of delirium is characterized by

Table 33.3. Drugs that can cause delirium in elderly patients with dementia

Sedatives	*Antihypertensives*
Benzodiazepines	β-blockers
Diazepam (Valium)	Methyldopa
Flurazepam (Dalmane)	Clonidine
Others	
Barbiturates	*Anticonvulsants*
Meprobamate (Miltown)	Phenytoin
Ethanol	Phenobarbital
Antihistamines	*Anti-inflammatories*
Diphenhydramine (Benadryl)	Indomethacin (Indocin)
Cimetidine (Tagamet)	Prednisone
Others	
	Anti-microbials
Anticholinergics	Cephalexin
Antiparkinsonian agents	Isoniazid
Benztropine (Cogentin)	Rifampin
Trihexyphenidyl (Artane)	Metronidazole
Others	
Antispasmodics	*Cardioglycosides*
Phenothiazines	Digoxin
Chlorpromazine (Thorazine)	Digitoxin
Thioridazine (Mellaril)	
Others	*Anti-arrhythmics*
Scopolamine patches	Quinidine
Tricyclic antidepressants	Procainamide
Amitriptyline (Elavil)	Disopyramide
Imipramine (Tofranil)	Mexiletine
Others	
	Stimulants
Dopaminergics	Amphetamines
Carbidopa/levodopa (Sinemet)	Methylphenidate
Bromocriptine (Parlodel)	
Others	*Topicals*
	Pilocarpine eyedrops
Analgesics	
Salicylates	*Miscellaneous*
Narcotics	Selegiline
Meperidine (Demerol)	Lithium
Others	

increased psychomotor activity with the patient exhibiting disruptive behavior, agitation and psychosis. While this form of delirium may be easily detected, the hypoactive variant is more difficult to recognize and is characterized by withdrawal and apathy. Simple bedside tests of attention and orientation may be useful in the diagnosis of delirium in the postoperative patient. Examples of such tests include digit span forward and backward, naming of the months of the year in the reverse order and serial subtraction of 7s from 100. In addition to these, a more

Table 33.4. Approach to the delirious postoperative patient

1. Detection is key; maintain high index of suspicion, especially for quiet, hypoactive delirious states. Consider bedside tests of memory and orientation or administration of more formal instruments such as Confusion Assessment Method (CAM).

2. Review all medications, including those that the patient may have been taking prior to hospitalization. Remember that several common medications have significant anticholinergic effects.

3. Focused physical examination to detect infection, comorbid conditions causing hypoxia and pain due to injury. Assess volume status and rule out fecal impaction and urinary retention. Neurological examination to detect new, focal deficits.

4. Further laboratory evaluation, as clinically appropriate may include complete blood count, serum electrolytes, pulse oximetry/arterial blood gas analysis and urinalysis. Consider chest X-ray to rule out pneumonia.

5. Management strategies include environmental modifications, supportive measures and pharmacological treatment.

formal cognitive assessment of the patient may help in early detection of the delirium and its treatment. Such evaluation may be especially useful if a formal assessment of mental status was also performed prior to surgery, so as to detect subtle abnormalities early on in the postoperative period. Several rating and assessment instruments are commonly used in clinical practice in the diagnosis of delirium. The confusion assessment method (CAM) is a convenient, algorithm-based instrument that can be used for the diagnosis of delirium. Another example is the confusion rating scale, which is based on assessment of key components of confusional behavior such as disorientation, inappropriate behavior, inappropriate speech, and hallucinations.[74]

A thorough history obtained from the family or caregiver is invaluable in the diagnosis of delirium. In the hospitalized patient, preoperative evaluation of the patient may already have documented all medications that the patient was taking. Particular attention must be paid to a history of alcohol abuse as delirium tremens may present a serious, life-threatening complication. In the elderly patient with or without pre-existing dementia, anticholinergic medications are especially likely to cause cognitive dysfunction, even at low doses.[77,78] Moreover, exposure to anticholinergic medications has been shown to be independently and specifically associated with the severity of delirium in the hospitalized patient.[79] Several commonly used medications in the elderly have known anticholinergic effects. These include the tricyclic antidepressants, benzodiazepines, neuroleptics, opiates, antihistamines, benztropine,

and belladonna alkaloids. Besides these, there are other commonly prescribed medications that are not traditionally considered to be anticholinergic, but may have potential anticholinergic effects. Examples of such drugs include ranitidine, codeine, nifedipine, and warfarin.[80] Other medications commonly associated with postoperative delirium include antiparkinsonian medications such as levodopa/carbidopa, beta-blockers, diuretics, antibiotics such as cephalosporins, anticonvulsants, anti-inflammatory agents including steroidal and non-steroidal preparations, and oral hypoglycemic agents.[81]

Physical examination of the delirious patient must be directed at identifying a source of infection, ascertaining the fluid status, detecting the presence of injury resulting in pain and the presence of comorbid conditions such as congestive heart failure or chronic obstructive pulmonary disease. Fecal impaction and urinary retention are common causes of postoperative confusion in the elderly and must be addressed in the physical examination. Patients with cognitive impairment may not be able to verbalize complaints of pain efficiently and may require more frequent assessment of pain/discomfort in the postoperative period. This is especially important, as effective control of postoperative pain has been shown to be associated with reduction in the incidence of delirium.[82] While the recognition of pain in the demented postsurgical patient is of practical significance, it must be remembered that the use of some analgesics in the postoperative period is also associated with delirium.[83] Both the scenarios constitute a good example of the importance of using appropriate clinical judgment in the approach to the delirious patient. A complete neurological examination to detect new, focal deficits is an important component of the physical examination. Laboratory evaluation that may be useful in the detection of an underlying cause for delirium includes a complete blood count and serum electrolytes that may help detect acid–base abnormalities or acute renal failure. Pulse oximetry and/or arterial blood gas measurement may be useful in the detection of hypoxia and confirmation of acid–base abnormalities. Chest X-ray may be performed upon suspicion of underlying pneumonia. Similarly, urinalysis may be indicated when urinary tract infection is suspected. Electroencephalography (EEG) may be a useful investigation when the diagnosis of delirium is in doubt,[84] especially in conditions such as non-convulsive status epilepticus.[85]

The phenomenon of "sundowning" refers to the recurring onset of confusion or agitation in the elderly during evening hours.[86] Sundowning is more common in the elderly patient with dementia and shares some similarities with delirium. Unlike delirium however, it lasts longer, and is not associated with acute medical illnesses or increased mortality. Its occurrence at specific times of the day has led to suggestions that it may reflect a disorder of circadian rhythm in the elderly.[87]

Management of delirium: environmental modification and supportive measures

The prompt treatment of delirium in the postoperative period is of paramount importance and must be instituted even while the search for an underlying cause is in progress. All non-essential medications should be held and the need for centrally acting medications, re-evaluated. Wherever possible, they should be replaced with peripherally acting equivalents. Attention must be paid to environmental modification and supportive measures in the treatment of delirium.[88] These include clear and concise communication between the caregivers and patient, providing repeated verbal reminders to the patient of the time, day, location and identity of relatives and members of the treatment team. Aids to help orientation may include signposting the patient's location and provision of a clock or calendar in the room. Ensuring adequate lighting in the room to reduce misperception and control of excessive noise are other examples of simple measures that can help provide an unambiguous environment to the delirious patient. Other useful strategies include measures to increase competence of the patient. Examples include the provision of an interpreter if necessary, ensuring that the patient has his glasses, hearing aid or dentures. Rescheduling visits by members of the treatment team so as to allow maximum periods of uninterrupted sleep is a simple intervention that is extremely useful in the treatment of the delirious patient. Mobilization of ambulatory patients and performing full range of movements in the non-ambulatory patient are also beneficial.[88]

Management of delirium: pharmacological treatment

The decision to use pharmacological interventions in the management of delirium must be made only after careful consideration of the potential adverse effects of such treatment. The delirious patient may require such treatment in order to prevent injury or to allow further diagnostic work-up or treatment.

Antipsychotics are the most commonly used drugs in the management of delirium. The use of neuroleptics in the treatment of delirium may be associated with serious and potentially life-threatening complications. This is especially true in patients with Lewy body dementia who are very sensitive to these drugs and may manifest worsening parkinsonism, cognitive decline, and features of neuroleptic-malignant syndrome.[89] The older neuroleptics such as haloperidol are particularly likely to cause adverse reactions in these patients and must be avoided.

The newer, atypical antipsychotics may be safer therapeutic options in the pharmacological management of delirium in the elderly patient.[90–93] Although large, randomized studies comparing their efficacy and safety to conventional neuroleptics are lacking, smaller studies have indicated that they may be used safely and effectively in the elderly patient with cognitive impairment.[94,95] Their main advantage is the relatively lower incidence of extrapyramidal side effects. The atypical antipsychotic risperidone has been shown to cause fewer extrapyramidal side effects and somnolence in comparison to haloperidol in elderly patients with dementia.[94,95] Similarly, the novel antipsychotic, quetiapine has been recently used in the treatment of delirium in hospitalized patients and may be associated with fewer extrapyramidal effects than older antipsychotics.[93] Some of the newer, atypical antipsychotics may also have fewer adverse effects on cognition in elderly patients with dementia, thus making them more useful in the management of delirium in these patients.[96] The use of the novel antipsychotic ziprasidone, as an injectable agent in the treatment of acute agitation in psychotic patients, has also been reported and may offer a useful treatment option in the delirious patient with agitation.[97]

When delirium occurs in the setting of seizures or alcohol withdrawal, benzodiazepines are the preferred choice of pharmacologic agents in treatment. Lorazepam has a rapid onset and short duration of action and can be given both by oral and parenteral routes in dosages ranging from 0.5 mg every 12 hours to 1 mg every 8 hours. It must be remembered that the long-term use of benzodiazepines in the elderly is often associated with a higher risk of adverse events, including falls and cognitive deficits.[98,99] Their use in the elderly patient for longer durations must hence be exercised with caution.[100]

Emerging research suggests that augmenting cholinergic neurotransmission may be a novel approach in the treatment of delirium both in conditions associated with a primary deficit in cholinergic pathways as well as in delirium due to other causes. For example, the acetylcholinesterase inhibitor, donepezil has been used in the treatment of delirium in patients with dementia due to Lewy bodies.[88] Similarly, donepezil has also been used in the treatment of post-operative delirium in Alzheimer's disease.[89,90] Another cholinesterase inhibitor, rivastigmine has been used in the treatment of delirium due to lithium intoxication.[91] Although most of these studies are single case reports, they highlight the importance of further research into a novel approach to the pharmacotherapy of delirium.

Summary

Owing to a growing population of the elderly, increasing numbers of older patients with dementia undergo major surgery. Dementia is a major risk factor for surgical morbidity and mortality. A careful evaluation of the elderly surgical patient is needed to both diagnose and further evaluate cognitive impairment. Particular attention must be paid to the detection of comorbid conditions that may worsen both cognitive functioning and outcome after surgery. The practicing physician must be familiar with the ethical and legal issues associated with the care of the demented patient. Worsening of cognitive function, both in the immediate postoperative period and in the long-term are common adverse outcomes of surgery in the elderly patient. The elderly surgical patient is particularly prone to develop life-threatening delirium in the early postoperative period. Increased vigilance, early detection and prompt treatment can reverse this condition and ensure better long-term prognosis.

REFERENCES

1. Meyer, J. Age: 2000. *US Census Bureau, Census 2000 Brief*, C2KBR/01–12, Washington, DC.

2. Schoenberg, B. S., Kokmen, E., & Okazaki, H. Alzheimer's disease and other dementing illnesses in a defined United States population: incidence rates and clinical features. *Ann. Neurol.* 1987; **22**: 724–729.

3. Rocca, W. A., Cha, R. H., Waring, S. C. *et al.* Incidence of dementia and Alzheimer's disease: a reanalysis of data from Rochester, Minnesota, 1975–1984. *Am. J. Epidemiol.* 1998; **148**: 51–62.

4. Kukull, W. A., Higdon, R., Bowen, J. D. *et al.* Dementia and Alzheimer disease incidence. A prospective cohort study. *Arch. Neurol.* 2002; **59**: 1737–1746.

5. Bachman, D. L., Wolf, P. A., Linn, R. T. *et al.* Incidence of dementia and probable Alzheimer's disease in a general population: the Framingham Study. *Neurology* 1993; **43**: 515–519.

6. Ganguli, M., Dodge, H. H., Chen, P. *et al.* Ten-year incidence of dementia in a rural elderly US community population: the MoVIES Project. *Neurology* 2000; **54**: 1109–1116.

7. Rocca, W. A., Amaducci, L. A., & Schoenberg, B. S. Epidemiology of clinically diagnosed Alzheimer's disease. *Ann. Neurol.* 1986; **19**: 415–424.

8. Jorm, A. F., Korten, A. E., & Henderson, A. S. The prevalence of dementia: a quantitative integration of the literature. *Acta Psychiatr. Scand.* 1987; **76**: 465–479.

9. Evans, D. A., Funkenstein, H. H., Albert, M. S. *et al.* Prevalence of Alzheimer's disease in a community population of older persons. Higher than previously reported. *J. Am. Med. Assoc.* 1989; **262**: 2551–2556.

10. Valcour, V. G., Masaki, K. H., Curb, J. D. *et al.* The detection of dementia in a primary care setting. *Arch. Int. Med.* 2000; **160**: 2964–2968.

11. Erkinjuntti, T., Autio, L., & Wikstrom, J. Dementia in medical wards. *J. Clin. Epidemiol.* 1988; **41**: 123–126.

12. Parry, A. J., Giannopoulous, N., Ormerod, O. *et al.* An audit of cardiac surgery in patients aged over 70 years. *Quart. J. Med.* 1994; **87**: 89–96.

13. Salameh, J. R., Myers, J. L., & Mukherjee, D. Carotid endarterectomy in elderly patients. low complication rate with overnight stay. *Arch. Surg.* 2002; **137**: 1284–1287.

14. Inouye, S. K., Schlesinger, M. J., & Lydon, T. J. Delirium: a symptom of how hospital care is failing older persons and a window to improve quality of hospital care. *Am. J. Med.* 1999; **106**: 565–573.

15. US Bureau of the Census. *Statistical Abstract of the United States: 1996*. 116th edn. Washington, DC, 1996; 165.

16. American Psychiatric Association. *Diagnostic and Statistical Manual of Mental Disorders*, 3rd edn., revised. Washington, DC: American Psychiatric Association, 1994.

17. Nyenhuis, D. L. & Gorelick, P. B. Vascular dementia: a contemporary review of epidemiology, diagnosis, prevention, and treatment. *J. Am. Geriatr. Soc.* 1998; **46**: 1437–1448.

18. Perry, R. H., Irving, D., Blessed, G. *et al.* Senile dementia of Lewy body type. A clinically and neuropathologically distinct form of Lewy body dementia in the elderly. *J. Neurol. Sci.* 1990; **95**: 119–139.

19. McKeith, I. G., Galasko, D., Kosaka, K. *et al.* Consensus guidelines for the clinical and pathologic diagnosis of dementia with Lewy bodies (DLB): report of the consortium on DLB international workshop. *Neurology* 1996; **47**: 1113–1124.

20. Ratnavalli, E., Brayne, C., Dawson, K. *et al.* The prevalence of frontotemporal dementia. *Neurology* 2002; **58**: 1615–1621.

21. Neary, D., Snowden, J. S., Northen, B. *et al.* Dementia of frontal lobe type. *J. Neurol. Neurosurg. Psychiatry* 1988; **51**: 353–361.

22. Cummings, J. & Benson, D. *Dementia: A Clinical Approach*, 2nd edn. Boston: Butterworth-Heinemann, 1992: 1–17.

23. Arnold, S. E. & Kumar, A. Reversible dementias. *Medi. Clin. North Am.* 1993; **77**: 215–230.

24. Clarfield, A. M. The reversible dementias: do they reverse? *Ann. Intern. Med.* 1988; **109**: 476–486.

25. Weytingh, M. D., Bossuyt, P. M. M., & van Crevel, H. Reversible dementia: more than 10% or less than 1%? *J. Neurol.* 1995; **242**: 466–471.

26. Mayeux, R., Foster, N. L., Rossor, M., & Whitehouse, P. J. *The clinical evaluation of patients with dementia*. In Whitehouse, J., ed. *Dementia*. Philadelphia: F. A. Davis, 1993: 92–129.

27. Jorm, A. F., Scott, R., Cullen, J. S. *et al.* Performance of the informant questionnaire on cognitive decline in the elderly (IQCODE) as a screening test for dementia. *Psychol. Med.*

1991; **21**: 785–790. (The Short IQCODE can be downloaded and reproduced without copyright restrictions from the web at: http://www.anu.edu.au/iqcode/)

28. Fuh, J. L., Teng, E. L., Lin, K. N. *et al.* The Informant Questionnaire on Cognitive Decline in the Elderly (IQCODE) as a screening tool for dementia for a predominantly illiterate Chinese population. *Neurology* 1995; **45**: 92–96.

29. Senanarong, V., Assavisaraporn, S., Sivasiriyanonds, N. *et al.* The IQCODE: an alternative screening test for dementia for low educated Thai elderly. *J. Med. Assoc. Thailand* 2001; **84**: 648–655.

30. de Jonghe, J. F. Differentiating between demented and psychiatric patients with the Dutch version of the IQCODE. *Int. J. Geriatr. Psych.* 1997; **12**: 462–465.

31. Mackinnon, A. & Mulligan, R. Combining cognitive testing and informant report to increase accuracy in screening for dementia. *Am. J. Psych.* 1998; **155**: 1529–1535.

32. Visser, P. J., Verhey, F. R., Ponds, R. W. *et al.* Distinction between preclinical Alzheimer's disease and depression. *J. Am. Geriatr. Soc.* 2000; **48**: 479–484.

33. Alexopoulos, G. S., Meyers, B. S., Young, R. C. *et al.* The course of geriatric depression with "reversible dementia": a controlled study. *Am. J. Psych.* 1993; **150**: 1693–1699.

34. Burt, D. B., Zembar, M. J., & Niederehe, G. Depression and memory impairment: a meta-analysis of the association, its pattern and specificity. *Psychol. Bull.* 1995; **117**: 285–305.

35. Lyness, J. M., Noel, T. K., Cox, C. *et al.* Screening for depression in elderly primary care patients: a comparison of the Center for Epidemiologic Studies – depression scale and the geriatric depression scale. *Arch. Intern. Med.* 1997; **157**: 449–454.

36. Moller, J. T., Cluitmans, P., Rasmussen, L. S. *et al.* Long-term postoperative cognitive dysfunction in the elderly: ISPOCD1 study. *Lancet* 1998; **351**: 857–861.

37. Newman, M. F., Kirchner, J. L., Phillips-Bute, B. *et al.* Longitudinal assessment of neurocognitive function after coronary-artery bypass surgery. *N. Engl. J. Med.* 2001; **344**: 395–402.

38. Paganini-Hill, A., Clark, L. J., Henderson, V. W. *et al.* Clock drawing: analysis in a retirement community. *J. Am. Geriatr. Soc.* 2001; **49**: 941–947.

39. Sunderland, T., Hill, J. L., Mellow, A. M. *et al.* Clock drawing in Alzheimer's disease. A novel measure of disease severity. *J. Am. Geriatr. Soc.* 1989; **37**: 725–729.

40. Tuokko, H., Hadjistavropoulos, T., Miller, J. A. *et al.* The clock test: a sensitive measure to differentiate normal elderly from those with Alzheimer's disease. *J. Am. Geriatr. Soc.* 1992; **40**: 579–584.

41. Wolf-Klein, G. D., Silverstone, F. A., Levy, A. P. *et al.* Screening for Alzheimer's disease by clock drawing. *J. Am. Geriatr. Soc.* 1989; **37**: 730–734.

42. Kuslansky, G., Buschke, H., Katz, M. *et al.* Screening for Alzheimer's disease: the memory impairment screen versus the conventional three-word memory test. *J. Am. Geriatr. Soc.* 2002; **50**: 1086–1091.

43. Folstein, M. F., Folstein, S. E., & McHugh, P. R. "Mini-mental state": a practical method for grading the cognitive state of patients for the clinician. *J. Psychiatry. Res.* 1975; **12**: 189–198.

44. Anthony, J. C., LeResche, L., Niaz, U. *et al.* Limits of the "Mini-mental state" as a screening test for dementia and delirium among hospital patients. *Psychol. Med.* 1982; **12**: 397–408.

45. Faustman, W. O., Moses, J. A., & Csernansky, J. G. Limitations of the Mini-mental state examination in predicting neuropsychological functioning in a psychiatric sample. *Acta Psychiatr. Scand.* 1990; **81**: 126–131.

46. Pfeiffer, E. A short portable mental status questionnaire for the assessment of organic brain deficit in elderly patients. *J. Am. Geriatr. Soc.* 1975; **23**: 433–441.

47. Jacobs, J. W., Bernhard, M. R., Delgado, A. *et al.* Screening for organic mental syndromes in the medically ill. *Ann. Intern. Med.* 1977; **86**: 40–46.

48. Mattis, S. *Dementia Rating Scale Professional Manual.* Odessa, FL: Psychological Assessment Resources, 1973.

49. Roman, G. C. Vascular dementia may be the most common form of dementia in the elderly. *J. Neurol. Sci.* 2002; **203–204**: 7–10.

50. Kurlan, R., Richard, I. H., Papka, M. *et al.* Movement disorders in Alzheimer's disease: more rigidity of definitions is needed. *Mov. Disord.* 2000; **15**: 24–29.

51. Perl, D. P., Olanow, C. W., & Calne, D. Alzheimer's disease and Parkinson's disease: distinct entities or extremes of a spectrum of neurodegeneration? *Ann. Neurol.* 1998; **44**: S19–S31.

52. McKeith, I. G., Galasko, D., Kosaka, K. *et al.* Consensus guidelines for the clinical and pathologic diagnosis of dementia with Lewy bodies (DLB): report of the consortium on DLB international workshop. *Neurology* 1996; **47**: 1113–1124.

53. Mori, E., Shimomura, T., Fujimori, M. *et al.* Visuoperceptual impairment in dementia with Lewy bodies. *Arch. Neurol.* 2000; **57**: 489–493.

54. Hesdorffer, D. C., Hauser, W. A., Annegers, J. F. *et al.* Dementia and adult-onset unprovoked seizures. *Neurology* 1996; **46**: 727–730.

55. Mendez, M. F., Catanzaro, P., Doss, R. C. *et al.* Seizures in Alzheimer's disease: clinicopathologic study. *J. Geriatr. Psychiatry Neurol.* 1994; **7**: 230–233.

56. Korczyn, A. D. Dementia in Parkinson's disease. *J. Neurol.* 2001; **248**(3): 1–4.

57. Hijdra, A. Vascular dementia. In Bradley, W. G., Daroff, R. B., Fenichel, G. M., & Marsden, D. C., ed. *Neurology in Clinical Practice*, 3rd edn. Boston: Butterworth-Heinemann, 2000: 1721–1729.

58. Knopman, D. S., DeKosky, S. T., Cummings, J. L. *et al.* Practice parameter: diagnosis of dementia (an evidence-based review). Report of the Quality Standards Subcommittee of the American Academy of Neurology. *Neurology* 2001; **56**: 1143–1153.

59. Marson, D. C., Hawkins, L., McInturff, B. *et al.* Cognitive models that predict physician judgments of capacity to consent in mild Alzheimer's disease. *J. Am. Geriatr. Soc.* 1997; **45**: 458–464.

60. Cruzan v. Director, Missouri Department of Health, 1990 US Lexicus 3301 (US June 25, 1990).

61. Iserson, K. V. Nonstandard advance directives: a pseudo-ethical dilemma. *J. Trauma* 1998; **44**: 139–142.

62. Hornbostel, R. Legal and financial decision making in dementia care. In Whitehouse, P. J., ed. *Dementia*. Philadelphia: FA Davis Co., 1993: 417–432.

63. Rudman, D. & Feller, A. G. Protein-caloric undernutrition in the nursing home. *J. Am. Geriatr. Soc.* 1989; **37**: 173–183.

64. Allison, S. P. & Kinney, J. M. Nutrition and ageing. *Curr. Opin. Clin. Nutr. Metab. Care* 2001; **4**: 1–4.

65. Nourhashemi, F., Andrieu, S., Rauzy, O. *et al.* Nutritional support and aging in preoperative nutrition. *Curr. Opin. Clin. Nutr. Metab. Care* 1999; **2**: 87–92.

66. Taggart, D. About impaired minds and closed hearts. *Br. Med. J.* 2002; **325**: 1255–1256.

67. Van Dijk, D., Keizer, A. M., Diephuis, J. C. *et al.* Neurocognitive dysfunction after coronary artery bypass surgery: a systematic review. *J. Thorac. Cardiovasc. Surg.* 2000; **120**: 632–639.

68. Bedford, P. D. Adverse cerebral effects of anaesthesia on old people. *Lancet* 1955; **269**: 259–263.

69. Dodds, C. & Allison, J. Postoperative cognitive dysfunction in the elderly surgical patient. *Br. J. Anaesth.* 1998; **81**: 449–462.

70. Galanakis, P., Bickel, H., Gradinger, R. *et al.* Acute confusional state in the elderly following hip surgery: incidence, risk factors and complications. *Int. J. Geriatr. Psychiatry* 2001; **16**: 349–355.

71. Popkin, M. K., Mackenzie, T. B., & Callies, A. L. Psychiatric consultation to geriatric medically ill inpatients in a university hospital. *Arch. Gen. Psychiatry* 1984; **41**: 703–707.

72. Parikh, S. S. & Chung, F. Postoperative delirium in the elderly. *Anesth. Analg.* 1995; **80**: 1223–1232.

73. Elie, M., Cole, M. G., Primeau, F. J. *et al.* Delirium risk factors in elderly hospitalized patients. *J. Gen. Intern. Med.* 1998; **13**: 204–212.

74. Rummans, T. A., Evans, J. M., Krahn, L. E. *et al.* Delirium in elderly patients: evaluation and management. *Mayo Clin. Proc.* 1995; **70**: 989–998.

75. Francis, J., Martin, D., & Kapoor, W. N. A prospective study of delirium in hospitalized elderly. *J. Am. Med. Assoc.* 1990; **263**: 1097–1101.

76. Cole, M. G., McCusker, J., Bellavance, F. *et al.* Systematic detection and multidisciplinary care of delirium in older medical patients: a randomized trial. *CMAJ* 2002; **167**: 753–759.

77. Berggren, D., Gustafson, Y., Eriksson, B. *et al.* Postoperative confusion after anesthesia in elderly patients with femoral neck fractures. *Anesth. Analg.* 1987; **66**: 497–504.

78. Sunderland, T., Tariot, P. N., Cohen, R. M. *et al.* Anticholinergic sensitivity in patients with dementia of the Alzheimer type and age-matched controls: a dose–response study. *Arch. Gen. Psychiatry* 1987; **44**: 418–426.

79. Han, L., McCusker, J., Cole, M. *et al.* Use of medications with anticholinergic effect predicts clinical severity of delirium symptoms in older medical inpatients. *Arch. Intern. Med.* 2001; **161**: 1099–1105.

80. Tune, L., Carr, S., Hoag, E. *et al.* Anticholinergic effect of drugs commonly prescribed for the elderly: potential means for assessing risk of delirium. *Am. J. Psychiatry* 1992; **149**: 1393–1394.

81. Winawer, N. Postoperative delirium. *Med. Clin. North Am.* 2001; **85**: 1229–39.

82. Lynch, E. P., Lazor, M. A., Gellis, J. E. *et al.* The impact of postoperative pain on the development of postoperative delirium. *Anesth. Analg.* 1998; **86**: 781–785.

83. Marcantonio, E. R., Juarez, G., Goldman, L. *et al.* The relationship of postoperative delirium with psychoactive medications. *J. Am. Med. Assoc.* 1994; **272**: 1518–1522.

84. Brenner, R. P. Utility of EEG in delirium: past views and current practice. *Int. Psychogeriatr.* 1991; **3**: 211–229.

85. Litt, B., Wityk, R. J., Hertz, S. H. *et al.* Nonconvulsive status epilepticus in the critically ill elderly. *Epilepsia* 1998; **39**: 1194–1202.

86. Vitiello, M. V., Bliwise, D. L., & Prinz, P. N. Sleep in Alzheimer's disease and the sundown syndrome. *Neurology* 1992; **42**: 83–93.

87. Bliwise, D. L., Carroll, J. S., Lee, K. A. *et al.* Sleep and "sundowning" in nursing home patients with dementia. *Psychiatry Res.* 1993; **48**: 277–292.

88. Meagher, D. J. Delirium: optimising management. *Br Med. J.* 2001; **322**: 144–149.

89. Ballard, C., Grace, J., McKeith, I. *et al.* Neuroleptic sensitivity in dementia with Lewy bodies and Alzheimer's disease. *Lancet* 1998; **351**: 1032–1033.

90. Sipahimalani, A. & Masand, P. S. Olanzapine in the treatment of delirium. *Psychosomatics* 1998; **39**: 422–430.

91. Sipahimalani, A. & Masand, P. S. Use of risperidone in delirium: case reports. *Ann. Clin. Psychiatry* 1997; **9**: 105–107.

92. Beuzen, J. N., Taylor, N., Wesnes, K. *et al.* A comparison of the effects of olanzapine, haloperidol and placebo on cognitive and psychomotor functions in healthy elderly volunteers. *J. Psychopharmacol.* 1999; **13**: 152–158.

93. Schwartz, T. L. & Masand, P. S. Treatment of delirium with quetiapine. Primary Care Companion. *J. Clin. Psychiatry* 2000; **2**: 10–12.

94. De Deyn, P. P., Rabheru, K., Rasmussen, A. *et al.* A randomized trial of risperidone, placebo, and haloperidol for behavioral symptoms of dementia. *Neurology* 1999; **53**: 946–955.

95. Lane, H. Y., Chang, Y. C., Su, M. H. *et al.* Shifting from haloperidol to risperidone for behavioral disturbances in dementia: safety, response predictors and mood effects. *J. Clin. Psychopharmacol.* 2002; **22**: 4–10.

96. Byerly, M. J., Weber, M. T., Brooks, D. L. *et al.* Antipsychotic medications and the elderly: effects on cognition and implications for use. *Drugs Aging* 2001; **18**: 45–61.

97. Daniel, D. G., Potkin, S. G., Reeves, K. R. *et al.* Intramuscular (IM) ziprasidone 20 mg is effective in reducing acute agitation associated with psychosis: a double-blind, randomized trial. *Psychopharmacology* 2001; **155**: 128–134.

98. Herings, R. C., Stricker, B. H., de Boer, A. *et al.* Benzodiazepines and the risk of falling leading to femur fractures. Dosage more important than elimination half-life. *Arch. Intern. Med.* 1995; **155**: 1801–1807.

99. Golombok, S., Moodley, P., & Lader, M. Cognitive impairment in long-term benzodiazepine users. *Psychol. Med.* 1988; **18**: 365–374.

100. Wang, P. S., Bohn, R. L., Glynn, R. J. *et al.* Hazardous benzodiazepine regimens in the elderly: effects of half-life, dosage, and duration on risk of hip fracture. *Am. J. Psychiatry* 2001; **158**: 892–898.

101. Kaufer, D. I., Catt, K. E., Lopez, O. L. *et al.* Dementia with Lewy bodies: response of delirium-like features to donepezil. *Neurology* 1998; **51**: 1512.

102. Wengel, S. P., Burke, W. J., & Roccaforte, W. H. Donepezil for postoperative delirium associated with Alzheimer's disease. *J. Am. Geriatr. Soc.* 1999; **47**: 379–380.

103. Wengel, S. P., Roccaforte, W. H., & Burke, W. J. Donepezil improves symptoms of delirium in dementia: implications for future research. *J. Geriatr. Psychiatry Neurol.* 1998; **11**: 159–161.

104. Fischer, P. Successful treatment of nonanticholinergic delirium with a cholinesterase inhibitor. *J. Clin. Psychopharmacol.* 2001; **21**: 118.

34

Neuromuscular disorders

Jaffar Khan

Emory University School of Medicine, Lawrenceville, GA

Myasthenia gravis

Of all the neuromuscular diseases, myasthenia gravis probably has the most significant implications for surgical patients.[1] It is caused by an autoimmune attack on the acetylcholine receptors of the postsynaptic (muscle) side of the neuromuscular junction. Characteristic clinical features include fluctuating weakness and fatigue, usually involving the extraocular muscles and eyelids (producing diplopia and ptosis). Weakness of the limbs can be severe, sometimes resulting in almost total paralysis. Sensation and deep tendon reflexes are normal. Respiratory muscle weakness is common and can be fatal. The introduction of practical mechanical ventilation has resulted in a dramatic decrease in the mortality rate.

Although the clinical features of myasthenia gravis are sufficiently characteristic in some cases, confirmatory tests are usually necessary.[2] The acetylcholine receptor (AchR)-antibody level is elevated in over 80% of patients with myasthenia gravis. Elevated levels of this antibody are extremely specific for this disease.[3] As a result the AchR-antibody serum test is typically the first step in confirming the diagnosis, and the presence of elevated levels eliminates the need for additional confirmatory testing. In antibody negative patients or when faced with an acutely symptomatic patient, the edrophonium test is often used. The strength of a specific weak muscle should be determined before and after the intravenous administration of 8 mg of edrophonium. A test dose of 2 mg of edrophonium should always be given first and atropine should be available in case significant bradycardia develops. Electrodiagnostic studies (repetitive nerve stimulation and single fiber electromyography) are often useful, particularly in antibody negative patients or patients with cardiac disease or asthma, in whom edrophonium is relatively contraindicated. The characteristic finding on 2- to 3-Hz repetitive motor nerve stimulation is a progressive decrease in the amplitude of the motor response. Single fiber electromyography may reveal the presence of jitter or blocking (a difference in the timing of activation or a failure of neuromuscular transmission in one of a pair of muscle fibers within a motor unit).

Many effective therapies have been developed for myasthenia gravis.[4] Acetylcholine esterase inhibitors increase the concentration of acetylcholine near the impaired receptors. This provides symptomatic relief of weakness. Pyridostigmine (Mestinon) is used most commonly and is generally given at a dosage of 60 mg every 3 to 6 hours, depending on the patient's response.

Immunosuppression with prednisone frequently is efficacious. Patients beginning prednisone therapy should be cautioned that weakness might increase during the first 10 to 14 days before the beneficial effect becomes apparent. Azathioprine[5,6] and cyclosporine[7,8] are effective and are often used in patients who do not respond to other treatments or are at increased risk for complications from prednisone. Mycophenolate mofetil (CellCept) is used with success in severe refractory myasthenia.[9] The rapid onset of therapeutic effect, safe side effect profile and patient tolerability make this drug a desirable candidate for future investigation in the treatment of myasthenia gravis.[10]

Thymectomy is recommended as an option for patients with non-thymomatous generalized myasthenia, except at the extremes of age.[11] However, about 10% of patients with myasthenia have a thymoma and their prognosis is worse, even if the tumor is removed. The incidence of thymoma increases with age and the tumor may develop at any time during the course of the illness. Chest computed tomography should be performed at the time of

Medical Management of the Surgical Patient: A Textbook of Perioperative Medicine, ed. M. F. Lubin, R. B. Smith, T. F. Dobson, N. Spell, H. K. Walker. 4th edn. Published by Cambridge University Press. © Cambridge University 2006.

diagnosis. Thymectomy produces permanent remission in about 50% of patients, although remission may not occur for many months after surgery.

Hyperthyroidism is found in 5% of patients with myasthenia gravis. Hypothyroidism also is more common in these patients than in the general population. Treatment of the thyroid abnormality usually improves muscle strength.

The term *myasthenic crisis* refers to progressive respiratory or bulbar weakness. Intubation usually should be done when the vital capacity falls to about 15 ml/kg. Causes of myasthenic crisis include infection, thyroid dysfunction, and medications that adversely affect neuromuscular transmission. The most common pharmacologic offenders are aminoglycosides, quinine, quinidine, magnesium, and neuromuscular blocking agents. Many medications are reported to exacerbate myasthenia occasionally, including most antiarrhythmic agents. Hypokalemia is a common cause of increased weakness in patients with myasthenia, especially those who are taking prednisone. As a precautionary measure, potassium replacement is advisable in these patients. In addition to correcting any precipitating factor, the most effective treatment for myasthenic crisis is plasma exchange, which almost always has a dramatic effect over a few days. High-dose intravenous immunoglobulin (400 mg/kg daily for 5 days) is also efficacious.[12]

Issues relevant to surgical patients

Thymectomy is often performed in patients with myasthenia gravis to remove thymomas, if present, and to attempt to induce remission. Patients should not undergo this surgery until medical management has been used to increase their strength, particularly in the respiratory muscles. If respiratory function remains significantly impaired (vital capacity 20 ml/kg or less) after maximal medical improvement, a course of intravenous immunoglobulin (400 mg/kg daily for 5 days) should be given. Patients who undergo surgery with significant respiratory weakness are more likely to require prolonged postoperative mechanical ventilation. After sternotomy, accurate measurement of the vital capacity usually is not possible because of incisional pain. If the use of medications with neuromuscular blocking potential is avoided during surgery, a normal potassium level is maintained, and preoperative medication regimens are resumed, problems with extubation are unlikely. Intravenous pyridostigmine (Mestinon) can be given but the dosage used (1 to 4 mg) should be one thirtieth to one fifteenth the oral dosages

(60 to 90 mg every 4 to 6 hours) because of the lack of first-pass hepatic metabolism. After surgery, remission may occur within a few weeks but can be delayed for several months. Medical therapy can gradually be withdrawn on an outpatient basis according to the patient's clinical status. The prednisone dosage can often be tapered over 6 to 8 weeks. A dose of pyridostigmine can be omitted during the day to determine whether the drug is still needed.

Patients occasionally develop weakness as a result of unsuspected myasthenia gravis during hospitalization for a surgical procedure. This is most often related to the administration of a medication with neuromuscular blocking activity,[13] although hypokalemia, hypermagnesemia, and infection are also capable of unmasking myasthenia gravis.[14] Intravenous magnesium should not be used in patients with myasthenia, except when life-threatening hypomagnesemia exists.[15] The use of aminoglycosides, quinine, quinidine, and intraoperative neuromuscular blocking agents also should be avoided. In addition, lincomycin, clindamycin, polymyxin, and colistin are capable of exacerbating myasthenia. Other antibiotics and antiarrhythmic drugs have been implicated rarely but are not considered to be contraindicated. These include erythromycin, penicillins, sulfonamides, tetracyclines, ciprofloxacin, vancomycin, procainamide, calcium channel blockers, and beta-blockers. There are anecdotal reports of numerous medications that have been associated with worsening of myasthenia, and it is prudent to suspect any newly added medication in this setting.

Lambert–Eaton syndrome

Lambert–Eaton syndrome is a rare disorder of neuromuscular transmission caused by autoantibodies directed against calcium channels in the presynaptic terminal.[16] This impairs acetylcholine release. Patients have proximal muscle weakness but it differs from myasthenia gravis in that extraocular muscles are rarely involved and deep tendon reflexes are reduced. About half of patients are eventually found to have small cell carcinoma of the lung. Repetitive nerve stimulation is necessary to make the diagnosis and shows a characteristic increase in the potential recorded over a muscle after exercise or rapid repetitive stimulation.

Immunosuppressant agents that are useful in myasthenia gravis are also useful in Lambert–Eaton syndrome but pyridostigmine (Mestinon) is not as helpful. The response to treatment of small cell carcinoma is unpredictable. Medications that exacerbate myasthenia gravis may also exacerbate Lambert–Eaton syndrome.

Prolonged neuromuscular blockade

Neuromuscular blocking agents are frequently used to facilitate mechanical ventilation. Although routine use of these agents typically does not result in any complications, some patients may develop persistent weakness for up to 1 week after the drugs are discontinued. This is more common in patients with renal or hepatic dysfunction in which the metabolism of the medications may be reduced or with the concomitant use of drugs that potentiate the action of neuromuscular blocking agents.[17] The diagnosis can be confirmed with repetitive nerve stimulation. A typical decrement of the motor response occurs when neuromuscular blockade is present, although in patients with severe weakness, the motor response may be absent. If the weakness persists beyond 10 days, the repetitive nerve stimulation should be repeated and a diligent search for another etiology of the weakness should be pursued. Otherwise, supportive care should be maintained until the pharmacologic effects of the paralytics have resolved.

Peripheral neuropathy

Mononeuropathy

Peripheral neuropathy may be generalized (polyneuropathy), focal (mononeuropathy), or multifocal (multiple mononeuropathy). All three syndromes may cause clinically significant problems for surgical patients. Mononeuropathies present as the dysfunction of an individual peripheral nerve and are common in patients undergoing surgical procedures. Compression neuropathies are probably the most frequent disorders. Patients with diabetes and other conditions associated with polyneuropathy are predisposed to the development of compressive neuropathy.[18] Patients who are undergoing general anesthesia are at risk because they may be positioned in such a way that continuous pressure is applied to a nerve. This is analogous to the well-known "Saturday night palsy," in which a person awakens from alcohol-induced anesthesia with a wristdrop.[19] The arm may have been draped over an object, resulting in damage to the radial nerve in the spiral groove of the humerus. Continuous pressure over the mid-humerus also can occur during surgery or be associated with impaired mobility before or after surgery. There is weakness of wrist extension and the brachioradialis with a normal triceps. Intrinsic hand muscles appear to be weak because they cannot be effectively activated without adequate wrist

extension. There may be loss of sensation over the dorsum of the hand in the web space between the thumb and index finger. The prognosis is good, with recovery usually occurring over weeks to months. A splint should be used to keep the hand in a more functional position and prevent contracture.

Ulnar neuropathy resulting from compression at the elbow is a common problem.[20] Pressure over the medial elbow is the usual cause when this condition develops during surgery. There is numbness of the fifth and medial portion of the fourth digits and palm. In more severe cases, weakness of abduction and, sometimes, flexion of the ulnar digits may be seen. Recovery is usual when the condition is mild but some permanent disability is common in severe cases. Patients should be advised to avoid pressure over the elbow and prolonged elbow flexion (which stretches the nerve across the ulnar groove).

The other common pressure palsy involves the peroneal nerve as it passes behind the head of the fibula.[21] Pressure behind the knee, resulting from prolonged leg crossing or squatting, is the usual cause, and patients who have recently experienced significant weight loss are predisposed. This also can occur during surgery when pressure is applied to that area. There is weakness of ankle dorsiflexion and often eversion, without weakness of ankle inversion. There may be sensory loss in the web space between the first two toes and, sometimes, the anterolateral foot and leg. The prognosis is good, with most patients recovering in 3 to 8 weeks. A brace (ankle–foot orthosis) improves the ability to walk by relieving footdrop.

Infrequently, obturator, lateral femoral cutaneous, peroneal, and sciatic neuropathies may result when a patient is placed in the lithotomy position during surgery. These compression neuropathies are more likely to occur if the position is maintained for more than 2 hours.[22] Numerous neuropathies are reported as a complication of cardiac surgery.[23] These neuropathies are usually a consequence of intraoperative positioning or a direct result of the surgical procedure. The phrenic nerve is at risk for injury during the internal mammary artery dissection and intraoperative hypothermia. Rarely, the recurrent laryngeal neuropathy may develop as a result of intraoperative hypothermia, tracheal intubation, central venous catheter placement or surgical dissection. Numbness and pain along the medial calf to the great toe can result from an injury to the saphenous nerve during a vein harvest.

In addition to the pressure palsies, mononeuropathies related to the trauma of an invasive procedure are commonly encountered in surgical patients. The femoral nerve is often damaged after femoral artery catheterization.[24] This usually is related to pressure from a hematoma, although inaccurate needle placement also is a potential cause. A hematoma may be evident on physical examination or it may lie proximal to the inguinal ligament and escape detection by physical inspection. Computed tomography or magnetic resonance imaging through the pelvis is necessary in this setting because evacuation of the hematoma can be beneficial. Femoral neuropathy is also a relatively common complication of hysterectomy or other gynecologic surgery, probably because of traction on the nerve. Femoral neuropathy causes weakness of knee extension that often is not recognized until patients begin to ambulate. The knee jerk is reduced or absent and there may be loss of sensation over the anterior thigh and medial leg (the saphenous branch of the femoral nerve provides sensory innervation to the medial leg). When they are severe, these nerve injuries commonly result in prolonged or permanent disability, although significant recovery is possible even after 1 year.

Damage to the spinal accessory nerve is a common complication of lymph node biopsy. An incision over the lateral neck puts this nerve at risk as it crosses the sterno-cleidomastoid muscle. Patients often develop insidious shoulder pain that increases with continued use of the shoulder joint. There is weakness of the trapezius, which causes scapular winging and instability of the shoulder joint. The winging is most evident when patients abduct the shoulders to 90 degrees. Testing for weakness of the shoulder shrug is rarely useful because muscles other than the trapezius also serve this action. Depending on the level of injury, there may be weakness of the sternocleidomastoid muscle. This can be recognized by asking patients to turn their heads in the opposite direction against resistance. This injury commonly results in long-term disability because this slender nerve is usually severed and reanastomosis is difficult. Range-of-motion exercises prevent frozen shoulder but strenuous use of the joint should be avoided because it may hasten the development of degenerative arthritis.

Polyneuropathy

Polyneuropathy occasionally requires diagnostic or therapeutic intervention in surgical patients. Typical clinical features include distal numbness, tingling, or burning; weakness of distal muscles; and reduced deep tendon reflexes. Numerous metabolic, toxic, inflammatory, and hereditary causes are known. The most common etiologies are diabetes and alcoholism. Neuropathies can be conveniently divided into two categories: (a) those in which peripheral axons are primarily damaged (axonal neuropathies), and (b) those in which peripheral myelin is the primary target (demyelinating neuropathies). Secondary damage to myelin or axons can occur in either type but they can often be differentiated with nerve conduction studies and electromyography. Demyelinating neuropathies show a greater degree of conduction velocity slowing and conduction block than do axonal neuropathies.

Virtually all toxic and metabolic neuropathies are axonal, as is the neuropathy caused by vasculitis. Additionally, neuropathy may result as a complication of critical illness and sepsis. Demyelinating neuropathies are either inflammatory (Guillain–Barré syndrome or chronic inflammatory demyelinating polyneuropathy) or hereditary (most commonly the dominantly inherited Charcot–Marie–Tooth disease).

Guillain–Barré syndrome commonly occurs after an infection but may also develop during the postoperative period.[26,27] The reason for these associations is unknown. Patients usually develop tingling or numbness in the feet and hands, followed by weakness of the lower and then the upper extremities, the respiratory muscles, and the facial muscles. Deep tendon reflexes are lost or reduced and mild distal sensory loss is common. There is frequently autonomic nerve involvement, which results in fluctuations in blood pressure and pulse rate. Atypical clinical patterns are fairly common, with asymmetry, greater involvement of upper extremity or facial muscles, and a predilection for the proximal muscles occurring in individual cases. Muscle and back pain is common and the creatine kinase level is sometimes elevated (although usually less than 1000 U/l). This sometimes mimics polymyositis. The cerebrospinal fluid cell count is usually normal and the protein level elevated, although the latter is frequently normal during the first week of illness. Progression to maximum weakness usually occurs during the first few weeks but quadriplegia with respiratory paralysis may be seen as early as the first day of illness. Spontaneous recovery is the rule over several weeks to months, although a significant minority of patients retain some permanent disability.

Plasma exchange and intravenous immunoglobulin are proven to be beneficial.[28,29] Although some authorities believe that plasma exchange is still the treatment of choice because it has a longer track record, a recent study determined that plasma exchange and intravenous immunoglobulin are equally efficacious in Guillain–Barré syndrome.[30] Furthermore, this study found that both therapies used in combination were no more effective than each therapy used alone.

Careful attention to respiratory and autonomic function is probably the most important aspect of therapy for

Guillain–Barré syndrome. In patients with actively progressing disease, respiratory function should be monitored at least twice a day. When the vital capacity reaches about 15 ml/kg, elective intubation should usually be performed. Inspiratory force can be estimated by asking patients to forcefully inhale through the nose (sniff) and vital capacity can be approximated by asking them to inhale and forcefully exhale. Patients should be instructed to cough to assess their ability to clear the airway and prevent aspiration. Patients with impending respiratory failure related to neuromuscular disease typically take rapid, shallow breaths and become diaphoretic. Blood gas analysis is usually consistent with hyperventilation initially, with carbon dioxide retention being a late, preterminal finding. Patients frequently develop autonomic dysfunction. Symptoms and signs of cardiac arrhythmias, labile blood pressure, urinary retention, and gastrointestinal dysfunction should be identified and appropriately managed.

Possibly more common than Guillain–Barré syndrome, is a neuropathy associated with critical illness and sepsis. This diagnosis is usually considered when a patient "fails to wean" from the ventilator. Critical illness polyneuropathy (CIP) is characterized as an acute flaccid quadriplegia with sensory loss. The facial muscles may be mildly involved. There is weakness of the diaphragm and respiratory muscles. The reflexes are often reduced or absent. Typically the ocular muscles are spared. Compared to the Guillain–Barré syndrome, dysautonomia is not a feature of CIP. Sepsis is the major risk factor for the development of this polyneuropathy. Electrophysiologic testing and sural nerve biopsy demonstrates extensive axonal loss, distinguishing this neuropathy from the typical Guillain–Barré syndrome.[31–33] Treatment is generally supportive involving respiratory support, physical therapy and splinting weak extremities. Care should be given to protecting possible sites of nerve entrapment and thereby preventing superimposed compression neuropathies. The use of immunosuppression, plasma exchange or intravenous immunoglobulin has not led to a significant improvement in the final outcome. Overall, the prognosis for recovery is good; however, incomplete recovery with permanent neurologic residual is common.[34]

Multiple mononeuropathy

Multiple mononeuropathy is occasionally encountered after surgery. It is most commonly associated with open heart surgery, and there is a predilection for involvement of the shoulder girdle and other upper extremity nerves. The brachial plexus is susceptible to stretch injury during sternal retraction. Traction on the nerves may be responsible in some instances but the involvement of nerves distant from the incision suggests that embolic occlusion of small vessels with nerve ischemia also may be contributory. A hematoma secondary to a fracture of the first rib may compress the nearby plexus and result in a similar injury.[23] Neuralgic amyotrophy (Parsonage–Turner syndrome) is a form of multiple mononeuropathy involving an upper extremity.[35] Pain in the shoulder region is followed after a few days by weakness resulting from multiple lesions in the brachial plexus or peripheral nerves. It has occurred after viral illness and immunization, and also is seen occasionally during the postoperative period. The prognosis for multiple mononeuropathies after surgery is good, with most patients recovering after several weeks or months.

Median, ulnar, and radial nerve injury may occur in combination after placement of a shunt in the upper extremity for hemodialysis. These patients present with an acute, painful, weak arm soon after the procedure. The distal forearm and hand muscles are usually affected. There is wrist drop with additional weakness of wrist flexion and the intrinsic hand muscles. Sensation of the hand is reduced or absent. Although hematoma formation, the surgical procedure, or anesthetic technique are possible causes, ischemic injury to the peripheral nerve as a result of diversion of blood flow by the shunt is commonly implicated. Diabetic patients with peripheral neuropathy and small vessel disease appear to be at high risk for this complication. Early recognition of the problem is important because patients may improve after prompt ligation of the shunt.[12]

Myopathy

Primary myopathies rarely present clinical problems in patients undergoing surgical procedures, with the notable exception of malignant hyperthermia.[36] This causes life-threatening muscle rigidity and is precipitated by potent inhaled anesthetics and depolarizing neuromuscular blocking agents. Severe episodes are characterized by combined metabolic and respiratory acidosis (inability to ventilate because of rigidity), tachycardia, cardiac arrhythmias and myoglobinuria. Extreme hyperthermia may be a late sign. The potential for this reaction should be anticipated in anyone with a personal or family history of malignant hyperthermia. This is usually an inherited disorder with a variable pattern of inheritance. The responsible genetic defect occurs in the calcium release channel, known as the ryanodine receptor. When triggered by the anesthetic agent, there is an efflux of calcium through this channel into the sarcoplasm, which results in contraction of the muscle fiber.[37] Although the ryanodine receptor has a major role, there are multiple genetic alleles and loci where a mutation may result in an increased susceptibility for the development of malignant hyperthermia.[38] Dantrolene is a calcium channel blocker used to treat an episode. Rapid recognition of the syndrome, discontinuation of the inciting medications and treatment with dantrolene has significantly reduced the mortality. It is given at a rate of 2 mg/kg every 5 minutes to a total dose of 10 mg/kg. There appears to be an increased incidence of malignant hyperthermia in patients with other myopathies, most notably central core disease (a congenital myopathy) and Duchenne muscular dystrophy. Patients with myotonic dystrophy occasionally experience transient rigidity after the administration of succinylcholine but the mechanism for this is probably different and treatment usually is not required. Safe anesthetic agents for these patients include nitrous oxide, thiopental, opiates, droperidol, and pancuronium.

Similar to, and often confused with, the polyneuropathy that develops in the context of critical illness and sepsis, acute quadriplegic myopathy may result in the surgical patient who has a prolonged course in the intensive care unit. It usually is considered when the patient "fails to wean" from the ventilator. The patient develops weakness of respiration and the extremities with retained sensation. The deep tendon reflexes may be normal or slightly reduced. In severe cases the reflexes may be absent. Important features that distinguish the myopathy from the polyneuropathy, such as retained sensation, may be difficult to identify due to coexisting encephalopathy and mechanical ventilation. The myopathy occurs in conjunction with asthma, the use of corticosteroids, non-depolarizing neuromuscular blocking agents and aminoglycosides.[39] In addition, this myopathy may occur during critical illness and sepsis in the absence of treatment with corticosteroids or non-depolarizing neuromuscular blocking agents.[40] In ideal situations nerve conduction studies reveal low amplitude motor nerve responses with normal sensory nerve responses. Electromyography may reveal acute denervation potentials and myopathic motor unit potentials with early recruitment. Although the underlying mechanism for the development of the myopathy is not known, a plausible explanation is a multi-factorial process that includes a combination of steroids, sepsis, pharmacological or immunological denervation of muscle and the patient's immobilization due to the critical illness.[41] Some investigators convincingly showed that electrical inexcitability of muscle tissue occurs in acute quadriplegic

myopathy.[42,43] Steroids and humeral changes that occur during sepsis are theorized to result in the changes in the electrical properties of neural tissue. Overall, the prognosis for the return of neurologic function is good if the concurrent medical illness resolves. Specific treatment for acute quadriplegic myopathy is largely supportive. Mechanical ventilation, physical therapy and protection of common sites of nerve compression should be performed as needed.

REFERENCES

1. Johns, T. R. & Howard, J. F., eds. Myasthenia gravis. *Semin. Neurol.* 1982; **2**: 193–280.
2. Phillips, L. H. & Melnick, P. A. Diagnosis of myasthenia gravis in the1990's. *Semin. Neurol.* 1990; **10**: 62–69.
3. Somnier, F. E. Clinical implementation of anti-acetylcholine receptor antibodies. *J. Neurol. Neurosurg. Psychiatry* 1993; **56**: 496–504.
4. Finley, J. C. & Pascuzzi, R. M. Rational therapy of myasthenia gravis. *Semin. Neurol.* 1990; **10**: 70–82.
5. Bromberg, M. B., Wald, J. J., Forshew, D. A., Feldman, E. L., & Albers, J. W. Randomized trial of azathioprine or prednisone for initial immunosuppressive treatment of myasthenia gravis. *J. Neurol. Sci.* 1997; **150**: 59–62.
6. Myasthenia Gravis Clinical Study Group. A randomized clinical trial comparing prednisone and Azathioprine in myasthenia gravis. Results of the second interim analysis. *J. Neurol. Neurosurg. Psychiatry.* 1993; **56**: 1157–1163.
7. Tindall, R. S., Phillips, J. T., Rollins, J. A., Wells, L., & Hall, K. A clinical therapeutic trial of cyclosporine in myasthenia gravis. *Ann. NY Acad. Sci.* 1993; **681**: 539–551.
8. Tindall, R. S., Rollins, J. A., Phillips, J. T., Greenlee, R. G., Wells, L., & Belendiuk, G. Preliminary results of a double-blind, randomized, placebo-controlled trial of cyclosporine in myasthenia gravis. *N. Engl. J. Med.* 1987; **316**: 719–724.
9. Hauser, R. A., Malek, A. R., & Rosen, R. Successful treatment of a patient with severe refractory myasthenia gravis using mycophenolate mofetil. *Neurology* **51**: 912–913.
10. Ciafoloni, E., Massey, J. M., Tucker-Lipscomb, B., & Sanders, D. B. Mycophenolate mofetil for myasthenia gravis: an open-label pilot study. *Neurology* **56**: 97–99.
11. Gronseth, G. S. & Barohn, R. J. Practice parameter: thymectomy for autoimmune myasthenia gravis (an evidence-based review). *Neurology* 2000; **55**: 7–15.
12. Arsura, E. L., Bick, A., Brunuer, N. C. *et al.* High-dose intravenous immunoglobulin in the management of myasthenia gravis. *Arch. Intern. Med.* 1986; **146**: 1365–1368.
13. Wittbrodt, E. T. Drugs and myasthenia gravis: an update. *Arch. Intern. Med.* 1997; **157**: 399–408.
14. Howard, J. F. Adverse drug effects on neuromuscular transmission. *Semin. Neurol.* 1990; **10**: 89–102.
15. Krendel, D. Hypermagnesemia and neuromuscular transmission. *Semin. Neurol.* 1990; **10**: 42–45.

16. Pascuzzi, R. M. & Kim, Y. I. Lambert–Eaton syndrome. *Semin. Neurol.* 1990; **10**: 35–41.

17. Murray, M. J., Cowen, J., De Block, H. *et al.* Clinical practice guidelines for sustained neuromuscular blockade in the adult critically ill patient. *Crit. Care Med.* 2002; **30**: 142–156.

18. Upton, R. M. & McComas, A. J. The double crush in nerve entrapment syndromes. *Lancet* 1973; **11**: 359–362.

19. Stewart, J. D. The radial nerve. In Stewart, J. D., ed. *Focal Peripheral Neuropathies.* New York: Elsevier Science Publishing, 1987: 194–210.

20. Stewart, J. D. The ulnar nerve. In Stewart, J. D., ed. *Focal Peripheral Neuropathies.* New York: Elsevier Science Publishing, 1987: 163–193.

21. Stewart, J. D. The common peroneal nerve. In Stewart, J. D., ed. *Focal Peripheral Neuropathies.* New York: Elsevier Science Publishing, 1987: 290–306.

22. Warner, M. A., Warner, D. O., Harper, C. M., Schroeder, D. R., & Maxson, P. M. Lower extremity neuropathies associated with lithotomy positions. *Anesthesiology* 2000; **93**: 938–942.

23. Sharma, A. D., Parmley, C. L., Sreeram, G., & Grocott, H. P. Peripheral nerve injures during cardiac surgery: risk factors, diagnosis, prognosis and prevention. *Anesth. Analg.* 2000; **91**: 1358–1369.

24. Stewart, J. D. The femoral and saphenous nerves. In Stewart, J. D., ed. *Focal Peripheral Neuropathies.* New York: Elsevier Science, 1987: 322–332.

25. Riggs, J. E., Moss, A. H., Labosky, D. A. *et al.* Upper extremity ischemic monomelic neuropathy: a complication of vascular access procedures in uremic diabetic patients. *Neurology* 1989; **39**: 997–998.

26. Hughes, R. A. C. Epidemiology. In Hughes, R. A. C., ed. *Guillain–Barré Syndrome.* London: Springer-Verlag, 1990: 101–119.

27. Arnason, B. G. & Asbury, A. K. Idiopathic polyneuritis after surgery. *Arch. Neurol.* 1968; **18**: 500–507.

28. Guillain–Barré Syndrome Study Group. Plasmapheresis and acute Guillain–Barré syndrome. *Neurology* 1985; **35**: 1096–1104.

29. Van der Meché, F. G. A. & Schmitz, P. I. M. A randomized trial comparing intravenous immune globulin and plasma exchange in Guillain-Barré syndrome. *N. Engl. J. Med.* 1992; **326**: 1123–1129.

30. Plasma Exchange/Sandoglobulin Guillain–Barré Syndrome Trial Group. Randomized trial of plasma exchange, intravenous immunoglobulin, and combined treatments in Guillain–Barré Syndrome. *Lancet* 1997; **349**: 225–230.

31. Bolton, C. F. Electrophysiologic studies of critically ill patients. *Muscle Nerve* 1987; **10**: 129–135.

32. Bolton, C. F., Gilbert, J. J., Hahn, A. F., & Sibbald, W. J. Polyneuropathy in critically ill patients. *J. Neurol. Neurosurg. Psychiatry* 1984; **47**: 1223–1231.

33. Bolton, C. F., Laverty, D. A., Brown, J. D., Witt, N. J., Hahn, A. F., & Sibbald, W. J. Critically ill polyneuropathy: electrophysiological studies and differentiation form Guillain-Barré syndrome. *J. Neurol. Neurosurg. Psychiatry* 1986; **49**: 563–573.

34. Witt, N. J., Zochodne, D. W., Bolton, C. F. *et al.* Peripheral nerve function in sepsis and multiple organ failure. *Chest* 1991; **99**: 176–184.

35. Rubin, D. I. Neuralgic amyotrophy: clinical features and diagnostic evaluation. *Neurologist* 2001; **7**: 350–356.

36. Gromert, G. A. Malignant hyperthermia. In Engel, A. C. & Bank, B. Q., eds. *Myology.* New York: McGraw-Hill, 1986: 1763–1784.

37. Baraka, A. S. & Jalbout, M. L. Anesthesia and myopathy. *Curr. Opin. Anaesthesiol.* 2002; **15**: 371–376.

38. Hogan, K. The anesthetic myopathies and malignant hyperthermias. *Curr. Opin. Neurol.* 1998; **11**: 469–476.

39. MacFarlane, I. A. & Rosenthal, F. D. Severe myopathy after status asthmaticus. *Lancet* 1977; **2**: 615.

40. Latronico, N., Fenzi, F., Recupero, D. *et al.* Critical illness myopathy and neuropathy. *Lancet* 1996; **347**: 1570–1582.

41. Hund, E. Myopathy in critically ill. *Crit. Care Med.* 1999; **27**: 2544–2547.

42. Rich, M. M., Bird, S. J., Raps, E. C., Mc Cluçkey, L. F., & Teener, J. W. Direct muscle stimulation in acute quadriplegic myopathy. *Muscle Nerve* 1997; **20**: 665–673.

43. Trojaborg, W., Weimer, L. H., & Hays, A. P. Electrophysiologic studies in critical illness associated weakness: myopathy or neuropathy – a reappraisal. *Clin. Neurophysiol.* 2001; **112**: 1586–1593.

35

Perioperative management of patients with Parkinson's disease

Jorge L. Juncos

Emory University School of Medicine, Atlanta, GA

Introduction and overview of Parkinson's disease

Patients with Parkinson's disease (PD) face surgery more often than their age-matched counterparts due to injuries provoked by the gait and balance difficulties that characterize the advanced stages of this illness. Recent advances in neurosurgical techniques and an improved understanding of the pathophysiology of motor symptoms in PD has led to a renewed interest and an increase in the number of patients under going various neurosurgical procedures for PD. This chapter provides an overview of the principles and preoperative management of patients with Parkinson's disease (PD) and other parkinsonian states.

Parkinson's disease is an adult-onset neurodegenerative disorder characterized by progressive slowness of movement (bradykinesia), muscular rigidity, tremor, short stepped and stooped gait, and varying degrees of cognitive impairment. It affects close to 1 million mostly elderly Americans with an annual incidence of 20 new cases per 100 000 and a prevalence of 130 cases per 100 000. Its primary pathology is limited to the brain and consists of selective degeneration of the nigrostriatal dopaminergic pathway and the presence of Lewy bodies and Lewy neurites in surviving mesencephalic dopamine neurons, as well as in other brainstem and cortical neurons. Biochemically, the denervation results in striatal dopamine depletion which is linked to the above signs and symptoms. The cause of selective neuronal death, and therefore the etiology of PD is unknown, although hereditary and environmental factors are thought to play a role.

Given the motor symptoms of PD, it is not surprising that they can interfere in the operative and perioperative management of PD. Tremor can make the electrocardiographic or electroencephalographic monitoring of patients difficult in the awake patient (e.g., regional or spinal anesthesia; stereotactic neurosurgery). General anesthesia will instead suppress tremor. The rigidity of PD can involve the chest wall limiting ventilatory reserve increasing the risk of hypoventilation and atelectasis during the postoperative period. Although swallowing is not generally affected in the early stages of PD, acute dysphagia can result from abrupt withdrawal of antiparkinsonian medications during the perioperative period. Vasomotor instability and autonomic dysfunction affects many patients with PD. For instance, asymptomatic orthostatic hypotension can become clinically significant under the influence of anesthetics, analgesics, benzodiazepines and antiemetics, a situation compounded by any unanticipated delay in resuming antiparkinsonian medications after surgery. Other autonomic defects include urinary hesitancy, severe constipation and paroxysmal autonomic discharges with profuse sweating and flushing. Postoperatively these defects can lead to urinary retention, obstipation, ileus, and dehydration.

Parkinsonian symptoms with more severe forms of autonomic failure suggest alternate diagnosis like multiple systems atrophy (MSA) also known as Shy–Drager syndrome. These patients typically have a history of orthostatic syncope, are at high risk of complications and require special planning of anesthesia and surgery.

Cognitive slowing can parallel the slowing of motor function and make patients with PD particularly sensitive to psychoactive drugs and anesthesia leading to postoperative confusion and hallucinations. This risk is particularly high in patients with PD and dementia and dementia can affect up to 80% of patients with advanced PD. The severity of dementia in PD is highly variable. Nonetheless, even mildly demented patients have a significantly increased risk of postoperative delirium. The most common forms of dementia in PD are due to

Medical Management of the Surgical Patient: A Textbook of Perioperative Medicine, ed. M. F. Lubin, R. B. Smith, T. F. Dobson, N. Spell, H. K. Walker. 4th edn. Published by Cambridge University Press. © Cambridge University 2006.

coexisting senile dementia of the Alzheimer type (SDAT), to dementia with Lewy bodies, and a combination of both. These dementias can be differentiated with the help of detailed neuropsychologic tests a review of which is beyond the scope of this chapter. Nonetheless, the principles outlined here apply to all forms of dementia in PD.

Finally, up to 50% of patients with PD have comorbid affective illnesses ranging from cyclothymia, and major depression, to anxiety disorders with panic. Unrecognized active symptomatology in these domains can impair cognition and increase the risk of perioperative complications in PD.

Symptomatic treatment of PD aims to re-establish dopamine transmission in the striatum. This strategy involves: (a) enhancing the cerebral availability of levodopa, the precursor amino acid of dopamine, (b) using direct dopamine agonists (ropinirole, pramipexole, cabergoline, pergolide or bromocriptine) to stimulate post-synaptic dopamine receptors directly, (c) blocking the peripheral breakdown of levodopa by the enzyme cathechol-O-methyl transferase (COMT) using COMT inhibitors like entacapone or tolcapone, and (d) blocking the oxidative breakdown of dopamine at the synapse with the selective monoamine oxidase A (MAO-A) inhibitor selegiline and rasagiline. Adjunctive therapy includes anticholinergics like trihexyphenidyl and benztropine, and amantadine, a weak glutamate (N-methyl-D-aspartame or NMDA) receptor antagonist with anticholinergic properties. These drugs are likely to contribute to postoperative confusion and delirium as the many other drugs that have been identified as risk factors for postoperative delirium in the elderly. As noted above, abrupt discontinuation of antiparkinsonian medications in preparation for surgery can also lead to acute confusion. In this center our impression is that this reaction is more likely with higher doses of antiparkinsonian drugs and appears to be a dose dependent phenomenon.

Drug-induced increases in parkinsonian signs and symptoms can be transient or chronic. It may involve the antiparkinsonian drugs, parkinson-promoting drugs or other drug interactions as noted below. Transient aggravation of symptoms is typified by motor fluctuations which result from the interaction between disease progression and the chronic use and schedule of antiparkinsonian therapy. Motor fluctuations range from the premature or sudden termination of drug effects ("off spells"), to an excessive and aberrant sensitivity to therapy (i.e., "denervation hypersensitivity") that leads to dyskinesias and dystonias ("on" symptomatology). The fluctuations are mediated in part by the progressive loss of dopamine nerve end terminals which destroys the ability of the

striatum to buffer fluxes in dopamine availability. In PD the cerebral availability of dopamine is subject to fluctuations in plasma levodopa levels. These in turn reflect levodopa's short half-life (about 2 hours when given with carbidopa) and its intermittent oral administration. Because levodopa is absorbed primarily in the proximal small intestine, its availability is also subject to the vagaries of gastric emptying, a function of a myriad of other factors including the timing, quantity and composition of meals.

Chronic toxicity from antiparkinsonian drug therapy may also involve affective and cognitive functions. These include visual hallucinations, sleep disturbances (insomnia and hypersomnia), sleep phenomena such as vivid dreams (rapid eye movement-related behavioral disturbances such as screaming and punching during sleep) and nocturnal myoclonus (leg jerking). More subtle and insidious are personality changes that evolve over weeks to months. These consist of increasingly demanding and selfish attitudes, intolerance to any discomfort, and a seeming unawareness of impositions on other family members. It is important to recognize these early signs because their presence suggests that the threshold for postanesthetic delirium is low. In a delirious PD patient, motor symptoms respond poorly to drug therapy, and increasing drug therapy will only aggravate the delirium. Abrupt discontinuation of antiparkinsonian therapy also carries the risk of a reaction as detailed under dopamine withdrawal syndrome.

Preoperative management

General medical considerations

The preoperative medical evaluation of patients with PD, regardless of age, is not unlike that of other elderly patients. Areas that require special attention in PD are outlined below.

In PD mild pharyngeal dysfunction leads to decreased spontaneous swallowing, accumulation of saliva in the posterior pharynx and sialorrhea. With sedating this otherwise minor dysfunction may worsen acutely and result in aspiration during the immediate postoperative period. To avoid this, frequent and extended suctioning is needed. Pharyngeal dysfunction may predispose PD patients to severe laryngospasm if all antiparkinsonian therapy is removed abruptly and the staff should be prepared to provide the extra care necessary.

Pulmonary status also needs special attention since pulmonary function tests often reveal restrictive pulmonary deficits even in asymptomatic PD patients. These abnormalities are partially relieved by levodopa therapy. Their restrictive qualities are due to the postural abnormalities (stooping, scoliosis), the rigidity of the chest wall musculature, and the advanced spinal osteoarthritis often associated with the illness. If asymptomatic, the patient does not need more than a routine preoperative evaluation consisting of a good history, chest exam and roentgenogram. If the pulmonary reserve is in doubt, abbreviated pulmonary function tests with arterial blood gases should be considered. Patients with PD do poorly once they develop pneumonia. This is due to easy fatigability, decreased respiratory capacity, and a weak cough reflex.

The autonomic nervous system is of particular interest in PD. Although PD patients technically do not have autonomic failure, they can have autonomic instability and special sensitivity to drugs that may cause hypotension, including antiparkinsonian drugs. Constipation is a universal problem and is taken for granted by many patients. Many have a tendency to delay evacuation and to rely on suppositories and enemas to do so. Constipation may be a source of abdominal distention, ileus or obstruction. Distention of the rectosigmoid may be a source of urinary retention and lead to urinary tract infection. These problems need to be detected before surgery because they can be compounded by the anesthesia and by the postoperative opiate analgesia.

Neurologic considerations

PD is the most common of a host of neurologic illnesses that look like, but are not idiopathic PD. These disorders present special management problems that need to be anticipated. Perhaps the two most important disorders to differentiate from PD are multiple systems atrophy (MSA) and progressive supranuclear palsy (PSP). Like PD they are both progressive neurodegenerative disorders of unknown etiology where slowness, rigidity and gait impairment are prominent. In contrast to PD, tremor is often absent, the course is more rapid and the response to therapy is poor. MSA features prominent autonomic failure which may influence the surgical decision and the strategy of anesthesia. Signs of autonomic failure include impotence, unexplained urinary dysfunction, postural hypotension, abnormal conduction or repolarization on electrocardiography and impaired sweating.

PSP features loss of supranuclear gaze control (e.g., decreased vertical and later horizontal gaze) described by patients as "trouble reading" not related to a refraction error. Patients note trouble walking downstairs (failure of down gaze), and when advanced, difficulty looking for items on a table. In addition, patients develop axial dystonia out of proportion to the appendicular rigidity which is the opposite of what is normally encountered in PD. Rigidity of the neck may make endotracheal intubation difficult and does not respond well to the usual perioperative muscle relaxants. Patients with MSA and PSP may be more prone to sleep apnea and other respiratory abnormalities than PD patients, and so may be more sensitive to sedatives and hypnotics. This diagnostic outline is meant to raise an index of suspicion for MSA and PSP when evaluating preoperative parkinsonian patients. Appropriate neurologic consultation should be sought when these entities are suspected.

Cervical spondylosis is not infrequent in PD, in part due to the affected age group and the accelerated osteoarthritic changes that stem from akinesia. Clinically significant cervical spondylosis may be adversely affected by a difficult intubation. Although not a contraindication to intubation, it may influence the route (nasotracheal versus oral) and preparation. Clinical signs of cervical spondylosis include neck and shoulder pain, pain radiating down the arms, leg and gait spasticity, hyperactive reflexes in the legs, brisk to patchy reflexes in the arms and extensor plantar responses. Of note is that similar findings due to cerebral rather than cervical pathology are common in PSP.

The presence of dementia significantly increases the risk of perioperative confusion and delirium. As mentioned earlier, dementia is found in approximately 15 to 20% of patients with PD and remains undetected in its early stages. The Mini Mental Status (MMS) exam is a simple, expeditious but unfortunately relatively insensitive tool to screen for dementia. Early on, a history of ill-defined occupational, personal and financial difficulties, loss of interest in hobbies, vague memory complaints and personality changes may be more sensitive indicators of dementia than the MMS. Pseudodementia due to depression is probably a more common cause of these complaints than SDAT. Depression affects >40% of patients at some point in the illness and is usually accompanied by vegetative signs such as poor sleep and appetite, weight loss and asthenia.

Pharmacotherapeutic issues

Drug interactions which may have been tolerated preoperatively may become critical postoperatively and thus need to be identified in the initial evaluation. The following is a brief review of parkinsonian drug therapy and how it may need to be altered perioperatively. Table 35.1 lists commonly prescribed drugs which may aggravate

Table 35.1. Drugs contraindicated in Parkinson's disease

Drug category	Generic name
Dopamine antagonists	
• antipsychotics	- haloperidol
	- perphenazine
	- chlorpromazine
	- triflouperazine
	- flufenazine
	- thiothixene
	- thioridazine
	- loxapine
• antiemetics	- compazine
	- metoclopramide
	- thiethylperazine
	- droperidol
Antidepressants	- combinations of perphenazine and amitriptyline (Triavil™, Etrafon™)
	- phenelzine (MAO inhibitor)
	- tranylcypromine (MAO inhibitor)
Narcotics	- meperidine
	- fentanyl
Antihypertensives and miscellaneous postoperative medications	- reserpine
	- tetrabenazine
	- alpha methylparatyrosine
	- rauwolfia serpentina
	- rauverid
	- wolfina
	- deserpine
	- rescinnamine
	- rauwiloid
Drugs with lesser potential to aggravate symptoms	- alpha-methyldopa
	- phenytoin
	- lithium carbonate
	- buspirone

Note:

MAO = monoamine oxidase

parkinsonian signs and which should be avoided in parkinsonian patients.

The mainstay therapy of PD is still levodopa. It is administered in the form of carbidopa/levodopa to minimize the incidence of peripheral side effects such as nausea and hypotension. Carbidopa is a peripheral dopa decarboxylase inhibitor which blocks the conversion of levodopa to dopamine. Peripheral conversion of levodopa to dopamine is believed to be responsible for many of levodopa's side effects. To effectively block peripheral dopa decarboxylase, doses of carbidopa should be 75 mg/day, that

is, three tablets of carbidopa/levodopa (25/100) or two tablets of controlled release carbidopa/levodopa (50/200) [Sinemet CR¨]. Dopamine agonists are more potent than levodopa but not as effective at alleviating symptoms, particularly when used as monotherapy (e.g., bromocriptine, pergolide)

The hypotensive effect of levodopa is probably due to a central mechanism and may be more pronounced in patients with high baseline blood pressures. The hypotensive effect of dopamine agonists is caused by several mechanisms: (a) relaxation of vascular smooth muscle in splanchnic and renal circulation, (b) inhibition of noradrenergic nerve endings, and (c) central inhibition of sympathetic activity. Dopamine agonists have a higher incidence of severe hypotension and other side effects than levodopa. Accordingly, and unlike levodopa, administration of dopamine agonists can be halted the night prior to surgery and not resumed until the patient is stable.

As noted, levodopa and dopamine agonists can also precipitate cardiac arrhythmias and delirium. When used in chronic, stable doses and stopped before surgery, these complications tend to be minor and manageable and do not require routine discontinuation of the drugs. If concerns over perioperative hypovolemia exist, dopamine agonists should be reduced over 2 to 3 weeks before considering reductions in the levodopa dose. If the baseline dose of levodopa is high (e.g., >800 mg/d), it too may be decreased slowly to approximately 300–400 mg/day. This should be attempted only if the risks of hypovolemia outweigh the postoperative discomfort the patient is likely to experience as a consequence of increased symptoms.

Ancillary antiparkinsonian therapy such as anticholinergics and amantadine may increase the risk of postoperative delirium but should not be stopped abruptly or withheld for extended periods. Abrupt withdrawal of these and other antiparkinsonian medications may result in acute exacerbation and relative unresponsiveness of parkinsonian symptoms. If the individual is not demented nor exhibits signs of drug-induced delirium, the likelihood of this complication is small thus the drugs need not be changed. If dementia or delirium is suspected, these drugs should be tapered or stopped over 2 to 4 weeks.

Special consideration should be given to the use of selegiline, an MAO B inhibitor devoid of the hypertensive reactions to tyramine and other amino acids characteristic of non-selective MAO A or AB inhibitors (see Table 35.1). Selegiline is used to enhance the efficacy of levodopa but it can also accentuate its side effects. Because of its long biologic half-life, it can be discontinued without tapering. The concomitant use of meperidine and selegiline should be avoided due to potentially serious adverse reactions (delirium). Based on studies in laboratory animals, selegiline should also be avoided in patients with active peptic ulcer disease. The use of non-selective MAO inhibitors in combination with the selective serotonin reuptake inhibitor (SSRI), fluoxetine, can lead to acute "serotonergic" reactions characterized by delirium, rigidity and fever. A similar interaction with selegiline has not been reported. In PD, however, fluoxetine may aggravate parkinsonian symptoms, and in combination with selegiline, may lead to acute mania.

Non-selective MAO inhibitors should be discontinued at least 2 weeks before surgery. Selegiline probably does not need to be stopped preoperatively for the reasons mentioned above. Nonetheless, as a general precaution we recommend stopping selegiline 1 week prior to surgery to minimize the risk of perioperative drug interactions. The symptomatic effect of selegiline on PD symptoms is rather modest compared to that of levodopa and dopamine agonists, thus stopping the drugs over a few days generally does not result in serious motor deterioration.

In the case of prolonged cerebral stereotactic procedures performed with the patient awake, consideration should be given to providing small doses orally with minuscule amounts of water or to providing an intraduodenal infusion of carbidopa/levodopa to maintain patient comfort (as described below).

Anesthesia management

The specific choice of anesthetics is made by the anesthesiologist in consultation with the treating neurologist. The choice of general over regional anesthesia should be determined by the usual considerations. When appropriate, local or regional anesthesia is preferred over general anesthesia with the provision that the first two provide less control of parkinsonian or drug-induced hypoventilation than the latter. Neuroleptanesthesia is not recommended due to the use of agents (e.g., droperidol) that antagonize dopamine transmission in the brain and elsewhere. Experience has shown that the potential arrhythmogenic and myocardial depressant effects of chronic dopamine-induced depletion of myocardial catecholamines is rather small. In brief, the anesthetic strategy should maintain a balance between inadequate anesthesia with its accompanying autonomic nervous system stimulation, and a needlessly deep anesthesia with its concomitant cardiopulmonary depressant effects.

Good anesthetic control of PD patients has been reported using thiopental or diazepam induction followed by enflurane and nitrous oxide for anesthesia/analgesia. More recently Hyman et al. reported a favorable experience using nitrous oxide and sufentanil infusion anesthesia and vencuronium for muscle relaxation in patients undergoing autologous transplantation of adrenal medulla to brain. Fentanyl analgesia should be used with caution since it can increase muscle tone, a problem already present in PD patients. General precautions such as anticipating tachycardias in response to pancuronium or hypotension in response to d-tubocurare are particularly important in patients with PD. Intraoperatively, the appearance of a fine body tremor may be misinterpreted as ventricular fibrillation on cardiac monitor since the typical parkinsonian tremor may be absent from the limbs.

Intra- and perioperative nasogastric suction may help reduce the risks and consequences of nausea and vomiting, particularly in PD patients where most antiemetics are contraindicated. Following surgery competitive muscle relaxants must be fully reversed to avoid compromising ventilatory function.

Postoperative management

General medical considerations

The postoperative care of PD patients is much like that of other elderly patients. Special emphasis should be placed on airway protection, chest physiotherapy with incentive spirometry and postural drainage, early mobilization and avoiding aspiration. PD patients may require more time to wake up from anesthesia but should be awake by the evening of the day of surgery. Surgical and postsurgical complications such as pain, infection and blood loss can lead to a protracted, poor response to antiparkinsonian medication. This poor response is also seen in ambulatory patients with mild medical problems such as urinary tract infections. The mechanisms in both cases are unknown but attempts to fine tune symptoms at this time are futile and ill-advised. Patients generally recuperate on their own within days to weeks after surgery without a change in medication.

Postoperative psychosis can develop upon awakening from anesthesia or the onset can be delayed as long as 5 to 7 days with many patients exhibiting the first signs after returning home. Immediate postoperative delirium may be caused by the intraoperative use of atropine, by acute metabolic derangement, or by the withdrawal reactions noted above. Delayed onset delirium does not appear to be related to a particular anesthetic or to the choice of anti-parkinsonian drug therapy and clears spontaneously within three days.

Parkinsonian motor symptoms, including so called "off" spells, can be severely debilitating following surgery. Although the symptoms can mimic other postoperative problems, they should not be assumed to be due to par-kinsonism until medical and surgical postoperative complications have been ruled out. "Off" symptoms include profound feelings of "weakness", shortness of breath (air hunger), urinary retention, anxiety and intense tremor. These "adrenergically charged" reactions, if persistent, can be arrhythmogenic. "On" spells consist of abnormal involuntary movements and muscle contractions termed dykinesias and dystonias. The latter can be particularly painful.

Constipation which should have been dealt with aggres-sively preoperatively, needs to be managed gingerly post-operatively when vital signs may be unstable. Aggressive treatment of constipation postoperatively with enemas or disimpaction can elicit vagal reflexes with concomitant bradycardia and hypotension. Several articles elaborate on specific interventions that address these and other important nursing issues.

Postoperative dysphagia or unconsciousness may make oral antiparkinsonian therapy impractical or nearly impossible. With excellent nursing care, patients with mild to moderate PD who were on small doses of medica-tion can probably remain unmedicated for a week or longer if necessary. Past this time they lose the long dura-tion response to levodopa and may reach levels of disabil-ity that may compromise their respiratory function and overall recovery. If the gastrointestinal tract is functional, levodopa can be given directly into the duodenum using a levodopa/carbidopa solution fed through a silastic tube with a weighted mercury tip. This technique is discussed under pharmacologic interventions below. In patients with a functional gastrointestinal tract, with advanced disease and who require high doses of medication, enteral administration of liquid carbidopa/levodopa should be started as soon as possible after surgery.

Dopamine withdrawal syndrome

Sudden withdrawal of all antiparkinsonian therapy in PD can lead to a dopamine withdrawal syndrome which clini-cally resembles the better known neuroleptic malignant syndrome (NMS). The onset of this potentially fatal syn-drome is usually 24 to 72 hours following abrupt with-drawal dopaminomimetic drug. It is thought to be mediated by acute cerebral dopamine depletion. NMS in

contrast has been linked to an aberrant and acute antag-onism (blockage) or cerebral dopamine receptors for which there may be individual (genetic?) predisposition. Fully developed, it is characterized by alterations in men-tal status (delirium to coma), hyperpyrexia, autonomic instability, muscular rigidity, acidosis, rhabdomyolysis and renal failure. Prompt resumption of antiparkinsonian therapy is key. Other therapeutic measures are discussed below under pharmacologic management. The differen-tial diagnosis includes malignant hyperthermia from exposure to anesthetics, sepsis, exposure to antiemetics and drugs used to alleviate gastric paresis (metoclopra-mide), tricyclic antidepressants with lithium, stimulants (cocaine, amphetamines), and some anticonvulsants.

Pharmacotherapeutic management

Liquid levodopa was mentioned above and has been used in numerous patients with PD to treat motor fluctuations. It has been administered either by constant enteral infu-sion or by intermittent oral bolus. Postoperative PD patients may also benefit from these delivery strategies when intubated or unconscious. The solution can be pre-pared by pulverizing and dissolving ten tablets of regular carbidopa/levodopa 10/100 in 1000 ml of tap water with one gram of ascorbic acid to yield a 1 mg/ml solution of levodopa. Depending on how well the tablet is pulverized, the solution may need to be filtered (using a regular coffee filter) to remove particulate matter. The solution is stable for at least 24 hours when refrigerated and protected from light. Levodopa is relatively insoluble in a basic medium and will not dissolve at concentration >2 mg/ml. Ascorbic acid serves to acidify the solution and prevent the oxida-tion of levodopa and dopamine. Carbidopa is much less soluble than levodopa but apparently enough gets into solution to block nausea and vomiting. Dosing guidelines can be extrapolated from the following example: if the patient uses 100 mg of levodopa every 4 hours, the infu-sion rate can start at 25 ml/h and then be adjusted accord-ing to the clinical response.

Postoperative patients with a non-functional gastro-intestinal tract have few options to treat PD symptoms. Repeated parenteral injection of anticholinergics such as benztropine has been advocated, but their use can lead to a slower recovery of gastrointestinal function, and in the elderly, to delirium. Subcutaneous injections and infusion of soluble dopamine agonists like apomorphine and lisur-ide have been used successfully in Europe and Canada for this purpose. Unfortunately these drugs are not available in the U.S. and their use is limited by the need to orally administer a peripheral dopamine blocker to control the nausea they produce. Domperidone is the antiemetic of choice for this purpose. It is a peripheral dopamine blocker which improves gastric emptying. Its approval for use in this country is under consideration by the FDA, but it is unclear whether it will be available in oral as well as parenteral forms.

The management of postoperative emesis presents another dilemma in PD patients. In mild cases nasogastric suctioning and small doses of benadryl or benzodiazepines (weak antiemetics) may work at the expense of sedating the patient. Conventional antiemetics may aggravate parkinsonism by virtue of their dopamine antagonisms. Other limiting side effects include sedation, dysphoria and hallucinations. In patients with mild PD where nasogastric suctioning fails, and who are not psychotic, the short-term use of these agents in low doses may be tolerated with only modest aggravation of parkinsonian signs. In this case we favor the cautious use of metoclopramine and thiethylperazine before compazine or droperidol. Patients with advanced disease, or with marked dystonic clinical features may not tolerate even small doses of these agents.

Nausea and vomiting in levodopa treated patients is thought to be mediated by the stimulation of dopamine receptors in the area postrema of the brainstem. In contrast, perioperative emesis is multifactorial. Ondansetron, a selective 5-HT3 serotonin receptor blocker, is effective in the treatment of perioperative nausea and vomiting in non-parkinsonian patients. Although ondansetron does not block dopamine receptors, it may be effective in treating postoperative emesis in PD through alternate mechanisms. Unlike conventional antiemetics, a recent report suggests ondasetrom may be devoid of extrapyramidal side effects in PD. Finally domperidone may be another promising candidate to alleviate postoperative nausea in PD without aggravating parkinsonism.

In PD patients meperidine should be avoided as noted above.

Postoperative situations unique to PD

Transient antiparkinsonian treatment failure

PD patients often experience transient periods of poor response to therapy following surgery, as noted above. This phenomenon is poorly understood, but like emesis, is probably also multifactorial. Suspected causes include a lingering depressant effect of general anesthetics and analgesics, and a slowing of gastric emptying which results in delayed and incomplete levodopa absorption. These partial explanations notwithstanding, there is, at best, a modest correlation between the complexity, duration and smoothness of the operative procedure and the patients' postoperative antiparkinsonian response. It seems that the stress of anesthesia makes the clinical heterogeneity of the illness more apparent. Patients with parkinson-like disorders (i.e., MSA, PSP, PD/SDAT) tend to do less well than patients with idiopathic PD. Other than good medical care and reassurance, no other specific neurologic measures need to be taken since the patients generally return to baseline within one to two months. A few complain they never return to their preoperative level of parkinsonian function, an unexplained situation that may be due to unmasking of disease progression.

Postoperative delirium

Delirium is a major concern in the postoperative care of PD patients and the elderly in general. As noted above, antiparkinsonian drugs may act synergistically with the various anesthetics and analgesics to promote a protracted alteration in mental status. The use of intraoperative atropine is another source of delirium. In most patients the delirium is quiet and manifested only by confusion and hallucinosis without agitation. In these cases observation and supportive care by staff and family may be sufficient. Polypharmacy, in particular antiparkinsonian polypharmacy should be avoided or simplified using the above guidelines. Although levodopa therapy should not be withdrawn entirely, ancillary therapy such as anticholinergics, amantadine and selegiline can be withdrawn as the situation warrants. If additional intervention is necessary, dopamine agonists can also be reduced or withdrawn over a few days while remaining vigilant for signs of the dopamine withdrawal syndrome.

If the above actions fails, or if the patient is in danger of hurting himself or others, a low potency neuroleptic like mesoridazine, molindone or thioridazine should be considered. These compounds are used for their sedative, anxiolytic and antipsychotic effects. Mesoridazine offers the advantage of being available in parenteral (25 mg/ml) and liquid (1 mg/ml) forms. It can be started at low doses (1 to 2 mg/d) and quickly titrated to control behavior while monitoring vital signs and extrapyramidal motor function. Molindone is available in 5 mg, 10 mg and larger tablet sizes, and should be used in the lowest possible dose. Hypotension associated with low potency neuroleptics is mostly orthostatic and thus less of a problem in bedridden patients. Other neuroleptics such as haloperidol and fluphenazine are more potent, less likely to alter vital signs, but more likely to worsen parkinsonian signs.

Clozapine has been used successfully for the treatment of psychosis in PD. Its use in PD has not been approved by the FDA, and it carries the risk of agranulocytosis. Its introduction may be associated with several days of increased confusion, hypotension, significant sedation, and the onset of antipsychotic action can be delayed for days. Its use is therefore more appropriate in the chronic outpatient setting. Psychotic PD patients respond poorly or adversely to general sedatives such as benzodiazepines and barbiturates. The onset of action of bupropion is too long (>5 days) to be useful in an acute situation. Diphenhydramine and promethazine, both in doses of 12.5 to 25 mg repeated up to every 6 hours may be useful as a general sedative. Promethazine can cause worsening of parkinsonian symptoms, and though a weak dopamine blocker, has no antipsychotic properties.

Ondansetron was recently reported to attenuate or eliminate hallucinosis in seven patients with PD. The drug was well tolerated with no worsening of cognition or parkinsonian signs as the oral dose was gradually increased up to 12–20 mg/d. Ondansetron is also available parenterally. Although the authors conclude this may be a safe alternative to the unsatisfactory choices outlined above, the results needs to be confirmed in a larger group of patients using a controlled design.

Dopamine withdrawal syndrome – management

Proper management of the dopamine withdrawal syndrome requires early recognition and transfer to a critical care unit for monitoring. Management involves aggressive cooling measures, vigorous hydration and stabilization of the cardiovascular and renal systems. Immediate withdrawal of any dopamine antagonists (see table under antiemetics) and resumption of antiparkinsonian therapy are critical. If a patient does not respond to levodopa within the first few hours, bromocriptine can be considered as it has been shown to be effective in the management of selected nonparkinsonian patients with the neuroleptic malignant syndrome. In this setting, doses as high as 100 mg/d have been recommended. In a critically ill PD patient the acute introduction of more than 20 to 40 mg of bromocriptine cannot be advocated, however. Even at these doses patients face the potential complications of severe nausea, emesis, hypotension and psychosis. Alternatives to consider include muscle relaxant such as diazepam (3 to 5 mg by i.v. bolus), and dantrolene (1 mg/kg by rapid I.V. push repeated every 1 to 3 minutes as needed up to maximum of 10 mg/kg). For patients with severe peripheral vasoconstriction, nitroprusside drip has been recommended (0.5 to 1 mg/kg/min

by constant infusion). Management also requires careful monitoring of renal function, cardiac function, rhabdomyolisis, myoglobinuria, acidosis and the continuing threat of superimposed infection.

The perioperative management of parkinsonian patients undergoing neurosurgical procedures such as fetal mesencephalic transplantation, stereotactic thalamotomy and pallidotomy involves the same principles outlined above as well as other subspecialty considerations which are beyond the scope of this chapter. For the interested reader, two references are provided that cover the overlapping topic of the perioperative and intensive care unit management of general neurology patients.

FURTHER READING

Alvir, J. M. J., Lieberman, J. A., Safferman, A. Z. et al. Clozapine-induced agranulocytosis. Incidence and risk factors in the United States. N. Engl. J. Med. 1993; **329**: 162–167.

Barr, A. The Shy–Drager syndrome. In Vinken, P. J., Bruyn, G. W., & Klawans, H. L., eds. Handbook of Clinical Neurology (vol 38). New York: Elsevier-North Holland, 1979: 233–256.

Berry, P. & Ward-Smith, P. A. Adrenal medullary transplant as a treatment for Parkinson's disease: perioperative considerations. J. Neurosci. Nurs. 1988; **20**: 356–361.

Brindle, G. F. Anesthesia in the patient with Parkinsonism. Primary Care 1977; **4**: 513–528.

Brod, T. M. Fluoxetine and extrapyramidal side effects. Am. J. Psychiatry 1989; **146**: 399–400.

Broussolle, E., Marion, M. H., & Pollack, P. Continuous subcutaneous apomorphine as replacement for levodopa in severe parkinsonian patients after surgery. Lancet 1992; **340**: 860.

Cohen, G. The pathobiology of Parkinson's disease: biochemical aspects of dopamine neuron senescence. J. Neural Transm. 1983; **19**: 89–103.

Cummings, J. L. Intellectual impairment in Parkinson's disease: clinical, pathologic, and biochemical correlates. J. Geriatr Psychiatry Neurol. 1988; **1**: 24–36.

Delgado, J. M. & Billo, J. M. Care of the patient with Parkinson's disease: surgical and nursing interventions. J. Neurosci. Nurs. 1988; **20**: 142–150.

Folstein, M. F., Folstein, S. E., & McHugh, P. R. "Mini-mental state." A practical method for grading the state of patients for the clinician. J. Psychiatry Res. 1975; **12**: 189–198.

Forno, L. S. Pathology of Parkinson's disease. In Marsden, C. E. & Fahn, S., eds. Movement Disorders. London: Butterworths, 1982: 25–40.

Frankel, J. P., Lees, A. J., Kempster, P. A., & Stern, G. M. Subcutaneous apomorphine in the treatment of Parkinson's disease. J. Neurol. Neurosurg. Psychiatry 1990; **53**: 96–101.

Golden, W. E., Lavender, R. C., & Metzer, W. S. Acute postoperative confusion and hallucinations in Parkinson disease. Ann. Int. Med. 1989; **111**: 218–222.

Guze, B. H. & Baxter, L. R. Neuroleptic malignant syndrome. *N. Engl. J. Med.* 1985; **313**: 163–166.

Hornykiewicz, O. and Kish, S. J. Biochemical pathophysiology of Parkinson's disease. *Adv. Neurol.* 1987; **45**: 19–34.

Hyman, S. A., Rogers, W. D., Smith, D. W. *et al.* Perioperative management for transplant of autologous adrenal medulla to the brain for Parkinsonism. *Anesthesiol.* 1988; **69**: 618–622.

Irwin, R. P., Nutt, J. G., Woodward, W. R. *et al.* Pharmacodynamics of the hypotensive effect of levodopa in Parkinsonian patients. *Clin. Neuropharmacol.* 1992; **15**: 365–374.

Jansen Steur, E. N. H. Increase of Parkinson disability after fluoxetine medication. *Neurology* 1993; **43**: 211–213.

Jenner, P., Dexter, D. T., Sian, J. *et al.* Oxidative stress as a cause of nigral cell death in Parkinson's disease and incidental Lewy body disease. *Ann. Neurol.* 1992; **32**(suppl): 82–87.

Juncos, J. L. Levodopa: pharmacology, pharmacokinetics and pharmacodynamics. *Neurol. Clin. N. Amer.* 1992; 487–509.

Juncos, J. L. Diet and related variables in the management of Parkinson disease. In Schneider, J. S. & Gupta, M., eds. *Current Concepts in Parkinson's Disease.* Toronto: Hogrefe & Huber, 1993: 365–402.

Kaufman, C. A. & Wyatt, R. J. Neuroleptic malignant syndrome. In Meltzer, H., ed. *Psychopharmacology: The Third Generation of Progress.* New York: Raven Press, 1987.

Kurlan, R., Nutt, J. G., Woodward, W. R. *et al.* Duodenal and gastric delivery of levodopa in parkinsonism. *Ann. Neurol.* 1988; **22**: 589–595.

Lipowski, Z. J. Delirium in the elderly patient. *N. Engl. J. Med.* 1989; **320**: 578–582.

Mayeux, R., Stern, Y., Rosenstein, R. *et al.* An estimate of the prevalence of dementia in idiopathic Parkinson's disease. *Arch. Neurol.* **45**: 260–262.

Mayeux, R., Stern, Y., Rosen, *et al.* Depression, intellectual impairment and Parkinson's disease. *Neurology* 1981; **31**: 645–650.

Merli, G. J. & Bell, R. D. Preoperative management of the surgical patient with neurologic disease. *Med. Clin. N. Amer.* 1987; **71**: 511–527.

Mier, M. Mechanisms leading to hypoventilation in extrapyramidal disorders, with special reference to Parkinson's disease. *J. Am. Geriatr. Soc.* 1976; **15**: 230–238.

Mitchelson, F. Pharmacological agents affecting emesis. A review (Part 1). *Drugs* 1992; **43**: 295–315.

Nobrega, F. T., Glattre, E., Kurland, L. T., & Okazaki, H. Comments on the epidemiology of parkinsonism including prevalence and incidence statistics for Rochester, Minnesota, 1935–1966. In Barbeau, A. & Brunette, J. R., eds. *Progress in Neurogenetics.* Amsterdam: Excerpta Medica, 1969.

Paulson, G. & Tafrate, R. Some "minor" aspects of Parkinsonism, especially pulmonary function. *Neurology* 1970; **20**: 14–17.

Pfeiffer, R. F., Kang, J., Graber, B. *et al.* Clozapine for psychosis in Parkinson's disease. *Movement Dis.* 1990; **5**: 239–242.

Rajput, A. H., Offord, K. P., Beard, C. M., & Kurland, L. T. Epidemiology of parkinsonism: incidence, classification, and mortality. *Ann. Neurol.* 1984; **16**: 278–282.

Reed, A. P. & Han, D. G. Intraoperative exacerbation of Parkinson's disease. *Anesth. Analg.* 1992; **75**: 850–853.

Ropper, A. H., ed. *Neurological and Neurosurgical Intensive Care.* New York, NY: Raven Press, 1993.

Sage, J. I., Schuh, L., Heikkila, R. E., & Duvoisin, R. C. Continuous duodenal infusions of levodopa: plasma concentrations and motor fluctuations in Parkinson's disease. *Clin. Neuropharmacol.* 1988; **11**: 36–44.

Scuderi, P., Wetchler, B., Sung, Y.-F. *et al.* Treatment of post-operative nausea and vomiting after outpatient surgery with the 5-HT3 antagonist ondansetron. *Anesthesiology* 1993; **78**: 15–20.

Steele, J. C. Progressive supranuclear palsy. *Brain* 1972; **95**: 693–704.

Suchowersky, O. & deVries, J. Possible interactions between deprenyl and fluoxetine. *Canad. J. Neurol. Sci.* 1990; **17**: 352–353.

Tanner, C. M. Epidemiology of Parkinson's disease. *Neurol. Clin. N. Amer.* 1992; **10**: 317–327.

Vincken, W. G., Bauthier, S. G., Dohlfuss, R. *et al.* Involvement of upper airway muscles in extrapyramidal disorders. A cause for airflow limitation. *N. Engl. J. Med.* 1984; **311**: 438–442.

Zoldan, J., Friedberg, G., Goldberg-Stern, H., & Melamed, E. Ondansetron for hallucinosis in advanced Parkinson's disease. *Lancet* 1993; **341**: 562–563.

36

Delirium in the surgical patient

Neil H. Winawer

Emory University School of Medicine, Atlanta, GA

Introduction

The acute confusional state known as delirium is the most common cause of altered mental status in surgical patients. Despite its common occurrence, delirium can often go unrecognized, leading to delays in treatment. This can have significant implications as patients with delirium suffer from higher mortality, postoperative complication rates, longer lengths of stay and delayed functional recovery.[1]

Delirium is usually acute in onset but may develop gradually. It can persist for hours to days and can fluctuate throughout the course of a day. The cardinal feature of delirium is an alteration in the level of consciousness that fluctuates over time. Patients may also display hyperalert, irritable, or agitated behavior. The sleep–wake cycle is often markedly disrupted. Sleep is usually fragmented, with restlessness and agitation. Psychomotor abnormalities may range from hyperactivity to lethargy, stupor, obtundation, and catatonia. Most cases of delirium improve or resolve within 1 to 4 weeks if sufficient attention is given to correcting the underlying disorder causing the cerebral dysfunction. Nonetheless, the development of delirium serves as a marker for those patients at risk of progressive functional decline.[2]

Multiple signs and symptoms may accompany delirium. Patients may be grossly psychotic with severe perceptual distortions that can include hallucinations (tactile, auditory, visual, olfactory), paranoia, delusions, thought disorganization and language incoherence resembling schizophrenia. Signs of cognitive dysfunction such as disturbances in memory, attention, concentration, and orientation are usually the first to be recognized. Behavioral abnormalities such as agitation, disinhibition, and combativeness may also occur.

Given the significant morbidity and mortality associated with delirium it is important for the preoperative consultant to identify those patients at increased risk. Age, comorbid medical conditions and the type of surgery all contribute to the incidence, which can be highly variable (ranging as high as 70% in susceptible patients).[3]

Pathogenesis

Although much is known about the pathogenesis of delirium, its exact biologic mechanisms remain poorly understood. Delirium is a difficult disorder to study, as it is transient, fleeting, and is often difficult to predict. Early studies noted that most episodes were characterized by specific electrocephalographic changes (abnormal slow wave activity), implying that the disorder was one of global cortical dysfunction.[4] The ability to reverse the process in certain conditions led researchers to suspect that delirium was a disorder of cerebral oxidative metabolism. However, other investigations have supported a role of subcortical structures, based on the observation that patients with infarcts in the thalamus and basal ganglia are at increased risk of developing delirium. Nonetheless, most patients who develop delirium have no identifiable abnormalities on imaging studies.

Several examples suggest that cholinergic pathways play a significant role in the pathogenesis of delirium. It has been observed that hypoxia and hypoglycemia are associated with decreased acetylcholine production in the central nervous system; the level of which correlates with the degree of cognitive decline.[5] Medications that decrease the level of acetylcholine in the CNS frequently cause confusion in the elderly. These drugs include neuroleptics, tricyclic antidepressants, benzodiazepines, and opiates (Table 36.1). Alzheimer's disease, characterized by a loss of cholinergic neurons, also increases the risk of developing delirium. Other neurotransmitters such as serotonin

Table 36.1. Drugs commonly associated with delirium

Class	Examples
Anticholinergic drugs	tricyclic antidepressants, neuroleptics antihistamines, benztropine, belladonna alkaloids
Opioids	morphine, codeine, meperidine
Benzodiazepines	diazepam, lorazepam, tenazepam
Antiparkinsonian agents	levodopa/carbidopa, amantadine, pergolide bromocriptine
Histamine-2 receptor blockers	ranitidine, cimetidine, famotidine, nizatidine
Cardiovascular agents	beta-blockers, digoxin, diuretics, calcium channel blockers
Antibiotics	penicillin, cephalosporins, gentamycin
Anticonvulsants	phenytoin, carbamezapine
Anti-inflammatory agents	prednisone, non-steroidal agents, cyclosporine, OKT3
Oral hypoglycemics	glyburide, glipizide, glimepiride

and norepinephrine have also been implicated given their effects on arousal and sleep. Cytokine activation may also play a role in specific disorders (e.g., sepsis).

Diagnosis

Although delirium can develop at any time during hospitalization, it typically presents early in the postoperative period. The diagnosis of delirium is usually suspected when a patient becomes acutely agitated, uncooperative, and confused. The quiet, withdrawn patient may not attract the same degree of attention or may be erroneously diagnosed as having a psychiatric illness.

Nursing observations often provide the earliest and best sources for suspecting delirium, especially for assessing the degree to which mental status fluctuates over a 24-hour period. Behaviors that nurses often note are: agitation, restlessness, disorientation, inability to focus, wandering out of bed, etc. This is often in stark contrast to the lucid behavior that patients may display at other times. If delirium is suspected, initial evaluation should focus on eliciting the elements that characterize the disorder. The hallmark features of delirium as defined in the *Diagnostic and Statistical Manual of Mental Disorders* (DSM-IV) are as follows:[6]

1. Disturbance of consciousness (i.e., reduced clarity of awareness of the environment) with reduced ability to focus, sustain, or shift attention.
2. A change in cognition (e.g., memory deficit, disorientation, language disturbance) or the development of a perceptual disturbance that is not accounted for better by a pre-existing, established, or evolving dementia.
3. Disturbance develops during a short period (usually hours to days) and tends to fluctuate during the course of the day.
4. Varies based on cause (see specific disorders for discussion).

Patients with delirium typically have difficulty with attention. They are unable to focus and have decreased levels of awareness. Often, these derangements are subtle and may be overlooked by the treating physician. Delirious patients may exhibit a variety of cognitive defects including disorientation, memory loss and difficulty with language and speech (rambling, incoherent or difficult to follow). While assessing the patient's degree of cognitive impairment, it is also vital to have established a baseline for comparison. Hence, a thorough preoperative evaluation should include a formal cognitive assessment (e.g., Folstein mini-mental status exam; see Fig. 36.1) in those at risk of developing delirium.

Clinicians face two diagnostic challenges in the evaluation of delirium. The first is recognizing that the disorder is present, and the second is evaluating the patient for suspected medical conditions that may have precipitated the episode. Despite advances in medical technology, the cornerstone in the evaluation of delirium remains the history and physical examination. After a thorough evaluation, further testing may be warranted; however, over-reliance on laboratory testing and diagnostic imaging can minimize the importance of the bedside examination and lead to increased costs.

Clinicians who apply the DSM-IV criteria at the bedside are more likely to make an accurate diagnosis. Initial evaluation should focus on the patient's level of consciousness. Patients should be assessed for their level of orientation and questioned on routine items to assess for any deficits in memory. Often, conversation may reveal a disorganized thought process or be devoid of any real content. If the clinician does not know the patient's baseline mental status, relatives or caregivers often can relay information that may aid in the patient's assessment.

Several formal cognitive tests are useful in identifying delirium. While these tests are valuable tools in establishing the diagnosis, it is important to realize that a normal examination does not necessarily rule out delirium, as patients can perform relatively well during lucid intervals. Therefore, if delirium is suspected, the examination should be repeated periodically. A simple and commonly used tool in the study of delirium is the Confusion Assessment Method (CAM) (see Fig. 36.2). Examples of CAM questions include "Did the patient's behavior fluctuate throughout

Orientation

1. Ask for year, season, date, day, month. Then ask specifically for parts omitted. One point for each correct. (0–5)
2. Ask in turn for name of state, county, town, hospital or place, floor or street. One point for each correct. (0–5)

Registration

Ask the patient whether you may test his or her memory. Then say the names of three unrelated objects, clearly and slowly, about 1 sec for each. After you have said all three, ask the patient to repeat them. This first repetition determines his or her score (0–3) but keep saying them until he or she can repeat all three up to six trials. If the patient does not eventually learn all three, recall cannot be meaningfully tested.

Attention and calculation

Ask the patient to begin with 100 and count backward by 7. Stop after five subtractions (93, 86, 79, 72, 65). Score total number of correct answers, one point for each. (0–5)

If the patient cannot or will not perform this task, ask him or her to spell the word world backward. The score is the number of letters in correct order, e.g., dlrow = 5. (0–5)

Recall

Ask the patient whether he or she can recall the three words you previously asked him or her to remember. (0–3)

Language

Naming: Show the patient a wrist watch and ask him or her what it is. Repeat for pencil. (0–2)
Repetition: Ask the patient to repeat this phrase after you: "no ifs, ands, or buts." Allow only one trial. (0 or 1)
Three-stage command: "Take a piece of paper in your right hand, fold it in half, and put it on the floor." Give the patient a piece of blank paper and repeat the command. Score 1 point for each part correctly executed. (0–3)
Reading: On a blank piece of paper print the sentence "Close your eyes," in letters large enough for the patient to see clearly. Ask him or her to read it and do what it says. Score 1 point only if the patient actually closes his or her eyes. (0–1)
Writing: Give the patient a blank piece of paper and ask him or her to write a sentence for you. Do not dictate a sentence; it is to be written spontaneously. It must contain a Subject and verb and be sensible. Correct grammar and punctuation are not necessary. (0–1)
Copying: On a clean piece of paper, draw intersecting pentagons, each side about 1 inch, and ask him or her to copy it exactly as it is. All 10 angles must be present and 2 must intersect to score 1 point. Tremor and rotation are ignored. (0–1)
Estimate the patient's level of sensorium along a continuum, from alert on the left to coma on the right.

Total possible score is 30 points. Patients with a total of 23 points or less are highly likely to have a cognitive disorder.

Fig. 36.1. Mini-Mental Status Examination: Instructions for Administration and Scoring.[13]

the day?" "Does the patient have difficulty focusing", etc. Validation of the CAM at two centers revealed a sensitivity of 94% to 100% and a specificity of 90% to 95%.[7]

Cause

Once the diagnosis of delirium is established, efforts should focus on identifying an underlying cause, since many of these are treatable. The medical history should begin by searching for the risk factors that can precipitate delirium. Of importance is the patient's age and the existence of underlying brain disease (e.g., cerebrovascular accident, dementia), psychiatric illness, or other underlying medical conditions (e.g., congestive heart failure, liver disease, renal failure, chronic obstructive pulmonary disease). The patient's medication list should be reviewed carefully, looking for agents that may cause altered mental status (e.g., benzodiazepines, antidepressants; see Table 36.1). The details of the surgery should be reviewed because patients with longer durations of anesthesia are at increased risk. Some types of surgery (e.g., cardiac, orthopedic, ophthalmologic) also increase the risk.

Physical examination should focus on vital signs, fluid status, and the appearance of localizing signs of infection. A brief focused neurologic examination should assess the patient's level of consciousness and look for the presence of focal neurologic findings. Routine head computed

Feature 1:   Acute onset and fluctuating course

This feature is usually obtained from a family member or nurse and is shown by positive responses to the following questions: Is there evidence of an acute change in mental status from the patient's baseline? Did the (abnormal) behavior fluctuate during the day, that is, tend to come and go, or increase and decrease in severity?

Feature 2:   Inattention

This feature is shown by a positive response to the following question: Did the patient have difficulty focusing attention, for example, being easily distractible, or having difficulty keeping track of what was being said?

Feature 3:   Disorganized thinking

This feature is shown by a positive response to the following question: Was the patient's thinking disorganized or incoherent, such as rambling or irrelevant conversation, unclear or illogical flow of ideas, or unpredictable switching from subject to subject?

Feature 4:   Altered Level of Consciousness

This feature is shown by any answer other than "alert" to the following question: Overall, how would you rate this patient's level of consciousness? (alert [normal], vigilant [hyperalert], lethargic [drowsy, easily aroused], stupor [difficult to arouse], or coma [unarousable])

The diagnosis of delirium by CAM requires the presence of features 1 and 2 and either 3 or 4.

Fig. 36.2. The confusion assessment method (CAM) diagnostic algorithm.[6]

tomography (CT) or magnetic resonance imaging (MRI) is not recommended. Although neuroimaging may uncover chronic abnormalities that can precipitate delirium, it rarely reveals reversible causes.[8]

Laboratory analysis should consist of a complete blood count (CBC), looking for evidence of infection, and serum electrolytes looking for evidence of hypernatremia/hyponatremia, acidosis/alkalosis, or acute renal failure. Pulse oximetry is a quick, non-invasive way to rule out underlying hypoxia. An arterial blood gas should also be performed if acid–base derangements are suspected or if pulse oximetry is unreliable. A chest radiograph and urinalysis are indicated if pneumonia or urinary tract infection is suspected. Blood and urine cultures should also follow if clinical suspicion warrants. An electrocardiogram should be performed in all patients who are at risk for myocardial ischemia.

As previously noted, there are several risk factors that have been identified with developing delirium after surgery. Age appears to place patients at greatest risk. Elderly patients take the most medications yet have decreased ability to metabolize drugs. They may often have visual and hearing impairments that predispose to disorientation. Postoperative hypoxia is more common in the elderly, given the higher incidence of cardiovascular, respiratory and cerebrovascular diseases in this age group.

Patients with pre-existing central nervous system disorders such as dementia and Parkinson disease have higher rates of postoperative delirium. Other central nervous system abnormalities such as epilepsy and head trauma can also place patients at increased risk. The association between depression and delirium has been well documented.

The type of surgery can also influence the development of delirium. Procedures that are longer in duration place patients at increased risk for intraoperative hypoxemia. Cardiac surgery can result in hypoperfusion and micro-emboli formation resulting in cerebral ischemia. Orthopedic procedures, most notably femoral neck fracture repair have been associated with high rates of delirium. These patients are also at higher risk for fat emboli. Patients undergoing cataract surgery often experience delirium due to vision loss and the use of ophthalmic drugs with anticholinergic side effects.

A variety of metabolic insults can cause delirium. These include dehydration, hyponatremia, hyperglycemia, hypoglycemia, acid–base disorders, hypercalcemia, hyperphosphatemia, hepatic, renal and endocrine diseases. Hypoxia, whether from anesthetics, pulmonary emboli, pneumonia, or other underlying respiratory/cardiac disease, may cause altered mental status.

Postoperatively, patients are at increased risk of developing infections. Pneumonia, urinary tract infections,

Table 36.2. Risk factors for developing postoperative delirium

- Age
- Preexisting central nervous system disease (e.g., dementia, Parkinson disease)
- Type and duration of surgery
- Sensory impairment (e.g., visual and hearing deficits)
- Hypoxia
- Metabolic derangements (e.g., hyponatremia, hyperglycemia, acid–base disorders, etc.)
- Infections
- Uncontrolled pain
- Chronic alcoholism
- Benzodiazepine dependence

intra-abdominal and wound infections can all cause confusion in susceptible patients. Delirium may be the only clinical clue, as systemic symptoms such as fever, chills, cough, purulent sputum and leukocytosis may often be absent.

Postoperative patients, in unfamiliar surroundings, can become disoriented. Additionally, the sensory overload associated with an ICU setting can lead to sleep deprivation, which is a risk factor for developing delirium. Often patients may have postoperative pain that is either uncontrolled or unaddressed. Pain, in several studies, has been shown to increase delirium rates.[9]

Patients who abuse alcohol can often become delirious secondary to withdrawal symptoms. Chronic alcoholics may also have end-organ damage such as cerebral atrophy and liver disease, which can predispose to encephalopathy. Patients with anxiety or sleep related disorders may become dependent upon benzodiazepines. The withdrawal symptoms associated with these agents are similar to those of alcohol withdrawal.

Treatment

During the preoperative evaluation, all efforts should be made to identify those patients at risk for developing delirium postoperatively (see Table 36.2). Data from several studies have revealed that delirium, in part, is preventable by intervening in several crucial areas.[10] These include identifying and addressing underlying medical problems; eliminating all medications that can precipitate delirium (e.g., sedative hypnotics, anticholinergics); optimizing the patient's fluid status; aggressively treating pain; promoting early ambulation; and ensuring a familiar, tranquil postoperative care setting. When delirium occurs, efforts

should focus on identifying the precipitating factors and treating the underlying cause.

Owing to the potential morbidity and mortality associated with delirium, patients should be urgently assessed with a brief history and focused physical exam. If no cause is readily apparent, supportive care should be provided. Although there are few studies in this regard, it appears that preventing iatrogenic functional decline will improve the chances of recovery. Several simple measures if implemented early and often can result in significant benefits. Providing a room with a window view can help orient the patient and correct sleep cycles. Large calendars, clocks or familiar objects (such as family photographs) are useful to help connect patients to the outside world. In this regard, family members or sitters should be allowed at the bedside to provide frequent orientation. The use of immobilizing devices, such as bladder catheters and restraints, should be minimized. Although the use of restraints often is touted as being in the patient's best interests, it can lead to increased agitation, social isolation, and increased morbidity.[11]

Delirious patients may require pharmacologic treatment to prevent injury or to allow further evaluation or treatment. Antipsychotic medications have traditionally been used as these agents not only control psychotic symptoms but also decrease agitation and provide sedation. Haloperidol (Haldol) is the most commonly used agent as it is potent and has minimal hemodynamic or respiratory side effects. It can be given orally for maintenance therapy or intravenously/intramuscularly when a faster onset of action is desired. Because the peak action of intramuscular haloperidol occurs 30 minutes after administration, patients can be reevaluated within the first hour and repeated doses can be given hourly if rapid tranquilizing is desired.[12] Peak action after oral ingestion occurs within 2 to 4 hours. After patients are adequately sedated, doses can be given orally or intramuscularly every 4 to 6 hours (see Table 36.3). Extrapyramidal symptoms (parkinsonian side effects, akathisia, dystonic reactions, and tardive dyskinesia) are the main side effects of treatment. The newer neuroleptics (e.g., respiridone, olanzapine) appear to have similar efficacy with fewer side effects; however, there is currently less evidence to support their use.

Benzodiazepines (e.g., diazepam, lorazepam) are the drugs of choice in alcohol and sedative withdrawal syndromes. They have a quicker onset of action than the neuroleptics (5 minutes intravenously) but can cause oversedation, hypotension, and respiratory depression, which can be life threatening. Benzodiazepines may be useful adjuncts to neuroleptics as they provide sedation without the risk of extrapyramidal side effects.

Table 36.3. Treatment guidelines for the use of intravenous haloperidol in the intensive care setting.[12]

Degree of agitation	Starting dose (mg)
Mild	0.5–2.0
Moderate-severe	2.0–10

Titration and maintenance

Allow 20–30 minutes before the next dose.

If agitation is unchanged, administer double dose every 20–30 minutes until patient begins to calm.

If patient is calming down, repeat the last dose at next dosing interval.

Adjust dose and interval to patient's clinical course. Gradually increase the interval between doses until the interval is 8 hours, then begin to decrease dose.

Once stable for 24 hours, give doses on a regular schedule and supplement with as-needed doses.

Once stable for 36 hours, begin attempts to taper dose.

When agitation is very severe, very high boluses (up to 40 mg) may be required.

Source: From Goldstein, M. G. Intensive care unit syndromes. In Stoudemire, A. & Fogel, B. S., eds. *Principles of Medical Psychiatry.* Orlando: Grune & Stratton, 1987: 412.

REFERENCES

1. Inouye, S. K., Rushing, J. T., & Foreman, M. D. Does delirium contribute to poor hospital outcomes? A three-site epidemiologic study. *J. Gen. Int. Med.* 1998; **12**: 234–242.

2. Francis, J. & Kapoor, W. N. Prognosis after discharge of elderly medical patients with delirium. *J. Am. Geriat. Soc.* 1992; **40**: 601–606.

3. Dyer, C. B., Ashton, C. M., & Teasdale, T. A. Postoperative delirium. *Arch. Intern. Med.* 1995; **155**: 461–465.

4. Romano, J. & Engel, G. L. Delirium: I. Electroencephalographic data. *Arch. Neurol. Psychiatry* 1944; **149**: 41.

5. Tune, L. E., Holland, A., Folstein, M. F., *et al.* Association of postoperative delirium with raised serum levels of anticholinergic drugs. *Lancet* 1981; **2**: 651–653.

6. American Psychiatric Association. *Diagnostic and Statistical Manual*, 4th edn. Washington, DC: APA Press; 1994.

7. Inouye, S. K., van Dyck, C. H., Alessi, C. A. *et al.* Clarifying confusion: the confusion assessment method. *Ann. Intern. Med.* 1990; **113**: 941–948.

8. Koponen, H., Hurri, L., Stenback, U. *et al.* Computed tomography findings in delirium. *J. Nerv. Ment. Dis.* 1989; **177**: 226.

9. Lynch, E. P., Lazor, M. A., & Gellis, J. E. The impact of postoperative pain on the development of delirium. *Int. Anesth. Res. Soc.* 1998; **86**: 781–785.

10. Inouye, S. K., Bogardus, S. T., Charpentier, P. A. *et al.* A multicomponent intervention to prevent delirium in hospitalized older patients. *N. Engl. J. Med.* 1999; **340**: 669–676.

11. Evans, L. & Strumpf, N. E. Tying down the elderly: a review of the literature on physical restraint. *J. Am. Geriatr. Soc.* 1989; **36**: 65–74.

12. Stoudemire, A. Delirium. In Lubin, M. F., Walker, H. K., & Smith, R. B. III, eds. *Medical Management of the Surgical Patient*, 3rd edn. Philadelphia: J. B. Lippincott, 1995: 378–387.

13. PR. "Mini-mental state": A practical method for grading the cognitive state of patients for the clinician. *J. Psychiatry Res.* 1975; **12**: 189.

Surgery in the elderly

37

Surgery in the elderly

Michael F. Lubin

Emory University School of Medicine, Atlanta, GA

Introduction

Surgical and anesthetic care have improved markedly in the last half century. It is likely that the greatest benefit of this improvement has been for the elderly population. Older patients can benefit from surgery that would not have been contemplated in the past; thus, patients are living longer and with a better quality of life than ever before.

The literature in surgical care of the elderly patient is extensive, growing rapidly and indicates that, with careful planning and care, the elderly can undergo surgery safely and with approximately the same risk as many younger patients. This section discusses the following topics as they pertain to the elderly population: (a) physiologic decrements of aging, (b) risks of surgery, (c) preoperative evaluation, (d) anesthesia, (e) common surgical procedures and (f) postoperative care.

Physiologic decrements of aging

Although physicians see many elderly patients who appear old and sick with many underlying health problems, a large percentage of the elderly population is quite well. These people can function entirely normally and have no limitations to their activities. Despite this degree of functional normality, however, all older people experience various decrements in physiologic function that are of importance in planning their care, particularly when they are under stresses such as surgery.[1-3] These decrements make even healthy older patients more fragile and more likely to suffer postoperative complications and death than their younger counterparts. Physicians must take them into account in their evaluations.

The cardiovascular system has been studied and reviewed extensively.[4-7] Although the ability of aging heart muscle to contract is unaffected, diastolic function deteriorates. Other important changes include decreases in maximal heart rate and cardiac output with exercise. The decreases in output are, in great part, the result of increased afterload because of increased stiffness of the arteries and decreased responsiveness to catecholamine stimulation. These changes are important when patients undergo the stresses of surgery.

Although there is evidence in population studies for an increase in blood pressure with age, there is great controversy about its cause. Some feel that this truly is an age-related change; others feel that it is the result of atherosclerotic changes in the vessels, a specific disease process that can be prevented.

Age-related decreases in pulmonary function are quite marked and have important physiologic consequences in patients undergoing surgery. The elasticity of the lung tissue decreases and compliance increases.[8] These changes result in an increase in residual volume and uneven ventilation. Increases in closing volume also result in ventilation/perfusion abnormalities.

Because of the uneven ventilation, arterial oxygen tension decreases in a predictable way. Sorbini and colleagues found a linear relationship with age; pO_2 of those less than 30 years of age was 94 mm Hg, while it was only 74 mm Hg for those over 60.[9] The authors were able to estimate pO_2 by using the following equation: pO_2 (mm Hg) $= 109 - 0.43 \times$ (age).

Other pulmonary changes are measurable on standard pulmonary function testing. There is a linear decrease in vital capacity of approximately 25 ml/yr beginning in the third decade.[10] Measurements of airflow decrease as well, with decrements in maximum minute ventilation, FEV_1, and maximum mid-expiratory flow rate. It is not

Medical Management of the Surgical Patient: A Textbook of Perioperative Medicine, ed. M. F. Lubin, R. B. Smith, T. F. Dobson, N. Spell, H. K. Walker. 4th edn. Published by Cambridge University Press. © Cambridge University 2006.

surprising that pulmonary complications are among the most frequent and important in this population.

The effects of aging on the kidney are important because of the kidney's function in maintaining tonicity and water and salt balance. They also perform a crucial role in the elimination of many drugs.[11,12] Grossly, the kidneys decrease 20% to 30% in weight from age 30 to 80. There is a significant decrease in the number of glomeruli and an increase in interstitial fibrosis.

Along with these anatomic changes comes an important decrease in creatinine clearance. Because of concomitant decrease in the lean mass of the body, however, there is generally no increase in the serum creatinine, which can be misleading to those unaware of these changes. Two groups have developed estimates of creatinine clearance (C_{cr}) as a function of age. The following equations can be used:[13,14]

$$C_{cr}\,(ml/min) = \frac{(140 - age) \times weight\,(kg)}{72 \times Cr_s}$$
$$or$$
$$C_{cr}\,(ml/min) = 135 - 0.84 \times age$$

These decreases in clearance in the absence of increases in serum creatinine must be taken into account when administering drugs primarily excreted by the kidney.

In addition to decreases in creatinine clearance, tubular function is also affected by age, and there are decreases in concentrating and diluting ability, which can lead to over-hydration, dehydration, hypernatremia, or hyponatremia if careful attention is not paid to fluid administration. Other important physiologic changes affect water balance. These include a decrease in thirst perception so that elderly patients who are volume depleted drink less and more slowly to replete the deficit. Data suggest that certain disorders in antidiuretic hormone (ADH) physiology pre-dispose at least some apparently normal elderly patients to excessive ADH secretion, resulting in unexpected hyponatremia.

Although the cardiovascular, pulmonary, and renal systems are vital in the survival of surgical patients, other systems undergo important physiologic changes that affect the patient's recovery as well. Osteoporosis is quite common, most severely in white women. Care must be taken in transferring patients to avoid fracture of brittle bones. Skin changes are equally as important and are often overlooked. The epidermis and dermis undergo degenerative changes, and the possibility for pressure ulcers is quite high if care is not taken to reposition the patient frequently. This may even need to be done in the operating room if the procedure is long.

Admission to the hospital may be the greatest danger to elderly patients.[15] Bedrest causes deconditioned muscles

in all patients and this is particularly problematic in elderly patients with little muscle reserve anyway. Loss of muscle power begins almost immediately and in elderly patients can result in the inability to transfer, toilet and even walk independently. Loss of these functions will result in the loss of the ability to live independently.

The final important areas of altered physiology are the distribution, metabolism, and elimination of drugs. Drug distribution is affected by the alterations in body composition. Lean body mass, plasma volume, and total body water decrease. Extracellular water decreases by 40%, and body fat increases by about 35%. These changes will alter drug action depending on the water and lipid solubility of the agent. For water-soluble drugs, there is a smaller volume of distribution, resulting in a higher concentration at the same dose. For lipid-soluble drugs, there may be relatively larger volume; this often results in prolonged action of the drug.

Drug metabolism in the liver is altered for some drugs. These changes are quite variable and not easily predicted. Some important drugs that have a decreased metabolic clearance in the elderly are the benzodiazepines, warfarin, and phenytoin. Renal clearance is invariably decreased in all older patients because of the changes in renal function already discussed. Thus, drugs such as digoxin, antibiotics, and others cleared primarily by the kidney must be adjusted for this decrease.

Risks of surgery

The safety of surgery in the elderly has been discussed for over 40 years. In a 1967 lecture entitled, "Is risk of indicated operation too great in the elderly?" Alton Ochsner said, "In 1927 as a young professor of surgery at Tulane Medical School, I practiced and taught that an elective operation for inguinal hernia in a patient over 50 years old was not justified".[16] Now the literature has titles such as "Surgery for aortic stenosis in severely symptomatic patients older than 80"[17] and "Open heart surgery in the elderly: results for a consecutive series of 100 patients aged 85 years or older".[18]

The first reports of the results of surgery in geriatric patients appeared in the late 1930s. These studies reported an overall mortality of about 20%, while the rate for abdominal surgery was over 30%. Recent reviews have reported mortality rates for elective surgery at 0%–5.4% and rates for emergency surgery vary from 13%–30%.[19] In more recent years there have been reports of surgical series of patients in their 80s and 90s having surgery.[20–23] Reports of mortality range from 10%–20% for emergency

Table 37.1.

Year	Mortality (%)
1931–1940	11.0
1941–1950	5.0
1951–1960	7.3
1961–1970	9.2
1971–1980	9.5

surgery down to an average of about 3%–7% for elective surgery. A paper looked at major surgery in a nursing home population and found a mortality rate of only 4%; all of the deaths occurred in patients undergoing emergency surgery.[24] There have also been a number of papers reporting small series of selected patients over the age of 100 who have successfully had surgical procedures.[25–26]

The profusion of reports in the literature prompted Linn and Linn in 1982 to review 108 studies of surgery in the elderly from 1930 to 1980.[27] They found flaws and omissions in many of the studies. There were differences in lower age limits, methods used to calculate mortality, lengths of follow-up, mixes of emergency vs. elective operations, and types of operations. They came to two main conclusions: emergency surgery is much riskier than elective surgery and, since 1941, the trend has been toward increasing mortality for elective, but not emergency, procedures.

It is quite clear that the first conclusion is true; Linn and Linn found an overall mortality of 28% for general emergency surgery and 43% for specialty emergency procedures. Elective surgery rates averaged about 9%. These basic findings have been shown in a large number of papers.

Their second conclusion is much more controversial and certainly misleading. The authors divided the studies by decade, which yielded the rates shown in Table 37.1.

They proposed two possibilities for this trend toward increasing mortality. The first is that surgical care is deteriorating, and the second is that surgeons are taking patients with greater risks; they did not indicate that one was more likely than another. However, it is clear from Dr. Ochsner's earlier comment, and from the subsequent titles listed, that surgeons are doing more extensive operations on sicker patients.

The extent of the increase in risk for older patients related to age alone is uncertain. There have been many papers that have examined this issue. The first of these papers was published in 1977 by Goldman and colleagues in the *New England Journal of Medicine*.[28] They studied over 1000 patients, 324 of whom were over 70. They found

an independent, statistically significant increase in risk for those over 70. Sikes and Detmer did a study comparing the mortality for different age groups from birth to 94 years.[29] They found that rates increased slowly from 2.6% in those below 64 years of age to 3.5% in those aged 70 to 74 years. From there, however, the rates increased from 4.4% to 10.3% for those aged 90 to 94 years. The authors did an adjusted mortality rate for procedure; they did not, however, adjust for comorbidity.

Other studies have separated some important factors in the mortality among elderly patients. In 1978 Turnbull and associates studied mortality in patients over 70 and found only a 4.8% mortality for procedures.[30] There were 193 deaths in the group; 79 patients died of metastatic disease from the original tumor or from treatment, and 48 were felt to have died of the tumor directly. Therefore, 25% died of cancer even though they were included in the surgical mortality. They then calculated the mortality for procedures if those patients who died of far advanced cancer and "multiple organ decompensation" were excluded and found a rate of only 2.8%. Only six of 4050 patients died intraoperatively or in the first 24 hours after surgery – three of cardiorespiratory failure and three of uncontrolled bleeding.

In another study of 75 patients 90 years and older, 11 patients died; 3 had extensive carcinomas for an adjusted death rate of 10.6%.[31] The other causes of death were two bowel perforations and peritonitis, two pneumonias, one myocardial infarction, one stroke, and one sudden death (presumed myocardial infarction or pulmonary embolism). Of 42 elective cases there was only one death, a 2.3% mortality. Of 32 urgent cases, 5 died (16% mortality, and of the 11 emergencies, 5 died (45% death rate).

It should be clear that comparing crude death rates can be very difficult. Seymour and Pringle suggested that, in comparing mortality, "non-viable" cases should be separated from potentially viable patients. In their study, mortality decreased from 12% to 5.8%.[32] This must be done for the younger population as well for proper comparison, but it is clear that the effect on mortality rates in the elderly will be much larger than the effect on younger patients.

Additional studies have concluded that surgery is safe and effective for cardiopulmonary bypass,[33,34] resection of abdominal aneurysms,[35,36] lung resection,[37,38] abdominal surgery,[39–42] orthopedic procedures,[43] and major gynecologic surgery.[44] Finally, a study in Canada looked at almost 9000 patients over 65 who had a surgical procedure. Using correlation and multiple regression analysis, they found that severity of illness was a much better predictor of outcome than age.[45] It is clear that a strong case can be made for the safety of surgery even in the very old if appropriate precautions are taken.

Another strong argument in favor of surgery was demonstrated by Andersen and Ostberg.[46] They compared the survival rates of 7922 surgical patients over age 70 with a matched sample of the general population. They found improved survival over 2 to 16 years of follow-up study, demonstrating that surgery appears to result in long-term improvement in survival. Another more recent study found the same results in an elderly population followed at the Mayo Clinic.[47] It is certainly clear that there is no negative effect on overall long-term survival as a result of surgical intervention.

Another important question has been raised by a number of authors. Can, could, or should physicians turn some of the emergency surgical cases into elective procedures? It has been shown that the elderly can have emergency surgery and return to their previous living situation.[48] The mortality in emergency procedures, however, is much higher than in elective ones. Seymour and Pringle reviewed this question, using hernias, peptic ulcers, and colorectal carcinomas as pertinent areas of study.[49] They found that 17% of surgical procedures in persons aged 45 to 64 years were emergencies. In those over age 75, however, emergencies accounted for 37% of the group. Femoral hernias showed a large increase in emergency procedures; inguinal hernias were increased as well. Peptic ulcers showed the same kind of trends as the hernias, although not quite as striking. Finally, the same kind of result is found in colorectal carcinoma, so that the rate of emergency operations for rectal carcinoma is highest in the oldest age group.

From these data, the authors did a prospective study of 74 emergency operations. They felt that the emergency procedure could have been avoided in one third of the patients. Eight of 10 patients with strangulated hernias had been diagnosed before the emergency. Nine of 36 patients with an acute abdomen had a disease that might have been amenable to surgical therapy, and seven of 22 with cancer had symptoms for 3 months before their emergency operations. Although their conclusions were based on speculation rather than on statistics, it seems fair to say that at least some elderly patients are not having elective surgery for known or diagnosable conditions until they have become emergencies, with much increased mortality.

There are recent studies confirming the increased mortality of emergency surgery in older patients. Keller and colleagues found a 20% mortality in emergency surgery vs. a 2% mortality in elective surgery.[50] In another study by Schoon and Arvidsson studying surgery in patients over 80, only one of 43 deaths within 30 days of surgery occurred after elective surgery.[51]

Barriers to early surgery

There are a number of causes for the reticence to take elderly patients for elective surgery. The first is the mistaken belief among physicians that elderly people in general are not good candidates. This can be disproved easily and convincingly as we have shown above. The second problem is that there are sick elderly patients who have higher mortalities, not so much because of their age but because of comorbid conditions; however, this is true in younger patients as well. The most common problems in the elderly are dementia, chronic obstructive pulmonary disease, diabetes, coronary artery disease, heart failure, and hypertension. It is clear that the increased risk from these and other diseases must be evaluated, therapy instituted in those whose condition can be improved, and surgery avoided in those patients who are at a risk that appears to be unacceptable to the medical team and patient.

The last reason is the patient's reluctance to undergo surgery. Many elderly patients are quite frightened of having surgery, feeling that they have little chance of survival. Often, families have the same concerns. This, physicians can assure them, is definitely not true. The elderly are frequently concerned that surgery will not improve their quality of life, will make them more dependent on others, or will cause them to have to live in a care facility.[52–54] In addition, they often do not want to undergo the anticipated pain, discomfort, and rigors of surgery and the recovery period to treat a process that may not bother them very much, if at all. This obstacle is often difficult, if not impossible, to overcome.

Postoperative mortality

Although it is clear that the elderly can undergo surgery without undue risk, it is still unfortunately true that some patients do die. There are no surprises in the disease processes that cause the mortality, but it is helpful in evaluating patients preoperatively and in caring for them postoperatively to know which complications might be prevented or need to be treated.

Palmberg and Hirsjarvi reviewed a large number of surgical cases in elderly patients to study the mortality statistics.[55] They found that 33% died of pulmonary emboli, 20% died of pneumonia, 11% died of "cardiac collapse" (with no pathologic evidence of myocardial infarction), and 9% of the primary illness. Aspiration, strokes, and gastro-intestinal bleeding each contributed 6%, and myocardial infarction contributed only 2%.

Other papers have found similar results, although the rates of myocardial infarction are usually in the 20% to 30% range. Pneumonia is the cause of death in about 15% to 30%, while pulmonary emboli contribute 10% to 20%. Sepsis is also seen regularly.[30] The highest death rates are for those patients having abdominal procedures, particularly those with perforation, obstruction, or bowel infarction.

Statistics for those with comorbid diseases are interesting.[55] Mortality in those with dementia was a surprising 45%. This is likely to be the result of patient selection, since only absolutely necessary or life-threatening surgery is likely to be done in the patients. In addition, demented patients cannot cooperate very well in postoperative care. Those with diabetes had a 26% rate, and those with cardiac disease died 17% of the time. Although the rate for cardiac disease seems relatively low compared with other disease states, unfortunately cardiac disease is very common. For this reason, those with cardiac disease alone, or in combination with diabetes, gangrene, dementia or pulmonary disease, accounted for 44 of the 54 deaths.

Preoperative evaluation

In many ways, the preoperative evaluation of the elderly differs little from the workup of younger people. Basically, a good history and physical must be done; but the elderly do present unique problems in preoperative evaluation.

First, physicians must remember all the expected physiologic decrements. Although elderly patients can often withstand the initial stresses of surgery, once a complication ensues, they have less reserve and are less likely to survive. Wilder and Fishbein found the mortality among those with complications was 62% but only 13% among those who appeared to be having a smooth postoperative course.[56] The most important decrements are in cardiac, pulmonary, and renal function as we have seen. These are the systems that sustain the most postoperative problems. Any underlying disease in these organ systems markedly diminishes the patient's ability to survive a complication.

Evaluating an older patient's history is fraught with difficulties. Some elderly patients are less than patient with long, meticulous histories, so history-taking should be to the point. In addition, elderly patients are often hard of hearing, and their memory of, and attention to, specific symptoms may be less than ideal. The elderly often minimize their symptoms out of fear of the consequences of the disease or because they feel that old age is necessarily accompanied by infirmity.

Symptoms may be less apparent and less specific than in younger patients, particularly in regard to infections and pain, which can be especially difficult to document.[57] Often, patients or their families complain of non-specific problems such as confusion, malaise, incontinence, falls, or refusal to eat.

Even specific complaints may be confusing. The presence of angina may be represented by prominent shortness of breath or epigastric discomfort rather than by classic substernal chest pain. Chest pain may be a manifestation of intra-abdominal processes rather than cardiac in origin. Abdominal pain is often poorly localized and may seem to be less severe than one would expect. Thus this misdirection can delay the diagnosis in such important diseases as appendicitis, mesenteric insufficiency, and perforations of ulcers or diverticuli.

Fever can be absent in many disease states that in younger people are manifest as febrile illness, and these diseases may present in the elderly as malaise or delirium. This is commonly true with pneumonia and urinary tract infection. Many patients complain of dyspnea for which an etiology cannot be found; it is important, however to make the diagnosis of heart failure or coronary disease if either of these is the etiology of the dyspnea. A heavy smoking history and symptoms of chronic bronchitis or emphysema are also quite important to elicit. Similarly, large numbers of elderly patients present with urinary and bowel complaints, and the physician must be aware of the possibilities of urinary obstruction and the increased risk of colon cancer. A careful history of medications is crucial: substantial numbers of elderly patients go to more than one doctor; they often take a number of over-the-counter drugs; and increasing numbers of patients are taking herbs and other complementary treatments that may have important clinical effects.

Taking note of visual and hearing impairments is important to help to provide sensory stimuli for patients who are at high risk for delirium, which presents great problems in providing postoperative care. Confused and disoriented patients, i.e., those with postoperative delirium, remove nasogastric tubes and intravenous lines, disrupt wounds, fall from beds and break bones. Studies have shown that these people have a much greater in-hospital mortality and decreased quality of life and life expectancy after discharge.[55–59]

Physical examination also presents difficult problems. An acutely ill elderly patient may cooperate poorly;

the examination should be direct and performed as expeditiously as possible. Nutritional assessment including the state of hydration is a primary area of concern that is often overlooked or addressed in a cursory fashion.[60] Chapter 2 provides a good way to assess nutritional status. It can be very difficult to assess fluid status in these patients. The most important pitfalls are found in evaluating skin turgor and peripheral edema. Turgor is hard to assess because of senile skin changes; I believe that the skin over the forehead is the most reliable area to check. Neck veins can be helpful particularly if they are clearly distended or flat. Peripheral edema can be quite misleading since many elderly patients have venous insufficiency and are often sedentary, accumulating dependent fluid. Patients are frequently quite unhappy with edema and wish it to be treated; unfortunately, many physicians are disturbed by edema as well and frequently treat it despite its usual benign nature. Vigorous diuresis to remove the edema may leave the patient significantly intravascularly depleted, predisposing to intraoperative hypotension and renal failure. Blood urea nitrogen:creatinine (BUN/Cr) ratio can also be quite helpful in those who are not malnourished. While there are other causes of an increased ratio (e.g., steroid therapy and gastrointestinal bleeding), any BUN/Cr ratio above 10 should result in a careful assessment, looking for intravascular volume depletion.

Protein-calorie malnutrition has also been shown to increase postoperative complications and decrease survival; hyperalimentation can decrease complications and increase survival[61] (see Chapter 2). From the ages of 65 to 94, the percentage of underweight men increases from 20% to 50% and the percentage of underweight women increases from 20% to 55%.[62] Elderly patients are often malnourished for a multitude of reasons: underlying disease states such as heart disease, diabetes, or pulmonary disease; drugs that interfere with digestion, absorption, appetite, and taste or smell; inadequate dentition; physical disability causing an inability to shop, cook or feed oneself; and poverty.

The recognition, evaluation, and therapy of protein-calorie malnutrition is therefore a very important part of the preoperative evaluation.[60] Recognition and evaluation can be carried out in the same manner as in younger patients. In addition, it has been shown by Kaminski and colleagues that older patients can tolerate aggressive enteral and parenteral hyperalimentation as well.[63] Decisions regarding hyperalimentation should be made by assessing the patient and the problem, not by looking at age.

Skin changes in elderly patients also add to the risks of hospitalization and surgery. Subcutaneous tissue decreases and the epidermis thins and becomes much more fragile. Pressure ulcers can occur with rather short episodes of bedrest and lack of position change. Pressure ulcers are an important cause of increased morbidity and frequently result in institutionalization of patients.

Biochemical deficiencies also occur with increased frequency. Elderly patients have often been shown to be deficient in vitamin A, pyridoxine, and calcium and iron. The latter two are absorbed less well in the elderly. Vitamin C and zinc appear to have a role in wound healing, and some studies indicate that at least some patients have decreased levels. Some surgeons routinely supplement both in operative patients.

Cardiac status, particularly in reference to signs of heart failure, needs careful evaluation. Systolic murmurs are quite common, and are frequently benign; significant aortic stenosis, however, is important to identify because it is an important risk factor. Low systolic blood pressure, narrow pulse pressure, enlarged and sustained PMI pulsation, and left ventricular hypertrophy on the electrocardiogram can be helpful in identifying patients who may have significant stenosis. There continues to be a great degree of controversy about the management of carotid bruits. Bruits that are accompanied by ischemic symptoms should be evaluated before surgery. Cerebral arterial bruits in the absence of symptoms, on the other hand, are a difficult problem and there are supporters of aggressive intervention and others who are much less aggressive and recommend no intervention without symptoms. This area of evaluation is discussed in detail in Chapter 32. My personal bias is not to evaluate patients without symptoms; there is still inadequate information to do diagnostic or therapeutic interventions routinely.[64] Evidence of underlying pulmonary disease will help to identify those at risk for atelectasis and pneumonia. The final significant examination should be for evidence of dementia and confusion, since patients so afflicted do so poorly after surgery. Patients with dementia are at much higher risk of delirium from both hospitalization and the surgical procedure. In Palmberg's study, mortality was 45% in those with dementia; in Wickstrom's study, seven of eleven patients who died had senile dementia.[55,65]

Laboratory assessment, as in all other patients, is still controversial. For a detailed discussion of preoperative testing see Chapter 3. Some authors still recommend all the "standard" laboratory tests: complete blood counts, electrolytes, chemistry panels, urinalysis, chest X-ray, and electrocardiogram. Some recommend routine pulmonary function tests, and Del Guercio and colleagues in a commonly cited study and others in more recent papers recommended routine use of diagnostic Swan–Ganz catheterization.[66] This view is not supported by good evidence.

For the well elderly, most geriatricians believe that there are few preoperative tests that need to be done. These recommendations include an hematocrit, a test of renal function, usually creatinine, an electrocardiogram and a chest X-ray. There is increasing evidence that, even in the elderly, only clinically indicated tests need to be done.[67] Many elderly patients have underlying diseases and take many medications, including over-the-counter drugs and therefore many patients will have indications for a significant number of preoperative tests. For indications for preoperative testing, see Chapter 3.

Seymour and colleagues did a study of electrocardiograms in 222 surgical patients over 65.[68] Only 21% had a normal preoperative electrocardiogram, and 53% had a major abnormality. Twenty-seven patients had a postoperative cardiovascular complication, including 22 cases of heart failure, three definite myocardial infarctions, and two suspected myocardial infarctions. Of interest, however, is that, in men, there was no correlation between preoperative abnormalities and postoperative complications, while in women there did seem to be some minor predictive value; they were not, however, clinically helpful. There were a large number of nonspecific changes in the electrocardiograms after surgery. The authors suggested that preoperative electrocardiograms should be done as a baseline measure to aid in interpretation of postoperative electrocardiographic changes. A recent study has again shown the lack of predictive value of an electrocardiogram.[69]

A study of chest X-rays was done by Tornebrandt and Fletcher.[70] They studied 100 consecutive patients over 70 for elective surgery. Of 91 chest X-rays, 43 were abnormal: 28 had cardiomegaly, 11 pulmonary hypertension, 7 chronic pulmonary disease, and one a pleural effusion. Of the 27 patients without an indication, 10 had abnormal findings: 5 had cardiomegaly, 2 atelectasis, and one each with emphysema, pulmonary hypertension, and tracheal deviation. Ten percent of the patients developed a postoperative complication, for which a comparison film was helpful. The authors did not attempt to see if the abnormal findings were predictive of postoperative complications, and it is hard to determine whether the routine use of chest X-rays really makes a difference in care. Because of the high incidence of cardiopulmonary complications, however, a recent chest X-ray is probably useful for comparison when a postoperative chest X-ray is necessary.

Although some authors recommend routine pulmonary function testing,[71,72] there are no definitive studies supporting its routine use. It seems reasonable to use the same indications employed for younger patients (see Chapter 9). Arterial blood gases, however, may be more important. As discussed in the physiology section, P_aO_2 falls progressively from an average P_aO_2 of 94 mm Hg for those under 30 to only 74 mm Hg for those over 60 in normal non-smoking patients. There is, however, a wide range of normal in elderly patients and it is impossible to know if a given patient's baseline P_aO_2 is 74 or 92 mm Hg. Those with a smoking history or evidence of chronic obstructive pulmonary disease are obviously affected even more. Since there is such a high incidence of postoperative cardiopulmonary complications, many patients may benefit from having a baseline P_aO_2 to help with diagnosis and therapy postoperatively.

Although specific management of disease states is beyond the scope of this chapter, some unique points must be emphasized in pulmonary care. Patients should stop smoking before the procedure. It has been shown that stopping smoking for 8 weeks before surgery is important to significantly decrease the incidence of postoperative complications. They should also be educated about incentive spirometry, coughing, and deep breathing. Finally, meticulous attention to pulmonary toilet both before admission and after surgery will help to reduce complications postoperatively.

The indications for invasive monitoring are still debated; most experts, however, do not believe that routine use is beneficial. Del Guercio and Cohn studied 148 consecutive patients who had been "cleared" for surgery by routine assessment.[66] The authors used a staging system that required Swan–Ganz catheterization in all patients and multiple cardiopulmonary function measurements. They reported that many patients had unsuspected abnormalities that put them at increased risk, and they were able to find a very high risk group for mortality although these patients had been "cleared" for surgery. Surgery was canceled or modified in some, and all of those who underwent the original procedure died.

The study, however, does not help to decide which patients need this kind of invasive testing. First, it was not controlled. The authors also included a number of young patients who were diseased, whom they called "physiologically old"; about one-third of the patients were under 60 and approximately half were under 70. From the data, it seems clear that some patients can benefit from this type of invasive evaluation; it is not clear from this study which patients do benefit. In addition, complications from procedures must be considered.

A later study by Schrader and colleagues has shown that routine use is often unnecessary.[73] They looked at 46 patients, over the age of 90, who had surgery. None of their patients had invasive monitoring and underwent 51 procedures, many of which were major surgery. There were seven major complications; only one of the major complications might have been predicted by the pre-operative use of Swan–Ganz catheterization. Most importantly, there were no perioperative deaths in their entire series. While it seems clear that there are patients who need intensive monitoring and evaluation preoperatively, it is also clear that age alone is not a primary indication for these tests.

Anesthesia

Although specifics of anesthetic care are beyond the scope of this chapter, some information is interesting and helpful to the non-anesthesiologist. There is a continuing debate over the choice of regional or general anesthesia. There appear to be arguments, both pro and con, for each. It seems clear that there is no appreciable difference in mortality.[65,74–77]

General anesthesia has a number of advantages. The patient is unconscious and therefore prevents unwanted movement. There is no anxiety during the procedure. In addition, control of respiration through endotracheal intubation is felt by some to be helpful in the elderly because of decreased respiratory function. There appear to be some drawbacks, however. It appears that there is an increased incidence of pulmonary complications. There may be an increased incidence of mental disturbances in those who undergo general anesthesia;[74] there have also been some small studies that have not found differences.[78] The extent of this effect is uncertain, but if present, is probably not large and may be outweighed by other considerations.

Regional methods have advantages as well. Some patients prefer being awake for their procedure. Some anesthesiologists believe that there is less suppression of respiration, less hypoxia, and perhaps fewer respiratory complications, but this is unclear.[74] Disadvantages include difficulties with moving of anxious patients and a somewhat higher incidence of intraoperative and postoperative hypotension.[75] In Hole's study of epidural versus general anesthesia in hip surgery, an equal number of patients in each group (four of 29 and four of 31) did not want the same kind of anesthesia if they were to be operated on for the other hip.[74] A recent Cochrane review of anesthesia in hip fracture reached similar conclusions about the lack of a significant difference between methods.[79]

Evaluation of risk

There have been a number of people who have attempted to find ways to quantify the risks of surgery from the data gleaned from history, physical examination and laboratory data. As with all other patients assessment of preoperative risk can begin with indices of cardiac risk by Goldman or Detsky discussed in Chapter 6.[28,80] The factors identified by these two groups have continued to be identified as important contributors to cardiac morbidity and mortality. They include recent myocardial infarction, severe or unstable angina, congestive heart failure, significant aortic stenosis, arrhythmia, poor general medical status, and emergency operations.

While the Goldman and Detsky indices identified important risk factors, they both have limited sensitivity and miss a considerable percentage of patients who have complications who were calculated to be at low risk. Gerson found that supine bicycle exercise was a way to increase sensitivity.[81] He found that the inability to increase heart rate above 99 beats per minute during 2 minutes of exercise was predictive of increased risk in the elderly population. A second paper by Gerson and colleagues found that this test was also useful for identifying elderly patients who were at risk for pulmonary complications.[82] This method has not been used by many people.

The most commonly used system to identify cardiac risk has been that devised by the American Heart Association in conjunction with the American College of Cardiology.[83] This system is addressed in detail in Chapter 6. Some of the major conclusions of the system are of interest. The most influential conclusion is that evaluation for pre-operative revascularization should generally be limited to those patients who have indications for evaluation even without surgery unless the surgery involves major vascular procedures in patients with limited mobility. Another important factor limiting the need for evaluation is the ability of the patient to exercise; most patients who can exercise at the 4 MET level (e.g., walking on level ground at a 4 mph pace) will not need preoperative evaluation.

Common surgical problems in the elderly

Cardiovascular surgery

General considerations

There is no doubt that cardiovascular surgery is feasible in the elderly patient. Many studies have been done to show that coronary bypass, valve replacement, and vascular surgery can be done in the elderly with acceptable mortality.[84–86] This can be true, even in those with severe cardiovascular disease, since the mortality from the underlying disease is very high. As discussed earlier, however, should these patients require emergency surgery, the mortality is much higher, frequently in the 80% range.

Coronary bypass surgery

There are now many studies of elderly patients who have undergone coronary artery bypass grafting procedures.[87,88] Many of these studies have been done on those between 80 and 90 years of age. Those patients who have no other underlying diseases and who are undergoing elective procedures have quite low mortality, perhaps a few percent, comparable with a younger population. Those with unstable angina, recent MI, reduced cardiac function and left main disease, are at higher risk, and perhaps higher than younger patients, at the 10%–12% level. As expected, however, there are more complications in these elderly patients because of their decreased reserve.

A number of studies have been done in those who are in NYHA Class IV. Even these patients should be considered for CABG procedures despite mortality rates in the 15%–20% range, since their prognosis without surgery is quite bad. Those who have particularly high mortality are those undergoing emergency procedures and those requiring intraaortic balloon pulsation.

Other very important factors in deciding to do surgery are the long term survival and functional improvement if surgery is done. Both of these areas have been studied and there are good data to show that the elderly have increased survival and are able to function at a higher level after surgery in a large percentage of those who survive surgery. Considerable numbers of patients have been shown to go from NYHA Class IV to NYHA Classes I and II. The latest innovation in bypass surgery has improved results even more. Off pump bypass procedures lead to fewer complications, shorter hospitalizations and lower costs.[89,90] Mortality rates are lower as well.[91]

Valvular surgery

There are many elderly patients who have significant valve pathology, particularly aortic stenosis and mitral insufficiency. The results of surgical procedures in these patients are mixed.[92–95] Again, there can be great benefit to these patients if they are properly selected and well cared for.

Aortic valve replacement can be a life-saving and life-sustaining procedure. When found early enough, particularly before the onset of significant myocardial dysfunction, elderly patients can have remarkable results from aortic valve replacement. Studies have shown increases in long-term survival and impressive increases in functional capacity. Operative mortality in those without severe myocardial dysfunction can be as low as a few percent.

Overall mortality for those with aortic valve replacement has been in the 10% range. Patients who do survive have had excellent results from their surgery. Their long-term survival is excellent; in one study 5-year survival was 70% (including operative mortality) compared to published 5-year survival of about 20% in those without surgery. Additionally, functional improvement is often dramatic with some studies showing almost all patients improving to NYHA Classes I and II. Recent studies confirm these basic principles.[96]

Mitral valve replacement is, unfortunately, not as successful.[97] Patients with mitral valve disease often can go for long periods of time without symptoms and, even after symptoms begin, they can be controlled reasonably well with medication. Thus, by the time the usual elderly patient is considered for surgery, there is often a good deal of underlying myocardial dysfunction. Mortality in mitral valve surgery is often in the 20% range and can be as high as 50% in those with significant heart failure, previous mitral procedures (valvulotomy), and pulmonary hypertension. Most patients appear to die of low output states accompanied by multiple organ failure. There is good evidence, however, that if patients survive surgery, their survival is approximately that of the population in general. There is a clearcut difference in mortality between those with mitral stenosis who do better, and those with mitral regurgitation who do less well.

Results of combined surgical procedures show an increase in mortality as well. Those who get aortic and mitral valves have a modestly increased mortality. Those who have coronary bypass procedures and mitral valve replacement appear to have a greatly increased risk of death and some authors suggest that this combination of procedures should be avoided if possible.

Vascular surgery

Since atherosclerosis is a disease of aging, many elderly patients are candidates for vascular surgery. A number of different procedures have been studied, particularly aortic aneurysm repair and carotid endarterectomy.

Many studies have been done for aortic aneurysms.[98,99] It is abundantly clear that emergency aneurysmectomy is a deadly procedure. Mortality ranges from 40%–80%, usually in the upper range. Alternatively, mortality for elective procedures generally is in the 5%–10% range. Symptomatic aneurysm repair usually falls in the middle of these.

It appears clear that patients who have diagnosed abdominal aneurysms larger than 6 cm should be seriously considered for elective aortic replacement if they do not have a high risk of mortality because of underlying diseases. There is a high risk of rupture in these patients and high mortality from emergency replacement surgery.

Results of surgery in older patients with carotid artery disease are still not clearcut. Cerebrovascular disease is discussed in detail in Chapter 32. As in younger patients, there are few clearcut definitive surgical indications for patients with carotid disease. It is clear that many elderly patients, particularly those with transient hemispheric symptoms can get relief of those symptoms, with acceptable, but somewhat increased, morbidity (perioperative stroke) and mortality. Surgery can be performed with low morbidity and mortality in the right hands, but clearcut benefits for those without symptoms are not obvious.[100] Most papers indicate that a lot of the morbidity from stroke appears to result from the presence of significant intracranial vascular disease that is obviously more prevalent in this aged population.

Peripheral arterial reconstructions in the elderly can be helpful procedures that can be done with little increase in morbidity and mortality compared to younger patients. There is still the continued higher risk of perioperative myocardial infarction, since coronary disease is so prevalent in those with peripheral vascular disease. The procedures usually result in increases in functional state and can prevent loss of limbs.

Orthopedic surgery

General considerations
Arthritis, particularly of the hip, is a very important factor limiting the mobility and independence of elderly patients. Fractures are also an important cause of morbidity and mortality. They are also very important as causes of immobility, dependency, and institutionalization.

Hip fracture
There are approximately 250 000 hip fractures in the USA each year. Elderly patients account for the vast majority of these fractures. Many of these patients are women who have substantial degrees of osteoporosis.

The care of these patients is clearly operative if at all possible. Morbidity from the procedure in unselected populations is quite low (approximately 5%) considering that significant proportions of these patients have chronic diseases and are debilitated. While mortality is not particularly high for the procedure and perioperative period, these patients often suffer a great loss of mobility and become more dependent on others for a variable length of time. It has been shown that the functional state depends heavily on the functional state of the patient before the fracture and not on chronological age. About 70% of those who were able to walk before the fracture are able to walk in some way after the operation. While there are some patients who must be admitted to nursing homes after the procedures, most patients who lived independently or with some assistance before the fracture are able to live independently or with some assistance after the procedure as well.

There are a number of important factors in the postoperative morbidity and mortality of femoral fracture patients. The procedures themselves are neither elective nor emergent. It is quite important that patients have adequate preoperative care to assure that they have had appropriate fluid resuscitation and that cardiopulmonary physiology is optimized. On the other hand, there are many studies showing that the sooner the operation is undertaken, the better the results.

Many patients have some degree of delirium postoperatively and this complication must be anticipated. Many patients suffer postoperative pulmonary complications so that, as much as possible, pre- and postoperative preparation and prophylactic measures should be taken. Another common, difficult and avoidable problem is that of pressure ulcers. These need to be avoided if at all possible since they contribute to increased lengths of stay, perioperative mortality, and admission to nursing homes instead of more independent living arrangements.

Elective hip replacement
The case for elective hip replacement is also strong, particularly since this can be performed with good results in a well selected population.[101] Most of these selected patients have very painful and disabling joint disease. In one study of 100 patients in their 80s, 92 returned home. In this population, there were only two deaths, one from MI and the other from PE.[102] DVT and UTI were the most common postoperative complications, as in most studies of hip repair. The vast majority of the patients have good to excellent results and have been happy to have had the surgery done.

Other elective joint replacement surgery has been done in the elderly population. Knee joints are commonly affected by osteoarthritis. Because the elderly are less mobile than younger patients, they in some ways are better candidates for replacement, since loosening with use is a major problem with this procedure. Ankle, shoulder, and elbow replacements have all been done in selected patients with good results.

The evaluation of rehabilitation units for geriatric patients with orthopedic problems is just beginning. There is some evidence to show that these units can be helpful in getting patients to be more self-sufficient and independent. Units have been developed for rehabilitation of hip fracture and replacement and amputations. The most important obstacle to rehabilitation is alteration in mental status; those with signs of dementia do poorly.

Abdominal surgery

General considerations

A great deal of work has been done to evaluate abdominal surgery in the elderly population since this is a major site for operations. More importantly, the morbidity and mortality from abdominal surgery can be high depending on a number of factors. The following factors are significantly associated with poorer prognosis: increasing age; emergency procedures; malignancy; poor physical status; and the site of surgery in the abdomen. Factors of aging, emergency surgery, malignancy and poor physical status have been addressed earlier in this chapter; they will be addressed only where there is significant additional information. One other factor that appears to be very important in abdominal surgery for these patients is infection. The risks of infection are much higher in abdominal surgery than in most other sites; the elderly seem to have a higher risk of infection than younger patients and they have much more difficulty in handling these infections.

Gall bladder disease

One of the more common problems in the elderly is the question of what to do with the discovery of gallstones. This decision is made more (or less) difficult by the findings of the results of emergency surgery for acute cholecystitis. Patients who must undergo emergency surgery for gall bladder disease have a mortality that ranges from 12%–20%. The corresponding mortality for those who have elective surgery is between 3% and 5%. Thus emergency surgery appears to be something to avoid as we have seen earlier.[103,104] One study has suggested that there is no indication for emergency cholecystectomy in the elderly; it suggests that patients should be stabilized if at all possible with fluids and antibiotics before the patient goes to the operating room. This is not a proven concept, and others believe that the only therapy for symptomatic gall bladder disease is immediate surgery. There is general agreement, however, that medical therapy alone is not an option in these patients.

Many elderly patients who present with symptomatic gall bladder disease already have gangrene and empyema;

a significant number have been found to have perforations, which can lead to subphrenic abscesses as well. This is not surprising since these patients often present with fewer and less severe symptoms, despite more severe disease.

Complications of importance in those having surgery for gall bladder disease are not surprising. Many patients have sepsis with common Gram-negative organisms, wound infections, and pulmonary complications as expected in those having upper abdominal surgery.

The advent of laparoscopic procedures for gall bladder disease has been a great boon for elderly patients. The risks of the surgery, particularly pulmonary complications, are much lower by this approach and therefore an elective operation can be undertaken with the expectation that there will be a good result. A number of studies have shown better results with this approach.[105–107]

Appendicitis

Appendicitis is one of the most frequently missed diagnoses in the elderly population. This can be of great consequence, since the disease can be fatal and, importantly, can be cured if the diagnosis is made in time.[108,109] The reason that the diagnosis is frequently missed is because it is never considered. Any elderly patient with abdominal pain should have appendicitis in the differential diagnosis. While symptoms are usually less severe than in younger patients, the elderly still most frequently present with the symptoms of abdominal pain, nausea and fever. They will frequently have abdominal tenderness as well.

A significant number of elderly patients has already perforated the appendix before operation. Although there are often delays in the diagnosis because of non-specific and muted symptoms, there are other factors involved. The appendix atrophies with age and the walls thin. In addition, the blood supply to the organ is also compromised with age. Thus, with infection, and increased pressure in the appendix, blood supply is quickly impeded, and the thinned wall more easily perforates.

Mortality in this disease depends heavily on the state of the patients underlying health, and even more importantly, on the progression of the disease. In those operated on early, mortality is quite low. If the diagnosis can be made before complications, the laparoscopic approach can be used as well with lower risks.[110] However, as perforation, abscess and sepsis appear, the mortality rates increase from 5% up to 20%–25%.

Colon resection

Elective resection of the colon is a reasonably safe procedure in the elderly. While most resections are for carcinoma which will be addressed later, other indications include diverticular disease, polyps, and other benign disorders. Mortality for elective resections is usually below 5%.[111] The laparoscopic approach has been used for colon resection as well with excellent results.[112]

Gynecologic surgery

General considerations

Major gynecologic surgery has been done for many years in elderly women.[113,114] Elective vaginal hysterectomy for such indications as prolapse has been shown to be very safe with mortality rates in the range of 1%. Abdominal hysterectomy has a higher mortality rate, in the 5% range. Studies have shown that elderly women who have surgery for pelvic malignancies have substantial survival after surgery so that age alone should not be considered a contraindication for surgery for pelvic cancers. Laparoscopic procedures have been used for gynecologic disease with good results in properly selected cases.

Cancer surgery

General considerations

Since cancer risk increases with age, the elderly have a disproportionate number of cancers and surgery is still the primary treatment modality for most forms of this disease process. The decision to perform cancer surgery in the elderly patient, however, also rests on a number of factors. The first is the combination of the life expectancy of the patient without surgery and the natural history of the underlying cancer. Radical surgery for a prostate cancer in an ill 90-year-old man is probably not indicated; alternatively, resection of a bowel cancer in a vigorous 70-year-old woman is clearly indicated. The second factor is the availability of non-surgical therapy. The final factor is the risk of the proposed surgery in relation to the chance of cure or life prolongation.

Lung cancer

Most lung cancers occur in the older age group. Since there is no curative non-surgical therapy, resection is the therapy of choice, if possible.[115,116] Given equivalent levels of pulmonary function, in general, the elderly do quite well in comparison with younger patients with lung resections. Mortality from surgery in elderly patients overall is in the 10%–15% range. Five-year survival in a group of patients over 70 years of age in one study was 32%, which is quite good.[117] Important to note is the fact that none of the patients in that study had other underlying severe disease. Some studies of patients treated without operation have had 0% 1 year survival.

Colon cancer

Most colon surgery in the elderly is for cancer. As with lung cancer, there is no curative non-surgical therapy for these patients. A number of studies have been done in the over 75 age group; these studies have shown the mortality for colon resection is between 2% and 9%, most in the lower range since most operations are elective.[118–120] In one study, all nine patients in their 90s survived the surgery. Laparoscopic procedures have been used effectively for colon cancer in properly selected cases with very good results.[121] Most patients who are admitted from home are able to return, and most importantly, postsurgical survival compares well with younger patients with bowel cancer. Because of the relatively long natural history of bowel cancers in general, the survival of older patients may not differ from their normal disease-free cohort, since they often die from other causes.

Other cancers

Esophageal cancer is a deadly disease that cannot be treated without surgery. One study from Japan showed that surgical results are reasonably good in the elderly.[122] This study showed a moderate increase in mortality in the elderly that appeared to result from an increase in pulmonary complications. The survival of the elderly group followed for 5 years is approximately 25%, essentially identical to those less than 60 years of age. A more recent study continues to support operative therapy if possible.[123]

Similar results have been found in a number of studies of gastric cancer.[124,125] Mortality is often somewhat greater in the elderly; however, many of their cancers are found at a later stage of disease. Their survival rates compare favorably with a younger population, and since non-surgical therapy offers nothing, surgical intervention is clearly indicated if the perioperative mortality is deemed to be reasonable.

Studies of the therapy of breast cancer have shown that 5-year survivals have been in the 50% range.[126] Since the risks of curative surgery are quite low in this disease process, operation should be offered to most patients.[127]

Postoperative care of the elderly patient

As with preoperative care, the postoperative management of the elderly patient is basically the same as for the younger patient. However, meticulous attention to detail and awareness of potential problems give these patients a better chance of survival and less opportunity for postoperative complications.

Even in the recovery room, attention to details of care is important. Hypothermia is common because of cool operating rooms, room temperature intravenous infusions, and cold blood transfusions.[128,129] Some elderly patients are particularly susceptible because of faulty temperature regulation. Hypothermia itself depresses the heart. In addition, on rewarming, the increased metabolic activity and cardiac output needed puts an added stress on the heart.

Narcotic-induced ventilatory depression can last longer than usual in the elderly. Particularly in patients who have had general anesthesia, there can be a significant drop in P_aO_2 after surgery.[130] This appears to be caused by a combination of shunting and an increase in ventilation–perfusion mismatching; this effect increases with increasing age. Campbell has stated that, in those in whom postoperative complications are expected, the continued use of mechanical ventilation into the postoperative period may help to prevent some of these complications.[71] In this way, adequate ventilation even in the face of narcotic analgesics and good tracheobronchial toilet can be provided. There is no objective evidence to support or refute this method of care.

It is clear, however, that it is quite important for elderly patients to be up in a chair and moving as soon as possible after surgery. This allows for increases in ventilation and easier clearing of secretions and results in less atelectasis. An important factor in avoiding pulmonary complications is adequate pain relief as well. Patients in pain, particularly from thoracic or abdominal surgery, are less likely to cough, breathe deeply, and cooperate with respiratory therapy.

Postoperative delirium is common in elderly patients, and those who manifest these changes have a mortality about twice that of patients who do not have delirium.[58,131] It has been estimated that 20%–30% of elderly patients become delirious following surgery; Bedford reported that 33% of 4000 patients who exhibited delirium during their hospital admission died within 1 month.[58,132]

Some authors feel that this complication in postsurgical patients is caused by the general anesthetic's effects on the cerebral cortex. Blundell did a study of 86 surgical patients over 70 years of age.[133] She found that the main effects were on memory and intellectual abilities that require organization of thought; these effects often lasted for several weeks after that.

Hole and coworkers feel that the effect may be on oxygenation of the brain. They argue that there is a decrease in cardiac output with positive pressure ventilation and that hyperventilation with resulting hypocapnia causes a further decrease in blood flow from the resulting cerebral

vasoconstriction.[74] Others feel that it may be an effect of the anesthetic agents themselves.

Some interesting factors appear to influence these changes. Those who have regional anesthesia appear to be affected to a lesser degree; those who have shorter procedures are often less affected; those who are febrile and are given other drugs are more frequently affected.

The prevention of postoperative delirium has been studied and there are data to support a variety of methods to decrease the incidence of this important complication. Marcantonio and colleagues looked at a group of patients having hip surgery and intervened in a number of different areas.[134] These included: oxygenation; fluids and electrolyte balances; pain; medications; bowel and bladder functions; nutrition; mobilization; observation and treatment for complications; and environmental factors like lighting and sensory stimulation. They were able to decrease the incidence of delirium from 50% to 32%.

Heart failure and myocardial infarction are two important and deadly postoperative complications. Heart failure can be prevented, at least in part, by meticulous attention to intravenous infusions and urine output. At times, it will be essential to use invasive monitoring by Swan–Ganz catheterization. As discussed above, clinical judgment must be used to decide which patients are likely to need this monitoring method.

Although physicians are unable to prevent myocardial infarction, it is possible to anticipate its occurrence and to be able to recognize its unusual presentations in the elderly. In a study of 387 patients over the age of 65, Pathy found that the "classic" presentation was seen in only 19% of the total. The most common presentations were sudden dyspnea or exacerbation of heart failure (20%). Other presentations were acute delirium (13%), strokes, peripheral emboli, and weakness.

Pulmonary embolism is a frequent complication that is theoretically preventable. Chapter 19 covers the discussion of DVT and pulmonary embolism prophylaxis in detail. There is evidence that, for most procedures, low-dose heparin before and after surgery is helpful. This method is not helpful in orthopedic procedures and low molecular weight heparin or coumadin prophylaxis should be used; intermittent compression stockings are used in neurosurgery and open prostatectomy, where anticoagulation is dangerous.

Because of their frailty and decreases in physiologic reserve, older patients who have complications have a greatly increased mortality, so that prevention and early intervention are crucial to their well being. As in all care of the elderly, careful attention to detail in all aspects of postoperative management will result in lower morbidity and mortality.

REFERENCES

1. Boss, G. R. & Seegmiller, J. E. Age-related physiological changes and their clinical significance. *West. J. Med.* 1981; **135**: 434–440.

2. Abrass, I. B. The biology and physiology of aging. *West. J. Med.* 1990; **153**: 641–645.

3. Evers, B. M., Townsend, C. M., & Thompson, J. C. Organ physiology of aging. *Surg. Clin. North Am.* 1994; **74**: 23–39.

4. Gerstenblith, G., Lakatta, E. G., & Weisfeldt, M. L. Age changes in myocardial function and exercise response. *Prog. Cardiovasc. Dis.* l976; **19**: 1–21.

5. Weisfeldt, M. L. Aging of the cardiovascular system. *N. Engl. J. Med.* 1980; **303**: 1172–1173.

6. Port, S., Cobb, F. R., Coleman, R. E., & Jones, R H. Effect of age on the response of the left ventricular ejection fraction to exercise. *N. Engl. J. Med.* 1980; **303**: 1133–1137.

7. Strahlman, E. R., ed. Clinical conferences at the Johns Hopkins Hospital: Presbycardia. *Johns Hopkins Med. J.* 1981; **149**: 203–208.

8. Kent, S. The aging lung. Part 1. Loss of elasticity. *Geriatrics* 1978; **33**(2): 124–130.

9. Sorbini, C. A., Grassi, V., Solinas, E., & Muiesan, G. Arterial oxygen tension in relation to age in healthy subjects. *Respiration* 1968; **25**: 3–13.

10. Muiesan, G., Sorbini, C. A., & Grassi, V. Respiratory function in the aged. *Bull. Physio.-Pathol. Respir.* 1971; **7**: 973–1007.

11. McLachlan, M. S. F. The aging kidney. *Lancet* 1978; **2**: 143–146.

12. Friedman, S. A., Raizner, A. E., Rosen, H., Solomon, N. A., & Sy, W. Functional defects in the aging kidney. *Ann. Intern. Med.* 1972; **76**: 41–45.

13. Cockcroft, D. W. & Gault, M. H. Prediction of creatinine clearance from serum creatinine. *Nephron* 1976; **16**: 31–41.

14. Hollenberg, N. K., Adams, D. F., Solomon, H. S. *et al.* Senescence and the renal vasculature in normal man. *Circ. Res.* 1974; **34**: 309–316.

15. Creditor, M. Hazards of hospitalization of the elderly. *Ann. Intern. Med.* 1993; **118**: 219–223.

16. Ochsner, A. Is risk of indicated operation too great in the elderly? *Geriatrics* 1967; **22**: 121–130.

17. Gilbert, T., Orr, W., & Banning, A. P. Surgery for aortic stenosis in severely symptomatic patients older than 80 years: experience in a single UK centre. *Heart* 1999; **82**: 138–142.

18. Rosengart, T. K., Finnin, E. B., Kim, D. Y. *et al.* Open heart surgery in the elderly: results from a consecutive series of 100 patients aged 85 or older. *Am. J. Med.* 2002; **112**: 143–147.

19. Pofahl, W. E. & Pories, W. J. Current status and future directions of geriatric general surgery. *J. Am. Geriatr. Soc.* 2003; **51**: S351–S354.

20. Liu, L. L. & Leung, J. M. Predicting adverse postoperative outcomes in patients aged 80 years or older. *J. Am. Geriatr. Soc.* 2000; **48**: 405–412.

21. Leung, J. M. & Dzanic, S. *J. Am. Geriatr. Soc.* 2001; **49**: 1080–1085.

22. Polanczyk, C. A., Marcantonio, E., Goldman, L. *et al.* Impact of age on perioperative complications and length of stay in patients undergoing noncardiac sugery. *Ann. Intern. Med.* 2001; **134**: 637–643.

23. Michel, S. L., Stevens, L., Amodeo, P., & Morgenstern, L. Surgical procedures in nonagenarians. *West. J. Med.* 1984; **141**: 61–63.

24. Keating, H. J. III. Major surgery in nursing home patients: procedures, morbidity and mortality in the frailest of the frail elderly. *J. Am. Geriatr. Soc.* 1992; **40**: 8–11.

25. Katlic, M. Surgery in centenarians. *J. Am. Med. Assoc.* 1985; **253**: 3139–3141.

26. Cogbill, T. H., Strutt, P. J., & Landercasper, J. Surgical procedures in centenarians. *Wisc. Med. J.* 1992; **91**: 527–529.

27. Linn, B. S. & Linn, M. W. Evaluation of results of surgical procedures in the elderly. *Ann. Surg.* 1982; **195**: 90–96.

28. Goldman, L., Caldera, D. L., Nussbaum, S. R. *et al.* Multifactorial index of cardiac risk in noncardiac surgical procedures. *N. Engl. J. Med.* 1977; **297**: 845–850.

29. Sikes, E. D. & Detmer, D. E. Aging and surgical risk in older citizens of Wisconsin. *Wisc. Med. J.* 1979; **78**: 27–30.

30. Turnbull, A. D., Gundy, E., Howland, W. S., & Beattie, E. J. Surgical mortality among the elderly. An analysis of 4050 operations (1970–1974). *Clin. Bull.* 1978; **8**: 139–142.

31. Adkins, R. B. & Scott, H. W. Surgical procedures in patients aged 90 years and older. *South. Med. J.* 1984; **77**: 1357–1364.

32. Seymour, D. G. & Pringle, R. A new method of auditing surgical mortality rates: application to a group of elderly general surgical patients. *Br. Med. J.* 1982; **284**: 1539–1542.

33. Alexander, K. P., Anstrom, K. J., Muhlbaier, L. H. *et al.* Outcomes of cardiac surgery in patients greater than or equal to 80 years: results from the National Cardiovascular Network. *J. Am. Coll. Cardiol.* 2000; **35**: 731–738.

34. Craver, J. M., Puskas, J. D., Wintraub, W. W. *et al.* 601 octogenarians undergoing cardiac surgery: outcome and comparison with younger age groups. *Ann. Thorac. Surg.* 2000; **69**: 317–318.

35. Alonso-Perez, M., Segura, R., Pita, S. *et al.* Operative results and death predictors for nonruptured abdominal aortic aneurysms in the elderly. *Ann. Vasc. Surg.* 2001; **15**: 306–311.

36. Huynh, T. T., Miller, C. C., Estrera, A. L. *et al.* Thoracoabdominal and descending thoracic aortic aneurysm surgery in patients aged 79 years or older. *J. Vasc. Surg.* 2002; **36**: 469–475.

37. Conti, B., Brega Massone, P. P., Lequaglie, C. *et al.* Major surgery in lung cancer in elderly patients? Risk factors analysis and long term results. *Minerva Chir.* 2002; **57**: 317–321.

38. Hanagiri, T., Muranaka, H., Hashimoto, M. *et al.* Results of surgical treatment of lung cancer in octogenarians. *Lung Cancer* 1999; **23**: 129–133.

39. Reiss, R., Deutsch, A. A., & Nudelman, I. Abdominal surgery in elderly patients: statistical analysis of clinical factors prognostic of mortality in 1,000 cases. *Mt. Sinai J. Med.* 1987; **54**: 135–140.

40. Sandler, R. S., Maule, W. F., Baltus, M. E. *et al.* Biliary tract surgery in the elderly. *J. Gen. Intern. Med.* 1987; **2**: 149–154.

41. Pigott, J. P. & Williams, G. B. Cholecystectomy in the elderly. *Am. J. Surg.* 1988; **155**: 408–410.

42. Rørbæk-Madsen, M. Herniorrhaphy in patients aged 80 years or more: a prospective analysis of morbidity and mortality. *Eur. J. Surg.* 1992; **158**: 591–594.

43. Terai, T., Henmi, T., Kanematsu, Y. *et al.* Clinical evaluation of aged patients who underwent surgery for femoral neck fractures – comparative study of clinical results according to age. *J. Orthop. Surg.* 2002; **10**: 23–28.

44. Susini, T., Scambia, G., Margariti, P. A. *et al.* Gynecologic oncologic surgery in the elderly: a retrospective analysis of 213 patients. *Gynecol. Oncol.* 1999; **75**: 437–443.

45. Dunlop, W. E., Rosenblood, L., Lawrason, L. *et al.* Effects of age and severity of illness on outcome and length of stay in geriatric surgical patients. *Am. J. Surg.* 1993; **165**: 577–580.

46. Andersen, B. & Ostberg, J. Long term prognosis in geriatric surgery: 2–17 year follow-up of 7922 patients. *J. Am. Geriatr. Soc.* 1972; **20**: 255–258.

47. Hosking, M. P., Warner, M. A., Lobdell, C. M. *et al.* Outcomes of surgery in patients 90 years of age and older. *J. Am. Med. Assoc.* 1989; **261**: 1909–1915.

48. Salem, R., Devitt, P., Johnson, J., & Firmin, R. Emergency geriatric surgical admissions. *Br. Med. J.* 1978; **2**: 416–417.

49. Seymour, D. G. & Pringle, R. Surgical emergencies in the elderly: can they be prevented? *Health Bull.* 1981; **41**: 112–131.

50. Keller, S. M., Markovitz, L. J., Wilder, J. R. *et al.* Emergency and elective surgery in patients over the age 70. *Am. Surg.* 1987; **53**: 636–640.

51. Schöön, I. M. & Arvidsson, S. Surgery in patients aged 80 years and over. *Eur. J. Surg.* 1991; **157**: 251–255.

52. Pomorski, M. E. Surgical care for the aged patient: the decision-making process. *Nurs. Clin. North Am.* 1983; **18**: 365–372.

53. Neugent, M. C. Social and emotional needs of geriatric surgery patients. *Soc. Work Health Care* l981; **6**: 69–75.

54. Reiss, R. Moral and ethical issues in geriatric surgery. *J. Med. Ethics* 1980; **6**: 71–77.

55. Palmberg, S. & Hirsjarvi, E. Mortality in geriatric surgery. *Gerontology* 1979; **25**: 103–112.

56. Wilder, R. J. & Fishbein, R. H. The widening surgical frontier. *Postgrad. Med.* 1961; **29**: 548–551.

57. Samiy, A. H. Clinical manifestations of disease in the elderly. *Med. Clin. North Am.* 1983; **67**: 333–344.

58. Hodkinson, H. M. Mental impairment in the elderly. *J. Roy. Coll. Phys. Lond.* 1973; **7**: 305–317.

59. Heijmeriks, J. A., Dassen, W., Prenger, K. *et al.* The incidence and consequences of mental disturbances in elderly patients post cardiac surgery – a comparison with younger patients. *Clin. Cardiol.* 2000; **23**: 540–546.

60. Corish, C. A. Pre-operative nutritional assessment in the elderly. *J. Nutr. Health Aging* 2001; **5**: 49–59.

61. Mullen, J. L., Buzby, G. P., Matthews, D. C. *et al.* Reduction of operative morbidity and mortality by combined preoperative and postoperative nutritional support. *Ann. Surg.* 1980; **192**: 604–613.

62. Master, A. M. & Lasser, R. P. Tables of average weight and height of Americans aged 65 to 94 years. *J. Am. Med. Assoc.* 1960; **172**: 658–662.

63. Kaminski, M. V., Nasr, N. J., Freed, B. A., & Sriram, K. The efficacy of nutritional support in the elderly. *J. Am. Coll. Nutr.* 1982; **1**: 35–40.

64. Berens, E. S., Kouchoukos, N. T., Murphy, S. F. *et al.* Preoperative carotid artery screening in elderly patients undergoing cardiac surgery. *J. Vasc. Surg.* 1992; **15**: 313–323.

65. Wickstrom, I., Holmberg, I., & Stefansson, T. Survival of female geriatric patients after hip fracture surgery: a comparison of 5 anesthetic methods. *Acta Anaesth. Scand.* 1982; **26**: 607–614.

66. Del Guercio, L. R. M. & Cohn, J. D. Monitoring operative risk in the elderly. *J. Am. Med. Assoc.* 1980; **243**: 1350–1355.

67. Dzanic, S., Pastor, D., Gonzalez, C. *et al.* The prevalence and predictive value of abnormal preoperative laboratory tests in elderly surgical patients. *Anesth. Analg.* 2001; **93**: 301–308.

68. Seymour, D. G., Pringle, R., & MacLennan, W. J. The role of the pre-operative electrocardiogram in the elderly surgical patient. *Age Aging* 1983; **12**: 97–104.

69. Liu, L. L., Dzanic, S., & Leung, J. M. Preoperative electrocardiogram abnormalities do not predict postoperative cardiac complications in geriatric surgical patients. *J. Am. Geriatr. Soc.* 2002; **50**: 1186–1191.

70. Tornebrandt, K. & Fletcher, R. Pre-operative chest X-rays in elderly patients. *Anaesthesia* 1982; **37**: 901–902.

71. Campbell, J. C. Detecting and correcting pulmonary risk factors before operation. *Geriatrics* 1977; **32**: 54–57.

72. Tisi, G. M. Preoperative evaluation of pulmonary function. *Am. Rev. Resp. Dis.* 1979; **119**: 293–310.

73. Schrader, L. L., McMillen, M. A., Watson, C. B. *et al.* Is routine preoperative hemodynamic evaluation of nonagenarians necessary? *J. Am. Geriatr. Soc.* 1991; **39**: 1–5.

74. Hole, A., Terjesen, T., & Breivik, H. Epidural versus general anesthesia for total hip arthroplasty in elderly patients. *Acta Anaesth. Scand.* 1980; **24**: 279–287.

75. Guillen, J. & Aldrete, J. A. Anesthetic factors influencing morbidity and mortality of elderly patients undergoing inguinal herniorrhaphy. *Am. J. Surg.* 1970; **120**: 760–763.

76. Miller, R., Marlar, K., & Silvay, G. Anesthesia for patients aged over ninety years. *NY State J. Med.* 1977; August: 1421–1425.

77. Davis, F. M., Woolner, D. F., Frampton, C. *et al.* Prospective, multi-centre trial of mortality following general or spinal anaesthesia for hip fracture surgery in the elderly. *Br. J. Anaesth.* 1987; **59**: 1080–1088.

78. Asbjørn, J., Jakobsen, B. W., Pilegaard, K. *et al.* Mental function in elderly men after surgery during epidural analgesia. *Acta Anaesthesiol. Scand.* 1989; **33**: 369–373.

79. Parker, M. J., Urwin, S. C., Handoll, H. H. G. *et al.* Regional versus general anesthesia for hip surgery in older patients: does the choice affect patient outcome? *J. Am. Geriatr. Soc.* 2002; **50**: 191–194.

80. Detsky, A., Abrams, H., McLaughlin, J. *et al.* Predicting cardiac complications in patients undergoing non-cardiac surgery. *J. Gen. Intern. Med.* 1986; **1**: 211–219.

81. Gerson, M. C., Hurst, J. M., Hertzberg, V. S. *et al.* Cardiac prognosis in noncardiac geriatric surgery. *Ann. Intern. Med.* 1985; **103**: 832–837.

82. Gerson, M. C., Hurst, J. M., Hertzberg, V. S. *et al.* Prediction of cardiac and pulmonary complications related to elective abdominal and noncardiac thoracic surgery in geriatric patients. *Am. J. Med.* 1990; **88**: 101–107.

83. Eagle, K. A., Berger, P. B., Calkins, H. *et al.* ACC/AHA guideline update for perioperative cardiovascular evaluation for non cardiac surgery: a report of the American College of Cardiology/American Heart Association task force on practice guidelines 2002 American College of Cardiology website http://www.acc.org/clinical/guidelines/perio/dirIndex.htm.

84. Mannion, J. D., Armenti, F. R., & Edie, R. N. Cardiac surgery in the elderly patient. *Cardiovasc. Clin.* 1992; **22**: 189–207.

85. Kolh, P., Kerzmann, A., Lahaue, L. *et al.* Cardiac surgery in octogenarians: peri-operative outcome and long-term results. *Eur. Heart J.* 2001; **22**: 1235–1243.

86. Mittermair, R. P. & Muller, L. C. Quality of life after cardiac surgery in the elderly. *J. Cardiovasc. Surg.* 2002; **43**: 43–47.

87. Ko, W., Gold, J. P., Lazzaro, R. *et al.* Survival analysis of octogenarian patients with coronary artery disease managed by elective coronary artery bypass surgery versus conventional medical treatment. *Circulation* 1992; **86**(suppl): II191–197.

88. Glower, D. D., Christopher, T. D., Milano, C. A. *et al.* Performance status and outcome after coronary artery bypass grafting in persons aged 80 to 93 years. *Am. J. Cardiol.* 1992; **70**: 567–571.

89. Hoff, S. J., Ball, S. K., Coltharp, W. H. *et al.* Coronary artery bypass in patients 80 years and over: is off-pump the operation of choice? *Ann. Thorac. Surg.* 2002; **74**: S1340–S1343.

90. Al-Ruzzeh, S., George, S., Yacoub, M. *et al.* The clinical outcome of off-pump coronary artery bypass surgery in the elderly patient. *Eur. J. Cardio-Thorac. Surg.* 2001; **20**: 1152–1156.

91. Demaria, R. G., Carrier, M., Fortier, S. *et al.* Reduced mortality and strokes with off-pump coronary artery bypass grafting surgery in octogenarians. *Circulation* 2002; **106**(12 Suppl 1): I5–I10.

92. Olsson, M., Granstrom, L., Lindblom, D. *et al.* Aortic valve replacement in octogenarians with aortic stenosis: a case-control study. *J. Am. Coll. Cardiol.* 1992; **20**: 1512–1516.

93. Pasic, M., Carrel, T., Laske, A. *et al.* Valve replacement in octogenarians: increased early mortality but good long-term result. *Eur. Heart J.* 1992; **13**: 508–510.

94. Davis, E. A., Gardner, T. J., Gillinov, M. *et al.* Valvular disease in the elderly: influence on surgical results. *Ann. Thorac. Surg.* 1993; **55**: 333–338.

95. Nair, C. K., Biddle, W. P., Kaneshige, A. *et al.* Ten-year experience with mitral valve replacement in the elderly. *Am. Heart J.* 1992; **124**: 154–159.

96. Bouma, B. J., van Den Brink, R. B., van Der Meulen, J. H. *et al.* To operate or not on elderly patients with aortic stenosis: the decision and its consequences. *Heart* 1999; **82**: 143–148.

97. Goldsmith, K., Lip, G. Y., Kaukuntla, H. *et al.* Hospital morbidity and mortality and changes in quality of life following mitral valve surgery in the elderly. *J. Heart Valve Dis.* 1999; **8**: 702–707.

98. Tabayashi, K., Ohmi, M., Syohji, Y. *et al.* Thoracic aortic operations in patients aged 70 years or older. *Ann. Thorac. Surg.* 1992; **54**: 279–282.

99. Dean, R. H., Woody, B. A., Carn, E. *et al.* Operative treatment of abdominal aortic aneurysms in octogenarians: when is it too much too late? *Ann. Surg.* 1993; **217**: 721–728.

100. Ommer, A., Pillny, M., Grabitz, K. *et al.* Reconstruction surgery for carotid artery occlusive disease in the elderly – a high risk operation? *Cardiovasc. Surg.* 2001; **9**: 552–558.

101. Ekelund, A., Rydell, N., & Nilsson, O. S. Total hip arthroplasty in patients 80 years of age and older. *Clin. Orthop.* 1992; **281**: 101–106.

102. Phillips, T. W., Grainger, R. W., Cameron, H. S. *et al.* Risks and benefits of elective hip replacement in the octogenarian. *CMAJ* 1987; **137**: 497–500.

103. Harness, J. K., Strodel, W. E., & Talsma, S. E. Symptomatic biliary tract disease in the elderly patient. *Am. Surg.* 1986; **52**: 442–445.

104. Margiotta, S. J., Horwitz, J. R., Willis, I. H. *et al.* Cholecystectomy in the elderly *Am. J. Surg.* 1988; **156**: 509–512.

105. Pessaux, P., Tuech, J. J., Derouet, N. *et al.* Laparoscopic cholecystectomy in the elderly: a prospective study. *Surg. Endosc.* 2000; **14**: 1067–1069.

106. Mayol, J., Martinez-Sarmiento, K., Tamayo, F. J. *et al.* Complications of laparoscopic cholecystectomy in the ageing patient. *Age Ageing* 1997; **26**: 77–81.

107. Brunt, L. M., Quasebarth, M. A., Dunnegan, D. L. *et al.* Outcomes analysis of laparoscopic cholecystectomy in the extremely elderly. *Surg. Endosc.* 2001; **15**: 700–705.

108. Smithy, W. B., Wexmer, S. D., & Dailey, T. H. The diagnosis and treatment of acute appendicitis in the aged. *Dis. Colon Rectum* 1986; **29**: 170–173.

109. McCallion, J., Canning, G. P., Knight, P. V. *et al.* Acute appendicitis in the elderly: a 5-year retrospective study. *Age Aging* 1987; **16**: 256–260.

110. Hui, T. T., Major, K. M., Avital, I. *et al.* Outcome of elderly patients with appendicitis: effect of computed tomography and laparoscopy. *Arch. Surg.* 2002; **137**: 995–1000.

111. Cohen, H., Willis, I., & Wallack, M. Surgical experience of colon resection in the extreme elderly. *Am. Surg.* 1986; **52**: 214–217.

112. Stewart, B. T., Stitz, R. W., & Lumley, J. W. Laparoscopically assisted colorectal surgery in the elderly. *Br. J. Surg.* 1999; **86**: 938–941.

113. Schneider, J. & Benito, R. Extensive gynecologic surgical procedures upon patients more than 75 years of age. *Surg. Gynecol. Obstet.* 1988; **167**: 497–500.

114. Lichtinger, M., Averette, H., Penalver, M. *et al.* Major surgical procedures for gynecologic malignancy in elderly women. *South. Med. J.* 1986; **79**: 1506–1510.

115. Roxburgh, J. C., Thompson, J., & Goldstraw, P. Hospital mortality and long-term survival after pulmonary resection in the elderly. *Ann. Thorac. Surg.* 1991; **51**: 800–803.

116. Thomas, P., Sielezneff, I., Ragni, J. *et al.* Is lung cancer resection justified in patients aged over 70 years? *Eur. J. Cardio-Thorac. Surg.* 1993; **7**: 246–251.

117. Sioris, T., Salo, J., Perhoniemi, V. *et al.* Surgery for lung cancer in the elderly. *Scand. Cardiovasc. J.* 1999; **33**: 222–227.

118. Whittle, J., Steinberg, E. P., Anderson, G. F. *et al.* Results of colectomy in elderly patients with colon cancer, based on Medicare claims data. *Am. J. Surg.* 1992; **163**: 572–576.

119. Fitzgerald, S. D., Longo, W. E., Daniel, G. L. *et al.* Advanced colorectal neoplasia in the high-risk elderly patient: is surgical resection justified? *Dis. Colon Rectum* 1993; **36**: 161–166.

120. Colorectal Cancer Collaborative Group. Outcomes in older people undergoing operative intervention for colorectal cancer. *Lancet* 2000; **356**: 968–974.

121. Vara-Thorbeck, C., Garcia-Caballero, M., Salvi, M. *et al.* Indications and advantages of laparoscopy-assisted colon resection for carcinoma in elderly patients. *Surg. Laparosc. Endosc.* 1994; **4**: 110–118.

122. Sugimachi, K., Inokuchi, K., Ueo, H. *et al.* Surgical treatment for carcinoma of the esophagus in the elderly patient. *Surg. Gyn. Obstet.* 1985; **160**: 317–319.

123. Xijiang, Z., Xizeng, Z., Xishan, H. *et al.* Surgical treatment for carcinoma of the esophagus in the elderly patient. *Ann. Thorac. Cardiovasc. Surg.* 1999; **5**: 182–186.

124. Coluccia, C., Ricci, E. B., Marzola, G. G. *et al.* Gastric cancer in the elderly: results of surgical treatment. *Int. Surg.* 1987; **72**: 4–10.

125. Matsushita, I., Hanai, H., Kajumura, M. *et al.* Should gastric cancer patients more than 80 years of age undergo surgery? Comparison with patients not treated surgically concerning prognosis and quality of life. *J. Clin. Gastroenterol.* 2002; **35**: 29–34.

126. Amsterdam, E., Birkenfeld, S., Gilad, A. *et al.* Surgery for carcinoma of the breast in women over 70 years of age. *J. Surg. Oncol.* 1987; **35**: 180–183.

127. Grube, B. J., Hansen, N. M., Ye, W. *et al.* Surgical management of breast cancer in the elderly patient. *Am. J. Surg.* 2001; **182**: 359–364.

128. Vaughn, M. S., Vaughn, R. W., & Cork, R. C. Postoperative hypothermia in adults: relationship of age, anesthesia, and shivering to rewarming. *Anesth. Anal.* 1981; **60**: 746–751.

129. Heymann, A. D. The effect of incidental hypothermia on elderly surgical patients. *J. Gerontol.* 1977; **32**: 46–48.

130. Lipowski, Z. J. Transient cognitive disorders (delirium, acute confusional states) in the elderly. *Am. J. Psychiatry* 1983; **140**: 1426–1436.

131. Bedford, P. D. General medical aspects of confusional states in elderly people. *Br. Med. J.* 1959; **2**: 185–188.

132. Blundell, E. A psychological study of the effects of surgery on eighty-six elderly patients. *Br. J. Soc. Clin. Psychol.* 1967; **6**: 297–303.

133. Marcantonio, E. R., Flacker, J. M., Wright, R. J. *et al.* Reducing delirium after hip fracture: a randomized trial. *J. Am. Geriatr. Soc.* 2001; **49**: 516–522.

134. Pathy, M. S. Clinical presentation of myocardial infarction in the elderly. *Br. Heart J.* 1967; **29**: 190–199.

Obesity

38

Obesity

John G. Kral

SUNY Downstate Medical Center, Brooklyn, New York

Introduction

The increasing prevalence of obesity among adults and children, new insights into the pathogenesis of obesity, and significant changes in the practice of surgery through adoption of less traumatic laparoscopic approaches, all justify up-dating this chapter from the third edition (published in 1995, containing references through 1993).

Prevalence

The age-adjusted prevalence of obesity was 30.5% in 2000 according to a national examination survey,[1] while the prevalence of overweight was 64.5%. The largest telephone survey in the USA reported a prevalence of 20.9% for obesity in 2000[2] giving an indication of the validity of telephone surveys related to this topic. Regardless of their relative validity, all studies unequivocally document disturbingly rapid yearly increases ($P < 0.001$) in obesity and overweight and their related serious diseases: diabetes, hypertension, dyslipidemia, asthma, etc. Class 3 obesity (BMI $\geq$ 40) tripled from 1990 to 2000, reaching a prevalence of 6% among black women, causing the authors of the study to conclude: "the incidence of various diseases will increase substantially in the future."[3] Increasing prevalences of childhood and adolescent overweight and obesity are especially troubling: adolescent overweight is a strong predictor of adult illness.[4]

Two large epidemiological studies published in January 2003 comprising 3457 subjects (The Framingham Heart Study[5]) and 23 659 subjects[6] confirmed that obesity and overweight in adulthood markedly decrease life expectancy. Fontaine *et al.* determined that younger adults generally had greater number of years lost than did older adults[6] and Peeters *et al.* found the decreases in life expectancy to be comparable to those seen with smoking.[5]

The metabolic syndrome of obesity (Syndrome X; the insulin resistance syndrome[7]), a cluster of findings including central obesity, glucose intolerance, dyslipidemia and hypertension, and an increasing list of components has similarly increased to epidemic proportions in both children[8] and adults.[9] There is a dose–response relationship between body fat and risks of diabetes, coronary heart disease, hypertension[10] and cancer mortality.[11] The proportion of the prevalence of type 2 diabetes (T2DM) attributable to obesity is 60%, emphasizing the need to consider obesity and diabetes together in medical management of the surgical patient. It is not unusual for T2DM to be detected in conjunction with a surgical procedure in overweight patients.

Pathogenesis

Discovery of ob protein, the leptin gene, in 1994[12] is a turning point in the study of obesity and, indeed, in the perception of the disease by the lay public as well as by the medical profession. The promise of a practical treatment for obesity has not been fulfilled, but numerous new mechanisms have been discovered governing energy expenditure, nutrient partitioning, eating behavior, gluco- and lipotoxicity, as well as psycho-neuro-immunological precursors of obesity and its sequelae.

Obesity is a multifactorial, predominantly polygenic disease requiring effortless access to food to express itself. The "success" of industrialization, labor-saving devices, improvements in production and distribution of food, and the massive marketing of palatable food products are beginning to undermine progress in prevention and

Medical Management of the Surgical Patient: A Textbook of Perioperative Medicine, ed. M. F. Lubin, R. B. Smith, T. F. Dobson, N. Spell, H. K. Walker. 4th edn. Published by Cambridge University Press. © Cambridge University 2006.

treatment of disease that followed the discovery of anti-biotics, sophisticated drugs and advanced diagnostic tools for screening and early detection of disease in the twentieth century.

Practice of surgery

Refinement of laparoscopic techniques has transformed the quality of postsurgery recovery and the quantity of complications after the surgeons' learning curve becomes linear and horizontal. Generically, obese patients have benefited the most from these minimally invasive techniques. The laparoscopic approach dramatically improves access and visibility, key problems in severely obese patients, and does away with large incisions contributing to the trauma, cytokine and chemokine release, and postoperative pain encumbering breathing, mobilization, and rehabilitation.[13,14] Attendant reductions in length-of-stay have limited exposure of obese patients to the unhealthy environment of limited physical activity and prevalent pathogens in hospitals.

The purpose of this chapter is to sensitize the reader to surgery-related risks associated with obesity, identify relevant pathophysiological mechanisms, and suggest strategies for optimizing pre- and postoperative medical care.

Morbidity

The new-found "legitimacy" of obesity with substantial marketing investments from the drug- and device-producers has increased public and professional interest in the disease. In parallel with the rising prevalence of obesity, a striking increase in the numbers of related morbidities, conditions, symptoms, and complications has been recorded: more than 50 in a review in 2001.[15] Although identifiable primary endocrine abnormalities are unusual causes of obesity, adipose tissue is now recognized as an endocrine organ, arguably the body's largest.

A conceptual framework for classifying obesity-related conditions is useful for understanding the medical management of obese candidates for surgery. The Venn diagram in Fig. 38.1 separates obesity into two overlapping categories: metabolic vs. weight-related obesity, based on pathophysiological mechanisms. Many of the associated diseases and conditions are treated surgically as is obesity itself, while others contribute to perioperative complications and side effects. Table 38.1 enumerates obesity-related surgical diseases.

Pathophysiology

Obesity is an independent risk factor for numerous serious systemic and organ-specific diseases and has a primary

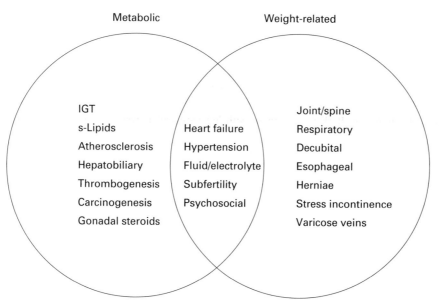

Fig. 38.1. Metabolic and weight-related obesity with overlapping conditions. IGT = impaired glucose tolerance comparising insulin resistance and type 2 diabetes mellitus.

Table 38.1. Obesity-related surgical diseases

Weight related

Orthopedic	*Vascular*
Joint disease	Varicose veins
Disk prolapse	Thromboembolism
Blount's disease	
Fractures	*Dermal*
	Decubitus ulcers
Gastrointestinal	Intertrigo
Esophageal reflux	
Hemorrhoids	*Gynecologic*
Herniae	Urinary incontinence

Metabolic

Gastrointestinal	*Genitourinary*
Cholelithiasis	Urolithiasis
Neoplasia	Neoplasia
Esophageal	Renal
Colo-rectal	Endometrial
Biliary	Cancer
Cirrhosis	Fibroids
Vascular	Prostate
Atherosclerotic	*Breast*
Gynecologic	Cancer
Caesarian sections	Fibroadenoma

role in the development of some forms of diabetes, hypertension, congestive heart failure, even cancer. The distribution of adipose tissue is a significant concomitant of complications of obesity, although the mechanism is unknown. Visceral or abdominal fat is more metabolically active than subcutaneous or peripheral fat. Its preferential drainage into the portal system is considered to contribute to the pathogenesis of metabolic obesity. The metabolic syndrome associates non-insulin-dependent diabetes, hypertension, dyslipidemia (low HDL, high triglyceride), and obesity with a central (visceral, abdominal, upper body) distribution of fat. A series of studies by Barker *et al.* demonstrated the importance of early growth in adult distribution of adipose tissue and the development of comorbid conditions.[16]

Initially, various simple anthropometric measures were shown to differentiate between upper body, central, or android, obesity, and femoral-gluteal, or gynoid, obesity. One of the simplest is the waist/hip ratio, which is obtained by dividing the minimum girth at the waist by the maximum girth below the waist in the standing position. There are no published normal, control, or reference values for the waist/hip ratio that can be applied to evaluate risk in particular patients. As a general rule, however, ratios greater than 0.82 in women and 0.92 in men

indicate greater risk of present or future morbidity. Computed tomography and MRI have been used in research studies to measure the amount of intra-abdominal or "visceral" adipose tissue compared with the amount of subcutaneous adipose tissue,[17] leading to refinements in the predictive power of the relative distribution of fat in identifying the risks for developing comorbid conditions. Data indicate that the absolute amount of visceral fat rather than the relative distribution of fat, the total amount of body fat, or the body weight is the strongest predictor of risk.[18,19] There has been considerable controversy over the "best" measure for risk evaluation in individual patients and in population studies. The simplest measure of them all, waist circumference, has recently been demonstrated to have higher predictive capacity than body mass index (BMI) for assessing medical costs.[20]

Cardiovascular complications of obesity

Cardiomegaly; increased cardiac output, stroke volume, and blood volume; and excess extracellular fluid, all increase the surgical risk of obese patients. It has been suggested that the hyperdynamic circulation of these patients reflects an adaptation to increased metabolic needs of the excess tissue. This adaptation leads to increased cardiac index and output, stroke volume, and left and right ventricular work; higher right and left heart filling pressures; and increased pulmonary artery pressure.[21]

Whereas hemodynamic variables are in the upper normal range in obese patients before operation, significant decreases in cardiac index and in right and left ventricular stroke work occur during operation and continue during the postoperative period.[22] However, these effects are substantially attenuated by laparoscopic approaches, which are associated with reductions in the cytokine cascade triggered by the trauma of large incisions.[14]

Obese patients react to the stress of anesthesia and surgery with left ventricular dysfunction. Intraoperative depression of cardiac output that persists after operation and is not followed by a normal elevation of these parameters predicts poorer outcome in trauma victims not stratified for weight. This response pattern may explain the increased operative risk of obese patients undergoing elective surgery, who often manifest left ventricular dysfunction at rest.[23]

It is not known whether fat distribution is a determinant of perioperative morbidity although there is reason to expect that increased visceral fat may be deleterious. Left, right, and biventricular cardiac dysfunction are prevalent among asymptomatic candidates for obesity surgery, and are significantly more common in patients with visceral than with peripheral fat distribution.[24] The increased cardiac size, from increased filling and wall thickness (resulting from greater stroke work causing hypertrophy) is associated with elevated systemic arterial pressure. Ventricular hypertrophy is part of the "cardiopathy of obesity" manifested in a predisposition to tachyarrhythmia or prolonged QTc intervals on the ECG.[25] The cardiopathy is independent of hypertension and underlying heart disease and is virtually totally reversible by weight loss.[26] Recent work has demonstrated an independent effect of insulin resistance on left ventricular mass in normotensive subjects.[27] Untreated obese patients are at risk because of their limited reserves to withstand the operative stresses of pain and hypoxia.[28] Laparoscopic approaches, once again, have proved invaluable in reducing these stresses.

Pulmonary compromise

The cardiac abnormalities described occur in conjunction with pulmonary dysfunction. Isolated cor pulmonale, however, is uncommon in severe obesity and seems to be caused by pulmonary embolization rather than progressive insufficiency.[29] The diminished cardiorespiratory fitness of obesity contributes significantly to the increased mortality of obesity.[30] Overweight, a body mass of $\geq 25\,kg/m^2$, increases the relative risk of postoperative pulmonary complications of abdominal surgery.[31]

The sheer mechanical burden of excess adipose tissue on the chest wall and in the abdomen, pushing on the diaphragm, compresses the lungs and leads to increased intrathoracic pressure.[32] The combined effects of decreased chest wall compliance and increased adipose tissue lead to the typical reduction of functional residual capacity and total lung volume that is seen in severe obesity. Increased weight causes hypoventilation with hypoxic pulmonary vasoconstriction, increased pulmonary artery pressure and peripheral resistance.[33] Sugerman et al. have demonstrated the importance of increased intra-abdominal pressure, an "intra-abdominal compartment syndrome", as a contribution to pulmonary and cardiac dysfunction.[34,35]

Of immediate perioperative concern are the two pulmonary syndromes, sleep apnea and obesity hypoventilation.[36] The restrictive respiratory pattern caused by excess fat that leads to obesity hypoventilation is often found in patients with other pulmonary risk factors, such as smoking, asthma, or fibrosis, and can occur alone or in conjunction with sleep apnea. The relationship between asthma and obesity has been rather controversial through the years. The respective roles of allergic reactions of airway mucosa, tonsillar swelling, obesifying effects of

steroids and other antiasthmatic medications, and even psychological correlates of asthma, have all obscured the understanding of any primary importance of obesity in the etiology of asthma. Only recently has it been recognized that asthma and pulmonary fibrosis may be manifestations of gastroesophageal reflux disease (GERD), another symptom of the increased intra-abdominal pressure of obesity.[35,37,38] The epidemic increase in pediatric asthma, in parallel with the increase in obesity has focused attention on childhood obesity as a strong independent risk factor for adult-onset asthma.[39]

Sleep apnea is clearly weight related, sometimes appearing at a threshold level of weight. It can be peripheral (obstructive) or, rarely, central in origin and contributes significantly to the increased prevalence of sudden death in obese patients. The obstruction can be caused by a large tongue or tonsils, or sometimes by a deviated nasal septum or other nasopharyngeal pathology. Loud snoring is the hallmark of this condition. Disordered sleep often leads to severe daytime somnolence, headaches, and even depression. Sleep apnea is exquisitely responsive to modest weight loss.

The increased blood volume in obesity is not associated with a commensurate increase in chest volume, so the relative increase in central circulation causes alveolar compression. There is an increased venous admixture from the ventilation-perfusion mismatch caused by atelectatic lung. Chronic hypoxemia in turn leads to polycythemia, a harbinger of thromboembolism.

Thromboembolism

The most prevalent serious complication of surgery in obese patients is thromboembolism. Tables 38.2 and 38.3 outline factors of pathogenetic importance for the increased incidence of pulmonary embolism and thrombotic conditions in obese patients. Many of these factors are inter-related; cause and effect cannot be determined. For example, several chemical abnormalities are associated with type II diabetes,[40–42] yet may be caused by fatty infiltration of the liver, which in turn is more prevalent in type II diabetes and the metabolic syndrome.[43] In principle, obesity is associated with elevated levels of thrombosis-promoting factors and decreases in fibrinolysis. These changes are significantly related to abdominal fatness.[44] In addition, hemodynamic abnormalities associated with comorbid conditions (hypertension), as well as mechanical (intra-abdominal pressure) and possibly behavioral factors (smoking, sedentary lifestyle), all contribute to explaining the high incidence of thromboembolism in obese patients.

Table 38.2. Comorbid conditions contributing to thromboembolism in obesity

Condition	Chemical abnormality
Dyslipidemia	↑ Serum triglycerides
	↑ Serum low-density lipoprotein cholesterol
	↓ Serum high-density lipoprotein cholesterol
	↑ Blood-viscosity
Diabetes	↑ Serum antithrombin III
	↑ Serum fibrinogen
	↑ Serum fibronectin
	↓ Tissue plasminogen activity
Hypertension	
Renal failure	

Table 38.3. Increased body fat mass predisposes to thromboembolism in obesity

↑ Intra-abdominal pressure
  Varicose veins

↑ Blood volume/intrathoracic pressure
  Cardiopulmonary failure
  Polycythemia

↑ Serum-free fatty acids
  Glucose intolerance/hyperinsulinemia
  Fatty liver

↓ Locomotion
  Hypostasis

The metabolic syndrome is extensively linked with thromboembolism and hypercoagulability has been suggested as one of the major components of the syndrome.[45] Plasminogen activator inhibitor-1 (PAI-1), a prothrombotic peptide abundant in adipose tissue,[46] is significantly related to insulin resistance[47] and is likely the most important mediator of obesity-related thromboembolism. Furthermore, important pathogenetic links between thrombosis and atherosclerosis[48] and malignancy have recently been elucidated.

Kidney failure

Both functional and morphologic renal abnormalities have been described in obese patients.[49] Just as with other obesity-related morbidity, it is difficult to separate the contributing factors. Thus, glucose intolerance and frank diabetes as well as hypertension are associated with glomerular hyperfiltration and with renovascular hypertrophy and fibrosis.[50,51] Gout is prevalent in obese patients and is a cause of renal

pathology. Several reports describe nephrosis in severely obese patients but there are no data implicating obesity as an independent risk factor for kidney failure.

The prevalence of obesity among kidney transplant recipients does not reflect the overall prevalence of kidney failure among obese patients because many transplant centers exclude these patients from their programs and nephrologists are reluctant to refer them. Some studies have demonstrated poorer outcome in obese patients after renal transplantation compared with control patients of normal weight[52] while others have obtained similar outcomes.[53] Regardless of perioperative results long-term graft survival associated with weight gain is poorer in obese patients. Reasons for poorer graft survival and higher mortality in obese patients may include impaired glucose metabolism associated not only with obesity but also with the administration of steroids and cyclosporin A, which may act synergistically with obesity.

Fluid and electrolyte abnormalities

Extracellular water increases with expanding fat mass through unknown mechanisms.[54] Irreversibility of the elevated ratio of extracellular to intracellular fluid with massive weight loss implies an intrinsic abnormality[55] unrelated to right ventricular failure or edema.[56] The increase in extracellular fluid influences distribution volumes of medications as well as volume status.[57]

Obese patients often have histories of diuretic use, either for surreptitious treatment of "swelling" or as part of legitimate therapy for hypertension. This use of diuretics as well as repeated bouts of fasting, low-calorie diets, or even bulimia may contribute to the depletion of total body potassium levels. Such depletion is not obvious from serum concentrations, in which a reduction from 4 to 3 meq/l may be associated with a body loss of 1000 meq of potassium.

Once again, comorbid conditions such as type II diabetes (hyperinsulinemia)[58] and hypertension can contribute to electrolyte abnormalities, although one study suggests the presence of an intrinsically low total body potassium level in obese patients.[59] Fatty liver, a corollary of hyperinsulinemia, is associated with decreased protein synthesis[60] and may be accompanied by reductions in serum albumin, which in turn predispose to fluid and electrolyte abnormalities.

Susceptibility to infection

Obese patients are at greater risk for wound infection than are patients of normal weight.[61] Studies on absenteeism have suggested that obese patients are more prone to other infections, too, but it is not known whether there is a primary immune defect in obesity. Intuitively, susceptibility to pneumonia from respiratory compromise and to cellulitis from intertriginous changes under an abdominal panniculus or in the edematous skin of the lower leg would be reasonable to expect without postulating any immune compromise. Evidence exists, however, for impaired immunocompetence in obese patients, although the mechanisms are not known.[62] Abnormalities in the leptin-proopiomelancortin (POMC) system,[63,64] elevated adipose tissue levels of the cytokine TNF α[65] and hypercortisolism have been proposed. Obesity-related impairment in glucose metabolism may be implicated: defective leukocyte function has been demonstrated in the prediabetic state.[66,67] Patients with diabetes are notorious for their susceptibility to infections, so it is possible that such susceptibility in obese patients is a reflection of the intrinsically deranged glucose metabolism in obesity, regardless of severity.

Insulin resistance

Diabetes is covered extensively in Chapter 26 to which the reader is referred. The common form of type 2 diabetes in obesity is widely regarded to evolve through a sequence starting with impaired fasting glucose (IFG), progressing to impaired glucose tolerance (IGT) with hyperinsulinemia and insulin resistance onward to beta-cell failure requiring insulin treatment.[68] There is controversy over the primary defect leading to this sequence including candidate mechanisms such as a primary (genetic) beta-cell lesion, tissue resistance to the effects of insulin involving liver, adipose tissue or muscle, adipose-tissue-derived molecules,[69] and substrate overload causing lipo- or glucotoxicity affecting the pancreas or other tissues. It is not likely that this controversy will be resolved until broad-based population studies determine the existence of subgroups with different primary mechanisms.

I believe that a prevalent cause of "diabesity" is substrate overload related to rapid and excessive eating[70] exceeding the substrate–product equilibrium "normally" balanced by energy expenditure. Although heritable susceptibility genes, commonly referred to as "thrifty genes",[71] can explain some of the variance, and "hunger genes" governing appetitive behavior might explain other portions, I am convinced that epigenetic mechanisms dominate. Only through early identification and active early intervention, will it be possible to curb the "diabesity epidemic."

Table 38.4. Obesity Severity Index I: physiological

Male sex	1[a]	Neck:thigh > 0.70	2
Age > 40 years	1	Cardiomegaly	2
Smoker	2	Uncontrolled blood pressure	2
Sleep apnea history	1	Hemoglobin >15 g/liter	1
Thromboembolism	1	$_pCO_2 > 45$ mm/Hg	1
Diabetes	1	Hyperinsulinemia	2
BMI 35–40 = 2; BMI $> 40 = 3$			

Note:
[a] Arbitrary units reflecting risk. Maximum 20 points.

For the practical management of the obese surgical patient, it is important to recognize that approximately 5% of obese patients may have gene polymorphisms causing defective impulse control leading to binge-eating disorder[72] and the metabolic syndrome.[73] In the future, such patients will likely benefit from preoperative treatment with medications currently being developed to counteract the deleterious effects of the gene polymorphisms.[74]

Evaluation of obese patients

Because of their size, obese patients pose a significant diagnostic challenge for purely physical reasons. In severe obesity, there is considerable occult pathology that may become manifest only during the added challenge of an operation. Limited physiologic reserves elude detection during routine activities of daily living that have gradually been adapted to the constraints imposed by excess weight. Thus, patients' histories may be noncontributory. In addition, risk factors for obesity must be considered:

- male gender
- adult onset
- visceral distribution of fat (increased waist)
- smoking
- manifest comorbid conditions (e.g., diabetes, hypertension, asthma)
- family history of complicated obesity (e.g., myocardial infarction, stroke, diabetes).

I have constructed an Obesity Severity Index as a prognostic indicator to assist in risk assessment of obese patients undergoing surgery, mainly antiobesity surgery.[75] Most existing physiologic scoring systems such as APACHE II and III, POSSUM, and the ASA classifications do not include obesity-specific indicators. Body weight or BMI alone are insufficient predictors. Table 38.4 presents a point system for risk assessment. Preoperative optimization should strive to down-stage modifiable risk factors, many of which are responsive to weight loss.

Basic preoperative evaluation

The goal of the preoperative evaluation is to detect any pre-existing pathology in order to optimize a patient's physical condition. It can also provide a baseline for the interpretation of postoperative findings. Lastly, it serves as a predictor, allowing the team to focus its monitoring efforts on potentially critical areas.

In the performance of standard electrocardiograms, chest radiographs, blood counts, and electrolyte levels, some specific findings that require particular attention may be overlooked in routine practice. A prolonged QT interval is an electrocardiographic marker of sudden cardiac arrest. A prolonged QT interval was found in retrospect in most severely obese patients who died of malignant arrhythmias in one study.[76] Similar findings have been associated with fatal[77] and non-fatal[78] dieting. Electrocardiographic signs of left ventricular hypertrophy also carry an increased risk of sudden cardiac death,[79,80] with an increased prevalence of ventricular ectopy in obese patients.[81]

Obtaining a routine chest radiograph in obese patients can be difficult for reasons of sheer size. Attention must be paid to achieving adequate penetration and evaluation of the whole lung. Obtaining well-penetrated images of both bases, in which small amounts of pleural fluid would indicate incipient heart failure, sometimes requires an extra set of films.

Standard blood tests are often challenging to obtain in obese patients because venepuncture is difficult. Prolonged stasis during sampling and the stress of pain from multiple needlesticks may influence such parameters as serum potassium, hematocrit, and blood glucose levels. A spurious elevation in the potassium level may raise an otherwise low level into the normal range. Among other routine blood tests, it is noteworthy that a leukocyte count in the high-normal range (greater than 9000/µl) is a strong predictor of risk for acute myocardial infarction independent of tobacco smoking.[82] Obese patients commonly have high–normal white blood cell counts and seem to have exaggerated postoperative elevations of the white blood cell count, likely attributable to cytokine release associated with the trauma of the incision.

Elevations of liver enzyme levels are common among obese patients and do not indicate severe liver disease but rather fatty infiltration of the liver.[83] Nevertheless, a fatty liver is more vulnerable than is a normal one, and this must be considered in anesthetic management.[84]

Special tests

Cardiopulmonary evaluation is particularly important in obese surgical patients who are at least 40% overweight. With or without histories indicative of cardiac or pulmonary disease, routine arterial blood gas determinations should be obtained with patients in the supine position and breathing room air. Peak flow spirometry, or simply having patients blow out a match at arm's length, are practical tests for evaluating pulmonary reserve to determine whether more complex testing is indicated, while routine performance of standard spirometry has been questioned in one cost/benefit analysis.

Indications for abbreviated sleep studies (i.e., without polysomnography and electroencephalography) should be broad in obese patients who have histories of snoring and daytime somnolence and any witnessed episode of apnea. Evaluation should include otorhinolaryngologic consultation to rule out nasopharyngeal pathology.

The issue of cardiovascular compromise is particularly important in obese patients. Standard diagnostic techniques such as exercise testing and echocardiography are limited in severely obese patients, who simply are unable to achieve prerequisite levels of exercise stress to make such studies meaningful. Excess adipose tissue limits the sensitivity of ultrasound of the chest, although intraesophageal echocardiography is helpful. In lieu of exercise testing, dipyridamole-thallium can be used to achieve stress levels of myocardial perfusion and detect areas of reduced flow in patients unable to use a bicycle ergometer or treadmill. Other quantitative radionuclide cardiographic techniques are able to detect abnormalities of ventricular function, although it has not been determined whether such abnormalities are predictors of outcome. Calibration standards and dosimetry present problems in the most obese patients. In spite of these difficulties, echocardiography has been valuable in demonstrating cardiac abnormalities in severely obese patients.[23,85]

Thorough preoperative lipid evaluations are important. In addition to elevated levels of serum cholesterol, decreased levels of high-density lipoproteins and increased levels of serum triglycerides are markers of coronary heart disease risk.[86] The controversy over the importance of triglycerides as an independent risk factor for coronary heart disease notwithstanding, their association with impaired glucose metabolism in obesity increases the significance of elevated levels.

Treatment and prevention

Weight loss

It is logical to recommend nutritionally sound weight loss before elective operation, particularly if this would correct comorbid conditions such as sleep apnea, diabetes, congestive heart failure, or respiratory insufficiency. As with smoking cessation, however, which is doubly important for obese patients, it is unrealistic to expect full cooperation with this recommendation. Nevertheless, the consistently poor results of obese patients in achieving and maintaining weight loss in daily life should not deter physicians from urging preoperative weight loss. This cannot be a universal requirement because weight loss may be detrimental to some diseases being treated. Care must be taken to avoid imposing a catabolic state and adding to the catabolism of surgery. Evidence to support preoperative weight loss via a prospective randomized trial is not feasible since weight loss is beneficial in optimizing selected patients who thus cannot be randomized to a non-treatment arm.

The increasing numbers of severely obese patients and the improved outcome of antiobesity ("bariatric") surgery, particularly through the laparoscopic approaches, have been accompanied by wider adoption of surgical treatment of obesity.[87] Standards for the performance of such surgery have been promulgated and generally emphasize the necessity of having a competent interdisciplinary team, of providing pre- and postoperative education and support, and making great efforts to maintain follow-up for monitoring of nutritional state and potential complications.

Candidates for antiobesity surgery have body mass index (BMI) of 35 kg/m^2 or greater in the presence of one or more complications of obesity. Personally, I do not feel that such surgery should be performed unless the candidate has had 3 months' preparation with opportunities to obtain second opinions, to have meetings with other "successful" and "unsuccessful" patients, and to involve significant others in the educational process.

Because of the severity of obesity and the relative safety of bariatric surgery, it is important to consider referring candidates for such surgery as part of a preoperative work-up when other procedures are being considered. An obvious example is the severely obese candidate for hip replacement, where deferral of the intended surgery until after weight-loss surgery would improve the perioperative and long-term outcome of the hip replacement.

There are three bariatric procedures that are predominant: gastric bypass, laparoscopic adjustable gastric banding and biliopancreatic diversion. All three can be performed laparoscopically at centers specializing in this type of surgery. Gastric bypass is the most commonly performed procedure in the USA, while gastric banding is more common in Europe, Japan, and Australia.[88]

Physical and respiratory therapy

Increasing physical activity, preferably through an exercise program, is an excellent preventive measure in sedentary obese patients. Combined with smoking cessation and chest physical therapy, exercise training dramatically reduces the risks of postoperative pulmonary complications. Patients with sleep apnea benefit from nasal continuous positive airway pressure (CPAP), which is preferable to tracheostomy.[37,89] As already mentioned, patients with upper airway obstruction experience great improvement with weight loss. Although surgical correction of a deviated nasal septum may be beneficial, there is little role for uvulopalatopharyngoplasty in obese patients who have snoring and intermittent hypercapnia.

Thrombosis prophylaxis

Several measures can be taken to help prevent thromboembolism. Before elective operations, the administration of low-dose warfarin can restore levels of antithrombin III and should be considered in obese patients with a prior history of thrombosis.[90] The routine use of mini-dose or fractionated heparin (dose adjusted for body weight), intermittent venous compression leggings, and early extubation and ambulation has drastically reduced the prevalence of thromboembolism in severely obese patients. The infusion of dextrose solutions in the postoperative period to suppress free fatty acid release has also been recommended, although the antilipolytic effects of insulin may be just as effective. Some surgeons treating severely obese patients administer excess fluid before operation to achieve hemodilution to rheologically optimal hematocrit levels (28% to 32%) as a potential antithrombotic measure. Theoretically, this could lead instead to a hypercoagulable condition resulting from the dilution of thrombolytic factors.[91] This has not been demonstrated, however, in any of the large series of obesity operations in which fluid loading has been performed consistently.

Infection control

Postoperative infections can be prevented effectively through several approaches, used alone or in

Table 38.5. Perioperative risk reduction in obese patients

Rule out treatable conditions
Congestive heart failure
Respiratory insufficiency
   Obstructive sleep apnea
   Hypercapnia
Diabetes out of control
Smoking
Coronary heart disease
Chronic skin infection

Treat complicating conditions
Diuresis
Weight loss
Glycemic control
Airway obstruction
Antibiotics – local control of skin infections
Malnutrition

Prevent known risks
Pulmonary
   Breathing exercises
   Early ambulation/physical theraphy
   Oxygen
   Elevate head and upper body
Thrombosis
   Intermittent compression stockings
   Ambulate
   Fluid load
   Heparin
Infection
   Prophylactic
      Showers
      Antibiotics
   Irrigation
   Paper drapes
   Technique
      Avoid drains
Others
   Aspiration
      Elevate head and upper body
      Nasogastric intubation
      Gastric acid suppression
   Monitor
      Central venous pressure
      Arterial blood gases
      Swan-Ganz

Miscellaneous
Access
   Antecubital/internal jugular/subclavian veins
Acid–base
Glycemic control
   Chemstrips
   Humulin (subcutaneous)
Nutritional support
   Total parenteral nutrition/lipids?
   Fluid volume

combination. Local treatment of skin infections and routine use of antibacterial soap for showering and shampooing the evening before and morning of surgery are simple first steps. The routine use of prophylactic antibiotics (such as 1 to 2 g of cefazolin, adjusted for weight) is justified to prevent wound infections in obese patients regardless of the type of operation planned. The efficacy of paper drapes, vigorous irrigation, and local antibiotics has not been evaluated in prospective, randomized trials in obese patients but has been demonstrated historically in operations with a high risk of infection. Sutures and drains should not be placed in the subcutaneous adipose tissue, since they have been demonstrated to increase wound infection rates.

Table 38.5 summarizes steps that can be taken to reduce surgical risks in obese patients. Specific anesthesiological measures are not considered in this chapter but have been outlined elsewhere.[92,93]

Postoperative care

It is particularly important that obese patients be mobilized as soon as possible after operation to prevent thromboembolism, atelectasis, and other pulmonary complications. Similarly, earliest possible extubation, adhering to stringent extubation criteria, helps to activate patients, promoting coughing and deep breathing. Having patients walk and perform knee bends within 4 hours of extubation significantly reduces the risk of postoperative pulmonary complications.

Early ambulation also has great psychological importance for obese patients because they frequently are sedentary. When they realize that they are able to ambulate without excessive pain, it helps them to overcome their intrinsic fear of moving and the common tacit assumption that they must remain in bed. Postponing ambulation to the first postoperative day may disproportionately prolong the recuperative process and length of hospitalization.

Anecdotally, it seems as if patients who are mobilized early require less pain medication, although it is difficult to separate cause and effect. Nevertheless, pain medications and sedatives may have profound depressive effects on respiration in obese patients, who have marginal respiratory reserves. It is difficult to balance the requirement for increased doses of narcotics adjusted for increased body mass to facilitate beneficial ambulation against the risk of sedating patients and increasing the risk of hypercarbia, hypoxia, and acidosis.

Summary

Obesity is an increasingly prevalent disease in industrialized nations and is associated with numerous conditions that require operation. For example, 14% of cancer deaths in men and 20% in women are attributable to obesity. Obese patients are at greater risk for perioperative complications than are patients of normal weight. Laparoscopic surgical approaches have substantially reduced complication rates and improved postoperative recovery. Severe obesity should not contraindicate necessary surgery. Just as pharmacogenomics has become a valuable tool to differentiate between responders and non-responders to positive as well as negative effects of drug treatment, it is conceivable that genome analysis might allow identification of complication–prone subgroups of obese patients. Identifying risk factors in obese patients, understanding the pathophysiology of their disease, and exhibiting compassion toward obese patients rather than the punitive attitude that is still common among healthcare practitioners will significantly enhance the quality of care these patients receive.

REFERENCES

1. Flegal, K. M., Carroll, M. D., Ogden, C. L. *et al.* Prevalence and trends in obesity among US adults, 1999–2000. *J. Am. Med. Assoc.* 2002; **288**: 1723–1727.

2. Mokdad, A. H., Ford, E. S., Bowman, B. A. *et al.* Prevalence of obesity, diabetes, and obesity-related health risk factors, 2001. *J. Am. Med. Assoc.* 2003; **289**: 76–79.

3. Freedman, D. S., Khan, L. K., Serdula, M. K. *et al.* Trends and correlates of class 3 obesity in the United States from 1990 through 2000. *J. Am. Med. Assoc.* 2002; **288**: 1758–1761.

4. Must, A., Jacques, P. F., Dallal, G. E. *et al.* Long-term morbidity and mortality of overweight adolescents: a follow-up of the Harvard Growth Study of 1922 to 1935. *N. Engl. J. Med.* 1992; **327**: 1350–1355.

5. Peeters, A., Barendregt, J. J., Willekens, F. *et al.* Obesity in adulthood and its consequences for life expectancy: a life-table analysis. *Ann. Intern. Med.* 2003; **138**: 24–32.

6. Fontaine, K. R., Redden, D. T., Wang, C. *et al.* Years of life lost due to obesity. *J. Am. Med. Assoc.* 2003; **289**: 187–193.

7. Hansen, B. C. The metabolic syndrome X. *Ann. NY Acad. Sci.* 1999; **892**: 1–24.

8. Sinha, R., Fisch, G., Teague, B. *et al.* Prevalence of impaired glucose tolerance among children and adolescents with marked obesity. *N. Engl. J. Med.* 2002; **346**: 802–810.

9. Ford, E. S., Giles, W. H., & Dietz, W. H. Jr. Prevalence of the metabolic syndrome among US adults: findings from the Third National Health and Nutrition Examination Survey. *J. Am. Med. Assoc.* 2002; **287**: 356–359.

10. Lakka, H.-M., Laaksonen, D. E., Lakka, T. A. *et al.* The metabolic syndrome and total and cardiovascular disease mortality in middle-aged men. *J. Am. Med. Assoc.* 2002; **288**: 2709–2716.

11. Calle, E. E., Rodriguez, C., Walker-Thurmond, K., & Thun, M. J. Overweight, obesity and mortality from cancer in a prospectively studied cohort of US adults. *N. Engl. J. Med.* 2003; **348**: 1625–1638.

12. Zhang, Y., Proenca, P., Maffei, M. *et al.* Positional cloning of the mouse obese gene and its human homologue. *Nature* 1994; **372**: 425–432.

13. Gupta, A. & Watson, D. I. Effect of laparoscopy on immune function. *Br. J. Surg.* 2001; **88**: 1296–1306.

14. Nguyen, N. T., Ho, H. S., Palmer, L. S. *et al.* A comparison study of laparoscopic versus open gastric bypass for morbid obesity. *J. Am. Coll. Surg.* 2002; **191**: 149–155.

15. Kral, J. G. Morbidity of severe obesity. In Sugerman, H. J., ed. *Obesity Surgery. Surg. Clin. North Am.* 2001; **81**:1039–1061.

16. Law, C. M., Barker, D. J. P., Osmond, C. *et al.* Early growth and abdominal fatness in adult life. *J. Epidemiol. Commun. Health* 1992; **46**: 184–186.

17. Shen, W., Wang, Z., Punyanita, M. *et al.* Adipose tissue quantification by imaging methods: a proposed classification system. *Obes. Res.* 2003; **13**: 15–16.

18. Sjöström, L. A CT based multicompartment body composition technique and anthropometric predictions of lean body mass, total and subcutaneous adipose tissue. *Int. J. Obes.* 1991; **15**(Suppl. 2): 19–30.

19. Folsom, A. R., Kushi, L. H., Anderson, K. E. *et al.* Associations of general and abdominal obesity with multiple health outcomes in older women: the Iowa Women's Health Study. *Arch. Intern. Med.* 2000; **160**: 2117–2128.

20. Cornier, M.-A., Tate, C. W., Grunwald, G. K. *et al.* Relationship between waist circumference, body mass index and medical care costs. *Obes. Res.* 2002; **10**: 1167–1172.

21. Alexander, J. K. Obesity and cardiac performance. *Am. J. Cardiol.* 1964; **14**: 860–865.

22. Agarwal, N., Shibutani, K., San Fillipo, J. *et al.* Hemodynamic and respiratory changes in surgery of the morbidly obese. *Surgery* 1982; **92**: 226–234.

23. Zarich, S. W., Kowalchuk, G. J., McGuire, M. P. *et al.* Left ventricular filing abnormalities in asymptomatic morbid obesity. *Am. J. Cardiol.* 1991; **68**: 377–381.

24. Tang, S., Kral, J. G., Barnard, J. T. *et al.* Android fat distribution predicts ventricular dysfunction in obese women. *Eur. J. Clin. Invest.* 1988; **18**: A10.

25. Alpert, M. A., Terry, B. E., Cohen, M. V. *et al.* The electrocardiogram in morbid obesity. *Am. J. Cardiol.* 2000; **85**: 908–910.

26. Alpert, M. A., Terry, B. E., Hamm, C. R. *et al.* Effect of weight loss on the ECG of normotensive morbidly obese patients. *Chest* 2001; **119**: 507–510.

27. Iacobellis, G., Ribando, M. C., Zappaterreno, A. *et al.* Relationship of insulin sensitivity and left ventricular mass in uncomplicated obesity. *Obes. Res.* 2003; **11**: 518–524.

28. Biring, M. S., Lewis, M. I., Liu, J. T. *et al.* Pulmonary physiological changes of morbid obesity. *Am. J. Med. Sci.* 1999; **318**: 293–297.

29. Alexander, K. L., Amad, K. H., & Cole, V. W. Observations on some clinical features of extreme obesity with particular reference to the cardiorespiratory effects. *Am. J. Med.* 1962; **32**: 512–524.

30. Wei, M., Kampert, J. B., Barlow, C. E. *et al.* Relationship between low cardiorespiratory fitness and mortality in normal-weight, overweight and obese men. *J. Am. Med. Assoc.* 1999; **282**: 1547–1553.

31. Brooks-Brunn, J. A. Predictors of postoperative pulmonary complications following abdominal surgery. *Chest* 1997; **1111**: 564–571.

32. Pelosi, P., Croci, M., Ravagnan, I. *et al.* The effects of body mass on lung volumes, respiratory mechanics and gas exchange during general anesthesia. *Anesth. Analg.* 1998; **87**: 654–660.

33. Sugerman, H. J., Baron, P. L., Fairman, R. P. *et al.* Hemodynamic dysfunction in obesity hypoventilation syndrome and the effects of treatment with surgically induced weight loss. *Ann. Surg.* 1988; **207**: 604–613.

34. Sugerman, H. J., Windsor, A., Bessos, M. *et al.* Intraabdominal pressure, sagittal abdominal diameter and obesity comorbidity. *J. Intern. Med.* 1997; **241**: 71–79.

35. Sugerman, H. J. Effects of increased intra-abdominal pressure in severe obesity. *Surg. Clin. North Am.* 2001; **81**: 1063–1075.

36. Sugerman, H. Pulmonary function in morbid obesity. *Gastroenterol. Clin. North Am.* 1987; **16**: 225–237.

37. Balsiger, B. M., Murr, M. M., Mai, J. *et al.* Gastroesophageal reflux after intact vertical banded gastroplasty: correction by conversion to Roux-en-Y gastric bypass. *J. Gastrointest. Surg.* 2000; **4**: 276–281.

38. Mercer, C. D., Rue, C., Hanelin, L. *et al.* Effect of obesity on esophageal transit. *Am. J. Surg.* 1985; **149**: 177–181.

39. Camargo, C. A. Jr., Weiss, S. T., Shang, S. *et al.* Prospective study of body mass index, weight change, and risk of adult-onset asthma in women. *Arch. Int. Med.* 1999; **159**: 2582–2588.

40. Dejgard, A., Andersen, T., & Gluud, C. The influence of insulin on the raised plasma fibronectin concentration in human obesity. *Acta Med. Scand.* 1986; **220**: 269–272.

41. Rillaerts, E., Van Gaal, L., Xiang, D. Z. *et al.* Blood viscosity in human obesity: relation to glucose tolerance and insulin status. *Int. J. Obes.* 1989; **13**: 739–745.

42. Gabriely, I., Yang, X. M., Cases, J. A. *et al.* Hyperglycemia induces PAI-1 gene expression in adipose tissue by activation of the hexosamine biosynthetic pathway. *Atherosclerosis* 2002; **160**: 115–122.

43. Marceau, P., Biron, S., Hould, F. S. *et al.* Liver pathology and the metabolic "syndrome X" in severe obesity. *J. Clin. Endocrinol. Metab.* 1999; **84**: 1513–1517.

44. Hansson, P. O., Eriksson, H., Welin, L. *et al.* Smoking and abdominal obesity: risk factors for venous thromboembolism among middle-aged men: "the study of men born in 1913". *Arch. Intern. Med.* 1990; **159**: 1886–1890.

45. Reaven, G. M. Syndrome X: six years later. *J. Int. Med.* 1994; **236**(Suppl. 736): 13–22.

46. Alessi, M. C., Peiretti, F., Morange, P. *et al.* Production of plasminogen activator inhibitor by human adipose tissue. *Diabetes* 1997; **46**: 860–867.

47. Juhan-Vague, I., Thompson, S. G., & Jespersen, J. Involvement of the hemostatic system in the insulin resistance syndrome: a study of 1500 patients with angina pectoris. *Arterioscler. Thromb.* 1993; **13**: 1865–1873.

48. Prandoni, P., Bilora, F., Marchiori, A. *et al.* An association between atherosclerosis and venous thrombosis. *N. Engl. J. Med.* 2003; **348**: 1435–1441.

49. Cohen, A. H. Massive obesity and the kidney. *Am. J. Pathol.* 1975; **81**: 117–130.

50. Carr, S., Mbanya, J. C., Thomas, T. *et al.* Increase in glomerular filtration rate in patients with insulin-dependent diabetes and elevated erythrocyte sodium–lithium countertransport. *N. Engl. J. Med.* 1990; **322**: 500–505.

51. Schmeider, R. E., Messerli, F. H., Garavaglia, G. *et al.* Glomerular hyperfiltration indicates early target organ damage in essential hypertension. *J. Am. Med. Assoc.* 1990; **264**: 2775–2780.

52. Gill, I. S., Hodge, E. E., Steinmuller, D. R. *et al.* The impact of obesity on renal transplantation. *Transplant Proc.* 1992; **25**: 1047.

53. Howard, R. J., Thai, V. B., Patton, P. R. *et al.* Obesity does not portend a bad outcome for kidney transplant recipients. *Transplantation* 2002; **73**: 53–55.

54. Waki, M., Kral, J. G., Mazariegos, M. *et al.* Relative expansion of extracellular fluid in obese versus non-obese women. *Am. J. Physiol.* 1991; **26**: E199–E203.

55. Mazariegos, M., Kral, J. G., Wang, J. *et al.* Body composition and surgical treatment of obesity: effects of weight loss on fluid distribution. *Ann. Surg.* 1992; **216**: 69–73.

56. Raison, J., Achimastos, A., Asmar, R. *et al.* Extracellular and interstitial fluid volume in obesity with and without associated systemic hypertension. *Am. J. Cardiol.* 1986; **57**: 2223–2226.

57. Shenkman, Z., Shir, Y., & Brodsky, J. B. Perioperative management of the obese patient. *Br. J. Anaesth.* 1993; **70**: 349–359.

58. De Fronzo, R. A., Cooke, R. E., & Andres, R. The effects of insulin and renal handling of sodium, potassium, calcium, and phosphate in man. *J. Clin. Invest.* 1975; **55**: 845–855.

59. Colt, E. W. D., Wang, J., Stallone, F. *et al.* A possible low intracellular potassium in obesity. *Am. J. Clin. Nutr.* 1981; **34**: 367–372.

60. Kral, J. G., Lundholm, K., Sjöström, L. *et al.* Hepatic lipid metabolism in severe human obesity. *Metabolism* 1977; **26**: 1025–1031.

61. Benoist, S., Panis, Y., Alves, A. *et al.* Impact of obesity on surgical outcomes after colorectal resection. *Am. J. Surg.* 2000; **179**: 275–281.

62. Weber, D. J., Rutala, W. A., Samsa, G. P. *et al.* Impaired immunogenicity of hepatitis B vaccine in obese persons. (Letter) *N. Engl. J. Med.* 1986; **314**: 1393.

63. Friedman, J. B. Obesity in the new millennium. *Nature* 2000; **404**: 632–634.

64. Smith, A. I. & Funder, J. W. Proopiomelanocortin processing in the pituitary, central nervous system, and peripheral tissues. *Endocr. Rev.* 1988; **9**: 159–179.

65. Hotamisligil, G. S., Arner, P., Caro, J. F. *et al.* Increased adipose tissue expression of tumor necrosis factor-α in human obesity and insulin resistance. *J. Clin. Invest.* 1995; **95**: 2409–2415.

66. Krishnan, E. C., Trost, L., Aarons, S. *et al.* Study of function and maturation of monocytes in morbidly obese individuals. *J. Surg. Res.* 1982; **33**: 89–97.

67. Kolterman, O. G., Olefsky, J. M., Kurakara, C. *et al.* A defect in cell-mediated immune function in insulin-resistant diabetic and obese subjects. *J. Lab. Clin. Med.* 1980; **96**: 535–543.

68. Felber, J.-P. & Golay, A. Pathways from obesity to diabetes. *Int. J. Obes.* 2002; **26**(Suppl. 2): S39–S45.

69. Wang, Y.-X., Lee, C.-H., Tiep, S. *et al.* Peroxisome-proliferator-activated receptor δ activates fat metabolism to prevent obesity. *Cell* 2003; **113**: 159–170.

70. Kral, J. G., Buckley, M. C. Kissileff, H. R., & Schaffner, F. Metabolic correlates of eating behavior in severe obesity. *Int. J. Obes.* 2001; **25**: 258–264.

71. Neel, J. V. Diabetes mellitus: a thrifty genotype rendered detrimental by progress? *Am. J. Hum. Genet.* 1962; **14**: 353–362.

72. Branson, R., Potoczna, N., Kral, J. G., Lentes, K. U., Hoehe, M. R., & Horber, F. F. Binge eating is a major phenotypic characteristic of melanocortin-4 receptor gene mutations. *N. Engl. J. Med.* 2003; **348**: 1096–1103.

73. Farooqui, I. S., Keogh, J. M., Yeo, G. S. H. *et al.* Clinical spectrum of obesity and mutations in the melanocortin 4 receptor gene. *N. Engl. J. Med.* 2003; **348**: 1085–1095.

74. Hamilton, B. S. & Doods, H. N. Chronic application of MT II in a rat model of obesity results in sustained weight loss. *Obes. Res.* 2002; **10**: 182–187.

75. Kral, J. G. Side-effects, complications and problems in antiobesity surgery: introduction of the obesity severity index. In Angel, A., Anderson, H., Bouchard, C., Lau, D., Leiter, L., & Mendelson, R., eds. *Progress in Obesity Research:7.* London: John Libbey, 1996: 655–661.

76. Drenick, E. J. & Fisler, J. S. Sudden cardiac arrest in morbidly obese surgical patients unexplained after autopsy. *Am. J. Surg.* 1988; **155**: 720–726.

77. Isner, J. M., Sours, H. E., Paris, A. L. *et al.* Sudden unexpected death in avid dieters using the liquid-protein modified-fast diet: observations in 17 patients and the role of the prolonged Q–T interval. *Circulation* 1979; **60**: 1401–1412.

78. Drenick, E. J., Blumfield, D. E., Fisler, J. S., & Lowy, S. Cardiac function during very low calorie reducing diets with dietary protein of good and poor nutritional quality. In Blackburn, G. L. & Bray, G. A., eds. *Management of Obesity by Severe Caloric Restriction.* Littleton, MA: PSG Publishing, 1985: 223–234.

79. Messerli, H., Ventura, H. O., Elizardi, D. J. *et al.* Hypertension and sudden death: increased ventricular ectopic activity in left ventricular hypertrophy. *Am. J. Med.* 1984; **77**: 18–22.

80. Spirito, P., Bellone, P., Harris, K. M. *et al.* Magnitude of left ventricular hypertrophy and risk of sudden death in hypertrophic cardiomyopathy. *N. Engl. J. Med.* 2000; **342**: 1778–1785.

81. Messerli, F. H., Nunez, B. D., Ventura, H. O. *et al.* Overweight and sudden death: increased ventricular ectopy in cardiopathy of obesity. *Arch. Intern. Med.* 1987; **147**: 1725–1728.

82. Ernst, E., Hammerschmidt, D. E., Bagge, U. *et al.* Leukocytes and the risk of ischemic diseases. *J. Am. Med. Assoc.* 1987; **257**: 2318–2324.

83. Palmer, M. & Schaffner, F. Effect of weight reduction on hepatic abnormalities in overweight patients. *Gastroenterology* 1990; **99**: 1408–1413.

84. Vaughan, R. W. Biochemical and biotransformation alterations in the obese. In Brown, B. R. Jr., ed. *Anesthesia and the Obese Patient.* Philadelphia: FA Davis Co, 1982: 55.

85. Terry, B. E. Morbid obesity: cardiac evaluation and function. *Gastroenterol. Clin. North Am.* 1987; **16**: 215–223.

86. Criqui, M. H., Heiss, G., Gohn, R. *et al.* Plasma triglyceride level and mortality from coronary heart disease. *N. Engl. J. Med.* 1993; **328**: 1220–1225.

87. Kral, J. G., Brolin, R. E., Buchwald, H. *et al.* Workshop summary: research considerations in obesity surgery. *Obes. Res.* 2002; **10**: 63–64.

88. Sugerman, H. J., ed. Obesity surgery. *Surg. Clin. North Am.* 2001; **81**(5): 1001–1198.

89. Rennotte, M. T., Baele, P., Aubert, G. *et al.* Nasal continuous positive airway pressure in the perioperative management of patients with obstructive sleep apnea submitted to surgery. *Chest* 1994; **102**: 367–364.

90. Bern, M. M., Bothe, A. Jr., Bistrian, B. *et al.* Effects of low-dose warfarin on antithrombin III levels in morbidly obese patients. *Surgery* 1983; **94**: 78–83.

91. Janvrin, S. B., Davies, G., & Greenhalgh, R. M. Postoperative deep vein thrombosis caused by intravenous fluids during surgery. *Br. J. Surg.* 1980; **67**: 680–693.

92. Vaughan, R. W. Anesthesia and morbid obesity. In Björntorp, B. & Brodoff, J. B., eds. *Obesity.* Philadelphia: JB Lippincott Co, 1992; 720–730.

93. Brown, B. R. Jr., ed. *Anesthesia and the Obese Patient.* Philadelphia: FA Davis, 1982.

Psychiatric disorders

39

Depression

Edward R. Norris[1] and Charles L. Raison[2]

[1]Department of Psychiatry, Lehigh Valley Hospital & Health Network, Allentown, PA
[2]Department of Psychiatry & Behavioral Sciences, Atlanta, GA

Depressive disorders are the most common psychiatric problem seen in medical–surgical patients. The point prevalence rate for depression is 10%–36% for general medical inpatients. The presence of depression has a significant effect on the patient's morbidity and mortality. Patients with depression following a myocardial infarction are 3.5 times more likely to die in the next 6 months than patients without depression.

The causes of depression in medically ill patients are multiple, including dealing with loss, helplessness, pain, lowered self-esteem, and financial and marital strain after illness. In many cases, depressive symptoms may result from the underlying physical illness or medications used in treatment.

Most depressive reactions in medical–surgical patients are relatively short, resolve after surgery, and do not cause major disturbances in social, occupational, interpersonal, physical, or psychological functioning. If depressive symptoms persist, they become major depression.

Major depression is characterized by a markedly depressed mood or loss of interest or pleasure in life (see Table 39.1). This depressed mood lasts longer than 2 weeks and causes significant disruptions in patient's occupational, social, and interpersonal functioning. Physical symptoms of depression can include sleep disturbances, appetite disturbance or weight change, fatigue, and physical feelings of being slowed down. Emotional symptoms can include disinterest, apathy, low self-esteem, hopelessness, helplessness, and guilt. Some patients will have suicidal thoughts or active plans for suicide. When severe, depression in the medically ill may give rise to psychotic symptoms, including paranoia, hallucinations, delusions (including somatic delusions of insect infestation), and obsessive–compulsive behavior. When depression involves psychosis or suicidal ideation, a psychiatric consultation is warranted. It is important to distinguish psychotic depression from delirium in the medically ill.

Assessment of suicide risk

Several factors help to identify patients who are at increased risk for suicide. Older men and persons who live alone, those who have suffered a recent major loss, those who have a chronic debilitating illness, or people with previous histories of depression or suicide attempts are at greater risk. Women attempt suicide more often, but men more often succeed in their attempts. Table 39.2 lists major risk factors for suicide.

A misconception about the assessment of suicide risk is that asking about suicidal ideation will bring the idea to the patient's mind and increase the risk of suicide. Actually, the opposite is true; an open discussion regarding suicide allows patients to express their possible motives, ideas and specific plans and to defuse a planned or potential suicide attempt. An open, thorough, and detailed questioning regarding suicidal ideation should be a part of every assessment of a depressed patient.

In addition to direct patient information, collateral history obtained from family members often reveals those patients who have already made up their minds and want no one to intervene. These patients often set their affairs in order, make out a will, and "get better" suddenly as they have figured a way out of their situation. In questioning potential suicidal patients it is important to ask about the method of suicide and evaluate the chance of rescue. Plans that involve guns, hanging, or carbon monoxide leave little chance for rescue. Patients with illnesses that impair cognition (such as schizophrenia, delirium, dementia, and substance abuse) are more likely to commit suicide due to poor judgment and impulsiveness.

Medical Management of the Surgical Patient: A Textbook of Perioperative Medicine, ed. M. F. Lubin, R. B. Smith, T. F. Dobson, N. Spell, H. K. Walker. 4th edn. Published by Cambridge University Press. © Cambridge University 2006.

Table 39.1. *Diagnostic and Statistical Manual of Mental Disorders*, 4th edn., text revision (DSM-IV TR) criteria for major depressive episode

A. Five (or more) of the following symptoms have been present during the same 2-week period and represent a change from previous functioning; at least one of the symptoms is either (1) depressed mood or (2) loss of interest or pleasure. *Note:* Do not include symptoms that are clearly due to a general medical condition, or mood-incongruent delusions or hallucinations.
   1. Depressed mood most of the day, nearly every day, as indicated by either subjective report (e.g., feels sad or empty) or observation made by others (e.g., appears tearful)
   2. Markedly diminished interest or pleasure in all, or almost all, activities most of the day, nearly every day (as indicated by either subjective account or observation made by others)
   3. Significant weight loss when not dieting or weight gain (e.g., a change of more than 5% of body weight in a month), or decrease or increase in appetite nearly every day
   4. Insomnia or hypersomnia nearly every day
   5. Psychomotor agitation or retardation nearly every day (observable by others, not merely subjective feelings of restlessness or being slowed down)
   6. Fatigue or loss of energy nearly every day
   7. Feelings of worthlessness or excessive or inappropriate guilt (which may be delusional) nearly every day (not merely self-reproach or guilt about being sick)
   8. Diminished ability to think or concentrate, or indecisiveness, nearly every day (either by subjective account or as observed by others)
   9. Recurrent thoughts of death (not just fear of dying), recurrent suicidal ideation without a specific plan, or a suicide attempt or a specific plan for committing suicide
B. The symptoms do not meet criteria for a mixed episode
C. The symptoms cause clinically significant distress or impairment in social, occupational, or other important areas of functioning
D. The symptoms are not due to the direct physiologic effects of a substance (e.g., a drug of abuse, a medication) or a general medical condition (e.g., hypothyroidism)
E. The symptoms are not better accounted for by bereavement; i.e., after the loss of a loved one, the symptoms persist for >2 months or are characterized by marked functional impairment, morbid preoccupation with worthlessness, suicidal ideation, psychotic symptoms, or psychomotor retardation

Depressed patients with anxiety, excessive guilt, low self-esteem, and feelings of helplessness and hopelessness are at extremely high risk.

If a significant suicide risk exists, immediate psychiatric consultation is needed before patients are discharged from the hospital. Steps should also be taken to protect the patient in the current hospital setting by utilizing family and friends or hospital staff to ensure that the

Table 39.2. Major risk factors for suicide

Older, divorced, or widowed man
Caucasian race
Unemployed
Poor physical health
Past suicide attempts
Family history of suicide
Psychosis
Alcoholism or drug abuse
Chronic painful disease
Sudden life changes
Living alone
Anniversary of significant loss

Table 39.3. Criteria for hospital admission for suicidal patients

Patients show no improvement with medication and interviews.
Patients improve but remain so psychotic that they cannot care for their daily needs.
Patients pose a physical threat to themselves or others.
Patients are having command hallucinations.
Physicians are in doubt of the severity of the illness.
Patients are toxic from drugs, alcohol, or prescribed medications.
Patients are psychotic and have exhausted caregivers and all external support.

patient is not left alone prior to psychiatric assessment and disposition. Psychiatric hospitalization is often accepted voluntarily by patients who realize that they need additional care. In cases where patients must be hospitalized against their wills, the broad grounds for psychiatric commitment usually state that the patient must have a mental illness and be either a danger to themselves or to others, or be unable to care for themselves as a result of a psychiatric condition. Psychiatric commitment procedure varies from state to state and psychiatric consultation is recommended before pursuing this option. Table 39.3 lists criteria for hospital admission for suicidal patients.

Pain and depression

In general, pain medications tend to be underused in the acute surgical setting. The reasons for this practice include exaggerated fear of addiction, underestimations of effective doses, and overestimation of the duration of narcotic action. In actual practice, there is little chance that a patient who is experiencing postoperative pain will become addicted to narcotics unless there is a history of narcotic abuse. Addiction should not be a concern in any terminally ill patient.

The relationship between pain, chronic pain, and depression arises frequently in medical–surgical patients. High rates of pain complaints have been observed in depressed patients, including headaches, abdominal pain, joint pain, back pain and chest pain. These somatic pain complaints in the presence of an obviously depressed mood have been described as masked depression and the symptoms as depressive equivalents.

Sometimes depression is masked by a patient's denial or limited ability to verbalize feelings. Patients with limited educational backgrounds may be especially prone to "somatizing" depression and have complaints referable to almost every organ system along with more classic neurovegetative signs of depression.[32] This somatic form of depression is a major way that patients present in the outpatient medical setting. Physicians, in this setting, should not accept patients' denial of depressed mood as excluding the diagnosis. After a reasonable medical evaluation has been completed, a therapeutic trial of antidepressant medication may be in order.

Secondary mood disorders

Medical conditions and medications may induce depression or at least mimic the neurovegetative symptoms of depression. This possibility should be ruled out before attributing a patients' depression to a psychiatric cause. Table 39.4 lists the major causes of secondary depressive disorders in medical patients.

Indications for psychopharmacologic treatment of depression

The indication for antidepressant drugs is clearest in patients who meet the criteria for major depression as listed in Table 39.1. These prominent somatic and vegetative signs and symptoms of depression are clear indications of an underlying biologic disruption in central nervous system mood regulation.

The number of antidepressants continues to expand each year and include the selective serotonin reuptake inhibitors (SSRIs), modern atypical antidepressants such as bupropion (Wellbutrin), venlafaxine (Effexor) and mirtazapine (Remeron), tricyclic antidepressants, and monoamine oxidase (MAO) inhibitors. The dose ranges and

Table 39.4. Major causes of depressive disorders in patients due to medications and general medical conditions

Medications
Antihypertensives (reserpine, methyldopa, propranolol)
Antineoplastic drugs (interferon, procarbazine, vincristine, tamoxifen)
Barbiturates
Corticosteroids
Levodopa
Opiates

Infectious diseases
HIV, HSV, Lyme disease, syphilis, rabies, prions

Neurological
Meningitis, seizures, demyelination, cerebrovascular disease, Parkinson's disease, Huntington's disease, Wilson's disease

Nutritional
Niacin, thiamine (B_1), cobalamin (B_{12})

Metabolic
Hepatic encephalopathy, renal insufficiency, hypoglycemia, porphyria, ketoacidosis, hypercalcemia, hypocalcemia

Endocrine
Thyroid, parathyroid, adrenal dysfunction

Neoplasm
Brain tumors, paraneoplastic syndromes, lymphomas, pancreatic

general properties of the antidepressants are shown in Table 39.5. In general, medications should be started at low doses and increased every 3 days as tolerated until a maintenance dose is reached.

A lag time of 4 to 6 weeks is typically seen before full symptomatic improvement is seen with antidepressants. Patients should be counseled to not expect overnight improvement. Improvement in some biologic abnormalities such as sleep disturbance, anxiety, and agitation may be seen early on and precede positive effects on mood or anxiety.

The duration of therapy with these drugs after the antidepressant effect is achieved is at least six to twelve months. Medications should be gradually tapered, while observing for signs of depression relapse.

Minimizing adverse effects

Safe administration of antidepressants involves management of potential side effects. Several general principles will enhance safety and compliance. These include the following.

Table 39.5. Properties of selected antidepressants

Drug	Sedation	Anticholinergic	Hypotension	Hypertension	Tachycardia	Conduction slowing	Dose range (mg/day)
Antidepressants (cyclics)							
Amitriptyline (Elavil)	+++	+++	+++	−	+++	yes	75–300
Amoxapine (Asendin)	+	+	+++	−	+	yes	75–600
Clomipramine (Anafranil)	+++	+++	+++	−	+++	yes	100–250
Desipramine (Norpramin)	+	+	+++	++	+	yes	75–150
Doxepin (Sinequan)	+++	+++	+++	−	+++	yes	75–300
Imipramine (Tofranil)	++	++	+++	−	++	yes	75–300
Maprotiline (Ludiomil)	++	+	++	−	+	yes	150–200
Nortriptyline (Pamelor)	+	+	+	−	+++	yes	40–150
Protriptyline (Vivactil)	+	+++	++	−	+++	yes	20–60
Trimipramine (Surmontil)	+++	++	++	−	++	yes	50–300
Antidepressants (SSRIs)							
Citalapram (Celexa)	−	−	−	−	−	−	20–60
Fluoxetine (Prozac)	−	−	−	−	−	−	20–60
Fluvoxamine (Luvox)	+	−	−	−	−	−	50–200
Paroxetine (Paxil)	++	−	−	−	++	−	20–60
Sertraline (Zoloft)	−	−	−	−	−	−	50–200
Antidepressants (MAOIs)							
Phenelzine (Nardil)	+	+	+++	+	−	−	45–60
Tranylcypromine (Parnate)	+	+	++	+	−	−	30–40
Antidepressants (Other)							
Bupropion (Wellbutrin)	+	−	−	−	−	−	150–450
Nefazodone (Serzone)	++	−	+	−	−	−	200–600
Trazodone (Desyrel)	+++	−	++	−	−	yes	200–600
Venlafaxine XR (Effexor XR)	+	−	−	++	−	−	37.5–225
Mirtazapine (Remeron)	++	+	+	−	−	−	15–45

Note:

Key: +, weak; ++, moderate; +++, strong.

1. Anticipate with the patient the probable side effects; include a review of the most common side effects. Reassure the patient that there are strategies to minimize the adverse effects of medications.
2. Select drugs that have the smallest chance of exacerbating current medical problems. Use the lowest effective dose and gradually titrate the dose. This may minimize side effects because side effects are often dose related.
3. **"Start low, go slow,"** especially in elderly, neurologically impaired, and medically ill patients.
4. Manage side effects with adjunctive agents rather than switching to another agent which may delay therapeutic response.
5. Reassure the patient; side effects frequently improve over time.
6. Educate the patient regularly that psychiatric symptoms often mirror common medication side effects. Clearly written patient instructions will increase medication compliance. Symptoms that begin after medication initiation or worsen with dose escalation are likely to be medication related.

Side effects

Psychiatric illness is regularly complicated by medical symptoms and disorders. The more severe the medical illness, the more frequent is the impact on psychiatric disorders. In a fashion similar to primary psychiatric disorders, proper management of many combined medical and psychiatric disorders requires use of medications. Physicians have long feared the effects of psychotropics in medically ill patients; they continue to be wary of them in severely medically compromised patients. Historically, many psychotropics have been recognized for their potential adverse effects on the cardiovascular (CV) system and on other organ systems. Knowledge of side effects and their prevalence is a requirement for safe and effective treatment of all patients.

Orthostatic hypotension (OH) is of greatest concern for the elderly, for those on antihypertensive medications, and for patients with cardiovascular disease. OH is correlated with the proclivity of an antidepressant to interfere with alpha-noradrenergic receptor activity. Many antidepressants, especially tricyclic antidepressants (TCAs) and monoamine oxidase inhibitors (MAOIs), cause OH. The maximum effect appears after 3–4 weeks, and OH can subside after 6 weeks. Among other antidepressants, nefazodone and mirtazapine are associated with a low incidence of OH, while fluoxetine, sertraline, paroxetine, citalopram, bupropion, fluvoxamine, and venlafaxine are not associated with OH. However, data indicate that SSRI-treated patients may have as many falls as TCA-treated patients. The mechanism is unknown and the topic is still under debate.

Essential hypertension may arise with use of some medications. Venlafaxine occasionally produces a dose-related elevation of supine diastolic BP in 7% of patients taking doses of 200–300 mg/day. It occurs in up to 13% in those with daily doses greater than 300 mg/day. Buspirone in combination with an MAOI or other serotoninergic drug can cause hypertension. Psychostimulants, especially at higher doses, can aggravate hypertension.

The hypertensive crisis, a potentially fatal interaction, is characterized by an elevation of BP, severe headache, nausea, vomiting, and diaphoresis. It occurs when patients on MAOIs ingest large amounts of tyramine-containing foods or take medications that influence the sympathetic nervous system. Hypertensive crisis requires immediate medical attention to reduce BP with the alpha-1-adrenergic antagonist phentolamine. Another potentially fatal interaction, serotonin syndrome, is characterized by hypertension, tachycardia, delirium, agitation, and hyperreflexia, and occurs when MAOIs and serotonergic agents, such as SSRIs, clomipramine, or buspirone, are coadministered.

The cardiac conducting system is affected by TCAs, which can cause tachycardia, prolong both atrial and ventricular depolarization, and prolong the QT interval. All TCAs should be avoided in patients with ventricular arrhythmias. MAOIs, bupropion, venlafaxine, fluoxetine, sertraline, citalopram, paroxetine, and fluvoxamine appear to have very few or no cardiac conduction effects.

The central nervous system is also affected by antidepressants. A high-frequency tremor can occur as a side effect of TCAs, SSRIs, and MAOIs. The use of low-dose beta-blockers (e.g., propranolol 10 mg t.i.d.) or low-dose benzodiazepines can minimize the tremor. Increased anxiety and jitteriness may be seen during the initiation of TCAs, SSRIs, venlafaxine, and bupropion. These symptoms often remit within a few weeks and they can be minimized by starting at low doses or by using benzodiazepines. Akathisia is characterized by the subjective feelings of restlessness or the appearance of restlessness. Besides dose reduction or a change of medication, use of beta-adrenergic blocking drugs and benzodiazepines is often helpful. Some patients on SSRIs experience an akathisia-like motor restlessness that may respond to low-dose propranolol or benzodiazepines.

Fatigue and sedation can be manifestations of psychiatric symptoms or medication side effects. TCAs, MAOIs, trazodone, nefazodone, mirtazapine, and antipsychotics are each likely to produce sedation. The side effect of sedation can be used to induce sleep in some patients. Sleep disturbances can be related to antidepressant treatment and may improve if the medication is moved to earlier in the day. Insomnia can occur with SSRIs, bupropion, venlafaxine, and MAOIs. Reducing caffeine, eliminating daytime naps, and practicing sleep hygiene (e.g., restricting activities in the bedroom to sleep or sexual relations) can be effective.

Hypomania or mania related to antidepressant use occurs in less than 1% of patients without a history of bipolar disorder. Patients with bipolar disorder are at much higher risk. Mania induction and/or induction of rapid-cycling between manias and depressions have been reported with all antidepressants, but appear to be most common with TCAs.

Nausea and dyspepsia are common side effects and can be relieved by the use of divided dosing or dosing with meals. Adjuvant treatment includes over-the-counter antacids, bismuth salicylate, and H_2 blockers. Diarrhea is more commonly seen with use of newer serotonergic antidepressants, such as the SSRIs, that lack anticholinergic activity. Management strategies include the use of antidiarrheal agents. Constipation is common with TCAs but can be seen with all antidepressants. In the elderly, severe constipation and paralytic ileus can be a serious health risk.

Weight gain is a common cause of medication noncompliance and is most strongly associated with tertiary amine TCAs (amitriptyline, imipramine, doxepin), MAOIs (phenelzine) and mirtazapine. Weight gain may be related to the antihistaminic or serotonergic effects of the agents. The SSRIs, bupropion, venlafaxine, and nefazodone are less likely to cause weight gain. If weight gain occurs, dietary modification and increased exercise are frequently effective countermeasures. There is little experience with the combination of weight loss agents and antidepressants.

Sexual dysfunction occurs in roughly one-third of patients treated with antidepressants. Sexual dysfunction is underreported unless it is specifically asked about. Sexual dysfunction can lead to medication non-compliance if not addressed by the physician. Decreased libido can also be a symptom of depression or medication. If it persists after improvement of mood symptoms, a medication effect should be suspected. Erectile dysfunction may result from the anticholinergic or anti-alpha-adrenergic effects of medications. Priapism can occur with antidepressants or antipsychotics. It is most frequently reported with trazodone use (1 in 1000 men). All men who receive trazodone should be warned that priapism is a medical emergency that requires evaluation by a urologist. Delayed orgasm and anorgasmia may be serotonergically mediated. These symptoms have been associated with TCAs, MAOIs, SSRIs, and atypical antidepressants. Recent evidence suggests that sildenafil successfully reverses antidepressant-induced sexual dysfunction in many cases.

Knowledge of the risk of side effects is a requirement for the safe and effective treatment of all patients. One should anticipate the side effects likely to develop and select drugs that have the smallest chance of exacerbating medical problems. The lowest effective dose should be used and gradually titrated to an effective dose.

Use of electroconvulsive therapy in the medically ill

Electroconvulsive therapy (ECT) is the treatment of choice for patients who cannot tolerate the side effects of antidepressants, who have severe melancholic, psychotic, or delusional symptoms, or who are so acutely suicidal that the waiting time for antidepressants to take effect would be dangerous. Contraindications to ECT include the presence of central nervous system mass lesions, recent myocardial infarction, or a history of unstable ventricular arrhythmia. ECT usually causes reflex bradycardia immediately after seizure onset, followed by tachycardia, and increases in systolic and diastolic blood pressure. These reactions are adrenergic mediated and can be safely blunted with the use of beta-blockers.

With modern anesthesia to induce sedation and muscle relaxation to keep the seizure centrally focused, ECT is a relatively benign procedure and is the safest and most effective treatment for many patients.

REFERENCES

1. Wells, C. E. Pseudodementia. *Am. J. Psychiatry* 1979; **136**: 895–890.

2. McAllister, T. W. Overview: pseudodementia. *Am. J. Psychiatry* 1983; **140**: 528–533.

3. Dubin, W. R. Psychiatric emergencies: recognition and management. In Stoudemire, A., ed. *Clinical Psychiatry for Medical Students*. Philadelphia: J. B. Lippincott, 1990; 497–526.

4. Marks, R. M. & Sachar, E. J. Undertreatment of medical inpatient with narcotic analgesics. *Ann. Intern. Med.* 1973; **78**: 173–181.

5. Goldberg, R. J. Acute pain management. In Stoudemire, A. & Fog, B. S., eds. *Psychiatric Care of the Medical Patient*. New York: Oxford University Press, 1993: 323–339.

6. Knorring, L. The experience of pain in depressed patients. *Neuropsychobiology* 1975; **1**: 155–165.

7. Hameroff, S. R., Cork, R. C., Scherer, K. *et al.* Doxepin effects chronic pain, depression and plasma opioids. *J. Clin. Psychiatry* 1982; **43**: 22–27.

8. Ward, N. G., Bloom, V. L., & Friedel, R. O. The effectiveness of tricyclic antidepressants in the treatment of coexisting pain and depression. *Pain* 1979; **7**: 331–341.

9. Portenoy, R. K. Chronic pain management. In Stoudemire, A. & Fogel, B. S., eds. *Psychiatric Care of the Medical Patient*. New York: Oxford University Press, 1993: 341–366.

10. Stoudemire, A. Organic mental disorders. In Stoudemire, A. *Clinical Psychiatry for Medical Students*. Philadelphia: J. B. Lippincott, 1990: 72–103.

11. Carroll, B. J. Dexamethasone suppression test: a review of temporary confusion. *J. Clin. Psychiatry* 1985; **46**: 13–24.

12. Glassman, A. H., Johnson, L. L. O., Giardina, E. G. V. *et al.* The use of imipramine in depressed patients with congestive heart failure. *J. Am. Med. Assoc.* 1983; **250**: 1997–2001.

13. Veith, R. C., Raskind, M. A., Caldwell, J. H. *et al.* Cardiovascular effects of tricyclic antidepressants in depressed patients with chronic heart disease. *N. Engl. J. Med.* 1982; **306**: 954–959.

14. Siris, S. G. & Rifkin, A. The problem of psychopharmacotherapy in the medically ill. *Psychiatr. Clin. North Am.* 1981; **4**: 379–390.

15. Robinson, D. S., Nies, A., Corcella, J. *et al.* Cardiovascular effects of phenelzine and amitriptyline in depressed outpatients. *J. Clin. Psychiatry* 1982; **43**: 8–15.

16. Zisook, S. A clinical overview of monoamine oxidase inhibitors. *Psychosomatics* 1985; **26**: 240–251.

17. Stoudemire, A., Fogel, B. S., Gulley, L. R., & Moran, M. G. Psychopharmacology in the medically ill. In Stoudemire, A. & Fogel, B. S., eds. *Psychiatric Care of the Medical Patient*. New York: Oxford University Press, 1993: 155–206.

18. Katon, W. & Raskind, M. Treatment of depression in the medically ill elderly with methylphenidate. *Am. J. Psychiatry* 1980; **137**: 963–965.

19. McKenna, G., Engle, R. P., Brooks, H. *et al.* Cardiac arrhythmias during electroshock therapy: significance, prevention and treatment. *Am. J. Psychiatry* 1970; **127**: 530–533.

20. Weiner, R. ECT in the physically ill. *J. Psychiatr. Treat. Eval.* 1983; **5**: 457–462.

21. Weiner, R. D. & Coffey, C. E. Electroconvulsive therapy in the medical and neurologic patient. In Stoudemire, A. & Fogel,

B. S., eds. *Psychiatric Care of the Medical Patient*. New York: Oxford University Press, 1993: 207–224.

22. Alpert, J. E., Bernstein, J. G., & Rosenbaum, J. F. Psychopharmacologic issues in the medical setting. In Cassem, N. H., Stern, T. A., Rosenbaum, J. F., & Jellinek, M. S., eds. *The Massachusetts General Hospital Handbook of General Hospital Psychiatry*, 4th edn. St. Louis: Mosby, 1997: 249–303.

23. Glassman, A. H., Rodriguez, A. I., & Shapiro, P. A. The use of antidepressant drugs in patients with heart disease. *J. Clin. Psychiatry* 1998; **59**(Suppl. 10): 16–21.

24. Goff, D. C. & Shader, R. I. Non-neurological side effects of antipsychotic agents. In Hirsch, S. R. & Weinberger, D. R., eds. *Schizophrenia*. Oxford: Blackwell Science, 1995: 566–578.

25. Grebb, J. A. General principles of psychopharmacology. In Kaplan, H. I. & Sadock, B. J., eds. *Comprehensive Textbook of Psychiatry VI*, 6th edn. Baltimore: Williams and Wilkins, 1995: 1895–1915.

26. Hyman, S. E., Arana, G. W., & Rosenbaum, J. F. *Handbook of Psychiatric Drug Therapy*, 3rd edn. Boston: Little, Brown, 1995.

27. Smoller, J. A., Pollack, M. H., & Lee, D. K. Management of antidepressant-induced side effects. In Stern, T. A., Herman, J. B., & Slavin, P. S., eds. *The MGH Guide to Psychiatry in Primary Care*. New York: McGraw-Hill, 1998: 483–496.

28. Tesar, G. E. Cardiovascular side effects of psychotropic agents. In Stern, T. A., Herman, J. B., & Slavin, P. S., eds. *The MGH Guide to Psychiatry in Primary Care*. New York: McGraw-Hill, 1998: 497–517.

29. Thapa, P. B., Gideon, P., Cost, T. W., Milam, A. B., & Ray, W. A. Antidepressants and the risk of falls among nursing home residents. *N. Engl. J. Med.* 1998; **339**: 875–882.

30. Stoudemire, A. Depression. In Lubin, M. F., Walker, H. K., & Smith, R. B., eds. *Medical Management of the Surgical Patient*. Philadelphia, PA: J. B. Lippincott Company, 1995: 430–437.

31. Norris, E. R. & Cassem, N. Cardiovascular and other side effects of psychotropic medications. In Stern, T. & Herman, J., eds. *Psychiatry Update and Board Preparation*, New York: McGraw-Hill Publishers, 2000: Chapter 39.

32. Guggenheim, F. Somatoform disorders. In Sadock, B. J. & Sadock, A. V., eds. *Comprehensive Textbook of Psychiatry*. Philadelphia, PA: J. B. Lippincott, Williams and Wilkins, 1999: 1504–1532.

*This is an updated chapter of a previous one of Alan Stoudemire.

Anxiety and somatoform disorders

Edward R. Norris and Charles L. Raison*

Department of Psychiatry, Lehigh Valley Hospital & Health Newtork, Allentown, PA

Department of Psychiatry & Behavioral Sciences, Atlanta, GA

Anxiety

Anxiety is a non-specific symptom, and many patients are justifiably anxious in reaction to the diagnosis of illness and the performance of diagnostic tests and surgical procedures. Most of these anxious reactions dissipate when the illness resolves but anxiety may be chronic if uncertainty exists about the course and prognosis of their illness. Stressful treatment options also can create chronic anxiety problems.

Patients with anxiety should be given periodic opportunities to express their questions, fears and concerns. Physicians should be open, attentive, empathetic, and supportive of patients' concerns; additionally, physicians should provide information, advice, encouragement, and reassurance. Caution should be taken not to "sugarcoat" responses, as this would suppress the fears and feelings that patients may need to express.

As with depression, underlying medical conditions and medications should be considered before patients' symptoms of anxiety are attributed to psychiatric factors. Medical conditions and medications that cause anxiety are varied and listed in Table 39.6. Careful optimization of these conditions should reduce or eliminate the anxiety that patients experience.

If patients have significant anxiety, agitation, or if their level of anxiety interferes with their social interactions or medical treatment, the short-term use of benzodiazepines may be considered, as long as several key points are kept in mind. First, benzodiazepines should be used in relatively low doses for short periods of time (2 to 4 weeks). If more than 1 month of benzodiazepine treatment is contemplated, psychiatric consultation or referral may be warranted. In addition, depression should be ruled out first to ensure that the patients' symptoms of anxiety are not secondary manifestations of mood disorders.

The half-life of benzodiazepines ranges from short (5 to 15 hours: alprazolam, lorazepam, oxazepam) to long (20 to 100 hours: diazepam). The details of dosing and half-lives of benzodiazepines are shown in Table 39.7. Lorazepam and oxazepam are primarily metabolized by glucuronide conjugation and are not as affected by the presence of liver

Table 39.6. Medical conditions and medications that can cause anxiety

Medical conditions
Hyperthyroidism
Hypercalcemia
Hypoglycemia
Hypoxia
Pulmonary failure
Cardiac arrhythmias
Mitral valve prolapse
Angina
Vitamin B_{12} deficiency

Medications
Caffeine
Psychostimulants
Theophylline
Alcohol and benzodiazepine withdrawal
Initiation of SSRIs
Anticholinergic medicines
Dopaminergic medicines

Table 39.7. Dosing equivalencies and half-lives of benzodiazepines

Drug	Peak plasma level (h)	Mean elimination half-life (h)	Approximate dose equivalent (mg)
Alprazolam (Xanex)	1–2	11 (6–16)	0.5
Chlordiazepoxide (Librium)	0.5–4	10 (5–30)	10
Clonazepam (Klonopin)	1–4	23 (18–50)	0.25
Clorazepate (Tranxene)	1–2	73 (30–100)	7.5
Diazepam (Valium)	1–2	43 (20–70)	5
Estazolam (ProSom)	2	14 (10–24)	1.0
Flurazepam (Dalmane)	0.5–2	74 (36–120)	5
Lorazepam (Ativan)	1–2	14 (10–25)	1.0
Midazolam	5 min i.v.	68 min	1–2 mg i.v.
Oxazepam (Serax)	2	7 (5–15)	15
Temazepam (Restoril)	1–1.5	13 (8–20)	15
Triazolam (Halcion)	1–2	2	0.25

disease, age, or the concurrent use of medications that prolong the half-lives of medications due to interactions with the P450 microsomal oxidation pathways in the liver. Diazepam and prazepam are primarily metabolized by microsomal oxidation and should be avoided in liver disease, old age, or when multiple medications are present. If intramuscular administration is required, lorazepam and midazolam are the only benzodiazepines that are reliably absorbed through this route. In patients who have received high doses or long-term treatment with benzodiazepines, abrupt discontinuation can cause a withdrawal syndrome in which seizures can develop. Thus, when tapering benzodiazepines, dosages should be tapered slowly.

Panic attacks

Panic attacks (or anxiety attacks) may present with a constellation of symptoms including hyperventilation, dizziness, choking sensations, tachycardia, palpitations, gastrointestinal distress, numbness, tingling, sweating, hot or cold flushes and feelings of impending doom, losing ones mind or depersonalization. These panic attacks usually are abrupt in onset, last for 5 to 10 minutes, and usually come on "out of the blue." Often agoraphobia, the fear of closed spaces where escape is not possible, develops in these patients. Panic attacks and agoraphobia have been found to respond to medications including SSRIs, tricyclic antidepressants, and monoamine oxidase inhibitors. The diagnosis may be important if patients are noted to be particularly phobic about surgery. Depression frequently accompanies panic disorder, and these patients should be referred to treatment by a psychiatrist.

For other physicians, benzodiazepines and SSRIs (e.g., paroxetine, sertraline, citalopram) are the drugs of choice for the pharmacolgic treatment of patients in the primary care setting. The long-acting benzodiazepine clonazepam (Klonopin) is preferred to the short-acting benzodiazepine alprazolam (Xanex) as there appear to be fewer problems with withdrawal reactions. Benzodiazepines can be used during the initiation phase of SSRIs as the serotonin antidepressants take 3 to 6 weeks to be fully effective against panic attacks. When SSRIs are initiated, doses should be low initially (10 mg/day) and increased slowly over weeks because patients with panic disorder are exquisitely sensitive to transient exacerbations of their anxiety symptoms when these drugs are first administered. Once patients are in remission, treatment must continue for at least 12 months before medication dosages can be tapered. Behavioral therapy may be useful in the treatment of panic disorder. Any medications that can interfere with anxiety should be discontinued if possible.

Insomnia

One of the most common complaints all physicians hear is insomnia. Many patients experience anxiety and insomnia during hospitalization and require medications to help them sleep. Many medications exist to help patients initiate and maintain sleep. Benzodiazepines are generally the drugs of choice in this situation because they are effective in inducing and maintaining sleep, have little likelihood in inducing respiratory depression, and have a wide safety margin. Flurazepam (Dalmane), temazepam (Restoril), triazolam (Halcion), and estazolam (ProSom) are benzodiazepines that have been developed primarily as soporifics. These drugs differ primarily in their half-lives. The dosages are given in Table 39.7.

Two recent medications zolpidem (Ambien) and zaleplon (Sonota) have been developed that are non-benzodiazepine hypnotics that bind to the benzodiazepine receptor. These drugs have a much lower abuse potential than benzodiazepines. The usual starting dose for both medications are 5 mg at bedtime. Neither should be used for more than 2 weeks in a row due to the development of tolerance.

Somatoform disorders, factitious disorders, and malingering

Several other psychiatric disorders may be seen in medical and surgical patients, although the emphasis here is on their recognition because their treatment, when and if possible, is usually difficult and requires psychiatric consultation. The importance of appropriate recognition is underscored by the fact that these patients often are a great burden on the medical system and tend to receive many unnecessary medications, tests, and surgery.

Somatoform disorders include hypochondriasis, somatization disorder, conversion disorder, and body dysmorphic disorder. Hypochondriasis is diagnosed when patients develop fixed illnesses despite repeated tests and reassurances to the contrary. This fear of being ill causes clinically significant distress, so much so that most patients may "doctor shop" and frustrate both their physicians and themselves. The neuropsychology of hypochondriasis is unknown, but it is important to realize that patients are not malingering or fabricating their symptoms. Patients with hypochondriasis are best managed through regular periodic office visits that are scheduled irrespective of the presence or severity of symptoms, thereby enabling them to maintain contact with physicians. In addition, physicians should take care to validate the symptoms and structure

their interactions to improve the quality of life of patients. Psychiatric comorbidity exists in over 60% of patients with hypochondriasis, thus psychiatric symptoms of depression and anxiety should be explored. Recent studies demonstrate that cognitive behavioral therapy is helpful in improving patients' lives. Preliminary data suggest that there may be some benefit of the serotonin antidepressants.

Somatization disorder is similar to hypochondriasis, although patients with somatization disorder typically have less insight into the psychological/psychiatric contributions to their illness. Although patients may chronically complain of many physical symptoms affecting almost every organ system, they usually are not obsessed with the idea of having life-threatening illnesses. These patients tend to focus their emotional distress into somatic symptoms. The goals of treatment include supportive care and containment of medical utilization by prevention of unnecessary tests, procedures, and surgeries. A referral to a psychiatrist should always be considered.

In diagnosing hypochondriasis and somatization disorder, physicians should be careful not to overlook an underlying depression or anxiety disorder because depression and anxiety often present with prominent somatization, somatic obsessions and preoccupations, and hypochondriacal concerns. Psychiatric consultation may be helpful in sorting such patients with masked depressions because the prognosis for improvement is much better if a mood disturbance is the primary problem.

Conversion disorder refers to the loss or alteration of a physical function usually referable to neurologic dysfunction that cannot be explained on the basis of known anatomic or pathophysiologic mechanisms. It may be more common in patients with histrionic personalities and reflects the repression of unconscious drives, feelings, or conflicts over dependency, aggression, and sexuality.

The diagnosis of factitious disorders and malingering should be contrasted. Factitious disorders are psychiatric conditions in which patients self-induce or manufacture symptoms with the intent of gaining medical attention. Examples are patients who present to numerous hospitals with chest or abdominal pain and submit to repeated tests, procedures and surgery. Other patients may self-inject feces and surreptitiously warm thermometers to create the appearance of fever. In factitious disorders, there is no clear goal or reward involved other than seeking to be a patient and to maintain the sick role. In contrast, malingerers fabricate symptoms with clearly identified goals in mind (i.e., disability or financial compensation), and their behavior is sociopathic.

Finally, body dysmorphic disorder (BDD) involves distortion in body image in which patients become excessively and obsessively preoccupied with the perception that some aspect of their body are ugly or defective. To neutral observers, the so-called bodily defects are considered trivial or inconsequential but to patients they are a source of extreme distress. Such patients are likely to seek corrective surgery from cosmetic surgeons with unrealistic expectations. Patients are rarely satisfied with corrective procedures, therefore, recognition of this condition is essential for specialists such as plastic surgeons and dermatologists, who are most likely to encounter these patients. Preliminary data suggest that the fluoxetine may be useful in the treatment of BDD.

FURTHER READING

Barsky, A.J. The patient with hypochondriasis. *N. Engl. J. Med.* 2001: **345**(19), 1395–1399.

Berlin, R.M. The management of insomnia in hospitalized patients. *Ann. Intern. Med.* 1984; **100**: 398–404.

Brown, J.T., Mulrow, C.D., & Stoudemire, A. The anxiety disorders. *Ann. Intern. Med.* 1984; **100**: 558–564.

Folks, D.G., Ford, C.V., & Houck, C.A. Somatoform disorders, factitious disorders, and malingering. In Stoudemire, A., ed. *Clinical Psychiatry for Medical Students.* Philadelphia: J.B. Lippincott, 1990: 237–268.

Folks, D.G. & Houck, C.A. Somatoform disorders, factitious disorders and malingering. In Stoudemire, A. & Fogel, B.S., eds. *Psychiatric Care of the Medical Patient.* New York: Oxford University Press, 1993: 267–288.

Goldberg, R.J. & Posner, D. Anxiety in the medically ill. In Stoudemire, A. & Fogel, B.S., eds. *Psychiatric Care of the Medical Patient.* New York: Oxford University Press, 1993: 87–104.

Goldberg, R.J. & Posner, D.A. Anxiety in the medically ill. In Stoudemire, A., Fogel, B.S., & Greenberg, D.B., eds. *Psychiatric Care of the Medical Patient.* New York: Oxford University Press, 2000: 165–180.

Greenblatt, D.J., Shader, R.I., & Abernathy, D.R. Current status of benzodiazepines. *N. Engl. J. Med.* 1983; **309**: 410–416.

Phillips, K.A., Albertini, R.S., & Rasmussen, S.A. A randomized placebo-controlled trial of fluoxetine in body dysmorphic disorder. *Arch. Gen. Psychiatry* 2002: **59**(4), 381–388.

Schuckit, M.A. Anxiety related to medical disease. *J. Clin. Psychiatry* 1983; **44**: 31–37.

Stoudemire, A., Fogel, B.S., Gulley, L.R., & Moran, M.G. Psychopharmacology in the medically ill. In Stoudemire, A. & Fogel, B.S., eds. *Psychiatric Care of the Medical Patient.* New York: Oxford University Press, 1993: 155–206.

Stoudemire, A. Anxiety and somatoform disorders. In Lubin, M.F., Walker, H.K., & Smith, R.B., eds. *Medical Management of the Surgical Patient.* Philadelphia, PA: J.B. Lippincott, 1995: 438–443.

Psychological and emotional reactions to illness and surgery

Edward Norris and Charles Raison[*]

Department of Psychiatry, Lehigh Valley Hospital, Allentown, PA
Department of Psychiatry & Behavioral Sciences, Atlanta, GA

Patients who are faced with major physical illness and surgery are beset by numerous basic stresses that may challenge their psychological equilibrium. Patients not only anticipate and fear the prospect of pain, disability, and perhaps even death but also must struggle with other stresses that may threaten their sense of personal control, autonomy, identity, and independence. Patients who are admitted to hospitals suddenly enter highly regimented bureaucratic and technologically oriented systems over which they have little control and which they do not fully understand. Their personal and physical privacy is suddenly invaded by questions, examinations, and procedures. Patients must temporarily relinquish a great deal of control over their lives to the hospital routine, which they find bewildering, confusing, anxiety-provoking, and at times even humiliating.

In addition, patients are separated from their loved ones and family and may be geographically far away from home. Elderly patients in particular may not have family readily available, older patients with cognitive impairment may become confused, disoriented, and agitated. Patients may face considerable financial strain if their insurance coverage is limited or if they will be out of work. Finally, uncertainty about the diagnosis and prognosis of their conditions may exacerbate the anxiety and fear that patients experience.

Patients who are facing extensive surgical procedures that involve ostomy formation, amputation or other types of surgery that result in some form of disfigurement are concerned about their appearance and body image and about the way in which the surgery will affect their sexual functioning and attractiveness. For example, women undergoing mastectomy may fear losing love and sexual desirability. Patients undergoing ostomy placement may react to surgery by fearing that they will appear ugly and repulsive and will be rejected. Patients undergoing urologic procedures may face the prospect of sexual dysfunction or impotence. Grief reactions manifested by depressive symptoms may be encountered as patients "mourn" the loss of body image, body parts, or physical functioning and mobility.

*This is an updated chapter of a previous one of Alan Stoudemire.

The reaction to these stresses varies among patients and depends on several factors, including pre-existing psychological strength, amount of family support available, financial resources, type and extent of illness, surgical procedures involved, and overall prognosis. Despite the stressful nature of illness, hospitalization, and surgery, most patients may be expected to do well. Physicians should be alert, however, for signs and symptoms suggesting that a patient's ability to adapt to the stress of illness is being overwhelmed, indicating some degree of psychological decompensation.

Behavioral regression

A helpful concept to consider in assessing psychological reactions to illness, especially with they appear to be maladaptive or pathologic, is the concept of behavioral regression. This regression means that patients, in reaction to the stress of illness and enforced dependency on others, may resort to more infantile and childlike ways of thinking, feeling and behaving. In most situations, this regression is limited as patients recover and adapt to their illness. Under certain circumstances, however, patients may undergo more severe and prolonged regression, particularly those with little or no social support, marginal abilities to cope under severe stress, or pre-existing psychiatric disorders. Regressive behavior is characterized by withdrawal, helplessness, clinging, excessive dependency, and fear. Patients may also whine and complain and be angry, irritable, and demanding. Serious forms of regression may lead to profound emotional withdrawal, passivity, depression, and occasionally, overtly psychotic behavior. Even the strongest and most psychologically healthy person may at times be overwhelmed emotionally in the context of severe stress, resulting in regressive forms of behavior.

Understanding the concept of behavioral regression under stress and its behavioral manifestations is helpful in the physician's management of these reactions. Because regression involves the display of frightened and child-like behavior, patients' reactions to physicians may resemble those of children to frustrated parents. Physicians, in the patients' view, may take on the roles of powerful and authoritative parent figures. Although such dependency may make some patients compliant with treatment and thankful for the physician's help, other more difficult reactions may occur. Patients may displace their anger, fear and frustration on the physicians and become resistant, difficult, defiant, ungrateful, and critical; they may even threaten litigation. Reasonable limits should be set for such behavior, and physicians ideally should attempt to help patients understand the feelings that usually underlie such behavior and empathize with those feelings as much as possible rather than respond with anger and defensiveness.

Physicians must give steady and consistent emotional support to patients who are in regressive emotional turmoil by providing information, advice, encouragement, and realistic reassurance. These efforts, termed *ego support*, are directed toward preventing extensive behavioral regression by suppressing anxiety and strengthening patients' psychological defenses and coping mechanisms. Severe regression should be prevented by encouraging patients to pursue rehabilitation efforts, helping them to become as independent as possible, and allowing them to participate as much as is reasonable in decisions regarding their care. The last approach gives patients some sense of control over their treatment.

One of the more common difficulties for physicians is managing patients who exhibit profound emotional reactions to an illness, such as crying or becoming deeply depressed, helpless, and dependant. Physicians who are uncomfortable with these types of intense emotions may actively discourage patients from talking about their feelings, avoid such patients, or offer unrealistic or patronizing reassurance. Such intense emotions, however, are often best handled with carefully titrated brief periods of catharsis by allowing patients to ventilate, "blow off steam," or cry and by empathizing with the patients' feelings. Such periods of emotional catharsis are usually transient and provide relief for patients by reassurance that physicians are interested and open to their feelings. Severe regressive behaviors that are persistent or accompanied by evidence of severe depression, anxiety, or significant psychopathologic reactions (especially those that create conflict or tension in the doctor-patient relationship) are indications for psychiatric referral.[1]

Identification of high-risk groups

Several characteristics place patients at relatively higher risk for the development of psychiatric complications during illness or surgery. Although no particular patient profile is totally predictive, there are criteria for identifying and monitoring high-risk patients.

Groups of psychologically high-risk patients have been delineated by Baudry and Weiner,[2] subsequently developed by Strain,[3] and modified by Stoudemire.[10] High-risk groups include the following:

- patients with histories of psychotic decompensation, delirium, or psychiatric consultation during previous physical illnesses or surgeries

- patients who refuse or are resistant to undergo surgery or who threaten to leave the hospital against medical advice or refuse to sign a consent form
- patients with histories of difficult or hostile relationships with nursing, medical or surgical staff
- patients with unrealistic or magical expectations of their surgery, including excessive denial
- patients who present special diagnostic problems, such as histories of multiple surgeries for questionable or vague indications with negative results (malingering, hysterical, factitious, or hypochondriacal patients)
- patients who show blasé, apathetic reactions or lack of appropriate concern and anxiety
- patients with histories of alcohol and substance abuse or those who are taking multiple psychotropic or analgesic agents
- elderly patients with cognitive impairment who are at risk for postoperative delirium
- patients with histories of medical litigation or questionable disability suits
- patients with histories of chronic pain complaint of obscure cause.

Value of preoperative psychological assessment

Numerous studies have demonstrated the potential value of preoperative preparation of the patient to promote increased tolerance to the stresses of the surgical procedure.[3] Education efforts provide patients with information that helps them anticipate surgery and tend to diminish uncertainty and alleviate anxiety. Patients who receive information and are familiar with the staff and the medical–surgical routine are better able to anticipate and prepare for whatever discomfort the procedure may entail. Such preparation is particularly important for children. In two studies, preoperative preparation by the anesthesiology staff resulted in a reduction in requests for narcotics and earlier discharge from the hospital among the patients involved compared to other patients.[4,5] Other investigations have reported decreased postoperative delirium in groups of patients who receive preoperative preparation by a psychiatrist.[6,7] Several additional studies have claimed improved recovery rates in patients who received instruction designed to facilitate coping with the stress

of surgery.[8,9] Although surgeons may have a limited amount of time to devote to extensive educational efforts, some programs can be administered by ancillary medical or nursing personnel with the aid of audiovisual guides.

Although significant methodological problems exist for most studies that claim effectiveness of psychiatric and behavioral interventions in improving postoperative outcomes, data suggest that appropriate screening and evaluation of high-risk patients and provision of adequate information to decrease anticipatory anxiety and postoperative confusion will yield therapeutic benefits and perhaps decrease the likelihood of major psychiatric complications.

REFERENCES

1. Green, S. A. Principles of medical psychotherapy. In Stoudemire, A. & Fogel, B. S., eds. *Psychiatric Care of the Medical Patient*. New York: Oxford University Press, 1993: 3–18.
2. Baudry, F. & Weiner, A. The surgical patient. In Strain, J. & Grossman, S., eds. *Psychological Care of the Medically Ill: A Primer in Liaison Psychiatry*. New York: Appleton-Century-Crofts, 1975: 123–137.
3. Strain, J. The surgical patient. In Cavenar, J., ed. *Psychiatry*. Philadelphia: J. B. Lippincott, 1986: 1–11.
4. Egbert, L. D., Battit, G. E., Welch, C. D., & Bartlett, M. K. Reduction of postoperative pain by encouragement and instruction of patient. *N. Engl. J. Med.* 1964; **270**: 825–827.
5. Egbert, L. D., Bartlet, G. E., Taldorf, H., & Beecher, H. K. The value of preoperative visits by the anesthetist. *J. Am. Med. Assoc.* 1963; **185**: 553–555.
6. Layne, O. L. Jr. & Yudofsky, S. C. Postoperative psychosis in cardiotomy patients: the role of organic and psychiatric factors. *N. Engl. J. Med.* 1971; **284**: 518–520.
7. Lazarus, H. R. & Hagens, T. H. Prevention of psychosis following open-heart surgery. *Am. J. Psychiatry* 1968; **124**: 1190–1195.
8. Andrew, J. M. Recovery from surgery, with and without preparatory instruction, for three coping styles. *J. Pers. Soc. Psychol.* 1970; **15**: 223–226.
9. Reading, A. E. The short-term effects of psychological preparation for surgery. *Soc. Sci. Med.* 1979; **13A**: 641–654.
10. Stoudemire, A. Psychologic and emotional reactions to illness and surgery. In Lubin, M. F., Walker, H. K., & Smith, R. B., eds. *Medical Management of the Surgical Patient*. Philadelphia, PA: J. B. Lippincott Company, 1995: 427–429.

40

Substance abuse

Ted Parran, Jr.

Case Western Reserve University School of Medicine, Cleveland, OH

Problems of drug and alcohol abuse are ubiquitous in hospitalized patient populations. A prevalence study at Johns Hopkins Hospital in 1986 demonstrated active alcoholism in 23% of surgical patients, with subgroup rates ranging from 14% in patients on the urology service, 28% in those on the orthopedic service, to 43% in those on the otorhinolaryngology service.[1] Although this study did not evaluate the prevalence of drug abuse, consideration of the abuse of drugs other than alcohol could only increase the overall rate of affected patients on surgical services. Detection rates by physician staff of patients with substance abuse problems are low in general and lowest on surgery and obstetrics-gynecology services. Data indicate that under 25% of affected patients are identified on these specialty services. In addition, less than half the substance-abusing patients who are identified receive any form of intervention, counseling, or even a medical treatment plan that addresses the substance abuse issues. Therefore, only about 10% of surgical patients with substance abuse problems have their abuse addressed in any way by their physicians.

In a few special populations of surgical patients, problems of substance abuse are of even greater magnitude. Trauma service data indicate that between 30% and 75% of all injured patients have positive results on toxicology testing for legal levels of alcohol intoxication or for drugs of abuse at the time of hospital admission.[2–5,37] Our experience after a year of testing each consecutive level 1 trauma admission indicates an alcohol intoxication rate of 63%, an illicit drug use rate of 48%, and a combined rate of 78%. Follow-up interviews with these patients reveal that most have serious drug and alcohol abuse or dependence, with only 8% being substance users who happened to suffer a major trauma.

A significant literature is emerging that examines the potential for increased morbidity, mortality, and hospitalization costs associated with drug and alcohol abuse in surgical patients. Although there are some conflicting reports and a vast diversity of research design, a consensus appears to be emerging that these patients do carry an increased burden of morbidity, mortality, and cost associated with their treatment. Some of them have been shown to have increased intraoperative and postoperative complication rates (i.e., neurosurgical patients with alcoholism and subdural hematoma, patients with alcoholism who undergo transurethral prostatectomy, patients with alcoholism and drug dependency who undergo plastic surgery and burn treatment, and patients with alcoholism who undergo bowel resection or hysterectomy).[6–10] They have also been shown to have increased postoperative morbidity and, in many studies, increased mortality. Finally, theoretic and actual anesthesia risks in surgical patients who abuse drugs and alcohol have recently been reviewed.[11]

Clinically important issues involved in the treatment of substance abuse in surgical patients are considered further in the following order: screening and diagnosis strategies, medical therapy considerations by drug class, brief intervention and treatment planning, and postoperative pain management issues.

Screening approaches

The need for better and more widespread screening for substance abuse problems in hospitalized patients is obvious.[12–24] Because the prevalence of these patients is between 20% and 40% on surgical services, and because the diagnosis is overlooked in 50% to 80% of cases, the need for active screening of all patients is indisputable. A good screening test should be clinically powerful (with high sensitivity and an acceptable level of specificity), simple to use, and easy to master and remember, and should have a high degree of patient and physician acceptability. Several good approaches have been developed and tested over the past 20 years, and three are perhaps most

Medical Management of the Surgical Patient: A Textbook of Perioperative Medicine, ed. M. F. Lubin, R. B. Smith, T. F. Dobson, N. Spell, H. K. Walker. 4th edn. Published by Cambridge University Press. © Cambridge University 2006.

Table 40.1. CAGE Questionnaire[a]

Have you ever felt the need to <u>C</u>ut down on your drinking?

Have people <u>A</u>nnoyed you by criticizing your drinking[a]?

Have you ever felt bad or <u>G</u>uilty about your drinking[a]?

Have you ever had a drink first thing in the morning to steady your nerves or to get rid of a hangover (<u>E</u>ye opener)?

The family CAGE (f-CAGE) involves asking if "anyone in your family" has felt the need to …

Note:

[a] Many clinicians substitute "drinking or drug use" when using the CAGE questionnaire.

Table 40.2. Trauma Scale Questionnaire

Since your 18th birthday,

Have you had any fractures or dislocations of your bones or joints?

Have you been injured in a road traffic accident?

Have you injured your head?

Have you been injured in a non-sports-related assault or fight?

Have you been injured after drinking?

appropriate to surgical settings: the CAGE questionnaire, the Trauma Survey, and toxicology testing.[12,15,16]

The CAGE questions were first published in the early 1970s and have been widely studied in various patient populations (Table 40.1). The questions are easy to remember and simple to ask, tend not to engender defensiveness and discomfort in patients or physicians, and are far more sensitive and specific in identifying clinically important substance abuse problems than are typical questions regarding amount and frequency of use. The CAGE questionnaire also can be used to ask family members about patients, especially when patients are unable to be meaningfully interviewed. In hospitalized patients, each positive response to a CAGE question indicates a 30% to 40% likelihood of a substance abuse problem. Therefore, two positive responses to four questions indicates an 80% sensitivity and specificity for substance abuse.

It is thought that young men tend to produce false-negative results when they are tested with the CAGE questionnaire. Skinner and colleagues[16] observed that young men with substance abuse problems often suffer repetitive traumatic injury. They developed the Trauma Survey (Table 40.2) for use in this population, and positive responses to two of its five categories indicate the likelihood of a substance abuse problem. The Trauma Survey is more clinically useful than are the results of laboratory tests (i.e., liver tests or the mean corpuscular volume) or standard questions regarding the amount and frequency of use, especially in populations of young men.

"For cause" rather than random or universal toxicology testing is one accepted strategy to screen for and assess addictive disease in hospitalized patients. For cause is a term that relates to toxicology testing which is prompted by clinical data indicating a significant chance of the presence of a substance abuse disorder. This clinical data can either be epidemiological data indicating a high prevalence rate in certain patient populations, or other screening information indicating a potential diagnosis. Most risk

management experts consider this "for cause" toxicology testing to be justified even without special informed written consent by patients. The prevalence of positive results on toxicology testing at the time of hospital admission is startlingly high in some surgical patient populations, especially trauma patients. A consensus has emerged among trauma services that the use of routine admission toxicology testing is a reasonable trauma protocol standard. Toxicology testing is the single most clinically useful laboratory test after positive results have been obtained with a CAGE questionnaire or Trauma Survey.

Substance abuse screening tools are available and are practical, clinically powerful, and easy to use. Their use should be extended into patient care in general and into surgical populations in particular. Once the use of effective screening is more widespread, detoxification management, referral for counseling and treatment, and management of special considerations such as postoperative pain become critical for the surgical team and its medical consultants.

Medical considerations by drug class

The medical considerations involved in caring for surgical patients with substance abuse problems are vast. The primary areas addressed here are basic pharmacology, management of intoxication and toxicity, management of withdrawal, and other considerations (e.g., nutritional, metabolic).[17] The various drugs are discussed by class: alcohol and sedative–hypnotics, cocaine and stimulants, and opiates.

Alcohol and sedative–hypnotics

Alcohol and sedative–hypnotic agents (e.g., benzodiazepines, barbiturates) are involved in most of the substance abuse that is encountered in surgical patients.[18] Intoxication with these agents is associated with dose-related and tolerance-related disinhibition, loss of judgment, delay in psychomotor coordination, decrease in cognitive ability, and impairment of short-term memory

Table 40.3. Alcohol and sedative–hypnotic withdrawal[a]

Class	Signs and symptoms	Time onset	Course[b] duration
Class 1	Increased heart rate, blood pressure, and reflexes Diarrhea, nausea, and vomiting Tremor, anxiety, and insomnia	12–24 h	72–96 h
Class 2	Visual > auditory hallucinations	12–24 h	72–96 h
Class 3	Grand mal seizures	12–96 h	6–24 h
Class 4	Class I signs with disorientation, hallucinations, anxiety, insomnia	3–6 d	72–96 h

Notes:

[a]Applies to alcohol and short-acting sedative–hypnotics. See text for time course differences with long-acting sedative–hypnotics.

[b]Onset relates to initiation of syndrome after last use of the involved drug.

formation. At high levels of intoxication, consciousness, the gag reflex, respiratory drive, and cardiovascular function are all depressed.[17] Signs of acute toxicity are altered mental status, lethargy and stupor, dilated pupils, slowed respiration, and decreased reflexes. The mixing of different types of sedative–hypnotics can markedly potentiate their toxicity, resulting in a dramatically narrowed toxic/therapeutic ratio and even death. This should be considered in the management of agitated behavior, the treatment of withdrawal, or the consideration of anesthesia or analgesia. The necessity of obtaining accurate blood alcohol content and urine toxicology screening for drugs of abuse, for use in perioperative management decisions cannot be overemphasized. The treatment of toxicity involves cardiovascular and respiratory monitoring and support, the cessation of gastrointestinal absorption, and attempts to increase drug excretion. Some investigators have used high doses of naloxone (Narcan) in these patients, with mixed results.

The alcohol and sedative–hypnotic withdrawal syndromes are similar and can be considered in terms of four categories of symptoms and signs (Table 40.3). Category 1 withdrawal involves increases in heart rate, blood pressure, and reflexes accompanied by tremors, diaphoresis, headache, nausea or diarrhea, insomnia, and anxiety. Category 2 withdrawal is benign alcohol hallucinosis, a clinical picture of visual, tactile, or auditory hallucinations coupled with a clear sensorium. Category 3 withdrawal is the so-called rum fits or withdrawal seizures. These grand mal seizures can be single or multiple discrete seizures, can progress to status epilepticus in the case of barbiturate and perhaps short-acting benzodiazepine (aprazolam) withdrawal, and tend to be of short duration with accordingly short post-ictal periods. Category 4 withdrawal is a delayed-type withdrawal that is also known as delirium tremens, or DTs. This

is characterized by the hyper-autonomic signs and symptoms of category 1 withdrawal symptoms, coupled with a state of delirium consisting of global confusion, hallucinations, and agitation.

The first three categories of withdrawal tend to begin within 12 to 24 hours of the last drink or sedative hypnotic drug ingestion, rapidly escalate to peak symptoms in another 12 to 24 hours, and ease over an additional 48 to 72 hours. Delayed withdrawal or DTs begin 3 to 5 days after the last use and then follow a similar time frame. The only significant exceptions to this involve the long-acting benzodiazepine medications such as diazepam, chlordiazepoxide, clorazepate (Tranxene), and clonazepam (Klonopin). Because of their extended half-lives or active metabolites, the onset of withdrawal from these agents can be delayed for 3 to 6 days after cessation of use, and symptoms often persist for an additional 10 to 21days.

The likelihood that patients will experience one or more categories of withdrawal symptoms is dependent on their previous withdrawal experience. Patients who have not had previous withdrawal symptoms upon abrupt discontinuation of alcohol or sedative hypnotic drug use, are unlikely to go through withdrawal during their hospitalization for surgery. Patients who have had category 3 withdrawal seizures in the past have as much as a 30% risk for recurrent seizures during each subsequent withdrawal episode. The easiest way to predict which patients are at risk for significant withdrawal (and hence which patients require moderate to vigorous withdrawal prophylaxis while they are hospitalized on a surgical service) is to closely interview patients and their families and to review the medical records for data regarding the presence or absence of previous withdrawal symptoms.

The treatment of alcohol withdrawal varies among hospital services. One approach that we recommend for

Table 40.4. Strategies for alcohol withdrawal management

Withdrawal symptoms	Pulmonary or hepatic function	
Symptoms	*Impaired*	*Not impaired*
Mild class I symptoms	Low-dose short-acting benzodiazepine: protocol A	Low-dose, long-acting benzodiazepine: protocol C
Severe Class I, class II, III, or IV symptoms	Intensive short-acting benzodiazepine: protocol B	Intensive long-acting benzodiazepine: protocol D

Table 40.5. Alcohol withdrawal protocols

Protocol A: Lorazepam 0.5 mg p.o., i.m., or i.v. each 4–8 hours per specific signs or symptoms of withdrawal. Discontinue after 72–96 hours.

Protocol B: Lorazepam 0.5 to 2 mg p.o./i.m. or i.v. each 1–4 hours until specific signs or symptoms of withdrawal are suppressed or patient is sleepy. Restart protocol if withdrawal reemerges.

Protocol C: Diazepam 5 mg p.o. or i.v. each 4–8 hours per specific signs or symptoms of withdrawal. Discontinue after 72–96 hours.

Protocol D: Diazepam 10 mg p.o. or i.v. each 1 hour until specific sign of withdrawal is suppressed or patient is sleepy. Restart protocol if withdrawal reemerges.

Protocol E: Sedative–hypnotic withdrawal protocol. Phenobarbital 90 mg p.o. or i.m. each 2–4 hours until therapeutic (antiseizure) blood level is achieved. Then titrate daily phenobarbital dose to maintain a therapeutic blood level.

surgical patients is to first evaluate pulmonary function, liver function, and previous withdrawal symptomatology. If patients have reasonable liver function (i.e., the prothrombin time is less than 1.3 times control) and pulmonary function (i.e., the FEV is greater than 1.5 l), we suggest the use of long-acting benzodiazepines to treat withdrawal symptoms (Table 40.4). If either hepatic or pulmonary function is impaired beyond the above parameters, the use of short-acting benzodiazepines is urged. It also is useful to assess the intensity of withdrawal signs and symptoms. In patients with mild category 1 or 2 symptoms, the low-dose intermittent use of "as needed" or prn benzodiazepines is reasonable. If the symptoms are intense or severe in any category a higher-dose intensive benzodiazepine regimen is strongly suggested (Table 40.5). There is no role for the use of alcohol in the management of surgical patients experiencing alcohol withdrawal.

Periodically, patients are seen who have been chronically prescribed large doses of benzodiazepines or barbiturates as outpatients. In this case, therapy with these medications either should be maintained without change during the surgical hospitalization, or discontinued and replaced with phenobarbital. The mixing of acute doses of benzodiazepines and phenobarbital is strongly discouraged because of the risk of iatrogenic overdose and respiratory depression. One phenobarbital dosing schedule is outlined in Table 40.5, and can be applied to the treatment of alcohol or sedative–hypnotic withdrawal.

Several electrolyte and nutritional issues must be considered when patients with alcoholism are treated on the surgical service. Thiamine deficiency is seen in this population and can have catastrophic and permanent neurologic consequences. Thiamine should be given intramuscularly or by mouth at a dosage of 100 mg immediately, and then per day for 3 days. In addition, patients with alcoholism frequently have vitamin C, vitamin B complex, and folic acid deficiencies. These should be supplemented by the oral, intravenous, or intramuscular route. Multiple electrolyte abnormalities occur in this population and careful evaluation and management of the serum sodium, potassium, phosphorus, glucose, and magnesium levels is essential. Abnormalities in each of these electrolytes as well as elevated serum ammonia levels can lead to altered mental status, seizures, or cardiac arrhythmias.

A review of all the medical complications of alcohol abuse and dependence is beyond the scope of this chapter but a few problems deserve special mention. Hematologic problems include alcohol-associated anemias, thrombocytopenia, and clotting factor abnormalities. Alcohol-associated liver disease can complicate the selection and dosage of anesthetics. Infectious diseases including especially TB, but also viral hepatitis B and C, and HIV can be encountered more commonly in alcoholic patients than the general population. Finally, it is important to screen for congestive heart failure symptoms related to alcoholic cardiomyopathy before surgery is undertaken.[19]

Table 40.6. Stimulant withdrawal

	Symptoms and signs	Duration
Binge	Repetitive compulsive self administration of cocaine; dilated pupils; increased pulse, increased blood pressure, decreased sleep, decreased eating; restlessness, grandiosity, pressured thoughts	Hours to several days
Agitated phase	Intense dysphoria, excitement, agitation, paranoia, rare cardiovascular instability	Up to several hours
Phase I ("crash")	Restlessness, anxiety, mood lability	12 to 72 hours
Phase II ("cravings")	Mood swings, concentration difficulties, strong urges regarding cocaine	Weeks to months

Cocaine and other stimulants

Cocaine is the most commonly abused stimulant, although the various schedule II, III, and IV amphetamines are still abused by some patient populations and methamphetamine (known as crystal, crystal-meth, or ice) has begun to be heavily abused in some regions of the country. Common properties of stimulants involve inhibition of the reuptake of norepinephrine systemically and dopamine centrally.[17] This produces systemic effects of markedly elevated heart rate, blood pressure, reflexes, and level of smooth muscle spasticity.[20] Cardiac arrhythmias; brain, heart, intestinal, uterine, and muscular ischemia; and seizures are common during stimulant binges and are thought to be caused by norepinephrine surges. Of special medical significance in patients who abuse cocaine is the markedly increased risk for trauma, sexually transmitted diseases, tuberculosis (including resistant strains), and the human immunodeficiency virus as a result of intravenous drug use or multiple sexual encounters.[21]

Centrally, the excess levels of dopamine and norepinephrine associated with cocaine and other stimulant use produce intense feelings of euphoria, stamina, power, and control associated with sleeplessness, loss of appetite, and physical restlessness.[20] These effects rapidly abate and are replaced by dysphoric and depressive feelings. The evanescent nature of the "high" associated with stimulant use results in frequent repeated administration of the drugs, and the typical binge/crash pattern of stimulant addiction. Urine toxicology testing for cocaine and metabolites remains positive in proportion to the duration and intensity of use. Toxicology often reveals casual use for 18 to 24 hours, whereas serial screenings (i.e., every 12 hours) after a several day binge can remain positive for as long as 4 days. Toxicology testing for amphetamine use often produces false-positive results in patients who are taking non-prescription cold preparations. These results should be confirmed with gas chromatography.

Toward the end of a binge, which can last from 12 to 72 hours, patients typically report more and more intense feelings of agitation, depression, and even paranoia that may last for several hours. It is during this unstable, agitated phase that much of the violence associated with stimulant abuse occurs. It is these agitated hypervigilant and paranoid patients who are often seen in emergency rooms with trauma, and who need urgent sedation to avoid violent episodes. Following this "postbinge" agitated period or "cocaine psychosis", patients then crash and begin a period of several hours to a few days of hypersomnia and hyperphagia (Table 40.6). This has been called phase 1 withdrawal. Phase 2 withdrawal is characterized by restlessness, edginess, mood swings, sleep disturbance, and stimulant cravings. These phase 2 withdrawal symptoms can affect patients intermittently for several weeks to months.

The symptoms of category 2 withdrawal are thought to be mediated on the basis of dopamine depletion. Therefore, the primary interventions include the administration of dopaminergic agents such as amantadine or bromocriptine, or antidepressant drugs such as desipramine. Although each of these medications has been studied for efficacy in cocaine withdrawal and shown to produce statistically significant decreases in symptoms, none has been demonstrated to clinically decrease relapse rates. Recent reports indicate that propanolol, 20 mg by mouth twice a day for several weeks may decrease relapse rates to a clinically significant degree. Cocaine associated symptoms that must be urgently medicated are those seen during the period of agitated paranoia at the end of a binge. At this point, patients tend to respond to intramuscular sedatives, ranging from 100 mg of hydroxyzine for relatively mild cases to 2 mg of lorazepam or 2 ml of droperidol for more agitated patients as a one-time dose.

Table 40.7. Strategies for opiate withdrawal management

Receptors	Actions	Agonists	Antagonists
mu	Supraspinal analgesia, euphoria, sedation, respiratory depression, physical withdrawal with drug cravings, myosis, constipation	Morphine Meperidol Methadone Oxycodone Codeine Propoxyphene Hydromorphone Buprenorphine[a] Heroin	Naloxone Naltrexone Pentazocine Nalbuphine
kappa	Spinal analgesia, myosis, sedation, physical withdrawal without drug cravings	Pentazocine Nalbuphine Butorphanol	Naloxone Naltrexone

Note:
[a] Partial agonist for indicated receptor.

Finally, the implications of a stimulant binge should be considered in planning anesthesia. Patients with recent stimulant binging and major trauma often have not had much to eat or drink for several hours to days. Their urinalyses commonly show maximally concentrated specimens with ketones, traces of protein, and much sediment. Serum creatinine and blood urea nitrogen determinations frequently do not reflect the true degree of volume depletion secondary to starvation effects. Therefore, accurate assessment of volume status with orthostatic checks or even a central line prior to induction of anesthesia is important. Another concern in undertaking surgery in these patients is the possible existence of a catecholamine-depleted state following a prolonged cocaine or amphetamine binge. Although no empiric evidence exists on this subject, catecholamine-stimulating pressors may not be as effective in these patients. Ruling out severe volume depletion, binge-associated cardiac ischemia, arrhythmia, pneumothorax, and rhabdomyolysis is important before surgery.[21] Other than taking these precautions into account, there is no indication to routinely cancel surgery in cocaine using patients purely on the basis of a positive toxicology screen.

Opiates

All opiates are abused by some patients, including propoxyphene, codeine, hydrocodone, oxycodone, meperidine, methadone, hydromorphone, morphine, heroin, opium, pentazocine, butorphanol, nalbuphine, and buprenorphine (Table 40.7). All opiates (except for methadone and perhaps buprenorphine) are rapidly metabolized and cleared, so their presence is rarely identified by urine toxicology testing performed more than 24 hours after the last use. Based on their observed actions, opiates are classified into two categories: mu-agonists and kappa-agonists.[22] The mu-agonists produce supraspinal anesthesia; euphoria; myosis; sedation; dose-related respiration, pulse, and blood pressure depression; tolerance; physiologic dependence; and a withdrawal syndrome associated with drug cravings. The kappa-agonists produce spinal anesthesia and physiologic tolerance. These drugs cause significantly less euphoria, myosis, and sedation. Respiratory depression, bradycardia, and hypotension are also less frequent with kappa-agonists. Withdrawal syndromes from mu-agonists are associated with much more drug craving. The kappa-agonists also act as mu-receptor antagonists, precipitating withdrawal in mu-agonist-dependent patients. At higher therapeutic doses, kappa-agonists tend to demonstrate more dysphoric symptoms, which limits their usefulness in the treatment of severe pain.

Opiate intoxication produces a clinical picture of transient nausea; dry mouth; constipation; sleepiness; euphoria; a feeling of tranquility; constricted pupils; warm, dry skin; and depressed respirations, heart rate, and blood pressure. Opiate toxicity presents as depressed mentation ranging from obtundation or coma to myotic pinpoint pupils, bradycardia, hypotension, apnea, and death.[17] This toxic state can be easily reversed by the administration of naloxone (Narcan). The intravenous administration of 0.4 mg usually produces a response in vital signs and pupillary dilation, although patients with greater degrees of intoxication sometimes require multiple doses. The duration of intoxication with most opiates is 1 to 3 hours, and the duration of naloxone's antagonistic effect is 20 to 40 minutes, so close patient observation and repeated dosing is important. Methadone has a much longer duration of intoxication and toxicity, and patients who have overdosed on this drug must be monitored for at least 12 to 24 hours. Naltrexone (Trexan) is an oral form of naloxone that has a half-life of 18 to 24 hours. It occasionally is useful in patients with toxicity, especially if methadone is involved. Because naloxone and naltrexone are mu-receptor and kappa-receptor antagonists, their administration in the proper dosage not only reverses opiate toxicity but can also precipitate opiate withdrawal in patients who are physically dependent. This withdrawal syndrome lasts for only 20 or 30 minutes in the case of naloxone but can last for as long as 24 hours after the administration of naltrexone.

By stage, the signs and symptoms of opiate withdrawal are as follows:

1. lacrimation, rhinorrhea, diaphoresis, yawning, restlessness, insomnia

2. mydriasis, piloerection, muscular fasciculation, myalgia, arthralgia, abdominal pain

3. tachycardia, hypertension, tachypnea, fever, anorexia, nausea, extreme restlessness

4. diarrhea, emesis, dehydration, hyperactive bowel sounds, orthostatic-hypotension, fetal position.

These withdrawal symptoms vary in intensity depending on the type of opiate used, the dose taken, and the duration of use. The symptoms of craving, restlessness, and insomnia tend to be especially long-lasting.[23] Non-methadone opiate withdrawal generally begins 6 to 12 hours after the last use, progresses to a peak within 36 hours of initiation, and resolves over an additional 48 hours. Thus most non-methadone opiate withdrawal symptoms resolve within 4–5 days of the last drug use. Methadone withdrawal begins about 48 hours after the last use, gradually builds for a week or so, and then abates over another 7 to 14 days.

The treatment of opiate withdrawal can involve the use of clonidine, methadone, buprenorphine or tramadol.[23–25,33,34] The following clonidine protocol has been used extensively in patients with mild to moderate opioid physical dependence who are hospitalized in detoxification units.

- Administer clonidine, 0.1 mg orally every 4 hours for 36 hours.
- Administer clonidine, 0.1 mg orally every 6 hours for 24 hours.
- Administer clonidine, 0.1 mg orally every 8 hours for 24 hours.
- Administer clonidine, 0.1 mg orally every 12 hours for 24 hours.
- Discontinue clonidine therapy.

Do not administer clonidine if patients are asleep or if the systolic blood pressure is less than 90 mmHg. Adjunct medications are often helpful, including ibuprofen and acetaminophen for myalgia, dicyclomine for abdominal symptoms, hydroxyzine for anxiety, and amitriptyline with diphenhydramine for sleep. Patients with hemodynamic instability, advanced age, or acute or chronic pain syndromes often do not tolerate this clonidine regimen.

It is in these patients that methadone has historically been used.[23] Difficulties with methadone therapy include the need to first stabilize patients on it and then taper them off relatively slowly, legal issues surrounding the outpatient prescription of methadone for the management of addiction, and the challenge of referral to methadone maintenance programs – with historically very long waiting lists – for patients who have begun such treatment in the hospital. Methadone has 30% more bioavailability when it is given intramuscularly than when it is given orally. Therefore, patients who cannot take oral methadone should be given two-thirds of their usual daily oral dose in two divided intramuscular injections every 12 hours. Methadone is administered as follows.

- Administer 5 to 10 mg of methadone orally every 12 hours.
- Monitor for ablation of withdrawal symptoms. Increase the dose by 5 to 10 mg until symptoms are suppressed (stabilization dose).
- Taper the methadone over 5 to 20 days by decreasing the dose by 5% to 20% per day.
- Treat re-emergent withdrawal symptoms with oral or transdermal clonidine.

The advent of short-term, inpatient buprenorphine tapering protocols has markedly decreased the number of patients in whom methadone therapy must be initiated during their hospitalization.[25,26]

1. Administer buprenorphine, 0.2 to 0.5 mg subcutaneously every 4 hours for 48 hours.
2. Administer buprenorphine, half the above dose every 4 hours for 48 hours.
3. Administer buprenorphine, one half the second dose every 4 hours for 48 hours.
4. Discontinue buprenorphine administration.

It appears that the withdrawal syndrome from buprenorphine, especially when it is given in this short-term, low-dose tapering method, is mild and often clinically trivial. Therapy is begun at a dosage designed to relieve withdrawal symptoms (and pain if appropriate) without making patients sleepy or sedated. Because 0.3 mg of buprenorphine is equivalent to 10 mg of morphine, we usually start with doses between 0.2 and 0.4 mg. Once this initial therapeutic dose is identified, it is relatively easy to taper drug treatment gradually over 5 or 6 days, often mirroring the decrease in acute pain experienced by the postoperative surgical patient. The administration of buprenorphine, a schedule V opioid, for the sole purpose of opioid detoxification for longer than 72 hours is problematic given the 1970 Federal Controlled Substances Act. Fortunately, in the postoperative surgical patient there are nearly always acute pain diagnoses present, making this short-term prescribing for pain relief and withdrawal management consistent with both the spirit and letter of the law.

Tramadol has recently begun to be used in a few centers for the management of acute opioid withdrawal.[33,34] The protocol reported in the literature involves the administration of tramadol 100 mg p.o. every 4 hours for 24 hours, then 100 mg every 6 hours for 24 hours, then 100 mg every 8 hours for 24 hours, then 50 mg every 6 hours for 24 hours, and finally 50 mg every 8 hours for 24 hours. This regimen is supplemented with the above-mentioned adjunctive medications, and even with occasional "rescue" doses of buprenorphine for severe breakthrough of withdrawal symptoms. With surgical patients it is perhaps optimal to initially treat with buprenorphine, providing acute pain relief and opioid withdrawal management. This buprenorphine can be continued until any similar postoperative surgical patient would be switched to oral analgesics. At this point the switch from buprenorphine to tramadol can occur and the tramadol taper can be carried out in the outpatient setting.[33,34]

Common medical complications in patients who are dependent on opiates are related to the degree of opiate tolerance and the delivery system used. The degree of tolerance that patients have for opiate effects can markedly affect decisions relating to anesthesia and analgesia management (see later discussion). A significant proportion of the estimated 1.1 million opiate-dependent persons in our country use, at least intermittently, the intravenous route. Careful observation for track marks, abscesses, and cellulitis is critical. Viral hepatitis is a ubiquitous problem, with seropositivity for hepatitis B and especially for hepatitis C being the rule rather than the exception. Current "best practices" suggest withholding interferon therapy for hepatitis C-positive patients with drug addiction, until the patient has documentation of 6 months of sobriety. Human immunodeficiency virus seropositivity also is high, ranging from 6% to 60% depending on the metropolitan area being studied. Other infectious problems include endocarditis, osteomyelitis, bacterial pneumonia, and tuberculosis. In some urban areas, patients who abuse intravenous drugs have a 35% positive rate on PPD testing. All intravenous drug users who are hospitalized require hepatitis testing, human immunodeficiency virus testing (with consent), and PPD testing with an anergy panel. Finally, many opiate-dependent patients have ignored or self-treated many symptoms before coming to the hospital. As they come out from under their self-induced opiate anesthetic, serious and at times far-advanced illnesses often emerge. It is important to perform a thorough baseline evaluation and to investigate all emerging symptom complexes.

Presenting the diagnosis and forming a treatment plan
After detoxification has been accomplished, physicians are often reluctant to address important issues in patients with substance abuse problems.[27] There are many reasons for this, including discomfort with this disease in general, lack of training in dealing with these types of patients, lack of institutional and departmental support, and a prevailing sense of therapeutic futility. This feeling of hopelessness and of being overwhelmed by the magnitude of

skills needed to treat chemically dependent patients is not supported by recent research. Data from brief intervention studies indicate that traditional skills used in presenting other difficult diagnoses to patients (i.e., cancer, acquired immunodeficiency syndrome) are also effective when presenting the diagnosis of substance abuse.[28]

Simple and effective strategies for presenting the diagnosis of alcohol or drug dependence are being taught in most medical schools and many residency programs. Two such strategies are the Eight Basic Actions outlined by Barker and Whitfield,[29] and the SOAPE mnemonic by Clark.[30] The primary points of these and other strategies include the need to be clear, concise, and specific about the diagnosis; to appear comfortable during the discussion; to avoid blaming patients; to show support for their present or future willingness to work toward sobriety; to be optimistic about eventual success; and to urge a treatment plan based on abstinence with close follow-up and reinforcement.[31]

Several specific pitfalls should be avoided when presenting the diagnosis and forming a treatment plan. The discussion should be kept extremely brief if patients are intoxicated and followed up at a later date. Patients often try to direct the discussion into various reasons or explanations for their problems. Efforts should be made to keep the discussion focused on the diagnosis itself and to avoid speculations about the cause or origin of substance abuse. Because arguments tend to be fruitless, an attempt should be made to defuse them with empathy, respect, and a thorough explanation of the disease as a chronic, progressive illness. Outpatient prescribing of controlled anxiolytics is strongly discouraged in all substance abusing populations and outpatient prescribing of opiate analgesics should be for a specific, self-limited period. Finally, physicians should strive to be clear, comfortable and caring.[31]

In many cases, this simple approach is unsuccessful. Consultation is often needed for these more complicated situations. Given the prevalence of substance abuse problems in surgical patients, it is reasonable for departments of surgery to insist that chemical dependency consultation services be provided by their hospital systems. With the prevalence exceeding 50% on some trauma services, substance abuse consultation is essential for adequate patient care at any level I or level II trauma center in North America.[5]

Pain management strategies

The management of acute and chronic pain is a difficult and complicated area of patient care that cannot be summarized in this chapter. Physicians have varying philosophies and beliefs about pain management, the prescription of opiate analgesics, and the use of pain management consultants. In contrast, the commonalities of addictions are strong, and patients who develop difficulties with the use of one mood-altering drug commonly develop problems with other mood-altering drugs to which they are exposed. Patients with substance abuse problems who are prescribed controlled drugs on a chronic basis create significant problems for physicians. Issues concerning the prescribing of controlled drugs are the leading cause for state medical boards to investigate and take action against physicians.[35] Despite the current state of disagreement nationally regarding indications for the prescribing of chronic opioids in chronic pain, most experts strongly encourage the prescribing of opioids for the short-term management of moderate to severe acute self-limited pain syndromes, even in patients with addiction histories. Several basic management principles can be outlined to help guide prescribing practices.[36]

Before opiate analgesics are prescribed for all patients, and especially for patients with substance abuse problems, a clear diagnosis must be identified. Then a therapeutic plan with specific treatment goals, methods of monitoring symptoms, and expected time course must be outlined and documented in the chart.[32,35,36] Several important factors should be considered once a decision to prescribe has been reached. First, the provision of reasonable relief for acute, self-limited pain is a justifiable expectation for all patients, regardless of their chemical dependency status. Second, patients who have misused mood-altering chemicals in the past may have higher medication tolerance than other patients, and thus may well require higher doses of medication. Third, patients with substance abuse problems may misuse their prescription analgesics. Fourth, physicians should always avoid the use of poly-pharmacy if at all possible – in other words the concomitant prescribing of multiple different classes of controlled drugs to a patient with an addiction history. Therefore, it is important to prescribe adequate dosages of analgesics, while at the same time limiting the amount of drug dispensed, providing no refills on any controlled prescription, and refusing to prescribe more medication than originally intended unless the diagnosis changes. Frequent brief visits to renew the prescription, monitor the response to treatment, and maintain patient commitment to discontinuing opiate therapy at the predetermined time is an appropriate pattern of management. The more common practice of providing large prescriptions and rare follow-up appointments often results in patient attempts to obtain early refills. When opiate analgesics are prescribed for patients with previous opiate dependence, physicians should attempt to use medications from a different class than the one previously abused. For example, a former heroin (mu-agonist) user who requires opiate-type analgesia should be treated with kappa-agonists if at all possible. This provides adequate pain relief with less risk of rekindling the former addiction.

The appropriate chronic use of opiate analgesics is widely discussed and debated in the treatment of chronic pain, especially if the pain is of unclear origin and even more so if it is chronic cryptogenic pain in patients with histories of substance abuse. Opiate therapy should be initiated in this setting with great reluctance and can be considered to be at least relatively contraindicated. In cases in which long-term opiate therapy has already been initiated in patients with chronic cryptogenic pain and substance abuse, it is reasonable to gradually taper the medication at a rate of 5% to 10% per week. Many practitioners ask their patients to sign a treatment plan or contract in which they agree to be admitted to the hospital for detoxification if this type of medication tapering regimen is not completed successfully. Patients who refuse such interventions present difficult choices; some authorities suggest that they be referred to methadone maintenance programs or to a physician licensed to provide office based buprenorphine maintenance. These management decisions are extremely difficult and influenced by many factors, including the personalities and philosophies of patients and physicians, and the rules and regulations of medical boards and state legislatures. Although treatment approaches are never clear-cut, the considerations outlined can help guide the decision-making process.

REFERENCES

1. Moore, R. D. & Levine, D. M. Prevalence, detection, and treatment of alcoholism in hospitalized patients. *J. Am. Med. Assoc.* 1989; **261**: 403–407.
2. Clark, D. E., McCarthy, E., & Robinson, E. Trauma as a symptom of alcoholism. *Ann. Emerg. Med.* 1985; **14**: 274–277.
3. Antti-Poika, I. Heavy drinking and accidents. *Br. J. Accid. Surg.* 1988; **19**: 198–204.
4. Anda, R. H. Alcohol and fatal injuries among U.S. adults. *J. Am. Med. Assoc.* 1988; **260**: 2529–2532.
5. Soderstrom, C. S. A National Alcohol and Trauma Center survey. *Arch. Surg.* 1987; **122**: 1067–1071.
6. Sonne, N. M. & Tonnesen, H. The influence of alcoholism on outcome after evaluation of subdural hematoma. *Br. J. Neurosurg.* 1992; **6**: 125–130.
7. Tonnesen, H. Influence of alcoholism on morbidity after transurethral prostatectomy. *Scand. J. Urol. Nephrol.* 1988; **22**: 175–177.

8. Brezel, B. S. & Stein, J. M. Burns in substance abusers. *J. Burn Care Rehabil.* 1988; **9**: 169–171.

9. Felding, C. F., Jensen, L. M., & Ronnesen, H. Influence of alcohol intake on postoperative morbidity after hysterectomy. *Am. J. Obstet. Gynecol.* 1992; **166**: 667–670.

10. Tonnesen, H. & Petersen, K. R. Postoperative morbidity among symptom-free alcohol misusers. *Lancet* 1992; **340**: 334–337.

11. Wood, P. R. & Soni, N. Anaesthesia and substance abuse. *Anaesthesia* 1989; **44**: 672–680.

12. Hays, J. T. & Spickard, W. A. Alcoholism: early diagnosis and treatment. *J. Gen. Intern. Med.* 1987; **2**: 420–427.

13. Rydon, P. & Reid, A. Detection of alcohol related problems in general practice. *J. Stud. Alcohol* 1992; **53**: 197–202.

14. Lewis, C. M. Perioperative screening for alcoholism. *Ann. Plast. Surg.* 1992; **28**: 207–209.

15. Ewing, J. A. Detecting alcoholism. *J. Am. Med. Assoc.* 1984; **252**: 1905–1907.

16. Skinner, H. A. Identification of alcohol abuse using a history of trauma. *Ann. Intern. Med.* 1984; **101**: 847–851.

17. Kantzian, E. J. & McKenna, G. J. Acute toxic and withdrawal reactions associated with drug abuse. *Ann. Intern. Med.* 1979; **40**: 361–372.

18. Turner, R. C. & Lichstein, P. R. Alcohol withdrawal syndromes. *J. Gen. Intern. Med.* 1989; **4**: 432–444.

19. Eckardt, M. J., Hartford, T. C., & Kaelber, C. T. Health hazards associated with alcohol consumption. *J. Am. Med. Assoc.* 1981; **246**: 648–666.

20. Gavin, F. H. & Ellinwood, E. H. Cocaine and other stimulants. *N. Engl. J. Med.* 1988; **318**: 1173–1182.

21. Cregler, L. L. & Marck, H. Medical complications of cocaine abuse. *N. Engl. J. Med.* 1988; **315**: 1495–1500.

22. Jaffe, J. H. & Martin, W. R. Opioid analgesics and antagonists. In Gilman, A. G., Goodman, L. S., Rall, T. W., & Murad, F., eds. *Pharmacological Basis of Therapeutics.* New York: MacMillan, 1985: 491–531.

23. Fultz, J. M. & Senay, E. C. Guidelines for the management of hospitalized narcotic addicts. *Ann. Intern. Med.* 1975; **82**: 815–818.

24. Gold, M. S., Pottash, C. A., & Kleber, H. D. Opiate withdrawal using clonidine. *J. Am. Med. Assoc.* 1980; **243**: 343–346.

25. Parran, T. V. & Jasinski, D. R. Buprenorphine detoxification of medically unstable narcotic dependent patients. *Substance Abuse* 1990; **11**: 197–202.

26. Bickel, W. K. & Johnson, R. E. Clinical trial of buprenorphine. *Clin. Pharmacol. Ther.* 1989; **43**: 72–78.

27. Clark, W. D. Alcoholism: blocks to diagnosis and treatment. *Am. J. Med.* 1981; **71**: 275–286.

28. Babor, T. F. & Good, S. P. Screening and early intervention. *Aust. Drug Alcohol Rev.* 1987; **6**: 325–339.

29. Barker, L. R. & Whitfield, C. L. Alcoholism. In Barker, L. I. Z., Burton, J. R., & Zieve, P. D., eds. *Principles of Ambulatory Medicine.* Baltimore: Williams & Wilkins, 2002: 258–259.

30. Clark, W. D. The medical interview: focus on alcohol problems. *Hosp. Pract.* 1985; **20**: 59–68.

31. Parran, T. V. Developing a treatment plan for the chemically dependent primary care patient. In Bigby, J. A., ed. *Substance Abuse Education* in *General Internal Medicine: A Manual for Faculty.* Society of General Internal Medicine and the Ambulatory Pediatric Association, Bureau of Health Professions HRSA, 1993: 1–11.

32. Parran, T. V. & Bigby, J. A. Prescription drug abuse. In Bigby, J. A., ed. *Substance Abuse Education in General Internal Medicine: A Manual for Faculty.* Society of General Internal Medicine and the Ambulatory Pediatric Association, Bureau of Health Professions HRSA, 1993: 1–35.

33. Tamaskar, R., Parran, T., & Grey, S. Tramadol v. buprenorphine in the management of heroin withdrawal. *J. Addic. Dis.* (in press).

34. Sobey, P., Parran T., Adelman, C., Grey, S., & Yu, J. Tramadol v. clonidine in the management of heroin withdrawal. *J. Addic. Dis.* (in press).

35. Parran, T. Prescription drug abuse: a question of balance. *Med. Clin. North Am.*, 1997; **81**(4): 967–978.

36. Longo, L. & Parran, T. Addiction: Part II. Identification and management of the drug seeking patient. *Am. Family Phys.* 2000; **61**(8): 2121–2128.

37. Blondel, R. D. & Looney, S. W. Characteristics of intoxicated trauma patients. *J. Addic. Dis.* 2002, **21**: 1–12.

Peripartum patients

41

Care of the peripartum patient

Clyde Watkins

Emory University School of Medicine, Atlanta, GA

Introduction

The past two decades have brought a greater understanding of pregnancy along with advances in the recognition and management of disorders that are unique to pregnancy or complicate pregnancy. Increasingly, generalist physicians are being asked to assist in the management of medical conditions that develop prior to or as a result of pregnancy. Coverage of the breadth of medical disorders that can complicate pregnancy is the topic of several excellent textbooks. Instead, this chapter focuses on the medical care of several conditions that are unique to pregnancy or influenced by the physiologic changes that occur around late pregnancy, labor, delivery and the immediate postpartum period.

Normal physiologic changes in pregnancy

Knowledge of the normal physiologic changes that occur with pregnancy is important to understand the effect that existing maternal disease has on maternal and fetal health. A few of the more important physiologic changes associated with pregnancy are listed in Table 41.1.

The hemodynamic adaptations are some of the most significant physiologic changes that occur during pregnancy. Soon after implantation systemic vascular resistance (SVT) falls. This adaptation, mediated by gestational hormones, prostaglandins and the creation of a low resistance circulation in the uterus and placenta, reaches its nadir at 20 weeks gestation.[1] During the latter half of pregnancy, the SVR rises, reaching near normal levels at term. Cardiac output rises 30%–50% during pregnancy. An increased stroke volume, a result of expanded blood volume, accounts for the majority of the

increase in CO in the early stages of pregnancy. An increase in the resting heart rate is responsible for maintaining the CO elevation throughout the latter stages of pregnancy. Total blood volume expands 30%–60% during pregnancy. This expansion is a result of an approximately 50% increase in plasma volume and 25% increase in red cell volume.

Further hemodynamic changes occur during labor and delivery. Autotransfusion of up to 500 ml of blood into the maternal circulation occurs with each uterine contraction.[2] Pain, which stimulates the sympathetic nervous system and the vigorous valsalva maneuver with pushing leads to increases in heart rate, blood pressure and myocardial oxygen demand.[2] Finally, intravascular volume is increased as a result of the release of IVC compression by the uterus.

Hypertensive disorders of pregnancy

The hypertensive disorders are the most common medical complication of pregnancy.[1] Though infrequent, these disorders carry an increased risk of perinatal morbidity and mortality for both the mother and fetus.[1] The American College of Obstetrics and Gynecology defines four categories of hypertension during pregnancy (Table 41.2).

Pre-eclamsia

Pre-eclampsia complicates approximately 5% of pregnancies. It is typically a disease of the late pregnancy, rarely occurring before 20 weeks' gestation and more commonly after 36 weeks' gestation. Classically defined as a syndrome characterized by hypertension, proteinuria and edema, pre-eclampsia is a multisystem disorder. It can,

Medical Management of the Surgical Patient: A Textbook of Perioperative Medicine, ed. M. F. Lubin, R. B. Smith, T. F. Dobson, N. Spell, H. K. Walker. 4th edn. Published by Cambridge University Press. © Cambridge University 2006.

Table 41.1. Normal physiologic changes during pregnancy[7]

Parameter	Physiologic change
Systemic vascular resistance	Decreases
Cardiac output	Increases
Blood volume	Increases: approximately 40%
Plasma volume	Increases: approximately 50%
Red cell volume	Increases: approximately 25%
Tidal volume	Increases
FEV1	No change
FVC	No change
Peak expiratory flow	No change
TSH	Decreases early in pregnancy, later returns to baseline.
Free T4	No change
Creatinine clearance	Increases
Glomerular filtration rate (GFR)	Increases
Glucose	Variable
Platelets	Decreases
Hematocrit	Decreases
Coagulation factors II, VII, IX, X	Increases
Fibrinogen	Increases
Protein S	Decreases
Fibrinolytic system	Inhibited

Table 41.2. Classification of the hypertensive disorders of pregnancy[3]

1. Chronic hypertension
2. Pre-eclampsia–eclampsia
3. Pre-eclampsia superimposed upon chronic hypertension
4. Gestational hypertension
   - transient hypertension
   - chronic hypertension

however, present in its most severe form with, or without, mild degrees of hypertension or edema.

Those at risk of developing pre-eclampsia include women with their first pregnancies, twin gestation, of African-American descent, a personal or family history of pre-eclampsia, diabetes, chronic hypertension, renal disease, and obesity.

The exact cause of pre-eclampsia is unclear. Though clinically manifest predominantly in the latter half of pregnancy, evidence shows the pre-eclamptic process begins early in pregnancy. The primary defect in pre-eclampsia is thought to be a failure in the trophoblastic invasion of the uterine spiral arteries leading to placental hypoperfusion, decreased production of PGI2, and widespread vasospasm.[4] Recent research suggests the defect in placental implantation may be related to an abnormal immune response at the maternal – placental interface.[3,5]

The clinical features of pre-eclampsia are few, nonspecific and tend to appear late in the course of the disease. A high index of suspicion is the key to early diagnosis. Scotomas and scintillations characterize the visual disturbances associated with pre-eclampsia. Headaches are frontal and are similar to migraines in quality. Epigastric discomfort associated with pre-eclampsia is thought to be due to hepatic edema and stretching of the hepatic capsule.[5] Edema, present in 30% of pregnant women, is not a reliable sign of pre-eclampsia but should prompt the clinician to look for other signs of pre-eclampsia. Hypertension, a cardinal feature of pre-eclampsia, may be absent in up to 33% of all cases of pre-eclampsia. Retinal disease in the form of retinal vasospasm, edema, hemorrhage and retinal detachment can be seen on fundoscopic examination. Papilledema is rare in pre-eclampsia.

Proteinuria is the most prominent laboratory abnormality associated with pre-eclampsia. Its presence should prompt a search for other features of pre-eclampsia but is not diagnostic of itself. A rising uric acid level suggests the diagnosis of pre-eclampsia. Liver enzyme and platelet abnormalities are indicative of severe pre-eclampsia.

Deaths from pre-eclampsia are rare with appropriate management. The only cure for pre-eclampsia is delivery. A caveat of therapy is that delivery is always good for the mother but not always good for the fetus.[1] Key in the management of pre-eclampsia is early recognition. Blood pressure elevation during the latter half of pregnancy should prompt consideration of pre-eclampsia. The clinical course of pre-eclampsia is unpredictable and often deteriorates rapidly, therefore if pre-eclampsia is suspected hospitalization is recommended. Symptoms suggestive of pre-eclampsia should be sought along with repeat blood pressure measurements and measurement of urinary protein, complete blood count, platelets, serum chemistry, uric acid, and liver enzymes.

There is agreement that persistent diastolic blood pressure levels above 110 mm Hg should be treated. However, many experts now advocate that treatment begin at 105 mm Hg.[3] The goal of treatment is to reduce the diastolic blood pressure to the 90–100 mm Hg range. Existing evidence does not show that lowering the diastolic blood pressure below 110 mm Hg improves maternal or fetal outcomes but many experts believe that the risk for seizure, placental abruption and cerebral hemorrhage are diminished by lowering blood pressure to mildly hypertensive levels.[5]

Currently, the drug of choice for acute hypertension in pregnancy is hydralazine. Hydralazine, a direct arteriolar dilator, has a long history of safety and efficacy when used in pregnancy. Potential adverse effects include reflex tachycardia, flushing, and rare reports of neonatal thrombocytopenia.[6] Parenteral labetalol is an effective second-line agent. Labetalol, a combined alpha and beta blocker, has been shown to be effective in the treatment of acute hypertension in pregnancy. Sodium nitroprusside is rarely needed to control hypertension in the obstetric patient but can be used when all other medications have failed.[6] Because of its potency, rapid onset of action, and short half-life, nitroprusside should be given as a constant infusion and blood pressure should be monitored by arterial catheter.[6] Nitroprusside crosses the placenta and as a result a risk of fetal cyanide poisoning has been described.[5,6] It is recommended that nitroprusside not be used for more than 4 hours and that maternal thiocyanate level must be followed.

Once the diagnosis of pre-eclampsia is established anticonvulsant therapy is indicated to prevent seizures. The drug of choice for seizure prophylaxis in pregnancy is magnesium sulfate. Not an intrinsic anticonvulsant, magnesium sulfate is thought to exert its anticonvulsant effects in pre-eclampsia through its action as a cerebral vasodilator.[5] It is usually given as an intravenous bolus of 4–6 g followed by a continuous infusion of 1–4 g/h to attain a therapeutic plasma level of 4–7 mmol/l.[5] In the event that an eclamptic seizure occurs while on magnesium prophylaxis, an intravenous benzodiazepine may be used to terminate the seizure activity and phenytoin is added to the regimen.

Pre-eclampsia and eclampsia may present or worsen during the postpartum period. It is advisable to continue anticonvulsant prophylaxis 2–4 days postpartum. Complete blood count, platelets, serum creatinine and liver enzymes should be monitored. Blood pressure may remain elevated up to 3 months postpartum. Care should be taken not to prematurely discontinue antihypertensive medication.

Chronic hypertension

Chronic hypertension is defined as either a history of hypertension before pregnancy, repeated blood pressure elevations greater than or equal to 140/90 mm Hg before 20 weeks gestation, or hypertension that is diagnosed for the first time during pregnancy and does not normalize postpartum.[3,7] The perinatal risks associated with chronic hypertension include intrauterine growth retardation, abruptio placentae, prematurity, stillbirth, and superimposed pre-eclampsia.[8] Despite many risks, the majority of pregnant women with chronic hypertension go on to have uncomplicated pregnancies.[1]

Classified as either mild or severe, with severe hypertension defined as a blood pressure 160/110 mm Hg or higher, there is good evidence that treatment of pregnant women with severe hypertension is beneficial and little evidence to support the treatment of mild hypertension.[9] Treatment of mild hypertension does not decrease the frequency of superimposed pre-eclampsia, preterm delivery, abruptio placentae or perinatal death but the data are unclear on whether treatment of mild hypertension prevents progression to severe hypertension.[4,8] As a result of the physiologic decrease of blood pressure during pregnancy, some women are able to discontinue their antihypertensive medications. Therapy should be reinstituted when blood pressure levels exceed 150 mm Hg systolic or 100 mm Hg diastolic. Methyldopa to date has not been associated with any short-term or long-term effects on the neonate or infant and as a result is considered first-line therapy in treating chronic hypertension of pregnancy.

Hydralazine and labetalol are both well studied and considered safe; however hydralazine has been infrequently associated with neonatal thrombocytopenia.[4] Beta-blockers are generally considered safe for use in pregnancy. There is a suggestion that beta-blockers prescribed early in pregnancy (specifically atenolol) may be associated with growth restriction.[3] The data on the use of calcium channel blockers outside of the third trimester are limited. Angiotensin converting enzyme (ACE) inhibitor and angiotensin II receptor blocker (ARBs) use are contraindicated in pregnancy as a result of their association with fetal growth retardation, oligohydramnios, neonatal renal failure and neonatal death. Recent data suggest that diuretic use is safe in women with chronic hypertension, especially when started prior to conception. Lingering questions around the association of diminished plasma volume expansion and its potential effect on fetal growth suggest that diuretics should not be used as first-line antihypertensive agents.

Pre-eclampsia superimposed on chronic hypertension

The greatest risk of chronic hypertension is of superimposed pre-eclampsia. Superimposed pre-eclampsia comprises the greatest risk to both mother and fetus.[1,10] The incidence of superimposed pre-eclampsia ranges from 10%–52% with the greatest risk being in women with renal insufficiency, hypertension for at least 4 years duration or pre-eclampsia in a previous pregnancy.[3] The

Table 41.3. Diagnosis of superimposed pre-eclampsia[3]

Superimposed pre-eclampsia is likely with the following findings:

1. new-onset proteinuria in women with hypertension and no proteinuria early in pregnancy (<20 weeks);
2. in women with hypertension and proteinuria before 20 weeks' gestation;
3. sudden increase in proteinuria;
4. a sudden increase in blood pressure in a woman whose hypertension has previously been well controlled;
5. thrombocytopenia (platelet count <100 000 cells/mm³);
6. an increase in ALT or AST to abnormal levels.

diagnosis of superimposed pre-eclampsia is often difficult, therefore a high index of suspicion is necessary. (Table 41.3).

Gestational hypertension

Gestational hypertension is a non-specific term that is applied to women who have blood pressure elevations for the first time after midpregnancy without proteinuria.[3] Because pre-eclampsia remains in the differential diagnosis in women with gestational hypertension, a final diagnosis is not assigned until the postpartum period. It can be determined that the mother suffers from transient hypertension provided that pre-eclampsia has not developed and blood pressure elevations have returned to normal by 12 weeks postpartum. If the blood pressure elevation has not normalized by 12 weeks postpartum, the diagnosis of chronic hypertension is assigned.[3]

Peripartum cardiomyopathy

Peripartum cardiomyopathy is a rare form of dilated cardiomyopathy affecting previously healthy women during the last month of pregnancy or the first 6 months after delivery in which no other cardiovascular cause is found. Peripartum cardiomyopathy occurs in 1 of every 3000 to 15 000 pregnancies.[11] Women at higher risk include those of advanced maternal age, multiparous, with twin gestation, or of African descent.[2,11] Though the etiology of peripartum cardiomyopathy is currently unknown; current evidence suggests that peripartum cardiomyopathy is a type of myocarditis of either an infectious, autoimmune or idiopathic process.[11] Current diagnostic criteria for peripartum cardiomyopathy are listed in Table 41.4.

Presenting symptoms of patients with peripartum cardiomyopathy are similar to those of other patients with left ventricular systolic dysfunction. Dyspnea, fatigue, pedal

Table 41.4. Diagnostic criteria for peripartum cardiomyopathy[2]

1. Development of cardiac failure in the last month of pregnancy or within 5 months after delivery.
2. No other etiology of heart failure.
3. The absence of heart disease before the last month of pregnancy.
4. Impairment of left ventricular systolic function on echocardiography.

edema, jugular venous distention, and palpitations are common findings in healthy pregnant women; therefore, the clinician must carefully evaluate the patient for clues that peripartum cardiomyopathy is present.[11] If peripartum cardiomyopathy is suspected, the diagnosis should be confirmed with echocardiography.[7]

Therapy with diuretics, digitalis, beta-blockers, and afterload reducing agents should be started as soon as possible. Antepartum afterload reduction should be achieved with hydralazine and low dose nitroglycerin. Angiotensin-converting enzyme (ACE) inhibitor and angiotensin II receptor blocker (ARBs) use are contraindicated in pregnancy as a result of their association with fetal growth retardation, oligohydramnios, neonatal renal failure, and neonatal death. ACE inhibitors or angiotensin receptor blockers can be substituted during the postpartum period if no other contraindication to their use exists. Diuretics should be used with caution to avoid dehydration and serum digoxin levels should be monitored.[1] The benefits of beta-blockers are well established; however, long-term use of beta-blockers during pregnancy may be associated with low birthweight babies. Thromboembolic complications are common; therefore, thromboprophylaxis with heparin is indicated. Warfarin use during pregnancy is contraindicated: a result of increased risks of fetal and neonatal hemorrage, placental abruption and a characteristic pattern of birth defects. Warfarin may be substituted postpartum.

Therapeutic anticoagulation should be started if there is evidence of mural thrombus or with an ejection fraction of less than 35%.[2]

Fifty percent of patients will have improvement or resolution of their symptoms and LV function within 6 months of presentation. The future prognosis for these patients is favorable. Cardiomyopathy that persists 6 months after presentation is likely irreversible and is associated with a worse survival.[1,12] The risk of recurrence in future pregnancies is greater in women with persistent LV dysfunction, and pregnancy is relatively contraindicated in this group of patients. Those who fully recover LV function tend to have successful future pregnancies; however, this set of patients may have a suboptimal response to future hemodynamic stress, which includes future pregnancy.[13]

Venous thromboembolic disease

Venous thromboembolic disease (VTE) is an uncommon complication of pregnancy occurring in 0.5–3.0 in 1000 pregnancies. It is the leading non-obstetric cause of maternal death during pregnancy and the purperium; therefore appropriate diagnosis and treatment is critical.

Pathophysiology

The risk of VTE is five to six times higher in pregnant women than in non-pregnant women of similar age.[14] The source of this increased risk is multifactorial. Obstetric risk factors include prolonged bed rest, instrument-assisted or c-section delivery, hemorrhage, sepsis, multiparity, and advanced maternal age. The most constant risk is related to venous stasis. A result of hormonally mediated venous distensibility and compression by the gravid uterus, the venous system of the lower extremities is particularly vulnerable to thrombus.

Normal pregnancy is associated with marked changes in the coagulation and fibrinolytic systems (Table 41.1). The platelet count decreases throughout pregnancy and the immediate postpartum period. Coagulation factors II, VII, IX, and X increase substantially by the middle of pregnancy.[14] Fibrinogen levels increase markedly during the antepartum period. Protein S levels decrease throughout pregnancy; though Protein C levels remain unchanged. Finally, the fibrinolytic system is inhibited during pregnancy, most substantially in the third trimester.[14] Factor V Leiden mutation, a major risk factor for VTE in pregnancy, is thought to have a bearing in 40%–70% of cases of venous thrombosis in pregnancy.[15] A point mutation on the factor V gene, factor V Leiden inhibits the deactivation of factor Va by activated protein C (APC resistance).

Diagnosis

The clinical diagnosis of DVT and PE is most difficult. Given that leg pain, edema, shortness of breath, and palpitations are common complaints during pregnancy, the diagnosis of VTE is quite difficult.

Compression ultrasonography (CUS) is the non-invasive test of choice for the diagnosis of DVT during pregnancy. CUS is most sensitive for detecting proximal DVT and a positive finding is enough to begin anticoagulation. CUS however is very insensitive for calf vein and iliac vein DVT. Repeat CUS, plethesmography or limited venography may be indicated if calf DVT is suspected. Magnetic resonance imaging has shown value in detecting iliac vein DVT.[14,16]

Ventilation–perfusion lung scanning is the diagnostic test of choice for pregnant patients with suspected PE. Normal or high probability studies can reliably rule in or rule out PE in pregnant women and should guide therapy decisions. Given the high prevalence of PE in patients with non-diagnostic, indeterminate, or intermediate probability scans, additional work up is warranted. CUS is used to evaluate for lower extremity thrombosis; if negative, pulmonary angiogram should be done to reliably exclude PE.[15] The effects of radiation exposure on fetal development are always a concern of both physicians and pregnant women when performing radiologic studies during pregnancy. The outlined diagnostic strategy would expose the fetus to approximately 0.5 rad of radiation.[15] This amount of radiation is well below the 5.0 rad limit that is recommended by the National Commission on Radiation Protection (NCRP).[15]

Treatment

The acute treatment of VTE in pregnancy is essentially no different from that in non-pregnant patients. The major differences in pregnancy involve the choice of anticoagulant, its dose, and duration.

Heparin is the anticoagulant of choice for use in pregnancy. Heparin's major advantage is that it does not cross the placenta, making it safe for the fetus.[15,16] Maternal risks include bleeding, heparin-induced thrombocytopenia, heparin-induced osteoporosis, and inadequate anticoagulation. The risk of inadequate anticoagulation should not be underestimated. The heparin requirements in pregnant women to prolong and maintain a therapeutic PTT may be significantly increased.

Low molecular weight heparin (LMWH) is considered equally efficacious in treating VTE in non-pregnant patients. Like unfractionated heparin, LMWH does not cross the placental barrier. LMWH has better bioavailability, a longer half-life and requires less monitoring (factor Xa levels).[17] LMWH is also associated with a lower risk of thrombocytopenia, osteoporosis and fewer platelet effects.[17] There are, however, few studies looking at acute treatment of VTE with LMWH in pregnancy. As a result, LMWH is only recommended for prophylaxis and in those who cannot tolerate unfractionated heparin.[15,17]

Warfarin should be avoided throughout pregnancy. Readily crossing the placental barrier, warfarin use in the first trimester is associated with a characteristic embryopathy. Additionally, the risks of fetal and neonatal hemorrhage along with placental abruption remain high with warfarin use throughout all phases of pregnancy.

Patients who develop venous thrombosis should initially receive 5–10 days of full dose intravenous heparin. This should be followed by adjusted dose subcutaneous heparin every 8–12 hours that prolongs the PTT 1.5 to 2.0 times control for at least 3 months.

Liver diseases unique to pregnancy

Liver disease is a rare but potentially tragic complication of pregnancy. Pregnant women are susceptible to a range of liver diseases. There are several liver diseases that are unique to pregnancy; these disorders will be the focus of this section.

Intrahepatic cholestasis of pregnancy

Intrahepatic cholestasis of pregnancy (ICP) typically occurs during the late second or third trimester with a mean incidence of 30 weeks' gestation. ICP is a rare disorder in most countries with an incidence ranging from 1 in 1000 to 1 in 10 000 deliveries.[18,19] Though the pathogenesis of ICP is unknown, indirect evidence suggests that estrogen has a strong role in the development of ICP. Risk factors include a personal or family history of the disease, genetic predisposition, a history of cholestasis while taking oral contraceptives, and twin gestation.

Maternal risks include poor weight gain, as a result of the accompanying anorexia and nausea. ICP has been associated with a 70% incidence of postpartum hemorrhage as a result of malabsorption of fat soluble vitamins, specifically vitamin K.[18] Fetal risks include increased rates of prematurity, stillbirth, intrapartum distress and thick meconium. Perinatal mortality ranges from 3.5% to 11%.[18]

Pruritis is the hallmark clinical finding in ICP. Usually starting in the palms and soles, pruritis may later spread to the trunk, extremities, and in severe cases the face and neck. Pruritis tends to be most severe at night, often leading to sleep deprivation and fatigue. Jaundice develops in 20%–60% of women 1 to 4 weeks after the onset of itching.[20,21] Elevation of serum bile acid levels is the most specific laboratory evidence of ICP. A 10–100-fold increase in serum bile acid concentration may precede the onset of symptoms by several weeks.[18,22] Moderate increases in serum aminotransferase values (two- to tenfold), bilirubin (<10 mg/dl), and alkaline phosphatase (fourfold) are also seen. GGTP and 5′ nucleotidase values are not elevated in ICP. Liver biopsy, though rarely needed to make the diagnosis, shows cholestasis with minimal or no inflammatory changes.[20]

The only cure for ICP is delivery. Pruritis and jaundice resolve within days of delivery and all other laboratory values typically normalize within 4 to 6 weeks of delivery. The antepartum challenge in managing ICP is alleviating pruritis. Ideally, successful treatment of ICP would alleviate pruritis and lower the serum bile acid concentration. Cholestyramine is widely used to treat pruritis in ICP. It has been shown to improve pruritis, but has no effect on serum bile acid concentration. Cholestyramine may, however, worsen vitamin K malabsorption increasing the risk of postpartum hemorrhage. Patients treated with cholestyramine are recommended to receive parenteral vitamin K and monitoring of the prothrombin time. Several small studies have noted an improvement in pruritis in up to 50% of patients taking phenobarbital.[18] Ursodeoxycholic acid (UDCA), a naturally occurring hydrophilic bile acid, has shown promise in the treatment of ICP. In several small case series UDCA was found to significantly deduce pruritis, bile acid levels and transaminases.[18] No maternal side effects were noted in these studies.[18] The safety of UDCA on the developing fetus is a concern and the focus of further study.

Acute fatty liver of pregnancy

Acute fatty liver of pregnancy (AFLP) is a rare disorder occurring in approximately 1 in 13 000 deliveries.[20,23] The characteristic picture of AFLP is of microvesicular fat infiltration within the hepatocytes. Patients with AFLP typically present in the third trimester at a mean of 36 weeks' gestation. There have been rare cases that have presented as early as 28 weeks. The pathogenesis of AFLP has been elusive. There is considerable evidence that the pathogenesis involves a mutation in the gene that codes for long chain 3-hydroxyl-acyl Co-A dehydrogenase (LCHAD), an enzyme involved in the intramitochondrial beta oxidation of fatty acids. The risk appears greatest in women with heterozygous defects of the LCHAD gene who carry a fetus with either a homozygous defect or compound heterozygous defects of the LCHAD gene.[24]

Initial clinical findings include nausea or vomiting, malaise, jaundice, and abdominal pain.[25,26] Pruritis is rare in AFLP. Encephalopathy, hypoglycemia, DIC, seizures, and coma may characterize severe cases. Liver size is usually normal or small. Aminotransferase levels are elevated but usually less than 1000 U.[27] Thrombocytopenia is usual in AFLP and is not always associated with other signs of DIC. The course of AFLP is noted for its rapid progression to coma and death.

The only treatment for AFLP is delivery. Because of the potential for rapid progression to coma and death, AFLP is considered an obstetric emergency. Before 1980 both the maternal and fetal mortality rates of AFLP were about 85%. Improved recognition of AFLP has lowered the maternal mortality to <10% and early delivery has lowered fetal mortality to <20%.[20,25] Patients with severe hepatic dysfunction are best treated in an ICU setting before and after delivery.

Medical management of patients with AFLP is supportive. Blood sugar levels should be monitored and severe coagulation disorders treated with platelet and fresh frozen plasma transfusions. Improvement usually begins with delivery. Patients with severe hepatic injury remain at risk for respiratory failure, renal failure, GI bleeding and nephrogenic diabetes insipidus and should be closely monitored during the immediate postpartum period. The rare patient who progresses to fulminant hepatic failure can be treated by liver transplantation. Surviving patients generally recover with no hepatic sequelae. Future pregnancies are often uncomplicated, but patients remain at risk for recurrent AFLP.

HELLP syndrome

The HELLP syndrome is characterized by the presence of microangiopathic hemolysis, elevated liver enzymes that are typically elevated transaminase levels and thrombocytopenia (platelet count < 100 000). The HELLP syndrome occurs in the setting of severe pre-eclampsia in 20% of cases.[28,29] Seventy percent of cases of HELLP occur between the 27th and 36th week of gestation and up to one-third of cases occur postpartum.[20] Maternal complications of HELLP include postpartum hemorrhage, DIC (20%), abruptio placentae (16%), ARF (7%) and pulmonary edema (6%). The perinatal mortality ranges from 5%–35%.[20,28] The major risk to the fetus is a result of prematurity. Liver disease and thrombocytopenia tend not to be found in babies born to women with the HELLP syndrome.[27,30]

HELLP syndrome, pre-eclampsia and AFLP, entities unique to pregnancy, share several clinical and biologic similarities and differences. Both HELLP and AFLP frequently occur in the setting of pre-eclampsia, but are two distinct disease states. Pathologically, AFLP is manifest by microvesicular fat infiltration within the hepatocytes without signs of infiltration of inflammatory cells. Periportal fibrin deposition, hemorrhage, and infiltration of neutrophils characterize HELLP.[28] Similar to AFLP defects in the LCHAD gene have been suggested as an associated factor in the pathogenesis of HELLP.[24] HELLP differs from classic pre-eclampsia in two ways. HELLP occurs before term in over 80% of cases and more frequently afflicts older women, whites and multiparas in contrast to pre-eclampsia.[28,29]

The most common clinical features of the HELLP syndrome are RUQ or epigastric pain (65%–90%), malaise (9%), nausea or vomiting (36%–50%), headache (31%), or jaundice (5%).[20] Typical physical examination findings include RUQ tenderness (80%) and weight gain with edema (60%). Hypertension may be absent in 20% of patients.[20] The differential diagnosis of HELLP syndrome includes acute fatty liver of pregnancy (AFLP), thrombotic thrombocytopenic purpura (TTP), hemolytic uremic syndrome (HUS), idiopathic thrombocytopenic purpura (ITP), and systemic lupus erythematosis (SLE).[31]

The only definitive treatment of pre-eclampsia and the HELLP syndrome is delivery. The management of HELLP is primarily supportive and anticipatory with the focus on determining the safest timing and route of delivery.[28] Seizure prophylaxis with magnesium sulfate should be instituted upon diagnosis and hypertension, if present, should be treated when severe.

The role of corticosteroids in HELLP syndrome is currently a focus of study. Small studies suggested that antepartum corticosteroid therapy might stabilize the disease or improve platelet count, liver enzymes, and LDH.[32] Studies of postpartum corticosteroid therapy in women with HELLP syndrome have accelerated recovery time when compared with women not treated with steroids.[33]

REFERENCES

1. Balk, M. A. & Watkins, C. Heart disease in pregnancy. In Branch, W. T., Alexander, R. W., Schlant, R. C., & Hurst, J. W., eds. *Cardiology in Primary Care.* New York: McGraw-Hill, 2000: 791–805.

2. Poppas, A., Carson, M. P., Rosene-Montella, K., & Powrie, R. O. Cardiovascular disease. In Lee, R. V., Rosene-Montelle, K., Barbour, L. A. *et al.* eds. *Medical Care of the Pregnant Patient.* Philadelphia: American College of Physicians, 2000: 345–386.

3. National High Blood Pressure Education Program Working Group Report on High Blood Pressure in Pregnancy. *Report of the National High Blood Pressure Education Program Working Group on high blood pressure in pregnancy.* NIH Publication # 00–3029, 2000: 1–38.

4. Roberts, J. M. & Redman, C. W. Preeclampsia: more than pregnancy-induced hypertension. *Lancet* 1993; **341**: 1447–1451.

5. Powrie, R. O. & Rosene-Montella, K. Hypertension and pre-eclampsia. In Lee, R. V., *et al.*, eds. *Medical Care of the Pregnant Patient.* Philadelphia, PA: American College of Physicians, 2000; 185–205.

6. Mabie, W.C. Management of acute severe hypertension and encephalopathy. *Clin. Obstet. Gynecol.* 1999; **42**(3): 519–531.

7. Watkins, C., Bernstein, L.B., & Higgins, S.M. Medical disorders of pregnancy. In Branch, W.T., ed. *Office Practice of Medicine*. 609–620 Philadelphia, PA: W.B. Saunders, 2000: 609–620.

8. Sibai, B.M. & Lindeheimer, M. Risk factors for preeclampsia, abruptio placentae and adverse neonatal outcomes among women with chronic hypertension. *N. Engl. J. Med.* 1998; **339**(10): 667–671.

9. Ferrer, R.L. & Sibai, B.M. Management of mild chronic hypertension during pregnancy: a review. *Obstet. Gynecol.* 2000; **96**(5): 849–860.

10. Garovic, V. Hypertension in pregnancy: diagnosis and treatment. *Mayo Clin. Proc.* 2000; **75**: 1071–1076.

11. Brown, C.S. & Bertolet, B.D. Peripartum cardiomyopathy: a comprehensive review. *Am. J. Obstet. Gynecol.* 1998; **178**(2): 409–414.

12. Beus, E., Mook, W.N.K.A., Ramsey, G. *et al.* Peripartum cardiomyopathy: a condition intensivists should be aware of. *Intens. Care Med.* 2003; **29**: 167–174.

13. Lampert, M.D. & Weinert, L. Contractile reserve in patients with peripartum cardiomyopathy and recovered left ventricular function. *Am. J. Obstet. Gynecol.* 1997; **176**(1): 187–195.

14. Toglia, M.R. & Weg, J.G. Venous thromboembolism during pregnancy. *N. Engl. J. Med.* 1996; **335**(2): 108–114.

15. Rosene-Montella, K. & Barbour, L.A. Thromboembolic disease and hypercoagulable states. In Lee, R.V. *et al.*, eds. *Medical Care of the Pregnant Patient*. Philadelphia: American College of Physicians, 2000: 423–448.

16. Spritzer, C.E., Evans, A.C., & Kay, H.H. Magnetic resonance imaging of deep venous thrombosis in pregnant women with lower extremity edema. *Obstet. Gynecol.* 1995; **85**: 603–607.

17. Ginsberg, J.A.S., Hirsh, J., Turner, D.C., *et al.* Risks to the fetus of anticoagulant therapy during pregnancy. *Thromb. Haemost.* 1989; **61**: 197–203.

18. Laurent, P., Dussarat, G.V., Bonal, J. *et al.* Low molecular weight heparins: a guide to their optimum use in pregnancy. *Drugs* 2002; **62**(3): 463–477.

19. Davidson, K.M. Intrahepatic cholestasis of pregnancy. *Semin. Perinatol.* 1998; **22**(2): 104–111.

20. Reyes, H. Intrahepatic cholestasis of pregnancy: estrogen related disease. *Semin. Liver Dis.* 1993; **13**: 289–301.

21. Knox, T.A. & Olans, L.B. Liver disease in pregnancy. *N. Engl. J. Med.* 1996; **335**(8): 569–576.

22. Reyes, H. The spectrum of liver and gastrointestinal disease seen in cholestasis of pregnancy. *Gastroenterol. Clin. North Am.* 1992; **21**: 905–921.

23. Heikkinen, J. Serum bile acids in the early diagnosis of intrahepatic cholestasis of pregnancy. *Obstet. Gynecol.* 1983; **61**: 581–587.

24. Pockros, P.J., Peters, R.L., & Reynolds, T.B. Idiopathic fatty liver of pregnancy: findings in ten cases. *Medicine* 1984; **63**: 1–11.

25. Ibdah, S.A., Bennett, M.J., Rinaldo, P., Zhao, Y. *et al.* A fetal fatty acid oxidation disorder as a cause of liver disease in pregnant women. *N. Engl. J. Med.* 1999; **340**(22): 1723–1731.

26. Bacq, Y. Acute fatty liver of pregnancy. *Semin. Perinat.* 1998; **22**(2): 134–140.

27. Riely, C.A. Gestational liver disease. In Lee, R.V., *et al.*, eds. *Medical Care of the Pregnant Patient*. Philadelphia: American College of Physicians, 2000: 585–598.

28. Saphier, C.J. & Repke, J.T. Hemolysis, elevated liver enzymes and low platelets (HELLP) syndrome: a review of diagnosis and management. *Semin. Perinatol.* 1998; **22**(2): 118–133.

29. Sabai, B.M., Ramadan, M.K., Usta, I. *et al.* Maternal morbidity and mortality in 442 pregnancies with hemolysis, elevated liver enzymes, and low platelets (HELLP syndrome). *Am. J. Obstet. Gynecol.* 1993; **169**: 1000–1006.

30. Hermis, K., Rath, W., Herting, E., & Kuhn, W. Maternal hemolysis, elevated liver enzymes and low platelet count, and neonatal outcome. *Am. J. Perinatol.* 1995; **12**: 1–6.

31. Egerman, R.S. & Sibai, B.M. Imitators of preeclampsia and eclampsia. *Clin. Obstet. Gynecol.* 1999; **42**(3): 551–562.

32. Magann, E.F. & Martin, J.N. Twelve steps to optimal management of HELLP syndrome. *Clin. Obstet. Gynecol.* 1999; **42**(3): 532–550.

33. Varol, F., Aydin, T., & Gucer, F. HELLP syndrome and postpartum corticosteroids. *Int. J. Gynecol. Obstet.* 2001; **73**: 157–159.

Part II

Surgical procedures and their complications

General surgery

42

Tracheostomy

David V. Feliciano

Emory University School of Medicine, Atlanta, GA

Historically, tracheostomy has been performed for relief of obstruction of the upper airway (trauma, epiglottitis); when prolonged ventilatory support for respiratory failure is likely; for control of secretions in patients with bulbar lesions or closed head injuries; or for sleep apnea. In many centers, open surgical tracheostomy has been replaced with bedside percutaneous dilational tracheostomy. In patients with acute airway obstruction, cricothyroidotomy ("high tracheostomy") is a better choice than tracheostomy, especially if the individual performing the procedure has little or no surgical training, if the procedure is being performed under less than ideal conditions in the emergency center or intensive care unit, or if there is impending asphyxiation. The delay until tracheostomy is performed in patients with prolonged endotracheal intubation varies from center to center, but prospective data demonstrate the advantage of doing the procedure after 7 to 10 days. Recent evidence also indicates that patients who cannot be weaned with endotracheal tubes in place can often be weaned rapidly after a tracheostomy is performed. Finally, newer devices are available that enable patients with sleep apnea to be managed without tracheostomies.

After instituting the delivery of 100% oxygen by mask, endotracheal tube, or ventilating bronchoscope, open tracheostomy is best performed in the operating room under local anesthesia supplemented by intravenous sedation. The patient's neck is hyperextended and a transverse incision is made over the second tracheal cartilage. The strap muscles are separated in the midline and the anterior trachea from the cricoid cartilage to the fourth tracheal cartilage is cleared, which often necessitates division of the thyroid isthmus between sutures. Either a vertical incision through the second and third cartilages or a three-sided superiorly based flap between the second and third cartilages is made. The tracheostomy tube is then inserted as the anesthesiologist removes the endotracheal tube.

Percutaneous tracheostomy is performed in the intensive care unit or in the operating room. After infiltration of the pretracheal skin with local anesthetic, a 1–2 cm superficial transverse incision is made midway between the cricoid cartilage and the sternal notch. The subcutaneous tissue over the trachea is spread with a hemostat and the trachea can then be palpated. After the anesthesiologist pulls the endotracheal tube cuff back to just below the vocal cords, a 16-gauge needle is directed posteriorly and inferiorly into the trachea. A flexible bronchoscope passed through the endotracheal tube confirms entry into the trachea. A plastic cannula over the needle is advanced into the trachea, the needle is removed, a guidewire is inserted through the cannula, and the cannula is then removed. After passage of a small dilator over the guidewire and dilatation of the anterior hole in the trachea, the dilator is removed and a plastic guiding catheter is placed over the guidewire. Progressively larger dilators are passed over the wire and guiding catheter. A tracheostomy tube fitted snugly over a 24-French dilator is then passed into the trachea. After removal of the dilator, guidewire, guiding catheter, and endotracheal tube, the airway is secure. The stress of tracheostomy can be considerable if it is performed as an emergent procedure or if there is poor coordination between the operating surgeon and the anesthesiologist. Tracheostomy can be performed in 3 to 5 minutes by an experienced surgeon in a sedated patient, but elective tracheostomy performed meticulously in the operating room often requires 20–25 minutes. Blood transfusions are never given.

Usual postoperative course

Expected postoperative hospital stay

The duration depends on the reason for the tracheostomy. In patients who are converted to tracheostomies to

Medical Management of the Surgical Patient: A Textbook of Perioperative Medicine, ed. M. F. Lubin, R. B. Smith, T. F. Dobson, N. Spell, H. K. Walker. 4th edn. Published by Cambridge University Press. © Cambridge University 2006.

enhance weaning, ventilatory support often is no longer necessary within 1 to 2 weeks.

Operative mortality

The hospital mortality rate for patients undergoing tracheostomy is 50% in some series. The mortality rate related directly to the procedure is under 1% and is always associated with hypoxia or hypoxia-induced cardiac arrhythmias.

Special monitoring required

Both oxygen saturation and end-tidal carbon dioxide monitoring are indicated when intubated and ventilated patients undergo tracheostomy.

Patient activity and positioning

The ventilator tubing should be positioned to prevent undue traction or angling of the tracheostomy tube.

Alimentation

Some patients have difficulty swallowing with a tracheostomy tube in place, presumably because of esophageal compression at the site of the balloon. Passage of a feeding tube with the balloon of the tracheostomy tube partially deflated is appropriate in such a situation.

Antibiotic coverage

Antibiotics are indicated only if the tracheostomy is performed for respiratory failure caused by pneumonia.

Procedural complications

Loss of airway

Failure to pass the tracheostomy tube into the distal trachea during open tracheostomy can occur due to poor visualization in the obese patient with a short deep neck.

Damage to posterior or lateral trachea

Overaggressive passage of or misplacement of dilators during percutaneous dilational tracheostomy may cause perforations of the posterior or lateral trachea mandating open repair.

Postoperative complications

In the hospital

Hemorrhage

Early bleeding from the soft tissues and thyroid gland near the tracheostomy site results from inadequate surgical hemostasis during open tracheostomy and can usually be controlled with packing around the stoma. Late transient arterial bleeding in the presence of a pulsating tracheal cannula is suggestive of a tracheal–innominate artery fistula, an extraordinarily rare event since the introduction of large volume–low pressure balloons on tracheostomy tubes. Hyperinflation of the cuff of the tube occludes the fistula and compresses the artery in most patients. The aspirated blood should be suctioned vigorously as the surgical team is mobilized. Operative therapy is mandatory and involves resection of the innominate artery and repair of the trachea.

Obstruction

Progressive hypoxia despite passage of a suction catheter through the tube suggests that the remainder of the lumen is occluded or there are thick secretions acting as a ball valve at the tip. If equal breath sounds are present and a tension pneumothorax is unlikely, the tracheostomy tube should be changed over a suction catheter.

Infection

Tracheitis, pneumonia, mediastinitis, and pneumonia have all been reported. Frequent suctioning through the tracheostomy tube using meticulous sterile technique should decrease the incidence of infection in the tracheobronchial tree. Loose closure of the skin wound and frequent suctioning around the tracheostomy tube should reduce the incidence of soft tissue infection.

Tracheoesophageal fistula

Increased secretions and tube feedings in the airway associated with severe coughing related to swallowing suggests the presence of a fistula. Once bronchoscopy and esophagoscopy have confirmed the diagnosis, operative repair involves closure of the holes in both organs and the interposition of a bulky vascularized muscle flap.

After discharge

Tracheal stenosis

The late development of stridor, wheezing, dyspnea on effort, or airway obstruction from secretions in patients with histories of prolonged tracheostomy placement mandates bronchoscopy. Strictures may occur at the level of the previous stoma, at the balloon site, or at the tip of the tracheostomy tube. Resection of the stricture and end-to-end anastomosis of the trachea are indicated.

FURTHER READING

Berrouschot, J., Oeken, J., Steiniger, L. *et al*. Perioperative complications of percutaneous dilational tracheostomy. *Laryngoscope* 1997; **107**: 1538–1544.

Friedman, Y., Fildes, J., Mizock, B. *et al*. Comparison of percutaneous and surgical tracheostomies. *Chest* 1996; **110**: 480–485.

Marx, W. H., Ciaglia, P., & Graniero, K. D. Some important details in the technique of percutaneous dilatational tracheostomy via the modified Seldinger technique. *Chest* 1996; **110**: 762–766.

Massick, D. D., Yao, S., Powell, D. M., *et al*. Bedside tracheostomy in the intensive care unit: a prospective randomized trial comparing open surgical tracheostomy with endoscopically guided percutaneous dilational tracheotomy. *Laryngoscope* 2001; **111**: 494–500.

Petros, S. & Engelmann, L. Percutaneous dilatational tracheostomy in a medical ICU. *Intens. Care Med.* 1997; **23**: 630–634.

43

Thyroidectomy

David V. Feliciano

Emory University School of Medicine, Atlanta, GA

Thyroidectomy is performed for nodules with suspicious cytology on fine-needle aspiration (follicular adenoma), biopsy-proven adenocarcinoma, large goiters with airway compromise or cosmetic concerns, or thyrotoxicosis. Given the 6% to 7% incidence of false-negative results on fine-needle aspiration for adenocarcinoma, nodules enlarging on medical therapy should also be treated with operation. Subtotal or total thyroidectomy continues to offer an immediate cure and the best chance of restoring a euthyroid state in certain subgroups of patients with thyrotoxicosis. Included among these are children and women of childbearing age with Graves' disease, those who have failed medical or radioiodine therapy for Graves' disease, those with toxic multinodular goiter (Plummer's disease), and those with toxic adenomas.

Preoperative preparation with antithyroid drugs, propranolol, and potassium iodide (SSKI) or propranolol alone is indicated in patients with thyrotoxicosis to prevent thyroid storm in the postoperative period. Vocal cord function is checked before the administration of paralytic agents by the anesthesiologist. Open thyroidectomy is usually performed under general anesthesia through a low collar incision, yielding excellent cosmetic results. Endoscopic thyroidectomy is also performed under general anesthesia with 3 mm and 5 mm instruments and an endoscope. After preliminary division of the superior thyroid vessels through a 1 cm lateral cervical incision, a 10 mm trocar is inserted through the incision and carbon dioxide is insufflated to a pressure of 10–12 mm Hg. After preliminary dissection through a 0 degree endoscope, a 30 degree endoscope and additional trocars are inserted to complete the dissection, mobilization, and removal of the ipsilateral lobe. The bilateral parathyroid glands, recurrent laryngeal nerves, and external branches of the superior laryngeal nerves are identified and preserved in both open and endoscopic thyroidectomies. Total thyroidectomy is indicated for patients with bilateral intrathyroidal (less than 1.5 cm) or extrathyroidal papillary cancer, follicular cancer with known pulmonary or osseous metastases, medullary cancer, Graves' disease, or large multinodular goiters.

Thyroidectomy imposes only a modest stress on patients, most procedures are completed in 1½ to 2½ hours, and transfusion is extremely uncommon.

Usual postoperative course

Expected postoperative hospital stay
Outpatient procedures are appropriate for solitary benign nodules and have been performed for thyrotoxicosis and thyroid cancer in some centers; otherwise, the hospital stay is 1 or 2 days.

Operative mortality
Under 0.1%.

Special monitoring required
Respiratory status should be carefully monitored if early postoperative stridor or difficulty in clearing secretions occurs. Patients with thyrotoxicosis who receive appropriate preoperative preparation should undergo routine monitoring.

Patient activity and positioning
The head should be elevated 30 to 45 degrees to minimize edema and venous oozing. Full activity is resumed the morning after operation.

Alimentation
Full liquids are permitted on the day of operation and a regular diet is resumed the next morning.

Medical Management of the Surgical Patient: A Textbook of Perioperative Medicine, ed. M. F. Lubin, R. B. Smith, T. F. Dobson, N. Spell, H. K. Walker. 4th edn. Published by Cambridge University Press. © Cambridge University 2006.

Antibiotic coverage

None indicated.

Drains

Closed suction drains are removed on the first postoperative day.

Postoperative complications

In the hospital

Hemorrhage

Although it is extremely rare (less than 0.5%), a hematoma in the area of resection may cause airway obstruction early in the postoperative period. Removal of the skin and strap muscle sutures and evacuation of the hematoma in the recovery room is preferable to tracheostomy. Patients are then returned to the operating room for irrigation of the operative site, control of hemorrhage, and repeat closure of the wound.

Hypoparathyroidism

Transient hypoparathyroidism is seen in 2% to 4% of all patients after thyroidectomy and in 20% to 22% of those who undergo total or repeated thyroidectomy. Permanent hypoparathyroidism occurs in under 0.6% of patients. Symptomatic hypocalcemia (less than 7.5 mg/dl) is characterized by anxiety, perioral or finger tingling, and a positive Chvostek's sign, usually developing 16 to 24 hours after surgery. Intravenous calcium is given to relieve acute symptoms in the hospital and oral calcium therapy is prescribed at the time of discharge.

Recurrent laryngeal nerve injury

Paralysis of one vocal cord causes hoarseness and difficulty in clearing secretions and usually is related to traction on the recurrent nerve and may resolve over a period of days to months. Permanent recurrent nerve palsy occurs in as many as 4.5% of all thyroidectomies, often resulting from intended sacrifice of a nerve involved with carcinoma.

Thyroid storm

This should not occur after surgery for thyrotoxicosis in adequately prepared patients, but it may be seen in patients with untreated thyrotoxicosis who are undergoing other operations. Symptoms of tremor, agitation, tachycardia, and hyperthermia are treated with intravenous fluids, propranolol, potassium iodide, and steroids.

After discharge

Recurrent benign nodule or goiter

Recurrence of a benign nodule or goiter can be prevented by the lifelong administration of thyroid hormone.

Recurrent thyroid cancer

To decrease the incidence of recurrent cancer in the neck, lungs, or bone, thyroid hormone replacement is delayed until radioactive iodine is administered.

Late or recurrent hyperthyroidism

Annual thyroid function tests are indicated in patients who are receiving thyroid hormone after operation for goiter or cancer and in those who are originally euthyroid after operation for Graves' disease.

"Permanent" hypoparathyroidism

Vitamin D is added to calcium replacement to enhance absorption. If serial parathyroid hormone levels begin to rise, first the vitamin D and then the calcium supplement should be tapered.

FURTHER READING

Feliciano, D. V. Everything you wanted to know about Graves' disease. *Am. J. Surg.* 1992; **164**: 404–411.

Feliciano, D. V. Image of the month. Toxic adenoma or solitary autonomous nodule (variant of Plummer's disease). *Arch. Surg.* 2001; **136**: 239–240.

Gagner, M. & Inabnet, W. B. Endoscopic thyroidectomy for solitary thyroid nodules. *Thyroid* 2001; **11**: 161–163.

Halsted, W. S. The operative story of goiter. *Johns Hopkins Hosp. Rep.* 1920; **19**: 171–257.

Inabnet, W. B. & Gagner, M. How I do it: endoscopic thyroidectomy. *J. Otolaryngol.* 2001; **30**: 41–42.

44

Parathyroidectomy

David V. Feliciano

Emory University School of Medicine, Atlanta, GA

Parathyroidectomy is performed most commonly in patients with primary hyperparathyroidism and those who are dialysis dependent and have symptomatic secondary hyperparathyroidism. In rare patients who have hypercalcemia on dialysis or after renal transplantation (tertiary hyperparathyroidism), operation is also indicated. A physical examination, chest radiograph, intravenous pyelogram (on unusual occasions), and modern parathormone assay distinguish between primary hyperparathyroidism and the hypercalcemia of sarcoidosis, metastases, or a paraneoplastic syndrome. A 24-hour urinary calcium test is occasionally indicated to rule out familial hypocalciuric hypercalcemia. Currently, virtually all preoperative patients undergo cervical ultrasonography or radionuclide scanning after the intravenous injection of ^{99m}Technetium-labeled sestamibi in order to allow for shortened operations through limited incisions.

Preoperative therapy to lower extraordinarily elevated serum calcium levels in patients with parathyroid comas or suspected carcinomas should include saline infusions, furosemide, and occasionally calcitonin. Parathyroidectomy is usually performed under general anesthesia through a low collar incision, although local anesthesia is appropriate for elderly and high-risk patients as well as those undergoing minimally radio-guided parathyroidectomy or "no frills" image-guided exploration.

There has been a rapid evolution in parathyroid surgery over the past 5–7 years. At present, there are at least five different operative approaches being utilized. Conventional parathyroid exploration performed through the standard low collar incision, in which the size of all four glands is assessed, is now accompanied by measurement of intraoperative intact parathyroid hormone levels. Basically, a drop $= 50\%$ from the highest preincision intact parathormone level 10 minutes after excision of a suspected adenoma on the immunochemiluminescent assay signifies that all hypersecreting tissue has been removed. Limited parathyroid exploration (one side) followed by measurement of intraoperative intact parathyroid hormone levels is appropriate when a preoperative sestamibi scan definitely localizes the enlarged adenoma. Minimally invasive radio-guided parathyroidectomy (MIRP) involves the injection of intravenous ^{99m}technetium-labeled sestamibi 1.5–2.5 hours before operation. Under local anesthesia and guided by a gamma probe, a 2.0–2.5 transverse incision is made over the area of highest gamma emission through the skin. The adenoma is localized by the gamma probe and removed, and the patient is discharged 1–2 hours later. The "no frills" image guided exploration proposed by surgeons at the Mayo Clinic involves preoperative sestamibi scanning with planar, oblique SPECT (single photon-emission CT). Under local anesthesia, the enlarged adenoma is removed and an intact parathormone assay is drawn in the recovery room. Failure of this limited approach as documented on the parathormone assay mandates a conventional cervical exploration 24 hours later. Finally, minimal access techniques such as endoscopic or video-assisted parathyroidectomy that involve the insertion of an endoscope or a trocar for insufflation of CO_2 and several small-sized operating ports for 2 mm instruments, are used in selected centers.

A solitary parathyroid adenoma is present in 80%–90% of patients and should be excised. Double adenomas are present in 2% to 4% of patients, and excision is appropriate along with biopsy of a normal gland. Sporadic hyperplasia (sestamibi scan does not localize) is best treated with subtotal parathyroidectomy (excision of 3½ glands). Patients with secondary or tertiary hyperparathyroidism who are unlikely to be candidates for renal transplantation or to have familial hyperparathyroidism or a multiple endocrine neoplasia (MEN) syndrome should undergo total parathyroidectomy with implantation of a diced half gland into the muscles of their nondominant forearm.

Medical Management of the Surgical Patient: A Textbook of Perioperative Medicine, ed. M. F. Lubin, R. B. Smith, T. F. Dobson, N. Spell, H. K. Walker. 4th edn. Published by Cambridge University Press. © Cambridge University 2006.

The surgical stress of parathyroidectomy is low and blood transfusions are almost never given.

Usual postoperative course

Expected postoperative hospital stay
Outpatient procedures are appropriate for the excision of solitary and double adenomas and have been used for all less than total parathyroidectomies in some centers; otherwise, the hospital stay is 1 day.

Operative mortality
Essentially 0%.

Special monitoring required
The serum calcium level should be measured daily.

Patient activity and positioning
The head should be elevated 30 to 45 degrees to minimize edema and venous oozing. Patients are out of bed on the day of the operation.

Alimentation
Full liquids are permitted on the day of operation, and a regular diet is resumed the next morning.

Antibiotic coverage
None indicated.

Drains
Many surgeons no longer place drains. If a closed suction drain is inserted, it is removed on the first postoperative day.

Postoperative complications

In the hospital

Hypoparathyroidism
Early postoperative hypocalcemia may occur in patients who have significant bone resorption before operation or in those who undergo excision of large adenomas or subtotal or total parathyroidectomy. Symptomatic hypocalcemia (less than 7.5 mg/dl) is characterized by anxiety, perioral or finger tingling, and a Chvostek's sign; it usually develops 16 to 24 hours after surgery. Intravenous calcium is given to relieve symptoms in the hospital, and oral calcium therapy may be necessary at the time of discharge in patients with dysfunction of a parathyroid remnant, severe "bone hunger," or total parathyroidectomy with

autotransplantation. In many centers in which patients are discharged shortly after operation, calcium supplementation is given at the time of discharge and continued until the patient returns to the clinic.

Hemorrhage, recurrent laryngeal nerve injury
Hemorrhage and recurrent laryngeal nerve injury occur in less than 0.3% of initial operations performed by experienced parathyroid surgeons.

After discharge

"Permanent" hypoparathyroidism
"Permanent" hypoparathyroidism occurs in only 0.6% to 2% of patients after subtotal or total parathyroidectomy or a second cervical exploration for persistent or recurrent hyperparathyroidism. Vitamin D is added to the calcium replacement to enhance absorption. If serial parathyroid hormone levels begin to rise, first the vitamin D and then the calcium supplement should be tapered.

Persistent or recurrent hyperparathyroidism
Persistent disease (failure of operation) or retrospective misdiagnosis occurs in only 2.5% to 5% of patients. The rate of recurrence after excision of an adenoma is under 1% but increases to 5% to 15% in patients with sporadic hyperplasia who undergo subtotal parathyroidectomy. In some series, the recurrence rate for hyperparathyroidism is 15% to 30% in patients with renal, familial, or MEN-associated disease who are treated with less than total parathyroidectomy. Symptomatic persistent or recurrent hyperparathyroidism should be evaluated first by a careful review of the original operative note and pathology report. Preoperative localization studies before reoperation include ultrasound of the neck, computed tomography or magnetic resonance imaging of the mediastinum, and sestamibi scanning. Reoperation by an experienced parathyroid surgeon, particularly after positive localization studies, results in an 85% to 90% cure rate.

FURTHER READING

Bauer, W. & Federman, D. D. Hyperparathyroidism epitomized: the case of Captain Charles E. Martell. *Metabolism* 1962; **11**: 21–29.

Edis, A. J., Beahrs, O. H., & van Heerden, J. A. "Conservative" versus "liberal" approach to parathyroid neck exploration. *Surgery* 1977; **82**: 466–473.

Goldstein, R. E., Billheimer, D., Martin, W. H. *et al.* Sestamibi scanning and minimally invasive radioguided parathyroidectomy without intraoperative parathyroid hormone measurement. *Ann. Surg.* 2003; **237**: 126–135.

Irwin, G. L., Molinari, A. S., Carneiro, D. M. *et al.* Parathyroidectomy: New criteria for evaluating outcome. *Am. Surg.* 1999; **65**: 1186–1189.

Monchik, J. M., Barellini, L., Langer, P. *et al.* Minimally invasive parathyroid surgery in 103 patients with local/regional anesthesia, without exclusion criteria. *Surgery* 2002: **131**: 502–508.

45

Lumpectomy and mastectomy

David V. Feliciano

Emory University School of Medicine, Atlanta, GA

Ductal carcinoma in situ (intraductal carcinoma) most commonly presents as microcalcifications on screening mammography; however, it may present as a mass or with nipple discharge. Because this cancer is confined to the ductal system and does not invade the basement membrane, there is no access to either lymphatic channels or nodes. Diagnosis is made by an image-guided biopsy in which a core of tissue is interpreted by a histopathologist. Wide excision of the area of ductal carcinoma in situ is the preferred therapy for smaller lesions, though obtaining tumor-free margins is often difficult because of the diffuse nature of the disease. Adjuvant irradiation to the remaining ipsilateral breast significantly lowers the risk of later ipsilateral invasive breast carcinoma.

Carcinoma of the breast is the most common invasive cancer in women and occurs with a 2½ times greater incidence than either colorectal or lung cancer. The risk of a woman in the USA developing breast cancer during her lifetime is about 10%. The surgical treatment of breast cancer has changed considerably since 1980, with a much greater emphasis on selective therapy. Patients with stage I (less than 2 cm) or smaller stage II (less than 4 cm) carcinomas diagnosed by fine needle aspiration or image-guided biopsy are treated most frequently with lumpectomy or quadrantectomy, sentinel lymph node biopsy (followed by formal axillary lymph node dissection if node contains metastatic cancer), and postoperative radiotherapy with 50 Gy (5000 rad). Data from numerous studies have documented that disease-free survival and actuarial survival rates of these patients at 8 to 10 years are equivalent to those of patients who undergo traditional mastectomy. Women with stage III breast cancer receive preoperative chemotherapy followed by lumpectomy modified radical mastectomy (pectoralis major and occasionally pectoralis minor muscles are preserved) and radiotherapy. All surgical specimens are sent for the appropriate hormone receptor assays after lumpectomy or mastectomy. Immediate reconstruction of the amputated breast using myocutaneous transposition flaps is also offered to most women who are likely to need a mastectomy. The surgical stress of a lumpectomy or mastectomy is modest. General anesthesia is used for both lumpectomy combined with axillary dissection and modified radical mastectomy, with each operation lasting about 1½ hours. The addition of breast reconstruction with a latissimus dorsi or transverse rectus abdominis pedicled flap after mastectomy adds another 3 to 5 hours to the operative time. Blood replacement is unusual.

Usual postoperative course

Expected postoperative hospital stay

2 or 3 days for lumpectomy and axillary dissection; 3 or 4 days for modified radical mastectomy.

Operative mortality

Under 1%.

Special monitoring required

The volume of postoperative bleeding through suction drains placed under the flaps of a mastectomy is monitored daily to aid in determining when the drains should be removed.

Patient activity and positioning

Patients may be out of bed on the day after the operation. Supervised exercises to maintain mobility of the shoulder on the side of the mastectomy also are begun on this day.

Alimentation

Liquids are ingested on the day of surgery with progression to a regular diet the next day.

Medical Management of the Surgical Patient: A Textbook of Perioperative Medicine, ed. M. F. Lubin, R. B. Smith, T. F. Dobson, N. Spell, H. K. Walker. 4th edn. Published by Cambridge University Press. © Cambridge University 2006.

Antibiotic coverage

Antibiotics are administered only on the day of operation.

Drains

Two or three closed suction drains are placed in the axilla and under the skin flaps if mastectomy has been performed to prevent fluid or blood accumulation and encourage adherence of the flap to the chest wall. Drainage is monitored as described earlier.

Psychological support

Visits from the group Reach to Recovery are of considerable value to patients who have undergone a mastectomy.

Postoperative complications

In the hospital

Wound infection

In obese patients, cellulitis of the mastectomy flaps or actual purulent drainage through suction drains occurs in 4% to 7% of cases. Antibiotics should be administered based on Gram stain, local heat applied, and infrequently a portion of the incision opened.

Necrosis of the edge of the skin flap

If the edges of the skin flaps are dissected too thin during a mastectomy, necrosis may result. Debridement and repeated closure are occasionally necessary.

After discharge

Wound seroma

Serum may accumulate under the skin flaps of a mastectomy if drains are removed prematurely. Needle aspiration and application of a pressure dressing are traditional outpatient treatments, but the use of a small incision and insertion of a soft rubber, open drain often prevents reaccumulation.

Edema of the upper extremity

Edema of the upper extremity occurs in less than 10% of women undergoing standard modified radical mastectomy even when postoperative radiotherapy is used. The primary exception is patients who have extensive nodal involvement around the axillary vein, causing it to become thrombosed in the postoperative period. Edema is treated with elevation and, if necessary, a fitted compression sleeve during the day and an external intermittent compression device at night.

Recurrent cancer

Postoperative radiotherapy administered to various axillary and chest wall ports reduces the incidence of local recurrence by about 15%. Nodules that recur in the old incision are locally excised, but are felt by many to be a marker of distant metastatic disease. Postoperative prophylactic combination chemotherapy is given to premenopausal women with positive lymph nodes. For postmenopausal women with positive lymph nodes and positive hormone receptors, tamoxifen or anastrozole is commonly prescribed. If distant metastases occur, other chemotherapeutic combinations or antihormonal therapy is administered depending on the site of the metastases and the age and hormonal status of the patient.

FURTHER READING

Fisher, B., Redmond, C., Poisson, R. *et al.* Eight-year results of a randomized clinical trial comparing total mastectomy and lumpectomy with or without irradiation in the treatment of breast cancer. *N. Engl. J. Med.* 1989; **320**: 822–828.

Ghafoor, A., Jemal, A., Ward, E. *et al.* Trends in breast cancer by race and ethnicity. *CA. Cancer J. Clin.* 2003; **53**: 342–355.

Haagensen, C. D. & Bodian, C. A personal experience with Halsted's radical mastectomy. *Ann. Surg.* 1984; **199**: 143–150.

Veronesi, U., Paganelli, G., Viale, G. *et al.* A randomized comparison of sentinel-node biopsy with routine axillary dissection in breast cancer. *N. Engl. J. Med.* 2003; **349**: 546–553.

Wong, S. L., Chao, C., Edwards, M. J. *et al.* Accuracy of sentinel lymph node biopsy for patients with T2 and T3 breast cancers. *Am. Surg.* 2001; **67**: 522–528.

46

Gastric procedures (including laparoscopic antireflux, gastric bypass, and gastric banding)

David V. Feliciano

Emory University School of Medicine, Atlanta, GA

Gastric procedures performed with the patient under general anesthesia include those done for complications of peptic ulcer disease (parietal cell vagotomy (PCV), vagotomy and pyloroplasty (VP), vagotomy and antrectomy (VA), hemigastrectomy alone); for benign neoplasms (proximal or distal gastrectomy); and for malignant neoplasms (extended subtotal or total gastrectomy). In the laparoscopic surgery era, antireflux procedures involving the fundus of the stomach and antiobesity procedures including gastric bypass or banding are commonly performed.

While open or laparoscopic PCV or denervation of the fundus and body of the stomach (parietal cell area) is rarely performed currently, open or laparoscopic VP and VA are still occasionally necessary for patients with life-threatening complications of duodenal ulcers – hemorrhage, perforation, or obstruction. Such patients usually have untreated *Helicobacter pylori* infections or a virulent ulcer diathesis of unknown cause. VP and VA involve cutting the vagal nerve trunks at the esophageal hiatus and rearranging or resecting the pylorus. With antrectomy, all the gastrin-secreting cells are removed as well and reanastomosis to the duodenum (Billroth I) or jejunum (Billroth II) is necessary. Preoperative decompression of the stomach for 5 to 7 days and antibiotic irrigation the night before operation is indicated in patients with gastric dilation from pyloric obstruction. Hemigastrectomy (removal of the ulcer and the distal stomach) is 96% curative for patients with uncomplicated and complicated gastric ulcers and 100% curative for those with benign tumors (leiomyomas). The stress of these procedures is moderate, they take 1½ to 2 hours to perform, and blood transfusion is required only in patients with anemia or active bleeding.

Extended subtotal gastrectomy (additional removal of the greater and lesser omentum, the celiac nodes, and occasionally the spleen) or total gastrectomy is reserved for patients with mid-stomach or proximal adenocarcinomas. With a leiomyosarcoma, only the gastrectomy is performed. Reconstruction is by a Roux (borrowed) limb of proximal jejunum. The stress of surgery is moderate, the procedure is performed in 3 hours, and blood transfusion may be necessary if neoplasms are adherent to the pancreas, liver, or retroperitoneum.

Open or laparoscopic anti-reflux procedures are performed in symptomatic patients who undergo extensive preoperative testing with esophagogastroduodenoscopy, 24-hour pH testing, and esophageal motility studies. In patients with normal esophageal motility, a laparoscopic Nissen fundoplication is the procedure of choice. Through five trocars placed in the upper abdomen, the fundus of the stomach is mobilized by division of the short gastric vessels. The previously mobilized gastroesophageal junction is then encircled with a short fundal wrap while a 52–60 French dilator is present in the esophagus to prevent narrowing. The stress of surgery is modest, the procedure is performed in less than 2 hours, and blood transfusion is unnecessary.

Open or laparoscopic gastric bariatric procedures are indicated in patients with a body mass index (BMI = weight in kilograms/height in meters^2) of 40 kg/m^2. They are also performed in patients with a BMI between 35 and 40 kg/m^2 if associated obesity conditions such as sleep apnea, Pickwickian syndrome, type II diabetes mellitus, or hypotension are present. Laparoscopic dissection and stapling in the upper abdomen creates a 15–30 ml proximal gastric pouch based on the lesser curve of the stomach. A Roux (borrowed) jejunal limb with a length of 75–150 cm based on the patient's BMI is then passed posterior (retrocolic) or anterior (antecolic) to the transverse colon and stapled to the small gastric pouch. The stress of surgery is modest, the procedure is performed in 1½–3 hours based on the operator's experience, and blood

Medical Management of the Surgical Patient: A Textbook of Perioperative Medicine, ed. M. F. Lubin, R. B. Smith, T. F. Dobson, N. Spell, H. K. Walker. 4th edn. Published by Cambridge University Press. © Cambridge University 2006.

transfusion is unnecessary. The need to convert to an open procedure in experienced centers is less than 5%–7%. Excess weight loss was 77% at 30 months in one recently published large series. The laparoscopic insertion of an adjustable gastric band to produce a calibrated outlet below a proximal gastric pouch of 15–30 ml has been performed for over 10 years, primarily in Europe. The advantages of this operation are that it is easier to perform than gastric bypass and that it preserves the normal gastrointestinal stream and absorption. There is less weight loss and more long-term regaining of weight with this procedure as compared to the laparoscopic gastric bypass. The stress of surgery is modest, the procedure is performed in 1–2 hours, and blood transfusion is unnecessary. Excess weight loss has been 45%–55% after 2 years in European studies.

Usual postoperative course

Expected postoperative hospital stay
7 to 10 days for VP, VA, or subtotal gastrectomy, and 12 to 14 days for total gastrectomy. Two days for laparoscopic antireflux procedure, gastric bypass, or adjustable gastric band.

Operative mortality
1% to 2% for elective VP, VA, and gastrectomy; 5% to 15% for emergency VP, VA, and gastrectomy; and 3% to 8% for elective total gastrectomy. Less than 1% for laparoscopic antireflux procedure, gastric bypass, or adjustable gastric band.

Special monitoring required
Nasogastric or nasojejunal tube drainage is monitored and replaced intravenously if it is excessive. Serum electrolytes also are measured and replaced as needed.

Patient activity and positioning
Patients may be out of bed on the day after the operation.

Alimentation
After operations for ulcer or neoplasm, patients are permitted clear liquids with the return of bowel function and food intake is advanced as tolerated. Patients with VAs or gastrectomies of any type are advised to eat slowly, drink less with meals, and avoid milk products in the early postoperative period as they adjust to the new size of their stomachs and loss of the pylorus. They are also advised to avoid large amounts of foods that are difficult to digest, including oranges, broccoli, and asparagus. Patients who have had total gastrectomies remain on distal enteral feedings or hyperalimentation until anastomoses are healed (discussed later).

Patients are permitted clear liquids on the first postoperative morning after laparoscopic antireflux procedure. If a Gastrografin contrast study is normal on the second postoperative day after gastric bypass, a clear liquid diet is started.

Antibiotic coverage
A cephalosporin or an advanced penicillin is administered preoperatively and for 24 hours postoperatively. If perforation of a duodenal or gastric ulcer is noted at surgery, the antibiotic is continued for 5 to 7 days postoperatively.

Antiemetics
Because of the risk of disruption of the fundoplication due to earlier postoperative vomiting, liberal use of antiemetics is encouraged.

Drains
After gastrectomy and reconstruction with a gastrojejunostomy, the duodenal stump is drained with a closed suction drain for 5 to 7 days. After total gastrectomy, the esophagojejunal anastomosis is drained by many surgeons until a healed anastomosis is demonstrated.

Upper gastrointestinal radiography
Upper gastrointestinal radiography is performed with water-soluble contrast 7 to 10 days after total gastrectomy to check healing of the esophagojejunal anastomosis. If a small leak is present, patients remain on distal enteral feedings or hyperalimentation until a repeat study is performed in 5 to 7 days. The gastric pouch and gastrojejunostomy after gastric bypass are evaluated by Gastrografin as described above.

Postoperative complications after open procedures

In the hospital

Wound infection
In patients with bleeding or perforated ulcers, gastric acid is neutralized by blood or food. This allows for overgrowth of bacteria, and open packing or delayed primary closure of the subcutaneous tissue and skin is appropriate after many emergency gastric procedures. If a wound infection does occur, treatment requires drainage and appropriate antibiotics.

Duodenal stump leak

Duodenal stump leak occurs in 1% to 2% of patients after gastric resection with gastrojejunostomy. Right upper quadrant pain, fever, tachycardia, and bilious drainage out of the suction drain placed beneath the stump are diagnostic. The leak is treated with prohibition of oral intake, insertion of a sump drain under fluoroscopy if needed, use of intravenous hyperalimentation, and administration of antibiotics and a somatostatin analogue (Sandostatin). Re-exploration is indicated only if sepsis does not resolve with insertion of the sump drain.

Stomal dysfunction

Slow gastric emptying occurs in less than 5% of patients after gastrectomy, particularly if gastrojejunostomy has been performed. If output through the nasogastric tube is excessive at 7 days after surgery, upper gastrointestinal radiography with water-soluble contrast is performed. If the agent does not pass through the anastomosis, a second study with barium is performed the next day. Passage of the barium is reassuring, and nasogastric tube decompression and hyperalimentation are continued for 2 to 3 more weeks as need. Failure of the barium to pass mandates endoscopy to rule out a mechanical obstruction.

After discharge

Nutritional disturbances

Megaloblastic anemia from loss of intrinsic factor and iron-deficiency anemia from unknown causes occur over time in many patients with previous gastrectomies. Life-long annual monitoring of hemoglobin levels is appropriate, with replacement therapy administered as needed. Calcium deficiency and steatorrhea also have occurred.

Dumping syndrome

The passage of a hypertonic food bolus directly into the duodenum or jejunum after an antrectomy may precipitate sweating, weakness, palpitations, nausea, vomiting, and diarrhea due to hormonal changes, as well as an outpouring of extracellular fluid into the upper gastrointestinal tract. Symptomatic dumping occurs in less than 15% of patients. Only 1% of patients may require remedial operations after failing to respond to a change in dietary habits (restriction of fluids, carbohydrates, and extra salt with meals).

Diarrhea

About 10% to 25% of patients have altered bowel movements after truncal vagotomy. Only 1% to 2% require remedial operations after failure to respond to a change in dietary habits (see earlier) or to the use of common medications such as codeine, diphenoxylate, or cholestyramine.

Gastric atony

Delayed gastric emptying is a persistent problem in 1% to 2% of patients and may respond to the administration of metoclopramide or erythromycin lactobionate. Remedial operation consists of near-total gastrectomy with Roux-en-Y gastrojejunostomy.

Marginal or recurrent ulcer

A marginal or stomal ulcer develops in about 1% of patients undergoing VA for duodenal ulcer, 4% to 6% of those undergoing gastrectomy for gastric ulcer, and 10–12% undergoing VP for duodenal ulcer – if postoperative anti-*Helicobacter pylori* therapy is not administered. A significantly elevated gastrin level is indicative of a previously undiagnosed Zollinger–Ellison syndrome or retained antrum syndrome after antral resection.

Other postgastrectomy complications

The afferent loop syndrome, efferent loop syndrome, and alkaline reflux gastritis occur infrequently, but remedial operations are available for correction.

Gastric stump carcinoma

Carcinomas of the gastric pouch develop in as many as 5% of patients who survive 10 to 15 years after gastrectomy. Late-developing symptoms of pain and anemia in patients who have previously done well after gastrectomy demand endoscopy with biopsy.

Postoperative complications after laparoscopic procedures

In the hospital

Failure of fundoplication to stay in place

This very rare complication is most often due to early postoperative vomiting, failure to divide the short gastric vessels, or improper fixation of the wrap to the crura of the diaphragm.

Wound infection

After laparoscopic gastric bypass, infection at port sites occurs in less than 2% of patients. Opening of the port site, irrigation, and open packing are appropriate treatment.

Leak from gastrointestinal tract

Leaks from the gastrojejunostomy or gastric pouch occurred in 14% of patients in one recent series. If asymptomatic, they can be observed. When there is excessive drainage through a Jackson–Pratt drain placed at surgery or peritonitis develops, laparoscopic reoperation is indicated.

After discharge

Late failure of fundoplication

In approximately 10% of patients, esophageal reflux recurs due to disruption of the hiatal repair, disruption of the fundoplication, or herniation of the fundoplication. Redo laparoscopic fundoplication is indicated and has an 80% success rate.

Prolonged nausea or vomiting after gastric bypass

In approximately 10% of patients, these symptoms occur. They spontaneously resolve in most patients.

Stricture of gastrojejunostomy after gastric bypass

Late strictures of the stapled gastrojejunostomy suture line occur in approximately 5% of patients and are treated with endoscopic balloon dilatation.

Iron deficiency anemia after gastric bypass

Because the majority of the stomach is bypassed by this procedure, iron deficiency anemia occurs in 20% of patients. Oral replacement of iron is the preferred therapy.

Need to reposition or deflate laparoscopic adjustable gastric band

Because of migration of the band, obstruction in patients with unrecognized esophageal dysmotility, gastric erosions, or patient non-compliance, the band will have to be moved or removed laparoscopically in 10–20% of patients.

FURTHER READING

Angrisani, L., Alkilani, M., Basso, N. *et al.* Italian Collaborative Study Group for the Lap-Band System. Laparoscopic Italian experience with the Lap-Band. *Obes. Surg.* 2001; **11**: 307–310.

Feliciano, D. V. Surgical options and results of treatment of perforated ulcers. *Curr. Probl. Surg.* 1987; **4**: 301–307.

Hunter, J. G., Swanstrom, L., & Waring, J. P. Dysphagia after laparoscopic antireflux surgery. The impact of operative technique. *Ann. Surg.* 1996; **224**: 51–57.

Nguyen, N. T., Goldman, C., Rosenquist, C. J. *et al.* Laparoscopic versus open gastric bypass: a randomized study of outcomes, quality of life, and costs. *Ann. Surg.* 2001; **234**: 279–289.

Schauer, P. R., Ikramuddin, S., Gourash, W. *et al.* Outcomes after laparoscopic Roux-en-Y gastric bypass for morbid obesity. *Ann. Surg.* 2000; **232**: 515–529.

47

Small bowel resection

David V. Feliciano

Emory University School of Medicine, Atlanta, GA

Small bowel resection is performed in a variety of settings, the most common of which are traumatic perforation, thrombotic or embolic infarction, regional enteritis, and concomitant colectomy. Less common indications for resection include benign or malignant neoplasms (leiomyoma, hemangioma, carcinoid, lymphoma, adenocarcinoma, sarcoma), fistula resulting from a previous repair or resection, symptomatic Meckel's diverticulum, neutropenic enterocolitis, and spontaneous perforation in patients with cancer who are receiving chemotherapy and corticosteroids.

The most significant change in the operative management of small bowel disease in recent years has been the increasing use of laparoscopic approaches. In patients with inflammatory small bowel disease, laparoscopic operations now include diversion for complex fistula, takedown of end or loop stoma, segmental resection, stricturoplasty, and lysis of adhesions. Conversion rates to an open approach have ranged from 2%–40% in series published since 1993. Such conversions are most often due to dense adhesions from prior operations and excessive inflammation.

Open segmental resection and end-to-end anastomosis with suture or staples usually can be performed in 20 minutes. Major laparoscopic resections, particularly those involving the colon in addition to the small bowel, generally take 3 to 5 hours. With the exception of those performed for a neoplasm in the adjacent right colon, most resections of the small bowel for trauma, infarction, or inflammatory bowel disease cause moderate to severe stress. General anesthesia is used, the duration of the procedure depends on the indication, and blood transfusions are necessary only in patients with trauma, extensive inflammation, or infiltrating neoplasms.

Usual postoperative course

Expected postoperative hospital stay
5 to 7 days.

Operative mortality
2% to 3% for elective resection, 12% for penetrating trauma with two other organ injuries, 25% for superior mesenteric artery embolism, and 60% for superior mesenteric artery thrombosis.

Special monitoring required
Many patients with major abdominal trauma or midgut infarction require postoperative hemodynamic monitoring with a pulmonary artery catheter. Serial measurements of arterial pH are also worthwhile if bowel with borderline viability is left in the abdomen at the first operation.

Patient activity and positioning
Patients may be out of bed on the day after the operation, depending on hemodynamic stability.

Alimentation
For routine procedures, clear liquids are begun with the return of bowel function and advanced as tolerated. In cases involving multiple intraabdominal injuries or major resection of the midgut secondary to infarction, intravenous hyperalimentation is begun as soon as patients are hemodynamically stable.

Antibiotic coverage
All patients receive cephalosporin or advanced penicillin preoperatively and for 24 hours postoperatively. In the presence of established peritonitis from infarction or

Medical Management of the Surgical Patient: A Textbook of Perioperative Medicine, ed. M. F. Lubin, R. B. Smith, T. F. Dobson, N. Spell, H. K. Walker. 4th edn. Published by Cambridge University Press. © Cambridge University 2006.

perforation of regional enteritis, a Meckel's diverticulum, neutropenic enterocolitis, or chemotherapy, the antibiotic is continued for 5 to 7 days postoperatively.

Postoperative complications

In the hospital

Wound infection
See Chapter 58.

Breakdown of enterotomy repair or small bowel anastomosis
See Chapter 58.

Recurrent infarction
If bowel with questionable viability is left in the abdomen or a borderline stoma is brought to the skin at the first operation, further ischemic changes may occur and necessitate reoperation. Many surgeons choose to close only the skin of the abdominal incision at the first operation and perform a second operation (second-look procedure) 12 hours later to reassess the questionably viable bowel. Others monitor the color of a stoma or serial arterial pH levels to assist in determining whether reoperation is necessary.

Prolonged ileus
Peristalsis may return slowly in patients with multiple intra-abdominal injuries, a superior mesenteric artery embolus or thrombus, chronic obstruction from enteritis or a neoplasm, or diffuse peritonitis from a perforation. Continuous nasogastric suction, intravenous hyperalimentation, and patience are indicated. If there is serious concern about a possible early mechanical small bowel obstruction instead of an ileus, the use of an oral colon-cleaning agent or barium is indicated as described in the chapter on "Lysis of adhesions."

After discharge

Obstruction
Early in-hospital adhesive small bowel obstruction occurs in 2% to 3% of patients who undergo small bowel resection. Late episodes of adhesive obstruction occur in 10% to 25% of patients.

Nutritional deficiency
Massive resection of the midgut may lead to chronic diarrhea and nutritional deficiencies, particularly if the ileocecal valve has been sacrificed. In-hospital and subsequent home hyperalimentation is indicated in such patients. Progressive hyperplasia of the lining of the remaining midgut may allow for resumption of enteral feedings over time.

FURTHER READING

Crohn, B. B., Ginzburg, L., & Oppenheimer, G. D. Regional ileitis: a pathologic and clinical entity. *J. Am. Med. Assoc.* 1932; **251**: 73–81.

Fazio, V. W., Marchetti, F., Church, J. M. *et al.* Effect of resection margins on the recurrence of Crohn's disease in the small bowel. A randomized controlled trial. *Ann. Surg.* 1996; **224**: 563–571.

Levy, P. J., Krausz, M. M., & Manny, J. Acute mesenteric ischemia: improved results: a retrospective analysis of ninety-two patients. *Surgery* 1990; **107**: 372–380.

Michelassi, F., Hurst, R. D., Melis, M. *et al.* Side-to-side isoperistaltic strictureplasty in extensive Crohn's disease: a prospective longitudinal study. *Ann. Surg.* 2000; **232**: 401–408.

Schmidt, C. M., Talamini, M. A., Kaufman, H. S. *et al.* Laparoscopic surgery for Crohn's disease: reasons for conversion. *Ann. Surg.* 2001; **233**: 733–739.

48

Appendectomy

David V. Feliciano

Emory University School of Medicine, Atlanta, GA

Appendectomy is performed for acute appendicitis (simple, suppurative, gangrenous, gangrenous with perforation); chronic or recurrent appendicitis; as an interval procedure after recovery from an appendiceal abscess; for small (less than 2.5 cm) carcinoid tumors or benign mucoceles; and prophylactically during laparotomy for other conditions. The accuracy of diagnosis in acute appendicitis has increased to over 90% in several recent series using diagnostic adjuncts such as graded-compression ultrasound and special CT protocols. In addition, percutaneous drainage of periappendiceal abscesses may allow for a subsequent single operation to remove the remnant of the perforated appendix (interval appendectomy).

With the patient under general anesthesia, appendectomy may be performed through a right lower quadrant muscle-splitting incision or by a laparoscopic approach using three ports. With simple, suppurative, or gangrenous appendicitis, the stress of operation is minimal. For patients with perforated gangrenous appendicitis and diffuse peritonitis or with a large intraabdominal abscess, stress can be moderate or major. The duration of a simple appendectomy is 45 minutes, but this increases to 60 to 75 minutes in obese patients with retrocecal appendicitis and rupture. In some of these patients, the usual 6- to 7-cm incision must be extended to gain exposure of the posterior cecum and ascending colon. Blood transfusion is never required.

Usual postoperative course

Expected postoperative hospital stay
1 to 2 days for simple, suppurative, or gangrenous (without rupture) appendicitis; 7 to 10 days for perforated appendicitis with diffuse peritonitis or an intra-abdominal abscess.

Operative mortality
0.1% for simple or suppurative appendicitis, 0.6% for gangrenous appendicitis, and 5% for perforated appendicitis.

Special monitoring required
Patients with sepsis syndrome or shock secondary to perforated appendicitis require postoperative hemodynamic monitoring with a pulmonary artery catheter.

Patient activity and positioning
Patients with appendicitis may be out of bed on the day of the operation and resume activity gradually during the first 2 weeks after hospital discharge.

Alimentation
Clear liquids are given on the day of operation, and food intake is advanced as tolerated in patients with nonperforated appendicitis. In those with perforated appendicitis, clear liquids are permitted with the return of bowel function and intake is advanced as tolerated.

Antibiotic coverage
All patients with suspected appendicitis receive a cephalosporin or advanced penicillin preoperatively. Those with simple or suppurative appendicitis require no further antibiotic coverage. All patients with gangrenous appendicitis receive antibiotics for 24 hours postoperatively, and those with perforated appendicitis and secondary peritonitis or intraabdominal abscess continue to receive antibiotics for 5 to 7 days postoperatively.

Drains
Closed suction drains are placed in well-defined abscess cavities in the pericecal or pelvic area for 5 to 7 days postoperatively. A decision for removal is based on clinical

Medical Management of the Surgical Patient: A Textbook of Perioperative Medicine, ed. M. F. Lubin, R. B. Smith, T. F. Dobson, N. Spell, H. K. Walker. 4th edn. Published by Cambridge University Press. © Cambridge University 2006.

findings, postoperative computed tomographic scan or a sinogram performed through the drains.

Wound closure

Open packing of the subcutaneous tissue and skin is indicated in adult patients with extensive gangrenous or perforated appendicitis. Delayed primary closure of the wound can be performed on the sixth postoperative day and has a 10% to 20% risk of infection.

Postoperative complications

In the hospital

Diffuse peritonitis

Diffuse peritonitis that is present at the time of appendectomy may lead to sepsis syndrome or septic shock in the early postoperative period or to intraabdominal abscess in the late postoperative period.

Wound infection

Wound infection occurs primarily when attempts are made to close the subcutaneous tissue and skin in patients with gangrenous or perforated appendicitis. Treatment includes the administration of antibiotics based on Gram stain results, the application of local heat, opening of a portion of the incision, and daily pack changes until healing by secondary intention occurs.

Intraabdominal abscess

Intraabdominal abscess may develop in up to 5%–15% of patients with gangrenous or perforated appendicitis. Diagnosis and treatment are by clinical examination and computed tomography followed by percutaneous drainage, transrectal drainage for pelvic abscess, or reoperation for paracecal or subphrenic abscess.

Fecal fistula

Less than 1% of patients experience blow-out of the appendiceal stump leading to a cecocutaneous fistula through the incision or a drain. Spontaneous closure usually occurs within 2 to 3 weeks.

After discharge

Late diagnosis of a carcinoid tumor or appendiceal carcinoma

A late pathology report may describe the presence of a carcinoid tumor larger than 2.5 cm or an appendiceal carcinoma in the resected specimen. Reoperation for a formal right hemicolectomy is indicated.

FURTHER READING

Fitz, R. H. Perforating inflammation of the vermiform appendix, with special reference to its early diagnosis and treatment. *Trans. Assoc. Am. Phys.* 1886; **1**: 107–144.

Frazee, R. C., Roberts, J. W., Symmonds, R. E. *et al.* A prospective randomized trial comparing open versus laparoscopic appendectomy. *Ann. Surg.* 1994; **219**: 725–728.

Mattei, P., Sola, J. E., & Yeo, C. J. Chronic and recurrent appendicitis are uncommon entities often misdiagnosed. *J. Am. Coll. Surg.* 1994; **178**: 385–389.

Puylaert, J. B., Rutgers, P. H., Lalisang, R. I. *et al.* A prospective study of ultrasonography in the diagnosis of appendicitis. *N. Engl. J. Med.* 1987; **317**: 666–669.

Rao, P. M., Rhea, J. T., Novelline, R. A. *et al.* Effect of computed tomography of the appendix on treatment of patients and use of hospital resources. *N. Engl. J. Med.* 1998; **338**: 141–146.

49

Colon resection

David V. Feliciano

Emory University School of Medicine, Atlanta, GA

Open or laparoscopic colon resection is performed for a variety of conditions, the most common of which are benign or malignant neoplasms (tubular or villoglandular adenomas, adenocarcinoma, carcinoid, lymphoma); complications of diverticular disease (perforation with peritonitis or abscess, stricture, bleeding); extensive traumatic perforations; angiodysplasia or arteriovenous malformation with lower gastrointestinal bleeding; and inflammatory bowel disease (ulcerative colitis, segmental colonic Crohn's disease, toxic megacolon). Less common indications for resection include volvulus of the sigmoid colon or cecum; thrombotic, embolic, or low-flow infarction; and premalignant conditions (familial polyposis, Gardner's syndrome).

Hemicolectomy for malignant neoplasms involves excision of the area of the tumor, at least 10 cm of normal proximal colon or small bowel, and 5 cm of normal distal colon as well as the regional lymphatics that accompany the major vessels. Therefore, a formal right hemicolectomy for carcinoma of the cecum would involve excision of 10 cm of distal ileum, the ascending colon, hepatic flexure, and right half of the transverse colon. In contrast, segmental resection for complications of diverticular disease, Crohn's disease, colonic volvulus, or infarction involves only grossly diseased bowel without excision of regional lymphatics. Subtotal abdominal colectomy with ileorectostomy is performed for patients with non-familial synchronous scattered benign or malignant neoplasms. It is also used in some patients with megacolon secondary to obstructing neoplasms of the sigmoid or rectosigmoid colon or of the upper rectum. A near-total abdominal colectomy with preservation of a seromuscular short rectal cuff and the sphincter muscles to preserve anal continence through the creation of an ileal pouch-anal anastomosis is indicated in patients with severe chronic ulcerative colitis, familial polyposis, or Gardner's syndrome.

Preoperative colon preparation involves gavage cleaning of the colon in combination with non-absorbable antibiotics (neomycin and erythromycin base at 1:00 pm, 2:00 pm, and 11:00 pm the day before operation). After colon resection as described above, a sutured or stapled anastomosis is performed. A difficult laparoscopic colectomy may become easier with a 4–8 cm incision to allow for insertion of one hand (hand-assisted). Because of the tedious nature of intracorporeal suture techniques in laparoscopic colon surgery, this limited incision made in the body wall will allow for the performance of an extracorporeal anastomosis. Emergency resections involving the right half of the colon – as might be performed for perforated cecal diverticulitis, angiodysplasia with bleeding, traumatic perforation, cecal volvulus, or low-flow infarction – are often reconstructed with an ileocolostomy, even without preoperative or intraoperative bowel preparation, because surgeons consider this to be a small bowel-type anastomosis. For the same reason, emergency resections involving the entire colon (for an unknown site of bleeding or megacolon secondary to an obstructing neoplasm of the sigmoid or rectosigmoid colon) are also reconstructed with an ileorectostomy by some surgeons. Emergency resections involving the transverse colon or left half of the colon are usually followed by creation of a proximal end colostomy and a mucous fistula (distal stoma in body wall) or Hartmann pouch (distal end of bowel closed and left in the abdomen).

Elective colon resection, even near-total colectomy, is a controlled operation with little blood loss and only moderate stress to the patient. Multiple studies have demonstrated that elective laparoscopic colectomies performed for complications of diverticulitis or for cancer result in less blood loss, less postoperative morbidity, shorter hospital stays, and earlier return to normal activities. Preliminary data suggest that the 5-year survival after

Medical Management of the Surgical Patient: A Textbook of Perioperative Medicine, ed. M. F. Lubin, R. B. Smith, T. F. Dobson, N. Spell, H. K. Walker. 4th edn. Published by Cambridge University Press. © Cambridge University 2006.

elective resection for colon cancer is improved when the procedure is performed laparoscopically as well. Emergency colon resection for perforated sigmoid diverticulitis, bleeding angiodysplasia, extensive traumatic perforation, toxic megacolon, or infarction from volvulus or low flow may be associated with moderate blood loss and is a significant stress, particularly in elderly patients.

Usual postoperative course

Expected postoperative hospital stay
4 to 7 days after laparoscopic procedures; 4–9 days after open procedures depending on protocol used.

Operative mortality
2% to 6% for elective resection in elderly patients; 4% to 9% for emergency right colon or subtotal resection with primary anastomosis; 10% to 20% for subtotal resection in the presence of a perforated toxic megacolon or unknown site of lower gastrointestinal hemorrhage.

Special monitoring required
Postoperative hemodynamic monitoring with a pulmonary artery catheter is necessary in many elderly patients with emergency resection of the colon and in younger patients with major abdominal trauma including injury to the colon.

Patient activity and positioning
Depending on hemodynamic stability and the presence of other injuries, patients may be out of bed on the day after the operation.

Alimentation
For routine procedures, patients are permitted clear liquids with the return of bowel function; intake of food is advanced as tolerated. Patients with emergency subtotal resection for obstruction, bleeding, toxic megacolon, or multiple intraabdominal injuries receive jejunal feedings or intravenous hyperalimentation when they are hemodynamically stable.

Antibiotic coverage
All patients receive intravenous cephalosporin, advanced penicillin, metronidazole, or a combination of antibiotics before and at least 24 hours after the procedure. Antibiotics are continued for 5 to 7 days postoperatively in patients with established peritonitis from perforated sigmoid or cecal diverticulitis, perforated toxic megacolon, gangrenous colon from volvulus or vascular catastrophe, or delayed operation for traumatic perforation.

Delayed wound closure
Open packing of the skin and subcutaneous tissue of the incision is indicated with gangrenous or perforated colon. Delayed primary closure is appropriate at 5 to 6 days in patients with clean, deep wounds that would otherwise require 6 to 12 weeks of dressing changes at home.

Drains
Colectomies above the peritoneal reflection are not drained unless a well-defined abscess cavity from a perforation is present. Many surgeons drain the deep pelvis after low anterior resection of the rectosigmoid colon or upper rectum.

Postoperative complications

In the hospital

Wound infection
See Chapter 58.

Breakdown of anastomosis
Disruption of an ileocolostomy or colocolostomy in the early postoperative period is a rare but potentially lethal complication. Patients with obvious fecal peritonitis require early reoperation. After 5 to 7 days, a partial leak leads to a contained perianastomotic or pelvic abscess or a colocutaneous fistula through a drainage site or the abdominal incision. Percutaneous drainage of an intraperitoneal abscess may be a worthwhile first step, although a fecal fistula is an obvious risk. Operative transrectal drainage is appropriate for a pelvic abscess that is palpable on rectal examination. Ileocolocutaneous or colocutaneous fistulas are treated with prohibition of oral intake, intravenous hyperalimentation, administration of a somatostatin analogue, and protection of the surrounding skin. In the absence of a foreign body, intraabdominal infection, a short tract (epithelialization), residual neoplasm, or distal obstruction ("FIEND"), the fistula is expected to close without reoperation.

Pseudomembranous enterocolitis
The sudden onset of tenderness over the remaining colon in association with diarrhea and systemic toxicity is strongly suggestive of pseudomembranous enterocolitis. A specimen of stool is sent for *Clostridium difficile*

enterotoxin and empiric vancomycin is administered intravenously.

After discharge

Change in bowel movements

Patients who have undergone resection of the ileocecal valve or an extensive portion of the left colon (left hemicolectomy, subtotal or total colectomy with anastomosis) have an increased number of bowel movements. These usually decrease over time; the average number of bowel movements in one series of patients with subtotal colectomy and ileorectostomy was two per day after 6 months.

Patients with total colectomy, creation of an ileal pouch, and an ileal pouch–anal anastomosis average five or six bowel movements in 24 hours. Complete daytime continence is present in 90%, even on long-term follow-up. Nighttime continence is present in 75% on long-term follow-up.

Recurrent tumor

After resection for colorectal carcinoma, the patient is monitored by colonoscopy every 6 months and carcinoembryonic antigen levels every 2 months for 2 years, after which time follow-up intervals may be lengthened. Reoperation is indicated if colonoscopy reveals recurrent tumor or the carcinoembryonic antigen level is increased but less than 10 ng/ml, and if no distant metastases are seen with positron emission tomography. The role of radio-labeled monoclonal antibody directed against tumor-associated antigens as a surveillance tool is being studied. Incisional or laparoscopic port site recurrences occur in 1%–2% of patients with resection for cancer.

FURTHER READING

Guller, D., Jain, N., Hervey, S. *et al.* Laparoscopic vs. open colectomy: outcomes comparison based on large nationwide databases. *Arch. Surg.* 2003; **138**: 1179–1186.

Lacy, A. M., Garcia-Valdecasas, J. C., Delgado, S. *et al.* Laparoscopy-assisted colectomy versus open colectomy for treatment of non-metastatic colon cancer: a randomized trial. *Lancet* 2002; **359**: 2224–2229.

Pahlman, L. Treatment of colorectal cancer. *Ann. Chir. Gynaecol.* 2000; **89**: 216–220.

Senagore, A. J., Duepree, H. J., Delaney, C. P. *et al.* Results of a standardized technique and postoperative care plan for laparoscopic sigmoid colectomy: A 30-month experience. *Dis. Colon Rectum* 2003; **46**: 503–509.

Weeks, J. C., Nelson, H., Gelber, S. *et al.* Clinical Outcomes of Surgical Therapy (COST) Study Group. Short-term quality-of-life outcomes following laparoscopic assisted colectomy vs. open colectomy for colon cancer: a randomized trial. *J. Am. Med. Assoc.* 2002; **287**: 321–328.

50

Abdominoperineal resection

David V. Feliciano

Emory University School of Medicine, Atlanta, GA

Abdominoperineal resection (Miles' operation) with excision of the rectum, anus, and sphincter muscles and creation of a permanent end colostomy is performed to remove malignant neoplasms of the mid or lower rectum or anus – adenocarcinoma, carcinoid, lymphoma, squamous cell carcinoma remaining after chemotherapy, cloacogenic carcinoma, basal cell carcinoma, and malignant melanoma – or extensive Crohn's disease with fistulas of the same areas. The operation is conducted with a transabdominal laparoscopic approach or through a low midline laparotomy incision and a circumferential perianal incision and is essentially a posterior exenteration of the pelvis. Included in the excision are the rectosigmoid colon, the rectum, the pelvic mesocolon, the lymph nodes associated with the three sets of hemorrhoidal vessels, the levator muscles out to the ischial tuberosities, the anus, and the perianal skin. As an alternate approach, many surgeons use low anterior transabdominal resection with an anastomosis in patients with adenocarcinoma of the upper or mid-rectum because it produces an essentially equivalent survival and precludes the need for a colostomy. The surgeon must be able to excise a 2 cm margin of normal bowel beyond the rectal tumor and to have enough rectum left at or above the levator muscles to allow the performance of a stapled or handsewn anastomosis.

A related approach is excision of the rectum alone (without the mesocolon or lymph nodes) and preservation of a seromuscular short rectal cuff to maintain anal continence through the creation of an ileal pouch–anal anastomosis in patients with severe chronic ulcerative colitis, familial polyposis, or Gardner's syndrome, but not in those with Crohn's disease. This operation is most commonly performed as part of a near-total abdominal colectomy and differs significantly from the exenterative rectal procedure described in this chapter.

If preoperative external-beam radiotherapy has been used to shrink a large rectal cancer and sterilize areas of adherence to the sacrum posteriorly or to the vagina or prostate gland anteriorly, abdominoperineal resection is delayed for 4 to 6 weeks. Preoperative colon preparation involves gavage cleaning of the colon in combination with non-absorbable antibiotics (neomycin and erythromycin base at 1 pm, 2 pm, and 11 pm the day before surgery). The ideal site for the permanent end colostomy in the left lower quadrant is marked by the surgeon or enterostomal therapy nurse the night before operation. The procedure is often performed by two surgical teams simultaneously. The team performing the laparoscopic approach or laparotomy mobilizes the rectosigmoid colon, rectum, and mesorectum with vessels and lymph nodes off the sacrum, divides the colon with a stapler, and creates a proximal end sigmoid colostomy. The second team excises the perianal skin, anus, and levator muscles out to the ischial tuberosities and removes the entire specimen through the perineum.

Extensive resection of a mid-rectal tumor may remove the pelvic peritoneum. Some surgeons leave the pelvis open and allow the small bowel to fall into the hollow of the sacrum, while others suture a sheet of absorbable mesh to replace the pelvic peritoneum and support the small bowel above the deep pelvic space. This is particularly useful if further postoperative radiotherapy is necessary because of tumor invasion of the pelvic side wall. Before the subcutaneous tissue and the skin of the perineal incision are closed, closed suction drains are inserted through the upper medial buttocks into the deep pelvic space for postoperative irrigation. In rare cases, the perineal wound must be left open because of sacral bleeding, requiring the insertion of pelvic packing, or because of extensive contamination associated with Crohn's disease of the anorectum.

Medical Management of the Surgical Patient: A Textbook of Perioperative Medicine, ed. M. F. Lubin, R. B. Smith, T. F. Dobson, N. Spell, H. K. Walker. 4th edn. Published by Cambridge University Press. © Cambridge University 2006.

A laparoscopic approach increases operative time by 50%–100% and the conversion rate (laparoscopic-to-open) is approximately 20% in experienced hands. Moderate blood loss can occur with either approach, particularly in patients in whom the neoplasm is affixed to the sacrum or prostate gland. Because the procedure involves two incisions and creates a large dead space in the posterior pelvis that takes time to heal, the stress is moderate to severe in all patients.

Usual postoperative course

Expected postoperative hospital stay
7 to 11 days.

Operative mortality
2%.

Special monitoring required
During a difficult procedure, postoperative hemodynamic monitoring with a pulmonary artery catheter may occasionally be necessary in elderly patients with excessive blood loss.

Patient activity and positioning
Patients may be out of bed on the day after the operation, depending on hemodynamic stability.

Alimentation
For routine procedures, patients are permitted clear liquids with the return of bowel function and food intake is advanced as tolerated.

Antibiotic coverage
All patients receive intravenous cephalosporin, advanced penicillin, metronidazole, or a combination of antibiotics preoperatively and for at least 24 hours postoperatively.

Delayed closure if the perineal wound has been left open
Once the pelvic packing has been removed or perineal cellulitis from previously resected Crohn's disease has resolved, delayed primary closure of the skin or transposition of gracilis muscle flaps by the plastic surgery service into the pelvic space and closure of the skin is performed.

Drains
Irrigation with normal saline at a rate of 1000 ml/12 h is performed through one perineal drain while continuous suction is applied to the other. When the effluent is clear, irrigation is discontinued, suction is applied to both drains for 12 to 24 hours, and drains are removed.

Bladder catheter
Attempts to remove the bladder catheter are begun 4 or 5 days after operation. Urinary retention is managed with reinsertion of the catheter for another 2 or 3 days.

Colostomy care
The patient is instructed in the care of the permanent end colostomy by an enterostomal therapist.

Postoperative complications

In the hospital

Wound infection
See Chapter 58.

Urinary tract complications
Operative injury to or deliberate excision of a portion of the ureter occasionally occurs in secondary pelvic surgery or during the excision of a large, bulky, or inflamed rectal neoplasm. Repair of the ureter or reimplantation into the dome of the bladder is best performed by an urologist. An unrecognized injury may present as a postoperative ureterocutaneous or cystocutaneous fistula with fluid containing high levels of creatinine leaking through the perineal wound or through drains. A retrograde cysto-ureterogram is necessary to localize the injury and the need for reoperation is determined by the urologist.

Urinary retention after removal of the catheter occurs more commonly in men than in women. Conservative treatment with reinsertion of the catheter succeeds in 70% of patients and transurethral resection of the prostate is necessary in the remainder after 2 to 3 weeks of outpatient observation with a catheter in place.

Intestinal obstruction
Even with insertion of an absorbable mesh to replace the pelvic peritoneum, adhesive obstruction of the small bowel in the pelvis may occur in the early postoperative period. On occasion, small bowel obstruction may also occur around the colon segment exiting the abdominal wall as a colostomy. Treatment is as described in Chapter 58.

Colostomy complications
Necrosis, retraction, prolapse, and parastomal abscess occur in 5% to 10% of patients and mandate reoperation.

Pelvic abscess

Pelvic abscess is a rare complication diagnosed by pelvic computed tomography and treated by reopening the perineal incision.

After discharge

Impotence

Impotence develops in 5% to 40% of men, depending on the level of the tumor and the extent of the resection.

Colostomy complications

Retraction, stricture, or fistula formation occurs in 7% to 8% of patients and late parastomal hernia occurs in 10% to 12%.

Tumor recurrence in the pelvis

Carcinoma recurs in as many as 32% of patients, with 70% of these cases developing within 2 years of operation. High histologic grade of the original tumor, local spread of the tumor, and metastases to pelvic nodes are ominous prognostic signs. Positron-emission tomography is used to determine the extent of the recurrence, and repeated transperineal excision, abdominosacral resection, pelvic exenteration, and further radiotherapy all have been used with moderate success to relieve pelvic pain and lengthen survival. In one recent study, potentially curative and palliative resections of recurrent rectal cancer resulted in median survivals of 20.4 and 8.4 months, respectively.

FURTHER READING

Fleshman, J. W., Wexner, S. D., Anvari, M. *et al.* Laparoscopic vs. open abdominoperineal resection for cancer. *Dis. Colon Rectum* 1999; **42**: 930–939.

Grumann, M. M., Noack, E. M., Hoffman, I. A. *et al.* Comparison of quality of life in patients undergoing abdominoperineal extirpation or anterior resection for rectal cancer. *Ann. Surg.* 2001; **233**: 149–156.

Hiotis, S. P., Weber, S. M., Cohen, A. M. *et al.* Assessing the predictive value of clinical complete response to neoadjuvant therapy for rectal cancer: an analysis of 488 patients. *J. Am. Coll. Surg.* 2002; **194**: 131–135.

Kakuda, J. T., Lamont, J. P., Chu, D. Z. J., & Paz, I. B. The role of pelvic exenteration in the management of recurrent rectal cancer. *Am. J. Surg.* 2003; **186**: 660–664.

Miles, W. E. A method of performing abdominoperineal excision for carcinoma of the rectum and of the terminal portion of the pelvic colon. *Lancet* 1908; **2**: 1812–1813.

51

Anal operations

David V. Feliciano

Emory University School of Medicine, Atlanta, GA

Anal operations, including hemorrhoidectomy, excision of anal fissure and lateral subcutaneous internal sphincterotomy, drainage of a perianal or ischiorectal abscess, anal fistulotomy, excision of condyloma acuminata, and excision of recurrent squamous cell carcinoma or perianal skin squamous carcinoma are among the most common operations performed by general surgeons.

Hemorrhoids are abnormally dilated veins of the hemorrhoidal venous plexus that are classified according to their location above (internal) or below (external) the dentate line. Most hemorrhoids cause minimal symptoms and are managed by sitz baths, topical anesthetics, stool softeners, and a high-fiber diet. In the absence of contraindications such as inflammatory bowel disease, portal hypertension, blood dyscrasias, local cellulitis, and uncontrollable diarrhea, hemorrhoidectomy is indicated for patients with persistent bleeding, pain, or prolapse. Patients with contraindications to operation are treated with injection of sclerosing agents or rubber band ligation (internal hemorrhoids only).

Fissures are usually posterior acute or chronic ulcers that cause painful defecation. Operative therapy is performed less frequently at this time because of the wide range of alternate therapies that relax the internal anal sphincter and promote healing. Included among these are the topical application of 1% isosorbide dinitrate ointment, 2% diltiazem cream, 1% bethanechol cream, or 2% glyceryl trinitrate ointment. Another conservative approach is the injection of 20 units of Botulinum toxin Type A into the internal sphincter muscle. The occasional chronic fissure that fails to respond to topical therapy or to Botox injection is excised, the area is closed with a Y–V local advancement flap, and an internal sphincterotomy is performed.

Perianal and ischiorectal abscesses are purulent collections thought to arise from extension of infection in an anal crypt. Perianal abscesses are painful when the patient sits or walks, but not always during defecation. Superficial abscesses present with erythema, swelling, induration, warmth, and tenderness to palpation, whereas deeper abscesses may cause rectal pressure and signs of sepsis. Prompt incision and drainage is the treatment of choice for these lesions, although fistulas result in 25%–50% of patients in some series.

Anal fistulas are openings in the perianal skin that drain purulent or feculent material. They arise from spontaneous or surgical drainage of abscesses originating in the anal crypts and may heal in some patients. Chronic or long fistulas are treated by fistulotomy, in which the fistula tract is unroofed by cutting through skin and portions of the sphincter muscles and the opened tract is allowed to heal by scarring.

Condyloma acuminata or anal warts caused by the human papilloma virus cause anal pain, soil underclothes, and may undergo degeneration into a squamous cell carcinoma if a giant condyloma is present (Buschke–Lowenstein tumor). Treatment is by excision with reconstruction of the anal margin with suture or by vaporization using electrocautery or the carbon dioxide laser.

Anal operations are performed under local, caudal, spinal, or general anesthesia, with the patient in the lithotomy, prone, or jackknife position. If local anesthesia is used, many surgeons add epinephrine to decrease blood loss. Most anal operations are performed in 30 to 60 minutes, blood loss is modest, there is minimal stress to the patient, and postoperative control of pain is critical.

Usual postoperative course

Expected postoperative hospital stay

Ambulatory procedures are routinely performed on patients with sphincterotomy for anal fissures, drainage

Medical Management of the Surgical Patient: A Textbook of Perioperative Medicine, ed. M. F. Lubin, R. B. Smith, T. F. Dobson, N. Spell, H. K. Walker. 4th edn. Published by Cambridge University Press. © Cambridge University Press 2006.

of perianal abscesses, and fistulotomies for fistulas in ano, as long as they are able to return to the surgeon's office on a regular basis in the early postoperative period. After an extensive hemorrhoidectomy, the hospital stay is 2–3 days.

Operative mortality
Under 0.1% in patients without portal hypertension.

Special monitoring required
The dressing is checked for bleeding every 4 hours during the immediate postoperative period.

Patient activity and positioning
Patients may be out of bed on the day of surgery. After removal of the pressure dressing on the first postoperative day, sitz baths of lukewarm water are permitted.

Alimentation
Clear liquids are permitted on the day of operation, and food intake is advanced as tolerated. Docusate sodium is often administered to soften stools.

Antibiotic coverage
Cephalosporin or advanced penicillin is given to patients undergoing operation for perianal or ischiorectal abscesses or fistulas in ano. Antibiotics are administered until the woody cellulitis surrounding the abscess or fistula tract resolves. All patients with valvular heart disease, prosthetic valves, or vascular grafts receive perioperative antibiotics because of the risk of infection from bacteremia.

Analgesia
Injections of a local anesthetic are frequently performed at the conclusion of anal procedures to relieve pain in the first 6 to 18 hours. Intramuscular narcotics are often administered until the patient has had the first bowel movement after hemorrhoidectomy.

Postoperative complications

In the hospital

Bleeding
Incomplete surgical hemostasis, particularly at the base of a resected hemorrhoid, may lead to postoperative bleeding. Ligation of the bleeding vessel may be possible only by reoperation because exposure at the bedside is too painful. On rare occasions, postoperative bleeding in a patient with cirrhosis may necessitate the use of balloon catheter tamponade followed by the injection of a sclerosing agent.

Urinary retention
Failure to void in the first 4 to 6 hours after operation delays discharge from the ambulatory surgical suite. In-and-out catheter insertion is usually all that is needed in the early postoperative period.

After discharge

Anal stricture
Excessive excision of anal skin during a hemorrhoidectomy or fissurectomy or suture closure of the remaining skin may cause an anal stricture as healing occurs. Progressive anal dilation usually solves the problem, although operative release of the stricture occasionally is necessary.

Anal incontinence
A fistula in ano extending into the high intermuscular or supralevator area should not be opened completely at the first operation because damage to the sphincters causes anal incontinence. If this has occurred, a late reoperation with reconstruction of the sphincter mechanism may be necessary.

FURTHER READING

Lysy, J., Israelit-Yatzkan, Y., Sestiere-Ittah, M. *et al.* Treatment of chronic anal fissure with isosorbide dinitrate: long-term results and dose determination. *Dis. Colon Rectum* 1998; **41**: 1406–1410.

Maria, G., Cassetta, E., Gui, D. *et al.* A comparison of botulinum toxin and saline for the treatment of chronic anal fissure. *N. Engl. J. Med.* 1998; **338**: 217–220.

Pfenninger, J. L. Modern treatments for internal haemorrhoids. *Br. Med. J.* 1997; **314**: 1211–1212.

Schouten, W. R. & van Vroonhoven, T. J. M. V. Treatment of anorectal abscess with or without primary fistulectomy. Results of a prospective randomized trial. *Dis. Colon Rectum* 1991; **34**: 60–63.

Vaizey, C. J., Kamm, M. A., & Nicholls, R. J. Recent advances in the surgical treatment of faecal incontinence. *Br. J. Surg.* 1998; **85**: 596–603.

52

Cholecystectomy

David V. Feliciano

Emory University School of Medicine, Atlanta, GA

Cholecystectomy is indicated for symptomatic calculous cholecystitis (acute or chronic); acalculous acute cholecystitis; a gallbladder that releases stones into the common bile duct (obstructive jaundice, gallstone pancreatitis, cholangitis); carcinoma of the gallbladder; and traumatic perforation of the gallbladder. It is also performed after right hepatic artery ligation for hepatic trauma and in preparation for infusion of the hepatic artery with chemotherapeutic agents for metastases. It is included as part of a pancreatoduodenectomy by some surgeons and may be necessary for exposure of the porta hepatis in occasional patients undergoing portacaval shunt procedures.

Cholecystectomy is routinely performed within 24 hours of admission for patients with acute cholecystitis documented on ultrasonography or radionuclide scanning (i.e., HIDA scan) unless general anesthesia is contraindicated. If patients with acute cholecystitis are observed for a longer period, the extent of inflammation may make a laparoscopic approach difficult. Patients with obstructive jaundice, gallstone pancreatitis, or cholangitis undergo cholecystectomy after observation to determine whether the bilirubin level will fall, when the amylase level returns to normal, and when hemodynamic stability has been restored, respectively.

General anesthesia is used for both open and laparoscopic cholecystectomy. Open procedures are completed in 1 to 1½ hours, blood transfusions are essentially never necessary, and the stress of the routine procedure is moderate. If gangrenous cholecystitis with perforation is present, the underlying disease causes severe stress during the perioperative period. Most patients are discharged from the hospital 2 to 4 days after operation and return to work in 4 to 6 weeks.

A laparoscopic approach is used in 90% to 95% of the more than 750 000 patients who undergo cholecystectomy in the USA each year. Rates of conversion to an open procedure are 5% to 10% for experienced laparoscopic general surgeons, with most conversions necessitated by adhesions, severe inflammation, confusing anatomy, or, rarely, bleeding. Laparoscopic procedures are completed in 1 to 1½ hours, blood transfusions are rarely necessary, and the stress of the routine procedure is modest. Most patients are discharged from the hospital the day after operation and return to work in 1 week. The major concern about this procedure has been the 0.2% to 0.5% incidence of injuries to the common bile duct, a figure slightly greater than that historically reported for open cholecystectomy. Continuing evidence suggests that the incidence of such injuries can be lowered by more use of intraoperative cystic duct cholangiography.

Usual postoperative course

Expected postoperative hospital stay

2 to 4 days for open cholecystectomy; 1 day for laparoscopic cholecystectomy.

Operative mortality

Under 0.1% for routine open or laparoscopic cholecystectomy, and 10% to 15% for cholecystectomy performed for empyema or gangrene of the gallbladder, emphysematous cholecystitis, or acalculous cholecystitis in a patient with recent major abdominal surgery or multisystem trauma.

Special monitoring required

Postoperative hemodynamic monitoring with a pulmonary artery catheter is necessary only in patients with sepsis from empyema or gangrene of the gallbladder, emphysematous cholecystitis, acalculous cholecystitis, toxic cholangitis, or associated hemorrhagic or necrotizing pancreatitis.

Medical Management of the Surgical Patient: A Textbook of Perioperative Medicine, ed. M. F. Lubin, R. B. Smith, T. F. Dobson, N. Spell, H. K. Walker. 4th edn. Published by Cambridge University Press. © Cambridge University 2006.

Patient activity and positioning

Patients may be out of bed on the day of surgery, depending on hemodynamic stability.

Alimentation

For patients undergoing routine open or laparoscopic cholecystectomy, clear liquids are allowed the evening after operation or the first postoperative morning. Patients with more complicated indications for cholecystectomy are permitted clear liquids with the return of bowel function and food intake is advanced as tolerated. Patients with associated hemorrhagic or necrotizing pancreatitis receive jejunal feedings or intravenous hyperalimentation as soon as they are hemodynamically stable.

Antibiotic coverage

Perioperative antibiotics such as a cephalolosporin or advanced penicillin are administered to patients who are undergoing cholecystectomy for cholelithias with chronic cholecystitis, acute cholecystitis, resolving acute cholecystitis, obstructive jaundice, known choledocholithiasis, or secondary toxic cholangitis. The duration of postoperative antibiotic administration depends on the underlying condition.

Postoperative complications

In the hospital

Wound infection

Subcutaneous wound infections occur in 1% to 5% of all patients undergoing open cholecystectomy, but in only 1% of those undergoing laparoscopic cholecystectomy.

Subhepatic biloma or abscess

A biloma that occurs from necrosis of the cystic duct stump or unrecognized division of a duct of Luschka (gallbladder–liver connection) is treated with percutaneous drainage. Subhepatic abscesses are extraordinarily rare and almost always occur when cholecystectomy is performed in conjunction with another intra-abdominal procedure.

Bile duct injury

An injury recognized during open or laparoscopic cholecystectomy is repaired with absorbable sutures, and a T-tube is inserted if an end-to-end anastomosis is required. An unrecognized injury during laparoscopic cholecystectomy leads to postoperative ileus and abnormal liver function test results. With early recognition in the postoperative period, immediate laparotomy is performed with biliary reconstruction as indicated. With delayed recognition in the presence of bile peritonitis, an endoscopic retrograde cholangiopancreatogram (ERCP) for diagnosis, biliary stent placement for decompression, and subhepatic drainage are performed before biliary reconstruction. Late reconstruction of the biliary system is best performed at experienced hepatobiliary centers.

Bowel injury

Injury to either the duodenum or the jejunum occurred in 0.3% of patients undergoing laparoscopic cholecystectomy in one series. Sepsis and ileus are usually present within 24 hours, and a laparotomy is performed with closure as indicated.

Bleeding

In one series, bleeding from the bed of the gallbladder or a branch of the cystic artery occurred in 0.3% of patients undergoing laparoscopic cholecystectomy. Either an open or a laparoscopic approach can be used to control the source of hemorrhage.

Retained or residual common bile duct stone

Failure to perform operative cholangiography may lead to a retained common bile duct stone after either open or laparoscopic cholecystectomy (see next section).

FURTHER READING

Davidoff, A. M., Pappas, T. N., Murray, E. A. *et al.* Mechanisms of major biliary injury during laparoscopic cholecystectomy. *Ann. Surg.* 1992; **215**: 196–202.

Flum, D. R., Cheadle, A., Prela, C. *et al.* Bile duct injury during cholecystectomy and survival in medicare beneficiaries. *J. Am. Med. Assoc.* 2003; **290**: 2168–2173.

Flum, D. R., Dellinger, E. P., Cheadle, A. *et al.* Intraoperative cholangiography and risk of common bile duct injury during cholecystectomy. *J. Am. Med. Assoc.* 2003; **289**: 1639–1644.

Lillemoe, K. D., Martin, S. A., Cameron, J. L. *et al.* Major bile duct injuries during laparoscopic cholecystectomy. Follow-up after combined surgical and radiologic management. *Ann. Surg.* 1997; **225**: 459–471.

Roslyn, J. J., Binns, G. S., Hughes, E. F. *et al.* Open cholecystectomy. A contemporary analysis of 42,474 patients. *Ann. Surg.* 1993; **218**: 129–137.

53

Common bile duct exploration

David V. Feliciano

Emory University School of Medicine, Atlanta, GA

Common bile duct exploration is indicated for radiologically confirmed (laparoscopic or open cholecystectomy) or palpable (open cholecystectomy) gallstones in the duct (choledocholithiasis) that are asymptomatic or causing obstructive jaundice, gallstone pancreatitis, or toxic cholangitis; to diagnose and treat obstructive jaundice from a benign or malignant stricture; to diagnose and treat stenosis of the sphincter of Oddi; or to repair an injury caused by operation or trauma. The need for open or laparoscopic common bile duct exploration has decreased significantly in recent years. In general, a preoperative ERCP with sphincterotomy to allow release of, or access to, common bile duct stones is cost effective if the risk of such stones is 80% or higher. Therefore, patients with resolved cholangitis, persistent jaundice, unresolving pancreatitis, or common bile duct stones documented by other tests are ideal candidates for preoperative ERCP.

General anesthesia is used for both open and laparoscopic common bile duct exploration. The procedure adds 60 minutes to a routine open cholecystectomy because of the need to expose and open the duct (choledochotomy), extract the stones and perform choledochoscopy, insert a T-tube, close the duct around the T-tube, and perform a completion T-tube cholangiogram. Laparoscopic common bile duct exploration also adds 30 to 60 minutes to a routine cholecystectomy. The ideal approach involves balloon dilation of the cystic duct, passage of a flexible fiberoptic endoscope (outer diameter = 3 mm) through the cystic duct, and basket extraction of common duct stones under direct vision. The major disadvantage of this approach is that the choledochoscope cannot be manipulated to retrieve stones from the hepatic ducts. Laparoscopic choledochotomy rather than transcystic exploration requires advanced laparoscopic fine suture skills, which are necessary to sew a T-tube into the common bile duct after removal of the stones. Success rates in removing stones with either laparoscopic approach are 90%–97%. Blood transfusion is essentially unnecessary with routine open or laparoscopic choledochotomy. In contrast, common bile duct exploration to diagnose and treat obstructive jaundice from a benign (i.e., previous operative injury) or malignant stricture often is associated with moderate blood loss that requires transfusion. Routine exploration creates modest stress for patients who also are undergoing cholecystectomy, whereas exploration for a benign or malignant stricture may cause severe stress from blood loss and extended duration of the procedure.

Usual postoperative course

Expected postoperative hospital stay
5 to 10 days.

Operative mortality
2% to 3% in elective operations; 15% and 30% for urgent and emergency operations, respectively, to relieve ascending cholangitis; 10% to 20% in patients undergoing exploration and biliary bypass to relieve obstructive jaundice from an unresectable malignant stricture.

Special monitoring required
Postoperative hemodynamic monitoring with a pulmonary artery catheter is necessary only in patients with toxic cholangitis, patients undergoing a complicated reoperation to correct a benign biliary stricture, and patients undergoing a biliary bypass procedure who are debilitated from an unresectable malignant stricture.

Patient activity and positioning
Patients may be out of bed on the day after operation, depending on hemodynamic stability.

Medical Management of the Surgical Patient: A Textbook of Perioperative Medicine, ed. M. F. Lubin, R. B. Smith, T. F. Dobson, N. Spell, H. K. Walker. 4th edn. Published by Cambridge University Press. © Cambridge University 2006.

Alimentation

For patients undergoing laparoscopic choledochotomy, clear liquids are permitted on the evening after operation or on the first postoperative morning. For those with open procedures, clear liquids are given with the return of bowel function and food intake is advanced as tolerated.

Antibiotic coverage

All patients undergoing common bile duct exploration receive a perioperative cephalosporin or advanced penicillin. Patients with toxic cholangitis are maintained on the appropriate antibiotic (determined by bile culture) until sepsis resolves and fever has been absent for 48 hours.

T-tube

The T-tube left in the common bile duct after an open choledochotomy is connected to gravity drainage. A T-tube cholangiogram is performed on postoperative day 6 or 7 to document the absence of retained stones and the free flow of contrast into the duodenum. About 12 hours after a normal cholangiogram, the portion of the T-tube outside the body is clamped or tied off, leaving 5–8 cm (2 to 3 in) of tubing covered with a piece of tape. The clamp or tie is released only if patients develop cholangitis, right upper quadrant pain, or a bile leak around the T-tube. A T-tube inserted at the time of a routine choledochotomy is removed in an outpatient setting 2 weeks after the exploration. Patients are warned to expect a small amount of bile leakage from the T-tube site for 2 or 3 days.

Postoperative complications

In the hospital

Wound infection

See chapter on "Cholecystectomy."

Subhepatic abscess

See chapter on "Cholecystectomy."

T-tube displacement

Early displacement of the T-tube may precipitate bile peritonitis that is not responsive to percutaneous drainage, and reoperation may be necessary. Late displacement when adhesions are present may be treated with insertion of a percutaneous drain near the choledochotomy site.

Retained or residual common bile duct stone

A retained stone is one which appears on a postoperative T-tube cholangiogram and is unexpected; a residual stone is one that the surgeon cannot remove at operation. A postoperative ERCP with sphincterotomy is indicated to allow for passage of the retained or residual stone if no T-tube has been left in the common bile duct at the first operation. If a T-tube is in place, early irrigation with heparinized saline or monoctanoin aids in the dissolution of cholesterol stones. Stones that do not respond to irrigation, attempted dissolution, or ERCP with sphincterotomy are approached through the T-tube tract by an interventional radiologist after 6 weeks.

Pancreatitis

Operative manipulation of the distal common bile duct may precipitate transient, mild postoperative pancreatitis. This is usually self-limited if the common bile duct has been cleared of stones.

After discharge

Stricture

Attacks of cholangitis manifested by pain, fever, jaundice, and elevation of the alkaline phosphatase level in the absence of choledocholithiasis are strongly suggestive of biliary stricture. The diagnosis is confirmed by ultrasound or computed tomography to rule out a neoplasm and by a transhepatic cholangiogram or endoscopic retrograde cholangiopancreatogram to localize the area of obstruction. Transhepatic balloon dilation of the area of stricture may obviate the need for reoperation with biliary reconstruction.

Common bile duct stone

In patients who are not of Asian descent, late cholangitis caused by a common bile duct stone is almost always the result of failure to clear stones from the common bile duct at the first operation. Either endoscopic sphincterotomy or transhepatic extraction is indicated. Patients of Asian descent have a much higher incidence of spontaneously formed intrahepatic ductal stones that may migrate into the common bile duct long after operation. In addition to endoscopic sphincterotomy, a variety of radiologic procedures for irrigation and extraction of impacted stones are usually attempted, although reoperation with a biliary–enteric bypass may be necessary.

FURTHER READING

Ammori, B. J., Birbas, K., Davides, D. *et al.* Routine vs "on demand" postoperative ERCP for small bile duct calculi detected at intraoperative cholangiography. Clinical evaluation and cost analysis. *Surg. Endosc.* 2000; **14**: 1123–1126.

Lilly, M. C. & Arregui, M. E. A balanced approach to choledocholithiasis. *Surg. Endosc.* 2001; **15**: 467–472.

Memon, M. A., Hassaballa, H., & Memon, M. I. Laparoscopic common bile duct exploration: the past, the present, and the future. *Am. J. Surg.* 2000; **179**: 309–315.

Traverso, L. W. A cost analysis of the treatment of common bile duct stones discovered during cholecystectomy. *Semin. Laparosc. Surg.* 2000; **7**: 302–307.

Urbach, D. R., Khajanchee, Y. S., Jobe, B. A. *et al.* Cost-effective management of common bile duct stones: a decision analysis of the use of endoscopic retrograde cholangiopancreatography (ERCP), intraoperative cholangiography, and laparoscopic bile duct exploration. *Surg. Endosc.* 2001; **15**: 4–13.

54

Major hepatic resection

David V. Feliciano

Emory University School of Medicine, Atlanta, GA

In addition to treating critical injuries, major hepatic resection is performed to remove malignant neoplasms (hepatoma, cholangiocarcinoma, metastases), benign neoplasms (liver cell adenoma, focal nodular hyperplasia, cavernous hemangioma), and cysts (congenital, multicystic disease, echinococcal). If the remaining hepatic tissue is normal, as much as 80% to 90% of the liver can be removed in children and adults.

Screening of high-risk individuals allows for earlier detection of hepatocellular carcinoma or hepatic metastases from colorectal cancer. In the former group, cirrhotics, hepatitis B carriers, and family members of patients with hepatocellular carcinoma should undergo yearly measurements of alpha-fetoprotein (AFP) and hepatic ultrasonography. In the latter group, measurements of carcinoembryonic antigen (CEA) and hepatic ultrasonography are indicated every 3–6 months in the first 3 years after resection of a colorectal cancer.

Preoperative screening before major resection is performed using MRI, which is very sensitive in detecting small nodules, showing the relationship between tumor nodules and major intrahepatic and retrohepatic blood vessels, and determining resectability. An indocyanine green clearance test is still used to assess functional reserve in patients with cirrhosis who need major hepatic resection.

Major hepatic resection is performed under general anesthesia through an upper abdominal incision using either vascular inflow occlusion (Pringle maneuver or clamping of the porta hepatis) or individual ligation of the lobar hepatic artery, portal vein, and right or left branch of the hepatic duct when lobectomy is planned. Division of the hepatic parenchyma is accomplished using finger fracture techniques, blunt knife handle dissection, or the ultrasonic vibrating-aspirating device. Blood loss depends on the extent of the resection and involvement of the retrohepatic vena cava. The median blood loss was 600 ml in one recent large series, and only 49% of patients were transfused at any time. The operative time is 4 hours in experienced hands, and the stress of a major hepatic resection is moderate to severe.

Usual postoperative course

Expected postoperative hospital stay
7 to 12 days.

Operative mortality
1% with hepatectomy only with <3 segments resected; 7% in complex hepatectomy with >3 segments resected. 25% to 30% in emergency resection for ruptured neoplasm. 25% to 50% in emergency resection for trauma.

Special monitoring required
Patients with known cardiac or pulmonary compromise and those who have undergone difficult resections associated with extensive blood loss require postoperative hemodynamic monitoring with a pulmonary artery catheter.

Patient activity and positioning
Patients may be out of bed on the day after the operation, depending on hemodynamic stability.

Alimentation
Hypoglycemia can usually be prevented by the infusion of a 10% glucose solution after extensive resection. Early nutritional support through the gastrointestinal tract is mandatory. Besides the theoretic benefit of lowering the incidence of gut-origin sepsis, use of the gastrointestinal tract appears to generate a hepatotrophic substance that

Medical Management of the Surgical Patient: A Textbook of Perioperative Medicine, ed. M. F. Lubin, R. B. Smith, T. F. Dobson, N. Spell, H. K. Walker. 4th edn. Published by Cambridge University Press. © Cambridge University 2006.

maintains the integrity of the liver. This is in contrast to the cholestasis and fatty infiltration that occurs in patients who are maintained on intravenous hyperalimentation for prolonged periods.

Antibiotic coverage

Perioperative coverage for 24 hours with cephalosporin or advanced penicillin is routine, although the precise benefit is unclear in patients without preoperative cholangitis.

Drains

Suction drains are left in the subphrenic and subhepatic spaces by some hepatic surgeons for 5 to 7 days or until drainage decreases to 30 to 50 ml/d.

Postoperative complications

In the hospital

Perihepatic abscess

Sterile perihepatic fluid collections or abscesses in the subphrenic or subhepatic area occur in 10% to 11% of patients and are treated with CT-guided percutaneous drainage.

Pleural effusion

Sympathetic pleural effusions occur in 8% to 10% of patients and are treated conservatively unless pulmonary compromise results.

Prolonged postoperative fever

This is a common problem in patients undergoing emergency resection in which mass ligation techniques are used. A CT scan with contrast should be used to monitor the viability of the remaining liver and rule out the presence of a perihepatic abscess.

Postoperative bleeding

A second laparotomy for bleeding from the raw edge of the remaining liver is necessary in only 1% to 2% of patients after elective operation and 5% to 7% of patients after emergency resection for severe hepatic injuries.

Hepatic failure

Metabolic failure characterized by progressive elevation of the transaminases, bilirubin, alkaline phosphatase and the INR occurs in 5% of patients after extensive resection and is usually reversible with enteral nutrition and support in the intensive care unit.

After discharge

Recurrent carcinoma

The median survival for patients without cirrhosis who undergo curative resection for hepatocellular carcinoma is about 24 months; this decreases by 11 to 12 months for patients with cirrhosis. The overall 5-year survival for elective resection of hepatocellular carcinoma is now nearly 45% in the Orient. The overall 5-year survival of patients undergoing hepatic resection for colorectal metastases is 30% to 40%. Patients with recurrent carcinoma usually have weight loss, abdominal distention, an abdominal mass, and progressive jaundice.

FURTHER READING

Fan, S. T., Ng, I. O. L., Poon, R. T. P. *et al.* Hepatectomy for hepato-cellular carcinoma: the surgeon's role in long-term survival. *Arch. Surg.* 1999; **134**: 1124–1130.

Feliciano, D. V. & Rozycki, G. S. Hepatic trauma. *Scand. J. Surg.* 2002; **91**: 72–79.

Jarnagin, W. R., Gonen, M., Fong, Y. *et al.* Improvement in peri-operative outcome after hepatic resection: analysis of 1,803 consecutive cases over the past decade. *Ann. Surg.* 2002; **236**: 397–406.

Lau, H., Man, K., Fan, S. T. *et al.* Evaluation of preoperative hepatic function in patients with hepatocellular carcinoma undergoing hepatectomy. *Br. J. Surg.* 1997; **84**: 1255–1259.

Sugihara, K. & Yamamoto, J. Surgical treatment of colorectal liver metastases. *Ann. Chir. Gynaecol.* 2000; **89**: 221–224.

55

Splenectomy

David V. Feliciano

Emory University School of Medicine, Atlanta, GA

Splenectomy is indicated for acquired thrombocytopenias (immune thrombocytopenic purpura (ITP) with or without a human immunodeficiency virus (HIV) infection, thrombotic thrombocytopenic purpura), congenital or acquired anemias (hereditary spherocytosis, hereditary elliptocytosis, autoimmune hemolytic anemia), chronic severe secondary hypersplenism with or without splenomegaly (non-Hodgkin's lymphoma, myelofibrosis, Felty's syndrome, hairy cell leukemia, chronic myelogenous or lymphocytic leukemia), splenic vein thrombosis with left-sided (sinistral) portal hypertension, most grade III and IV and all grade V traumatic ruptures, splenic artery aneurysms, and some splenic cysts. The primary indications for splenectomy on university surgical services are thrombocytopenia, anemia, and severe hypersplenism because staging for Hodgkin's disease and operative therapy of traumatic rupture have significantly decreased in frequency in the past 20 years.

General anesthesia is used for both open and laparoscopic splenectomy. Open procedures for routine thrombocytopenia, anemia, or isolated severe blunt rupture are completed in 1 to 1½ hours. A careful search for accessory spleens is mandatory in the first two groups of patients. Blood transfusions are almost never necessary for routine elective procedures, and platelets usually are not infused in patients with severe thrombocytopenia until the splenic artery has been ligated. The stress of the surgical procedure is modest even in patients with underlying HIV infection when the spleen is of normal size.

Laparoscopic procedures are performed through five ports placed in the epigastrium and left upper quadrant of the anterior abdomen. Operative times are 1–2 hours when a normal-sized spleen is removed and blood loss is under 100 ml. When splenomegaly (600 g or greater or craniocaudal length = 17 cm) was present, operative times increased to 3 hours and blood loss to 175 ml in one study while it was only 114 ml in another. Truly massive spleens can also be removed laparoscopically with a hand-assisted approach and with morcellation of the spleen in a specimen bag prior to removal through the abdominal wall. Conversion to an open procedure because of intraoperative bleeding or difficulty in extracting an intact spleen occurs in less than 4% of patients. The stress of the procedure in compromised patients with non-Hodgkin's lymphoma or leukemia and massive splenomegaly is modest with a laparoscopic approach.

All patients receive antipneumococcal vaccine before hospital discharge, but usually only children younger than 2 years and selected older adults are given anti-*Hemophilus* and anti-*Meningococcus* vaccines.

Usual postoperative course

Expected postoperative hospital stay
5 to 7 days for routine open splenectomy; 10 to 21 days for complex open splenectomy; 2 days for laparoscopic splenectomy.

Operative mortality
0% to 2% for elective routine splenectomy; 0% to 40% for trauma splenectomy, depending on associated injuries.

Special monitoring required
Platelet counts are monitored after splenectomy for thrombocytopenia and a complete blood count is obtained as necessary in patients with preoperative anemia or pancytopenia.

Patient activity and positioning
Depending on hemodynamic stability, patients may be out of bed on the day after the operation.

Medical Management of the Surgical Patient: A Textbook of Perioperative Medicine, ed. M. F. Lubin, R. B. Smith, T. F. Dobson, N. Spell, H. K. Walker. 4th edn. Published by Cambridge University Press. © Cambridge University 2006.

Alimentation

For routine or complex procedures, clear liquids are permitted with the return of bowel function and food intake is advanced as tolerated. For trauma patients with multiple associated injuries (usually Injury Severity Score is over 15), early institution of enteral or intravenous hyperalimentation is appropriate.

Antibiotic coverage

A cephalosporin antibiotic is administered for routine elective splenectomy. For trauma splenectomy, antibiotics are given for at least 24 hours after surgery in patients with associated perforations of the gastrointestinal tract.

Drains

Drains are not placed after elective routine or trauma splenectomy. If a trauma splenectomy is performed as part of a distal pancreatectomy, a closed suction drain is usually left in place for 7 to 10 days.

Postoperative complications

In the hospital

Left lower lobe atelectasis

This occurs in 15% to 20% of patients after open splenectomy and usually responds to nasotracheal suctioning and chest physiotherapy.

Left subphrenic abscess

Occurs in only 2% to 3% of patients who have elective routine or complex open splenectomy but in 5% to 7% of those who have trauma splenectomy. Only 2% to 3% of patients who undergo open splenorrhaphy (splenic repair) after trauma or iatrogenic injury develop this complication.

Rebound thrombocytosis

Aspirin therapy is suggested if the platelet count exceeds 1 million, but this complication is extremely rare.

Persistent thrombocytopenia

Thrombocytopenia persists in 10% to 30% of patients who undergo splenectomy for ITP. If a radionuclide scan with ^{111}I-labeled autogenous platelets was not performed before surgery, this study is used occasionally in the postoperative period to rule out residual accessory spleens not detected at the time of splenectomy. Positive results mandate reoperation if thrombocytopenia persists; patients with normal results should remain on immunosuppressive therapy. Splenectomy as a salvage procedure in patients with thrombotic thrombocytopenic purpura had a remarkable success rate of 88% in one recent laparoscopic series.

After discharge

Persistent thrombocytopenia

See earlier discussion.

Overwhelming postsplenectomy infection (OPSI)

Splenectomy usually is not performed in children younger than 2 years and is performed infrequently in children younger than 10 years because of the risk of OPSI with encapsulated pneumococci, meningococci, or *Hemophilus* organisms. Most episodes of OPSI occur in the first several years after splenectomy. The relative risk of developing OPSI is lowest when splenectomy is performed for trauma and increases progressively as splenectomy is performed for primary splenic disease, hematologic disease, incidental injury at other operation, and incidental injury at operation for malignancy. The long-term risk in adults is thought to be about 0.5% to 1.45%, and the mortality has decreased to 20%–30% with earlier recognition of the overwhelming bacteremias in patients with previous splenectomy. Neither the administration of antipneumococcal vaccine nor the development of antipneumococcal antibodies is uniformly protective against the development of OPSI.

FURTHER READING

Greene, A. K. & Hodin, R. A. Laparoscopic splenectomy for massive splenomegaly using a Lahey bag. *Am. J. Surg.* 2001; **181**: 543–546.

Heniford, B. T., Backus, C. L., Matthews, B. D. *et al.* Optimal teaching environment for laparoscopic splenectomy. *Am. J. Surg.* 2001; **181**: 226–230.

Kercher, K. W., Matthews, B. D., Walsh, R. M. *et al.* Laparoscopic splenectomy for massive splenomegaly. *Am. J. Surg.* 2002; **183**: 192–196.

Rosen, M., Brody, F., Walsh, R. M. *et al.* Hand-assisted laparoscopic splenectomy vs. conventional laparoscopic splenectomy in cases of splenomegaly. *Arch. Surg.* 2002; **137**: 1348–1352.

Schwartz, J., Eldor, A., & Szold, A. Laparoscopic splenectomy in patients with refractory or relapsing thrombotic thrombocytopenic purpura. *Arch. Surg.* 2001; **136**: 1236–1238.

56

Pancreatoduodenal resection

David V. Feliciano

Emory University School of Medicine, Atlanta, GA

Pancreatoduodenal resection (Whipple procedure) is performed for attempted cure of periampullary carcinomas (head of pancreas, ampulla of Vater, duodenal wall, or distal common bile duct); malignant islet cell neoplasms in the head of the pancreas; mucinous cystic neoplasms or mucinous cystadenocarcinoma of the head of the pancreas; benign masses from chronic pancreatitis in the head of the pancreas with secondary pancreatic duct, common bile duct, or duodenal obstruction; and, rarely, major trauma to the pancreatoduodenal complex.

Patients with obstructive jaundice (dilated hepatic ductal system) and no evidence of gallstones on ultrasound or computed tomography (CT) should undergo abdominal helical CT or MRI to determine whether there is a mass in the periampullary area and whether hepatic metastases or regional invasion has occurred. Further work-up to localize the area of obstruction in patients without a periampullary mass should include an MRCP and, if necessary, endoscopic retrograde cholangiopancreatogram or transhepatic cholangiogram. In patients in whom there is the need to differentiate between chronic pancreatitis and ductal carcinoma of the pancreas, PET scanning may be useful. Percutaneous preoperative pancreatic biopsy is not indicated in patients who are at low operative risk and who may have resectable tumors. In patients with suspected islet cell neoplasms, transduodenal ultrasound is helpful for localization.

Percutaneous transhepatic drainage of the obstructed biliary ductal system in the preoperative period is no longer performed because prospective trials have not demonstrated improvement in postoperative survival. The preoperative administration of parenteral vitamin K and the institution of intravenous or supplemental enteral alimentation are appropriate in patients with 10% loss of body weight, albumin levels less than 2.5 mg/dl, or anergy on delayed hypersensitivity skin testing.

After the induction of general endotracheal anesthesia, many younger surgeons first perform transduodenal needle biopsies if a solid mass is present to verify the presence of a malignant tumor. More experienced surgeons are usually comfortable performing pancreatoduodenal resection for local firm or cystic masses in the head of the pancreas with secondary biliary and duodenal obstruction in appropriately selected patients. The mass is staged before resection to verify the absence of hepatic, celiac nodal, and pelvic metastases or regional invasion into the portal vein, superior mesenteric vessels, inferior vena cava, or aorta. Traditional resection for cure includes the head, neck, and, sometimes, a portion of the body of the pancreas; the entire duodenum; the distal common bile duct; and the antrum of the stomach. Some surgeons also perform cholecystectomy and a truncal vagotomy as part of the procedure. Reconstruction is accomplished by anastomosis of the jejunum to the ends of the remaining pancreas, common bile duct, and stomach. An alternate and increasingly popular approach is the pylorus-preserving pancreatoduodenectomy in which the stomach and a 2 cm cuff of proximal duodenum are preserved to improve the patient's long-term nutritional status. Short- and long-term survival rates after this operation are similar to those with standard pancreatoduodenectomy, though a clear-cut long-term nutritional advantage remains to be proven.

Experienced surgical teams perform pancreatoduodenectomy in 4½ to 7 hours with a blood replacement of zero to four units. The procedure is extremely stressful because of the underlying disease, the duration of the operation, the complications that are encountered in 40%–50% of patients, and the nutritional problems that are associated with reconstruction of the upper digestive tract.

Medical Management of the Surgical Patient: A Textbook of Perioperative Medicine, ed. M. F. Lubin, R. B. Smith, T. F. Dobson, N. Spell, H. K. Walker. 4th edn. Published by Cambridge University Press. © Cambridge University 2006.

Usual postoperative course

Expected postoperative hospital stay
10–20 days, with a median of 17 days in one large series.

Operative mortality
In series reviewing operations performed between 1970 and 1980, the operative mortality rate was about 8% to 9%. Series since the early 1980s have reported an in-hospital mortality rate of 0% to 2.8%. A recent report described 145 consecutive pancreatoduodenectomies over a 33-month period with no operative mortality.

Special monitoring required
Patients with known cardiac or pulmonary compromise and those who have undergone difficult procedures associated with excessive blood loss require postoperative hemodynamic monitoring with a pulmonary artery catheter.

Patient activity and positioning
Depending on hemodynamic stability, patients may be out of bed on the day after operation.

Alimentation
Because of the magnitude of the procedure and the compromised nutritional state of many patients, enteral feedings are administered routinely beyond the pancreatic and biliary anastomoses. Clear liquids are permitted with the return of bowel function, and food intake is advanced as tolerated. Erythromycin, a known motilin agonist, is administered to improve gastric emptying in the postoperative period.

Antibiotic coverage
All patients receive an intravenous cephalosporin or advanced penicillin preoperatively and for at least 24 hours postoperatively.

Drains
Closed suction drains are usually placed posterior to the pancreatojejunostomy and choledochojejunostomy and are removed within 5 to 7 days if no fistula occurs. Some surgeons leave a plastic stent through the pancreatojejunostomy or a T-tube through the choledochojejunostomy, with the timing of removal based on personal preference.

Postoperative complications

In the hospital

Delayed gastric emptying
Delayed gastric emptying occurs in about 20% of patients after either standard or pylorus-preserving pancreatoduodenectomy. Intravenous erythromycin lactobinate appears to decrease the incidence of this complication, and nasogastric suction and intravenous hyperalimentation are indicated when it occurs.

Pancreatic fistula
A leak from the pancreatojejunostomy occurs in 8% to 15% of patients and is treated by prohibiting oral intake, continuing suction drainage, and, on some surgical services, administering 100 to 150 µg of somatostatin analogue (Octreotide) every 8 hours.

Intraabdominal abscess
An abscess occurs in 5% to 10% of cases and is caused by a leak from the pancreatojejunostomy or the choledochojejunostomy. The diagnosis is suggested by spiking temperatures, ileus, and leukocytosis, and CT-guided percutaneous drainage is the appropriate treatment.

Wound infections
See Chapter 58.

Hyperglycemia
Elevated glucose levels are frequently noted, particularly in elderly patients receiving hyperalimentation. Intravenous insulin is administered as necessary until an enteral diet is resumed. Long-term insulin rarely is required.

After discharge

Recurrent carcinoma
The median survival for patients with positive lymph nodes in the resected specimen of ductal adenocarcinoma of the pancreas is about 12 months. Patients with recurrent carcinoma usually have back pain, weight loss, an abdominal mass, and hepatic metastases, and pain control is often the most important palliation that can be offered.

Marginal ulcer
The incidence of an ulcer in the gastrojejunostomy generally ranges from 5% to 10% in long-term survivors.

Patients who are *Helicobacter*-negative and who survive long enough for a marginal ulcer to develop are best treated with H$_2$ blockers or omeprazole.

Pancreatic insufficiency

Even with a successful pancreatojejunostomy, pancreatic insufficiency may occur and is treated with exocrine replacement.

FURTHER READING

Adamek, H. E., Albert, J., Breer, H. *et al.* Pancreatic cancer detection with magnetic resonance cholangiopancreatography and endoscopic retrograde cholangiopancreatography: a prospective controlled study. *Lancet* 2000; **356**: 190–193.

Berberat, P., Friess, H., Kashiwagi, M. *et al.* Diagnosis and staging of pancreatic cancer by positron emission tomography. *World J. Surg.* 1999; **23**: 882–887.

Bradley, E. L., III. Pancreatoduodenectomy for pancreatic adenocarcinoma: triumph, triumphalism, or transition? *Arch. Surg.* 2002; **137**: 771–773.

Whipple, A. O., Parsons, W. B., & Mullins, C. R. Treatment of cancer of the ampulla of Vater. *Ann. Surg.* 1935; **102**: 765–779.

Yeo, C. J., Cameron, J. L. The treatment of pancreatic cancer. *Ann. Chir. Gynaecol.* 2000; **89**: 225–233.

57

Adrenal surgery

David V. Feliciano

Emory University School of Medicine, Atlanta, GA

Adrenalectomy is performed to remove functional masses such as adrenocortical hyperplasia (Cushing's disease), cortisol-secreting adenoma or adenocarcinoma (Cushing's syndrome), aldosterone-secreting adenoma (Conn's syndrome), pheochromocytoma, and adrenal causes of feminizing or virilizing syndromes. Non-functional masses that are also treated with adrenalectomy include adrenal adenocarcinoma, symptomatic adrenal cysts or angiomyolipomas, adrenal incidentalomas >4 cm discovered on imaging studies, and isolated adrenal metastases.

With functioning tumors confirmed biochemically, a CT or MRI is performed to determine the side of the neoplasm as well as its size, local invasion, and hepatic metastases. A ^{131}I-MIBG scan is also performed in patients with a diagnosis of pheochromocytoma to localize occult second tumors or metastatic disease to the liver, lung, or bone. Selective venous sampling from the adrenal veins and inferior vena cava is useful to confirm the diagnosis of an aldosterone-secreting adenoma verses bilateral adrenal micronodular hyperplasia of the zona glomerulosa.

Preoperative alpha and, occasionally, beta blockade is necessary before all adrenalectomies performed for pheochromocytomas. Preoperative administration of spironolactone may help reverse persistent hypokalemia in patients with aldosterone-secreting adenomas. Perioperative glucocorticoid supplementation is used in patients undergoing adrenalectomies for Cushing's disease or syndrome.

A laparoscopic approach with or without hand-assist under general anesthesia is used when non-malignant adrenal lesions under 10–12 cm are to be excised. An open anterior transabdominal, flank extraperitoneal, or posterior (with resection of the 12th rib) retroperitoneal approach under general anesthesia is used when adrenal adenocarcinoma, a mass >10–12 cm, extensive adhesions, or portal hypertension is present. Intermittent compression stockings are applied to the lower extremities before the operation begins.

For a right adrenalectomy, the patient is placed in the left lateral decubitus position and four laparoscopic trocars are placed extending from the epigastrium around and inferior to the right costal margin. The "open book" approach involves separation of the right lobe of the liver and the underlying adrenal gland, mobilization of the hepatic flexure of the colon, identification of the right lateral edge of the inferior vena cava, and double clipping and division of the right adrenal vein at the inferior vena cava before removal of the adrenal gland. For a left adrenalectomy, the "open book" approach involves separation of the spleen and the underlying left kidney, medial mobilization of the spleen, lateral and medial exposure of the adrenal gland, and double clipping and division of the left adrenal vein before removal of the gland.

An open anterior transabdominal approach used for a large carcinoma may be performed through an extended subcostal incision on the side of the mass or through a midline incision.

Laparoscopic adrenalectomies performed for reasonably sized lesions by experienced surgeons are associated with minimal blood loss, a conversion rate to an open procedure less than 5% of the time, a 1–2 hour operating time, and only modest stress. An open adrenalectomy performed for adrenocortical carcinoma may be associated with moderate blood loss, a 3–4 hour operating time, and moderate stress.

Usual postoperative course

Expected postoperative hospital stay

1–2 days after laparoscopic approach or open posterior approach; 7–10 days after open anterior approach.

Medical Management of the Surgical Patient: A Textbook of Perioperative Medicine, ed. M. F. Lubin, R. B. Smith, T. F. Dobson, N. Spell, H. K. Walker. 4th edn. Published by Cambridge University Press. © Cambridge University 2006.

Operative mortality

0.3% for laparoscopic approach; less than 5% for open anterior approach.

Special monitoring required

Patients undergoing bilateral adrenalectomy for Cushing's disease or for familial pheochromocytoma (MEN IIA or B) will require continued postoperative supplementation with glucocorticoids and mineralocorticoids and careful hemodynamic monitoring. Patients undergoing a unilateral adrenalectomy for a pheochromocytoma will need careful hemodynamic monitoring postoperatively, even with appropriate preoperative blockade.

Patient activity and positioning

Depending on hemodynamic stability, patient may be out of bed on the day of the operation after a laparoscopic approach.

Alimentation

For routine procedures patients are permitted clear liquids with the return of bowel function. After a laparoscopic approach, patients usually tolerate oral liquids on the evening after surgery.

Antibiotic Coverage

Not administered.

Drains

Not used.

Postoperative complications

In the hospital

Addisonian crisis

This may occur in patients receiving inadequate glucocorticoid replacement or supplementation after bilateral or unilateral adrenalectomy for Cushing's disease or syndrome, respectively.

Early postoperative hypotension

This may occur in patients who have had inadequate preoperative alpha blockade and inadequate intraoperative fluid resuscitation during adrenalectomy for a pheochromocytoma. Treatment is with fluid resuscitation based on central hemodynamic monitoring and vasopressors.

Wound infections or breakdown

In patients undergoing adrenalectomy for Cushing's disease or syndrome by an open approach, wound complications are not rare. In the past, the loss of bulk of abdominal wall muscles, thinning of the skin, and high glucose levels have been associated with both infections in the incision and dehiscence of closures of the anterior abdominal wall. Poor healing has also been noted with some posterior incisions.

After discharge

Recurrent tumor

If a unilateral adrenalectomy has been performed for a pheochromocytoma in a patient with a MEN IIA or B syndrome, the risk of a contralateral pheochromocytoma over time is at least 30%–50%. If an adrenalectomy has been performed for adrenocortical cancer, the optimistic 5-year survival has been reported to be 20%–25%; however, mean survival for most victims is only 24 months.

FURTHER READING

Brunt, L. M. The positive impact of laparoscopic adrenalectomy on complications of adrenal surgery. *Surg. Endosc.* 2002; **16**: 252–257.

Cushing, H. The basophil adenomas of the pituitary body and their clinical manifestations (pituitary basophilism). *Bull. Johns Hopkins Hosp.* 1932; **50**: 137–195.

Henry, J. F., Defechereux, T., Raffaelli, M. *et al.* Complications of laparoscopic adrenalectomy: results of 169 consecutive causes. *World J. Surg.* 2000; **24**: 1342–1346.

Siren, J., Tervahartiala, P., Sivula, A., & Haapiainen, R. Natural course of adrenal incidentalomas: seven-year follow-up study. *World J. Surg.* 2000; **24**: 579–582.

Thompson, G. B., Grant, C. S., van Heeden, J. A. *et al.* Laparoscopic versus open posterior adrenalectomy: a case-control study of 100 patients. *Surgery* 1997; **122**: 1132–1136.

58

Lysis of adhesions

David V. Feliciano

Emory University School of Medicine, Atlanta, GA

Adhesions from previous abdominal operations are the most common cause of mechanical small bowel obstruction in adults. In the past, attempts to limit the number and magnitude of postoperative adhesions through instillation of agents such as heparin and hydroxyethyl starch into the peritoneal cavity proved unsuccessful. In recent years, a number of newer compounds such as oxidized, regenerated cellulose or the combination of sodium hyaluronate/carboxymethyl cellulose were approved by the FDA and are now in widespread use.

Patients with adhesive small bowel obstruction present with either partial or complete obstruction. In patients who are still passing flatus and have only moderate cramping, minimal abdominal distention, and display no signs of peritonitis, a trial period of nasogastric tube suction, hydration, and observation is worthwhile. Laparotomy has been avoided in 40% of such patients with nasogastric tube decompression and in 70% to 90% with endoscopic placement of long intestinal tubes. Patients with a history of complete bowel obstruction or with closed loop obstruction (steady pain), elevated temperature, signs of peritonitis on examination, progressive leukocytosis, or a "stepladder" appearance of dilated intestinal loops on flat plate radiographs of the abdomen should undergo urgent operation. Ischemia and even gangrene of the obstructed bowel can occur in the absence of the classical symptoms and signs.

Dehydration and electrolyte abnormalities (hyponatremic hypokalemic metabolic alkalosis) are common in patients with repeated episodes of vomiting related to proximal obstruction of the small bowel. Preoperative correction of these problems is appropriate in all patients and assists in maintaining hemodynamic stability through the perioperative period.

When an open procedure is performed, rapid-induction general endotracheal anesthesia is used and adhesions are divided by the finger fracture technique, scissors, or electrocautery. A laparoscopic lysis of adhesions mandates the insertion of operating ports away from old incisions in the abdominal wall. An iatrogenic enterotomy increases postoperative morbidity because of the overgrowth of colonic-type bacteria in the obstructed loop. If this complication occurs, vigorous antibiotic irrigation and open packing of the skin and subcutaneous tissue of the laparotomy incision are appropriate. The procedure may last only 1 hour if a single adhesive band has caused the obstruction and from 4 to 6 hours in patients with multiple previous laparotomies and dense adhesions. The stress of the procedure depends on the duration of the obstruction, the magnitude of dehydration and electrolyte abnormalities, the type of adhesions, and the absence or presence of ischemia. In elderly patients with prolonged bowel obstruction and gangrene, stress is considerable because of sepsis. Administration of one or two units of blood may be needed during a difficult and prolonged lysis procedure.

Usual postoperative course

Expected postoperative hospital stay
7 to 10 days.

Operative mortality
Up to 5% overall; up to 15% for strangulation obstruction.

Special monitoring required
Hyponatremic hypokalemic metabolic alkalosis and dehydration may be present postoperatively if an emergency operation was necessary. In hypokalemic patients who are voiding, 15- to 20-meq aliquots of potassium chloride are administered every hour through a central venous line, if

necessary. Fluid replacement with 0.45% sodium chloride (approximates gastric juice) is based on central venous pressure and urine output. Rehydration is suggested by a urine output of 0.5 to 1 ml/kg per hour in adults.

Patient activity and positioning

Patients may be out of bed by the day after the operation. If significant abdominal distention is present, upright positioning aids in ventilation.

Alimentation

Nasogastric tube decompression may be prolonged in patients with marked preoperative dilation of multiple loops of bowel or severe perioperative electrolyte abnormalities as well as those who undergo difficult and lengthy operations. Once electrolyte abnormalities are corrected, postoperative intravenous hyperalimentation is started in patients with obvious nutritional deficiencies at the time of operation.

Antibiotic coverage

All patients receive cephalosporin or advanced penicillin preoperatively and 24 hours postoperatively. If the obstructed small bowel is seen to be gangrenous or perforated at the time of surgery, antibiotic administration is continued for 5 to 7 days postoperatively.

Postoperative complications

In the hospital

Prolonged ileus

As noted, peristalsis may return slowly in some patients. Because recurrent obstruction of the small bowel is always a concern, the administration of low volumes of a bowel-cleaning agent (e.g., GoLYTELY) in patients with bowel sounds after the first week may be useful. Passage of this agent rectally without severe cramping suggests that merely an adynamic ileus is present. Barium may also be administered to rule out a recurrent mechanical bowel obstruction but may be difficult to remove if the ileus persists after the study.

Wound infection

Patients who require prolonged preoperative in-hospital observation and those who have undergone a previous laparotomy during the same admission or had an enterotomy during the lysis of adhesions are at significantly increased risk for the development of a postoperative wound infection. Open packing of the subcutaneous tissue and skin at the time of the lysis is appropriate. Delayed primary closure of the wound can be performed on the sixth postoperative day, with a 10% to 20% risk of infection.

Breakdown of enterotomy repair or small bowel anastomosis

A variety of factors may lead to a leak from a repaired enterotomy site or small bowel anastomosis. An enterocutaneous fistula through the abdominal wound or drainage tract is treated with oral intake prohibition, sump drainage, intravenous hyperalimentation, antibiotics, and somatostatin analogue (Sandostatin). A low-output fistula (less than 500 ml/24 h) in the distal ileum has an excellent likelihood of closing with this management. If an intra-abdominal abscess occurs, either percutaneous drainage or another laparotomy is indicated.

After discharge

Recurrent obstruction

Repeated episodes of adhesive obstruction occur in 30% of patients within 10 years and should be managed as described.

FURTHER READING

Becker, J. M., Dayton, M. T., Fazio, V. W. *et al.* Prevention of postoperative abdominal adhesions by a sodium hyaluronate-based bioresorbable membrane: a prospective, randomized, double-blind multicenter study. *J. Am. Coll. Surg.* 1996; **183**: 297–306.

Gowen, G. F. Long tube decompression is successful in 90% of patients with adhesive small bowel obstruction. *Am. J. Surg.* 2003; **185**: 512–515.

Landercasper, J., Cogbill, T. H., Merry, W. H. *et al.* Long-term outcome after hospitalization for small-bowel obstruction. *Arch. Surg.* 1993; **128**: 765–770.

Nubiola, P., Badia, J. M., Martinez-Rodenas, F. *et al.* Treatment of 27 postoperative enterocutaneous fistulas with the long half-life somatostatin analogue SMS 201–995. *Ann. Surg.* 1989; **210**: 56–58.

Stewart, R. M., Page, C. P., Brender, J. *et al.* The incidence and risk of early postoperative small bowel obstruction. A cohort study. *Am. J. Surg.* 1987; **154**: 643–647.

59

Ventral hernia repair

David V. Feliciano

Emory University School of Medicine, Atlanta, GA

Ventral hernias encompass a wide variety of abdominal wall defects, including incisional, epigastric, umbilical, and spigelian types; for the purposes of this chapter, the term ventral hernia is restricted to the incisional type. A ventral hernia with a small ring predisposes patients to incarceration and possible strangulation of a segment of small or large intestine. Patients with significant ascites are at risk for rupture of a ventral hernia if there is only skin covering the defect. Those with large ventral hernias have difficulty wearing regular clothes and are often embarrassed by their appearance. For these reasons, elective repair of ventral hernias is indicated in patients who are healthy enough to undergo mechanical bowel cleaning and general anesthesia. Over 100 000 such repairs are performed in the USA each year.

At the time of ventral herniorrhaphy performed through an open approach, the thinned-out skin covering the hernia sac itself and all scar tissue back to normal-appearing rectus or other muscles of the abdominal wall are excised. Once the true size of the hernia defect is seen, a decision is made regarding primary repair versus insertion of a prosthetic patch. Primary repair is possible even with defects as wide as 5–6 cm using lateral divisions of the external oblique muscles from within the incision or the "components separation" technique. Because of the size of many ventral hernias after debridement, patches made of polypropylene (porous) or polytetrafluoroethylene (non-porous) are frequently inserted to fill the musculofascial defect.

Surgical stress is moderate because extensive lysis of adhesions and debridement of the sac are necessary when much of the linea alba has been chronically separated. General anesthesia is used in patients with defects exceeding 4 to 5 cm in diameter, the procedure may last as long as 2 to 3 hours, and blood transfusion is unnecessary.

Laparoscopic ventral herniorrhaphy is also performed under general anesthesia and is especially useful in obese patients with large hernia defects or multiple defects and in patients with recurrent hernias after prior open repair. After insufflation of CO_2 with an open technique that avoids the hernia site or prior incisions, dissection through laparoscopic trocars is performed to divide adhesions, reduce the contents of the peritoneal sac, and determine the number of defects or the size of the one large defect. Once the hernia defect is measured, a tailored polypropylene (porous) or polytetrafluoroethylene (non-porous) synthetic mesh sized 3 cm greater than the edge of the defect is inserted through a trocar or trocar site. The intraperitoneal mesh is anchored to the abdominal wall at one centimeter intervals with sutures or tacks. As noted above, general anesthesia is used for the laparoscopic approach, the procedure may last as long as 2 to 4 hours, and blood transfusion is unnecessary.

Usual postoperative course

Expected postoperative hospital stay
5 to 7 days for open procedures; 1–3 days for laparoscopic procedures.

Operative mortality
Under 1% for elective procedures not involving strangulated or gangrenous bowel.

Special monitoring required
Nasogastric tube drainage is monitored and replaced intravenously if it is excessive. Serial electrolytes are measured and replaced as needed. The volume of postoperative serum drainage through suction drains placed under the skin flaps in open procedures is monitored daily to aid in determining when the drains should be removed.

Medical Management of the Surgical Patient: A Textbook of Perioperative Medicine, ed. M. F. Lubin, R. B. Smith, T. F. Dobson, N. Spell, H. K. Walker. 4th edn. Published by Cambridge University Press. © Cambridge University 2006.

Patient activity and positioning

Patients may be out of bed on the day after the operation. Because of the risk of recurrence, heavy lifting is discouraged for 6 to 8 weeks.

Alimentation

Clear liquids are permitted with the return of bowel function and food intake is advanced as tolerated.

Antibiotic coverage

All patients receive antistaphylococcal antibiotics preoperatively to prepare for the insertion of a prosthetic mesh. If a mesh is inserted, the antibiotics are continued for 1 day after surgery.

Drains

Two large-bore closed suction drains are placed under the skin flaps at the end of open procedures to prevent fluid accumulation and encourage adherence of the flaps to the primary or mesh repair. Drainage is monitored as described earlier.

Postoperative complications

In the hospital

Wound infection

The incidence of wound infection is under 2% in patients undergoing elective open procedures but much higher in those undergoing concomitant resection of gangrenous small bowel or colon at the first operation. In such a situation, the surgeon should attempt a primary repair without mesh or a delayed laparoscopic insertion of mesh at a reoperation 5–6 days later. If a prosthetic patch of polypropylene or polytetrafluoroethylene has been used at the first operation, a postoperative wound infection may necessitate patch removal and result in failure of the repair. Treatment of a wound infection includes the administration of antibiotics based on Gram stain, the application of local heat, and the opening of a portion of the incision over the repair.

Wound seroma

If the subcutaneous tissue has been dissected extensively during an open repair or a large defect has been repaired laparoscopically, seromas often occur above the prosthetic patch. Even when closed suction drains have been placed above the patch in open repairs as described above, they can occur as well. Seromas are observed unless the patient is very symptomatic or has an elevated temperature associated with a leukocytosis. Aspiration of a seroma should only be performed in the operating room under sterile conditions.

After discharge

Hernia recurrence

Historically, open ventral herniorrhaphy with or without the insertion of mesh has been associated with a 10% to 15% recurrence rate on short-term follow-up. In one very recent disheartening study from Holland, the 10-year cumulative rate of recurrence was 63% after suture repair and 32% after mesh repair. Laparoscopic ventral herniorrhaphies performed by experienced surgeons have a 1–4% recurrence rate at this time on short-term follow-up.

FURTHER READING

Burger, J. W. A., Luijendijk, R. W., Hop, W. C. J. *et al.* Long-term follow-up of a randomized controlled trial of suture versus mesh repair of incisional hernia. *Ann. Surg.* 2004; **240**: 578–585.

Dumanian, G. A. & Denham, W. Comparison of repair techniques for major incisional hernias. *Am. J. Surg.* 2003; **185**: 1–7.

Heniford, B. T., Park, A., Ramshaw, B. J., & Voeller, G. Laparoscopic repair of ventral hernias: nine year's experience with 850 consecutive hernias. *Ann. Surg.* 2003; **238**: 391–400.

Reitter, D. R. Five year experience with the "four-before" laparoscopic ventral hernia. *Am. Surg.* 2002; **66**: 465–468.

Rosen, M., Brody, F., Ponsky, J. *et al.* Recurrence after laparoscopic ventral hernia repair: a five-year experience. *Surg. Endosc.* 2003; **17**: 123–128.

60

Inguinal hernia repair

David V. Feliciano

Emory University School of Medicine, Atlanta, GA

Inguinal herniorrhaphy is performed for indirect (lateral to the inferior epigastric vessels) or direct (medial to the inferior epigastric vessels in Hesselbach's triangle) groin hernias in over 750 000 patients in the USA each year. Elective procedures for symptomatic reducible hernias are preferred, but urgent and emergency operations are still required for irreducible hernias and strangulated (ischemic bowel) hernias, respectively.

Routine open inguinal herniorrhaphy through a transverse inguinal incision is performed under general, regional, or local anesthesia in an outpatient setting. Rectangular or oval pieces of permanent mesh are inserted in all adult patients to prevent recurrent hernias. Some surgeons also use a shuttlecock-shaped second prosthesis (plug) inserted under the flat sheet mentioned above. Patients are discharged home when they can void. General anesthesia is appropriate for patients with large hernias that are difficult to reduce, those with multiple recurrent hernias in whom orchiectomy is a consideration, and those who prefer to be asleep. The stress of a routine open inguinal herniorrhaphy performed in 1 hour is minimal, and blood transfusions are essentially never required. In contrast, an emergent repair of a strangulated inguinal hernia in which resection of the small bowel is necessary through a separate midline laparotomy incision may be life threatening to elderly patients because of the risk of perioperative sepsis.

Laparoscopic inguinal herniorrhaphy is performed under general anesthesia in an outpatient setting, as well. The three main operative approaches include intraperitoneal onlay of mesh, transabdominal preperitoneal approach, and the totally extraperitoneal approach. There is a learning curve for each of these procedures, operative time is slightly longer than with open repairs, and the operation is more expensive to perform because of the additional equipment. However, recovery time is significantly shorter.

Usual postoperative course

Expected postoperative hospital stay

Patients who undergo routine inguinal herniorrhaphy under local, regional, or general anesthesia are discharged on the day of operation. If gangrenous bowel was resected through a separate midline laparotomy incision during the procedure, a 7-day hospitalization is likely.

Operative mortality

Under 0.1% for elective procedures; increases to 5% to 10% for emergency procedures.

Special monitoring required

Postoperative hemodynamic monitoring may be required in elderly patients who have undergone emergency resection of gangrenous small bowel in a hernia sac.

Patient activity and positioning

Patients are ambulatory on the day of surgery. Most surgeons discourage the lifting of heavy objects for 4 to 8 weeks after non-prosthetic repair. When a prosthetic patch is used, most patients return to normal daily activities (modest lifting) within 7–14 days.

Alimentation

Patients receive a regular diet on the day of operation. If incarceration or strangulation was present preoperatively or bowel resection was necessary during the operation, oral liquids are begun when bowel sounds return.

Antibiotic coverage

As all patients now receive repairs with a prosthetic mesh, preoperative and postoperative doses of a cephalosporin antibiotic are administered. If strangulated bowel

Medical Management of the Surgical Patient: A Textbook of Perioperative Medicine, ed. M. F. Lubin, R. B. Smith, T. F. Dobson, N. Spell, H. K. Walker. 4th edn. Published by Cambridge University Press. © Cambridge University 2006.

is present or if there is a need for bowel resection during the herniorrhaphy, postoperative antibiotics are continued for 24 hours postoperatively if a controlled resection is performed or for 5 to 7 days if peritonitis is present.

Special care

A pressure dressing on the wound minimizes pain, and a scrotal support and ice bag to the scrotum may decrease edema.

Postoperative complications

In the hospital

Inability to void

Some men, including those undergoing operation with local or regional anesthesia, may be unable to void for the first 4 to 6 hours after operation. In-and-out bladder catheterization is indicated before discharge. Elderly patients with prostatism may occasionally require correction of this condition before discharge.

Scrotal hematoma

Extensive dissection of a large or recurrent hernia may lead to the slow development of a scrotal hematoma. Local treatment with ice and elevation is indicated but the need for surgical decompression is rare.

Wound infection

Under 2% in patients undergoing elective procedures but much higher in those undergoing concomitant resection of gangrenous small bowel. If a synthetic prosthetic patch has been used to complete the repair, a wound infection may result in removal of the patch and failure of the repair.

Delayed intestinal perforation

If strangulated bowel appears to recover intraoperatively after removal from the internal inguinal ring, it is returned to the abdominal cavity. On rare occasions, part of the wall of the returned bowel undergoes necrosis, leading to peritonitis. Immediate laparotomy with segmental resection of the involved loop is indicated.

Urinary leak

Unrecognized injury to the bladder has occurred occasionally after repair of a direct inguinal hernia. Leakage of clear fluid from the incision is pathognomonic and demands immediate operative repair.

After discharge

Hernia recurrence

Open repairs performed with insertion of a synthetic prosthetic mesh have a recurrence rate of only 0.5%–1.0% in recent years. Laparoscopic repairs performed with insertion of a synthetic prosthetic mesh have a recurrence rate of 5%–10%.

Migration of mesh plug

A mesh plug may rarely migrate into the peritoneal cavity and will need to be removed laparoscopically if it causes symptoms.

Testicular atrophy

Inadvertent ligation of the spermatic vessels or a significant scrotal hematoma may cause ipsilateral testicular atrophy. No treatment is possible.

FURTHER READING

EU Hernia Trialists Collaboration, Grant, A. Laparoscopic compared with open methods of groin hernia repair: systematic review of randomized controlled trials. *Br. J. Surg.* 2000; **87**: 860–867.

Halsted, W. E. The radical cure of inguinal hernia in the male. *Bull. Johns Hopkins Hosp.* 1893; **4**: 17–24.

Lichetenstein, I. J., Schulman, A. G., Amid, P. K., & Montllor, M. M. The tension-free hernioplasty. *Am. J. Surg.* 1989; **157**: 188–193.

Neumayer, L., Giobbie-Hurder, A., Jonasson, O. *et al.* Open mesh versus laparoscopic mesh repair of inguinal hernia. *N. Engl. J. Med.* 2004; **350**: 1819–1827.

Ramshaw, B., Shuler, F. W., Jones, H. B. *et al.* Laparoscopic inguinal hernia repair: lessons learned after 1224 consecutive cases. *Surg. Endosc.* 2001; **15**: 50–54.

Stylopoulos, N. A cost-utility analysis of treatment options for inguinal hernia in 1,513,008 adult patients. *Surg. Endosc.* 2003; **17**: 180–189.

61

Laparotomy in patients with human immunodeficiency virus infection

David V. Feliciano

Emory University School of Medicine, Atlanta, GA

The presence of infection with the HIV-1 RNA retrovirus, acquired immunodeficiency related complex, or full-blown acquired immunodeficiency syndrome is not a contraindication to major abdominal surgery. Judgment should be exercised, however, when the patient with AIDS has multiple opportunistic diseases in association with a CD4 T-cell count less than 200/mm³. As in patients without these disorders, indications for laparotomy include emergency abdominal conditions (perforation of the gastrointestinal tract, intestinal infarction, intra-abdominal hemorrhage); urgent abdominal conditions (acute inflammation, obstruction of the small or large intestine, acute gynecological lesion); and diagnosis and treatment of an abdominal malignancy, fever of unknown origin, or abdominal pain of unknown cause.

The diagnostic problem in immunocompromised patients with HIV infection and abdominal pain of unknown cause is the increased incidence of conditions related to the presence of unusual infectious agents (*Candida*, *Histoplasma*, *Mycobacterium avium*, *Cryptococcus*, cytomegalovirus) or uncommon malignancies (non-Hodgkin's lymphoma, Kaposi's sarcoma). Because of the hepatosplenomegaly, intra-abdominal inflammatory masses, retroperitoneal lymphadenopathy, and enterocolitis related to the processes listed above, diagnostic dilemmas are common in these patients.

Modestly invasive diagnostic procedures such as laparoscopy should be considered in patients with HIV infection and abdominal pain that is not typical of the usual emergent or urgent conditions requiring laparotomy.

Approach to the patient with HIV infection and abdominal pain (summarized from Barone and colleagues)

1. If diarrhea is present, search for an infectious cause of the pain and observe the abdomen.

2. In patients with organomegaly or ileus, abdominal pain may be related to these problems.

3. Common acute abdominal conditions (appendicitis, cholecystitis) occur in patients with HIV infection and should be treated appropriately.

4. If laparotomy is performed and enteritis is the only finding, mesenteric nodes should be excised for biopsy and culture.

For patients with cachexia from their HIV infection, preoperative enteral nutritional supplementation with a high calorie-high nitrogen diet is appropriate when an elective laparotomy is to be performed.

After laparotomy in the patient with HIV infection, universal precautions are used to protect the patient from hospital-acquired infections and to protect health-care workers from exposure. Pre-existing opportunistic diseases such as *Pneumocystis carinii* pneumonia or oropharyngeal or vulvovaginal candidiasis undergo continuing therapy. Presumed hospital-acquired infections are usually treated before final culture results are available. The resumption of antiretroviral therapy is based on recommendations from the infectious disease service.

Usual postoperative course

Wound healing does appear to be delayed in patients with HIV infection. Therefore, overly aggressive attempts to close skin incisions in the presence of significant intra-abdominal bacterial contamination or to perform delayed primary closure of open skin incisions 5–6 days after laparotomy usually fail.

The significant mortality recorded after emergency laparotomy in patients with HIV infection is believed to be related to their immunocompromised state and the

Medical Management of the Surgical Patient: A Textbook of Perioperative Medicine, ed. M. F. Lubin, R. B. Smith, T. F. Dobson, N. Spell, H. K. Walker. 4th edn. Published by Cambridge University Press. © Cambridge University 2006.

relentless progression of the opportunistic infections and neoplasms that are so prevalent in the last 8 to 12 months of their lives.

FURTHER READING

Barone, J. E., Gingold, B. S., Arvantis, M. L. *et al.* Abdominal pain in patients with acquired immune deficiency syndrome. *Ann. Surg.* 1986; **203**: 619–623.

Bizer, L. S., Pettorino, R., & Ashikari, A. Emergency abdominal operations in the patient with acquired immunodeficiency syndrome. *J. Am. Coll. Surg.* 1995; **180**: 205–209.

Wastell, C. & Davis, P. A. The surgery associated with HIV infection. In Morris, P. J. & Wood, W. C., eds. *Oxford Textbook of Surgery.* 2nd edn. Oxford; Oxford: University Press, 2000: 99–108.

Whitney, T. M., Brunel, W., Russell, T. R. *et al.* Emergent abdominal surgery in AIDS: experience in San Francisco. *Am. J. Surg.* 1994; **168**: 239–243.

Yequez, J. F., Martinez, S. A., Sands, D. R. *et al.* Colorectal malignancies in HIV-positive patients. *Am. Surg.* 2003; **69**: 981–987.

62

Abdominal trauma

David V. Feliciano

Emory University School of Medicine, Atlanta, GA

In patients with blunt abdominal trauma, emergent or urgent laparotomy is performed for hypotension and abdominal hemorrhage (frequently confirmed by diagnostic peritoneal lavage or surgeon-performed ultrasound), overt peritonitis, or obvious signs of abdominal visceral injury without the need for further advanced diagnostic studies. Included are patients with significant proctorrhagia after pelvic fracture; those with evidence of a ruptured hemidiaphragm or air in the peritoneal cavity or retroperitoneum on plain radiographs; and those with evidence of a ruptured duodenum, intraperitoneal rupture of the bladder, or significant injury to the renal artery or kidney on contrast-enhanced radiographs. All other stable patients whose abdominal examinations are compromised by an abnormal sensorium (related to alcohol, drugs, head injury), abnormal sensation (due to spinal cord injury), or adjacent injuries are best evaluated by abdominal helical computed tomography.

In patients with stab wounds to the abdomen, emergent or urgent laparotomy is performed for abdominal distention and hypotension, overt peritonitis, significant evisceration, or obvious signs of abdominal visceral injury without the need for further advanced diagnostic studies. Included in the last group are patients with hematemesis, proctorrhagia, or hematuria; those with evidence of diaphragmatic defect on finger palpation before insertion of a thoracostomy tube; and those with evidence of an injury to the kidney, ureter, or bladder on contrast-enhanced radiograph. All other stable and reasonably cooperative patients undergo local exploration of the stab wound to verify peritoneal penetration. In asymptomatic patients with peritoneal penetration, a 24-hour period of observation is appropriate. The diagnosis of intraabdominal injury is delayed 10–12 hours in patients with false-negative results on initial physical examination.

In the past, gunshot wounds thought to traverse the abdominal cavity on either physical examination or plain radiograph of the trunk were documented to cause visceral or vascular injuries 96% to 98% of the time. In recent studies, up to 30% of patients with gunshot wounds of the abdomen have been observed in certain high volume centers. This is presumably due to a broadening of the definition of the abdomen (flanks often included) and to the ever-increasing thickness of the subcutaneous tissue in obese Americans. Therefore, the indications for emergent or urgent laparotomies listed above for stab wounds now apply to gunshot wounds as well. In asymptomatic patients with gunshot wounds in proximity to the abdomen, either contrast-enhanced helical CT to document the track of the missile or actual abdominal injuries or diagnostic laparoscopy to document peritoneal penetration are used frequently at the present time.

General anesthesia is used for trauma laparotomy. After evacuation of blood and clot from the peritoneal cavity, areas of hemorrhage are controlled by manual compression, packing with laparotomy pads, or vascular clamps. Perforations in the gastrointestinal tract are then sealed with non-crushing clamps. The sequence of operative repairs or resections depends on the combination of injuries. Laparotomies for trauma are usually completed in 3 hours or less because longer procedures in previously hypotensive patients can lead to hypothermia, persistent metabolic acidosis, and coagulopathies. These complications can be minimized by performing a "damage control" operation in which shocky patients have control of hemorrhage and gastrointestinal contamination, only, at a first, shortened operation in which the abdominal incision is left open at completion. When the patient is stable, visceral reconstructions and closure of the abdominal wall are performed in a series of operations. The need for transfusion is extremely variable, ranging from less than 25% of patients with stab wounds to 50% of patients with gunshot wounds. The stress of the operative procedure

Medical Management of the Surgical Patient: A Textbook of Perioperative Medicine, ed. M. F. Lubin, R. B. Smith, T. F. Dobson, N. Spell, H. K. Walker. 4th edn. Published by Cambridge University Press. © Cambridge University 2006.

depends on the number of organs injured and the magnitude of blood loss in the perioperative period.

Usual postoperative course

Expected postoperative hospital stay

5 to 7 days after laparotomy for a stab wound and 7 to 9 days after laparotomy for a gunshot wound or blunt trauma, depending on associated injuries.

Operative mortality

In patients undergoing laparotomy for stab wounds of the abdomen, the mortality rate is 1% to 2%. The mortality increased to 3% in patients with routine gunshot wounds, to 25% in patients with major isolated vascular injuries, and to 48% in patients with multiple vascular injuries. Therefore, overall mortality for patients undergoing laparotomy for an abdominal gunshot wound is currently 15 to 17%. In patients requiring an emergency "damage control" laparotomy at a first operation because of profound shock, the mortality is 25% to 27%.

The mortality after laparotomy for blunt trauma is related to the presence of associated injuries to the head and chest and to the magnitude of intra-abdominal visceral injuries. For example, the mortality after laparotomy for major blunt hepatic injuries in referral trauma centers ranges from 14% to 31%.

Special monitoring required

Patients with known cardiac or pulmonary compromise and those who undergo difficult procedures associated with excessive blood loss require postoperative hemodynamic monitoring with a pulmonary artery catheter.

Patient activity and positioning

Patients may be out of bed the day after the operation, depending on hemodynamic stability.

Alimentation

Early enteral feeding through a nasojejunal tube or needle-catheter jejunostomy placed at laparotomy is the standard of care in many centers for patients with major abdominal injury (Penetrating Abdominal Trauma Index 15 to 40 or Injury Severity Score greater than 25 for blunt trauma). Full caloric requirements can be met at 2½ to 3 days in properly selected patients. Early enteral feeding has reduced septic morbidity after laparotomy for abdominal trauma in several studies.

In patients with extensive resection of the midgut, marked abdominal distention, or exposure of the midgut under a plastic silo (abdominal wall not closed), early intravenous hyperalimentation may be used in place of enteral feeding. Full caloric requirements can be met at 2 to 2½ days in properly selected patients. Disadvantages of intravenous feeding include the fixed rate of long-term catheter infection (3% to 10%), a higher overall rate of postoperative infection exclusive of catheter infection (possible gut-origin sepsis), and the development of hepatic cholestasis and fatty infiltration.

Antibiotic coverage

Postoperative antibiotics are not routinely administered to patients with blunt abdominal trauma unless rupture of the gastrointestinal tract is found at laparotomy or a chest tube is in place. A cephalosporin or advanced penicillin with aerobic and anaerobic coverage is continued for 24 hours in patients who have undergone laparotomy for a penetrating abdominal wound within 8 to 12 hours of injury. Patients with a long delay between injury and laparotomy and those with extensive fecal contamination are treated for 5 to 7 days for established peritonitis.

Drains

Suction drains are placed by most surgeons in patients who have undergone repair or resection of a major hepatic injury, repair of a major duodenal or renal injury, or distal pancreatectomy. The duration of drain placement depends on the injury, but typically ranges from 5 to 7 days in most centers.

Postoperative complications

In the hospital

Wound infection

Infection occurs in 2% to 3% of patients without colon injuries. If the colon is perforated and moderate to extensive contamination is present, the subcutaneous tissue and skin are packed open in the majority of patients. This decreases the wound infection rate in these high-risk patients to 5% to 6%.

Intraabdominal abscess

Abscesses occur in 2.5% to 3% of patients undergoing laparotomy for abdominal trauma, usually in those with perforation of the gastrointestinal tract (3.9% to 4% vs. 1% to 1.5%). Percutaneous drainage by an interventional radiologist is an appropriate first step, followed by reopening of an old drain tract or extraperitoneal surgical drainage if the percutaneous approach fails. Reopening of the midline incision is rarely necessary and carries the highest mortality.

Postoperative hemorrhage

Hemorrhage requiring reoperation occurs in 2% to 2.5% of patients, almost all of whom had severe hepatic injury or an intraoperative coagulopathy at the first procedure.

After discharge

Adhesive small bowel obstruction

Similar to those patients who have undergone elective abdominal procedures, late adhesive obstruction occurs in 10% to 25% of patients.

Incisional hernia

In patients who have undergone only skin closure of the abdominal wall or who have split-thickness skin grafts applied to the open abdomen before discharge, a significant ventral hernia results. Many such patients choose to have reconstruction of the abdominal wall 6–12 months after their original "damage control" procedure.

FURTHER READING

Chiu, W. C., Shanmuganathan, K., Mirvis, S. E. *et al.* Determining the need for laparotomy in penetrating torso trauma: a prospective study using triple-contrast enhanced abdominopelvic computed tomography. *J. Trauma.* 2001; **51**: 860–868.

Davis, T. P., Feliciano, D. V., Rozycki, G. S. *et al.* Results with abdominal vascular trauma in the modern era. *Am. Surg.* 2001; **67**: 565–570.

Demetriades, D., Velmahos, G., Cornwell, E. III *et al.* Selective nonoperative management of gunshot wounds of the anterior abdomen. *Arch. Surg.* 1997; **132**: 178–183.

Nicholas, J. M., Rix, E. P., Easley, K. A. *et al.* Changing patterns in the management of penetrating abdominal trauma: the more things change, the more they stay the same. *J. Trauma* 2003; **55**: 1095–1110.

Tremblay, L. N., Feliciano, D. V., Schmidt, J. *et al.* Skin only or silo closure in the critically ill patient with an open abdomen. *Am. J. Surg.* 2001; **182**: 670–675.

Cardiothoracic surgery

63

Coronary artery bypass procedures

Vinod H. Thourani and John D. Puskas

Emory University School of Medicine, Atlanta, GA

An estimated 12 million people have coronary artery disease (CAD) in the USA. While the majority of patients are treated conservatively with pharmacologic and percutaneous interventions (percutaneous transluminal coronary angioplasty (PTCA) and/or coronary stents) by cardiologists, over 1.4 million patients have undergone surgical revascularization for their CAD over the past decade. Coronary artery bypass grafting (CABG) is performed for the relief of anginal symptoms and to prolong life. Extended relief of angina can be expected in approximately 90% of those with reasonable distal vessel targets. Coronary artery bypass surgery is indicated in patients with angiographically proven CAD with unstable angina refractory to medical therapy or PTCA, positive results on exercise or thallium stress testing, significant left main coronary artery disease, or complex double or triple-vessel CAD. Coronary artery bypass, when compared with medical therapy, has been shown to provide a survival advantage in patients with left main coronary artery stenosis, triple-vessel disease, double-vessel disease with proximal left anterior descending (LAD) artery stenosis, and in patients with depressed left ventricular function. In those patients presenting with chest pain and an evolving myocardial infarction of less than 6 hours duration, either percutaneous or surgical revascularization are plausible treatment modalities. Intractable ventricular arrhythmias may be an additional indication for emergent surgical intervention, since control of arrhythmias and ultimate survival may occur despite the grave prognosis.

Besides routine preoperative laboratory assessment, other necessary specific tests include pulmonary function testing for patients with severe chronic obstructive pulmonary disease and carotid duplex examination in those patients greater than 70 years of age that have either left main coronary artery disease, symptomatic cerebrovascular disease or carotid bruits, or a previous history of cerebrovascular accident or carotid endarterectomy. Patients with poor left ventricular (LV) function (an ejection fraction [EF] less than 30%) and signs or symptoms of congestive heart failure (CHF) should have hypocontractile areas evaluated for viability utilizing positron-emission tomographic scanning with FDG imaging. Possible concomitant valvular heart disease should be evaluated with echocardiography.

Smooth induction of general anesthesia with opiates and inhalation agents is necessary to minimize the stress of intubation. The patient can undergo CABG either with the traditional on-pump approach utilizing cardiopulmonary bypass or by the off-pump (OPCAB) technique, the difference being in the use or avoidance of cardiopulmonary bypass in the completion of distal coronary anastomoses. In OPCAB, the utilization of latest generation coronary stabilizing devices allows a motionless coronary anastomosis with exact precision, while the remaining portions of the heart continue to beat. This procedure has been shown to avoid the inherent adverse consequences of cardiopulmonary bypass.

Following sterile preparation of the skin and draping from the chin to ankles, a median sternotomy is performed. While the left or both internal mammary arteries are harvested, the greater saphenous vein (SVG) and/or radial artery(s) is/are removed utilizing either open or endoscopic harvesting techniques. In the conventional on-pump operation, the ascending aorta and right atrium are cannulated after the patient is systemically heparinized. Prior to cannulation, epiaortic ultrasound is performed to rule out a heavily calcified or severely atheromatous ascending aorta. The patient is then placed on cardiopulmonary bypass and systemically cooled to a core temperature of $32\,^\circ$C to $34\,^\circ$C. An aortic crossclamp is placed proximal to the aortic cannulation site and myocardial arrest is achieved by utilizing antegrade aortic cold

Medical Management of the Surgical Patient: A Textbook of Perioperative Medicine, ed. M. F. Lubin, R. B. Smith, T. F. Dobson, N. Spell, H. K. Walker. 4th edn. Published by Cambridge University Press. © Cambridge University 2006.

blood potassium cardioplegia and topical cooling. Myocardial preservation is maintained by redosing cardioplegia via the aortic root every 20 minutes throughout the cross-clamp period (antegrade cardioplegia) or via intermittent or continuous infusion of cardioplegia into the coronary sinus (retrograde cardioplegia). During OPCAB, cardioplegia is not required, since the bypass operation is performed on the beating heart. Blood autotransfusion techniques are utilized to minimize transfusion of banked blood products.

Reversed saphenous grafts, free radial grafts, or free or in situ internal mammary artery grafts are anastomosed distal to the coronary artery stenoses; proximal anastomoses of the free grafts are performed to the ascending aorta. The operative strategy for first-time revascularization patients consists of a single left or bilateral internal mammary artery in situ graft(s) (LIMA and/or RIMA) to the LAD and most important lateral wall coronary target, as well as segments of reversed saphenous vein for the remaining required grafts. The radial artery free graft is routinely used in patients with >70% coronary artery stenosis and age less than 60 years. Ten-year patency rates may exceed 90% for the LIMA graft and 50%–70% for the reverse saphenous vein grafts.

Following completion of the grafts, the patient is warmed to normothermia and separated from cardiopulmonary bypass; during OPCAB, patients are maintained at normothermia. Following restoration of an autogenous heart rate, all cannulae are removed and systemic heparinization is reversed with protamine sulfate. In those patients that require hemodynamic support, inotropic agents or intra-aortic balloon pump may be necessary. In on-pump coronary bypass, temporary pacing wires may be placed; OPCAB patients do not routinely require temporary pacing wires. Thoracostomy tubes are used in the necessary pleural spaces and mediastinum. Following meticulous hemostasis, the patient's sternum is closed with interrupted stainless steel wires and the fascia and skin reapproximated. The operation usually takes 2 to 4 hours. Patients are transported to the intensive care unit on a respirator and generally extubated within 2–6 hours.

Usual postoperative course

Expected postoperative hospital stay
3 to 5 days.

Operative mortality
From 1 to 3% for primary CABG. Statistically significant independent predictors of poorer outcome include older age, female gender, prior heart surgery, diminished LV ejection fraction, percent stenosis of the left main coronary artery, number of coronary arteries with greater than 70% stenosis, and urgency of operation.

Special monitoring required
In the absence of complications, patients remain in the intensive care unit for 8 to 24 hours after operation. Healthy, young patients may be transferred to a monitored private room 4–6 hours after OPCAB in selected cases. Arterial blood pressure, electrocardiographic signs, central venous pressure or cardiac index (via Swan–Ganz catheter), urinary output, and chest tube drainage are monitored. Serum potassium and magnesium and hematocrit levels are obtained once on the day of surgery and postoperative day one. Arterial blood gases are monitored for extubation criteria. On postoperative day 1, the patient is transferred to a telemetry floor and most invasive monitoring devices are discontinued. The chest tubes are removed when chest drainage is less than 100 ml/tube per 8 hours. Bedside glucose monitoring is performed periodically and subcutaneous insulin administered to maintain a glucose level below 140 mg/dl.

Patient activity and positioning
On the day of operation and while intubated, patients remain on bedrest with the head elevated 30 degrees. After extubation, aggressive pulmonary toilet is performed, including turning from side-to-side every 2 hours and administration of bronchodilators and chest physiotherapy. The patient sits at the bedside with assistance as necessary to allow dependent chest tube drainage. On postoperative day 1, they are out of bed at mealtime and encouraged to ambulate in the hallway as tolerated.

Alimentation
Clear liquids are permitted after extubation, and food intake is advanced to a low fat, low cholesterol, 4 gram sodium diet as tolerated. A diabetic diet is provided when appropriate. Mild constipation or diarrhea and nausea are common.

Antibiotic coverage
Preoperative prophylaxis with a second-generation cephalosporin (cefuroxime), or vancomycin in penicillin-allergic patients, is continued for 24 hours after surgery.

Routine immediate medications
All patients are transferred to the telemetry floor with β-blockers (metoprolol 25 mg by mouth every 8 hours),

enteric-coated aspirin (81 mg by mouth every 8 hours), 2% mupirocin topical nasal gel every 12 hours, chlorhexidine mouthwash (15 milliters swish and spit every 12 hours), and simvastatin (20 mg by mouth every evening). Those patients undergoing OPCAB receive clopidogrel 75 mg by mouth every day.

Pulmonary toilet

Intensive pulmonary toilet post-extubation is performed to prevent atelectasis and pneumonia, including chest physical therapy every 4 hours, incentive spirometry every 1 hour, bronchodilators every 4 hours, and cough and deep breathe exercises every 2 hours while awake.

Postoperative complications

In the hospital

Perioperative myocardial infarction (MI)

Advances in intraoperative myocardial protection, including antegrade and retrograde cardioplegic protection, have significantly reduced the incidence of perioperative myocardial infarction (MI) over the last 20 years to a current rate well under 5%. Acute postoperative myocardial ischemia occurs infrequently, but may be seen in patients with acute coronary occlusion, early graft failure, or incomplete revascularization.

Low cardiac output

A cardiac index (CI) below 2.0 l/min per m^2 or a mixed venous oxygen saturation from the pulmonary artery catheter less than 65% are unacceptably low and generally will require therapeutic intervention. Common causes of postoperative low CI include decreased LV preload, pre-existing poor LV function, or acute right or left ventricular dysfunction. Other less common causes include postoperative myocardial ischemia or cardiac tamponade. Therapeutic interventions include administration of fluid or red blood cells, optimization of the heart rate to 90 to 100 beats/min (utilizing epicardial pacing or pharmacological means), or the administration of inotropic agents (epinephrine, dobutamine, milrinone, dopamine). If the initial therapeutic maneuvers are unsuccessful, transthoracic or transesophageal echocardiography should be performed to exclude the presence of cardiac tamponade. A final therapeutic step is the deployment of a percutaneous intraaortic balloon pump via the femoral artery to decrease afterload and augment diastolic coronary perfusion and cardiac index.

Arrhythmias

Transient conduction abnormalities are frequent following cardiac surgery. The most common aberrations are sustained tachycardia, atrial fibrillation or flutter, various degrees of atrioventricular blockade, as well as premature ventricular beats, sustained or non-sustained ventricular tachycardia and, less frequently, ventricular fibrillation. Contributing factors include the severity of CAD, duration of aortic cross-clamping and cardiopulmonary bypass, adequacy of myocardial protection, depth of myocardial hypothermia, patient age, severe LV dysfunction (EF less than 30%), and complex valvular or multiple valvular operations.

The most common conduction abnormality is sustained sinus tachycardia and is treated by correcting the underlying cause (pain, anxiety, low cardiac output, anemia, fever, or beta-blocker withdrawal). Postoperative ventricular arrhythmias range from occasional premature beats to bigeminy, trigeminy, sustained ventricular tachycardia, and ventricular fibrillation. Prophylactic correction of hypoxemia, acidosis, hypokalemia, and hypomagnesemia is particularly important in the immediate postoperative period. Ventricular tachycardia generally responds to beta-blockers and/or intravenous amiodarone. Immediate cardioversion followed by resuscitation and antiarrhythmic therapy is essential for sustained ventricular tachycardia and ventricular fibrillation. Rarely, patients may require an implanted automatic internal cardiac defibrillator prior to discharge.

Atrial fibrillation and atrial flutter occur in 10% to 30% of patients following cardiac surgery and are most commonly seen on the second postoperative day. Acidosis, hypokalemia, hypomagnesemia, or hypoxemia may contribute to the onset of this arrhythmia and should be corrected. The prophylactic use of beta-blockers or amiodarone has been shown to have a protective effect against the development of atrial fibrillation or flutter. Treatment in stable patients involves control of the ventricular rate and conversion to sinus rhythm utilizing beta-blocker therapy combined with intravenous infusions of either sotalol, diltiazem, or amiodarone. Immediate electrical cardioversion is recommended for unstable, symptomatic patients. Within 1 to 3 days, 80% of patients who develop postoperative atrial fibrillation will return to sinus rhythm with beta-blocker therapy alone; only approximately 10% require electrical cardioversion. Among those who do not convert to sinus rhythm prior to hospital discharge, most will revert to sinus rhythm during the next 3 months on coumadin and antiarryhthmic therapy. Despite atrial fibrillation, early and late mortality rates do not appear increased. However, patients who remain in atrial fibrillation require anticoagulation since there is a two- or threefold increase in the risk of stroke with long-term atrial fibrillation.

Pulmonary embolism

The incidence of pulmonary embolism following open heart surgery is minimal and ranges from 0.56% to 2%. The incidence of deep vein thrombosis is equally distributed between the donor leg and the opposite limb. Significant risk factors include prolonged pre- or postoperative bedrest, previous venous thromboembolism, obesity, and hyperlipidemia. Diagnosis is confirmed by duplex scanning. Hospital mortality in patients with pulmonary emboli ranges between 19% and 34%.

Pleural effusion

Blood or serous fluid may accumulate in the pleural cavities following thoracostomy tube removal prior to discharge from the hospital. Significant effusions should be treated by thoracentesis or thoracostomy tube in order to allow the lung to completely expand and to reduce the risk of infection in the compressed lung. Undrained pleural effusions may become organized and require thoracoscopic decortication.

Pneumonia/bronchitis

While 70% of patients undergoing cardiac surgery may develop postoperative atelectasis, pneumonia occurs in only 4%. The most important preoperative predictors for pneumonia include underlying pulmonary disease, COPD, ongoing smoking, and advanced age. Pain associated with sternotomy or chest tubes interferes with normal respiratory function and impairs deep breathing, possibly contributing to the development of atelectasis and/or pneumonia. The diagnosis is suspected in patients with postoperative fever, leukocytosis, and purulent sputum. Identification of pathogenic organisms by gram stain or culture of the sputum or blood and presence of an infiltrate on chest X-ray confirm the diagnosis. Immediate treatment with intravenous broad spectrum antibiotics is followed by organism-specific antibiotic therapy. Chest physiotherapy and pulmonary toilet are performed to facilitate clearance of pulmonary secretions. Preventive measures include incentive spirometry, antibiotic prophylaxis, bronchodilators (in patients with chronic bronchitis), and cessation of smoking.

Neurologic complications

Cognitive dysfunction, atypical behavior, and disorientation occur in up to 75% of patients in the immediate postoperative period, but nearly all patients regain full cognitive function within 6 months. However, 7% of patients may demonstrate moderate to severe psychometric abnormalities at late follow-up, and approximately 1% are unable to return to work and normal daily activities. Disabling stroke occurs in about 2% of patients while 3% experience transient ischemic events. The mechanisms associated with neurologic complications following open heart surgery include macroembolization of debris from aortic atheroma or left ventricular thrombus; microembolization of aggregates of granulocytes, platelets, and fibrin; air embolism; and cerebral hypoperfusion. Radiologic evaluation utilizing head CT is used to make the diagnosis. Focal neurologic deficits resulting from intraoperative events are usually noted within the first 24 to 48 hours and are treated with measures to decrease intracerebral pressure and expectant, supportive care. Massive intraoperative air embolism may be effectively treated with emergency hyperbaric therapy. It is hoped that OPCAB techniques may reduce the incidence of neurologic dysfunction after CABG.

Phrenic nerve injury

Although the exact incidence of phrenic nerve injuries following coronary surgery is difficult to quantify, approximately 2% of patients appear to be affected. The etiology may include stretch injuries from prolonged, extreme opening of the chest retractor, direct injury during harvest of the internal mammary artery, or cold injury from topical ice slush. The diagnosis is usually suspected by a high diaphragmatic shadow on chest roentogram. Nerve conduction and fluoroscopic studies are used to confirm the diagnosis. Clinical sequelae of unilateral phrenic nerve paralysis include atelectasis, dyspnea on exertion, and pneumonia, while bilateral phrenic paralysis may lead to prolonged respiratory dependence and could necessitate tracheostomy. Most phrenic nerve injuries resolve over a 6 to 18-month period.

Gastrointestinal symptoms

Following CABG, gastrointestinal (GI) complications range from 0.41% to 2%. These are generally thought to be a consequence of an overall low flow state resulting from decreased cardiac output and are often associated with respiratory and renal failure. Macroembolism or thrombosis of mesenteric vessels may also be an important etiology. The severity of symptoms are masked by metabolic disturbances and the inability of the sedated, intubated patient to complain, leading to a delay in diagnosis. Early recognition and treatment is imperative for control of GI complications.

Gastrointestinal bleeding

The incidence of GI bleeding following CABG ranges from 0.35% to 3%, usually occurring during the first postoperative month. Although gastritis or peptic ulcer are the most common sources, other causes include esophagitis, ischemic bowel disease, diverticulitis, and A–V malformations. Advanced age and a prior history of GI bleeding are the most reliable preoperative predictors of postoperative bleeding. While melena is the most common symptom, hematemesis may occur. Upper GI bleeding sources present more commonly; therefore upper GI endoscopy should be initially performed to guide therapy. GI bleeding following CABG is associated with a high mortality ranging up to 75%.

Perforated ulcer

A perforated duodenal or gastric ulcer following CABG occurs in 0.02% to 0.08% of patients and is usually diagnosed by free abdominal air on a routine upright chest X-ray. Some patients complain of upper abdominal pain and many patients have a previous history of ulcer disease. Most are treated with an omental patch surgical repair. Mortality ranges from 30% to 50%, reflecting the frequent delay in diagnosis, with subsequent sepsis.

Biliary complications

The incidence of cholecystitis following CABG ranges from 0.2% to 0.5%. These patients usually develop symptoms 5 to 15 days after operation and complain of fever, nausea, and vague, diffuse abdominal pain. Abdominal ultrasonography and HIDA scanning are the most common tests utilized. If the patient is stable, cholecystectomy often is necessary. Percutaneous cholecystostomy and broad-spectrum antibiotics may be more appropriate in severely unstable, septic patients.

Pancreatitis

Although 25% to 30% of patients may have asymptomatic hyperamylasemia, only 1% to 2% develop symptomatic pancreatitis, and even less (0.13% to 0.6%) have necrotizing pancreatitis. Pancreatitis generally occurs within a few days after operation with symptoms of fever, nausea, epigastric pain, and a leukocytosis with elevated serum amylase and lipase levels. The diagnosis is confirmed by a computed tomography scan. Patients with mild pancreatitis are treated with intravenous fluids, nasogastric drainage, and bowel rest until serum amylase levels return to baseline. Necrotizing pancreatitis requires enteral feeding and immediate surgical debridement of the pancreas with wide drainage. Mortality of necrotizing pancreatitis may exceed 50%.

Ischemic colitis

The incidence of ischemic colitis after CABG is estimated to be 0.02% to 0.3% and typically presents 6 or more days after operation. Older age, generalized peripheral vascular disease, need for emergency surgery, and a period of perioperative hypotension may contribute to the development of ischemic colitis. Signs and symptoms include abdominal distention, severe abdominal pain, abrupt distention, vomiting, extreme leukocytosis, and melena. Sigmoidoscopy, laparoscopy, and arteriography may be used for diagnosis and/or treatment. If surgical intervention is performed, the necrotic bowel is excised. The overall mortality for this population ranges between 50% and 95%. Early diagnosis and surgical intervention is essential for a successful outcome.

Diverticulitis

Following open-heart surgery, the incidence of this condition is 0.13% to 0.25%. The majority of patients have a prior history of diverticulosis or diverticulitis. Perioperative splanchnic hypoperfusion is believed to be a contributing factor. Clinical symptoms include fever, leukocytosis, left lower quadrant pain, and abdominal distention. Endoscopy or computed tomography scanning aid in the diagnosis. Intravenous antibiotics and bowel rest are recommended for treatment of non-perforated diverticulitis; segmental colectomy and diverting colostomy are performed for perforated diverticulitis. The overall mortality for those with perforated diverticulitis nears 25%.

Hepatic derangements

Serum levels of hepatic enzymes are transiently elevated following cardiopulmonary bypass in approximately 15% to 20% of patients between the second and fourth postoperative days. This rise in enzymes is plausibly related to blood trauma, hepatic congestion, and hypoperfusion during bypass. Despite the rise in hepatic enzymes, less than 0.5% of patients develop significant hepatic dysfunction as a feature of multisystem organ failure.

Postoperative renal insufficiency

Approximately 15% of patients develop evidence of renal dysfunction following cardiac surgery. Renal blood flow and glomerular filtration rate may be reduced by 25% to 75% during cardiopulmonary bypass, with partial recovery in the first postoperative day. While many patients suffer mild, transient renal dysfunction, severe renal failure requiring dialysis occurs in 1.5% to 3.0% of patients and is intimately related to preoperative renal function, postoperative cardiac output, ischemic periods during operation, preoperative administration of radiographic contrast materials, and toxic drugs. Treatment requires optimization of cardiac output, management of fluid balance, avoidance of nephrotoxic drugs, and prevention of infection. Venovenous hemofiltration may be used to correct fluid and electrolyte imbalances and is not dependent on cardiac output. Renoprotective agents used to prevent or treat renal ischemia include mannitol, lasix, renal dose dopamine, and fenoldopam. The mortality among patients who develop severe, acute renal failure is approximately 45%.

Postoperative metabolic disorders

Hypokalemia

This commonly occurs following cardiac surgery and has important effects on the electrical activity of the heart. The large and rapid fluid shifts during and after cardiac surgery are in part responsible for these aberrations. Hypokalemia is treated with intravenous KCl at a rate of no more than 10–15 Meq/h to maintain a serum level of at least 4.5 Meq/l.

Hypomagnesemia

Mimicking potassium in its effects on the electrical activity of the heart, this generally occurs following cardiac surgery. Preoperative use of loop diuretics, thiazides, digoxin, or alcohol may also be causes. Patients with hypomagnesemia have an increased risk of atrial and ventricular dysrhythmias, leading to decreased stroke volume and cardiac index. Intravenous magnesium sulfate should be administered to raise the serum levels to 2 Meq/l.

Hyperglycemia

The inherent surgical stress associated with CABG leads to a rise in blood glucose levels because of increased glucose mobilization related to elevations in cortisol, catecholamine, and growth hormone levels, and the apparent failure of insulin secretion during hypothermia. These mechanisms are present in non-diabetics and are exaggerated in the diabetic patient. A strict protocol utilizing insulin drips and sliding scale supplementation are utilized to maintain blood glucose less than 140 mg/dl.

Mediastinal bleeding

Two to three percent of patients require re-exploration for bleeding following open-heart surgery. Thoracostomy tubes are placed in the pleural space(s) and mediastinum and are monitored carefully after operation. When moderate postoperative mediastinal bleeding occurs, the platelet count, partial thromboplastin time, prothrombin

time, INR, thromboelastogram (TEG), and fibrinogen levels are measured. An elevated prothrombin time or INR indicates a defect in the extrinsic coagulation pathway and is treated with fresh frozen plasma. Secondary to the functional deficit in most of the circulating platelets following cardiopulmonary bypass, platelet transfusions are prescribed in bleeding patients for counts under 80 000/μl. Supplemental cryoprecipitate is administered if the fibrinogen is below 200. Additional maneuvers include warming the patient, increasing the PEEP on the ventilator to 10–15 cm H_2O in an attempt to tamponade venous bleeding sites, and aggressive control of hypertension. Although expensive, recombinant Factor VII has recently become commercially available and acts on both the intrinsic and extrinsic pathways to promptly restore normal coagulation in cases of severe coagulopathy unresponsive to more conventional therapy. Re-exploration is indicated if sudden massive bleeding occurs or if excessive chest tube drainage persists during the first few hours after operation. In approximately two-thirds of patients who are re-explored no surgical bleeding source is found, and the bleeding is secondary to coagulopathy. Patients undergoing OPCAB have been shown to have significantly less postoperative mediastinal bleeding and blood product transfusion.

Infection

Sternal wound complications represent a serious morbidity associated with coronary surgery and occur in 0.5% to 4% of cases, with multiple risk factors including pneumonia, emphysema/chronic obstructive pulmonary disease, prolonged mechanical ventilation (especially with tracheostomy), emergency operations, postoperative hemorrhage with mediastinal hematoma, early re-exploration, obesity, diabetes mellitus, and use of bilateral internal mammary grafts.

Deep sternal wound infections include acute mediastinitis with sternal dehiscence and osteomyelitis of the sternum. The incidence of deep wound infection following sternotomy ranges from 0.4% to 4% and is usually apparent 2 to 4 weeks postoperatively. Presenting signs and symptoms include wound drainage, fever, sternal instability, excessive wound pain, leukocytosis, and dehiscence. Any drainage from the wound should be cultured. The clinical signs and character of wound drainage usually suffice for both the diagnosis and localization of the infected tissues; CT scan is infrequently necessary. Appropriate antibiotics are given intravenously before and up to 4 or 6 weeks after the wound is opened and drained. Although debate continues regarding the most appropriate initial treatment, our institution prefers plastic surgical closure with an immediate pectoralis myocutaneous advancement flap.

Patients who have had a CABG rarely experience leg wound infections that necessitate extra care. Leg infections seem to occur more frequently in obese women, especially if the thigh veins are harvested. The routine use of endoscopic vein harvest has been associated with a significant reduction in incidence of this complication.

After discharge

Constrictive pericarditis

Following cardiac surgery, this condition complicates approximately 0.2% to 0.3% of all operations. While the etiology of the process remains unclear, the disease may progress to a fibrotic, pericardial shell. Patients complain of dyspnea with minimal exertion, fatigue, and peripheral edema and may present from 2 weeks to 17 years after surgery. Symptoms and signs are non-specific, and the ECG often shows non-specific ST segment changes. The chest X-ray may show cardiomegaly. Echocardiography, MRI, and CT scan all demonstrate pericardial thickening and occasional pericardial calcium. The most common echocardiographic findings show biatrial dilatation, small to normal ventricular size, and a shell of pericardium. Corticosteroids and non-steroid anti-inflammatory agents generally are ineffective in preventing constrictive pericarditis in patients with the postpericardiotomy syndrome, but a tapered dose of corticosteroids is recommended in patients with constrictive pericarditis within two months of operation. Persistent symptoms after 2 weeks of steroids, presentation after 2 months, or compromised hemodynamic condition are indications for reoperation. In the majority of cases, immediate improvement in performance is appreciated after subtotal pericardiectomy.

Incisional pain

Usually can be controlled with oral analgesics. Parasternal numbness may persist for up to 12 months after IMA harvesting.

Sternal problems

Sternal mobility (clicking) is increased with exertion and coughing. This generally resolves in 6 to 12 weeks as the sternum heals. Infrequently, a sterile non-union may develop and the sternum may need to be rewired. Occasionally, patients complain of a painful sternal wire in the absence of inflammation or infection, which can be treated with removal of the wire (or all wires) during brief general anesthesia using small skin incision(s) over each offending wire. If purulent discharge is encountered, proper evaluation for deep sternal wound infection is performed.

Leg edema

The majority of patients are discharged from the hospital with some degree of lower leg edema either from the saphenous vein harvest and/or fluid retention. The excess fluid is controlled with leg elevation, support hose, and diuresis, generally resolving within a few months.

Peripheral nerve injuries

The reported incidence of upper extremity peripheral nerve injuries ranges from 2% to 18%. Most are attributed to stretch or compression during sternal retraction and involve brachial plexus roots C8 and T1. Other causes include injury from the fractured end of a first rib or by needle trauma from a jugular vein cannulation. Ulnar or, more rarely, radial neuropathies may occur after general anesthesia, even when appropriate precautions with arm positioning, padding, and protection are taken. Most of these injuries become apparent in the first postoperative week when the patient complains of numbness, decreased sensation, or motor strength of the affected part. Such deficits usually resolve spontaneously over 6 weeks to 6 months. Injuries slow to resolve require further evaluation by a neurologist.

Peripheral nerve injuries in the lower extremities may occur from saphenous vein harvest trauma and are often attributed to injury of the saphenous nerve. The sensory deficit includes diminished sensation to the medial forefoot and ankle and usually improves within 1 to 3 months. Injuries to the sciatic, femoral, or common peroneal nerves may occur from needle puncture, compression, or lack of protection over the head of the fibula and may result in considerable disability.

Recurrent angina

Incomplete revascularization, graft closure, or progression of native coronary disease causes this condition. Unless contraindicated, all patients are administered daily aspirin after CABG to prolong graft patency. Repeat coronary angiography may be necessary to evaluate the source of angina. Repeat angioplasty or bypass surgery is rarely required early after the initial procedure.

Postcardiotomy syndrome

The incidence of the postcardiotomy or postpericardiotomy syndrome is approximately 18% and decreases with advancing age. Although not well understood, the etiology appears to be an autoimmune inflammatory phenomenon. Symptoms usually develop within the first month after operation and the most common presentation includes fever, pleuritic pain, malaise, and a pericardial friction rub. Some patients develop pleural or pericardial effusions or painful swallowing. The disease may progress to pericardial effusion and infrequently constrictive pericarditis. The differential diagnosis includes atelectasis, pneumonia, endocarditis, and wound infection. A mild leukocytosis may be present and the ECG may show diffuse non-specific ST segment elevation. The disease is self-limited, with a mean duration of symptoms lasting one month; up to 20% of patients develop a recurrence. Patients are encouraged to limit activity and are prescribed analgesics for pain and NSAIDs for anti-inflammatory effects. Severe symptoms may require a tapered dose of corticosteroids.

FURTHER READING

Brown, W. M. & Jones, E. L. First operation for myocardial revascularization. In Edmunds, L. H. Jr., ed. *Cardiac Surgery in the Adult*, 1st edn. New York, NY: McGraw-Hill, 1997: 535.

Eagle, K. A., Guyton, R. A., Davidoff, R. *et al*. ACC/AHA Guidelines for coronary artery bypass graft surgery: a Report of the American College of Cardiology/American Heart Association Task Force on Practice Guidelines (committee to revise the 1991 guidelines for coronary artery bypass graft surgery). *J. Am. Coll. Cardiol.* 1999; **34**: 1262.

Guyton, R. A. Coronary artery bypass. In Morris, P. J. & Wood, W. C., eds. *Oxford Textbook of Surgery*, 2nd edn. Oxford, UK: Oxford University Press, 2000: 40.8.3.

Lytle, B. W. Coronary bypass surgery. In Fuster, V., Alexander, R. W., & O'Rourke, R. A., eds. *Hurst's The Heart*, 10th edn. New York, NY: McGraw-Hill, 2001: 1507.

Puskas, J. D., Williams, W. H., Duke, P. G. *et al*. Off-pump coronary artery bypass grafting provides complete revascularization with reduced myocardial injury, transfusion requirements, and length of stay: a prospective randomized comparison of two hundred unselected patients undergoing off-pump versus conventional coronary artery bypass grafting. *J. Thorac. Cardiovasc. Surg.* 2003; **125**: 797.

Puskas, J. D., Thourani, V. H., Marshall, J. J. *et al*. Clinical outcomes, angiographic patency, and resource utilization in 200 consecutive off-pump coronary bypass patients. *Ann. Thorac. Surg.* 2001; **71**: 1477.

64

Cardiac rhythm management

Omar M. Lattouf

Emory University School of Medicine, Atlanta, GA

Therapeutic, device-aided cardiac rhythm management is useful in patients with a variety of rhythm and rate related abnormalities, leading to reduction of symptoms of cardiac dysfunction and improvement in quality of life. Single-chamber atrial pacing has been commonly utilized in the treatment of patients with sinus pauses, sick sinus syndrome, and bradycardia–tachycardia syndrome. As long as AV synchrony is maintained and there is no AV block, this method has been noted to be efficacious and safe. If AV block does develop, atrial pacing will not prevent bradycardia. For prevention of atrial fibrillation, dual-site atrial pacing has been shown to be valuable as an adjunct to drug therapy in reducing the incidence of paroxysmal atrial fibrillation.

Single-chamber ventricular pacing has been utilized in patients with high-grade AV block, Mobitz type II, or third-degree heart block, and is usually reserved for such patients who are not candidates for dual chamber AV pacing due to other comorbid factors that significantly reduce life expectancy or physical abilities. A major limiting factor for the utilization of this method is the occasional development of pacemaker syndrome, which occurs due to retrograde electrical current conduction through the AV node to the atria, causing discordant premature contraction of the atria during closed phase of the AV valve with resultant decreased cardiac output. Weakness, dizziness, or even frank syncope are symptoms of this condition.

Currently, dual-chamber pacing is the most commonly applied method and involves sensing and pacing both the right atrium and the right ventricle in accordance with specific programming dictated by the existing rhythm and conduction disturbances. Indications for dual-chamber pacing include:

(a) sick sinus syndrome;
(b) sinus pauses;
(c) bundle branch block with prolonged His bundle-ventricular interval;
(d) alternating bundle branch block;
(e) bifasicular block with His bundle-ventricular interval greater than 100 ms;
(f) symptomatic third-degree AV block;
(g) asymptomatic third-degree AV block;
(h) asymptomatic type II AV block;
(i) post-AV nodal ablation;
(j) autonomic nervous system dysfunction, with drug refractory and vasovagal syncope;
(k) symptomatic carotid hypersensitivity, confirmed by either bradycardia (greater than 3 sec sinus pause) or greater than 50 mm drop in blood pressure, or both.

Another group of patients that have been reported to benefit from right ventricular pacing are those with hypertrophic obstructive cardiomyopathy and documented left ventricular outflow tract gradient.

In dual chamber pacing, native atrial activity is sensed and transmitted through the atrial lead into the pacemaker unit, initiating an appropriate ventricular stimulating signal down the ventricular wire into the right ventricle in accordance with a preprogramed time interval. In the absence of a sensed atrial signal, the dual chamber pacer will initiate coordinated timed signals to the atrium and subsequently to the ventricle, resulting in coordinated and specifically timed atrial ventricular contraction.

Cardiac resynchronization therapy

More recently, trichamber pacemaker technology has been shown to significantly improve the clinical status and functionality of patients suffering from congestive heart failure that display ejection fractions that are $<35\%$ associated with widened QRS complex and left bundle branch block of 120 msec or more. This atrial–biventricular resynchronization technique with optimization of AV delay appears to improve systolic function, overall cardiac function, and reduce mitral regurgitation.

Medical Management of the Surgical Patient: A Textbook of Perioperative Medicine, ed. M. F. Lubin, R. B. Smith, T. F. Dobson, N. Spell, H. K. Walker. 4th edn. Published by Cambridge University Press. © Cambridge University 2006.

Automatic implantable cardiac defibrillator

Implantable cardiac defibrillators are indicated and are increasingly utilized in the management of patients with sudden cardiac death and other serious ventricular dysrhythmias. Patients who are acceptable candidates for AICD implantation are those at high-risk of ventricular arrhythmia, such as patients with non-sustained ventricular tachycardia with decreased left ventricular (LV) function due to coronary artery disease; those with poor LV function and an ejection fraction less than 30% due to prior myocardial infarction; and those with a prior history of aborted sudden death due to cardiac dysrhythmia.

Operative technique for implantation of cardiac rhythm management devices

Percutaneous transvenous radiographic guided lead placement has essentially replaced the thoracotomy-based approach in pacemaker insertion procedures, though a minithoracotomy or thoracoscopic technique may be used for lead implantation in rare cases where the transvenous route is inaccessible due to unfavorable anatomy, thrombosed subclavian vein, or persistent left superior vena cava. After the appropriate leads have been positioned in the targeted cardiac chambers, the energy source is usually implanted in the left infraclavicular area either subcutaneously or in the sub pectoral region. For atrial sensing and pacing, an atrial lead is typically positioned in the right atrial appendage. The right ventricular lead is positioned in the ventricular apex. In cases of biventricular resynchronization, the preceding two leads are combined with a third lead that is inserted transvenously into the coronary sinus for pacing the left ventricle. With the impulse delivered at the lateral left ventricular wall, this lead will pace the left ventricle.

AICD placement has likewise become technically straightforward and is similar to pacemaker implantation. As with the previous method, the procedure is done with strict antiseptic technique under local anesthesia with additional intravenous sedation. The right ventricular lead (sensing, pacing, and defibrillation) is inserted via the subclavian or cephalic vein and directed toward the apex. A right atrial lead is inserted as needed in the usual fashion. Prior to completion of the procedure the device is tested for sensing, defibrillation, and pacing.

Local anesthesia and intravenous sedation are commonly used for these procedures. Occasionally, general anesthesia with double lumen intubation is required if thoracotomy or thoracoscopy are utilized for lead placement.

Usual postoperative course

Expected postoperative hospital stay
Discharge on the same or following day after uncomplicated course.

Operative mortality
Postprocedure deaths rarely occur from cardiac chamber perforation, but overall mortality is more related to the underlying heart condition.

Special monitoring required
Postoperative chest X-ray and EKG are routinely performed.

Patient activity and positioning
Ambulated the same day.

Alimentation
Patient's usual diet is allowed.

Antibiotic coverage
Perioperative antibiotic coverage for 24 hours with cephalosporin or, in case of penicillin allergy, with vancomycin.

Postoperative visits
Cardiology follow-up for interval evaluation of cardiac rhythm maintenance.

Postoperative complications

In the hospital

Infection
Bleeding, hemothorax or pericardiac tamponade
Pneumothorax

After discharge

Lead erosion
Lead fracture with conduction abnormality
Over- and under-sensing
AICD inappropriate shock for atrial fibrillation or sinus tachycardia
Lead displacement
Diaphragmatic stimulation
Generator failure
Subclavian vein thrombosis

FURTHER READING

Abraham, W., Fisher, W. G., Smith, A. L. *et al.* Cardiac resynchronization in chronic heart failure. *N. Engl. J. Med.* 2002; **346**: 1945–1953.

Buxton, A. E., Lee, K. L., Fisher, J. D., Josephson, M. E., Prystowsky, E. N., & Hafley, G. A. Randomized study of the prevention of sudden death in patients with coronary artery disease. *N. Engl. J. Med.* 1999; **341**(25): 182–190.

Connelly, D. T. Implantable cardioverter-defibrillators. *Br. Med. J. Heart* 2001; **86**: 221–228.

Gregoratos, G., Cheitlin, M. D., Conill, A. *et al.* ACC/AHA Guidelines for implantation of cardiac pacemakers and anti-arrhythmia devices: a report of the American College of Cardiology/American Heart Association Task Force in Practice Guidelines (Committee on Pacemaker Implantation). *J. Am. Coll. Cardiol.* 1998; **31**(5): 1175–1209.

Kappenberger, L., Linde, C., Daubert, C. *et al.* Pacing for hypertrophic cardiomyopathy. *Eur. Heart J.* 1997; **18**(8): 1249–1256.

Kass, D. (ed.) Pathophysiology of physiologic cardiac pains: advantages of leaving well enough alone. *J. Am. Med. Assoc.* 2002; **288**: 3159–3161.

Kenny, R. A., Richardson, D. A., Steen, N., Bexton, R. S., Shaw, F. E., & Bond, J. Carotid sinus syndromes: a modified risk factor for non-accidental falls in older adults. *J. Am. Coll. Cardiol.* 2001; **38**(5): 1491–1496.

Kusumoto, F. Device therapy for cardiac arrhythmias. *J. Am. Med. Assoc.* 2002; **287**(14): 1848.

Lau, C. P. Pacing for atrial fibrillation. *Br. Med. J. Heart* 2003; **89**: 106–112.

Mansour, K. A. & Connoly, M. W. Permanent pacemaker implantation. In Lubin, M. F., Walker, K. C., & Smith, R. B., eds. *Medical Management of the Surgical Patient.* Philadelphia, PA: J. B. Lippincott, 1995.

Maron, B. J. Assessment of dual-chamber pacing as a treatment for drug refractory symptomatic patients with obstructive hypertrophic cardiomyopathy: a randomized, double-blind, cross-over study. *Circulation* 1999; **99**: 2927–2933.

Moss, A. J., Hall, W. J., Cannom, D. S. *et al.* Improved survival with an implanted defibrillator in patients with coronary disease at high risk for ventricular arrhythmia. *N. Engl. J. Med.* 1996; **335**(26): 1933–1940.

Moss, A. J., Zareba, W., Hall, W. J. *et al.* Prophylactic manipulation of a defibrillator in patients with myocardial infarctions and reduced ejection fraction. *N. Engl. J. Med.* 2002; **346**(12): 877–883.

Olshensky, B. Indications for internal cardioverter defibrillators. In Kusumoto, F. M. & Goldshlager, N., eds. *Cardiac Pacing for the Clinician.* Philadelphia, PA: Lippincott, Williams and Wilkins, 2001.

Sutton, R., Brignole, M., Menozzi, C. *et al.* Dual-chamber pacing with treatment of neurally mediated tilt-positive cardioinhibitory syncope. *Circulation* 2000; **102**(3): 294–299.

65

Aortic valve surgery

Jason M. Budde and William A. Cooper

Emory University School of Medicine, Atlanta, GA

Aortic stenosis

Etiologies of aortic stenosis (AS) are almost evenly divided between rheumatic fever (RF) (40%), usually with concomitant mitral valve pathology, and congenital bicuspid anatomy (40%), with the remainder of cases due to senile, calcific degeneration. The classic triad of symptoms in AS includes angina, syncope, and congestive heart failure (CHF), each of these independently predicting a limited life expectancy: 5 years, 3 to 4 years, and 1½ to 2 years, respectively. Sudden death may occur in 15%–20% of cases, and the onset of symptoms, particularly near the age of 60, usually heralds precipitous decline leading to death. Therefore, operation is indicated at the onset of these symptoms, as well as in selected asymptomatic patients with estimated transvalvular gradients exceeding 50 mm Hg or valve orifice areas less than 0.8 cm. The orifice area is calculated using the Gorlin equation, which takes into account the cardiac output and square root of the transvalvular gradient.

Aortic regurgitation

Aortic regurgitation (AR) is caused in 50% of cases by RF, with remaining etiologies being endocarditis, myxomatous changes, rheumatoid arthritis, lupus, and a host of causes of aortic root dilatation (tertiary syphilis, Marfan's syndrome, Ehlers–Danlos, osteogenesis imperfecta, aortic dissection). Emergent operation may be indicated in acute aortic regurgitation as a result of aortic dissection, and is seen primarily in patients with uncontrolled hypertension, ascending aortic aneurysms, annuloaortic ectasia, and Marfan's syndrome. In this setting, operation may require replacement or resuspension of the aortic valve plus ascending aortic reconstruction with a tube graft.

Chronic AR is typically asymptomatic and can be difficult to diagnose by history and physical examination alone; over time the heart compensates via elevated end-diastolic pressure (EDP), ventricular dilatation, and decreased wall tension. The net effect of these compensatory changes allows for a positive aortic gradient and forward aortic ejection. Heart failure negatively impacts patient mortality and long-term outcomes. Therefore, operation is indicated at the earliest sign of development of failure – seen clinically by CHF symptoms, S3 gallop, or left ventricular EDD (end diastolic diameter) of 70 mm or more. Unfortunately, statistics still indicate that 40% of patients are in CHF – with 53% in NYHA classes III or IV – at the time of surgery.

Endocarditis

Indications for operation in endocarditis include failure to eradicate infection, severe regurgitation, evidence of perivalvular extension, and repeated significant embolic episodes. As with mitral surgery, preoperative preparation includes coronary angiography for patients over 50 years of age or those with angina, periodontal evaluation in the case of oral infection, and therapeutic antibiotics prior to skin incision.

Aortic valve repair

Seldom performed, aortic valve repair is reserved for a select group of patients with limited cuspal prolapse or enlarged annulus. Postrepair persistent regurgitation is as high as 17%, with reoperation required in half of these patients. Direct repair may be suitable for children or patients who cannot be anticoagulated or who have an exceedingly small annulus or outflow tract.

Aortic valve replacement

The issues of anticoagulation and durability are of paramount importance in the decision-making process for aortic valve replacement surgery. The majority of replacement valves (60%) in the aortic position are bioprosthetic and

Medical Management of the Surgical Patient: A Textbook of Perioperative Medicine, ed. M. F. Lubin, R. B. Smith, T. F. Dobson, N. Spell, H. K. Walker. 4th edn. Published by Cambridge University Press. © Cambridge University 2006.

require only 6 to 12 weeks of postoperative anticoagulation or no anticoagulation at all. Reoperation for valve degeneration occurs in 15% at 10 years and 35% at 15 years, primarily due to structural valve deterioration. Mechanical valves (36%) are more durable, require permanent coumadin therapy, and increase the incidence of hemolysis – typically subclinical and manifested by mild anemia. The bileaflet-disk type demonstrates the least shear stress but has the highest regurgitant fractions. The optimal candidates for mechanical valves are young adults and patients with small aortic roots, although patients with smaller annula may also benefit from the improved durability of newer-generation bioprosthetic valves designed for supraannular seating. Cryopreserved homografts (human allograft) (2.6%) represent a very attractive option due to superior valve performance and no need for anticoagulation, but are limited in use by scarce supply, rigorous preservation and thawing protocols, and by the technical demands of implantation. The use of autologous pulmonic valve in the aortic position ("Ross procedure") represents the maximization of flow dynamics, durability (15% reoperative rate at 24 years), resistance from infection and thrombosis, and affords valve growth in children. The main obstacles have been difficulties with sizing, explantation, and opposition to the creation of new right-sided valve disease, although freedom from reoperation due to pulmonic regurgitation has been as high as 81% at 20 years.

Perioperative monitoring includes pulmonary arterial and upper extremity arterial line as well as large-bore venous access. Operative exposure is via median sternotomy. Cardioplegic techniques are customary and depend upon institutional and surgeon preference; however, in cases of surgery for AR, the ostia of the coronary arteries require direct cannulation, with meticulous attention to avoid obstruction or calcific embolization. The valve is accessed via transverse aortotomy followed by valve excision and debridement of calcifications from the annulus, which is usually where the replacement valve is seated. Aortic cross-clamp time averages 80 minutes, total bypass time 112 minutes, and total operative time 180–240 minutes. Great attention is paid to de-airing of the patient, accomplished by left ventricular and aortic venting, slow side-to-side rocking of the table, and real-time surveillance of air bubbles with transesophageal echocardiography (TEE).

Usual postoperative course

Expected postoperative hospital stay
On the average, approximately 8 days, which may be shorter if anticoagulation is not required.

Operative mortality
Three percent overall for primary aortic surgery and below 5% for patients under 80 years of age. Outcomes for AS are generally better than for AR. Reoperation increases mortality 6% to 10%, and depressed left ventricular function can increase 5-year mortality by 50%.

Special monitoring required
The patient's intensive-care stay continues until ventilation is discontinued, mental status is near normal, and inotropic and antiarrhythmic drips are no longer required. Routine floor care includes 24 to 48 hours of telemetry monitoring, early ambulation, and aggressive pulmonary toilet.

Patient activity and positioning
Up to chair after extubated. Early ambulation is encouraged.

Alimentation
Diet advanced as tolerated.

Antibiotic coverage
Antibiotic selection and duration depends upon the clinical situation.

Postoperative complications

In the hospital

Cardiac rhythm disturbances
Perioperative complications include atrial arrhythmias in 40% of patients with an incidence of atrial fibrillation of 24.6%, which usually resolves spontaneously in those with preoperative sinus rhythm. Bradyarrhythmias are common, with up to 10% of postop patients experiencing heart block and half of these requiring permanent pacing.

Bleeding
Reexploration for bleeding occurs in 3.7% of patients and may be related to several factors: early elevated partial thromboplastin time from residual heparin, thrombasthenia from the extracorporeal bypass circuit, or surgically correctible factors such as intercostal vessel hemorrhage or leaking or disrupted aortotomy suture line. Despite corrective and resuscitative measures, persistent hourly chest tube output greater than 200 ml, falling hematocrit levels, and hemodynamic compromise mandate urgent reexploration. Pericardial tamponade is life threatening and requires formal operative or bedside emergent re-exploration.

Cerebrovascular accident

Stroke is reported in 3.5% of patients, half of whom will experience permanent deficit. Aortic atherosclerotic debris is the frequent source of embolic stroke; however, ventricular and mitral thrombi, and, less commonly, valve thrombus should be considered as well. Carotid atherosclerotic disease is a significant risk factor for stroke, but should be properly assessed and treated as indicated in the preoperative period.

Impaired ejection fraction

Low cardiac output is generally reported as the most common cause of death in the early postoperative period. Workup starts with optimization of preload – which may need to be higher than usual, with pulmonary capillary wedge pressure of 16–18 mm Hg in the hypertrophied ventricle of aortic stenosis – and of rate and rhythm, using external pacing if necessary. Intraaortic balloon pump is required in 2.8% of patients, with only 0.5% placed preoperatively and 0.5% placed postoperatively. Perioperative myocardial infarction has a reported incidence of 0.3%.

Wound infection

Deep sternal wound infection is a costly, morbid, and often fatal complication that nearly doubles mortality. Fortunately, it occurs in only 0.4% of isolated aortic valve surgeries. Preoperative Hibiclens scrub to the chest, surgeon double-gloving, perioperative prophylactic antibiotics, and adhesive surgical draping serving to block contact of skin flora with the wound have all contributed to low infection rates. Treatment includes tailored antibiotic regimens, early operative drainage and debridement, and tissue defect coverage with pectoral muscle and omental flaps.

After discharge

Endocarditis

The appearance of this valve-related complication within several months after discharge typically represents initial surgical contamination or residual infection and is best treated with aggressive surgical management, which can halve the high (50%–75%) mortality rate. Infection beyond 3 months usually results from an invasive procedure-related bacteremia, emphasizing the importance of life-long antibiotic prophylaxis. Mechanical and bioprosthetic valves demonstrate nearly equal reinfection rates – between 6% and 8% rate at 10 years with the peak at 1 month – which is approximately 1/50th as common in

homografts. Autograft infections are usually reported as zero in larger studies.

Thromboembolism and bleeding

These are the most commonly documented complications encountered with prosthetic valves. In mechanical valves in the aortic position, thromboembolism is reported at 0.7–4.7 events per patient–year, and anticoagulant related bleeding at 0.7 to 7.9 events. In bioprosthetics, the values are 0.7–1.2 and 0.3–0.8, respectively. Patient selection and education are most effective in preventing these problems, but consideration may be given to re-replacement of mechanical with bioprosthetic material after repeated and significant episodes of hemorrhage in anticoagulated patients.

Mechanical failure

Regurgitation or periprosthetic leaks can occur in all valves for many reasons, including annuloprosthetic size mismatch, suture error, calcification, infection, or inadequate fibrous ingrowth. Structural deterioration in bioprosthetic valves occurs at an expected rate, usually at 0.4–1 event per year, and 20%–25% need replacement at 20 years. Calcification of tissues often followed by cusp rupture is the predominant mechanism, which is accentuated in patients less than 30 years of age. Failure of mechanical valves has a much lower incidence and is typically attributable to thrombus, pannus ingrowth, or the presence of long chordal tissue or unraveled sutures, all of which may interfere with disk closure. Homografts have demonstrated nearly equivalent endurance rates to bioprosthetic porcine grafts, which are greatly augmented by increased cell viability of the implanted graft. Autograft pulmonic valves require reoperation at about half this rate.

FURTHER READING

Baue, A. E., Geha, A. S., Hammond, G. L. *et al.*, eds. *Glenn's Thoracic and Cardiovascular Surgery*. 6th edn. Stamford, CT: Appleton and Lange, 1996.

Gott, J. P., Thourani, V. H., Wright, C. E. *et al.* Risk neutralization in cardiac operations: detection and treatment of associated carotid disease. *Ann. Thorac. Surg.* 1999; **68**(3): 850–856.

McGiffin, D. C., Galbraith, A. J., McLachlan, G. J. *et al.* Risk factors for death and recurrent endocarditis after aortic valve replacement. *J. Thorac. Cardiovasc. Surg.* 1992; **104**: 511–520.

Moon, M. R., Miller, D. C., Moore, K. A. *et al.* Treatment of endocarditis with valve replacement: the question of tissue versus mechanical prosthesis. *Ann. Thorac. Surg.* 2001; **71**(4): 1164–1171.

Society of Thoracic Surgeons Database, Fall 2001.

66

Mitral valve surgery

Jason M. Budde and William A. Cooper

Emory University School of Medicine, Atlanta, GA

Both in the USA and worldwide, the most common cause of mitral valve pathology in adults is rheumatic fever (RF). Postrheumatic structural changes to the mitral valve typically occur over the 2 to 10 years following infection, with symptoms appearing over the subsequent 5 to 10 years. In descending order, secondary etiologies include myxomatous degeneration, endocarditis, idiopathic annular calcification, connective tissue disorders (Marfan's and Ehlers–Danlos disease), and hypertrophic cardiomyopathy; however, mitral stenosis (MS) is almost exclusively attributable to rheumatic fever. The advent of decompensated heart failure in MS patients is typically presaged by decreased exercise tolerance with progressive dyspnea secondary to low cardiac output, pulmonary hypertension, and decreased lung compliance. Timely operative intervention early in the symptomatic period can completely reverse heart failure. Mitral regurgitation (MR), where the valve is almost purely regurgitant, is also caused by RF. Ischemic MR is present in up to 20% of patients with coronary artery disease (CAD) requiring operative coronary artery bypass (CAB), and infrequently involves the catastrophic event of ruptured papillary muscle.

Indications for operation depend upon the pathophysiologic condition present. In severe MS, symptoms and signs of worsening heart failure absolutely indicate surgery. Angiographic or echocardiographic estimation of a mitral orifice area of $2\,cm^2$ denotes mild to moderate disease, while $1\,cm^2$ denotes severe levels. Intervention should be undertaken prior to the appearance of heart failure, which significantly worsens outcome. Operative candidates with MR may be divided into two categories: those in which acute regurgitation is caused by either abrupt endocarditic cuspal tear or ischemic papillary rupture, resulting in an uncompensated heart that demands immediate surgery; and those with chronic MR that have a

well-compensated heart who can be stably situated in NYHA class I or II. Patients in the latter category may best be managed with medical therapy, especially if they are of advanced age with significant comorbidities. On the other hand, healthy young patients with mild to moderate disease and low expected risk should be strongly considered for surgery before the development of left ventricular failure. Operation in chronic MR is indicated mainly for NYHA class II or greater, pulmonary pathophysiology such as hemoptysis and hypertension, signs of right heart failure, and desired pregnancy in appropriately aged females with mild to moderate disease in whom increased flow across the valve during gestation could increase symptoms. Surgery for both MS or MR should occur either before or shortly after the onset of atrial fibrillation (AF) when left atrial architecture is sufficiently preserved and reversion to normal sinus rhythm can be reasonably expected. Operation for native valve endocarditis is indicated for failed eradication of infection, grade 4 angiographic regurgitation independent of failure, repeated significant embolic episodes, and infection with resistant organisms (fungus, *Pseudomonas*, *Serratia*, *Staphylococcus aureus*, *Herellia*). Threshold for operation should be lowered with valve vegetations larger than one centimeter; evidence of progression to perivalvular abscess or the ominous finding of AV block (signifying destruction of the AV node), should be considered a failure of non-operative management and operation undertaken immediately.

The choice of surgical repair or replacement is a complex decision that requires that the valve be examined by the surgeon. Mitral commissurotomy is a somewhat outdated technique indicated for rheumatic fusion of commissures in cases of either MR, MS, or a combination of both. Commissurotomy is typically performed with mitral annuloplasty and achieves an acceptable reoperative rate

Medical Management of the Surgical Patient: A Textbook of Perioperative Medicine, ed. M. F. Lubin, R. B. Smith, T. F. Dobson, N. Spell, H. K. Walker. 4th edn. Published by Cambridge University Press. © Cambridge University 2006.

of 13% at 10 years. Formal repair is indicated for more extensive structural damage, such as chordal rupture, cuspal tear, or limited cuspal perforation that encompasses well below 50% of the valve mechanism. For MR, repair is generally more feasible than replacement and is accomplished with decreased bypass and crossclamp times, hospital stays, and reoperative and mortality rates. However, those with preoperative shock or serious comorbidities should not be considered for repair; therefore, improved outcomes with repair may not only reflect technical advantage over replacement, but also less extensive disease and better preoperative conditions.

Mitral valve replacement is chosen for "sicker" patients and those with more extensive valvular destruction. Replacement should include preservation of the posterior leaflet and chordal mechanism to preserve ventricular systolic shortening and limit ventricular stress. Whether to use a mechanical or bioprosthetic valve relies essentially upon the risks of anticoagulation with mechanical valves versus the decreased durability of bioprosthetics. In the former (58% of replacements), mean valve longevity is approximately 20 years and anticoagulation is absolutely required. As for bioprosthetic valves (37% of mitral valve replacements), the most common type is the stented porcine xenograft, which has a mean durability of 10–15 years. Bioprosthetics show decreased shear stress compared to mechanical valves, but are more stenotic at smaller sizes and hence an inferior choice in those with a diminutive annulus. They are ideal when anticoagulation is contraindicated or unfeasible (gastrointestinal or central nervous system hemorrhagic potential), when pregnancy is desired (due to the teratogenicity and perinatal complications of Coumadin), and those over 30 years of age, after which the strong propensity towards calcification and structural failure begins to decrease. Promising new technologies such as valve treatment with alpha-amino oleic acid (Mosaic valve) seek to stem the process of calcific degeneration; the Mosaic valve has shown favorable 4-year performance data and may change the algorithm of valve choice. Anticoagulation with bioprosthetics is favored by most surgeons postoperatively for 6 to 12 weeks during the process of valve incorporation.

The choice of replacement valve for endocarditis depends mainly upon the site of infection: isolated cuspal involvement may be completely resected and allow for antibiotic penetration and thus feasibility of a mechanical valve; however, deep perivalvular extension may contraindicate placement of a synthetic material. Finally, the use of "minimally invasive" robotic techniques, for both repair

and replacement of mitral valves, has proven feasible with cardioplegic arrest. In the USA and in other countries, it has shown reduced bypass and crossclamp times and acceptable short-term morbidity and mortality; therefore, robotic methods may become more standard in the future.

Preoperative preparation routinely consists of coronary angiography for patients older than 50 years of age and is mandatory in any patient with angina or anginal equivalent. Periodontal evaluation is indicated, and those with endocarditis should receive therapeutic levels of appropriate antibiotics. In non-endocarditic surgery, a standard antistaphylococcal antibiotic regimen (cefazolin, or vancomycin for the penicillin-allergic) should be administered thirty minutes prior to skin incision.

The mitral valve is best accessed via a standard left atrial incision parallel to the interatrial groove, while a right atrial incision and transseptal access are used in scarred "redo" or calcified left atria or if tricuspid surgery is planned. Although a median sternotomy affords the least postoperative pain and pulmonary embarrassment, a right anterolateral thoracotomy provides for optimal exposure. Intraoperative transesophageal echocardiography (TEE) is standard and essential for real-time feedback regarding valve mechanics. Perioperative monitoring has been greatly simplified in recent years: thermister tip pulmonary artery (PA) catheters are standard as the use of left atrial catheters have been found to provide no advantage and are seldom applied. Myocardial preservation is customary and great care is taken to avoid harming the conduction system, left circumflex coronary artery, aortic valve apparatus, and particularly the atrioventricular groove, especially during debridement of infected or calcified annuli. Total operative time is typically 150 to 300 minutes and is generally shorter for mitral repair.

Usual postoperative course

Expected postoperative hospital stay
An average of 8.5 days (repair) to 12.5 days (replacement), with a portion of this time needed for anticoagulation.

Operative mortality
2.2% for repair and 5.9% for replacement. Mortality may increase to 10%–20% or higher in emergent operations, ischemic MR, or cardiogenic shock. NYHA class, increased ventricular chamber size, MR as opposed to MS, and duration of cross-clamp time are all predictors of poor outcome. All told, the rate of early major complication plus operative mortality is 13.1% for mitral repair and 24.7% for replacement.

Special monitoring required

Though most patients leave the operating room on one or more cardiotonic or vasotonic intravenous drips, most are weaned off and many extubated later the same postoperative day. Most patients not already taking beta-blocking medications are administered low-dose metoprolol for antiarrhythmic prophylaxis. If in a stable rhythm, epicardial pacing wires and telemetry monitoring are discontinued 48 hours postoperatively.

Patient activity and positioning

Patients are up at their bedsides on the day of extubation. Ambulation is encouraged early on, and incentive spirometry and other methods of pulmonary toilet are instituted.

Alimentation

Diet advanced as tolerated.

Antibiotic coverage

Perioperative antibiotic selection and duration depend upon the underlying diagnosis.

Postoperative complications

In the hospital

Cardiac rhythm disturbances

Atrial arrhythmias are the most common perioperative rhythm disturbance, occurring in 70% of mitral cases, with AF in 20% of all mitral replacement patients. Most patients in sinus rhythm preoperatively will ultimately revert spontaneously; until then, ventricular rate control is accomplished with short-acting beta blockade, calcium channel blockade, and digoxin therapy. Surgical ablation of chronic AF achieves lasting conversion to sinus rhythm in 96% of patients at up to 5 years. This can be performed at the time of mitral surgery, and is becoming the standard of care in patients with mitral disease and AF. Bradyarrhythmias and AV nodal block are common, usually transient, and best managed with pacing or occasionally with oral theophylline. Premature ventricular contractions (PVCs) are also typical and may be suppressed with atrial or atrioventricular pacing to a rate of 90 to 100 beats/minute, or simply corrected with electrolyte repletion.

Cerebrovascular accident

Perioperative stroke occurs in 10.9% of patients and is permanent in 2.4%. Intraoperative embolism of thrombus or of particles, including air, may be responsible; in the latter the use of hyperbaric oxygen may reverse the neurologic deficit up to 24 hours postoperatively.

Impaired ejection fraction

Postoperative low cardiac output, characterized by measured cardiac index less than $2\,l/min$ per m^2 and low mixed venous saturations, is initially treated by optimizing preload and heart rate (often requiring pacing to greater than, or equal to, 90 beats/min) and with pharmacologic inotropy (calcium, phosphodiesterase inhibitors such as milrinone, and catecholamines such as epinephrine). Intraaortic balloon pumps are used in 7.9% of patients, with approximately half of them placed preoperatively.

Severe cardiac dysfunction

Myocardial infarct is reported in 0.3% and cardiogenic shock in 3% of mitral operations. Sudden development of low ventricular output combined with equalizing chamber pressures as measured by PA catheter, should raise suspicion of cardiac tamponade and prompt either repeat TEE or, in the presence of overwhelming evidence, emergent re-exploration.

Wound infection

Deep sternal wound infections occur in 0.1% of patients and present a particularly precarious problem with a high mortality, especially in the setting of infected prosthetic valves.

After discharge

Bleeding and thrombosis

Late postoperative thromboembolism is reported in up to 1.7% of mitral operations and is most frequent in ball-in-cage type mechanical valves and, to a lesser degree, in tilting-disk types. There are no data to suggest any advantage with the maintenance of prothrombin times greater than 1.5 to 2 times normal. Bleeding occurs at 3% per patient–year, with a 0.2% patient–year mortality. Thorough patient education may reduce this rate, but repeated significant bleeding episodes may prompt consideration of re-replacement of the valve with a bioprosthetic.

Infection

Prosthetic valve endocarditis may be stratified into early and late cases. Those at less than six months postoperatively are typically due to intraoperative contamination and are better managed operatively (mortality rate 22%–46%) than non-operatively (65%). Earlier operation is key, especially to prevent new perivalvular abscess. Therefore, initial postoperative antibiotics should be immediately initiated, tailored to positive intraoperative cultures, and continued for six weeks. Late infections are usually related to dental or other procedures and can be successfully treated medically in the absence of perivalvular extension.

Valve failure

Need for reoperation is uncommon after mitral repair (around 2%), and is usually determined during initial operation, after separation from bypass, and during physiologic reassessment with TEE. Mitral re-replacement is most common with the use of bioprosthetics – 20 to 25% at 10 years, higher in patients less than 35 years of age – and is typically due to calcific degeneration with later cuspal tear. Malfunction of mechanical valves seldom occurs, though when it does it is chiefly due to pannus formation over time and requires reintervention in only 0.5% of patients. More acute appearance of mechanical valve dysfunction, often symptomatic, should raise suspicion of a thrombotic cause, and indicates more immediate therapy, either surgical thrombectomy or re-replacement.

FURTHER READING

Baue, A. E., Geha, A. S., Hammond, G. L. *et al.*, eds. *Glenn's Thoracic and Cardiovascular Surgery*. 6th edn. Stamford, CT: Appleton and Lange, 1996.

Choudhary, S. K., Dhareshwar, J., Govil, A. *et al.* Open mitral commissurotomy in the current era: indications, technique, and results. *Ann. Thorac. Surg.* 2003; **75**(1): 41–46.

Cox, J. L. Atrial transport function after the maze procedure for atrial fibrillation: a 10-year clinical experience. *Am. Heart J.* 1998; **136**(6): 934–936.

Duarte, I. G., MacDonald, M. J., Cooper, W. A. *et al.* In vivo hemodynamic, histologic, and antimineralization characteristics of the Mosaic bioprosthesis. *Ann. Thorac. Surg.* 2001; **71**(1): 92–99.

Nifong, L. W., Chu, V. F., Bailey, B. M. *et al.* Robotic mitral valve repair: experience with the da Vinci system. *Ann. Thorac. Surg.* 2003; **75**(2): 438–442.

Society of Thoracic Surgeons Database, Fall 2001.

Thomson, D. J., Jamieson, E. J., Dumesnil, J. G. *et al.* Medtronic mosaic porcine bioprosthesis: midterm investigational trial results. *Ann. Thorac. Surg.* 2001; **71**: S269–S272.

Trehan, N., Mishra, Y. K., & Sharma, M. Robotically controlled video-assisted port-access mitral valve surgery. *Asian CV Thorac. Ann.* 2002; **10**(2): 133–136.

67

Ventricular assist devices and cardiac transplantation

V. Seenu Reddy and J. David Vega

Emory University School of Medicine, Atlanta, GA

The first example of mechanical circulatory support is credited to Stuckey and colleagues who used an early heart–lung machine to support a patient suffering an acute myocardial infarction in 1957. In 1965, Spencer reported the use of a centrifugal pump in a patient with circulatory collapse after cardiac surgery. The management of cardiogenic shock and the ability to transiently support the heart was revolutionized by Kantrowitz and associates in 1968 with the clinical use of the intra-aortic balloon pump (IABP). Although the first ventricular assist devices (VAD) were pioneered in the 1970s, it wasn't until the late 1980s that the Thoratec, Novacor, and HeartMate assist devices attained widespread use as bridges to cardiac transplantation. In 1967, the treatment for end-stage heart disease was forever altered with the advent of heart transplantation. Currently in the USA, there are approximately 500 VADS placed each year and 2500 heart transplants performed in adults.

There are two goals associated with mechanical circulatory support. As with the IABP, the initial goal of the VAD is to stem the multiorgan dysfunction that ensues with poor perfusion secondary to cardiogenic shock; however, the long term goal of VAD therapy is to rehabilitate patients while awaiting cardiac transplantation. In some cases, VAD therapy has become the definitive treatment for a patient's end-stage heart disease. Mechanical support is both initiated and continued in the setting of optimized medical and pharmacological management of the failing heart patient. Usually temporary inotropic drug infusions combined with vasodilator therapy are routinely used in these patients.

Patient selection criteria for mechanical circulatory support includes but is not limited to postcardiotomy shock, acute myocardial infarction combined with cardiogenic shock, decompensated chronic heart failure, malignant cardiac dysrhythmias not amenable to chemical or electrical cardioversion, and acute myocarditis with hemodynamic compromise. In general, these patients have cardiac indices $<2 l/min$ per m^2, mean arterial pressures $<65 mmHg$, left or right atrial pressures >20, decreased urine output $<0.5 ml/kg$ per hour, and an elevated systemic vascular resistance of >2100 dynes s per cm^{-1}. Patient selection for heart transplantation requires an extensive multidisciplinary medical evaluation and institutional committee approval.

Contraindications to the initiation of mechanical circulatory support are relative to the patient's acute condition and clinical course and are designed to obviate the unnecessary utilization of valuable resources. Relative exclusion criteria include irreversible renal failure, severe peripheral vascular or cerebrovascular disease, malignancy, advanced hepatic dysfunction or coagulopathy, and advanced sepsis.

Usual postoperative course

Expected postoperative hospital stay

The average time on mechanical circulatory support depends upon whether the device is intended as a bridge to transplantation or is destination therapy for end stage heart disease. Patients are typically discharged 30 days after implantation of ambulatory devices while heart transplant patients are generally discharged seven to ten days after transplantation depending most often on whether the patient was hospitalized or an outpatient prior to transplantation.

Operative mortality

Two to four percent for heart transplantation. The operative mortality for mechanical support devices is highly variable, ranging from 10–20%.

Medical Management of the Surgical Patient: A Textbook of Perioperative Medicine, ed. M. F. Lubin, R. B. Smith, T. F. Dobson, N. Spell, H. K. Walker. 4th edn. Published by Cambridge University Press. © Cambridge University 2006.

Special monitoring required

Patients remain in the intensive care unit for 2 to 4 days following transplantation. Invasive monitoring initially consists of a pulmonary artery catheter and direct arterial pressure measurements. Other measurements include continuous pulse oximetry and occasionally co-oximetry, indwelling catheter for urinary output, chest tube drainage, and electrocardiography to monitor rate and rhythm. Periodic laboratory assays, including arterial blood gas and electrolyte and cell counts, are performed every 4 to 6 hours initially and then lengthened to daily. Immunosuppression levels are obtained each day and postoperative echocardiography is performed to evaluate graft function. The first endomyocardial biopsy to evaluate for rejection is performed 7 to 10 days after transplantation. Monitoring after VAD placement is similar but is typically of longer duration. An aggressive effort is made to remove all invasive monitoring lines as soon as possible. Anticoagulation may be necessary after VAD insertion.

Patient activity and positioning

Patients arrive at the ICU intubated and sedated. Standard ICU protocols regarding mobilization are followed with side to side turning. Efforts are made to extubate patients as soon as possible so that full mobilization out of bed is facilitated. Incentive spirometry, pulmonary hygiene, and ambulation with physical therapy are initiated early and continued until discharge.

Alimentation

Oral diet is begun with clear liquids after extubation and advanced slowly to a low-sodium diet. Postoperative ileus and nausea are common, especially since VAD drive lines are tunneled through the abdominal wall. Some patients, especially if intubated preoperatively, are continued on hyperalimentation and converted to enteral feedings when weaned from vasopressors. Aggressive nutritional support is an important element of the postoperative course for both transplant and VAD patients.

Antibiotic coverage

Prophylactic perioperative antibiotic coverage may be extended to cover invasive lines and devices.

Epicardial pacing wires and chronotropes

Temporary atrial and ventricular pacing wires are typically left in place in transplant patients until the first biopsy or until the patient is weaned from chronotropic agents such as isoproteronol or dobutamine.

Postoperative complications

In the hospital

Low cardiac output

Usually defined as cardiac index of less than $2\,l/min$ per m^2. In transplant patients, this is most often due to problems with myocardial preservation, right heart failure, or acute graft dysfunction and is treated with epicardial pacing (HR > 90) or with inotropic agents (milrinone, epinephrine or dobutamine). In VAD patients it is usually due to volume status, right ventricular dysfunction, or inadequate pump flows and is treated with transfusion of blood products, colloid, or crystalloid; inotropic support; possible temporary RVAD insertion; and adjustment of VAD flow rates.

Postoperative bleeding

Common complication (3%–8%) in both transplant and VAD patients since these are often reoperations after a primary operation such as CABG. Heart failure patients are routinely anticoagulated. Also, extensive suture lines and anastomoses between the VAD and native tissue are common bleeding points. If surgical bleeding is excluded, then repletion of clotting factors is paramount. When bleeding persists or leads to extensive mediastinal collection of clot (tamponade physiology), reexploration and washout may be indicated.

Arrhythmias

Very common in VAD patients and less frequent in transplant patients. Management includes aggressive repletion of electrolytes, temporary epicardial pacing, and anti-arrhythmic medications. Atrial arrhythmias occur in up to 15%–20% of transplant patients while ventricular arrhythmias are common in VAD patients, especially if the device is attached directly to the ventricle and the patients are managed with either beta-blockers, calcium channel blockers, or amiodarone. Electrical cardioversion may be required. RVAD support may be necessary for refractory ventricular dysrhythmias.

Pericarditis

Infrequently seen but presents with chest pain, fever, and occasional arrhythmias approximately 10–30 days post-cardiotomy. Pericardial rub is pathognomonic. Treated with indomethacin, NSAIDS, or in severe cases with steroids.

Thromboemboli (peripheral, pulmonary and cerebral)

Occurs in up to 5%–10% of VAD patients depending on length of time on the device and management of anticoagulation. Etiology includes air emboli, atheromatous debris, emboli from intracardiac sources, or thromboemboli directly from the VAD. Sequelae may include ischemic limbs requiring urgent embolectomy, pulmonary emboli requiring ventilatory support, and anticoagulation or cerebral infarcts.

Infection/sepsis (including pneumonia)

A serious complication in device and transplant patients alike, occurring in up to 15% of patients if pneumonia and wound infections are included. Bacterial source is common in early infections (*S. aureus* and *Streptococcus* species). Nosocomial infections also include *Pseudomonas* and *Candida* related to ventilators and indwelling catheters despite prophylactic antibiotics. All indwelling devices should be removed as soon as possible in these immunosuppressed patients.

Late infections are usually opportunistic organisms in transplant patients and include viral agents. Many transplant patients are maintained on prophylactic trimethoprim-sulfamethaxazole to guard against *Pneumocystis*, *Nocardia*, *Toxoplasma*, and *Legionella*. In VAD patients, a common site of infection is at the site of entry of the drive lines to the intracorporeal pump. Overwhelming sepsis, although infrequent, is a devastating complication with high mortality. Mediastinitis can occur in up to 10% of patients, which is treated with antibiotics if mild or with open debridement, drainage, and muscle flap closure if extensive.

Pleural/pericardial effusions

Occur in 5%–15% of patients, often within 30 days of the procedure. Present with shortness of breath or occult tamponade physiology. Definitive diagnosis is with chest radiographs or echo. If detected early, it can be managed with aggressive diuresis, but may require catheter directed drainage if persistent or a large volume. Only 2%–5% will recur.

Gastrointestinal complaints

Nausea, emesis, and postoperative ileus can occur in up to 30% of patients. GI bleeding is much less common. Patients should be on prophylactic acid suppression therapy, especially if receiving steroids and immunosuppression. If nausea and ileus persist, it should be determined if pancreatitis related to cardiopulmonary bypass or immunosuppressive agents is the cause.

After discharge

Rejection

The average transplant recipient experiences 1.3 rejection episodes in the first year. Endomyocardial biopsy is the usual method of evaluation and is graded against a standardized scale. The risk of rejection is greatest in the first month following transplantation and decreases significantly after the first year. Symptoms include fever, dysrhythmias, or signs of heart failure. Rejection is usually managed with modulation of immunosuppression, including pulse dosing of intravenous steroids. In cases of severe vascular rejection, inotropic or mechanical circulatory support may be required as well as cytolytic therapy.

Graft vasculopathy

Remains the primary cause of late mortality following transplantation. Symptoms include heart failure, arrhythmias, and occasionally angina. The process is diffuse and therefore difficult to treat with traditional therapies such as angioplasty or surgical revascularization. Retransplantation is usually the only recourse in severe cases.

FURTHER READING

Benza, R. L. & Tallai, J. Cardiac allograft vasculopathy (chronic rejection). In Kirklin, J. K., Young, J. B., McGiffin, D. C., & Shumway, N. E., eds. *Heart Transplantation*. 1st edn. Philadelphia, PA: Churchill Livingstone, 2002: 615.

Holman, W. L. & Kormos, R. L. Mechanical support of the failing heart. In Kirklin, J. K., Young, J. B., McGiffin, D. C., & Shumway, N. E., eds. *Heart Transplantation*. 1st edn. Philadelphia, PA: Churchill Livingstone, 2002: 252.

Martich, G. D. & Vega, J. D. Heart transplantation. In Grenvik, A., Ayres, S. M., Holbrook, P. R., & Shoemaker, W. C., eds. *Textbook of Critical Care*. 4th edn. Philadelphia, PA: W. B. Saunders, 2000: 1958.

Pennington, D. G., Oaks, T. E., Hines, M. H., & Lohmann, D. P. Use of mechanical circulatory support systems in critically ill patients. In Grenvik, A., Ayres, S. M., Holbrook, P. R., & Shoemaker, W. C., eds. *Textbook of Critical Care*. 4th edn. Philadelphia, PA: W. B. Saunders, 2000: 1070–1078.

Rayburn, B. K. Other long-term complications. In Kirklin, J. K., Young, J. B., McGiffin, D. C., & Shumway, N. E., eds. *Heart Transplantation*. 1st edn. Philadelphia, PA: Churchill Livingstone, 2002: 666.

68

Pericardiectomy

Joseph I. Miller, Jr.

Emory University School of Medicine, Atlanta, GA

The surgical indications for pericardiectomy are pericarditis with significant pericardial effusion and tamponade associated with several conditions. The most common types of pericarditis are idiopathic, uremic, infectious, posttraumatic, neoplastic, and chronic constrictive, and patients usually have marked cardiovascular compromise. The primary objective of the operation is to remove as much pericardium as possible to alleviate the altered vascular hemodynamics.

The operation represents significant surgical stress to a patient with an already compromised cardiovascular system. General endotracheal anesthesia is used. The procedure is usually carried out as a closed cardiac operation, except in patients with chronic constrictive pericarditis who have calcium impregnation into the pericardium. In such patients, the procedure should be done as a "pump standby" procedure, with cardiopulmonary bypass available in case of cardiac perforation. A subxiphoid, left anterior thoracotomy, or median sternotomy surgical approach can be used. The approach of choice in all patients except those with chronic constrictive pericarditis is a left anterior thoracotomy. The usual duration of pericardiectomy is 1½ hours; a more extended period is required in patients with chronic constrictive calcific pericarditis. Generally transfusion is unnecessary, although blood should always be available and three or four units may be given if cardiopulmonary bypass is performed.

Usual postoperative course

Expected postoperative hospital stay

From 5 to 7 days, depending on the extent of altered cardiovascular dynamics.

Operative mortality

1% to 5%.

Special monitoring required

Patients receive intensive care for 1 or 2 days, with monitoring of cardiovascular signs, respiratory status, and urinary output. Close cardiac monitoring is required to detect arrhythmias, particularly atrial arrhythmias, which are common after pericardiectomy. Most patients are given digitalis if they are not already taking it preoperatively.

Patient activity and positioning

Patients remain flat in bed for the first 24 hours, then are mobilized to a sitting position and assisted out of bed 24 hours later.

Alimentation

Liquids are allowed the morning after operation and food intake is advanced to a regular diet as rapidly as possible.

Antibiotic coverage

Broad-spectrum antibiotics are begun before operation and continued for 1 week afterward. Cephalosporin is the antibiotic of choice.

Pulmonary care

Patients are given mask oxygen for the first 48 hours after operation to assist oxygenation. Serial monitoring of arterial blood gases and close observation of the pulmonary status are vital. Daily chest radiographs are required until all chest tubes have been removed and again on the day before discharge from the hospital.

Medical Management of the Surgical Patient: A Textbook of Perioperative Medicine, ed. M. F. Lubin, R. B. Smith, T. F. Dobson, N. Spell, H. K. Walker. 4th edn. Published by Cambridge University Press. © Cambridge University 2006.

Thoracotomy tubes

Two chest tubes are left in place until significant drainage has ceased, which generally requires 4 days. The chest tubes are connected by water seal to 20 cm H_2O suction.

Postoperative complications

In the hospital

Congestive heart failure

Occurs in 30%–35% of patients who have chronic constrictive pericarditis. The heart is unable to adequately pump all the blood returning to it after release of the pericardium and patients may develop significant heart failure. This generally requires 6 weeks to 2 months to abate and must be carefully treated with digitalis preparations, diuretics, and a salt-restricted diet.

Arrhythmias

Occur in 15%–20% of patients and generally consist of atrial tachycardia, atrial flutter, or atrial fibrillation. Management is by digitalization.

Infection

Significant infection develops in 1%–3% of patients, occurring most often in patients who are unusually susceptible to superinfection because of immunosuppression, malignancy, or azotemia.

Postpericardiotomy syndrome

Reported in 15%–20% of patients and recognized by a pericardial friction rub, fever, and precordial chest pain radiating into the neck and back. Initial treatment is with salicylates or indomethacin; steroids may be required. The syndrome is usually short-lived, though there are rare cases where symptoms are prolonged.

Bleeding

Uncommon except in uremic patients who may have altered clotting mechanisms. In such cases, appropriate blood products should be available for postoperative administration.

After discharge

Arrhythmia

Chronic arrhythmia problems should be followed up at frequent intervals with electrocardiograms.

Persistent pericarditis

Patients with this complication should be observed closely and treated with salicylates and steroids, if indicated. Occasionally, steroid therapy must be maintained for an extended course and tapered gradually.

FURTHER READING

Chen, E. P. & Miller, J. I. Modern approaches and use of surgical treatment of pericardial disease. *Curr. Cardiol. Rep.* 2002; **4**, 41–49.

Churchill, E. D. Pericardial resection in chronic constrictive pericarditis. *Ann. Surg.* 1936; **104**: 516–529.

Engle, M. A., McCabe, J. C., Ebert, P. A., & Zabriskie, J. The postpericardiotomy syndrome and antiheart antibodies. *Circulation* 1974; **49**: 401–406.

Franco, K. L., Breckenridge, I., & Hammond, G. L. The pericardium. In Baue, A. E., Geha, A. S., Hammond, G. L. *et al.*, eds. *Glenn's Thoracic and Cardiovascular Surgery*, 5th edn., vol 2. Norwalk: CT; Appleton & Lange, 1991, 1985.

Hazelrigg, S. R., Mack, M. J., Landreneau, R. J. *et al*. Thoracoscopic pericardiectomy for effusive pericardial disease. *Ann. Thorac. Surg.* 1993; **56**: 792–795.

Kloster, F. E., Crislip, R. L., Bristow, J. D. *et al.* Hemodynamic studies following pericardiectomy for constrictive pericarditis. *Circulation* 1965; **32**: 415–424.

Miller, J. I. Surgical management of pericardial disease. In Schlant, R. C. & Alexandria, R. W., eds. *Hurst's The Heart, Arteries and Veins*. New York, NY: McGraw Hill, 1994: 1675–1680.

Miller, J. I., Mansour, K. A., & Hatcher, C. R. Jr. Pericardiectomy: current indications, concepts, and results in a university center. *Ann. Thorac. Surg.* 1982; **34**: 40–45.

69

Pulmonary lobectomy

Joseph I. Miller, Jr.

Emory University School of Medicine, Atlanta, GA

Pulmonary lobectomy is most often performed for benign and malignant neoplasms of the lung. It may also be required for pulmonary tuberculosis, refractory lung abscess, residual bronchiectasis, pulmonary sequestration, and other infectious processes.

General anesthesia is administered through an indwelling double-lumen endotracheal tube. In general, the operation does not require blood transfusion, although blood should always be available in case technical problems arise. Patients are usually placed in the lateral decubitus position with the operated side superior. The main operative steps after thoracotomy incision consist of control of the arterial supply and venous drainage of the respective lobe, followed by dissection of the fissures and division of the bronchus. The operation takes 1½ to 2 hours for a lower lobectomy and 2 to 2½ hours for an upper lobectomy. The procedure is generally well tolerated and is not a major surgical stress if patients have few associated medical problems and adequate pulmonary function.

Usual postoperative course

Expected postoperative hospital stay
Depending on their general condition and the degree of postoperative air leak, patients remain in the hospital for 5 to 7 days.

Operative mortality
1%–3% for elective surgery and 15%–25% for emergency intervention.

Special monitoring required
Intensive care unit observation is required for 1 day for careful monitoring of vital signs, chest tube drainage, arterial blood pressure, urinary output, renal function, and ventilatory status.

Patient activity and positioning
Patients generally remain in the semi-Fowler position for the first 24 hours and may sit on the side of the bed the morning after operation. They can move to a chair at 24 hours and begin ambulating at 48 hours.

Alimentation
Clear liquids are given the morning after operation and food intake is advanced to a regular diet as rapidly as tolerated.

Antibiotic coverage
Routine prophylactic antibiotics of the cephalosporin group are given before operation and continued for a minimum of 1 week afterward or until all chest tubes have been removed.

Thoracotomy tubes
Chest tubes are connected to wall suction at 20 cm H_2O until all air leaks have ceased, generally within 4 to 7 days. Air leaks may persist for a longer period in patients with infectious processes and those whose procedures involved technical difficulty. Once the leaks have ceased, the chest tubes are placed on underwater seal drainage and disconnected from suction. When there has been no leak for 24 hours, the chest tubes are removed on successive days, with the lower tube pulled first and the upper tube pulled second.

Pulmonary care
Chest physical therapy, ultrasonic nebulization, and incentive spirometry are begun on the day of operation and continued four times a day until patients have satisfactorily recovered.

Medical Management of the Surgical Patient: A Textbook of Perioperative Medicine, ed. M. F. Lubin, R. B. Smith, T. F. Dobson, N. Spell, H. K. Walker. 4th edn. Published by Cambridge University Press. © Cambridge University 2006.

Postoperative radiographs

Daily portable upright chest radiographs are obtained to observe lung reexpansion.

Postoperative complications

In the hospital

Arrhythmia

Atrial tachycardia, atrial flutter, and atrial fibrillation are the most frequently encountered arrhythmias. They occur in 5%–15% of patients and usually are recognized by a decrease in blood pressure or are noted on electrocardiographic monitoring in the intensive care unit.

Intrapleural space

A persistent intrapleural space may exist after lobectomy in 5%–15% of patients. The space results from technical problems or from disease in the residual lung that prevents it from filling the adjacent pleural cavity. In general, these cavities rarely become infected or cause major difficulties.

Prolonged air leak

Occurs in 3%–7% of patients and is defined as any air leak that persists longer than 7 days. The leak is detected by the bubbling of air through the underwater sealed chamber and is managed by continued chest tube suction.

Pleural empyema

Develops in 1%–3% of patients who undergo lobectomy and is generally managed by closed chest tube thoracostomy or open rib resection. Appropriate antibiotic therapy is administered based on culture and sensitivity reports.

Bronchopleural fistula

Approximately 1% of patients develop this complication. It generally becomes evident 7 to 14 days after resection and is manifested by fever, cough, and an increasing air leak. Therapy consists of closed chest tube thoracostomy or open rib resection, followed later by a definitive procedure.

Pulmonary embolism

The postoperative incidence of this complication is only 1%. Preventive measures include antiembolism stockings perioperatively and early mobilization postoperatively. All patients undergoing open thoracotomy are treated with minidose heparin unless contraindicated by other conditions.

Bleeding

Less than 1% of patients experience major postoperative bleeding, which usually becomes evident from excessive drainage through the chest tubes. The source can often be traced to injury of an intercostal artery or other blood vessel that resumes bleeding after surgery. Proper therapy includes transfusion and, if necessary, reoperation to achieve hemostasis. Reoperation is generally indicated if the blood loss amounts to 300 ml/h for 2 successive hours.

After discharge

Arrhythmias

Generally treated for a minimum of 3 months with the appropriate cardiac medications.

Intrapleural space

Should be observed by serial chest radiographs at monthly intervals for the first 6 months.

Bronchopleural fistula

After patients are stable, bronchopleural fistulas can be tracked on an outpatient basis with serial chest radiographs, volume determination of the size of the cavity, appropriate sinograms, and subsequent definitive operation.

FURTHER READING

Dart, C. H. Jr., Scott, S. M., & Takara, T. Six-year clinical experience using automatic stapling devices for lung resections. *Ann. Thorac. Surg.* 1970; **9**: 535–550.

Hood, R. M. *Techniques in General Thoracic Surgery*. Philadelphia, PA: W. B. Saunders, 1995.

Kirsh, M. M., Rotman, H., Behrendt, D. M. *et al.* Complications of pulmonary resection. *Ann. Thorac. Surg.* 1975; **20**: 215–236.

Martini, N. & Ginsberg, R. J. In Pearson, F. G., ed. *Lobectomy in Thoracic Surgery*. 2nd edn. New York, NY: Churchill Livingstone, 2002: 981–990.

Meade, R. H. *A History of Thoracic Surgery*. Springfield, IL: Charles C. Thomas, 1961.

Scannell, J. G. Pulmonary resection: anatomy and techniques. In Baue, A. E., Geha, A. S., Hammond, G. L. *et al.*, eds. *Glenn's Thoracic and Cardiovascular Surgery*. 5th edn. vol 1. Norwalk, CT: Appleton & Lange, 1991: 111.

Urschel, H. & Cooper, J. D., eds. *Atlas of Thoracic Surgery*. New York, NY: Churchill Livingstone, 1995.

70

Pneumonectomy

Joseph I. Miller, Jr.

Emory University School of Medicine, Atlanta, GA

The chief indication for pneumonectomy is a pulmonary neoplasm involving structures that render pulmonary lobectomy unfeasible. On rare occasions, pneumonectomy may be indicated for benign conditions, such as residual problems with pulmonary tuberculosis, lung trauma, or complications of a pulmonary lobectomy.

General endotracheal anesthesia is administered with the aid of an indwelling double-lumen tube to ensure proper inflation of the dependent lung and to protect it from blood or secretions draining down from the operated bronchus. Patients are placed in the lateral decubitus position. The procedure takes 1½ to 2 hours. While blood transfusion is rarely required in elective pneumonectomy, blood should always be available. The main operative steps consist of control of the pulmonary artery and superior and inferior pulmonary veins and secure closure of the bronchial stump. The procedure carries a high level of surgical stress and should only be performed in patients who have been demonstrated to have sufficient pulmonary reserve to tolerate the procedure. Therefore, results of preoperative pulmonary function tests comprise the main patient selection criteria for elective resection. Cardiac status should also be evaluated before operation using an exercise treadmill or thallium scan.

Usual postoperative course

Expected postoperative hospital stay
6 to 7 days.

Operative mortality
5%–12%.

Special monitoring required
Patients remain in the intensive care unit for 1 or 2 days to allow close observation for arrhythmias, pulmonary reserve, urinary output, and other vital functions. To monitor respiratory status, blood gases are assessed daily or, if necessary, more often.

Patient activity and positioning
The semi-Fowler position is maintained for the first 24 hours and patients are not allowed to turn onto their operated side. They are permitted to sit on the side of the bed the morning after operation and are moved to a chair 1 day later. Ambulation is begun the next day.

Alimentation
Since division of the vagal trunks frequently produces gastric retention, oral intake is prohibited for 3 days. Patients are allowed to consume liquids after 72 hours and food intake is rapidly advanced to a regular diet.

Antibiotic coverage
Broad-spectrum antibiotics of the cephalosporin group are first given 12 hours before resection and continued for 7 to 10 days afterwards.

Gastric decompression
An indwelling nasogastric tube is kept in place for 3 days to allow the postoperative gastric atony to resolve.

Postoperative radiographs
Portable upright chest radiographs are obtained regularly to monitor the filling of the pulmonary cavity, a process that generally requires 6 weeks. The hemogram is checked every other day for approximately 10 days to assess the hematologic response.

Thoracotomy tube
If a chest tube has been left in place connected to a clamped underwater seal bottle, it is removed within

Medical Management of the Surgical Patient: A Textbook of Perioperative Medicine, ed. M. F. Lubin, R. B. Smith, T. F. Dobson, N. Spell, H. K. Walker. 4th edn. Published by Cambridge University Press. © Cambridge University 2006.

48 hours after the procedure. Some surgeons prefer to remove the tube in the operating room after stabilization of the mediastinum.

Postoperative complications

In the hospital

Arrhythmias

Atrial tachycardia, atrial flutter, or atrial fibrillation develops in 25%–40% of patients as a result of increased vagal tone or hypoxia. All patients undergo routine prophylactic digitalization in the operating room when the decision is made to perform a pneumonectomy. Digitalis therapy is continued for a minimum of 6 months after operation. An alternative is to use a beta-blocker.

Empyema

Occurs in 2%–10% of patients in the early postoperative period, though it can also develop up to several years later. It is recognized by systemic signs of infection plus a change in the air–fluid level in the hemithorax or by the expectoration of brown, purulent material. Treatment of an empyema in the pneumonectomy space requires immediate tube thoracostomy drainage followed by a subsequent Clagett procedure or thoracoplasty.

Bronchopleural fistula

Develops in 3% of patients, generally between the 7th and 14th postoperative days, the weakest period of bronchial stump healing. It is manifested by fever, cough, drainage, or an air leak. Treatment consists of immediate tube thoracostomy followed by subsequent irrigation of the space with antibiotics and the performance of a delayed closure with muscle flaps.

Cardiac herniation

A rare complication that carries greater than 50% mortality. It can be prevented by adequate closure of the pericardium after intrapericardial pneumonectomy.

Bleeding

Less than 1% of patients who undergo pneumonectomy experience postoperative bleeding that is serious enough to require either immediate reexploration for control or subsequent evacuation of the pleural space. After operation, hemorrhage is recognized by immediate filling of the operated hemithorax and rapid deterioration of the vital signs.

Tension pneumothorax

Occurs in less than 1% of patients and results from a bronchial leak. It is recognized by a shift of the mediastinum accompanied by acute worsening of respiratory status. Treatment consists of immediate tube thoracostomy of the involved thorax.

After discharge

Empyema or bronchopleural fistula

Although these complications usually develop in the hospital, they can arise months to years after surgery. They are manifested by systemic signs of toxemia, fever, and cough, and are diagnosed by a chest radiograph that shows a decrease in the level of fluid in the chest or the presence of an air-fluid level. Treatment consists of immediate tube thoracostomy with subsequent definitive repair.

Arrhythmias

May persist after hospital discharge but generally respond to appropriate digitalis glycoside therapy.

Respiratory insufficiency

Respiratory insufficiency may be observed in patients with borderline pulmonary reserve after resection. They may remain severely dyspneic and be unable to function at previous levels of exercise tolerance, if borderline function was present before operation.

FURTHER READING

Allen, M. S., Jett, J. R., & Kozelsky, T. F. Stage II lung cancer. *Chest Surg. Clin. North Am.* 2001; **11**: 61–69.

Dart, C. H. Jr., Scott, S. M., & Takara, T. Six-year clinical experience using automatic stapling devices for lung resections. *Ann. Thorac. Surg.* 1970; **9**: 535–550.

Kirsh, M. M., Rotman, H., Behrendt, O. M. *et al.* Complications of pulmonary resection. *Ann. Thorac. Surg.* 1975; **20**: 215–236.

Meade, R. H. *A History of Thoracic Surgery.* Springfield, IL: Charles C Thomas, 1961.

Roviaro, G., Varolli, F., Vergani, C. *et al.* Techniques of pneumonectomy. *Chest Surg. Clin. North Am.* 1999; **9**: 419.

Scannell, J. G. Pulmonary resection: anatomy and techniques. In Baue, A. E., Geha, A. S., Hammond, G. L. *et al.*, eds. *Glenn's Thoracic and Cardiovascular Surgery.* 5th edn. vol 1. Norwalk, CT: Appleton & Lange, 1991: 111.

Walsa, G. L., Pistens, M. W., Steven, C. Treatment of Stage I lung cancer. *Chest Surg. Clin. North Am.* 2001; **11**: 17–39.

71

Hiatal hernia repair

Kamal A. Mansour and Daniel L. Serna

Emory University School of Medicine, Atlanta, GA

Indications for surgical repair of hiatal hernia include failure of strict medical management (intractability); reflux esophagitis with ulcerations, stricture, or bleeding; recurrent aspiration pneumonia; large sliding hernias; and all paraesophageal hernias. The purpose of surgery is twofold: to reposition the stomach below the diaphragm and to reestablish gastroesophageal competence. Three approaches (transabdominal, transthoracic, and laparoscopic) and three primary techniques (Belsey, Hill, and Nissen) are used, depending on the preference of the surgeon. If the procedure is performed well, the magnitude of surgical stress is low. General endotracheal anesthesia is typically used and the operative time is 2 to 3 hours. Intraoperative blood transfusions are rarely required.

Usual postoperative course

Expected postoperative hospital stay
Ranges from 7 to 10 days for open procedures and 2 to 5 days for the minimally invasive approach. Length of stay is also influenced by the age and associated medical condition of the patient.

Operative mortality
Under 1%.

Special monitoring required
Intraoperative assessment of the lower esophageal sphincter zone is performed by pressure manometric studies.

Patient activity and positioning
If a transthoracic approach is used, a chest tube is inserted and removed after 24 hours, after which ambulation is allowed.

Alimentation
A nasogastric tube is usually left in place for the first 24 hours. Patients are then given clear liquids and food intake is advanced to a soft diet, which is maintained until hospital discharge.

Antibiotic coverage
A second generation cephalosporin is given during the 24-hour perioperative period.

Chest physiotherapy
Chest physiotherapy is stressed, especially when the transthoracic approach is used, to minimize pulmonary complications.

Barium swallow
Done on the seventh postoperative day to assess the status of the surgical repair and to provide a baseline study for follow-up.

Postoperative complications

In the hospital

Pulmonary complications
Caused by retained secretions, which are less frequent following the laparoscopic approach. Pneumothorax is the most common complication of laparoscopic fundoplication.

Temporary dysphagia
Edema at the cardia may result in temporary dysphagia, which should improve with observation. The patient is maintained on a soft diet until this complication resolves.

Medical Management of the Surgical Patient: A Textbook of Perioperative Medicine, ed. M. F. Lubin, R. B. Smith, T. F. Dobson, N. Spell, H. K. Walker. 4th edn. Published by Cambridge University Press. © Cambridge University 2006.

Rupture of the stomach

This has been reported in cases in which a Nissen fundoplication was left in the chest or herniated into the chest postoperatively.

Ulceration

Some instances of bleeding peptic ulcer have occurred along the lesser curvature in association with a Nissen repair; their cause is not definitely known.

Splenic injury

Intraoperative splenic injury requiring splenorrhaphy or splenectomy may occur in association with Nissen fundoplication.

After discharge

Recurrence

Hernia recurrence is reported in 8% (Nissen) to 18% (Belsey) of patients following primary open repair. Results after laparoscopic repair compare favorably with open techniques. In the presence of symptomatic, radiologic, and endoscopic evidence of recurrent gastroesophageal reflux, another surgical repair is indicated.

Gas-bloat syndrome

Occurs in 15% of patients after Nissen fundoplication, results from overdistention of the stomach that is not relieved by belching or vomiting, and may require repeated esophageal dilatation or reoperation.

FURTHER READING

Bowrey, D. J. & Peters, J. H. Laparoscopic esophageal surgery. *Surg. Clin. North Am.* 2000; **80**(4): 1213–1242.

Fenton, K. N., Miller, J. I., Jr., Lee, R. B., & Mansour, K. A. Belsey Mark IV antireflux procedure for complicated gastroesophageal reflux disease. *Ann. Thorac. Surg.* 1997; **64**(3): 790–794.

Mansour, K. A., Burton, H. G., Miller, J. I., Jr., & Hatcher, C. R., Jr. Complications of intrathoracic Nissen fundoplication. *Ann. Thorac. Surg.* 1981; **32**(2): 173–178.

72

Esophagogastrectomy

Kamal A. Mansour and Daniel L. Serna

Emory University School of Medicine, Atlanta, GA

Esophagogastrectomy is usually performed for high-grade dysplasia or carcinoma of the esophagus, particularly of the middle and lower thirds. Less common indications for this procedure are nondilatable stricture of the distal esophagus requiring resection and rupture of the esophagus that is irreparable.

Two separate incisions are generally used: abdominal and right thoracic. A left thoracotomy or left thoracoabdominal incision may be used for carcinoma of the distal esophagus and the gastroesophageal junction. A combined laparoscopic/thoracoscopic approach is currently undergoing clinical evaluation but is still considered experimental, while the open approach remains the gold standard. To mobilize the stomach, the short gastric, left gastroepiploic, and left gastric arteries are sacrificed, and the blood supply through the right gastroepiploic and right gastric arteries is preserved. The distal line of resection in the proximal stomach is securely closed and an esophagogastric anastomosis is performed on the anterior surface of the stomach below the line of resection. Feeding jejunostomy with pyloroplasty or pyloromyotomy may be done. Surgical stress is great and the procedure has relatively high morbidity and mortality rates. Anesthesia is endotracheal, using a double lumen tube to allow the lung on the side of the operation to remain collapsed. The procedure takes 4 to 6 hours and requires 2 to 4 units of blood.

Usual postoperative course

Expected postoperative hospital stay
Seven to 10 days.

Operative mortality
The operative mortality rate is approximately 4%–5%.

Special monitoring required
Patients are observed in the intensive care unit with central venous pressure recordings and an arterial line. Urine output and chest tube drainage are recorded.

Patient activity and positioning
Patients may ambulate 24 to 48 hours after operation. While they are in bed, patients should be maintained with the head of the bed elevated to prevent gastric or bile reflux and aspiration.

Alimentation
Patients are kept n.p.o. and given intravenous nutrition for 2–3 days and then by jejunostomy tube. A nasogastric tube is connected to gravity drainage. On the seventh postoperative day, a barium swallow is obtained. If the anastomosis is satisfactory, oral feedings may be permitted.

Antibiotic coverage
Broad-spectrum antibiotics are administered for 1 week.

Chest tube management
To diminish the possibility that a leak might occur at the anastomosis, the chest tube is removed as soon as drainage is minimal and the chest radiograph is satisfactory.

Postoperative complications

In the hospital

Anastomotic leak
The physical signs of an anastomotic leak include undue pain, fever, tachycardia, tachypnea, or pleural effusion.

Medical Management of the Surgical Patient: A Textbook of Perioperative Medicine, ed. M. F. Lubin, R. B. Smith, T. F. Dobson, N. Spell, H. K. Walker. 4th edn. Published by Cambridge University Press. © Cambridge University 2006.

This must be investigated immediately by radiopaque contrast medium or barium swallow. If the leak is contained and drains back into the gastrointestinal tract, it may be observed; otherwise, immediate external drainage is indicated.

Gastric slough resulting from a vascular accident

Gastric slough may be fatal if the diagnosis is missed. Persistent tachycardia and a progressively rising white blood cell count are suggestive. In addition, the persistence of a foul or old blood-stained aspirate in the nasogastric tube after 48 hours may be an early sign of gastric necrosis. Prompt reoperation is mandatory.

After discharge

Dysphagia

Dysphagia is caused by stricture at the anastomotic site and may require repeated transesophageal dilatation.

FURTHER READING

Fernando, H. C., Luketich, J. D., Buenaventura, P. O., Perry, Y., & Christie, N. A. Outcomes of minimally invasive esophagectomy (MIE) for high-grade dysplasia of the esophagus. *Eur. J. Cardiothorac. Surg.* 2002; **22**(1): 1–6.

Headrick, J. R., Nichols, F. C. 3rd, Miller, D. L. *et al.* High-grade esophageal dysplasia: long-term survival and quality of life after esophagectomy. *Ann. Thorac. Surg.* 2002; **73**(6): 1697–1702; discussion 1702–1703.

Mansour, K. A., Thourani, V. H., & Cooper, W. A. As originally published in 1989: Esophageal carcinoma: surgery without preoperative adjuvant chemotherapy. Updated in 1998. *Ann. Thorac. Surg.* 1998; **65**(5): 1492–1493.

73

Colon interposition for esophageal bypass

Kamal A. Mansour and Daniel L. Serna

Emory University School of Medicine, Atlanta, GA

Indications for colon replacement of the esophagus include gastroesophageal malignancy, benign non-dilatable distal esophageal strictures caused by reflux esophagitis, extensive chemical strictures, benign tumors of the esophagus that are extensive or multiple and are not amenable to simpler measures, congenital atresia of the esophagus for which a primary anastamosis is impossible or impractical, rare cases of achalasia (megaesophagus) in which Heller myotomy fails or is complicated by malignancy, bleeding varices for which shunting fails or stricture formation follows disconnection operation, and rupture of the esophagus for which conservative repair fails or is impossible.

The right or left colon may be used, based on the right or left branch of the middle colic artery. Depending upon the surgeon's preference, the prepared colonic segment is passed through a retrosternal tunnel or brought into the posterior mediastinum through the right or left pleural cavity. An anastomosis is then constructed to the cervical esophagus. Regardless of the approach used, the procedure is of great magnitude. A general endotracheal anesthetic is administered and the procedure usually lasts 4 to 6 hours. Two to four units of blood are frequently required. Intensive preoperative preparation, including correction of fluid, caloric, and protein deficiencies, substantially improves outcome, particularly for elderly or debilitated patients. Careful mechanical and chemical bowel preparation is also required.

Usual postoperative course

Expected postoperative hospital stay
Approximately 2 weeks.

Operative mortality
Approximately 12%, depending on the age and condition of the patient and the vascularity of the interposed colonic segment.

Special monitoring required
Standard thoracotomy intensive care is provided for the first 2 or 3 days, including daily chest radiographs, electrolyte and arterial blood gas determinations, urinary output monitoring, and central venous pressure measurement.

Patient activity and positioning
Patients are ambulatory 24 to 48 hours after operation.

Alimentation
A nasogastric tube is left in the interposed colon and a feeding jejunostomy is performed at operation. Patients are supported by intravenous fluids for the first 2 to 4 days until bowel sounds are audible, at which time tube feedings are provided. On the ninth or tenth day, a barium swallow is performed to assess the colonic implant for any evidence of leakage. If the reconstruction is intact, patients are allowed oral liquid feedings and food intake is progressively advanced to a soft diet over several days.

Antibiotic coverage
A cephalosporin is given for 7 to 10 days and modified as indicated.

Physiotherapy
Chest physical therapy and vigorous pulmonary toilet are indicated.

Postoperative complications

In the hospital

Pulmonary complications
Pulmonary complications are often relatively minor but may become life-threatening in elderly patients or those with poor respiratory reserve.

Medical Management of the Surgical Patient: A Textbook of Perioperative Medicine, ed. M. F. Lubin, R. B. Smith, T. F. Dobson, N. Spell, H. K. Walker. 4th edn. Published by Cambridge University Press. © Cambridge University 2006.

Colonic necrosis

Massive necrosis of the colon must be diagnosed early and the involved bowel removed before the patient becomes moribund. The nasocolonic tube aspirate is carefully observed for its color and odor; foul or old blood-stained fluid continuing after 48 hours may be the earliest sign of bowel necrosis.

Minor leaks at the cervical anastomosis

This complication occurs in 14.8% of patients but usually resolves with simple drainage. A prolonged delay in oral feeding may be necessary. Patients may require a feeding gastrostomy or, ideally, a feeding jejunostomy.

After discharge

Fibrous stricture of the cologastric anastomosis

May require dilation or surgical revision.

Gastric ulceration

Usually occurs just proximal to the cologastric anastomosis on the lesser curvature. Medical therapy generally suffices but vagotomy and drainage may become necessary.

Redundancy of the colon above the diaphragm

Colonic stasis and a prolonged transit time may result from this condition, which may require surgical revision if it is severe.

FURTHER READING

DeMeester, T. R., Johansson, K.-E., Franze, I. *et al.* Indications, surgical technique, and long-term functional results of colon interposition or bypass. *Ann. Surg.* 1988, **208**: 460–474.

Mansour, K. A., Bryan, F. C., & Carlson, G. W. Bowel interposition for esophageal replacement: twenty-five-year experience. *Ann. Thorac. Surg.* 1997; **64**(3): 752–756.

Mansour, K. A., Hansen, H. A. II, Hersh, T. *et al.* Colon interposition for advanced nonmalignant esophageal stricture. *Ann. Thorac. Surg.* 1981; **32**: 584–591.

Vascular surgery

74

Carotid endarterectomy

Sunil S. Rayan and Thomas F. Dodson

Emory University School of Medicine, Atlanta, GA

Cerebrovascular accident (CVA) is the third leading cause of death and affects over 500 000 patients per year in the USA. The disability suffered by stroke victims places an enormous financial burden on the healthcare system. Carotid endarterectomy, an operation designed to prevent stroke, is the most common vascular procedure performed today. Over the last 15 years, the indications for carotid endarterectomy have been firmly established. Three large multicenter trials published in 1991 conclusively demonstrated the beneficial effects of surgical therapy of cerebrovascular disease over medical therapy in symptomatic patients. Endarterectomy for asymptomatic carotid stenosis in two large multicenter trials also showed a smaller but significant benefit of carotid endarterectomy for stroke prevention. Indications are not as conclusive and are considered on an individual basis for patients with stroke-in-evolution or with completed CVA and carotid stenosis. Since carotid endarterectomy is a preventive operation, the benefits from these studies apply to centers where the perioperative stroke rate is under 3%.

Carotid endarterectomy can be performed under local, regional, or general anesthesia, but we prefer local anesthesia and selective shunting. General anesthesia is reserved for those patients who may be anxious or in whom we anticipate difficult anatomy. The operation takes approximately two hours and involves a longitudinal incision in the lateral neck. The stages of the procedure are gentle exposure of the carotid bifurcation, heparinization, cross-clamping of the vessels, shunting if necessary, removal of the plaque, and usually closure with a Dacron patch angioplasty. Factors which may make the operation technically challenging include scarring from a prior operation or radiation, a high carotid bifurcation, or an atheromatous plaque that extends high into the internal carotid artery. Blood transfusions are rarely required.

Usual postoperative course

Expected postoperative hospital stay
Since complications typically occur within the first 12 to 24 hours, patients are usually discharged within the first 2 days following operation.

Operative mortality
Under 1% in patients with no symptoms, about 1% in patients having transient ischemic attacks, and 2% to 5% in patients with stroke-in-evolution or recently completed CVA.

Special monitoring required
Patients are monitored with an arterial line to assess fluctuations in blood pressure in the postanesthesia care unit for a period of 2 to 4 hours. If medications are required to maintain them normotensive, they are transferred to the intensive care unit for 24-hour monitoring.

Patient activity and positioning
Patients are usually kept at bed rest on the day of operation and encouraged to ambulate the next day.

Alimentation
Clear liquids are permitted the day of operation in the unlikely event of a need to return to the operating room. Patients are allowed to resume a regular diet the following day.

Medical Management of the Surgical Patient: A Textbook of Perioperative Medicine, ed. M. F. Lubin, R. B. Smith, T. F. Dobson, N. Spell, H. K. Walker. 4th edn. Published by Cambridge University Press. © Cambridge University 2006.

Antibiotic coverage

One dose of a cephalosporin is given before the operation and continued for a maximum of 24 hours.

Patient discomfort

Discomfort from the neck incision is usually minimal and patients often discontinue narcotics in favor of over-the-counter analgesics after the first day.

Postoperative complications

In the hospital

Nerve injury

The carotid artery is intimately associated with several cranial nerves, all of which are at risk for injury during the procedure. Transient deviation of the tongue toward the side of operation may result from injury or traction on the hypoglossal nerve. Transection of the hypoglossal is rare and may require urgent repair. Similarly, damage to the vagus nerve may result in either temporary or permanent hoarseness. Injury to the marginal mandibular branch of the facial nerve results in drooping at the corner of the mouth. Damage to the superior laryngeal nerve may cause fatigability of the voice and impairment in phonation. Trauma to the spinal accessory nerve is an uncommon complication of carotid endarterectomy, but the resulting shoulder dysfunction is troublesome. Fortunately, most cranial nerve injuries are transient and recovery can be expected in 6 to 12 months.

Bradycardia

A common complication that can be attributed to manipulation of the carotid sinus. Atropine is administered in the unlikely event that the bradycardia is persistent or is associated with hypotension.

Hematoma

Postoperative wound hematomas occur in about 5% to 10% of patients. Of these, a small fraction requires return to the operating room for evacuation. An expanding hematoma in the neck must be treated expeditiously to avoid airway compromise.

Cardiac complications

Patients with asymptomatic cervical bruits have a higher risk of cardiac ischemic events than of stroke, illustrating that vascular disease involves the entire vascular tree. Therefore, although the stress of carotid endarterectomy is low, patients are still at risk for myocardial ischemia perioperatively.

Cerebrovascular accident (CVA)

Although carotid endarterectomy is designed to prevent stroke, CVA is a recognized complication of the procedure that occurs approximately 2% of the time. Patients who present with neurologic deficit upon emergence from anesthesia or soon thereafter are promptly re-explored. The most common cause of these events is thrombosis at the operative site. Delayed neurologic events are best managed by ascertaining the diagnosis to provide specific treatment of the underlying etiology.

Cerebral hyperperfusion syndrome

This most feared complication of carotid surgery occurs in only 1% of cases but carries a mortality of over 30%. Hyperperfusion syndrome can cause severe headaches, seizures, neurologic deficits, and ultimately death from cerebral hemorrhage. It is associated with risk factors such as high-grade ipsilateral stenosis (>90%), contralateral carotid occlusion, recent history of CVA, and severe postoperative hypertension. Of these risk factors, only postoperative hypertension can be controlled. For this reason, the patient's blood pressure is monitored continuously via an arterial line in the perioperative period. Large fluctuations in blood pressure are treated in the intensive care unit with the appropriate vasopressors or vasodilators. If the patients develop hyperperfusion syndrome, they are treated supportively. Anticoagulants and antiplatelet agents are withheld. The prognosis after cerebral hemorrhage is poor.

After discharge

Peri-incisional hypesthesia

Patients may complain of numbness of the ear lobe if the greater auricular nerve has been damaged, and they frequently experience diminished sensation in the region of the neck incision because of the interruption of cutaneous cervical nerves.

Carotid restenosis

As many as 37% of patients develop greater than 50% carotid restenosis over time. Fortunately, most restenoses are asymptomatic and do not seem to carry the same neurologic threat as do primary atherosclerotic lesions. Reoperation is undertaken for the same indications as primary operation.

FURTHER READING

European Carotid Surgery Trialists' Collaborative Group: Medical Research Council European Carotid Surgery Trial. Interim results for symptomatic patients with severe (70–99%) or with mild (0–29%) carotid stenosis. *Lancet* 1991; **337**: 1235.

Hamdan, A. D., Pomposelli, F. B. Jr., Gibbons, G. W., Campbell, D. R., & LoGerfo, F. W. Perioperative strokes after 1001 consecutive carotid endarterectomy procedures without an electroencephalogram: incidence, mechanism, and recovery. *Arch. Surg.* 1999; **134**(4): 412.

Hobson, R. W. II, Weiss, D. G., Fields, W. S. *et al.* Efficacy of carotid endarterectomy for asymptomatic carotid stenosis. *N. Engl. J. Med.* 1993; **328**: 221.

Lattimer, C. R. & Burnand, K. G. Recurrent carotid stenosis after carotid endarterectomy. *Br. J. Surg.* 1997; **84**: 1206.

Mayberg, M. R., Wilson, S. E., Yatsu, F. *et al.* For the Veterans Affairs Cooperative Studies Program 309 Trialist Group. Carotid endarterectomy and prevention of cerebral ischemia in symptomatic carotid stenosis. *J. Am. Med. Assoc.* 1991; **266**: 3289.

North American Symptomatic Carotid Endarterectomy Trial Collaborators. Beneficial effect of carotid endarterectomy in symptomatic patients with high-grade carotid stenosis. *N. Engl. J. Med.* 1991; **325**: 445.

Pomposelli, F. B., Lamparello, P. J., Riles, T. S. *et al.* Intracranial hemorrhage after carotid endarterectomy. *J. Vasc. Surg.* 1988; **7**: 248.

The Executive Committee for the Asymptomatic Carotid Atherosclerosis Study. Endarterectomy for asymptomatic carotid artery stenosis. *J. Am. Med. Assoc.* 1995; **273**: 1421.

75

Abdominal aortic aneurysm repair

Sunil S. Rayan and Thomas F. Dodson

Emory University School of Medicine, Atlanta, GA

In the USA, where aortic aneurysm rupture is the tenth leading cause of death in men older than 55 years, recent evidence suggests that the death rate from abdominal aortic aneurysms has increased in the past several decades. Potential explanations for the apparent rise include an aging population, improved radiologic detection, and closer observation of families and first-degree relatives of patients with abdominal aortic aneurysms. The mortality in patients with ruptured aneurysms ranges from 78% to 94%, with half of those patients dying before they reach the hospital. Elective or non-emergent aneurysm repair carries a mortality rate 10 to 25 times lower than that in patients with ruptured aneurysms; hence, emphasis should be on detection, evaluation, and planned surgery, the key concept being that aneurysms are relatively easily and safely treated in the elective setting. Unfortunately, 12% of patients initially present with rupture.

After an aneurysm of the abdominal aorta is detected, whether by physical examination, plain radiography of the abdomen, computed tomography, magnetic resonance imaging, or B-mode ultrasonography, the urgency and timing of repair must be determined. According to Laplace's law, the likelihood of aneurysm rupture is proportional to maximal aneurysm diameter. The yearly risk of rupture is 1% to 4% for small aneurysms (less than 5 cm in diameter), 6% to 11% for aneurysms 5 to 7 cm, and over 20% for aneurysms greater than 7 cm. Because aneurysms usually enlarge annually by 0.3 to 0.5 cm, small aneurysms should be followed with ultrasound examinations every 6 to 12 months. When the aneurysm exceeds 5 cm in diameter, a vascular surgeon should be consulted regarding prompt operative intervention. All patients with symptomatic or ruptured aneurysms should be emergently treated. The risk of elective surgery is determined by the health of the patient and the anatomy of the aneurysm. As many as half of the patients with abdominal aortic aneurysms have some evidence of cardiac disease. Therefore, preoperative cardiac evaluation is an important step in risk stratification. Chronic obstructive pulmonary disease linked with aortic aneurysms must also be evaluated. Other associated problems include renal insufficiency and peripheral vascular disease. The relationship of the aneurysm to the renal arteries also influences the risk of operation. Suprarenal aneurysm repair is associated with a higher morbidity and mortality than infrarenal repair. Also, suprarenal aneurysms are currently not amenable to standard endovascular repair, making open repair the only option.

Operations

Two different methods exist to repair an abdominal aortic aneurysm.

Open surgical repair

The open method is the gold standard but poses a high surgical stress to the patient. It is the choice for patients without significant comorbidities who can tolerate aortic clamping and substantial intravascular volume shifts. Repair is usually performed through a midline incision, although flank or retroperitoneal exposures are occasionally preferred. Once the aneurysm is exposed, the patient is heparinized and the aorta is cross-clamped above and below the aneurysm, interrupting the blood flow to the lower body. The aneurysm is opened longitudinally and the intraluminal thrombus is evacuated. An interposition tube or bifurcated prosthetic graft is rapidly sewn into the normal vessels both proximally and distally. The aneurysm sac is then closed over the graft to prevent aortoenteric fistula and to assist in hemostasis.

Medical Management of the Surgical Patient: A Textbook of Perioperative Medicine, ed. M. F. Lubin, R. B. Smith, T. F. Dodson, N. Spell, H. K. Walker. 4th edn. Published by Cambridge University Press. © Cambridge University 2006.

The major concern with this operation is blood loss. Fortunately, the ability to recycle lost red blood cells by means of an auto-transfusion device has reduced the amount of exogenous blood products required. Nevertheless, transfusion is not uncommon in the post-operative period. Most open abdominal aortic aneurysm procedures are completed in 3 or 4 hours; patients then recover in the ICU.

Endovascular repair

The endovascular approach, by contrast, presents a much smaller surgical stress to the patient; however, since reliable data on its long-term efficacy is unavailable, this procedure is relegated to high-risk candidates. In addition to fulfilling risk criteria, patients must have suitable anatomy to be considered for an endograft. Up to 40% of patients are rejected for this procedure based on anatomy alone. Eligibility requirements include: aneurysm limited to the infrarenal aorta, presence of an adequate infrarenal "neck," acceptable calcification and tortuosity of the iliac vessels, and vessel diameters compatible with existing devices.

Endovascular aneurysm repair can be performed under general or local anesthesia with sedation. Bilateral groin cutdowns are used to gain arterial access in order to deploy each limb of the device and the patient is systemically heparinized. The device is then placed below the renal arteries with the aid of contrast arteriography or intravascular ultrasound. The arteriotomies are closed when an adequate seal has been obtained and communication between the aorta and the aneurysm sac is obliterated. The groin wounds are then repaired with layered absorbable sutures.

Usual postoperative course

Open surgical repair

Expected postoperative hospital stay
Most patients recover in the ICU for the first 1–3 days. Uncomplicated patients are usually discharged from the hospital in a week; however, return to a preoperative level of function may take several months. After discharge, patients are seen 6 weeks after operation and then yearly unless complications occur.

Operative mortality
Elective aneurysmectomy carries a mortality of 2%–5% and morbidity of 10%–30%.

Special monitoring required
Invasive monitoring in an ICU is required for continuous measurements of vital signs, urine output, and filling pressures. In patients with known cardiopulmonary dysfunction, a pulmonary arterial catheter is used to elucidate cardiac output and pulmonary capillary wedge pressure.

Patient activity and positioning
Patients are encouraged to resume activity as soon as possible and they are usually ambulatory within 2 days after operation.

Alimentation
Oral alimentation is withheld for the first few days after operation as the manipulation of the small bowel during the operation inevitably results in temporary adynamic ileus. Liquids are usually started the third day after operation and patients are eating normally by discharge. In patients with poor preoperative nutritional status or with prolonged ileus, intravenous hyperalimentation should be considered.

Antibiotic coverage
Cephalosporin administered immediately prior to the incision.

Endovascular repair

Expected postoperative hospital stay
An average of 2–3 days. In general, patients recover quickly and are grateful for the ease of the procedure. They return to their preoperative functional status within a few weeks.

Operative mortality
Ranges from 1%–3%, not significantly different from open repair. This is attributed to selection bias: the endovascular subgroup is much sicker than those undergoing open repair.

Special monitoring required
Invasive monitoring is employed in the operating room; however, it is discontinued once the patient leaves the postanesthesia recovery unit.

Patient activity and positioning
Patients are encouraged to ambulate the following day, though the pain from bilateral groin incisions may impair mobility somewhat.

Alimentation

Patients drink liquids the evening of surgery and eat the following day.

Antibiotic coverage

Cephalosporin administered immediately prior to the incision.

Postoperative complications

In the hospital

Open surgical repair

Vascular complications

Close attention to the abdominal and vascular examination is especially important to monitor for signs of bleeding or graft thrombosis. Transfusions of blood products are not uncommon with open repair as blood loss can be substantial. Hemorrhage is a primary cause of mortality. Close monitoring of the hematocrit and rapid reversal of any coagulopathy is essential in excluding significant postoperative bleeding. Persistent bleeding is an indication for urgent re-exploration. Graft infection in the perioperative period is extremely rare.

Cardiac complications

Open aortic aneurysm repair is a major hemodynamic stress to the patient. Because aortic cross-clamping and general anesthesia place strong demands on the myocardium, any unexpected clinical deterioration should prompt an immediate reevaluation of cardiac status with a 12-lead electrocardiogram, cardiac enzymes, and/or echocardiography. Careful preoperative cardiac evaluation stratifies patient risk, and therapy with beta-blockers and aspirin minimizes many postoperative cardiac complications except in poor-risk patients. Nonetheless, cardiac events such as myocardial infarction, congestive heart failure, and arrhythmias account for most of the morbidity in patients with vascular disease. Cardiac complications are the second most common cause of postoperative mortality after bleeding.

Pulmonary complications

In general, these patients recover similarly to others that have had major abdominal surgery. Postoperative pain can lead to decreased activity, shallow respirations, and subsequent atelectasis and pneumonia. This is most commonly observed in long-term smokers with underlying lung disease, so particular attention to pulmonary toilet is important for an uncomplicated recovery. In elderly, oversedated, and delirious patients, aspiration may contribute to lung injury. Judicious use of pain medication, including patient-controlled devices or epidural analgesia, is essential for patients to recover smoothly. Patients are encouraged to sit up, use incentive spirometry, and ambulate with assistance as soon as they are able.

Renal complications

The combination of significant blood loss and a major laparotomy produce wide swings in intravascular volume status. Generally, large intravascular fluid shifts occur in the first 12 to 48 hours; management after this period is usually somewhat easier. Acute renal failure after open repair may result from atheromatous embolization to the kidneys during clamping of the aorta or prerenal causes due to inadequate resuscitation, hypotension, or ongoing bleeding. Most renal dysfunction is transient, but a small minority of patients progress to temporary hemodialysis.

Gastrointestinal complications

Since adynamic ileus is common after laparotomy, oral feeding is started only when bowel function has returned. Colonic ischemia is a rare complication of aneurysm repair and can present as abdominal pain, distention, leukocytosis, acidosis, hematochezia, or shock. Sigmoidoscopy confirms the diagnosis; treatment requires urgent laparotomy and colon resection.

Minor complications

Local complications include hematomas and superficial wound infections. The groin is more frequently involved than the abdomen. These complications are usually short-lived and rarely require reoperation.

Endovascular repair

Device-related complications

Technical considerations regarding device deployment account for the majority of complications in this subgroup. In patients with excessive iliac tortuosity, calcification, or small vessel diameters, perforation of the native vessels and hemorrhage can occur. This can often be managed in an endovascular manner with an occlusion balloon and a covered stent; uncontrolled hemorrhage rarely mandates immediate conversion to open surgical repair. Device malfunction is rare but may necessitate conversion for removal of the device. Finally, kinking of the limbs of the endograft can result in early or late limb thrombosis requiring urgent revascularization. This can often be avoided by angioplasty and stenting of a kinked endograft limb during initial surgery. Conversion is considered a failure of endovascular repair but occurs less than 5% of the time. Inability to gain access to the aorta or persistent endoleak after endograft deployment does not mandate immediate conversion; instead, patients can recover from anesthesia and return at a later date for conventional open repair.

Cardiac complications

Since patients undergoing endovascular repair are generally in a poor-risk category, cardiac complications can have grave consequences. Patients are managed perioperatively with beta-blockers and aspirin and undergo cardiac screening prior to the procedure. Myocardial infarction, arrhythmias, and congestive heart failure account for the majority of fatal complications in these patients.

Renal complications

Acute renal failure caused by contrast nephrotoxicity is a complication frequently associated with endovascular aneurysm repair. In patients with known pre-existing renal insufficiency, acute tubular necrosis can be minimized by the use of iso-osmolar contrast or gadolinium. In addition, pretreatment with agents such as acetylcysteine may be indicated if contrast cannot be avoided. Intravascular ultrasound is used to guide device placement when contrast cannot be used.

Minor complications

Similar to open repair, hematomas, pseudoaneurysms, and superficial wound infections can occur after endovascular repair.

After discharge

Open surgical repair

Aortoenteric fistula

Patients with retroperitoneal prosthetic grafts are candidates for developing aortoenteric fistulas. This diagnosis should be suspected in all patients with either upper or lower gastrointestinal bleeding and prior aortic surgery. Occasionally, patients present with a herald bleed. Aggressive steps toward diagnosis and definitive treatment may be life saving before exsanguination occurs.

Graft infection

While uncommon, this complication is notoriously difficult to treat. The use of preoperative antibiotics reduces the incidence of graft infection to about 1%. Patients with prosthetic graft infection require removal of the infected prosthetic graft, extraanatomic bypass, and long-term antibiotic therapy. The mortality rate is approximately 20%.

Urologic complications

Sexual dysfunction is a well-documented complication of aortic operations and should be discussed with the patient before operation. Sympathetic arteries and nerves that course along the lateral walls of the aorta and supply the pelvis are at risk during aneurysm surgery. Thus, patients who are sexually active may complain of impotence and retrograde ejaculation. Urologic consultation should be sought if recovery does not occur within several months.

Psychiatric complications

In the elderly, a feeling of listlessness or fatigue often persists for weeks to months. Unless there are mitigating circumstances, these symptoms should gradually wane.

Endovascular repair

Endoleak

This is a complication unique to endovascular aneurysm repair that presents as persistent blood flow into the aneurysm sac after stent-graft placement. While it may result from an inadequate seal of the graft against the native arterial wall, it can also occur from retrograde perfusion via patent aortic side branches, leaks between connections of a modular graft, or defects in the graft material itself. Endoleak can develop during or at any time after the procedure and can lead to aneurysm growth and delayed rupture. Depending on the type and severity, patients may require treatment or observation. Most endoleaks requiring additional intervention can be addressed by endovascular techniques such as placement of an extension cuff, balloon angioplasty, or coiling of a branch vessel. Lifelong radiologic surveillance is mandatory for patients who have undergone endovascular repair to assess for the development of endoleak.

Device-related complications

Device migration and limb thrombosis are known complications after endovascular repair. Migration usually occurs caudally and may result in a proximal endoleak. This can usually be managed with deployment of an extension cuff. Late limb thrombosis can be managed with endovascular therapy, thrombectomy, or femorofemoral bypass. Graft infection is a rare complication that carries a high mortality.

Conversion to open surgical repair

Aneurysms that continue to enlarge in size represent a failure of endovascular therapy and may be secondary to persistent endoleak despite attempted treatment, endoleak that cannot be treated safely by endovascular methods, or radiologically undetectable endoleak. If the surgical risk is not prohibitive, these patients should undergo open repair.

Aneurysm rupture

Patients rarely present with aneurysm rupture after endovascular repair, though when they do it is most often due to an endoleak causing pressurization and enlargement of the aneurysm. Lifelong radiologic surveillance of endografts is essential to assess for development of new endoleaks and prevent aneurysm enlargement and rupture.

FURTHER READING

Bengtsson, H., Bergqvist, D., & Stemby, D. H. Increasing prevalence of abdominal aortic aneurysms: a necropsy study. *Eur. J. Surg.* 1992; **15**: 19–23.

Halett, J. W. Jr. Abdominal aortic aneurysm: natural history and treatment. *Heart Dis. Stroke.* 1992; **1**: 303–308.

Hollier, L. H., Taylor, L. M., & Ochsner, J. Recommended indications in operative treatment of abdominal aortic aneurysms: report of the Joint Council of the Society for Vascular Surgery and the North American Chapter of the International Society for Cardiovascular Surgery. *J. Vasc. Surg.* 1992; **15**: 1046–1056.

Katz, D. A., Littenberg, B., & Cronenwett, J. C. Management of small abdominal aortic aneurysms: early surgery vs. watchful waiting. *J. Am. Med. Assoc.* 1992; **268**: 2678–2686.

Nevitt, M. P., Ballard, D. J., & Halett J. W. Jr. Prognosis of abdominal aortic aneurysms: a population-based study. *N. Engl. J. Med.* 1989; **321**: 1009–1014.

Szilagyi, D. E., Smith, R. F., DeRusso, P. J. *et al.* Contribution of abdominal aortic aneurysmectomy to prolongation of life. *Ann. Surg.* 1960; **164**: 678–699.

76

Aortobifemoral bypass grafting

Victor J. Weiss

University of Mississippi, Jackson, MS

Aortobifemoral bypass is performed in patients with atherosclerotic disease primarily involving the infrarenal aorta and iliac arteries. This typically causes claudication of the hip and buttock and may produce vasculogenic impotence in men in severe cases (called LeRiche syndrome). On examination, patients have diminished or absent femoral pulses and are frequently younger – 10 years younger on average – than the typical patient with symptomatic femoropopliteal disease.

Preoperative assessment usually includes contrast angiography, which may be performed via a brachial arterial approach if there are no palpable femoral pulses. Since aortobifemoral bypass is a physically stressful operation, an assessment of the patient's overall medical condition is imperative; some evaluation of cardiac function is frequently a part of this preoperative evaluation. If the patient's condition is not suitable for aortobifemoral bypass, other less invasive options that are not quite as durable may exist, including axillary-bifemoral bypass or endoluminal angioplasty.

The procedure requires a general anesthetic, a laparotomy incision, and bilateral groin incisions. After clamping the infrarenal aorta, a prosthetic graft is sewn onto the aorta proximally. The limbs of the graft are then tunneled in a retroperitoneal plane and sewn onto the femoral arteries. The procedure typically takes 2–4 hours and often requires packed red blood cell transfusion or the use of a cell saver autotransfusion system.

Usual postoperative course

Expected postoperative hospital stay
7 to 10 days.

Operative mortality
The operative mortality for aortobifemoral bypass is 1% to 3%. The most common cause of death in the early postoperative period is due to myocardial infarction. Along with cardiac events, pulmonary (i.e., atelectasis, pneumonia), and renal complications are the major morbidities associated with the procedure.

Special monitoring required
Postoperatively, the patient typically spends at least the first night in the ICU. During this time, the vital signs, hemoglobin/hematocrit, ECG, and urine output are monitored. An epidural analgesia catheter is commonly employed for pain control. Central venous catheters are often employed for volume assessment, with Swan–Ganz catheters reserved for those with severe cardiac disease.

Patient activity and positioning
Patients are often kept with the head of the bed elevated to assist with pulmonary function. Postoperative mobility typically consists of allowing the patient to move from the bed to a chair on the first postoperative day, and ambulating with assistance on the following day.

Alimentation
Following laparotomy, an ileus is frequently present for 2–5 days. During this period of intestinal inactivity, nasogastric tube decompression may be used at the discretion of the surgeon. Peristalsis is heralded by the return of active bowel sounds, with the passage of flatus as an indication to begin liquids by mouth. The diet is advanced over the next day or two.

Medical Management of the Surgical Patient: A Textbook of Perioperative Medicine, ed. M. F. Lubin, R. B. Smith, T. F. Dobson, N. Spell, H. K. Walker. 4th edn. Published by Cambridge University Press. © Cambridge University 2006.

Antibiotic coverage

Perioperative antibiotics are imperative for patients having prosthetic graft material placed. The agent of choice is typically a first generation cephalosporin, with vancomycin reserved for those with a penicillin allergy. The dosing schedule begins with a preoperative dose prior to making the skin incision, and routinely extends for 24–48 hours or upon removal of invasive lines.

Prevention of pulmonary complications

Patients requiring aortobifemoral bypass are frequently active smokers, predisposing them to an increased risk of pulmonary complications. In order to minimize this risk, patients are counseled on the importance of smoking cessation. Despite this, the vast majority of patients will continue to smoke. Pre- as well as postoperative incentive spirometry, bronchodilator treatments, chest physical therapy, and early ambulation are all aimed at minimizing pulmonary complications. Quite possibly the greatest advance in this direction has been the use of epidural analgesia, providing patients with an improved ability to cough and breathe deeply with minimal discomfort.

Prevention of cardiac complications

Preoperative cardiac assessment aimed at diagnosing and treating coronary disease is the key to preventing cardiac complications. If indicated, coronary intervention takes precedence over elective lower extremity revascularization. Perioperative pharmacotherapy frequently consists of nitroglycerin and beta-blockers. ECG is often immediately performed postoperatively and then daily while the patient is in the ICU. Cardiac telemetry monitoring when out of the ICU can detect ischemic events that are otherwise silent.

Postoperative complications

In the hospital

Cardiac complications

Myocardial infarction is the most frequent cause of death in the early postoperative period. Arrhythmias and heart failure may occur, particularly as the patient experiences the usual postoperative fluid shifts.

Pulmonary complications

Atelectasis is a frequent postoperative finding, with pneumonia seen less commonly. Pulmonary embolus is an infrequent finding, although most patients receive some type of prophylaxis to prevent deep vein thrombosis.

Renal complications

The patient with underlying renal insufficiency is particularly prone to postoperative renal complications. Acute renal failure may have several different etiologies, including intraoperative renal embolization, renal ischemia from suprarenal cross-clamping, hypotension, and significant blood loss requiring large volume red cell transfusion.

Postoperative bleeding

Bleeding occurs in the immediate postoperative period and is infrequent after the first postoperative night. The source of bleeding may be from an anastomosis, the retroperitoneum, from within the peritoneal cavity, or along the tunnel leading to the femoral arteries. Assessment of bleeding is better evaluated by the hemoglobin/hematocrit rather than abdominal girth, as a large volume of blood can be lost before any significant increase in abdominal size can be measured.

Peripheral embolization

Embolization to the lower extremities may occasionally occur as an intraoperative event. Doppler signals at the dorsalis pedis and posterior tibial arteries are noted preoperatively. Loss of a signal may indicate embolization and require further evaluation. Microembolization may result in "trash foot" or ischemic changes to the skin with preservation of flow in the vessels at the ankle.

Acute graft occlusion

Graft occlusion in the early postoperative period is an uncommon event and typically results from a technical problem with an anastomosis, kinking, or extrinsic compression of the graft. This requires reoperation with identification and correction of the problem.

Wound infection

Infection of the abdominal incision is rare, but more common at the groins where the femoral arteries are exposed. Obese patients with a large panniculus which covers the groins and results in excessive moisture increases the risk of wound infection. Attention to hygiene and keeping the groins dry and covered with gauze may help prevent local wound complications.

After discharge

Delayed wound infection

This is an uncommon complication, typically occurring in the groin. Erythema, swelling, discharge, and warmth raise concern for graft infection and warrant further investigation.

Impotence

Retrograde ejaculation occurs in approximately 20% of male patients as a result of the disruption of sympathetic nerve fibers near the left common iliac artery. Erectile dysfunction is a rare complication of the procedure, but may be commonly seen in this population for a variety of reasons.

Graft occlusion

Occlusion of the graft most commonly occurs years after surgery, and involves one of the limbs of the bifurcated graft. This may result in a recurrence of preoperative symptoms or an acute onset of more severe symptomatology. Intervention consists of thrombolysis, thrombectomy, or femoral–femoral bypass.

Anastomotic pseudoaneurysm

A pulsatile mass in the groin following aorto-femoral bypass often signifies an anastomotic pseudoaneurysm. This may be due to infection or deterioration of the anastomosis years after graft implantation. Either etiology of pseudoaneurysm requires surgical repair.

Aortoenteric fistula

Aortoenteric fistula is an uncommon complication and most often results from erosion of the proximal aortic suture line into the duodenum. This may present with a small "herald" intestinal bleed, followed by massive blood loss. Treatment requires emergent exploration with repair of the intestinal defect and removal of the infected graft. A high index of suspicion should be maintained in anyone presenting with a GI bleed and a history of aortic graft placement.

Minimally invasive aortoiliac interventions

In addition to bypass, aortoiliac occlusive disease may also be treated by angioplasty with or without stent. The lesions best suited for this modality are focal stenoses of the common iliac arteries. Angioplasty and stent of the most ideal lesions can provide long-term patency comparable to bypass. Longer lesions, occlusions, and disease involving the external iliac arteries can be treated with angioplasty, although the long-term patency is diminished. Some believe these latter lesions are best managed by surgical revascularization.

The prime advantage of angioplasty is that it obviates the morbidity of aortobifemoral bypass. Complications are rare and primarily involve bleeding or pseudoaneurysm formation at the femoral arterial puncture site. The most common long-term problem is restenosis, which typically presents as a return of the preangioplasty symptoms.

FURTHER READING

Passman, M. A., Taylor, L. M., Moneta, G. L. *et al.* Comparison of axillofemoral and aortofemoral bypass for aortoiliac occlusive disease. *J. Vasc. Surg.* 1996; **23**(2): 263–269.

Powell, R. J., Fillinger, M., Walsh, D. B. *et al.* Predicting outcome of angioplasty and selective stenting of multisegment iliac artery occlusive disease. *J. Vasc. Surg.* 2000; **32**(2): 564–569.

Szilagyi, D. E., Elliot, J. P., Smith, R. F. *et al.* A thirty-year survey of the reconstructive surgical treatment of aortoiliac occlusive disease. *J. Vasc. Surg.* 1986; **3**: 421–436.

Timaran, C. H., Stevens, S. L., Freeman, M. B. *et al.* Predictors for adverse outcome after iliac angioplasty and stenting for limb-threatening ischemia. *J. Vasc. Surg.* 2002; **36**(3): 507–513.

77

Femoropopliteal bypass grafting

Victor J. Weiss

University of Mississippi, Jackson, MS

Femoropopliteal bypass is a procedure in which autogenous vein (typically the greater saphenous vein), a prosthetic conduit, or a combination of the two is used to improve the circulation of the lower extremity. This is most commonly performed for atherosclerotic disease of the superficial femoral and/or popliteal artery, though it is occasionally done to treat a popliteal aneurysm.

Indications for femoropopliteal bypass performed for chronic arterial insufficiency typically include severe, disabling short distance calf claudication, rest pain, ischemic non-healing ulcers, or gangrene. Not uncommonly, atherosclerotic obstructions of the superficial femoral artery can be asymptomatic and such lesions rarely if ever require treatment. Mild to moderate claudication symptoms are seldom treated with bypass, as the natural history of this condition infrequently progresses to threaten the limb and a failed bypass can significantly worsen the ischemic symptoms and may jeopardize the extremity.

In addition to a thorough history and physical examination, preoperative assessment typically includes Doppler measurement of the ankle-brachial index and imaging with contrast arteriography. Alternate imaging modalities such as ultrasound or MRA are occasionally performed, especially if the patient has renal insufficiency. The surgeon evaluates the imaging studies to verify that there are no significant lesions proximal to the femoral artery or distal to the popliteal artery that would compromise the success of the bypass. Prior to operative intervention, attention should be directed toward assessment of the heart, as a significant number of patients with lower extremity arterial occlusive disease have concomitant coronary artery disease.

Autogenous saphenous vein (in either a reversed or in situ location) is the ideal conduit for lower extremity bypass grafting. Autogenous alternatives to greater saphenous vein include lesser saphenous vein and upper extremity cephalic or basilic veins. Other possible conduits include polytetrafluoroethylene (PTFE), Dacron, human umbilical vein, or cryopreserved veins. Femoropopliteal bypass can be performed in 2–4 hours under general, spinal, or epidural anesthesia. The operation constitutes a moderate surgical stress, but seldom requires transfusion of blood.

Usual postoperative course

Expected postoperative hospital stay
4 to 6 days.

Operative mortality
2 to 4%.

Special monitoring required
Dorsalis pedis and posterior tibial pulses should be evaluated every 2 to 4 hours either by palpation or by Doppler assessment.

Patient activity and positioning
Patients may ambulate with assistance on the first postoperative day. If the patient is in a chair, the leg should be elevated to minimize the edema which is frequently encountered postoperatively.

Alimentation
The patient is made n.p.o. after midnight prior to surgery and a resumption of the usual diet begins the first postoperative day.

Antibiotic coverage
A first-generation cephalosporin is administered preoperatively and continued for 24 hours. A longer course with a variable antibiotic regimen may be required for patients with open or infected wounds.

Medical Management of the Surgical Patient: A Textbook of Perioperative Medicine, ed. M. F. Lubin, R. B. Smith, T. F. Dobson, N. Spell, H. K. Walker. 4th edn. Published by Cambridge University Press. © Cambridge University 2006.

Postoperative complications

In the hospital

Bleeding

As the most common immediate postoperative complication, bleeding may arise from the incision, the anastomoses, or from within the tunnel where the conduit is placed. Small hematomas may be observed and will resorb with time. Larger hematomas which cause pressure on the skin or the graft should be evacuated in the operating room.

Graft thrombosis

Graft thrombosis in the immediate postoperative period usually indicates a technical problem, either with the anastomoses, the inflow or outflow vessels, or with the conduit. Re-exploration, graft thrombectomy, and intraoperative angiography are typically indicated.

Leg edema

Postoperative leg edema is a nearly universal finding, although the severity may vary. The etiology can be multifactorial, with surgical disruption of lymphatic drainage as the principal cause. Improvement can be provided by elevation of the limb; spontaneous improvement is often seen within a few months from the bypass.

Wound infection

Infection is an uncommon but unsettling problem, particularly when a synthetic conduit has been used. If the synthetic graft material becomes infected, the patient may be at risk of limb loss. Wound infection overlying an autogenous vein graft is somewhat less critical since this conduit is less likely to become infected. Superficial infections may be treated by opening the wound to allow for the drainage of pus, applying dressings to promote healing, and systemic antibiotic therapy. Deeper infections that involve a synthetic graft or that leave a graft exposed necessitate graft removal and replacement with an autogenous conduit (typically saphenous vein). Exposed autogenous vein may require a sartorius muscle flap to be rotated into position to provide coverage of the graft. Amputation may ultimately be required in as many as 70% of patients with prosthetic bypass graft infection.

After discharge

Vein graft stenosis

Thrombosis of autogenous vein grafts occur in 10% to 15% of patients within the first two years following bypass. This most often is the result of a hyperplastic reaction, either within the vein or at the anastomosis, and can be detected by ultrasonographic surveillance. "Failing" grafts are usually asymptomatic and may not be detected simply by the measurement of ankle pressures. The natural history of a segmental stenosis discovered on routine ultrasound and repaired surgically is the same as if no narrowing were ever detected; that is, an excellent chance for prolonged patency. Once a vein graft actually occludes, the chances for durable patency are significantly diminished. Thus, routine duplex surveillance of the autogenous lower extremity bypass graft is imperative. Prosthetic material behaves differently and is not routinely followed with duplex examination.

Graft occlusion

Thrombotic occlusion of a bypass graft may occur suddenly, with an acute onset of symptoms. Such patients may develop a profoundly ischemic limb if the bypass had been performed for limb salvage, or may have a return of their prebypass claudication symptoms. If the patient presents soon after the graft occludes, a restoration of patency may be obtained by either surgical thrombectomy or by thrombolytic infusion. An investigation as to the cause of the occlusion is made, and the lesion must be treated to prevent recurrent thrombosis.

FURTHER READING

Abbott, W. M. Prosthetic above-knee femoral-popliteal bypass: indications and choice of graft. *Semin. Vasc. Surg.* 1997; **10**(1): 3–7.

Johnson, W. C. & Lee, K. K. A comparative evaluation of polytetrafluoroethylene, umbilical vein, and saphenous vein bypass grafts for femoral-popliteal above-knee revascularization: a prospective randomized Department of Veterans Affairs cooperative study. *J. Vasc. Surg.* 2000; **32**(2): 268–277.

Landry, G. J., Moneta, G. L., Taylor, L. M. Jr. *et al.* Long-term outcome of revised lower-extremity bypass grafts. *J. Vasc. Surg.* 2002; **35**(1): 56–62.

Mills, J. L. Sr., Wixon, C. L., James, D. C. *et al.* The natural history of intermediate and critical vein graft stenosis: recommendations for continued surveillance or repair. *J. Vasc. Surg.* 2001; **33**(2): 273–278.

Veith, F. J., Gupta, S. K., Acer, E. *et al.* Six-year prospective randomized comparison of autologous saphenous vein and expanded polytetrafluoroethylene grafts in infrainguinal reconstruction. *J. Vasc. Surg.* 1986; **3**: 104–114.

78

Lower extremity embolectomy

Sunil S. Rayan and Thomas F. Dodson

Emory University School of Medicine, Atlanta, GA

With mortality and amputation rates remaining over 20%, thromboembolic arterial disease continues to be a major health problem despite improvements in patient care. While embolic sources are primarily cardiogenic in 80%–90% of cases, other causes include atheroemboli from large vessels, tumors, paradoxical emboli, and aneurysmal debris. Classically, patients have a history of atrial fibrillation, myocardial infarction, or a prosthetic heart valve. The majority of emboli affect the lower extremity, most commonly in the femoropopliteal system, and occlude distal flow and collateral pathways by typically lodging at the bifurcations of vessels such as the femoral bifurcation.

Patients with thromboembolism of the extremities present with one or more of the "six classic P's of limb ischemia": pain, pallor, paresthesia, paralysis, pulselessness, and poikilothermia (cold limb). Since each patient has a critical window before irreversible tissue damage occurs, the duration of symptoms is important. Six hours is commonly considered to be the span before such damage begins. It cannot be overemphasized that immediate referral to a vascular surgeon is absolutely paramount if a patient presents with acute limb ischemia, as delays in triage or unnecessary imaging can ultimately compromise limb salvage. Diagnosis can usually be made by history and physical examination, though certain cases may require duplex ultrasonography or arteriography prior to definitive treatment.

The algorithm for treating patients with acute thromboembolism can be quite complex and takes into account duration and severity of ischemia, presence of pre-existing peripheral vascular disease, history of prior vascular surgery, and therapeutic modalities available to the treating surgeon. As a general rule, all patients are immediately anticoagulated with heparin. Subsequent treatment may include balloon embolectomy, thrombolytic therapy, or percutaneous mechanical thrombectomy. Originally described by Fogarty in 1962, balloon catheter embolectomy via a groin incision has become the mainstay of therapy for most surgeons. Thrombolytic therapy has not been shown to be superior to surgery but has a role in distal disease and ischemia of relatively short duration. Finally, a myriad of mechanical thrombectomy catheters are available that employ different principles to effect thrombus dissolution.

Usual postoperative course

Expected postoperative hospital stay

Following the procedure at our institution, patients are in the hospital for an average of five days, though this can vary with the patient's condition at presentation and the extent of surgery. Although patient recovery time is usually quite short, much of the postoperative hospital stay is spent in ascertaining the etiology of the embolus. Often, hematologists and cardiologists are involved in postoperative care. Transesophageal echocardiography, computed tomography, and angiography are tools that aid in diagnosing the source of emboli.

Operative mortality

The high hospital mortality rate of 20% to 30% is a reflection of the underlying disease process and overall health of this patient population, not the morbidity of the procedure itself.

Special monitoring required

Patients often recover in the intensive care unit for 24 hours and are placed on telemetry for cardiac monitoring. Frequent monitoring of peripheral pulses is essential as most recurrent thromboses happen in the earlypostoperative period. Assessment of motor and sensory

Medical Management of the Surgical Patient: A Textbook of Perioperative Medicine, ed. M. F. Lubin, R. B. Smith, T. F. Dodson, N. Spell, H. K. Walker. 4th edn. Published by Cambridge University Press. © Cambridge University 2006.

function after revascularization for severe ischemia is also imperative, with heightened suspicion for compartment syndrome. Measurement of renal function by urine output and serum creatinine determines renal injury that may result from myoglobinuria or contrast arteriography.

Patient activity and positioning

Most patients who undergo catheter embolectomy via a single femoral incision recover quickly and are encouraged to ambulate the following day.

Alimentation

Patients can resume normal diet the evening of surgery.

Antibiotic coverage

Cephalosporin is administered immediately prior to surgical procedure.

Postoperative anticoagulation

Patients must be converted to therapeutic levels of an oral anticoagulant prior to discharge, which can take several days. We inform patients about the risks of warfarin therapy, the need for lifelong monitoring of prothrombin time, and the advisability of purchasing Medic-Alert bracelets to notify medical professionals of this therapy in the event of an emergency.

Postoperative complications

In the hospital

Compartment syndrome

This is a dreaded consequence of acute limb ischemia. Edema of the revascularized tissue may exceed the perfusion pressure within the fascial compartments of the leg resulting in muscle necrosis, nerve damage, or thrombosis of the arteries and veins in the affected compartment. The anterior compartment of the lower leg is most frequently involved. Symptoms such as severe leg pain on dorsiflexion of the foot or diminished sensation and paresthesias in the first toe web space are strongly suggestive of anterior compartment syndrome. Early detection is the key to limiting the process, which can be accomplished by frequent assessment of the motor and sensory function or by measurement of compartment pressures. Once compartment syndrome is suspected, immediate decompressive four-compartment fasciotomy must be performed. Some surgeons prefer to perform fasciotomy at the time of initial revascularization if the duration of ischemia has been prolonged. Fasciotomy wounds can usually be closed secondarily after the edema subsides.

Renal failure

Can either result from contrast nephropathy if arteriography was employed or from myoglobinuria, which can occur after severe limb ischemia with muscle necrosis. Patients with prolonged ischemia should be monitored closely for acute renal insufficiency and treated aggressively with intravenous hydration. Alkalinization with sodium bicarbonate is essential to diminish precipitation of myoglobin in the renal tubules and prevent further renal tubular injury. Mannitol assists with both diuresis and prevention of reperfusion injury.

Metabolic acidosis

Another sign of severe ischemia that may indicate that embolectomy and revascularization was not effective. Occasionally, an emergency amputation is the only way to control continued metabolic acidosis and poor tissue perfusion. Hyperkalemia, another concern in cases of severe ischemia, results from cellular breakdown and release of potassium into the circulation. Again, maintenance of a brisk urinary output in the postoperative period is an important precaution.

Leg edema

Correlates with the degree of preoperative ischemia as well as the complexity of the revascularization. Elevation of the affected limb continues to be the mainstay of therapy and patients should be reassured that most edema subsides with time.

Recurrent embolization

Relatively uncommon when anticoagulation is strictly maintained after the initial procedure. However, it occasionally occurs and should be considered when patients develop worsening symptoms or signs of emboli to other vascular territories.

Hematomas

May occur with resumption of heparin therapy after operation, though it is a minor problem that rarely requires return to the operating room for evacuation. Some surgeons employ the use of a drain to minimize hematoma formation in the groin wound. Patients should be reassured that stable hematomas and ecchymosis will gradually resolve without sequelae.

After discharge

Peripheral nerve deficits

This is often the most disabling complication in those who present with severe ischemia. It can manifest as numbness in the sensory distribution of the affected nerve, loss of motor function, or painful neuropathy. Time and analgesics are the only treatments; in extreme cases, amputation may be required for symptom control.

Pseudoaneurysms

As a potential complication after any arteriotomy, they should be promptly treated if discovered. They typically present as an expansile mass, thrill, or bruit over the incision site. Duplex ultrasonography or CT scan with contrast confirms the diagnosis. Treatment options include open operation, ultrasound-guided compression, and thrombin injection.

Claudication or rest pain

This symptom complex may result if embolectomy is incomplete or collateral vessels undergo thrombosis before definitive therapy is achieved. Claudication is usually treated conservatively, whereas rest pain necessitates reevaluation of limb perfusion and an attempt to improve distal blood flow.

FURTHER READING

Abbott, W., Maloney, R., McCabe, C. *et al.* Arterial embolism in a 44-year perspective. *Am. J. Surg.* 1982; **143**: 460.

Fogarty, T., Cranley, J., & Krause, R. A method for extraction of arterial emboli and thrombi. *Surg. Gynecol. Obstet.* 1962; **44**: 557.

Fogarty, T., Daily, P., Shumway, N. *et al.* Experience with balloon catheter technique for arterial embolectomy. *Am. J. Surg.* 1971; **122**: 231.

Haimovici, H. Muscular, renal, and metabolic complications of acute arterial occlusions: myonephropathic-metabolic syndrome. *Surgery* 1979; **85**: 461.

Jivegård, L., Holm, J., & Sterstén, T. Acute limb ischemia due to arterial embolism or thrombosis: Influence of limb ischemia versus pre-existing cardiac disease on postoperative mortality rate. *J. Cardiovasc. Surg.* 1988; **29**: 32.

Matsen, F., Winquist, R., & Krugmire, R. Diagnosis and management of compartment syndromes. *J. Bone Joint Surg.* 1980; **62**: 286.

Ouriel, K., Shortell, C., DeWeese, J. *et al.* A comparison of thrombolytic therapy with operative revascularization in the initial treatment of acute peripheral arterial ischemia. *J. Vasc. Surg.* 1994; **19**: 1021.

Sharafuddin, M. & Hicks, M. Current status of percutaneous mechanical thrombectomy: Part II. Devices and mechanism of action. *J. Vasc. Interv. Radiol.* 1998; **9**: 15.

79

Treatment of chronic mesenteric ischemia

Karthikeshwar Kasirajan and Elliot L. Chaikof

Emory University School of Medicine, Atlanta, GA

Owing to the rich blood supply to the intestines, symptoms of chronic mesenteric ischemia are rare. The major vessels supplying the intestines are the celiac artery for the foregut, the superior mesenteric artery for the midgut, and the inferior mesenteric artery for the hindgut. Additionally, the inferior mesenteric artery receives a rich collateral flow from branches of both internal iliac arteries. In the event of chronic occlusion of one or more of the main arteries supplying the bowel, an extensive network of interconnecting branches ensures adequate collateral flow to the intestines. Hence, for symptoms of chronic mesenteric ischemia, stenosis or occlusion in two or more of the three major vessels is often necessary.

The diagnosis of chronic mesenteric ischemia can usually be suspected on clinical grounds alone. Postprandial pain is the most prevalent complaint, which may be accompanied by symptoms of bloating, weight loss, "food fear," nausea, vomiting, diarrhea, and/or constipation. The pain is typically dull and crampy, poorly localized to the midepigastric region or midabdomen, and usually occurs within the first hour after eating. The symptoms are often severe enough to cause the patient to restrict food intake ("food fear"). The weight loss may be so acute as to result in cachexia and prompt a work-up for an underlying neoplasm. In the only available natural history study of chronic mesenteric ischemia, 86% of the patients developed symptoms significant enough to attempt revascularization or they died due to bowel ischemia. The first clinical presentation may be acute mesenteric ischemia in 15% to 50% of the patients, with a mortality rate of about 15% to 70%. Unfortunately, the accurate diagnosis of chronic mesenteric ischemia continues to challenge physicians and a high index of suspicion is required in elderly patients with known cardiovascular risk factors.

A non-invasive duplex ultrasound exam is often used as the initial screening test, but angiography with selective mesenteric images remains the gold standard for diagnosis and planning of therapy. While magnetic resonance angiography and computed tomogram angiography hold promise as diagnostic adjuncts, they cannot presently supplement arteriography.

When the diagnosis of chronic mesenteric ischemia has been confirmed, patients are offered open surgical revascularization or percutaneous balloon angioplasty with or without stent placement. The choice of therapy is determined by patient and physician preference, associated comorbid factors, and status of the mesenteric vessels. Occlusions are best managed by open surgical revascularization, while stenoses in patients with significant comorbid conditions are best approached using percutaneous techniques. Open surgical revascularization has superior long-term patency, but at a cost of higher morbidity and mortality (Tables 79.1 and 79.2). In addition to routine preoperative labs and diagnostic studies, all patients should have a cardiac stress test and an evaluation of nutritional status (e.g., serum albumin and transferrin levels), and patients with a history of tobacco use should also have pulmonary function studies done. Although poor nutritional status is not easily correctable prior to intervention, it serves as a useful indicator of the success of revascularization during the follow-up period.

Since the postoperative course is significantly different for open surgical revascularization and balloon angioplasty, they are discussed separately.

Open surgery

Usual postoperative course

Expected postoperative hospital stay
8 to 10 days.

Medical Management of the Surgical Patient: A Textbook of Perioperative Medicine, ed. M. F. Lubin, R. B. Smith, T. F. Dobson, N. Spell, H. K. Walker. 4th edn. Published by Cambridge University Press. © Cambridge University 2006.

Table 79.1. Open surgical revascularization for mesenteric ischemia

Author	n	Success	Follow-up (months)	Long-term pain relief	Complications	Mortality	Patency
Kieny	60	100%	102	NA	NA	3.50%	75%
Cormier	32	100%	69	NA	NA	9%	91%
Cunningham	74	100%	71	86%	17.10%	12.20%	NA
McAfee	58	100%	60	90%	41%	10%	90%
Calderon	20	100%	36	100%	20%	0	100%
Christensen	90	100%	55	63%	NA	13%	NA
Gentile	26	100%	48	89%	NA	10%	89%
Johnston	21	100%	120	NA	19%	0	86%
Moawad	24	100%	60	78%	45%	4%	78%
Mateo	85	100%	36	87%	33%	8%	76%
Average	49	100%	66	85%	29%	7%	86%
S.D.	28		27	12%	12%		9%

Note:

n, number of patients; NA, not available; S.D., standard deviation.

Operative mortality

Varies widely, but averages 7% with complications noted in $29 \pm 12\%$ of patients (Table 79.1). The most frequent cause of mortality is cardiac disease, reflecting the need for cardiac work-up and optimization. Adverse cardiac events are noted in 15% of patients in the postoperative period. Pulmonary, gastrointestinal, and renal complications are the most frequently encountered non-fatal complications. Respiratory failure requiring prolonged ventilatory support is noted in 15% of patients, and prolonged ileus or renal failure is observed in 30% and 10% of patients respectively.

Special monitoring required

All patients are placed in the intensive care unit for monitoring and cardiac enzymes are routinely obtained. Preventing fluid overload (close monitoring of the pulmonary wedge pressure and central venous pressure), and continued pulmonary toilet (incentive spirometer, deep breathing, vigorous coughing, use of bronchodilators and mucolytic agents if required) pre- and post-extubation diminishes the incidence of pulmonary complications. Renal failure is best prevented by avoiding wide blood pressure fluctuations both intra- and postoperatively and by minimizing aortic cross clamp time.

Patient activity and positioning

May be mobilized out of bed when hemodynamically stable and off the ventilator.

Alimentation

Oral intake is withheld until postoperative ileus has resolved.

Antibiotic coverage

Broad spectrum antibiotic coverage should be extended until intestinal function returns.

Postoperative complications

In the hospital

Local complication

Complications may occur in the gastrointestinal system that are often difficult to diagnose and require a high index of suspicion. Hematocrit levels are followed closely and a rapid or continued downward trend may require transfusion, correction of any abnormal coagulation parameters, or reexploration. Nasogastric tubes are routinely used to minimize the problems that may result from a prolonged ileus. Early initiation of total parenteral nutrition may be required in patients with known preoperative nutritional depletion.

Abdominal pain

This complication may have a variety of causes ranging from ileus, bowel ischemia, intestinal edema and pancreatitis. Plain abdominal films and clinical exam should be sufficient to diagnose postoperative ileus. Intestinal ischemia/gangrene may be differentiated from bowel edema by an elevation in the white cell count and lactate, unexplained acidosis, and base deficit. Presence of any of these serum abnormalities warrants early reexploration to assess for bowel ischemia and exclude acute graft thrombosis.

Table 79.2. Percutaneous angioplasty and stenting for mesenteric ischemia

Author	n	Success	Follow-up (months)	Long-term pain relief	Complications	Mortality	Patency
Matsumoto	19	79%	25	52%	32%	0	NA
Hallisey	16	84%	27.6	75%	6%	6%	75%
Allen	19	95%	39	79%	5%	5%	NA
Maspes	23	90%	27	75%	9%	0	88%
Nyman	5	100%	21	80%	40%	0	40%
Sheeren	12	92%	15.7	75%	NA	8%	74%
Kasirajan	28	88%	36	66%	18%	11%	73%
Average	17	90%	27	72%	18%	4%	70%
S.D.	7	7%	8	10%	15%		18%

After discharge

Recurrent mesenteric ischemia

Restenosis/occlusion of the native artery or bypass graft may result in abdominal angina or acute mesenteric ischemia.

Balloon angioplasty

Usual postoperative course

Expected postoperative hospital stay
1 to 2 days.

Operative mortality
Mortality is observed in about 5% of patients and complications are seen in $18 \pm 15\%$ (Table 79.2). Mortality is often associated with gastrointestinal complications, especially bowel necrosis that may be seen in 5%–10% of patients. At 4%, cardiac and pulmonary events are less frequent. After percutaneous revascularization, the majority of encountered complications are local. Access complications include hematoma, bleeding, pseudoaneurysm, or access vessel thrombosis. Intra-abdominal complications may include vessel rupture, thrombosis, malpositioning of the stent, and distal embolization during angioplasty.

Special monitoring required
As systemic complications are far less frequent with percutaneous revascularization, patients do not need to be monitored in an intensive care unit. However, unlike many other peripheral angioplasty procedures, these patients are observed in the hospital overnight. Special attention is paid to maintenance of adequate hydration due to the added risk of using contrast agents. Fenoldopam may be used at 0.1 µg/kg per minute to decrease the incidence of renal failure in patients with pre-existing renal compromise.

Patient activity and positioning
Mobilize progressively as patient's condition permits.

Alimentation
Usually resume oral intake promptly.

Antibiotic coverage
Antibiotic administered prior to the intervention.

Postoperative complications

In the hospital

Local complications
Careful attention to access techniques should minimize the incidence of access vessel complications. Recent advances in endovascular devices, with smaller device profile and better capacity for tracking around acute angles, have helped eliminate many of the complications observed in the past. In former times, the acute downward angle of the mesenteric vessels off the abdominal aorta often required the use of a brachial approach to track the larger and stiffer devices. Historically, this resulted in a higher incidence of brachial complications. Currently, most mesenteric angioplasty procedures may be adequately performed via the femoral approach. Following angioplasty, patients are maintained on aspirin for life. In addition, they are placed on clopidogrel (Plavix) for a week before the procedure and continued for 3 months

afterwards. The use of these antiplatelet agents may help decrease the incidence of acute stent thrombosis.

After discharge

Abdominal pain

Elimination of postprandial abdominal pain is one of the primary indicators of the success of the procedure. Similarly, the recurrence of pain may be a reliable indicator of recurrent stenosis.

Nutritional status

Serum albumin and transferrin levels are monitored as a measure of the success of revascularization along with weight gain, which may be apparent within a few weeks of intervention.

Graft or stent restenosis

The treated vessel is routinely monitored for restenosis. Clinical symptoms may not be obvious until the stenosis is critical or results in thrombosis. Hence, we recommend surveillance with non-invasive imaging studies, such as duplex ultrasound, magnetic resonance imaging, or CT angiography. Typically, the bypass graft or stented vessel is assessed at 1 month, every 6 months for 2 years, and then annually for prompt diagnosis and correction of any subclincal restenosis.

FURTHER READING

Cho, J.-S., Carr, J. A., Jacobsen, G. *et al.* Long-term outcome after mesenteric artery reconstruction: a 37-year experience. *J. Vasc. Surg.* 2002; **35**: 453–460.

Kasirajan, K., O'Hara, P. J., Gray, B. H. *et al.* Chronic mesenteric ischemia: open surgery versus percutaneous angioplasty and stenting. *J. Vasc. Surg.* 2001; **33**: 63–71.

Kihara, T. K., Blebea, J., Anderson, K. M. *et al.* Risk factors and outcomes following revascularization for chronic mesenteric ischemia. *Ann. Vasc. Surg.* 1999; **13**: 37–44.

Moawad, J., McKinsey, J. F., Wyble, C. W. *et al.* Current results of surgical therapy for chronic mesenteric ischemia. *Arch. Surg.* 1997; **132**: 613–619.

Mohammed, A., Teo, N. B., Pickford, I. R. *et al.* Percutaneous transluminal angioplasty and stenting of celiac artery stenosis in the treatment of mesenteric angina: a review of therapeutic options. *J. Roy. Coll. Surg. Edin.* 2002; **45**: 403–407.

80

Inferior vena cava filters

Sunil S. Rayan and Thomas F. Dodson

Emory University School of Medicine, Atlanta, GA

Pulmonary embolism (PE) accounts for 150 000 to 200 000 deaths per year in the USA. Although anticoagulation is the standard of care for PE, up to 1.5% of patients on anticoagulation suffer a subsequent fatal PE. Recurrent PE despite adequate anticoagulation, contraindication to anticoagulation, and bleeding complications of anticoagulation therapy are all accepted indications for caval interruption. The introduction of inferior vena caval (IVC) filters have revolutionized interruption procedures, which have existed since the nineteenth century. Since the original Mobin–Uddin umbrella filter was described over 30 years ago there have been many technological advances, the most significant thus far being the Greenfield filter, introduced in 1973, which overcame many of the original device's shortcomings and is the most commonly used filter today.

IVC filters are now inserted percutaneously under local anesthesia via the femoral or jugular approach, usually in less than 30 minutes. The procedure consists of achieving central venous access, venography, and device deployment. Venography is usually accomplished with a minimum of contrast and is used to size the IVC, locate the renal veins, and identify possibly aberrant anatomy. Procedural morbidity is extremely rare and consists primarily of complications at the insertion site. Long-term complications are more significant and need to be considered when placing filters in young patients. Such complications include device migration, device fracture, caval thrombosis, and lower extremity edema.

Multiple permanent devices are currently approved by the Food and Drug Administration for use in PE prevention: Greenfield® (Boston Scientific, Natick, MA), Bird's Nest® (Cook Inc., Bloomington, IN), Trapease® (Cordis Endovascular, Warren, NJ), LGM Vena-Tech™ and Vena-Tech LP® (B. Braun, Evanston, IL) and Simon-Nitinol® (C. R. Bard, Murray Hill, NJ). Each of these devices possesses its own unique advantages and complication rates,

and all of them protect against PE in over 95% of cases. Our choice for filter placement is the stainless steel Greenfield® filter, which has the longest track record of any IVC filter. It boasts the lowest long-term complication rates and the over-the-wire version is extremely easy to deploy. Its main disadvantage is the requirement of a 12F sheath, the largest of the percutaneous filters; however, a lower-profile version is promised in the near future. We rarely use the Bird's Nest® filter as deployment can be difficult and high IVC thrombosis rates have been reported; however, it is the filter of choice for megacava. Our second choice for filter placement is the Simon-Nitinol® filter because of its low complication rates, ease of deployment, and small 9F sheath size. The Trapease® has the smallest introducer diameter but has been associated with isolated reports of caval thrombosis. Overall, IVC filters are quite successful in preventing recurrent pulmonary embolization with rates ranging from 1.9% to 2.4% and fatal PE occurring in only 0.3% of cases.

After being successfully used in Europe for years, retrievable filters have recently been introduced into the US marketplace. These devices may be ideal in patients who require temporary caval interruption before they can be safely anticoagulated, such as multitrauma and pregnant patients or patients undergoing bariatric surgery. Three retrievable filters are currently available: the Optease™ (Cordis Endovascular, Warren, NJ), the Günther Tulip™ (Cook Inc., Bloomington, IN) and the Recovery® (C. R. Bard, Murray Hill, NJ). The Optease™ and Günther Tulip™ must be removed within two weeks while, at the time of this writing, the Recovery® has an open-ended window for device retrieval. All three devices are remarkably easy to deploy and retrieve, utilize low-profile delivery systems, and should theoretically eliminate the long-term complications of filters such as IVC thrombosis and device migration. They may represent the gold standard in the future.

Medical Management of the Surgical Patient: A Textbook of Perioperative Medicine, ed. M. F. Lubin, R. B. Smith, T. F. Dobson, N. Spell, H. K. Walker. 4th edn. Published by Cambridge University Press. © Cambridge University 2006.

Usual postoperative course

Expected postoperative hospital stay

Depending upon associated medical problems, the patient can be released on the evening of the procedure. In order to minimize bleeding complications, we prefer to have the patient remain flat in bed for 4 hours after manual pressure of the insertion site is discontinued.

Operative mortality

Death from the procedure itself should approach 0%, but hospital mortality overall is substantial due to underlying medical/surgical conditions.

Special monitoring required

None.

Patient activity and positioning

Relates to the patient's condition otherwise, though the patient can often be ambulatory after 4 hours.

Alimentation

As tolerated.

Antibiotic coverage

One dose of antibiotics covering skin flora is administered prior to insertion.

Anticoagulation

If the patient requires anticoagulation, we prefer to resume heparin six hours after the procedure, especially if a large introducer sheath was used.

Postoperative complications

In the hospital

Insertion problems

Procedural morbidity is rare and is usually limited to local complications at the site of device insertion. Hematomas, ecchymosis, and bleeding from the puncture site occur infrequently and are usually controlled by gentle compression at the insertion site.

Deployment problems

Most serious immediate complications are due to operator error or device malfunction. Inadvertent misdeployment of the device into the iliac veins or suprarenal cava is a minor problem that simply requires insertion of another device in the correct location. Catheter and wire complications resulting in perforation of the vena cava or right atrium have been reported and require expedient management. Device malfunction resulting in incomplete device expansion or device migration can usually be successfully managed using endovascular techniques.

Infection

Extremely rare in terms of the device or insertion-site.

After discharge

Clinicians must be aware of the long-term complications of permanent IVC filters when considering their use in younger patients. IVC thrombosis is device-specific with rates ranging from 0 to 25%. The Greenfield® filter has the lowest rate of IVC thrombosis (0% to 3%); the Bird's Nest filter has the highest rates of thrombosis (5% to 21%). IVC thrombosis may lead to disabling clinical symptoms such as extensive lower extremity edema, venous ulceration, or phlegmasia cerulea dolens. Recurrent deep venous thrombosis is an uncommon problem (3% to 7%) after filter placement and probably reflects the underlying disorder rather than a complication of filter placement. When larger sheath sizes were used, venous thrombosis at the entry site was a relatively common occurrence but now occurs in approximately 2% of cases. Many believe that prevention of fatal PE by IVC filters outweighs the negative effects of delayed large vein thrombotic complications. In all cases of symptomatic venous thrombosis, anticoagulation is the treatment of choice unless otherwise contraindicated.

FURTHER READING

Becker, D. M., Philbrick, J. T., & Selby, J. B. Inferior vena cava filters: indications, safety, effectiveness. *Arch. Intern. Med.* 1992; **152**: 1985–1994.

Douketis, J. D., Kearon, C., Bates, S. *et al.* Risk of fatal pulmonary embolism in patients with treated venous thromboembolism. *J. Am. Med. Assoc.* 1998; **279**: 458–462.

Greenfield, L. J. & Proctor, M. C. Twenty-year clinical experience with the Greenfield filter. *Cardiovasc. Surg.* 1995; **3**: 199–205.

Greenfield, L. J., McCurdy, J. R., Brown, P. P. *et al.* A new intracaval filter permitting continued flow and resolution of emboli. *Surgery* 1973; **73**: 599–606.

Mohan, C. R., Hoballah, J. J., Sharp, W. J. *et al.* Comparative efficacy and complications of vena caval filters. *J. Vasc. Surg.* 1995; **21**: 235–246.

Roehm, J., Johnsrude, I., Barth, M. *et al.* The Bird's Nest inferior vena cava filter: progress report. *Radiology* 1988; **165**: 745–749.

81

Portal shunting procedures

Tarek A. Salam and Atef A. Salam

Emory University School of Medicine, Atlanta, GA

Decompressive portosystemic shunts play a significant role in the treatment of patients with portal hypertension and gastroesophageal varices. The main indication for portal shunting procedures is the prevention of recurrent variceal bleeding in patients with cirrhosis and portal hypertension after failure of endoscopic sclerotherapy. Portal shunting procedures are not indicated for prophylaxis against variceal bleeding in patients who have not yet bled. The ideal candidates for shunt procedures are patients at Child's class A or B risk levels who have favorable venous anatomy. The procedures themselves can be divided into two main categories:

Total shunts

With total shunts, the entire portal venous blood flow is shunted into the systemic venous circulation. This includes end-to-side and side-to-side portacaval shunts, central splenorenal shunts, Marion–Clatworthy mesocaval shunts, interposition mesocaval shunts, and the recently introduced transjugular intrahepatic portosystemic shunt (TIPS). The small graft portacaval interposition shunt is a modification designed to achieve partial rather than total diversion of portal venous flow.

Selective distal splenorenal (Warren) shunt

With the selective distal splenorenal shunt, the gastroesophageal varices are selectively decompressed by way of the upper stomach through the short gastric veins and the disconnected splenic vein into the left renal vein, while enough pressure is maintained in the portal and superior mesenteric veins to drive blood through the diseased liver. The spleen is not removed in this procedure.

Because it is associated with a lower incidence of encephalopathy and hepatic insufficiency, the distal splenorenal shunt is used in most patients. Although collateral veins develop over time after this shunting procedure, with progressive diversion of portal blood flow there is often no parallel progress of encephalopathy, which remains significantly less than that seen after rapid diversion of portal flow by a total shunt. Unlike portacaval shunts, distal splenorenal shunts do not complicate future liver transplantation. In some patients, however, adequate splenic or renal veins are not available to make this shunt feasible. The selective shunt is not recommended for patients with refractory ascites. A total shunt should be considered under these circumstances. If patients who require total shunts are potential candidates for liver transplantation, mesocaval rather than portacaval shunts should be chosen to preclude dissection in the liver hilus, which would complicate subsequent liver transplantation. All portal shunts cause severe surgical stress and may necessitate multiple perioperative transfusions.

Radiologic shunts (transjugular intrahepatic portosystemic shunts or tips)

In this procedure, access to the right hepatic vein is obtained using percutaneous guidewire and catheter techniques. A special needle pierces the liver tissue between the hepatic vessel and the right branch of the portal vein. The track thus created is balloon dilated and stented, establishing an intrahepatic portosystemic shunt between these two large veins.

TIPS are best used to protect cirrhotic patients who are transplant candidates awaiting a donor liver, and may also be used to treat resistant ascites in patients with intrahepatic portal hypertension. Hemodynamically, TIPS are a form of total shunt; hence they put the patient at risk for postshunt hepatic encephalopathy.

Medical Management of the Surgical Patient: A Textbook of Perioperative Medicine, ed. M. F. Lubin, R. B. Smith, T. F. Dobson, N. Spell, H. K. Walker. 4th edn. Published by Cambridge University Press. © Cambridge University 2006.

Liver transplant

Liver transplant is the treatment of choice for patients with advanced liver disease (Child's C). A successful liver transplant eliminates liver failure and variceal hemorrhage, the two main causes of death in cirrhotics. Organ shortage precludes wider application of this modality to include cirrhotics with adequate liver reserve. Therefore, shunts continue to be the preferred treatment when sclerotherapy fails to control variceal bleeding in this patient population.

Usual postoperative course

Expected postoperative hospital stay
Without complications, generally 7 to 10 days.

Operative mortality
Varies from 5% to 30%, depending on the Child's classification and the urgency of the procedure.

Special monitoring required
Intensive care unit observation is necessary for the first 2 or 3 days after surgery. Serial monitoring of vital signs, intake and output, central venous pressure, body weight, renal function, hematocrit, and liver function is essential.

Patient activity and positioning
Intensive pulmonary care and early ambulation starting on the first postoperative day are important to minimize atelectasis and subsequent pulmonary complications.

Alimentation
Oral intake is allowed when intestinal peristalsis returns, usually the third to fourth postoperative day. Free sodium intake should be minimized. Dietary protein is not restricted unless patients have signs of encephalopathy.

Antibiotic coverage
A first- or second-generation cephalosporin is usually administered for 24 to 48 hours after operation, especially if a prosthetic interposition graft has been implanted.

Reaccumulation of ascites
A common occurrence for several days after operation that should be monitored by daily weighing and abdominal girth measurements. Intravenous colloid solutions coupled with potassium-sparing diuretics (spironolactone, 25 mg three times daily) should be given to maintain a stable urinary output (30 to 50 ml/h).

Postoperative ultrasonography
Shunt patency should be evaluated with ultrasonography.

Postoperative complications

In the hospital

Gastrointestinal bleeding
Recurrence of bleeding after portal shunting can result from postoperative gastritis or peptic ulcer disease. However, variceal bleeding as a result of shunt occlusion must always be considered and angiographic evaluation of the shunt may be required.

Ascites
To a mild degree, a common complication in the early postoperative period. Persistent or massive ascites refractory to medical therapy may eventually require a peritoneovenous shunt. Chylous ascites may occur after distal splenorenal shunt placement because of disruption of intestinal lymphatics in the vicinity of the superior mesenteric vessels. A peritoneal tap is diagnostic in such cases, and treatment consists of cessation of oral intake and institution of parenteral hyperalimentation.

Hepatic encephalopathy
After total shunt procedures, the incidence of this complication ranges from 20% to 60%. The rate is significantly lower after distal splenorenal shunt placement because portal perfusion is maintained, particularly in patients without cirrhosis. Therapy consists of dietary protein restriction and the administration of drugs that alter colonic bacterial flora (lactulose, neomycin).

Hepatorenal failure
Serum bilirubin and liver enzyme levels are often mildly elevated during the first postoperative week but usually decline promptly to preoperative baseline levels if the hepatic reserve is adequate. Progressive deterioration of liver function coupled with hypovolemia secondary to dehydration, postoperative bleeding, or massive ascites can result in hepatorenal syndrome, which is associated with a high mortality once it is established.

Ascitic fluid leakage from the abdominal incision
If ascitic fluid leaks from the abdominal incision, the wound may need to be sutured again to prevent massive fluid losses and to reduce the risk of peritonitis.

After discharge

Shunt occlusion with recurrent variceal bleeding
Sclerotherapy or reoperation should be considered if shunt failure is confirmed by angiography.

Progressive hepatic failure
Progressive hepatic failure is the most common cause of late death in patients with cirrhosis who undergo shunt placement.

Ascites reaccumulation
Salt restriction and diuretic administration usually control ascites, but the possibility of shunt failure must be considered.

Chronic alcoholism
Continued alcoholism is generally associated with a poor prognosis for long-term survival.

FURTHER READING

Galloway, J. R. & Salam, A. A. Management of portal hypertension. In Geroulakos, G., Cherry, K. J. Jr., eds. *Diseases of the Visceral Circulation*. London, UK: Hodder Arnold, 2002.

Henderson, J. M., Kunter, M. H., Millikan, W. J. *et al.* Endoscopic variceal sclerosis compared with distal splenorenal shunt to prevent recurrent variceal bleeding in cirrhosis: a prospective randomized trial. *Ann. Intern. Med.* 1990; **112**: 262–269.

Jim, G. & Rikkers, L. F. Cause and management of upper gastrointestinal bleeding after distal splenorenal shunt. *Surgery* 1992; **112**: 719–727.

Richter, G. M., Noeldge, G., Palmaz, J. C. *et al.* Transjugular intrahepatic portacaval shunt: preliminary clinical results. *Radiology* 1990; **174**: 1027–1030.

Salam, A. A. Decompressive shunts for variceal hemorrhage. In Ernst, C. B. & Stanley, J. C., eds. *Current Therapy in Vascular Surgery*, 3rd edn. St. Louis, MO: Mosby, 1995.

Plastic and reconstructive surgery

82

Breast reconstruction after mastectomy

Alfredo A. Paredes, Jr. and T. Roderick Hester

Emory University School of Medicine, Atlanta, GA

Breast cancer continues to present an alarming health concern for women. As a treatment for breast cancer, mastectomy remains a common modality despite numerous advances in cancer therapy. Fortunately, breast reconstruction has become state-of-the-art plastic surgery, capable of restoring a woman's breast and sense of wholeness, while minimizing the negative psychological impact of mastectomy. Furthermore, "immediate" breast reconstruction – where reconstruction is performed directly following the mastectomy – has become a standard component of breast cancer treatment. Nowadays, after a mastectomy, women can expect a soft, natural-appearing, symmetric breast that will last a lifetime. Delayed reconstruction, performed months to years later, remains an excellent option for women who were not offered immediate reconstruction or simply were not ready for the adjunctive procedure.

Breast reconstruction can be divided into two types: autologous tissue reconstruction or implant-expander reconstruction.

Autologous tissue reconstruction

Various tissue donor sites on the female body can be used for reconstruction, including the backs, hips, gluteal area, and lateral thigh. However, skin and fat from the lower abdomen is the most common region used in what is known as TRAM (transverse rectus abdominis myocutaneous) flap reconstruction. Similar to a "tummy tuck" procedure, TRAM flap involves dissection of an elliptical pattern of skin and fat below the umbilicus that is transferred up to the breast defect on either a "pedicle" (still attached to the rectus muscle and superior epigastric artery) or as a "free" flap (where it is completely detached and then inset into the breast defect with a microvascular anastomosis of artery and vein using a microscope).

Preoperative preparation includes CBC, chemistry profile, PT/PTT, type and screen, pregnancy test, chest X-ray and, if indicated, an EKG. Blood transfusions are usually not needed, though the patient may donate blood preoperatively. The surgery usually lasts 2–4 hours; anesthesia is general, with epidural or PCA pump postoperation for pain control; and primary risk factors are obesity, hypertension, diabetes, history of radiation, and smoking.

Usual TRAM flap postoperative course

Expected postoperative hospital stay
3–5 days.

Operative mortality
Very rare (less than 1%).

Special monitoring required
Flap color and warmth are closely followed, especially in the first 24–48 hours. With free flaps, this may be hourly. Vital signs and Foley catheter are used to closely monitor fluid status.

Patient activity and positioning
Placed in "beach chair" position for several days postoperatively to reduce tension on abdominal wall closure. Encouraged to be out of bed 24 hours later and ambulating by second day. No heavy lifting or strenuous activity for 6 weeks.

Alimentation
Ice chips initially, then liquid diet if bowel sounds present on second postoperative day. Typically, regular diet by third or fourth day.

Medical Management of the Surgical Patient: A Textbook of Perioperative Medicine, ed. M. F. Lubin, R. B. Smith, T. F. Dobson, N. Spell, H. K. Walker. 4th edn. Published by Cambridge University Press. © Cambridge University 2006.

Antibiotic coverage

One dose preoperation, then continued while in-house and often for several days after discharge while drains are in place. Cephalexin or clindamycin are most commonly used and are intended to cover *Staphylococcus* and *Streptococcus* in the large areas of fascial dissection.

Drains

Placed on suction, usually left in place for 4–14 days (in breast, abdomen).

TRAM flap postoperative complications

In the hospital

Flap loss

Total flap loss is rare (less than 1%–2%), and partial flap loss only slightly higher. Careful flap monitoring may mitigate some of these losses.

Infection

Infrequent, typically a wound infection or urinary tract infection, less commonly a pulmonary source.

Hematoma

The large area of surgical dissection creates many potential pockets for hematomas. Drains are intended to prevent hematomas/seromas.

Pulmonary complications

The most serious complication is pulmonary embolus from deep vein thrombosis (less than 1%). Calf sequential compression boots and early ambulation are used as prophylaxis. Also, difficulty breathing early postoperation may be encountered due to tight fascial closures. Oxygen per nasal cannula is used in the first 24 hours, and incentive spirometry is encouraged. Pneumonia is possible but rare.

After discharge

Abdominal hernia

Infrequent (less than 10%), though the occurrence thereof often requires surgical correction. May be reduced with free flap or perforator flap techniques.

Additional surgery

2–3 months after the initial surgery, a patient may have revision of the reconstructed breast and nipple reconstruction, all in an outpatient setting. Tattoo for areolar recreation is then performed 2 months later.

Implant–expander reconstruction

Implant–expanders offer women a simpler technique for breast reconstruction with less recovery time than a TRAM flap; however, this method requires a permanent prosthesis placed within the tissues of the chest wall. In certain cases, particularly those of thin-skinned individuals or smokers, the latissimus muscle may be transferred from the back to provide additional coverage over the implant. An expander is typically placed in the mastectomy defect at the initial procedure, with an implant exchange months later. Preoperative preparation, anesthesia, blood transfusion issues, and primary risk factors are similar to that of TRAM flap.

Usual expander reconstruction postoperative course

Expected postoperative hospital stay
1–2 days.

Operative mortality
Rare and usually anesthesia related.

Special monitoring required
None.

Patient activity and positioning
No strenuous activity with the arms for 3–4 weeks.

Alimentation
Quickly advance diet the evening of surgery or next morning.

Antibiotic coverage
Prophylaxis with antibiotics (first generation cephalosporin) preoperation as well as for a few days afterwards.

Expander management
Beginning 1–2 weeks following operation, the expander is slowly inflated in the office over several weeks. In an outpatient procedure the expander is replaced with the final implant, either silicone gel or saline filled.

Drains
Placed on suction, usually left in place for 4–14 days (in breast, abdomen).

Expander reconstruction postoperative complications

In the hospital

Hematoma

Infrequent, but use of drains intended to prevent such collections.

After discharge

Implant complications

Implant extrusion through the mastectomy skin flaps, capsular contracture (which can create a hard, painful breast), breast asymmetry, and implant deflation can occur and may require reoperation.

FURTHER READING

Bostwick, J. *Plastic and Reconstructive Breast Surgery, Vol II.* St. Louis: Quality Medical Publishing, 2000.

Hartrampf, C. R., Anton, M. A., & Trimble Bried, J. Breast reconstruction with the transverse abdominal island (TRAM) flap. In Georgiade, G. S., Riefkohl, R., Levin, L. S., eds. *Plastic, Maxillofacial and Reconstructive Surgery*, 3rd edn. Baltimore: Williams & Wilkins, 1997.

Maxwell, P. G. & Hammond, D. C. Breast reconstruction following mastectomy and the surgical management of the patient with high risk breast disease. In Aston, S. J., Beasley, R. W., & Thorne, C. H. M. *Grabb and Smith's Plastic Surgery.* Philadelphia: Lippincott-Raven, 1997.

83

Facial rejuvenation

Steve Szczerba and T. Roderick Hester

Emory University School of Medicine, Atlanta, GA

Approaches to facial rejuvenation include non-surgical and surgical techniques. Non-surgical techniques such as dermabrasion, chemical peels, or laser skin resurfacing are often adjunctive to surgical procedures. Chemodenervation with botulinum A exotoxin (BOTOX) is another treatment modality for certain facial wrinkles or as an adjunct to operation. Injections are directed to areas of skin wrinkling caused by active muscle contraction such as frown lines and crow's feet. The paralytic effect of the injection has peak effect at 5–7 days and duration of 4–6 months with standard dosing.

Skin care regimens that focus on protection from sunlight, collagen stimulation with retinoid products, exfoliation and hydration are used preoperatively and postoperatively to enhance and prolong surgical rejuvenation procedures. Additional precautions include smoking cessation and strict avoidance of aspirin and non-steroidal anti-inflammatory agents for two weeks prior to the operation.

Surgical procedures for facial rejuvenation are typically performed on an outpatient basis. Postoperative monitoring can be done in a recovery suite, occasionally with an overnight stay in a hospital setting. General anesthesia provides reliable intraoperative patient comfort and allows quick postanesthetic recovery. For selected operations of short duration, local anesthesia with sedation is adequate; however, if multiple operations are planned during the same episode, general anesthesia is preferred.

The duration of the operation tends to vary with the number of procedures being performed: browlift surgery may take 30 minutes to 1 hour, surgery of the upper eyelid can be completed in approximately 30 minutes, and lower eyelid and cheek surgery as well as the standard facelift may each take 1–2 hours.

The traditional surgical approach to facial rejuvenation is the facelift, though advances in the understanding of facial aging have led plastic surgeons to view facial aging in terms of anatomical zones of the face.

Upper facial aging

Typical age-related changes of the upper third of the face consist of eyebrow descent and upper eyelid aging with skin redundancy and herniation of orbital fat.

Brow descent is addressed with a brow lifting procedure, with the endoscopic method involving three to five incisions behind the hairline being more prevalent than the open procedure. Dissection typically proceeds in a plane below the periosteum down to the orbital rim, after which the muscles that cause furrow lines in the mid-forehead between the eyebrows can be divided. The elevated scalp and forehead is then pulled back and fixed to the underlying bone with sutures or screws.

Upper eyelid aging is treated with upper eyelid blepharoplasty. After preoperatively evaluating for lid ptosis and other pathology, the operative correction of eyelid aging is performed through an elliptical incision in the upper eyelid. Bulging orbital fat is teased from beneath the underlying orbital septum and removed, and a predetermined amount of redundant skin and underlying muscle is resected and the skin and muscle are sewn closed. Correction of eyelid position secondary to ptosis can be addressed with an additional procedure.

Mid-facial aging

Aging changes of the mid-face area consists of laxity of both the lower eyelid orbital septum and overlying orbicularis muscle along with descent of the cheek. These changes are seen as descent of the eyelid to cheek junction, bulging of the lower eyelid tissues, wrinkling of the skin, and deepening of natural grooves in the midface area.

Medical Management of the Surgical Patient: A Textbook of Perioperative Medicine, ed. M. F. Lubin, R. B. Smith, T. F. Dobson, N. Spell, H. K. Walker. 4th edn. Published by Cambridge University Press. © Cambridge University 2006.

Several approaches to lower eyelid and cheek rejuvenation have been described. The authors' method starts with a skin incision just below the lateral lower eyelashes and extends out over the lateral orbital rim. The dissection proceeds directly through the muscle to the periosteum of lateral orbital rim, continuing with the aid of an endoscope deep along the facial skeleton into the cheek area. Once the entire cheek mass is mobilized, fixation of the cheek to an elevated position is performed with stitches between the cheek and the solid fascia just beyond the lateral orbital rim. In the fixation process, support for the lower eyelid is created with additional stitches to the lateral orbital rim. Excess skin and muscle are conservatively trimmed and the incision is closed.

Lower facial aging

Aging in the lower third of the face includes lateral facial wrinkles, jowls along the mandible, fat deposition in the neck and below the chin, and bands in the neck area from the platysma muscle.

The traditional facelift or rhytidectomy procedure treats age-related changes of the neck and lateral face. Rhytidectomy is performed through a preauricular incision that is continued under the earlobe and extends along the hairline of the mastoid area. Dissection of the soft tissues of the face and neck raises the areas that require correction. Plication sutures are often used to tighten the deeper fascial layers of the face. The elevated skin is then pulled in a lateral and superior vector, with the excess tissue then excised along the incisions.

Usual postoperative course

Expected postoperative hospital stay
Discharge can be the same day or the following one for the majority of patients undergoing facial rejuvenation surgery. Based on surgeon's preference or clinical indication, monitored postoperative recovery can be performed in a recovery suite or in a hospital. The patient typically returns for the first postoperative visit within 1 week. Another office visit is scheduled at approximately 2 weeks after surgery for screw, staple, or stitch removal.

Operative mortality
Under 1%.

Special monitoring required
None.

Patient activity and positioning
Head elevation, a facial pressure dressing, and icepacks to the eyes along with prophylactic treatment of nausea are crucial aspects of care for the immediate postoperative period. Many surgeons will place small drains under the facial flaps overnight to minimize blood collection under the skin. Strict avoidance of vigorous exercise for 2–3 weeks is emphasized to minimize swelling, hematoma formation, and bruising. Patients are prophylactically medicated for nausea as emesis may initiate postoperative bleeding.

Alimentation
Diet is routinely liquids with crackers for the first few hours after surgery to minimize nausea. A regular diet can be resumed the next day.

Antibiotic coverage
A preoperative dose followed by up to 5 days of postoperative broad spectrum antibiotics.

Postoperative complications

Hematoma
The significance of blood accumulation within previously dissected tissue varies considerably upon location. Retrobulbar hematoma after eyelid surgery is an extremely rare complication. Without emergent treatment consisting of release of the lateral canthus of the eye, visual loss can occur. Imbalances in the extraocular muscles secondary to edema or hematoma may lead to transient diploplia. Significant hematomas after a standard facelift procedure occur with a rate of approximately 4%. Prompt evacuation is recommended to avoid skin loss. Skin loss after facelift occurs in approximately 1%–3% of patients. Hematomas, thin skin flaps, and smoking contribute to skin loss risk.

Nerve injuries
After a browlift procedure, numbness or paresthesias in the forehead area occur in up to 30% of patients. Almost all are temporary and resolve completely within 4–6 weeks. Injuries to small sensory nerves are unavoidable and lead to transient numbness of the ear and cheek area for approximately 2 to 6 weeks. Injuries to the facial nerve during facelift surgery are a dreaded complication, but are extremely rare with a rate well under 1%.

Eyelid malposition

Complications of eyelid surgery center on lid malposition. Lagopthalmos (incomplete closure of the upper eyelid) may be associated with corneal exposure and its complications of drying, pain, or scarring. When lower eyelid blepharoplasty with or without cheeklift is performed, malposition of the lower lid is always a risk. Malposition of the lower lid ranges from mild scleral show to frank ectropion. Functional problems can range from swelling and irritation of the conjunctiva (chemosis) to complaints of corneal dryness.

Patient dissatisfaction

Crucial factors in patient satisfaction with rejuvenating procedure include proper selection of patients and full description of anticipated results along with identification of areas that will have little improvement.

FURTHER READING

Aston, S. J., Beasley, R. W., & Thorne, C. H. *Grab and Smith's Plastic Surgery*. Philadelphia: Lippincott-Raven, 1997: 633–648.

Barton, F. E. The aging face: rhytidectomy and adjunctive procedures. *Select Read Plast. Surg.* 2001; **9**: 19.

Hester, T. R. Jr., Codner, M. A., McCord, C. D. *et al.* Evolution of technique of the direct transblepharoplasty approach for the correction of lower lid and midfacial aging: maximizing results and minimizing complications in a 5-year experience. *Plast. Reconstr. Surg.* 2000; **105**: 393.

84

Liposuction

Ashley D. Gordon and T. Roderick Hester, Jr.

Emory University School of Medicine, Atlanta, GA

Liposuction or suction assisted lipectomy (SAL) is used to recontour specific areas of the face and body by removing unwanted deposits of fat, though it is not considered an alternative to weight loss. It is best performed on localized areas that do not respond well to diet and exercise. The ideal liposuction patient is healthy, exercises, eats a well-balanced diet, has good skin elasticity, desires treatment of minimal-to-moderate localized fat deposits, and is within 20%–30% of ideal body weight. A preoperative CBC is important when performing "mega" liposuctions in which a large blood volume may be lost. Clotting studies, electrolytes, urinalysis, EKG, and radiographs may also be indicated by patient age and medical history. A set of standard photographs should be taken prior to the procedure which can serve as an intraoperative guide and enable comparison of preoperative and postoperative results.

The procedure involves making small stab incisions with insertion of a cannula into the deep fat layer. Using the tumescent technique, the targeted area is first infused with a saline solution containing lidocaine and epinephrine. The cannula is then attached to a vacuum device that suctions out the targeted fat. This suctioning is repeated in a "to and fro pattern" through the layer, creating a radial pattern. Ultrasound-assisted liposuction (UAL) is similar in technique to SAL, except that it uses ultrasonic energy to fractionate or burst the fat cells. The fat is then removed with relatively low-volume suction, resulting in less trauma to the tissues, though the incisions are larger than those made for SAL. The incisions are closed with absorbable sutures, after which sterile dressings are applied. A fitted compression garment is placed over the treated areas. Operative time is usually 1–3 hours, depending on the amount of tissue to be removed. The surgery may be performed under local, epidural, or general anesthesia.

Usual postoperative course

Expected postoperative hospital stay
Most procedures are performed on an outpatient basis. Extremely large volume suctions (more than 6 liters) may require an overnight stay.

Operative mortality
Under 0.5%. Pulmonary embolism is the most common cause of death in these patients.

Special monitoring required
None.

Patient activity and positioning
Compression garments, which reduce swelling and bleeding, are worn over the treated area continuously for 2–6 weeks. Liquefied fat, injection fluid, and small amounts of blood may leak from the incision sites for about 24 hours and should be dressed appropriately. Patients may return to physical activities within a few days as their comfort allows. Full recovery from bruising and swelling may take up to 3 months.

Alimentation
Oral alimentation is provided immediately after operation.

Antibiotic coverage
Perioperative antibiotic coverage is usually provided with a single agent.

Medical Management of the Surgical Patient: A Textbook of Perioperative Medicine, ed. M. F. Lubin, R. B. Smith, T. F. Dobson, N. Spell, H. K. Walker. 4th edn. Published by Cambridge University Press. © Cambridge University 2006.

Postoperative complications

In the hospital

Volume depletion

May result from large volume suctions. These patients should be admitted for overnight monitoring and fluid replacement.

Pulmonary/fat embolus

Rarely occurs. If possible, patients are routinely placed in intermittent pneumatic compression garments before surgery. These should be continued until the subject is ambulating freely.

After discharge

Swelling and bruising

Temporary bruising, swelling, and/or soreness are expected and will resolve over time.

Hematomas/seromas

Compressive dressings minimize hematoma formation. Large hematomas or seromas may require evacuation with a large bore needle.

Wound infection

Early recognition and oral antibiotics are usually sufficient for treatment, although a very low incidence of necrotizing fasciitis has been reported.

Loss of sensation/paresthesias

May occur and usually resolves in a few months.

Cosmetic sequelae

The most common long term complication is contour irregularity. Rippling or bagginess of the skin may also occur. Skin color changes and skin necrosis are rare, but may occur with aggressive superficial UAL.

FURTHER READING

Klein, J. A. The tumescent technique. Anesthesia and modified liposuction technique. *Dermatol. Clin.* 1990; **8**(3): 425–437.

Pitanguy, I. Evaluation of body contouring surgery today: a 30-year perspective. *Plast. Reconstr. Surg.* 2000; **105**(4): 1499–1514; discussion 1515–1516.

Pitman, G. H. & Teimourian, B. Suction lipectomy: complications and results by survey. *Plast. Reconstr. Surg.* 1985; **76**(1): 65–72.

Teimourian, B. & Adham, M. N. A national survey of complications associated with suction lipectomy: what we did then and what we do now. *Plast. Reconstr. Surg.* 2000; **105**(5): 1881–1884.

85

Repair of facial fractures

Hisham Seify and T. Roderick Hester

Emory University School of Medicine, Atlanta, GA

The increased incidence of patients with facial fractures relates to the frequency of motor vehicle accidents. Management of these patients requires a team approach, as they usually present with multiple injuries. Proper treatment includes resuscitation, early care, and late reconstruction. Emergency management involves airway control, control of bleeding, and identification of occult injuries. As soon as the patient is stabilized, early care begins with a clinical examination that focuses on occlusion of the mandible, evaluation of sensory and motor nerves, assessment of the muscles of extra-ocular movement, and the identification of open fractures such as those involving the mandible. Next, radiographic imaging of the face is ordered to determine exact fracture patterns. Imaging studies may include CT scans, plain films, and specialized views such as Panorex films of the mandible; however, a CT scan with fine cuts of the face and mandible is the preferred modality.

Soft tissue injuries in the form of contusions, lacerations, and avulsions are identified and treated primarily. Treatment plans for the craniofacial skeleton are tailored to specific fracture patterns. Repair of facial fractures is indicated to restore both appearance and function, particularly in mandible and orbital floor fractures where such qualities are greatly at risk. The general principle of accurate reduction and proper fixation applies to facial injuries as well. Facial fractures are approached through a variety of incisions. Reduction is evaluated with mandible occlusion and direct visualization of bone segments. Fixation is performed with wires, plates, and screws and intermaxillary fixation. Recent advances in plating materials allows fixation of selected patients to be performed with absorbable material.

Specific fracture patterns

Facial fractures are classified as closed or open, as well as by anatomic region. Anatomic areas include the following.

Upper face

(frontal bone, frontal sinus, orbital fractures). It should be noted that fractures around the orbit require identification of globe or optic nerve injury as well as extraocular muscle entrapment. Frontal sinus fracture may involve the intracranial structures and could require a combined approach with the neurosurgery team.

Mid face

(maxillary and zygomaticus bone fractures). These injuries usually result in abnormal shape or malocclusion.

Mandibular fractures

Mostly affecting the angle of the mandible and condyle in children. Identification of abnormal occlusion is paramount.

Usual postoperative course

Expected postoperative hospital stay

2 to 5 days.

Operative mortality

Related to extent of the injuries, age, and comorbidities.

Patient activity and positioning

Elevation of the head of the bed is important to reduce facial swelling. Patient is encouraged to get out of bed on the first postoperative day.

Alimentation

Patients with mandibular fractures require pureed diet and liquids. Most other patients are comfortable with soft diets. Intermaxillary fixation requires instructing the patient to use a straw for alimentation.

Medical Management of the Surgical Patient: A Textbook of Perioperative Medicine, ed. M. F. Lubin, R. B. Smith, T. F. Dobson, N. Spell, H. K. Walker. 4th edn. Published by Cambridge University Press. © Cambridge University 2006.

Antiboiotic coverage

Prophylactic antibiotic coverage for both gram-positive and gram-negative organisms is provided for the first few days.

Postoperative complications

In the hospital

Aspiration

If intermaxillary fixation is used, aspiration could occur following vomiting. Suction should be readily available to patients throughout the hospital stay. Wire cutters should also be placed at bedside for rapid release of the wires in order to prevent aspiration.

Facial swelling

Swelling is generally maximal between 24 and 48 hours after surgery and resolves over 1 to 2 weeks.

Blindness

A retrobulbar hematoma is an extremely rare event following orbital fracture fixation, though it requires emergency treatment upon occurrence.

After discharge

Cosmetic sequela

Malocclusion, facial scarring, and residual asymmetry and disfigurement are unusual. Ectropion could be present early and should be managed conservatively for the first few weeks.

FURTHER READING

Manson, P. Facial injuries. In McCarthy, J. G., ed. *Plastic Surgery.* Philadelphia, PA: W. B. Saunders, 1990; vol. 2: 979–991.

Manson, P., Clark, N., Robertson, B., Crawley, W. A comprehensive management of pan facial fractures. *Craniofac. Trauma* 1995; **1**: 43–56.

86

Flap coverage for pressure sores

Dustin L. Reid and T. Roderick Hester

Emory University School of Medicine, Atlanta, GA

"Pressure sore" is the term used to describe ischemic tissue loss resulting from pressure, usually over a bony prominence. With an incidence of 1.5 to 3.0 million new cases in the USA annually, the condition is a common problem. Pressure sores typically arise in paralyzed or otherwise debilitated patients, usually occurring in the lower part of the body; the sacrum, heel, trochanters, and ischium are the most frequent sites. Since the etiology of these lesions is always unrelieved pressure, prevention remains the cornerstone of any management plan and includes minimizing stress over these prominences and meticulous skin care. The majority of pressure sores will heal, with non-operative wound management consisting of infection control, dead tissue debridement, pressure avoidance, and dressing changes. However, those instances involving significant tissue loss in which the sores will not readily close on their own do require surgical closure. Reconstruction should be performed only in patients who can avoid placing pressure on the affected areas in the future; otherwise, the problem will quickly recur. Thus, only a select few patients with pressure sores are appropriate candidates for operative reconstruction.

Prior to repair, pressure sores must be clean and free of infection. This may require hospital admission well in advance of operation for aggressive wound care. Other issues which must be addressed preoperatively include: optimization of nutrition status, with tube feeding or hyperalimentation if necessary; correction of anemia; alleviation of contributing spasm; and release of contractures. Once these issues are resolved, operation can be safely performed. Even in those with complete spinal injury, general anesthesia is always used to prevent reflex sympathetic response. Surgical management consists of complete excision of the ulcer and closure of the wound, often with local muscle or soft tissue flaps. Suction drains are usually placed below the flap to remove excess fluid.

Most procedures last 1 to 3 hours, and blood transfusion is usually avoided with careful hemostasis.

Usual postoperative course

Expected postoperative hospital stay
14 to 28 days.

Operative mortality
Less than 5%. The rare deaths that do occur are usually related to the poor general condition of the patient rather than the magnitude of the operation.

Special monitoring required
None.

Patient activity and positioning
The patient is moved directly from the operating table to an air-fluidized bed. The air-fluidized bed is used for a total of 3 weeks without allowing any pressure on the flap. Patients are then permitted to spend brief periods with pressure on the flap (15 minutes every 2 hours) for the next 2 months with the goal of returning slowly to the activities of daily living.

Alimentation
Diet may be restricted to liquids for several days.

Hygiene
Preoperative enemas and 3–4 days of postoperative narcotics can be used to prevent fecal soiling of the flap.

Drains
Closed suction drainage is maintained for 7–10 days.

Medical Management of the Surgical Patient: A Textbook of Perioperative Medicine, ed. M. F. Lubin, R. B. Smith, T. F. Dobson, N. Spell, H. K. Walker. 4th edn. Published by Cambridge University Press. © Cambridge University 2006.

Antibiotic coverage

The authors suggest culture-specific antibiotic coverage perioperatively, especially if there is underlying osteomyelitis.

Postoperative complications

In the hospital

Hematoma

This is the most common complication and its presence predisposes to the other complications. When recognized in the postoperative period, all hematomas should be immediately evacuated. Delayed closure may be necessitated.

Seroma

Closed suction drainage must be maintained for at least 7–10 days.

Wound infection

Wound infection occurs in 10%–20% of patients. Prompt diagnosis depends on the recognition of erythema, persistent spiking fevers, or purulent drainage from the wound. Early surgical drainage and broad spectrum antibiotics should be initiated to prevent systemic effects.

Flap loss or dehiscence

Partial flap loss or dehiscence is seen in 10%–20% of patients. This usually requires early debridement and further flap coverage or, more often, healing by secondary intention.

After discharge

Recurrence

Despite advances in surgical reconstruction, recurrence remains extremely high with an incidence of up to 70%. The reasons for recurrence are the same as those for the initial ulceration. Therefore, patient education is probably the most important element in the long-term management of these patients.

FURTHER READING

Colen, S. R. Pressure sores. In McCarthy, J. G., ed. *Plastic Surgery*, Vol 6. Philadelphia: W. B. Saunders, 1990: 3797–3837.

Meehan, M. Multisite pressure ulcer prevalence survey. *Adv. Wound Care* 1994; **7**: 27.

87

Muscle flap coverage of sternal wound infections

Joshua A. Greenwald and T. Roderick Hester, Jr.

Emory University School of Medicine, Atlanta, GA

The median sternotomy is the incision of choice for most patients undergoing coronary artery bypass grafting and heart valve surgery, as it provides unparalleled exposure of the heart and great vessels. Although sternal wound infections occur with a reported incidence of 5%, the associated morbidity and mortality is dramatically higher. In the early 1970s, treatment of these patients consisted largely of debridement, placement of catheters for antibiotic irrigation, and either primary or delayed primary closure of the rewired sternum. If the wound couldn't be closed, they were packed open and allowed to heal secondarily. Such management was associated with a mortality rate of 20%–50%, leading reconstructive and cardiothoracic surgeons to seek alternative treatment options. Fortunately, most institutions have abandoned these techniques with the advent of muscle flap surgery.

Wide debridement of all devitalized bone and soft tissues, removal of all foreign material (i.e., sternal wires) followed by immediate closure using various muscle and/or omental flaps is now widely performed and considered the standard of care for sternal wound infections. Typically, the overlying soft tissues are reapproximated following muscle flap transposition. When an omental flap is used for coverage, it is covered with a skin graft. The pectoralis major, rectus abdominus, and latissimus dorsi muscles are the structures of choice for mediastinal coverage and deadspace obliteration, with the patient's anatomy, wound status, and previous surgeries serving as the reconstructive surgeon's guide to proper flap selection. While initial debridement and delayed flap closure used to be routine, debridement and immediate reconstruction is now performed in the overwhelming majority of patients. Delayed muscle flap closure is typically reserved for the patient with complete sternal disruption and suppurative mediastinitis. Much of the

pioneering work in the treatment of this dreaded complication of cardiothoracic surgery has been performed by the Department of Plastic and Reconstructive Surgery at Emory University. The guidelines presented herein are taken from a 20-year experience of treating median sternotomy wounds at Emory University affiliated hospitals.

Usual postoperative course

Expected postoperative hospital stay

With one-stage debridement and closure, typically 10–14 days.

Operative mortality

Overall mortality in the Emory series of 409 patients was 8.1%.

Special monitoring required

Dependent on the clinical status of the patient. For the patient with frank sepsis, invasive hemodynamic monitoring and endotracheal intubation are often required preoperatively. For the patient with a draining sinus tract and no evidence of sepsis, large bore intravenous access may suffice.

Patient activity and positioning

Postoperatively, patients are mobilized as tolerated. If pectoralis major muscle flaps have been transposed, there are typically three large suction drains in place (one under each pectoralis muscle and one in the midline). These are maintained on low wall suction for at least 24 hours to evacuate fluid and obliterate dead space. Women with large breasts must have their breasts supported in order to avoid tension on the midline wound.

Medical Management of the Surgical Patient: A Textbook of Perioperative Medicine, ed. M. F. Lubin, R. B. Smith, T. F. Dobson, N. Spell, H. K. Walker. 4th edn. Published by Cambridge University Press. © Cambridge University 2006.

Alimentation

Diet is advanced as tolerated. Frequently, nutritional supplementation is needed in critically ill patients. If the abdominal cavity has been violated to harvest an omental flap, a nasogastric tube is left in place for 4–5 days until bowel function has returned.

Antibiotic coverage

Broad spectrum antibiotic coverage is initiated preoperatively in all patients. For patients with sternal osteomyelitis, antibiotic treatment is narrowed and continued for 6 weeks based on sternal bone cultures obtained intraoperatively. For patients without sternal osteomyelitis, a shorter course of antibiotics can be used with coverage based on intraoperative cultures.

Postoperative complications

In the hospital

Hematomas

7.8% of patients required re-exploration for evacuation of hematomas. Meticulous operative technique is needed to avoid this complication, as is the judicious use of blood products to correct coagulopathy and platelet abnormalities secondary to sepsis and/or medications (i.e. Coumadin® or warfarin and aspirin).

Wound problems

Wound dehiscence occurred in 6.1% of patients. If superficial, healing by secondary intention is usually obtained. More rapid healing of small areas of dehiscence may be achieved with the use of suction dressings.

Flap loss

Partial flap loss was reported in 3.8% of patients.

Prolonged ICU stay

A prolonged stay in the ICU can usually be determined by the patient's preoperative condition and is not directly attributable to the operative procedure.

After discharge

Hernias

Abdominal hernias developed in 2.8% of patients most frequently after rectus abdominus transposition and omental flap utilization.

Recurrent sternal infection

5.6% of patients required re-exploration for recurrent sternal wound infections.

FURTHER READING

Bryant, L. R., Spencer, F. C., & Trinkle, J. K. Treatment of median sternotomy infection by mediastinal irrigation with an antibiotic solution. *Ann. Surg.* 1969; **169**: 914.

Grossi, E. A., Culliford, A. T., Krieger, K. H. *et al.* A survey of 77 major infectious complications of median sternotomy: a review of 7,949 consecutive operative procedures. *Ann. Thorac. Surg.* 1985; **40**: 214.

Jones, G., Jurkiewicz, M. J., Bostwick, J. *et al.* Management of the infected median sternotomy wound with muscle flaps. The Emory 20-year experience. *Ann. Surg.* 1997; **225**: 766.

Jurkiewicz, M. J., Bostwick, J., 3rd, Hester, T. R., Bishop, J. B. & Craver, J. Infected median sternotomy wound. Successful treatment by muscle flaps. *Ann. Surg.* 1980; **191**: 738.

Nahai, F., Rand, R. P., Hester, T. R., Bostwick, J. 3rd, & Jurkiewicz, M. J. Primary treatment of the infected sternotomy wound with muscle flaps: a review of 211 consecutive cases. *Plast. Reconstr. Surg.* 1989; **84**: 434.

Sarr, M. G., Gott, V. L., & Townsend, T. R. Mediastinal infection after cardiac surgery. *Ann. Thorac. Surg.* 1984; **38**: 415.

88

Skin grafting for burns

Gary A. Tuma and T. Roderick Hester

Emory University School of Medicine, Atlanta, GA

The essential nature of a burn is the thermal, and or, chemical destruction of skin and underlying tissue. Skin grafting is always necessary for treating full thickness (third-degree) burns, but is only occasionally required for partial-thickness (second-degree) burns and rarely needed to repair superficial (first-degree) burns. In addition, the procedure is used to mitigate the functional and aesthetic damage caused by some burns.

Burn treatment consists of debridement of devitalized tissue followed by skin grafting. This should occur as soon as possible, depending on the stability of the patient. Attempts to preserve as much tissue as possible are initiated by tangential excision of the burn. Theoretically, the skin graft can be of varying thickness, but usually is of the split thickness type. It can be applied as sheet grafts or meshed grafts to increase surface area. All attempts are made to minimize the meshed ratio to improve cosmesis. If larger ratio meshing is needed for coverage because of a lack of donor availability, it is common to use a combination of autologous skin and cadaveric skin. The cadaveric skin is placed over the meshed skin, creating a closed wound that allows the meshed skin to heal underneath the cadaveric skin. After 3 weeks, the cadaveric skin undergoes necrosis and sloughs, leaving the healed autologous skin intact. The location of the burn and the total body surface area involved determine both the thickness and the location of the donor site. If the burn encompasses more than 60% of the total body surface, a small piece of skin is harvested and sheets of cultured epithelial cells are grown for coverage. These operations can be long in duration and can include such complications as excessive blood loss, fluid shifts, infection, and difficulty with body temperature control. Major skin grafts are most commonly performed under general anesthesia.

Usual postoperative course

Expected postoperative hospital stay

As a rule, one can expect the patient to stay in the hospital 1 day for each percent of total body surface area burned; therefore, a patient with 10% total body surface area involvement can expect at least 10 days in the hospital. This number varies with increasing age and comorbidities.

Operative mortality

Increases with percentage total body surface area injured. In addition, as age increases so does the morbidity and mortality.

Patient activity and positioning

The patient is limited in physical activity for at least the first 5–7 days, which helps reduce the loss of grafts secondary to shearing forces or infection. Once the graft has taken, physical therapy is initiated to start range-of-motion exercises. Initially, the most important aspect is to prevent the graft from being in a dependant position. Most commonly, the patient remains in the intensive care unit for some period of time.

Alimentation

Nutrition is the key to healing, which is why resumption of enteral feeding occurs as soon as possible.

Antibiotic coverage

Oral or intravenous antibiotics are given preoperatively. The most important coverage is gram-positive unless the patient has other immunocompromising states, requiring broader spectrum coverage.

Medical Management of the Surgical Patient: A Textbook of Perioperative Medicine, ed. M. F. Lubin, R. B. Smith, T. F. Dobson, N. Spell, H. K. Walker. 4th edn. Published by Cambridge University Press. © Cambridge University 2006.

Postoperative complications

In the hospital

Volume depletion

Fluid resuscitation is the most important goal initially as well as postoperatively. Once the skin is injured, it loses the ability to regulate fluid loss and temperature control. Urine output is the most reliable indicator of fluid resuscitation and serves as a guide in fluid management.

Graft site hematoma

The most common immediate cause of skin graft loss. Using a bolster dressing and/or meshing the skin graft minimizes the formation of hematoma.

Loss of graft

Since the three most common causes of graft loss are hematoma, infection, and motion, every attempt must be made to diminish the occurrence of these events. If the graft fails, such local treatment as keeping the wound clean and applying Silvadene® will generally suffice. Occasionally repeat grafting may be required.

After discharge

Scarring

Hypertrophic scarring can produce an unfavorable outcome. In addition, scar contracture can develop over time.

Silicone sheeting and compression garments attempt to lessen these complications. Once the grafts are healed, it is vital for physical therapy to begin range of motion exercises as soon as possible. There is also an increased risk of developing Marjolin's ulcer, which is a squamous cell carcinoma on the skin graft. This may occur years later, typically in areas of repeated trauma.

FURTHER READING

Hunt, J. L., Purdue, G. F., Pownell, P. H., & Rohrich, R. J. Acute burns, burn surgery and postburn reconstruction. In *Selected Readings in Plastic Surgery*. Vol. 8, 1997: 1–37.

Mlcak, R. Pre-hospital care and emergency management of burn victims. In Wolf, S. E. & Herndon, D. N., eds. *Handbook of Burn Care*. Georgetown, TX: Landes, 1999.

Robson, M. C. & Smith, D. J. Care of the thermal injured victim. In Jurkiewicz, M. J., Krizek, T. J., Mathes, S. J., & Ariyan, S., eds. *Plastic Surgery: Principles and Practice*. St. Louis: C. V. Mosby, 1990: 1355–1410.

Townsend, C. M. Jr., Beauchamp, R. D., Evers, B. M., & Mattox, K. L., eds. *Sabiston Textbook of Surgery*, 16th edn., Philadelphia, PA: W. B. Saunders, 2001: 355–356.

Gynecologic surgery

89

Abdominal hysterectomy

Hugh W. Randall

Emory University School of Medicine, Atlanta, GA

Hysterectomy is the most common gynecologic operation and the second most common major surgical procedure in the USA. The frequency of abdominal hysterectomy is 1 per 1000 in women younger than 25 years, but rises to 16 per 1000 in women older than 35 years. After the age of 35 years, women usually have completed their childbearing and also have a higher incidence of significant gynecologic disease. The mortality risk for hysterectomy in the USA has been studied by the Centers for Disease Control and Prevention, which reported 477 deaths among 317 389 women having abdominal hysterectomies from 1979 through 1980. The mortality rate for hysterectomy was higher for procedures associated with pregnancy and cancer than for procedures not associated with these conditions (29.2, 37.8, and 6.0 per 10 000 hysterectomies, respectively). Abdominal hysterectomy had a higher mortality rate than did vaginal hysterectomy. Excluding cases related to pregnancy or cancer, the mortality rate was 8.6 per 10 000 women for abdominal hysterectomy and 2.7 per 10 000 women for vaginal hysterectomy.

Simple total abdominal hysterectomy involves the removal of the uterine corpus and cervix through an abdominal incision and is performed for a variety of indications, including uterine leiomyomas, pelvic abscesses, endometriosis, and recurrent dysfunctional uterine bleeding. In addition, simple abdominal hysterectomy is performed for two malignant indications: adenocarcinoma of the endometrium and ovarian cancer. Invasive cancer of the cervix requires a radical abdominal hysterectomy. Transfusion for simple abdominal hysterectomy is rare and the operative time is 1/2 to 2 hours. General anesthesia is usually chosen, although spinal anesthesia can be used.

Usual postoperative course

Expected postoperative hospital stay
3 to 4 days.

Operative mortality
Under 1%.

Special monitoring required
No special monitoring is necessary.

Patient activity and positioning
Patients are out of bed the day of operation and ambulatory by the next day.

Alimentation
Clear liquids are permitted on the first postoperative day, with food intake progressing to a regular diet as the patient demonstrates good bowel sounds, toleration of solid food, and no distention.

Antibiotic coverage
Preoperative intravenous antibiotics aimed at polymicrobial contamination – covering most gram-negative rods, anaerobes, and gram-positive cocci – are administered. The use of prophylactic antibiotics has been shown to significantly reduce postoperative infectious morbidity and decrease the length of hospitalization in women undergoing abdominal hysterectomy.

Catheterization
Indwelling Foley catheter drainage is rarely required. Urinary retention is seen in 10% to 15% of patients but can be managed by intermittent self-catheterization.

Medical Management of the Surgical Patient: A Textbook of Perioperative Medicine, ed. M. F. Lubin, R. B. Smith, T. F. Dobson, N. Spell, H. K. Walker. 4th edn. Published by Cambridge University Press. © Cambridge University 2006.

Vaginal packing

Vaginal packing is not required.

Postoperative complications

In the hospital

Excessive vaginal bleeding

Postoperative vaginal bleeding predominantly occurs from three areas: the infundibulopelvic ligament when an oophorectomy has been performed, the uterine artery pedicle, and the uterosacral ligament pedicle. Vaginal cuff bleeding after abdominal hysterectomy is rare. A pelvic examination should be performed in the operating room and the vaginal cuff sutures removed. The structures of the broad ligament, the uterine artery pedicle, and the utero-sacral ligament pedicle can be exposed with long Allis clamps applied to the round ligament and to the uterosac-ral ligament. Bleeding can often be secured vaginally by re-exploration through the vaginal cuff incision, but those less experienced with vaginal surgery may need to reopen the abdominal incision. If bleeding occurs from the ovar-ian artery and vein located in the infundibulopelvic liga-ment, the vaginal approach is rarely successful and repeat laparotomy is required. The integrity of the ureters is always of concern after bleeding from the pedicles of the uterus is controlled. Indigo carmine dye should be injected intravenously and cystoscopy performed to ensure that the ureters are not obstructed.

Intraperitoneal bleeding is associated with tachycardia, low urinary output, and low blood pressure. There can be significant loss of blood into the peritoneal cavity before the abdomen becomes significantly distended.

Thromboembolic phenomena

Deep venous thrombosis may be manifested by an unex-plained fever and tachycardia. Some patients report swel-ling and pain in the legs; others do not. Duplex ultrasound evaluation assists in making the diagnosis, but equivocal results may require venography. The heparin challenge test, which consists of anticoagulation with heparin for 48 hours, produces a significant drop in fever and tachy-cardia if venous thrombosis is the correct diagnosis.

Dehiscence with or without evisceration

Patients displaying dehiscence, evidenced by the drainage of serosanguineous fluid through the abdominal incision, should be returned to surgery so that the rectus fascia can be resutured with a mass closure technique using a No. 1 synthetic absorbable suture; a running delayed synthetic absorbable suture has greater strength than the Smead–Jones suture formerly advocated for this problem. Dehiscence with evisceration should be managed first by wrapping the intestine in a sterile, moist towel. Once the patient is in the operating room, the incision is reopened, the intestine replaced in the abdominal cavity, and the wound resutured.

After discharge

Intestinal obstruction

The location of intestinal obstruction in patients who have undergone gynecologic surgery is almost exclusively in the terminal ileum near the ileocecal junction. Obstruction results predominantly from adhesions to a loop of bowel or from the terminal ileum entering an internal hernia and becoming incarcerated. Therapy with long-tube suction decompression can be efficacious. If this method fails, however, the patient should be taken to the operating room and reexplored for relief of the intestinal obstruction.

Acknowledgment

This chapter is based on material from: Abdominal hyster-ectomy by Clifford R. Wheeless, Jr., which appeared in the 3rd edition of *Medical Management of the Surgical Patient*.

FURTHER READING

Antibiotic prophylaxis for gynecologic procedures. *ACOG Practice Bulletin*, No. 23, January 2001. Washington, DC: American College of Obstetricians and Gynecologists.

Farquhar, C. M. & Steiner, C. A. Hysterectomy rates in the United States, 1990–1997. *Obstet. Gynecol.* 2002; **99**: 229–234.

Jones, H. W. III. Hysterectomy. In Rock, J. A. & Jones, H. W. III, eds. *Te Linde's Operative Gynecology*. 9th edn. Philadelphia, PA: Lippincott, Williams & Wilkins; 2003: 799–828.

Kelly, H. A. Ligature of the trunks of the uterine and ovarian arteries as a means of checking hemorrhage from the uterus and broad ligaments in abdominal operations. *Johns Hopkins Hosp. Rep.* 1891; **2**: 220–223.

Lee, R. A. Abdominal hysterectomy (simple). In Breen, J. L. & Osofsky, H. J., eds. *Current Concepts in Gynecologic Surgery*. Baltimore, MD: Williams & Wilkins; 1987: 151.

Lepine, L. A., Hillis, S. D., Marchbanks, P. A. *et al.* Hysterectomy surveillance – United States, 1980–1993. *Morb. Mortal. Wkly. Rep.* 1997; **46** (No. SS-4): 1–15.

Wingo, P. A., Huezo, C. M., Rubin, G. L. *et al.* The mortality risk associated with hysterectomy. *Am. J. Obstet. Gynecol.* 1985; **152**: 803–808.

90

Vaginal hysterectomy

Hugh W. Randall

Emory University School of Medicine, Atlanta, GA

Nearly 600 000 women undergo hysterectomy each year in the USA, and more than one-fourth of US women will have a hysterectomy – the second most frequent surgical procedure among reproductive-aged women – by the time they are 60 years old. The average annual rate of hysterectomy per 1000 women aged 15 years and older declined from 7.1 in 1980 to 6.6 in 1987, then holding at 5.5 from 1988 to 1993; the decline from 1987 to 1988 resulted from changes in the data collection used to define the survey. Conditions most often associated with hysterectomy are uterine leiomyomata, endometriosis, and pelvic organ prolapse.

The comprehensive study on hysterectomy published by Wingo and associates from the Centers for Disease Control and Prevention reported that there were 46 deaths among 119 972 women undergoing vaginal hysterectomy. The vaginal approach to hysterectomy was associated with a much lower mortality rate than the abdominal approach. Excluding pregnancy and cancer-related cases, the mortality rate for abdominal hysterectomy was 8.6 per 10 000 women while that for vaginal hysterectomy was 2.7 per 10 000 women. Therefore, hysterectomy should be considered a low-risk operation that can be performed to treat non-pregnant patients and those with benign gynecologic symptoms or disease. Vaginal hysterectomy can be used for many indications, including pelvic relaxation, cervical intraepithelial neoplasias, small leiomyoma, and recurrent dysfunctional uterine bleeding.

The success of a vaginal hysterectomy is directly related to the particular surgeon's experience. If their operative familiarity is insufficient to allow proper and safe performance of the vaginal method, surgeons shouldn't hesitate to open the abdomen and complete the hysterectomy through the abdominal route or to choose abdominal hysterectomy initially. The procedure generally takes 1 hour to perform and transfusion is rarely required. While spinal or epidural anesthesia is acceptable, general anesthesia is usually used.

Usual postoperative course

Expected postoperative hospital stay
The hospital stay varies from 2 to 3 days, depending on the age and associated medical problems of the patient.

Operative mortality
Under 1%.

Special monitoring required
Unnecessary.

Patient activity and positioning
Patients are ambulatory on the day of operation.

Alimentation
Postoperative food intake is permitted as desired.

Antibiotic coverage
Intravenous antibiotics should be administered immediately prior to induction of anesthesia and are directed at polymicrobial contamination covering gram-negative rods, anaerobes, and gram-positive cocci.

Catheterization
Patients who undergo anterior repair of the bladder should have an indwelling Foley catheter or suprapubic catheter for several days after surgery. Persistent urinary retention occurs in 10% to 15% of patients, but usually responds well to intermittent self-catheterization. Urinary retention should be resolved before the catheter is discontinued.

Medical Management of the Surgical Patient: A Textbook of Perioperative Medicine, ed. M. F. Lubin, R. B. Smith, T. F. Dobson, N. Spell, H. K. Walker. 4th edn. Published by Cambridge University Press. © Cambridge University 2006.

Vaginal packing
Not required.

Postoperative complications

In the hospital

Excessive vaginal bleeding
A uterine artery pedicle or uterosacral pedicle that has retracted outside the suture ligature, which can be very serious, are the most common sources of extreme bleeding, followed by bleeding from the posterior vaginal cuff between the uterosacral ligaments. A pelvic examination should be performed in the operating room and the vaginal cuff sutures removed. The structures of the broad ligament, the uterine artery pedicle, and the uterosacral pedicle can then be exposed with long Allis clamps applied to the round ligament and to the uterosacral ligament. Bleeding can often be controlled by suture ligature. For surgeons who are less experienced with vaginal surgery, a laparotomy may be required for secure control of bleeding. After bleeding from the uterine artery pedicle is controlled, cystoscopy should be performed with the intravenous injection of indigo carmine solution to ensure the integrity of the ureters. Bleeding from the posterior vaginal cuff is usually controlled with vaginal packing and hemostatic agents.

Intraperitoneal bleeding
Tachycardia, low urine output, and low blood pressure are encountered whenever either of the two vascular pedicles described earlier hemorrhages into the peritoneal cavity. Since the peritoneal cavity can contain several liters of blood before the abdomen appears to be distended, such bleeding is especially dangerous. If intraperitoneal bleeding is suspected, the patient should be returned to the operating room for exploratory laparotomy and bleeding control. Blood transfusions may be required.

Vaginal cuff abscess
If the vaginal cuff has been left open and its margin has been sutured, the development of a vaginal cuff abscess is rare. Most cases are seen in premenopausal women whose vaginal cuffs have been closed. If a vaginal abscess does occur, it should be drained and broad spectrum antibiotics administered.

Peroneal nerve injury
Manifested by footdrop and a steppage gait, this is caused by improper positioning of the patient's legs without the usual flexion of the hip and knees. While slow, recovery is almost always complete within 6 to 8 months. Physiotherapy is helpful and a foot brace should be prescribed.

Ureteral injury
May be asymptomatic but usually causes flank tenderness or spiking fever and should always be considered when there is persistent ileus or unexplained fever. A ureterovaginal fistula usually presents the 10th to 14th postoperative day. Patients with this complication should undergo immediate intravenous pyelography and cystoscopy to locate the site of the communication. If the fistula is identified in the first 2 or 3 postoperative days and there is no massive tissue necrosis or sepsis in the pelvis, ureteroneocystostomy should be performed. However, if the fistula is discovered in the second postoperative week when there is a large degree of cellulitis in the pelvis, most patients are better served having a percutaneous nephrostomy stent inserted by an interventional radiologist. After waiting 4 to 6 weeks to allow inflammation in the pelvis to subside, the surgeon should proceed with exploratory laparotomy and ureteroneocystostomy. Rarely, the percutaneous nephrostomy ureteral stent can be advanced past the ureteral fistula into the bladder. The fistula may then close without stricture and the problem is solved. Unfortunately, long-term results of ureteral fistula treatment with stents reveal a significant incidence of stenosis with obstruction, and most patients eventually require surgical correction.

Vesicovaginal fistula
Leakage of urine through the vagina is the principal symptom. Methylene blue instilled into the bladder is immediately present in the vagina. Cystoscopy usually confirms the location of the fistula above the ureteric ridge, high on the interior wall of the bladder. If there is no significant cellulitis, edema, or necrosis in the margin of the fistula, immediate repair can be performed and is successful in 80% of cases. With the discovery of necrosis or cellulitis in the margin of fistula, however, it is best to delay treatment until the process resolves, which is usually after 3 months. Foley catheter drainage of the bladder may reduce the distressing flow of urine through the fistula and occasionally allows small fistulas to heal.

After discharge

Granulation tissue of the vaginal vault
A more common occurrence when catgut suture was used, this condition has become a rare occasion with the advent of modern synthetic and absorbable suture material.

Tuboovarian abscess

Rare but usually associated with fever, pain, and a pelvic mass, it generally occurs 10 to 14 days after discharge from the hospital. Although the abscess can sometimes be drained by percutaneous needle and catheter insertion by an interventional radiologist, it often requires surgical incision and drainage.

Acknowledgment

This chapter is based on material from: Vaginal hysterectomy by Clifford R. Wheeless, Jr., which appeared in the 3rd edn of *Medical Management of the Surgical Patient*.

FURTHER READING

Dicker, R. C., Greenspan, J. R., Strauss, L. T. *et al.* Complications of abdominal and vaginal hysterectomy among women of reproductive age in the United States. *Am. J. Obstet. Gynecol.* 1982; **144**: 841–848.

Farquhar, C. M. & Steiner, C. A. Hysterectomy rates in the United States 1990–1997. *Obstet. Gynecol.* 2002; **99**: 229–234.

Jones, H. W. III. Hysterectomy. In Rock, J. A., Jones, H. W. III, eds. *Te Linde's Operative Gynecology*, 9th edn. Philadelphia, PA: Lippincott, Williams & Wilkins, 2003: 799–828.

Lepine, L. A., Hillis, S. D., Marchbanks, P. A. *et al.* Antibiotic prophylaxis for gynecologic procedures. ACOG Practice Bulletin Number 23, January 2001. Washington, DC, American College of Obstetricians and Gynecologists, Hysterectomy surveillance – United States, 1980–1993. *Morb. Mortal. Wkly. Rep.* 1997; **46** (No. SS-4): 1–15.

Montz, F. J., Bristow, R. E., & Del Carmen, M. G. Operative injuries to the ureter: prevention, recognition, and management. In Rock, J. A., Jones, H. W. III, eds. *Te Linde's Operative Gynecology*, 9th edn. Philadelphia, PA: Lippincott, Williams & Wilkins, 2003.

Wingo, P. A., Huezo, C. M., Rubin, G. L. *et al.* The mortality risk associated with hysterectomy. *Am. J. Obstet. Gynecol.* 1985; **152**: 803–808.

91

Uterine curettage

Hugh W. Randall

Emory University School of Medicine, Atlanta, GA

As the second most frequently performed gynecologic operation, uterine curettage is used for diagnostic and therapeutic considerations and for the following indications:

Polymenorrhea: menstrual cycle interval less than 21 days.

Oligomenorrhea: menstrual cycle interval more than 37 days.

Metrorrhagia: menstrual bleeding longer than 7 days, or interval bleeding.

Menorrhagia: excessive or prolonged menstrual bleeding.

Postmenopausal bleeding or uterine bleeding occurring more than 12 months after the last menstrual period in a menopausal woman.

Breakthrough bleeding or intermenstrual bleeding in a menstrual cycle that is the result of exogenous hormones.

Dysfunctional uterine bleeding: characterized by any abnormal uterine bleeding in the absence of pregnancy, neoplasm, infection, or uterine lesion.

Spontaneous abortion, fetal death in utero, septic abortion, legal termination of pregnancy, dilation and evacuation of gestational trophoblastic neoplasias, incomplete abortion, or inevitable abortion.

The most common of the above complications are incomplete abortion, postmenopausal bleeding, and dysfunctional uterine bleeding. Curettage of the uterus responds to these conditions by removing endometrial or endocervical tissue for histologic study and evacuating products of conception.

It is extremely important that dilation and curettage be performed correctly for the proper indications and with minimal morbidity, as serious complications and even death may result from poor and inappropriate application. While regional and local anesthesia may be used, general anesthesia is usually administered to allow more abdominal relaxation for optimal bimanual examination of the pelvic viscera. The operative time for dilation and curettage is less than 15 minutes. Transfusion is rarely indicated unless significant preoperative hemorrhage has occurred, usually associated with pregnancy. Formerly, uterine curettage was believed to be contraindicated in the presence of pelvic infection, pyometra, and septic abortion; however, when indicated and with the use of preoperative antibiotic coverage and drainage of the pyometra, dilation and curettage under septic conditions can remove the source of infection (e.g., septic abortion, pyometra) and provide valuable histologic information.

Various instruments, usually suction devices, have been devised to allow the sampling of endometrial tissue as an outpatient office procedure. In patients suspected of having adenocarcinoma, diagnostic confidence in these devices should be maintained only if the biopsy sample shows carcinoma. Otherwise, a classic dilation and curettage should be performed.

Usual postoperative course

Expected postoperative hospital stay
Typically, these procedures are performed on an outpatient basis. Inpatient hospitalization should be reserved for medical or surgical complications.

Operative mortality
Under 1% and almost always associated with an anesthetic complication.

Special monitoring required
Unnecessary.

Patient activity and positioning
Patients are ambulatory on the day of the procedure.

Medical Management of the Surgical Patient: A Textbook of Perioperative Medicine, ed. M. F. Lubin, R. B. Smith, T. F. Dobson, N. Spell, H. K. Walker. 4th edn. Published by Cambridge University Press. © Cambridge University 2006.

Alimentation

Food intake is permitted as tolerated on the day of surgery.

Antibiotic coverage

Preoperative antibiotic coverage is indicated for septic abortions and pyometra, and should be directed toward polymicrobial contamination (gram-negative rods, anaerobes, and gram-positive cocci).

Oxytocin

Should be administered to patients who have undergone abortion.

Postoperative complications

In the hospital

Perforation of the uterus

Most cases of uterine perforation are associated with the use of a sound or cervical dilators and occur in patients with acutely anteflexed or retroflexed uteri. Overnight observation in the hospital is usually required. The two principal dangers of uterine perforation are bleeding and trauma to adjacent abdominal viscera. Lateral perforation through the uterine vessels is especially dangerous. When serious damage from perforation is suspected, a diagnostic laparoscopy should be performed so that the damage may be assessed and repaired.

Hemorrhage

Bleeding may be obvious or concealed within the peritoneal cavity. Hemorrhage generally results from injury to the uterine vessels caused by a dilator or curette and requires immediate abdominal exploration, control of bleeding, and sometimes hysterectomy.

Intestinal perforation

Intestinal perforation is a rare complication that usually results from termination of pregnancy and evacuation of products of conception with a suction curette. Immediate laparotomy is required with repair or resection of the injured bowel.

After discharge

Bleeding and fever

If bleeding is copious and sustained, re-exploration of the endometrial cavity is indicated. If fever develops, a culture should be obtained from the endometrial cavity and broad spectrum antibiotics administered.

Asherman's syndrome

This is a pathologic condition of uterine adhesions which may occur as a consequence of puerperal D&C and can cause secondary amenorrhea. The diagnosis can be confirmed by a hysterosalpingogram and hysteroscopy. Lysis of adhesions can be done through the hysteroscope.

Acknowledgment

This chapter is based on material from: Uterine curettage by Clifford R. Wheeless, Jr., which appeared in the 3rd edn of *Medical Management of the Surgical Patient*.

FURTHER READING

Butler, W. J. Normal and abnormal uterine bleeding. In Rock, J. A., Jones, H. W. III, eds. *Te Linde's Operative Gynecology*, 9th edn. Philadelphia, PA: Lippincott, Williams & Wilkins; 2003: 457–481.

Speroff, L., Glass, R. H., & Kase, N. G. *Clinical Gynecologic Endocrinology and Infertility*. 6th edn. Philadelphia, PA: Lippincott, Williams & Wilkins, 1999.

Word, B. Current concepts of uterine curettage. *Postgrad. Med.* 1960; **28**: 450–456.

92

Radical hysterectomy

Jack Basil

Emory University School of Medicine, Atlanta, GA

Carcinoma of the uterine cervix is the third most common gynecologic malignancy in the United States, with an estimated 12 200 newly diagnosed cases and 4100 deaths in 2003. With the adoption of routine screening programs, the mortality from the condition has steadily decreased since the 1940s in this country, though the disease remains a significant problem in developing countries.

The disease is typically clinically staged, and all stages may be treated with radiotherapy or a combination of radiotherapy and chemotherapy. Traditionally, surgical treatment has been used in early stage disease. Microinvasive disease or stage IA1 can be adequately treated with a vaginal or simple abdominal hysterectomy. Radical hysterectomy, usually referred to as a type III hysterectomy, is a treatment modality utilized to treat early stage invasive carcinoma of the cervix (stages IA2 thru IIA). In addition to the radical hysterectomy, a pelvic and/or para-aortic lymphadenectomy is also performed as a component of this treatment. Wertheim and Meigs described variations of the radical hysterectomy that are most often employed today.

Whether patients are treated with radical hysterectomy and lymphadenectomy versus radiotherapy, treatment outcomes for early stage cervical cancer are similar. Patients undergoing surgery must consider the following operative risks: blood transfusion, perioperative infection, thromboembolic disorders, postoperative bladder and bowel dysfunction, fistula formation, nerve injury, and lymphedema.

Despite the risks, there are certain potential advantages to radical hysterectomy over primary radiotherapy. For premenopausal women, radical hysterectomy affords the opportunity for ovarian preservation. Metastatic disease to the ovaries is unusual, especially in squamous cell cancer of the cervix, and removal of the ovaries is not a routine part of the procedure. Also, most clinicians believe that radical surgery affects vaginal anatomy less than radiotherapy, in that the vaginal tissues are left more elastic and less stenotic and fibrotic. Finally, radical surgery allows for evaluation of nodal metastasis. Surgical staging of the disease is becoming more common in the USA and may aid the clinician in treatment planning.

Since the overall survival of early stage cervical cancer is similar between radical hysterectomy and radiotherapy, those patients who are poor surgical candidates due to severe medical illness or morbid obesity are probably best treated with primary radiotherapy. Advanced age is not a contraindication for radical hysterectomy, as the morbidity of elderly patients is no higher than that of younger patients. Preoperatively, surgical patients should have been ruled out for metastatic disease and have undergone routine bowel prep.

The primary goal of radical hysterectomy is removal of the cervical tumor with a sufficient surgical margin, which entails removal of the uterus, cervix, superior vaginal margin, and parametrial tissue. Removal of the latter involves extensive dissection of bladder, ureters, rectum, and lateral pelvic sidewalls. Operative time usually ranges from 2½ to 4 hours. General anesthesia, preoperative antibiotics, and venous thrombosis prophylaxis are customary. The estimated blood loss for the operation ranges from 800–1500 ml, with one-third to one-half of patients requiring blood transfusion. Intraoperative complications and their reported frequencies include: injury to major vessels, 1.8%; bladder injury, 1.3%; ureteral injury, 1.0%; injury to the obturator nerve, 0.3%; and rectal injury, 0.1%. Significant postoperative complications can include: thromboembolic disease, bladder dysfunction, urinary fistulas, peripheral nerve injury, lymphedema, and bowel obstruction.

Medical Management of the Surgical Patient: A Textbook of Perioperative Medicine, ed. M. F. Lubin, R. B. Smith, T. F. Dobson, N. Spell, H. K. Walker. 4th edn. Published by Cambridge University Press. © Cambridge University 2006.

Usual postoperative course

Expected postoperative hospital stay
Typically 3–4 days.

Operative mortality
Less than 1%, though this rate is greater than the mortality from primary radiotherapy.

Special monitoring required
Intensive care observation may be necessary for some postoperative patients; however, the majority can be monitored on the routine postsurgical floor.

Patient activity and positioning
Up to one-fourth of patients have been reported to experience thromboembolic events. Routine use of prophylaxis intraoperatively and postoperatively with intermittent pneumatic calf compression and/or heparin is the standard of care; this should be continued until the patient is fully ambulatory or at the time of hospital discharge. Even after patient discharge, the clinician should be alert to the possibility of thromboembolic events.

Alimentation
Bowel function usually returns within the first couple of postoperative days and diet may be advanced as tolerated.

Antibiotic coverage
Preoperative antibiotics aimed at polymicrobial contamination are administered.

Postoperative complications

In the hospital

Bladder dysfunction
Some denervation of the bladder occurs following radical hysterectomy, with the degree of dysfunction depending upon how extensive the dissection was. The majority of patients will experience some bladder dysfunction, though most will establish baseline voiding patterns within several weeks to a few months after surgery. Several options exist for immediate postoperative bladder care to prevent overdistention of the bladder and prolonged dysfunction. An indwelling urethral catheter may be placed for 7–10 days or until voiding becomes satisfactory. When the operation is performed, a suprapubic catheter can be placed that enables the patient to perform voiding trials in the immediate postoperative period. The suprapubic catheter has the advantage of comfort and less infectious morbidity. In well motivated patients, another option is intermittent self-catheterization until voiding returns to baseline.

Urinary fistula formation
In the immediate postoperative period up to 3 weeks, vesicovaginal and ureterovaginal fistula formation usually presents as a watery uriniferous vaginal discharge. With either catheter or ureteral stent placement, small fistulae may heal spontaneously, though those that do not heal can be surgically repaired. Generally, repair after several weeks to allow for resolution of edema and inflammation gives the best results.

Neural deficits
The majority of nerve injuries sustained after radical hysterectomy are transient and most patients will regain full sensory and motor function. Such injuries may be the result of the surgery itself or secondary to the use of retractors. Nerves at risk include: femoral, obturator, sciatic, genitofemoral, ilioinguinal, and lateral femoral cutaneous.

After discharge

Lymphedema
A consequence of disruption of the regional lymphatic channels after lymphadenectomy, this complication usually worsens if a patient undergoes postoperative adjuvant radiotherapy. The condition may be treated with elevation of the involved extremity along with the use of elastic stockings. Patients evincing this complication may also intermittently develop lymphangitis which can be treated with oral antibiotics.

Bowel obstruction
Though this is uncommon after radical hysterectomy, the incidence increases in those patients requiring postoperative adjuvant radiotherapy. Initially, intestinal obstruction is managed non-surgically with bowel rest and tube decompression, while re-exploration is reserved for those patients who fail conservative treatment.

FURTHER READING

Artman, L. E., Hoskins, W. J., Bibro, M. C. *et al.* Radical hysterectomy and pelvic lymphadenectomy for stage IB carcinoma of the cervix: 21 years experience. *Gynecol. Oncol.* 1987; **28**: 8–13.

Covens, A., Rosen, B., Gibbons, A. *et al.* Differences in the morbidity of radical hysterectomy between gynecological oncologists. *Gynecol. Oncol.* 1993; **51**: 39–45.

Jemel, A., Murray, T., Samuels, A. *et al.* Cancer Statistics, 2003. *CA Cancer J. Clin.* 2003; **53**: 5–26.

Levrant, S. G., Fruchter, R. G., & Maiman, M. Radical hysterectomy for cervical cancer: morbidity and survival in relation to weight and age. *Gynecol. Oncol.* 1992; **45**: 317–322.

Meigs, J. V. The Wertheim operation for carcinoma of the cervix. *Am. J. Obstet. Gynecol.* 1945; **49**: 542–553.

Piver, M. S., Rutledge, F., & Smith, J. P. Five classes of extended hysterectomy for women with cervical cancer. *Obstet. Gynecol.* 1974; **44**: 265–272.

Shuster, P. A., Barter, J. F., Potkul, R. K. *et al.* Radical hysterectomy morbidity in relation to age. *Obstet. Gynecol.* 1991; **78**: 77–79.

Walsh, J. J., Bonnar, J., & Wright, F. W. A study of pulmonary embolism and deep vein thrombosis after major gynaecological surgery using labeled fibrinogen-phlebography and lung scanning. *J. Obstet. Gynaecol. Br. Commun.* 1974; **81**: 311–316.

Wertheim, E. The extended abdominal operation for carcinoma uteri (based on 500 operative cases). *Am. J. Obstet. Gynecol.* 1912; **66**: 169–232.

93

Vulvectomy

Ira R. Horowitz

Emory University School of Medicine, Atlanta, GA

Vulvectomy is performed for both preinvasive and malignant conditions of the vulva. This procedure may vary in extent from a skinning procedure performed for multicentric intraepithelial neoplasia to a radical vulvectomy combined with bilateral inguinofemoral lymph node dissections for invasive carcinoma. The radical procedure has changed during the past decade and may range from hemivulvectomy with unilateral inguinofemoral lymph node dissection to an en bloc resection including bilateral inguinofemoral lymph nodes. Lateralizing stage T_1 lesions smaller than 2 cm are treated with a radical hemivulvectomy and ipsilateral lymph nodes dissection. For larger or midline lesions, attempts are made to perform a radical vulvectomy and bilateral inguinofemoral lymph node dissections through separate incisions (three incision technique). This generally results in fewer postoperative complications (e.g., wound infection) and a shorter hospital stay. Depending on the extent of resection, myocutaneous flaps may be needed to fill the operative defect. The time necessary for this operation is 2 to 5 hours and varies according to the extent of resection and reconstruction. General, regional, or combination anesthesia can be equally efficacious. Intraoperative transfusions are not routinely required during radical vulvectomy.

Usual postoperative course

Expected postoperative hospital stay

The duration of hospitalization ranges from 4 to 21 days, depending on the extent of resection, the required reconstruction, and the rate of wound healing.

Operative mortality
Under 1%.

Special monitoring required
Patients undergoing radical vulvectomy do not require specific monitoring. Because most patients are elderly, however, their medical condition, rather than the operative procedure itself, may necessitate intensive care monitoring.

Patient activity and positioning
Bed rest for 24 to 48 hours is recommended to allow the myocutaneous flaps or primary closure to begin healing before increased tension is placed on the suture lines.

Alimentation
Although a regular diet would be tolerated on the first postoperative day, clear liquids or a low-residue diet are recommended to decrease fecal soiling of the wound.

Antibiotic coverage
The perioperative administration of first- or second-generation cephalosporin in the first 24 hours may decrease the risk of wound infection. Some gynecologic oncologists prescribe doxycycline during the immediate postoperative period to reduce the incidence of cellulitis.

Thromboembolism
In the 1986 National Institutes of Health Consensus Report, the use of low-dose heparin and sequential pneumatic compression devices was recommended to decrease thromboembolic phenomena in patients with gynecologic malignancies. The Sixth ACCP (2000) guidelines concur with combination therapy in the high risk patient. Low molecular weight heparin can be substituted for unfractionated sodium heparin. This may result in fewer postoperative hematomas. If epidural anesthesia is used consult your anesthesiologist prior to prescribing low molecular weight heparin.

Medical Management of the Surgical Patient: A Textbook of Perioperative Medicine, ed. M. F. Lubin, R. B. Smith, T. F. Dobson, N. Spell, H. K. Walker. 4th edn. Published by Cambridge University Press. © Cambridge University 2006.

Perineal care

Various philosophies exist regarding perineal care in patients undergoing radical vulvectomy. Most surgeons agree, however, that the wound should be kept dry. This may be accomplished with a heat lamp or hair dryer.

Postoperative complications

In the hospital

Wound separation and necrosis

The most common complication of radical vulvectomy is wound separation and necrosis, which occurs in about 70% to 80% of patients. This complication has been significantly reduced by using the Three Incision Technique. Although the use of myocutaneous flaps and skin grafts can decrease the incidence of this problem, flaps frequently undergo necrosis at their distal margins. Skin necrosis is treated with aggressive debridement and frequent irrigation. It may take several weeks for complete wound healing to occur. These patients do not require additional skin grafting, and a complete radical vulvectomy can be allowed to granulate in with satisfactory results.

Wound hematoma/serosa

In a radical vulvectomy, the saphenous vein may be sacrificed, though some gynecologic oncologists attempt to spare the saphenous vein. This is felt to decrease some of the post operative leg edema. In addition, the various small branching arteries and veins from the femoral vessels may result in postoperative hematoma. Re-exploration may be necessary to evacuate the collection and achieve hemostasis.

Cellulitis

Cellulitis is the second most common complication of radical vulvectomy. Patients should be treated with doxycycline or broad-spectrum antibiotics effective against staphylococcal and streptococcal species.

Rupture of femoral vessels

Rupture of femoral vessels is a life-threatening complication that should be treated with local compression to control bleeding until patients can be returned to the operating room for repair of the damaged vessel. Transposition of the sartorius muscle to cover the femoral vessels during the initial operation has almost eliminated this complication. More conservative approaches of node dissection permit primary closure of the fascia that does not necessitate a sartorius muscle flap.

Femoral neuropathy

The femoral nerve lies lateral to the femoral artery and is only rarely injured during the inguinofemoral dissection.

After discharge

Edema of the lower extremities

Excision or interruption of the regional lymphatics frequently results in chronic lymphedema. Therapy consists of elastic support stockings and limb elevation. In more severe cases, pneumatic compression devices are used.

Lymphangitis and cellulites

Lymphangitis and cellulites require aggressive antibiotic coverage of proper duration.

Vaginal stricture

Cicatricial reaction around the introitus may result in dyspareunia. Vaginal dilators, and occasionally, surgical correction may be required to provide a normal vaginal caliber and restore the ability to have coitus.

Hernia formation

Inguinal and femoral hernias may develop if care is not exercised in closing the respective fascial planes. Using a sartorius flap at the initial procedure further decreases the incidence of this complication.

Incontinence

Urinary or fecal incontinence may occur after resection of the distal urethra or anal sphincter. Attempts should be made to train patients to achieve increased muscle tone. If efforts prove unsuccessful, or if the resection was extensive, reconstructive surgery is frequently warranted.

FURTHER READING

Daly, J. W. & Pomerance, A. J. Groin dissection with prevention of tissue loss and postoperative infection. *Obstet. Gynecol.* 1979; **53**: 395–399.

DiSaia, P. J., Creasman, W. T., & Rich, W. M. An alternate approach to early cancer of the vulva. *Am. J. Obstet. Gynecol.* 1979; **133**: 825–830.

Geerts, W. H., Heit, J. A., Clagett, G. P. *et al.* Prevention of thromboembolism. (Sixth ACCP Consensus Conference on Antithrombotic Therapy). *Chest* 2001; **119** (Suppl. 1): 1325–1755.

Hacker, N. F., Leuchter, R. S., Berek, J. S. *et al.* Radical vulvectomy and bilateral inguinal lymphadenectomy through separate groin incisions. *Obstet. Gynecol.* 1981; **586**: 574–579.

Horowitz, I. R. Gynecologic malignancies. In Wood, W. C., ed. *The Anatomic Basis of Tumor Surgery.* St. Louis, MO: Quality Medical Publishing, 1998.

Horowitz, I. R. & Basil, J. B. Postanesthesia and postoperative care. In Rock, J. A. & Jones, H. W., eds. *Te Linde's Operative Gynecology*, 9th edn. Philadelphia, PA: Lippincott, Williams & Wilkins, 2003.

Iverson, T., Abelet, V., & Aalders, J. Individualized treatment of stage I carcinoma of the vulva. *Obstet. Gynecol.* 1981; **57**: 85–89.

Podratz, K. C., Symmonds, R. E., & Taylor, W. F. Carcinomas of the vulva: analysis of treatment failures. *Am. J. Obstet. Gynecol.* 1982; **143**: 340–351.

Podratz, K. C., Symmonds, R. E., Taylor, W. F. *et al.* Carcinomas of the vulva: analysis of treatment and survival. *Obstet. Gynecol.* 1983; **61**: 63–74.

Rutledge, F. N., Smith, J. P., & Franklin, E. W. Carcinoma of the vulva. *Am. J. Obstet. Gynecol.* 1970; **106**: 1117–1130.

Stehman, F. B., Bundy, B. N., Ball, H. *et al.* Sites of failure and times to failure in carcinoma of the vulva treated conservatively. A Gynecology Oncology Group Study. *Am. J. Obstet. Gynecol.* 1996; **174**: 1128–1133.

Way, S. Results of a planned attack on carcinoma of the vulva. *Br. Med. J.* 1954; **2**: 780–782.

Wheeless, C. R., McGibbon, B., Dorsey, J. H., & Maxwell, G. P. Gracilis myocutaneous flap in the reconstruction of the vulva and female perineum. *Obstet. Gynecol.* 1979; **54**: 97–102.

Neurologic surgery

94

Craniotomy for brain tumor

Jeffrey J. Olson

Emory University School of Medicine, Atlanta, GA

New diagnostic systems and innovative surgical and adjuvant treatments have contributed to improved diagnostic and surgical accuracy and provide more treatment options in patients with brain tumors. Despite these advances, craniotomy is still an important component in the therapy of brain tumors and is particularly important when the lesion is symptomatic due to its size causing compression of surrounding brain. Craniotomy allows for diagnosis of the lesion, but open surgery is not mandatory to obtain tissue for histology as it can also be obtained by stereotactic needle biopsy. The latter technique is particularly useful where there is no need for craniotomy for decompression or if the lesion is deep or in functionally important tissue. Additionally, the less invasive stereotactic biopsy is useful in individuals with compromised systemic health. It has been difficult to show that aggressive resection of a tumor by craniotomy significantly impacts survival in patients with malignant tumors of the brain.

In most cases, the radiographic features of a brain tumor are usually sufficiently specific to proceed with a craniotomy. Improved MRI sequences and MR spectroscopy have made considerable information available to the treating physician preoperatively. However, even with such improved information, it may still be impossible to exclude mass lesions that would not ordinarily be treated by a craniotomy, such as cerebral infarction, multiple sclerosis, and viral infections.

Once the decision is made to perform a craniotomy, the surgeon uses the data obtained from diagnostic tests to plan the operative approach in order to obtain maximum access to the tumor at minimal risk to the patient. Medical preparation for craniotomy is generally straightforward. In cases with peritumoral vasogenic edema, oral systemic corticosteroids are usually administered to reduce mass effect and diminish intraoperative difficulties encountered as a result of cerebral edema. Clinically, the response to the corticosteroid effect on cerebral edema occurs within two days; longer periods of administration will not necessarily facilitate surgical resection further. Preoperative anticonvulsants are administered if the patient's presentation has included seizure activity of any kind. This decision and the length of time postoperative anticonvulsants are utilized is largely based on surgical judgment.

Once in the operating suite, peripheral or central venous access is obtained and an arterial line and a Foley catheter are inserted before final operative positioning. Pneumatic stockings are placed to reduce the incidence of venous thrombosis. These interventions can certainly be modified based upon the health of the patient, the extent of the procedure, and the experience of the surgical and anesthesia teams. A spinal drain may be inserted to allow cerebrospinal fluid (CSF) drainage during the operation. Once the patient is fully anesthetized, they are carefully positioned on the operating table with head firmly secured in a manner that affords the best exposure of the tumor. Patients who are placed in the sitting position are additionally monitored with a precordial Doppler stethoscope to detect air emboli.

The cranium is entered through burr holes, which are connected with a craniotome. The cranial bone flap is elevated from the field and epidural hematomas are prevented by securing the exposed dura to the periphery of the skull defect with sutures. A bulging or tense dura, indicative of raised intracranial pressure, is a common finding in patients with brain tumors. This is treated with elevation of the head to promote venous drainage, hyperventilation to reduce intracranial blood volume, or mannitol infusion to reduce the brain turgor due to cerebral edema. The dura is then incised. In intrinsic tumors an incision is made in the pia-arachnoid overlying the brain tumor. This can be aided by an image-guidance system to maximize accuracy

Medical Management of the Surgical Patient: A Textbook of Perioperative Medicine, ed. M. F. Lubin, R. B. Smith, T. F. Dobson, N. Spell, H. K. Walker. 4th edn. Published by Cambridge University Press. © Cambridge University 2006.

of the approach. Alternatively, cortical mapping can be carried out in the conscious patient to identify important regions of function and preserve them during surgery. A path is developed through the brain to the tumor if it is not externally visible. Once the tumor is encountered, tissue samples are submitted for frozen section to provide preliminary histologic confirmation and to narrow the differential diagnosis of the type of tumor. This information, combined with such parameters as site of the tumor, the age and condition of the patient, and the efficacy of alternate treatment options, is essential to deciding how extensive a resection should be undertaken. The tumor is partially or completely resected by a variety of sharp and blunt dissection techniques that are aided by ultrasonic aspirators and other methods when appropriate. When the resection is accomplished, hemostasis of the tumor bed is obtained, the dura is closed, and the bone flap is reattached to the surrounding skull defect. The stress of the procedure is moderate and largely dependent on the underlying health of the individual. Blood transfusion may be required.

Usual postoperative course

Expected postoperative hospital stay

2–5 days.

Operative mortality

Immediate operative mortality is rare. Mortality in the first 30 days is usually under 5% and is heavily dependent on the condition of the patient as well as the location, size, and type of tumor.

Special monitoring required

The first 12–24 hours after surgery are spent in the intensive care unit, a period that may be extended dependent on the need for management of tumor-induced or underlying respiratory or cardiac concerns. These situations include the need for continuous cardiac rhythm assessment, direct or indirect arterial pressure monitoring, central venous access for evaluation of volume, and delivery of compounds active in blood pressure and volume control. Those individuals that require active intracranial pressure control and ventriculostomy are clearly best monitored in an intensive care or intermediate care setting. Ongoing electroencephalographic monitoring is rarely needed and is reserved for cases of refractory postoperative seizure activity.

Patient activity and positioning

Bed rest is necessary until patients are fully conscious. In cases where intracranial pressure is a concern, the head of the bed is kept at 30 degrees. The level of activity is then increased as tolerated. Physical therapy, speech therapy, and occupational therapy are instituted if required.

Alimentation

A full, regular diet is provided as soon as possible and is initiated in a stepwise fashion beginning with clear liquids. In cases of tumors involving the brain stem, the ninth and tenth nerves, or where level of consciousness is depressed and cough and gag reflexes may be impaired, formal swallowing evaluation must be performed prior to oral intake to prevent aspiration. In cases with a significant swallowing impairment, temporary nasogastric tube placement or insertion of a gastrostomy or jejunostomy may be necessary.

Antibiotic coverage

Intravenous antibiotics with the ability to cover gram positive organisms and penetrate the central nervous system are given immediately prior to the scalp incision and for 24 hours after the surgery. In cases where there is need for ongoing invasive intracranial monitoring and where there might be significant concern about infection, prophylactic antibiotics may be continued. Ventriculostomies impregnated with antibiotics are now available and serve as an alternative and efficacious method of decreasing infection due to this form of monitoring.

Medications

Though associated with many toxicities, high dose corticosteroids are sometimes the only useful method of controlling cerebral edema. This edema is often exacerbated by the effects of surgery and will actually increase for approximately three days thereafter; therefore, high doses are administered for at least this period and then gradually tapered depending on individual circumstance. In cases where radiotherapy will follow soon after surgery, individuals are kept on corticosteroids for that therapy and beyond. Once cerebral edema improves, corticosteroids are tapered on an individual basis. Prophylactic antacids are used as needed. Anticonvulsants may also be used prophylactically in the immediate perioperative period in any case where cerebral cortical manipulation occurs. Agents that can be administered intravenously are preferred, as there may be a temporary period of inability to take oral medications after the surgery. In cases where a portion of the presentation was seizure activity, anticonvulsants are continued for the longer term.

Postoperative complications

In the hospital

Hemorrhage

Either immediately or in the early postoperative period, this potentially life-threatening complication usually results from bleeding from the tumor bed and can lead to the formation of an intracerebral hematoma. Because the tumor-associated blood vessels are abnormal, hemostasis is more difficult to achieve than with normal brain tissue. In addition, bleeding into the ventricular, subdural, epidural, or subgaleal spaces may occur. Systemic hypertension as can occur during arousal following anesthesia or that may have been present at baseline, can be a precipitating factor. Expectant control of hypertension is important to avoid this complication. If deemed necessary at the time of tumor resection, placement of an intracranial pressure monitor allows early detection of unfavorable changes. The diagnosis of hematoma is confirmed by computed tomographic scan. Selected hematomas may require surgical evacuation if they are causing mass effect and dysfunction of adjacent cerebral tissue due to compression.

Infection

Infections may be deep within the cerebral tissue or superficial in the scalp or craniotomy bone flap. Septic contamination may give rise to cerebritis, intracerebral abscess, meningitis, bone flap infection, subdural or epidural empyema, subgaleal effusion, or cellulitis of the scalp, all of which are serious complications. Treatment is enhanced by identification of the offending organism through microbiologic culture and drug sensitivity tests. This may only require culturing of wound discharge, but there should be no hesitation to utilize surgical methods to obtain samples and debride the area. This may include needle aspiration, even using stereotactic methods as necessary, or craniotomy for drainage and removal of devitalized tissue. Bone flap removal should be entertained if gross purulence is present. In cases where the infection is less intense in the surgeon's estimation, an antibiotic suction–irrigation system may be installed at the time of surgery, lying in either the sudural space, the subgaleal space, or both. The initial choice of antibiotic is dependent on the patient, craniotomy location (e.g., adjacent to the nasal sinuses vs. at the convexity), and individual institutional trends in bacterial infection.

Cerebral edema

Postoperative swelling of the brain may be a function of the brain tumor itself, the result of direct surgical manipulation of the brain tissue, or interruption of brain arterial supply or venous drainage. The swollen brain will malfunction, causing defects in performance originating from that area and, in more severe cases, exerting a mass effect that may compromise vital brain stem centers. Cerebral edema is usually well seen on a computed tomographic scan or on a postoperative MRI scan. Treatment includes the careful monitoring of systemic fluid balance to avoid overhydration, use of corticosteroids and three percent saline, and mannitol and hyperventilation in more severe cases. When hypertonic solutions or diuretics are used, it is important to follow serum osmolarity and sodium concentrations to avoid excessive dehydration and impairment of microvascular flow and renal and cardiac function. When any question arises about overall fluid status, central venous pressure monitoring is indicated.

Cerebral infarction

Interruption of the arterial blood supply may impair function or may destroy the brain tissue in that particular distribution. The clinical effects are largely dependent in the particular arterial region that is compromised. It is potentially lethal when arterial supply to the brain stem is jeopardized. Since the venous tributaries typically drain large areas of the brain, an extensive infarction may occur as a result of venous occlusion. Aggravating factors include a low cerebral perfusion pressure and hematocrit level as well as poor blood oxygenation. Careful control of blood pressure, volume status, and oxygenation are maintained before and after surgery to minimize these factors.

Seizures

Tumors that invade the cerebral cortex and the presence of cortical surgical scars are potentially epileptogenic. A seizure that occurs in the immediate postoperative period may raise the intracranial pressure, result in temporary hypoxia in already compromised brain, or induce hemorrhage in the tumor bed due to hypertension. Therefore, anticonvulsants are routinely administered as a safeguard before surgery, during anesthetic induction, or during the tumor resection. The choice of anticonvulsants may vary, though an agent that can be delivered intravenously is advantageous, particularly if postoperative obtundation or inability to swallow is expected. The duration of anticonvulsant therapy is partly dependent on tumor location and pathology. In cases where seizure risk is low, the anticonvulsant may be stopped 1 to 2 weeks after operation. If patients are at high risk for seizures or have experienced them as a portion of their presentation, the medication may be continued for a longer period of time.

Associated fluid and electrolyte imbalances

Brain tumors adjacent to the hypothalamus and pituitary gland pose special problems, with fluid and electrolyte imbalances related to the abnormal secretion of antidiuretic hormone. Excessive or insufficient amounts of antidiuretic hormone may result in the syndrome of inappropriate antidiuretic hormone or diabetes insipidus, respectively. These states are managed by a variety of drugs, hormone replacement, or strict fluid control. The use of high dose corticosteroids may also alter fluid balance, causing significant soft tissue retention and fluid space shifts. Sensitivity to corticosteroid effects varies from individual to individual and must be monitored by standard laboratory analysis to assure reasonable balance is maintained.

Cerebrospinal fluid leakage

Impairment of CSF reabsorbtion in the arachnoid granulations due to the effects of tumor debris, blood products, or diminished venous sinus outflow may occur postoperatively. Though this may be manifest as hydrocephalus when the coverings of the central nervous system are intact, it may lead to persistent drainage of CSF when closure is discovered not to be watertight. The creation of a fistula from the CSF space is of special concern when the paranasal sinuses or mastoid spaces are breached; this may result in CSF rhinorhea or otorrhea, respectively. Leakage may also occur if dural closure is impaired because of poor tissue quality or tumor induced dural destruction. Because of difficulty with persistent headache and risk of meningitis, treatment is necessary. Therapy may consist of elevation of the head of the bed, continuous CSF drainage via a lumbar drain in individuals without increased intracranial pressure, or a ventriculostomy in individuals with increased intracranial pressure. In recalcitrant cases, surgical obliteration of the fistula may be necessary. In cases with impaired CSF reabsorption and hydrocephalus, supplementation with long term ventriculoperitoneal shunting may also be required.

After discharge

Each of the above postoperative complications can occur after discharge. However, delayed hemorrhage, fluid and electrolyte imbalance due to new anatomic changes, and true cerebral infarction are unusual.

Infection

As a significant number of individuals with brain tumor are immunocompromised due to the effects of the tumor, the corticosteroid therapy, or prior chemotherapy or radiation therapy, they remain at risk for wound infection, meningitis, or brain abscess. Wound healing may be slowed and incomplete due to the effect of corticosteroids and prior therapies that leave the wound at risk for incursions of scalp flora. Progressive fever, wound erythema, tenderness, swelling, or new neurologic deficits not otherwise explained must be investigated as possible infection. Imaging with computerized tomography or MRI with and without enhancement will assist in defining the process. Identified infection should be treated with antibiotic therapy and, when necessary, surgical drainage and debridement as aggressively as in the initial postoperative period.

Cerebral edema

After surgery, corticosteroid taper is performed as soon as reasonably possible. In some instances, neurologic status declines or headache and nausea ensue which may be due to progressive or residual cerebral edema and can be confirmed by computerized tomography or MRI. Confirmation of proper electrolyte balance and treating for associated hyperglycemia are necessary. Therapy generally consists of avoidance of overhydration and institution of increased doses of corticosteroids. Subsequently, other causes for the increased edema such as tumor recurrence, infectious cerebritis, or impaired venous outflow must be considered and treated.

Hydrocephalus

As in the immediate postoperative period, ventricular enlargement may result from the obstruction of CSF flow along intracerebral pathways (noncommunicating hydrocephalus) or from the obstruction of CSF outflow at the level of the venous sinuses (communicating hydrocephalus) by tumor, hemorrhage, or surgical scars. This may manifest as progressive mental status changes, visual obscuration, headache, nausea, vomiting, or other new neurologic deficits. Placement of a ventriculoperitoneal shunt is the treatment of choice. If active intra-abdominal disease is likely to cause intraperitoneal adhesions or peritonitis is present, a ventriculoatrial shunt is a reasonable second choice.

Cerebrospinal fluid leakage

Though CSF reabsorption and wound healing may be initially adequate, the effects of postoperative radiation therapy, chemotherapy, and surgical scarring can have a negative impact over time, most notably resulting in wound breakdown. It is likely that a combination of these effects are mandatory for the onset of a delayed CSF leak. In a minority of circumstances, it may be controlled by lumbar drainage or ventriculostomy on a temporary basis. More often, permanent CSF diversion with a ventri-culoperitoneal shunt may be necessary. Evidence of meningitis or wound infection will require treatment with antibiotics while the CSF leak is being managed with a lumbar drain or ventriculostomy. Once the infection is controlled, a permanent shunt can be placed.

Tumor recurrence

Despite the use of surgery, radiation, and chemotherapy, highly malignant primary brain tumors almost inevitably recur. By itself this is not a postoperative complication. However, the onset of a new neurologic decline due to this event can be initially discerned as a complication of therapy. Depending on the clinical circumstance, it is important to investigate neurologic decline with a proper neurologic examination, laboratory studies, and imaging. The most reliable indicator of the likelihood of tumor recurrence is directly related to the aggressiveness of the histo-logic type and grade of the tumor, the patient's age, and their performance status. Once recurrence is identified, therapy is chosen based on the nature of the recurrence and may include reoperation, alternative forms of radi-ation, or a new chemotherapy regimen. When profound neurologic injury has occurred and is felt to be irreversible, simple supportive care or hospice may be chosen.

FURTHER READING

Barnett, G. H. The role of image-guided technology in the surgical planning and resection of gliomas. *J. Neuro-oncol.* 1999; **42**: 247–258.

Beaumont, A. & Whittle, I. R. The pathogenesis of tumour associated epilepsy. *Acta Neurochir. (Wien)* 2000; **200**: 1–15.

Bingaman, K. & Olson, J. J. Cranial bone flap infections and osteo-myelitis of the skull. In Osenback, R. K. & Zeidman, S. M., eds. *Infections of the Central Nervous System: Diagnosis and Management.* Philadelphia, PA: Lippincott-Raven; 1999: 65–84.

Cascino, G. D. Epilepsy and brain tumors: implications for treat-ment. *Epilepsia* 1990; **31**: S37–S44.

Chin, C. T. & Dillon, W. P. Magnetic resonance imaging of central nervous system tumors. In Prados, M., ed. *Brain Cancer.* Hamilton, Ontario, Canada: BC Decker, Inc.; 2002: 105–128.

Chin, L. S., Levy, L. M., & Appuzzo, M. L. J. Principles of stereotac-tic neurosurgery. In Youmans, J. R., ed. *Neurological Surgery*, 4th edn. Philadelphia, PA: W. B. Saunders; 1996: 767–785.

Cloughesy, T. F. & Black, K. L. Peritumoral edema. In Berger, M. S. & Wilson, C. B., eds. *The Gliomas.* Philadelphia, PA: W. B. Saunders; 1999: 107–114.

Davies, D. C. Blood–brain barrier breakdown in septic encephalo-pathy and brain tumors. *J. Anat.* 2002; **200**: 639–646.

Gildenberg, P. L. & Woo, S. Y. Multimodality program involving stereotactic surgery in brain tumor management. *Stereotactic Funct. Neurosurg.* 2000; **75**: 147–152.

Lote, K., Stenwig, A. E., Skullerud, K., & Hirschberg, H. Prevalence and prognostic significance of epilepsy in patients with gliomas. *Eur. J. Cancer.* 1998; **34**: 98–102.

Poon, W. S., Lolin, Y. I., Yeung, T. F. *et al.* Water and sodium disorders following surgical excision of pituitary region tumors. *Acta Neurochir.* 1996; **138**: 921–927.

Sawaya, R., Hammoud, M., Schoppa, D. *et al.* Neurosurgical out-comes in a modern series of 400 craniotomies for treatment of parenchymal tumors. *Neurosurgery* 1998; **42**: 1044–1055.

Wen, P. Y. & Marks, P. W. Medical management of patients with brain tumors. *Curr. Opin. Onocol.* 2002: **14**: 299–307.

95

Intracranial aneurysm surgery

Y. Jonathan Zhang, C. Michael Cawley, and Daniel L. Barrow

Emory University School of Medicine, Atlanta, GA

Intracranial aneurysms are a relatively common disorder with an autopsy prevalence of 2% to 5% in the general population. Nearly half of these aneurysms become symptomatic during the patient's lifetime, usually presenting as subarachnoid hemorrhage (SAH). In North America, approximately 28 000 cases of aneurysmal SAH occur each year, mostly in adults. As opposed to the fusiform aneurysms that are encountered in the extracranial peripheral vasculature, intracranial aneurysms are typically saccular with a well-defined neck and sac distinct from the lumen of the parent vessel, frequently at proximal intracranial arterial branching points. Although the pathophysiology of intracranial aneurysms is controversial, they are thought to arise from defects in the muscularis media which may be congenital or acquired. Once these aneurysms have developed, conditions like hypertension and tobacco smoking may increase the risk of rupture, leading to SAH. Unruptured aneurysms are believed to bleed at varying rates according to multiple factors, including their diameter at the time of diagnosis. Although evidence suggests that intracranial aneurysms are less likely to bleed if they are less than 7 to 10 mm, both angiographic and direct intraoperative observational studies have demonstrated that even smaller aneurysms may rupture. About 40% to 50% of patients die within the first month as a result of the initial hemorrhage and its complications. Of those who survive, approximately 20% succumb to rebleeding in the ensuing 2 weeks (50% in 6 months) if the aneurysms are not treated, with the highest rate of recurrent hemorrhage (4%) during the first 24 hours after initial rupture.

The most common presentation of intracranial aneurysms is SAH with or without an intraparenchymal hematoma or intraventricular blood. The peak age for aneurysmal SAH is 55 to 60 years with a slight female predominance. Less often, aneurysms may exert mass effect because of their location or size. A common example is an aneurysm of the posterior communicating artery that, by virtue of its intimate relationship with the oculomotor nerve, may expand and compress the latter, resulting in a partial or complete oculomotor nerve deficit. Rarely, a large aneurysm may accumulate thrombus, causing embolization and cerebral ischemia. The clinical features of SAH are sudden onset of a severe headache, usually described as the worst headache of the patient's life. It is often associated with nausea, vomiting, transient loss of consciousness, and neck stiffness with back pain. In as many as 50% of cases, there may be a history of minor rupture or symptoms referable to the aneurysm, typically within the 2 weeks prior to SAH.

After the initial history solicitation and physical examination, a computed tomographic (CT) scan of the head without intravenous contrast is obtained to confirm the diagnosis of SAH or intracerebral hematoma. A good-quality, contemporary, high-resolution CT scan can detect the subarachnoid blood in about 95% of cases if the study is performed within 48 hours of onset. In cases of a negative CT scan but with strong suspicion of SAH, lumbar puncture should be performed to detect xanthochromia of the cerebrospinal fluid (CSF), which may appear within six hours after the hemorrhage and is a hallmark of SAH. Four-vessel cerebral angiography is then performed to identify the aneurysm responsible for the hemorrhage and to search for multiple aneurysms, which occur in about 20% of cases. The quality of CT angiography has improved to the degree that it can be used for the diagnostic workup of selected aneurysms, avoiding the necessity of catheter angiography.

The two major potential complications of aneurysmal SAH are rebleeding and cerebral arterial vasospasm, both of which are responsible for significant morbidity and mortality. The incidence of rebleeding is estimated to be 4% in the first 24 hours and 1.5% per day over the next

Medical Management of the Surgical Patient: A Textbook of Perioperative Medicine, ed. M. F. Lubin, R. B. Smith, T. F. Dobson, N. Spell, H. K. Walker. 4th edn. Published by Cambridge University Press. © Cambridge University 2006.

13 days, although patients with worse neurologic status (graded by Hunt and Hess class) may rebleed at higher rates. The major supporting argument for early operation in suitable patients is that the risk of rebleeding can be eliminated by prompt and definitive clip ligation of the aneurysm. Vasospasm usually occurs between 4 and 10 days after SAH, becomes clinically apparent during this period as cerebral ischemia in 30% to 40% of patients, and is commonly manifested by a decrease in the level of consciousness followed by focal neurological deficits that may ultimately result in death. Patients with CT evidence of diffuse SAH in the basal cisterns or major cerebral fissures are at high risk for the development of vasospasm and should be treated accordingly. Antifibrinolytic agents, once widely used to reduce the risks of rebleeding, may also increase the risk of ischemic deficits caused by vasospasm but are used selectively in some patients to reduce the re-hemorrhage risks until definitive aneurysm treatment can be provided. Vasospasm is treated by the deliberate inducement of hypertension and hypervolemic hemodilution in an effort to increase cerebral blood flow. Nimodipine, a selective cerebral calcium channel antagonist, may improve long-term outcomes in patients at risk for vasospasm and is given orally for three weeks. Focal, medically refractory vasospasm in the proximal intracranial arteries may be treated by transluminal intracranial angioplasty in specialized neurovascular centers, with resultant dramatic clinical improvement in many cases. Angioplasty is contraindicated in patients with a recently ruptured but unsecured aneurysm.

Therapeutic intervention is dictated by the clinical conditions of the patient as assessed by the classification of Hunt and Hess, which grades the severity of meningismus and decreasing level of consciousness. If hydrocephalus is present on the CT scan and the patient is stuporous, judicious blood pressure and intracranial pressure control by external ventricular drainage is done prior to definitive treatment. The timing of aneurysm surgery is controversial and must be individualized. Patients with large intraparenchymal hematomas causing mass-effect are candidates for immediate operation. It has become fairly standard for patients who are not stuporous after initial stabilization (including treatment of hydrocephalus) to have surgical treatment as soon as feasible after SAH to achieve aneurysm obliteration and parent vessel preservation, thereby eliminating the risk of recurrent hemorrhage and allowing for aggressive treatment of possible cerebral vasospasm. Patients who have poor neurologic function or have presented more than 4 days after the hemorrhage may undergo delayed surgery after the risk of vasospasm has passed and/or the patient has improved.

During the operative procedure, mannitol, furosemide, mild hyperventilation, and meticulous microsurgical cerebral cisternal dissection are used to relax the brain and minimize retraction injury. Direct surgical exposure of the aneurysm is accomplished by atraumatic dissection of the aneurysm and its parent vessels, after which one or more occlusive clips are placed across the neck or base of the aneurysm. In the past, hypotensive anesthesia was used to reduce intraluminal pressure during dissection of the aneurysm, thereby decreasing the risk of intraoperative rupture. This technique has been surpassed by a more contemporary strategy of temporary clipping of afferent vessels during critical stages of dissection under moderate hypertension, mild hypothermia, and pharmacological cerebral protection with barbiturate-induced EEG-burst suppression.

An intraoperative angiogram is performed at many centers to confirm adequate clip placement and patency of parent vessel before closure; otherwise, angiography is performed before patients are discharged from the hospital.

Over the past decade, endovascular therapy has evolved into an alternative treatment for selected aneurysmal SAH patients, particularly patients with poor medical or neurological conditions. When the angioarchitecture of the aneurysm is favorable, endovascular neurosurgeons can access the lesion and pack thrombogenic materials – usually platinum microcoils – tightly into the aneurysm dome and neck while preserving parent vessel patency. This minimally invasive technique can markedly reduce the rebleeding rate in the acute phase of SAH. However, endovascular therapy has its limitations, including procedural risks, uncertain durability, and the necessity for long-term follow-up with angiography. Current endovascular techniques are not suitable for all aneurysms, and depend on size, location, angioarchitecture, and presence of intraluminal thrombus. Intense research and development are under way to define the role of endovascular therapy in aneurysmal SAH management.

Usual postoperative course

Expected postoperative hospital stay
At least 2 weeks for patients with SAH and 3–5 days for patients undergoing surgery for unruptured aneurysms.

Operative mortality
Ranges from 1% to 8% and is generally related to the patient's preoperative condition. Neurologic morbidity is often due to perforating vessel injuries and varies with

aneurysm location, ranging from 3% to 15%. There is strong evidence that volume–outcome relationships exist for aneurysm surgery.

Special monitoring required

Intensive care unit (ICU) observation is necessary, with frequent assessment of vital signs, neurologic status, intracranial pressure if ventriculostomy is placed, central venous pressure, intake and output, and cardiac monitoring for 48 to 72 hours. Serial transcranial Doppler study is conducted along with neurological examination to detect cerebral vasospasm in patients presenting with SAH. If vasospasm is present, 10 to 14 days in the ICU may be required.

Patient activity and positioning

Initially, the head of the bed should be elevated 30 degrees. Patients may get out of bed as soon as possible. If physical therapy is needed, it should commence soon after surgery.

Alimentation

Food intake should be advanced as tolerated. Nasogastric tube feedings may be given if patients are unable to eat or if they require supplementation.

Antibiotic coverage

No antibiotic coverage is needed other than usual perioperative prophylactic doses. When external ventricular drainage is required, frequent CSF surveillance is necessary to detect infection early.

Postoperative complications

In the hospital

Development of a focal neurologic deficit

This may be related to edema, contusion, infarction from brain retraction, or to damaged intracranial vessels or nerves. Aggressive investigation for treatable conditions should be conducted, including CT head scanning and intracranial pressure monitoring. Hyperosmolar therapy with mannitol or hypertonic saline and mild hyperventilation along with external ventricular drainage, should be used cautiously to treat intracranial hypertension. Cerebral vasospasm, detected by serial transcranial Doppler ultrasound, causes decreased cerebral perfusion and can also produce a focal neurologic deficit. If this is suspected, hypervolemic hypertensive hemodilution treatment should be instituted immediately and a catheter or CT cerebral angiogram obtained

to confirm the diagnosis and evaluate for possible transluminal angioplasty.

Subdural or epidural hematoma

These can occur after any craniotomy, but can be prevented by meticulous intraoperative hemostasis. They should be suspected when there is evidence of increased intracranial pressure in postoperative patients with neurological deterioration. Prompt neuroimaging can detect these problems early and appropriate surgical evacuation should minimize neurologic damage.

Acute hydrocephalus

This complication, which results from the prevention of either normal circulation or resorption of CSF by intraventricular or subarachnoid blood, is usually evident preoperatively and should be managed by judicious use of external ventricular drainage. About 20% of patients who have early acute hydrocephalus with subsequent ventricular drainage may eventually require CSF diversionary shunt procedures to optimize their recovery.

Cardiac problems

SAH may be associated with cardiac arrhythmia manifested by a wide variety of EKG changes in over 50% of cases. Occasionally, SAH may produce EKG or even echocardiogram abnormalities indistinguishable from an acute myocardial infarction ("stunned myocardium"). Most of these cardiac complications resolve spontaneously when the sympathetic surge following SAH subsides. Rarely, however, serious cardiac compromise may require invasive cardiac monitoring, inotropic agent use, and avoidance of hyperdynamic therapy for vasospasm.

Hyponatremia

Hypovolemia and hyponatremia frequently follow SAH as a result of natriuresis and diuresis. Symptoms can include an alteration in mentation or seizures, mimicking delayed cerebral ischemia from vasospasm. Care should be exercised when diagnosing such symptoms so that hyponatremia is not routinely attributed to the syndrome of inappropriate antidiuretic hormone (SIADH). Frequently, urinary loss of sodium after SAH is found to contribute to the development of hyponatremia (cerebral salt wasting, CSW). Differentiating CSW from SIADH is also important, since the former is treated with volume repletion, while the latter with fluid restriction. However, routine laboratory values in both conditions may be very similar, with the only difference evident in the patient's volume status. In CSW, the patient is hypovolemic, while in SIADH, the patient is either euvolemic or hypervolemic.

Seizures

Although seizure activity is often observed in the acute phase of SAH, which can be treated with antiepileptic medication, it rarely becomes a chronic condition. There is no evidence of benefit from prophylactic use of anticonvulsants. Therefore, medication can be tapered off shortly after recovery if the patient remains seizure-free.

After discharge

Chronic hydrocephalus

This is typically due to impaired CSF absorption. Acute hydrocephalus occurs in most patients with aneurysmal SAH, but only about 20% develop chronic hydrocephalus requiring a shunt. If patients do not achieve expected rehabilitation goals or even experience deterioration, efforts should be made to identify the possibility of chronic hydrocephalus or shunt malfunction.

Recurrence

With demonstration of surgical aneurysmal obliteration by appropriate intraoperative or postoperative angiograms, recurrence is extremely rare. Some patients may be predisposed to developing de novo intracranial aneurysms, especially if they have conditions known to be associated with aneurysms, e.g., autosomal dominant polycystic kidney disease, fibromuscular dysplasia, and other connective tissue disorders. If the aneurysm was occluded with endovascular embolization, serial angiographic and clinical follow-up is essential as recurrence is significantly more common.

FURTHER READING

Auer, L. M. & Mokry, M. Disturbed cerebrospinal fluid circulation after subarachnoid hemorrhage and acute aneurysm surgery. *Neurosurgery* 1990; **26**: 804–809.

Baker, C. J., Prestigiacomo, C. J., & Solomon, R. A. Short-term perioperative anticonvulsant prophylaxis for the surgical treatment of low-risk patients with intracranial aneurysms. *Neurosurgery* 1995; **37**: 863–871.

Drake, C. G. Management of cerebral aneurysm. *Stroke* 1981; **12**: 273–283.

Fisher, C. M., Kistler, J. P., & Davis, J. M. Relation of cerebral vasospasm to subarachnoid hemorrhage visualized by CT scanning. *Neurosurgery* 1980; **6**: 1–9.

Harrigan, M. R. Cerebral salt wasting syndrome: a review. *Neurosurgery* 1996; **38**: 152–160.

Hop, J. W., Rinkel, G. J., Algra, A. *et al.* Case-fatality rates and functional outcome after subarachnoid hemorrhage: a systematic review. *Stroke* 1997; **28**: 660–664.

Hunt, W. E. & Hess, R. M. Surgical risk as related to time of intervention in the repair of intracranial aneurysms. *J. Neurosurg.* 1968; **28**: 14–20.

Kassell, N. F., Boarini, D. J., Adams, H. P. *et al.* Overall management of ruptured aneurysm: comparison of early and later operation. *Neurosurgery* 1981; **9**: 120–128.

Kassell, N. F., Sasaki, T., Colohan, A. R. T. *et al.* Cerebral vasospasm following aneurysmal subarachnoid hemorrhage. *Stroke* 1985; **16**: 562–572.

Ogilvy, C. S. General management of aneurysmal subarachnoid hemorrhage. In Ojemann, R. G., Ogilvy, C. S., Heros, R. C., & Crowell, R. M., eds. *Surgical Management of Neurovascular Disease*. 3rd edn. Baltimore, MD: Williams & Wilkins, 1996: 111–122.

Ogilvy, C. S. & Rordorf, G. Mechanisms and treatment of coma after subarachnoid hemorrhage. In Bederson, J. B., ed. *Subarachnoid Hemorrhage: Pathophysiology and Management, Neurosurgical Topics*. Park Ridge, IL: The American Association of Neurological Surgeons, 1997; Chapter 9: 157–171.

Raymond, J. & Roy, D. Safety and efficacy of endovascular treatment of acutely ruptured aneurysms. *Neurosurgery* 1997; **41**: 1235–1246.

Winn, H. R., Richardson, A. E., & Jane, J. A. The long-term prognosis in untreated cerebral aneurysms. I. The incidence of late hemorrhage in cerebral aneurysm: a 10-year evaluation of 364 patients. *Ann. Neurol.* 1977; **1**: 358–370.

Winn, H. R., Richardson, A. E., & Jane, J. A. The long-term prognosis in untreated cerebral aneurysms. II. Late morbidity and mortality. *Ann. Neurol.* 1978; **4**: 418–426.

96

Evacuation of subdural hematomas

Praveen V. Mummaneni, Franklin J. Lin, and Valli P. Mummaneni

Emory University School of Medicine, Atlanta, GA

Anatomically, there are three distinct potential spaces between the skull and the surface of the brain where hematomas may accumulate: the epidural space is between the skull and the dura, the subdural space is between the dura and the arachnoid, and the subarachnoid space is between the arachnoid and the pia (which lines the cortical surface of the brain). Subdural hematomas (SDH) typically result from venous bleeding from torn bridging veins that traverse the potential space beneath the dura. SDHs can be subdivided into two groups: acute SDH and chronic SDH; the etiologies and the treatment options may vary between these two types.

Acute SDH

Etiology

Acute subdural hematomas most often occur soon after significant head trauma. Patients with acute traumatic SDH may also have other intracranial pathologic lesions contributing further to elevated intracranial pressure. Potential coexisting intracranial pathologies include: cerebral contusions, intraparenchymal hemorrhages, epidural hematomas, and/or subarachnoid hemorrhages.

Unlike epidural hematomas (which arise from brisk arterial bleeding), acute subdural hematomas may form over several hours after the injury from slow venous bleeding in the subdural space. Consequently, patients who accumulate large acute subdural hematomas may have a lucid interval of up to a few hours before becoming progressively confused or (in some cases) comatose.

Acute SDHs can also occur without any history of significant head trauma. For instance, patients with coagulopathies and/or vascular disorders are more prone to develop hematomas spontaneously or with even the slightest trauma to the head.

Neurosurgical intervention

In general, the factors that neurosurgeons take into account before deciding to evacuate an acute subdural hematoma include the size of the hematoma, the location of the hematoma, coexisting intracranial pathological lesions, the neurological status of the patient, and medical comorbidities (such as coagulopathy). Sizeable acute subdural hematomas causing significant mass effect with midline shift and with associated neurologic compromise may require emergent evacuation via craniotomy.

If a craniotomy is necessary, patients are often induced with propofol and maintained under general anesthesia with an inhalational anesthetic such as isoflurane and a muscle relaxant such as vecuronium. Intraoperative monitoring of blood pressure is typically performed with an arterial line. Intravenous access with two large bore i.v.s or a central line is preferred. Intraoperative maneuvers to decrease the intracranial pressure include the administration of mannitol and mild hyperventilation. Patients are also usually given dilantin before or during surgery to minimize the risk of seizures. Perioperative dosing of antibiotics (1 gram nafcillin or ceftriaxone) is standard to minimize the risk of infection. The average surgery typically lasts approximately 3 hours. Blood transfusion of 1 to 2 units of packed red cells may be necessary.

Chronic SDH

Unlike acute subdural hematomas, chronic subdural hematomas often develop over days or often weeks or months. Because of this slow accumulation of the hematoma, patients with chronic SDHs accommodate the hematoma well and often present with subtle and slowly

Medical Management of the Surgical Patient: A Textbook of Perioperative Medicine, ed. M. F. Lubin, R. B. Smith, T. F. Dobson, N. Spell, H. K. Walker. 4th edn. Published by Cambridge University Press. © Cambridge University 2006.

progressive neurologic symptoms. Some patients with chronic SDH accommodate the hematoma to the degree that they have no symptoms and their hematomas are found incidentally.

Etiology

Chronic SDHs are often the result of mild or even unnoticed head trauma and are seen most often in the elderly population. Because of their slowly expansive nature, these hematomas can grow quite large in elderly patients, who often have cerebral atrophy, before causing significant deficits or symptoms. Chronic SDHs may also occur spontaneously or following mild head trauma in patients with coagulopathy. Occasionally, patients may have an acute component of SDH in conjunction with a chronic SDH. This may be a result of repetitive head trauma.

Neurosurgical intervention

In patients with small chronic SDHs and no symptoms, neurosurgeons may elect not to evacuate the hematoma and to follow the patient with periodic cranial CT scans to ensure that the hematoma resolves. However, with large hematomas causing significant mass effect in association with neurologic symptoms, evacuation is recommended. Unlike acute SDHs, which tend to form a cohesive blood clot, chronic SDHs are typically liquefied, allowing for evacuation through burr holes. Occasionally conversion to a full craniotomy is warranted when the hematoma cannot be optimally drained or when complications arise.

If a patient requires burr holes for drainage of a chronic subdural hematoma, the operation usually takes approximately 60 minutes. Induction and general anesthetic agents are the same as those used for craniotomy. Patients usually are not given mannitol but are often given dilantin to prevent seizures and perioperative antibiotics to minimize the risk of infection. Excessive blood loss is rare, and patients typically do not require a blood transfusion. Use of an arterial line or a central line is usually unnecessary for these cases.

Usual postoperative course

Expected postoperative hospital stay
Depends upon severity of the head trauma and associated injuries.

Operative mortality

Acute SDH
Overall, mortality following evacuation of acute subdural hematomas in severe head injury can vary from 30% to 60%. Factors that influence mortality include mechanism of injury, initial Glasgow Coma Score (GCS), patient age, medical comorbidities, operative timing, coexisting traumatic injuries to other organ systems, coexisting intracranial pathologies (such as cerebral contusions and edema), and intracranial pressure (ICP) control. Of those that survive severe head injuries, functional recovery can vary widely and is also related to the above factors.

Chronic SDH
Outcomes of those with chronic subdural hematomas are better than those with acute SDH. Overall mortality in patients undergoing evacuation of chronic SDH is 10% and is usually secondary to postoperative medical complications. This is not surprising given that those with chronic SDH are often elderly and have significant medical comorbidities. Functional recovery for this group is likewise good with 75% of patients resuming activities of daily living.

Special monitoring required

Acute SDH
Those with acute subdural hematomas usually have prolonged ICU stays due to the severity of the head trauma and coexisting injuries. Patients with severe head injuries need to be monitored closely to avoid further brain injury from inadequate cerebral perfusion. Cerebral perfusion pressure (CPP) equals the difference between the mean arterial pressure (MAP) and the intracranial pressure (ICP). (i.e., CPP = MAP − ICP). Most neurosurgeons prefer to keep the CPP above 70 mm Hg. Close monitoring and treatment of blood pressure (both high and low) is necessary to optimize cerebral perfusion and to prevent further brain injury.

In those with severe head trauma the ICP is monitored via a ventriculostomy or intracranial pressure monitor. These patients also have arterial lines placed to accurately monitor MAP. In critically ill patients, neurologic exams are performed serially every hour.

Control of ICP is crucial. Patients with malignant elevations in ICP (over 30 mm Hg) require rigorous measures to reduce the ICP including draining CSF via ventriculostomy, heavy sedation, short-term hyperventilation (goal of 30–35 mm Hg pCO_2), and hyperosmolar therapy (mannitol 1 g/kg load then 0.25 mg/kg every 6 hours). Sedatives like benzodiazepines or propofol may be used in these cases. Paralytics such as vecuronium may also be used to minimize hypertension and sympathetic tone. Barbiturate coma (pentobarbital) may be induced as a last medical measure. However, sedatives block the opportunity to follow the patient's neurological exam.

Hypertonic saline (3%), which has been more popular in recent years, is bolused at 1–4 ml/kg and continued every 6 hours. Serum osmolarity is monitored closely and should not exceed 310 mOsm/l.

Frequently, closed system subdural drains are placed temporarily following subdural hematoma evacuation. The drains are placed for the purpose of minimizing recurrence and output is monitored for quantity and character of the fluid. Ideally, the output should return to a clear, cerebrospinal fluid (CSF) appearance. Drains are usually removed by 24–48 hours to minimize infection.

Chronic SDH

Typically, patients with acute or chronic SDH are monitored in the intensive care unit for at least 24 hours following evacuation. Those with chronic subdural hematomas usually are stable enough to be moved out of an ICU setting after 24 hours and usually do not require invasive monitoring of intracranial pressure.

Patient activity and positioning

Acute SDH

Following evacuation of acute subdural hematomas from head trauma, most authors recommend that the head be elevated at 30 to 45 degrees in the neutral position. This allows for venous outflow which can help to lower ICP without compromising cerebral blood flow. Excessively tight cervical collars, tracheostomy tape, and neck turning should be avoided to prevent kinking of the venous outflow. Typical ICU supportive care is often performed, including frequent turning and aggressive pulmonary physiotherapy as needed. However, in patients with refractory, malignant elevation in ICP (over 30 mm Hg), stimulation is kept to a minimum.

Chronic SDH

Positioning following evacuation of chronic subdural hematomas is quite different. The previously chronically compressed brain may be slow to return to its normal dimensions. Patients are kept flat for at least 24 hours to allow for re-expansion of the brain and maximal obliteration of the potential subdural space. Usually, the evacuated subdural fluid is replaced by air (pneumocephalus) until the brain re-expands to reoccupy the cranial vault. In cases with a large pneumocephalus, the patients may be temporarily placed on 100% non-rebreather oxygen therapy to help decrease the intracranial air.

When out of the ICU, mobilization with physical therapy should be expedited. Extended rehabilitation may be necessary.

Alimentation

Maintenance intravenous fluids should be isotonic. Oral diet should be resumed as soon as possible. For comatose patients, enteral or parenteral nutrition should begin by the third postoperative day. Patients with isolated head injuries are significantly hypermetabolic, and their caloric needs range from 120% to 250% of normal.

It is important to note that patients with head injuries often have hyperactive sympathetic responses and should receive antacids or H_2 blockers to control gastric acid secretion.

Antibiotic coverage and other therapy

Antibiotic coverage following evacuation of subdural hematomas is commonplace, the duration and type depending on the circumstances. If a subdural drain is placed, antibiotics are often continued until the drain is removed. Standard antibiotic therapy includes nafcillin 1 g every 6 hours or ceftriaxone 1 g every 24 hours. In uncomplicated cases, postoperative coverage does not extend beyond 24 hours.

Antiepileptic medication is given in almost all cases for at least one week. The most common therapy is a phenytoin 18–20 mg/kg load intravenously followed by maintenance doses of usually 200–600 mg per day (adjusted depending on serum phenytoin levels). In patients who have seizures, the antiepileptics may be continued for a longer period.

Corticosteroids are not indicated in the setting of head trauma and are not administered to patients with subdural hematomas.

Postoperative complications

In the hospital

Recurrence of hematoma

Factors such as inadequate hemostasis during surgery, the presence of subdural air following evacuation, and the existence of bleeding disorders may predispose patients to recurrence. Recurrence is countered by strategies such as good blood pressure control, correction of coagulopathies, and the temporary placement of a closed-system subdural drain at the close of the operation.

Intracerebral hemorrhages

Some occur as a result of underlying small intraparenchymal clots that expand upon evacuation of a subdural hematoma. As the underlying brain may be significantly injured, especially in cases of acute subdural hematomas, cerebral edema is seen in many cases.

Hydrocephalus

May develop following evacuation of subdural hematomas. If the neurological examination deteriorates following evacuation of the hematoma, a follow-up CT scan is often performed to assess for new or recurrent hemorrhages or for hydrocephalus.

Seizures

Most patients do not develop epilepsy and have only one or two isolated seizures. Therapy for seizures includes a single dose of a benzodiazepine and at least a 1-week course of antiepileptic therapy.

Electrolyte imbalances

Common and may precipitate seizures. Causes of electrolyte imbalances include the syndrome of inappropriate antidiuretic hormone release (SIADH), cerebral salt wasting, or diabetes insipidus, all of which are common following head injury.

Other complications

The rate of medical complications following evacuation of chronic subdural hematomas ranges from 10% to 20%. This includes pneumonia, sepsis, gastrointestinal bleeding, and deep venous thrombosis. Many of the above complications may occur in a delayed fashion after patient discharge and are treated similarly.

After discharge

Wound infections

Occur especially in the setting of contaminated wounds. Simple scalp infections can lead to bone flap infection, intracranial abscess, or meningitis if not managed with appropriate antibiotics and/or wound revision surgery.

Delayed hydrocephalus

Some patients develop hydrocephalus after discharge from the hospital and may require the placement of a ventriculoperitoneal shunt.

Seizure activity

Most patients do not have epilepsy following subdural hematoma evacuation. However, long-term antiepileptic therapy is warranted for late post-traumatic seizures, i.e., those occurring beyond 7 days post-injury.

FURTHER READING

Andrews, B. T. *Intensive Care in Neurosurgery.* New York, NY: Thieme Medical Publishers; co-publication of Thieme and the American Association of Neurological Surgeons; 2003.

Bullock, R., Chestnut, R. M., Clifton, G. *et al. Guidelines for the Management of Severe Head Injury.* The Brain Trauma Foundation, The American Association of Neurologic Surgeons, and the Joint Section of Neurotrauma and Critical Care, 1995.

El-Kadi, H., Miele, V. J., & Kaufman, H. H. Prognosis of chronic subdural hematomas. *Neurosurg. Clin. North Am.* 2000; **11**(3): 553–576.

Nakaguchi, H., Tanishima, T., & Yoshimasu, N. Relationship between drainage catheter location and postoperative recurrence of chronic subdural hematoma after burr-hole irrigation and closed-system drainage. *J. Neurosurg.* 2000; **93**(5): 791–795.

Rohde, V., Graf, G., & Hassler, W. Complications of burr-hole craniostomy and closed-system drainage for chronic subdural hematomas: a retrospective analysis of 376 patients. *Neurosurg. Rev.* 2002; (1–2): 89–94.

Tindall, G. T., Payne, N. S., & O'Brien, M. S. Complications of surgery for subdural hematoma. *Clin. Neurosurg.* 1976; **23**: 465–482.

Wilberger, J. E., Jr., Harris, M., & Diamond, D. L. Acute subdural hematomas: morbidity, mortality, and operative timing. *J. Neurosurg.* 1991; **74**(2): 212–218.

97

Stereotactic procedures

Michele M. Johnson and Robert E. Gross

Emory University School of Medicine, Atlanta, GA

As in all fields of surgery, the current trend in neurosurgery is towards less invasive procedures and the shorter hospital stays that result from them. Therefore, stereotactic techniques are an indispensable tool for the modern neurosurgeon and have been dramatically improved by the recent revolution in digital image guidance technology. These techniques provide a relatively straightforward, accurate, and safe method to approach intracranial targets that are defined by either anatomical or functional characteristics. Anatomically defined targets include brain tumors and abscesses as well as other structural lesions. Targeting for anatomical disorders relies entirely on patient-specific anatomy derived from radiographs (e.g., ventriculography) or tomograms (e.g., CT, MRI) for localization. Functionally defined structures include the various nuclei of the basal ganglia and thalamus that are targeted for pain and movement disorders (e.g., Parkinson's disease, essential tremor, and dystonia), as well as other conditions. Targeting for functional disorders combines computerized imaging with intraoperative electrophysiological mapping for localization.

Stereotactic brain biopsy – which is purely diagnostic and does not allow for tumor resection – has been used increasingly during the past decade to aid in the diagnosis and treatment of intracranial lesions, providing a definitive pathologic diagnosis in more than 90% of the patients with a low associated morbidity. On the day of operation, the patient undergoes a contrast-enhanced imaging study (MRI or CT) following the attachment to the cranium of the stereotactic base ring and localizer under local anesthesia and sedation. In the operating room, again using local anesthesia with light sedation, the cranium is entered using a twist drill and a small hole is made through which the biopsy is performed. The procedure is markedly facilitated by the use of neuronavigational computer workstations and can even be done using frameless

navigational technology. Generally, immediate feedback from an experienced neuropathologist is obtained from the initial specimen prior to the completion of the procedure. Therapeutic measures may also be performed simultaneously, such as aspiration of a cyst or abscess with possible instillation of antibiotics for abscesses or interstitial brachytherapy for specific tumors. The procedure typically lasts less than an hour, after which the patient is transferred to the postanesthesia care unit. Prior to leaving the unit, a postoperative computerized tomogram (CT) scan is performed in order to check for hemorrhage.

Stereotactic ablation and deep brain stimulator electrode implantation in the basal ganglia and thalamus have been used to alleviate pain as well as the symptoms of Parkinson's disease and other movement disorders. These procedures are for symptomatic relief to improve the patient's quality of life, but are not curative. Targeting of the contralateral internal segment of the globus pallidus, subthalamic nucleus, and thalamus has been approved for Parkinson's disease and other movement disorders. Overall, deep brain stimulation is a nondestructive and reversible procedure as it produces a functional rather than a structural lesion when compared with ablative procedures such as thalamotomy or pallidotomy. As with brain biopsies, the patient arrives on the day of operation and undergoes a CT or MRI after the stereotactic base ring and localizer are applied; some centers perform stereotactic ventriculography. The operative procedure is done under local anesthesia in the operating room. The cranium is entered through a burr hole in the pre-coronal region. Trajectory selection to avoid veins is important; some surgeons attempt to avoid penetration of the ventricles as well, although this is not critical. The initial path to the anatomical target is localized by identifying its spatial coordinates in a stereotactic atlas, and proceeds by correlating this point with patient-specific anatomy

Medical Management of the Surgical Patient: A Textbook of Perioperative Medicine, ed. M. F. Lubin, R. B. Smith, T. F. Dobson, N. Spell, H. K. Walker. 4th edn. Published by Cambridge University Press. © Cambridge University 2006.

derived from the preoperative MRI. The target is expressed as a set of intraoperative stereotactic coordinates. After opening the dura, electrodes are passed to the initial target to perform intraoperative electrophysiological confirmation while the patient is awake. Fine adjustments to the initial position are performed as necessary. After this is completed, the target is either ablated using radiofrequency electrocoagulation (e.g., thalamotomy, pallidotomy) or a deep brain stimulator electrode is implanted. Test stimulation is performed to assess symptom relief and to evaluate the threshold for adverse effects. This procedure takes several hours. The pulse generator for the implanted electrode is implanted on the ipsilateral chest wall just below the clavicle, either on the same day or later. The extension wire is tunneled subcutaneously and connected to the pulse generator with excess wire placed under the scalp. The patient is then placed under general anesthesia for implantation of the pulse generator. Postoperatively, the subject is transferred to the postanesthesia care unit, where a postoperative MRI scan is performed to rule out intracerebral hemorrhage prior to being transferred to the floor. Similar procedures are performed for functional disorders other than Parkinson's disease.

Usual postoperative course

Expected postoperative hospital stay
1 to 2 days.

Operative mortality
Less than 1%.

Special monitoring required
If the patient is monitored in the postanesthesia care unit for 1–4 hours with a postoperative scan reviewed prior to transfer to the floor, ICU observation is usually unnecessary.

Patient activity and positioning
Initially, the head of the bed is elevated to 30 degrees. Patients may get out of bed as soon as possible. Physical therapy is instituted if required.

Alimentation
A full, regular diet is provided as soon as possible.

Antibiotic coverage
Typically, intravenous antibiotics are given intraoperatively and 24 hours postoperatively.

Medications
Parkinson's disease medications are held after midnight if the pulse generator is to be programmed the following day.

Postoperative radiographic tests
Postoperative brain computed tomographic scan or magnetic resonance image in the postanesthesia care unit prior to transfer to floor.

Postoperative complications

In the hospital

Development of a focal neurologic deficit
This complication may be related to hemorrhage, edema, or infarction. The diagnosis is confirmed by an emergent head computed tomographic scan. A potentially life-threatening complication, hemorrhage usually results from bleeding along the surgical pathway and can lead to formation of an intracranial hematoma. In addition, bleeding may occur into the subdural, epidural, or subgaleal spaces. Selected hematomas or subdural or epidural collections may require surgical evacuation or placement of an external ventricular drainage system. Cerebral edema (swelling of the brain) may result from surgical manipulation of the brain parenchyma. Treatment includes hyperventilation, hyperosmolar therapy, furosemide, and possible placement of an intracranial pressure monitoring device or external ventricular drainage system. Cerebral infarction is potentially lethal if the arterial supply to the brain is compromised, placing that particular brain tissue at risk. An extensive infarction may also occur if venous drainage is interrupted or occluded. Care is taken to control blood pressure, volume status, and oxygenation to maintain cerebral perfusion pressure.

Seizure
A seizure that occurs intraoperatively or in the immediate postoperative period may lead to increased intracranial pressure. Thus, antiepileptic medications should be given immediately to stop the seizure, followed by routine maintenance doses for approximately 3 to 6 months. An emergent head computed tomographic scan should be performed to rule out possible intracranial pathology such as hemorrhage, though seizures can result from intracranial air.

Neuroleptic malignant syndrome
Parkinson's disease patients undergo operations in the "off medication" condition, which can be associated with a typical neuroleptic malignant syndrome. This must be

recognized early and is treated with anti-parkinsonian medication, fluid resuscitation, and/or dantrolene, as necessary.

After discharge

Infection

Infections may be superficial or deep. Skin erosions or cellulitis may be treated with appropriate oral or intravenous antibiotics, but severe infections may also require surgical debridement. Although rare, deep septic contamination may cause such potentially life-threatening complications as meningitis, cerebritis, intracerebral abscess, or subdural or epidural empyema. Treatment includes i.v. antibiotics, surgical debridement for abscesses, and possible hardware removal.

Sterile subcutaneous fluid collections

Postoperative subcutaneous fluid collections can occur weeks to months after surgery from CSF leaks or seromas. CSF leaks require surgical repair, and one should be suspicious of hydrocephalus in such cases. Sterile seromas may be drained by needle aspiration and seldom require surgical intervention.

Other device-related or stimulation-related deep brain stimulation complications

Hardware failure may be due to electrode or extension wire breaks, migration of the electrode, or pulse generator malfunction, which can be evaluated and repaired surgically. Adverse effects related to the stimulated target and its vicinity are common but expected. Stimulation of the internal segment of the globus pallidus may induce visual field disturbance, paresthesia, muscle contractions, confusion, and depression; stimulation of the thalamus may provoke paresthesia, muscle cramps, decreased fine motor skills, dysarthria, dizziness, and balance disturbances; and stimulation of the subthalamic nucleus may generate dyskinesia, dysarthria, paresthesia, eyelid-opening apraxia, hemiballismus, confusion, and changes in mental status. In the vast majority of instances, careful adjustments of stimulation parameters and reduction in medications will reverse these side effects.

FURTHER READING

Berstein, M. & Parrent, A. G. Complications of CT-guided stereotactic biopsy of intra-axial brain lesions. *J. Neurosurg.* 1994; **81**: 165–168.

Bhardwaj, R. D. & Bernstein, M. Prospective feasibility study of outpatient stereotactic brain lesion biopsy. *Neurosurgery* 2002; **51**: 358–364.

Hariz, M. I. Complications of deep brain stimulation surgery. *Mov. Disord.* 2002; **17**(3): S162–S166.

Higuchi, Y. & Iacono, R. P. Surgical complications in patients with Parkinson's disease after posteroventral pallidotomy. *Neurosurgery* 2003; **52**(3): 558–571.

Kulkarni, A. V., Guha, V., Lozano, A., & Bernstein, M. Incidence of silent hemorrhage and delayed deterioration after stereotactic brain biopsy. *J. Neurosurg.* 1998; **89**: 31–35.

Terao, T., Takahashi, H., Yokochi, F., Taniguchi, M., Okiyama, R., & Hamada, I. Hemorrhagic complication of stereotactic surgery in patients with movement disorders. *J. Neurosurg.* 2003; **98**: 1241–1246.

Umemura, A., Jaggi, J. L., Hurtig, H. I. *et al.* Deep brain stimulation for movement disorders: morbidity and mortality in 109 patients. *J. Neurosurg.* 2003; **98**: 779–784.

Warnick, R. E., Longmore, L. M., Paul, C. A., & Bode, L. A. Postoperative management of patients after stereotactic biopsy: results of a survey of the AANS/CNS section on tumors and a single institution. *J. Neuro-oncol.* 2003; **62**: 289–296.

98

Transsphenoidal surgery

Nelson M. Oyesiku

Emory University School of Medicine, Atlanta, GA

Transsphenoidal surgery is the preferred mode of therapy for most pituitary tumors. Tumors of the pituitary gland generally present with clinical findings related to an endocrinopathy or mass effect. Symptoms of endocrinopathy include the Forbes–Albright syndrome (amenorrhea–galactorrhea), infertility, and decreased libido from hyperprolactinemia; acromegaly (Marie's disease) or gigantism from excessive growth hormone (GH); and Cushing's disease from excessive adrenocorticotropic hormone (ACTH) resulting in hypercortisolism. Symptoms of mass effect include visual deficits, cranial nerve palsies, hypopituitarism, headaches, or rarely, obstructive hydrocephalus or hypothalamic dysfunction. Tumors causing mechanical compression are usually hormonally inactive. Diagnosis is made by history, clinical examination, laboratory tests, and neuroimaging (MRI). Several therapeutic options are available, including pharmacotherapy, radiotherapy, and surgery. The goal of treatment is to return hormone secretion to normal, remove the tumor and correct any mass effect.

Pharmacotherapy

Pharmacotherapy is a therapeutic option for functional tumors. Bromocriptine (Parlodel) and cabergoline (Dostinex), both oral dopamine agonists, are the primary options for prolactinomas. These drugs shrink prolactinomas in approximately 80% of patients, but they are tumorostatic rather than tumoricidal. If therapy is withdrawn, the tumor resumes growth; therefore, therapy is typically lifelong. Another disadvantage is that these drugs may cause tumor fibrosis, which reduces surgical cure rates, especially if patients take them for more than one year. Side effects include nausea, dizziness, headaches, and postural hypotension. For acromegaly, the drug options include bromocriptine or cabergoline, the somatostatin analogues octreotide (Sandostatin) or lanreotide (Somatuline), and the GH analogue pegvisomant (Somavert). Bromocriptine has been used with some success in acromegaly, but it is less effective than the somatostatin analogues. Octreotide is given subcutaneously (s.c.) three times a day or monthly intramuscularly (Sandostatin LAR, depot). Lanreotide (Somatuline LA) is available both as an intramuscular injection given every 7 to 14 days, or monthly depot. Octreotide and lanreotide reduce growth hormone levels to $<5\,\mathrm{mU/l}$ in $>50\%$ of patients, improving symptoms and sometimes shrinking the tumor. They are indicated for long-term maintenance therapy with inadequate response to surgery or radiation or if surgical resection is contraindicated. Drawbacks include cost, discomfort at the site, nausea, abdominal discomfort, flatulence, diarrhea, gallstones, hypo- or hyperglycemia. Pegvisomant is a new drug that is a recombinant GH analogue and a GH receptor antagonist. When given in daily s.c. doses, 97% of patients achieve a normal IGF-1 level during one year of treatment, accompanied by clinical improvement. Side effects include liver function abnormalities, pain, flu-like syndrome, diarrhea, nausea, and a rise in GH that could potentially increase the size of a tumor.

For Cushing's disease, drug therapy includes: steroid biosynthesis inhibitors (ketoconazole, metyrapone, mitotane, aminoglutethimide), neuromodulators (bromocriptine, cyproheptadine, valproic acid, octreotide), and glucocorticoid receptor antagonists (mifepristone, RU 486). Ketoconazole decreases cortisol, but side effects include headache, sedation, nausea and vomiting, hepatoxicity, gynecomastia, decreased libido, and impotence. Cyproheptadine decreases ACTH secretion and cortisol in 30%–50% of patients. It is poorly tolerated with side effects including somnolence, hyperphagia, weight gain, vomiting, hepatoxicity, gynecomastia, decreased libido, and impotence.

Medical Management of the Surgical Patient: A Textbook of Perioperative Medicine, ed. M. F. Lubin, R. B. Smith, T. F. Dobson, N. Spell, H. K. Walker. 4th edn. Published by Cambridge University Press. © Cambridge University 2006.

Radiotherapy

Radiotherapy (conventional external-beam therapy, fractionated stereotactic radiotherapy or stereotactic radiosurgery) is used for treatment of recurrent functional or non-secretory tumors or tumors invading the cavernous sinus. Stereotactic radiosurgery (linear accelerator or gamma-knife) is preferable to conventional external therapy when the tumor configuration relative to the chiasm and optic nerves is favorable. With radiosurgery, normalization of urine free cortisol occurs in about 50%–66% patients with Cushing's disease within 3–38 months. In acromegaly, 20%–30% of patients have GH and IGF1 levels in the normal range with a latency of 10–38 months. Prolactinomas rarely require radiotherapy. Hypopituitarism is the most common side effect of pituitary irradiation with an incidence of 13%–56%.

Surgery

Surgery is performed via the trans-sphenoidal approach in the majority of cases. Indications include: functional microadenomas for which pharmacotherapy is undesirable or ineffective; non-functional macroadenomas and other tumors of the pituitary region exhibiting mass effect that are not amenable to pharmacotherapy; tumors associated with cerebrospinal fluid rhinorrhea; tumors with extension into the sphenoid sinus or bone; cerebrospinal fluid fistulas involving the sphenoid sinus; and biopsy and excision of any lesion in the sphenoid and parasellar areas, including chordoma, nasopharyngeal carcinoma, and sphenoid mucocele or abscess.

Sellar and suprasellar tumors can be removed from the trans-sphenoidal approach by a sublabial, transseptal, or direct endonasal approach using the endoscope or microscope. Some surgeons insert a lumbar drain and instill saline to help bring down the suprasellar extension. C-arm radiographs or MRI image-guidance may be used to orient the surgeon intraoperatively. Relative contraindications to trans-sphenoidal surgery include: infectious process involving the sphenoid sinus; a dumbbell tumor, with narrowing at the junction of the sellar and suprasellar portions; a tumor with a large parasellar extension; and occasionally an extremely fibrous tumor. Trans-sphenoidal surgery is well tolerated in the treatment of most pituitary tumors. General anesthesia is required and the supine or semi-sitting position is used. The duration of the procedure ranges from 1–3 hours, depending on the size of the tumor and the experience of the surgeon. One unit of blood is ordinarily available for transfusion, but is rarely used. In most cases this is an elective procedure. If the patient is significantly hyper- or hypothyroid or hypocortisolemic preoperatively, surgery is usually delayed until the patient can begin thyroid or hydrocortisone replacement therapy. If vision loss is rapid or the adenoma is associated with hemorrhage or abscess, more urgent surgical treatment is needed. Transcranial approaches are preferred in patients with significant intracranial extension of pituitary tumors to the subfrontal, retrochiasmatic, or middle fossa regions.

In transsphenoidal surgery for prolactinomas, the results depend on tumor size and prolactin level. The higher the PRL level, the lower the chance of normalizing serum PRL. In experienced hands, surgery corrects PRL levels in 80% of patients with a serum PRL less than 250 ng/ml. In Cushing's disease remission is achieved in 70%–94% of patients with microadenomas and in 45%–58% of patients with macroadenomas; recurrence occurs in 2%–13% and 5%–20% of cases will have negative explorations where no adenoma is found. In patients with acromegaly, 60% with macroadenomas achieve a GH <5 ng/ml and 70%–80% of patients with microadenomas achieve a GH <5 ng/ml.

Usual postoperative course

Expected postoperative hospital stay
3–4 days.

Operative mortality rate
<0.5%.

Special monitoring required
Fluid balance, CSF rhinorrhea.

Patient activity and positioning
Coughing, sneezing, and blowing the nose are discouraged. A nasal decongestant is usually prescribed as needed to treat symptoms of congestion.

Alimentation
Clear liquids after surgery and food intake is advanced as tolerated.

Antibiotic coverage
Nafcillin 1 g intravenously is given just prior to operation.

Corticosteroid therapy
Patients are given perioperative corticosteroids to forestall adrenal insufficiency. Supplemental steroid therapy is continued until the second postoperative day and then

held that afternoon; an AM fasting cortisol level is drawn the next morning. Continuation of steroid therapy is based on laboratory data.

Postoperative complications

Significant complications from transsphenoidal surgery are not common. The incidence of rhinorrhea is about 5%. Approximately 10% of patients develop transient diabetes insipidus (DI); however, permanent DI is uncommon. Approximately 10% of patients have partial worsening of their hormone function. The chances of visual loss, stroke, and death are less than 1%.

In the hospital

Persistent diabetes insipidus

A likelihood for patients whose urinary output exceeds 300 ml/h and whose urine specific gravity levels are <1.010. The diagnosis is confirmed by measurement of serum sodium (>146 meq/l), serum osmolality (>300 mOsm/l), and urinary osmolality (<100 mOsm/l). Treatment consists of intramuscular or subcutaneous aqueous vasopressin (Pitressin; 5 U is the usual adult dose), which may be repeated as needed until homeostasis recovers. If DI persists, intranasal desamino D-arginine vasopressin (DDAVP) may be administered after discharge from the hospital.

Cerebrospinal fluid rhinorrhea

An uncommon complication. It can be treated successfully by a lumbar drain or, rarely, reoperation. If the condition is left untreated, meningitis may result.

After discharge

Delayed cerebrospinal fluid leak

Requires readmission to the hospital for lumbar drainage or reoperation.

Acute or chronic adrenal insufficiency

May occur from failure to take maintenance medications or to increase the dosage during periods of illness or stress.

FURTHER READING

Alleyne, C. H. Jr., Barrow, D. L., & Oyesiku N. M. Combined transsphenoidal and pterional craniotomy approach to giant pituitary tumors. *Surg. Neurol.* 2002; **57**: 380–390.

Ciric, I. Long-term management and outcome for pituitary tumors. *Neurosurg. Clin. North Am.* 2003; **14**(1): 167–171.

Liu, J. K., Weiss M. H., & Couldwell, W. T. Surgical approaches to pituitary tumors. *Neurosurg. Clin. North Am.* 2003; **14**(1): 93–107.

Oyesiku, N. M. & Tindall, G. T. Endocrine-Inactive adenomas: surgical results and prognosis. In Landolt, A. M., Vance, M. L., & Reilly, P. L., eds. *Pituitary Adenomas.* New York: Churchill-Livingstone, 1996: 377–383.

Oyesiku, N. M. & Tindall, G. T. Management of hypersecreting pituitary tumors. In Tindall, G. T., Cooper, P. R., & Barrow, D. L., eds. *The Practice of Neurosurgery.* Baltimore: Williams & Wilkins, 1996: 1135–1152.

Petrovich, Z., Jozsef, G., Yu, C., & Apuzzo M. L. Radiotherapy and stereotactic radiosurgery for pituitary tumors. *Neurosurg. Clin. North Am.* 2003; **14**(1): 147–166.

Singer, P. A. & Sevilla, L. J. Postoperative endocrine management of pituitary tumors. *Neurosurg. Clin. North Am.* 2003; **14**(1): 123–138.

Vance, M. L. Medical treatment of functional pituitary tumors. *Neurosurg. Clin. North Am.* 2003; **14**(1): 81–87.

99

Treatment of herniated disk

Maxwell Boakye and Regis W. Haid, Jr.

Emory University School of Medicine, Atlanta, GA

Herniated disks usually occur in the cervical and lumbar spine. The thoracic spine is relatively non-mobile and thus rarely affected by disk herniations. Herniated disks typically occur in younger patients between ages 30 and 50 years and present primarily with appendicular pain (arm, leg) as opposed to axial pain (neck, back). Cervical and thoracic disks may present with myelopathy but more commonly with radiculopathy. Ninety percent of patients with disk herniation obtain relief with conservative treatment. Herniated disks are initial manifestations of the continuum of degenerative disk disease later manifested by development of osteophytes.

Cervical level

Patients with cervical disk herniation typically come to operation because of arm and periscapular pain, often with weakness, numbness, or paresthesias in a nerve root distribution. Since the majority of patients improve with non-surgical therapeutic options such as cervical collar, active rest, and physical therapy, patients should be considered for operation only if they have failed a reasonable trial of conservative therapy.

Central disk herniations are treated via an anterior approach. Foraminal disk herniations can be treated by either an anterior or posterior cervical approach. Anterior cervical diskectomy and fusion is the most common procedure performed for cervical disk herniations. After cervical diskectomy the disk space may be replaced with allograft or autograft. Studies have shown that using allograft leads to fusion in approximately 90% of patients. Addition of a cervical plating system increases the fusion rate to 96%. Although adding a plating system raises the cost of the operation, it allows for faster return to work and obviates the use of a postoperative collar.

Anterior cervical diskectomy

Patients are placed supine after general endotracheal intubation has been established. An incision is made that typically extends from the midline to the anterior border of the sternocleidomastoid muscle. The medial border of the sternocleidomastoid muscle is identified and the adjacent fascial plane is developed. The carotid sheath is retracted laterally, the esophagus and trachea are retracted medially, and the prevertebral fascia is dissected. Radiographs are then taken to confirm the level of interest and the disk is removed with curettes and rongeurs. Decompression of the spinal cord and nerve root is accomplished. The choice of graft material is selected and placed. Plating may be added. If a decision is made to use autograft, an incision should be made in the anterior iliac crest approximately two fingerbreadths lateral to the anterior superior iliac spine. The dissection is carried to the bone and the graft is removed using a double oscillating saw and bone cutter. The graft site is then closed.

Posterior cervical diskectomy and foraminotomy

The posterior cervical diskectomy and foraminotomy procedure is indicated for patients with foraminal disk herniation. Cervical foraminotomy may be performed for patients with foraminal disk herniation or for patients with cervical spondylosis and foraminal osteophytes or narrowing. Patients with lateral or foraminal disk herniations will require diskectomy in addition to foraminotomy. Posterior diskectomy/foraminotomy is done under general anesthesia with the patient in a prone position and the head supported in a Mayfield clamp. The incision is made midline and the fascia and muscle are stripped laterally until the facet is exposed. Radiographs are taken. High-speed drills/Kerrison rongeurs are used to perform a foraminotomy and to expose the nerve

Medical Management of the Surgical Patient: A Textbook of Perioperative Medicine, ed. M. F. Lubin, R. B. Smith, T. F. Dobson, N. Spell, H. K. Walker. 4th edn. Published by Cambridge University Press. © Cambridge University 2006.

root. The herniated fragment is then removed following gentle mobilization of the nerve root. This procedure can be done by means of a minimally invasive approach using a tubular retractor, which splits the muscle and precludes the muscle trauma that accompanies muscle stripping in the open approach. The disk is removed through the retractor using specially designed microinstruments.

Usual postoperative course

Expected postoperative hospital stay
1 to 2 days.

Operative mortality
Rare.

Special monitoring required
None.

Patient activity and positioning
Patients can be out of bed ambulating as soon as tolerated. Postoperative X-rays are needed if grafting and plating are performed.

Alimentation
Diet is advanced as tolerated.

Antibiotic coverage
Typically for 12–24 hours.

Follow-up
For anterior cervical diskectomy with fusion, follow-up is necessary for 1 to 2 years to evaluate fusion.

Postoperative complications

In the hospital

Spinal cord or nerve root injury
May occur during disk removal or from graft placement. Risk of injury can be minimized by careful removal of the disk and posterior longitudinal ligament. In addition, the selected bone graft should be shorter than the depth of the disk space. Graft retropulsion may cause cord injury, which may be avoided by selecting an appropriate graft size and gently tapping the graft into the disk space.

Vertebral artery injury
May result from aggressive lateral dissection or aggressive foraminotomies, particularly in patients with aberrant vertebral arteries. If an injury occurs, the bleeding should be stopped, an angiogram performed to assess the situation, and a decision made as to whether the artery may need to be occluded endovascularly. If the bleeding cannot be arrested, the artery should be repaired intraoperatively.

Wound hematoma
Usually attributable to inadequate intraoperative hemostasis, especially in patients with history of aspirin use, occult bleeding disorder, or functional platelet disorder. Large symptomatic hematomas require emergent reexploration and evacuation of the clot. Using a postoperative drain may reduce the risk of postoperative hematoma.

Recurrent laryngeal nerve injury
This complication leads to ipsilateral vocal cord dysfunction and usually occurs as a result of retraction or dissection with the thermal cautery. Symptoms include hoarseness, dysphagia, and vocal cord fatigue.

Carotid artery injury
May result from retraction and manipulation and occurs rarely when the procedure is performed by an experienced neurosurgeon.

Cerebrospinal fluid fistula
May be difficult to repair intraoperatively, but is generally treated with the application of a fat or muscle graft and fibrin glue with or without postoperative lumbar drainage.

Esophageal or tracheal injury
Caused by retraction or from failure to adequately protect the esophagus during bovie dissection. If this complication is recognized intraoperatively, the esophagus should be repaired. Delayed injuries may manifest as odynophagia, dysphagia, and mediastinitis, and should be evaluated urgently by an otolaryngologist.

Airway compromise
More likely in obese patients and may be a result of wound hematoma or laryngeal edema. This complication should be recognized promptly and the patient should be reintubated immediately. A CT scan and/or MRI of the patient's cervical spine should be obtained emergently.

After discharge

Diskitis, graft infection, osteomyelitis
When these complications occur, appropriate radiological studies should be obtained and the wound should be

re-explored. Grafts may be removed and the patient should be treated with 6 to 12 weeks of intravenous antibiotics.

Graft extrusion, screw pullout, and plate abnormalities

These abnormalities typically present with dysphagia and require revision of the graft and/or plate.

Pseudoarthrosis

When pseudoarthrosis occurs, there may be a return or increase of preoperative symptoms, particularly neck pain. The graft may need to be revised. In addition, redo of anterior or posterior cervical fusion may be required.

Donor site infection

Iliac crest graft site infection should be re-explored, irrigated, washed out, and treated with 2 to 12 weeks of intravenous antibiotics.

Thoracic level

Patients with thoracic disk herniations may present with back pain, radicular pain, or myelopathy. Individuals with back pain should be treated conservatively. Those with radicular pain and intercostal neuralgia may benefit from a trial of intercostal nerve blocks. Since surgical approaches for thoracic disk are fairly major procedures with potential for blood loss and higher morbidity, surgery is indicated only in patients with progressive neurological deficit, myelopathy, or resistant, severe radicular pain. Surgical options include transpedicular, costotransversectomy, and transthoracic approaches. Minimally invasive methods using thoracoscopic techniques have also been successfully utilized. Transthoracic approaches require postoperative chest tube drainage.

Lumbar level

Patients with lumbar disk herniations typically present with buttock and leg pain. Weakness or paresthesias may also be present. Treatment involves lumbar diskectomy, microdiskectomy, or endoscopic microdiskectomy. Microdiskectomy utilizes the operating microscope, a smaller incision, and minimal bony removal. Both procedures require general anesthesia. The patient is placed in the prone position supported on an appropriate frame. A small midline incision is made and dissection is carried down to the spinous process. The fascia and paravertebral muscle are stripped off the spinous process and the lamina above and below the disk space exposed. Radiographs are obtained to confirm the level of interest. A hemilaminotomy is performed, ligament of flavum removed, and the nerve root identified and retracted medially. A rectangular incision is made in the disk and the disk is removed.

Recently, microendoscopic approaches for the removal of lumbar herniated disks have been described. The microdiskectomy is performed via a tubular retractor that splits the muscle, causing less muscle trauma and postoperative pain and possibly shorter hospital stays. A microscope or endoscope is used to visualize the disk and nerve root via the tubular retractor, which is docked on the lamina of interest after dilating to an adequate tube size. Specially designed microsurgical instruments are then used to remove the herniated disk. Large lumbar disk herniations may present with cauda equina syndrome with urinary retention and saddle anesthesia in addition to pain and weakness. These should be treated emergently using a larger laminectomy at the level of disk herniation.

Usual postoperative course

Expected postoperative hospital stay
1 to 2 days.

Operative mortality
Rare.

Special monitoring required
Unnecessary.

Patient activity and positioning
Advancement of ambulation as tolerated. No X-rays or brace is needed.

Alimentation
No restriction.

Antibiotic coverage
Typically for 12–24 hours.

Postoperative complications

In the hospital

Hematoma
May present with cauda equina syndrome and require prompt recognition and evacuation.

Diskitis/wound infection
This complication requires a CT scan/MRI to evaluate the disk space and to rule out bony involvement. The wound

should be re-explored and washed out. Wound cultures should be performed and the patient treated for 6 to 12 weeks with intravenous antibiotics appropriate to the offending organisms. The patient should be followed with serological tests such as erythrocyte sedimentation rate (ESR) and complement reactive protein (CRP).

Cerebrospinal fluid injury

This type of injury should be repaired intraoperatively. If it occurs postoperatively, an attempt can be made to treat the injury with flat bed-rest and lumbar drainage; however, the most effective method is to re-explore the wound and repair the leak as there is an increased risk of meningitis, arachnoiditis, and low-pressure head aches if the leak persists.

Nerve root injury

Should be avoided with careful dissection and gentle retraction during disk removal.

Vascular injury

Blood vessel injury may result from aggressive disk removal, violation of the anterior longitudinal ligament, and overzealous curettage of the anterior disk space with pituitary rongeurs. Most vascular injuries that occur with L4/5 diskectomies may be recognized intraoperatively by sudden blood in the operative field or the development of hemodynamic shock. This complication may also manifest early postoperatively, since bleeding can be concealed in the retroperitoneal space. Some patients may present years later with a persistent arteriovenous fistula. When the injury is recognized, emergent vascular surgery consultation should be obtained as the patient must be stabilized and prepared for an emergency laparotomy.

Recurrent disk herniations

While uncommon, this complication may occur and will require a second procedure and/or fusion.

Arachnoiditis

Develops as a complication of surgery, prior contrast injection, lumbar punctures, or cerebrospinal fluid leak. It is difficult to treat and reoperation is frequently ineffective.

Complications of surgical positioning

Compressive neuropathies of the peroneal and ulnar nerves result from difficulties in surgical positioning. Therefore, special care should be taken to ensure that elbows are padded and that there is no excessive pressure on the peroneal nerve during the operative procedure.

FURTHER READING

Anand, N. & Regan, J. J. Video-assisted thoracoscopic surgery for thoracic disc disease: classification and outcome study of 100 consecutive cases with a 2-year minimum follow-up period. *Spine* 2002; **27**: 871–879.

Daneyemez, M., Sali, A., Kahraman, S. *et al.* Outcome analyses in 1072 surgically treated lumbar disc herniations. *Minim. Invas. Neurosurg.* 1999; **42**: 63–68.

Kotilainen, E., Valtonen, S., & Carlson, C. A. Microsurgical treatment of lumbar disc herniation: follow-up of 237 patients. *Acta Neurochir. (Wien)* 1993; **120**: 143–149.

Moore, A. J., Chilton, J. D., & Uttley, D. Long-term results of micro-lumbar discectomy. *Br. J. Neurosurg.* 1994; **8**: 319–326.

Mummaneni, P. V., Rodts, G. E., Subach, B. R. *et al.* Management of thoracic disc disease. *Contemp. Neurosurg.* 2002; **23**(22): 1–8.

Perez-Cruet, M. J., Foley, K. T., Isaacs, R. E. *et al.* Microendoscopic lumbar discectomy: technical note. *Neurosurgery* 2002; **51**: 129–136.

Rosenthal, D. & Dickman, C. A. Thoracoscopic microsurgical excision of herniated thoracic discs. *J. Neurosurg.* 1998; **89**: 224–235.

Stillerman, C. B., Chen, T. C., Couldwell, W. T. *et al.* Experience in the surgical management of 82 symptomatic herniated thoracic discs and review of the literature. *J. Neurosurg.* 1998; **88**: 623–633.

Ophthalmic surgery

100

General considerations in ophthalmic surgery

Enrique Garcia-Valenzuela, G. Baker Hubbard, III, and Thomas M. Aaberg, Sr.

Emory University School of Medicine, Atlanta, GA

Numerous types of surgical intervention can be performed in the treatment of diseases of the eye and its adnexa. Owing to the great degree of technical skill required to execute these interventions, subspecialists perform a significant portion of ophthalmic surgeries. Microsurgery is involved in all procedures and most of the operations are limited to intervention into the eye and orbit with minimal risk to other organs. Ophthalmic surgery offers a high probability of success with a major positive impact on the quality of life. However, many patients with eye pathology are elderly and some have significant systemic illness, so the risk of elective intervention must be balanced against expected benefits. Optimal preoperative management of medical problems can make surgery safer and minimize patient discomfort.

Anesthesia

The large majority of ophthalmic interventions can be performed under local anesthesia with intravenous sedation. In some cases, even topical anesthetics are sufficient. Ophthalmic surgeries that require general anesthesia are those that involve significant extraocular manipulation in regions where a local anesthetic is not effective, and those that are prolonged as occurs in many vitreoretinal and orbital procedures as well as some cosmetic operations. General anesthesia is also indicated in younger patients and individuals who may not remain motionless during surgery and trauma cases with significant ocular laceration where administration of local anesthetics may raise intraorbital pressure with consequent extrusion of intraocular contents.

Several choices exist in the route of administration of local ophthalmic anesthesia for intraocular surgery. The most widely used approach is injection of 3 to 7 ml of a mixture of lidocaine and bupivocaine through a retrobulbar approach using a blunted needle (Atkinson needle) with or without a regional seventh nerve block to paralyze eyelid closure. While the incidence is small, the risks of local ophthalmic anesthesia can have significant consequences, including local damage through retrobulbar hemorrhage, extraocular muscle injury, or penetration of the globe or optic nerve, with the most serious complication being systemic damage through intravascular or subarachnoid injection of the anesthetic that can lead to hypertension, seizures, apnea, or death.

Musculoskeletal problems

Ophthalmic procedures require the patient to be comfortably motionless in a supine position. Many patients in need of eye surgery are elderly, some of whom may have associated ailments of the bones and joints that interfere with their ability to remain still for any length of time. Similarly, patients with nervous system diseases that cause involuntary movements or tremors may require more than local anesthetics. Depending on the patient and the situation, there are three standard choices of insuring stillness: increased use of sedatives and analgesics, an adjustment in the usual supine position, or general anesthesia.

Ventilation under anesthesia

Supplemental oxygen is usually administered during all ophthalmic procedures through nasal prongs or a mask. However, the combination of lying supine covered with surgical drapes and the natural anxiety from undergoing surgery may result in the perception of dyspnea during the operation. Ensuring that patients who suffer from true dyspnea or orthopnea are in the best possible ventilatory state is a major issue to be addressed prior to surgery.

Medical Management of the Surgical Patient: A Textbook of Perioperative Medicine, ed. M. F. Lubin, R. B. Smith, T. F. Dobson, N. Spell, H. K. Walker. 4th edn. Published by Cambridge University Press. © Cambridge University 2006.

Elective procedures may need to be postponed until severe chronic obstructive pulmonary disease, respiratory infections, congestive heart failure, or other major medical illnesses are optimally treated. Coughing spasms during ocular surgery increase venous pressure and may lead to intraocular hemorrhage in an eye that is open to atmospheric pressure, resulting in prolapse of intraocular tissues and blindness.

Patient cooperation

When using local anesthesia, ophthalmic operations rely on the strictest patient cooperation. When deciding between local and general anesthesia, every patient's potential for anxiety as well as the effect of any psychological disorder or psychiatric dysfunction need to be considered. The patient's internist may have valuable insight into this matter.

Arterial hypertension

Patients with known systemic arterial hypertension should take their oral antihypertensive medications on the morning of surgery. In spite of compliance with their medications, chronic hypertensive patients can experience acute elevation of their blood pressure during ophthalmic surgery that may result from normal anxiety, phenylephrine eye drops used for mydriasis, or poor preoperative hypertensive control. In addition to the usual concerns about the systemic effects, an acute increase in blood pressure during eye surgery may cause intraocular hemorrhage. Such an event in an open eye susceptible to atmospheric pressure can result in complications causing blindness. Therefore, it is essential that patients having elective ophthalmic surgery be evaluated for arterial hypertension and that their therapy be optimized. Patients should be instructed to faithfully continue their daily antihypertensive medications.

Coagulation

As mentioned earlier, orbital and intraocular hemorrhages pose a serious threat to vision. Normal coagulation makes ophthalmic surgery safer. If medically feasible, patients on chronic anticoagulation and antiplatelet medications should interrupt their therapy in advance to allow for clotting parameters to return to normal prior to operation. Usually, anticoagulant medications can be resumed immediately after the procedure.

In patients who cannot interrupt anticoagulation for a period of several days, transfusion of fresh frozen plasma and other blood elements immediately prior to surgical intervention can be considered. Some ophthalmic procedures can be modified to avoid the most hemorrhage-prone steps of surgery. For example, scleral buckling surgery can be executed without trans-scleral drainage, thereby avoiding incision through the extremely vascular choroid, and cataract surgery can be performed exclusively through corneal incisions that circumvent ocular structures that are vascular. Retrobulbar anesthesia can be replaced by general anesthesia or, in some instances, by a combination of topical anesthesia and administration of retrobulbar and/or peribulbar anesthesia with a blunt cannula.

Infection

Fortunately, intraocular infection is a rare event that usually occurs within days of the operation. If the causative agent is a slow-growth bacteria or a fungus, it may not present until weeks or months later. Infection often leads to profound visual loss and even loss of the globe itself if not recognized early enough. To combat this possibility, most ophthalmologists inject subconjunctival antibiotics at the end of the procedure and prescribe prophylactic topical antibiotics during the early postoperative period.

Intraocular infections are typically treated with intravitreous antibiotics and, when severe, with vitrectomy as well. Since most systemic antibiotics do not achieve significant intraocular concentration they are usually not administered, unless the ocular infection is associated with a systemic infectious origin. It is unlikely that intraocular surgery and even infection will cause significant bacteremia and associated fever. Intraocular surgery also does not require prophylactic systemic antibiotics to prevent endocarditis.

Ophthalmic medications

Dilation of the pupil is usually required prior to intraocular surgery. A combination of a topical sympathomimetic such as phenylephrine and a parasympatholytic such as cyclopentolate, atropine, or others is administered. Postoperatively, a topical parasympatholytic is often given to prevent discomfort from spasm of the ciliary body and a topical steroidal to minimize ocular inflammation. While the topical steroidals have virtually only ocular side effects, phenylephrine can lead to arrhythmia, arterial hypertension, and palpitations, and atropine and other parasympatholytics can result in headaches, constipation, restlessness, delirium, and urinary retention.

Occasionally ophthalmic surgery causes acute elevation of intraocular pressure in the early postoperative period. Patients typically complain of eye pain accompanied by a vagal response with nausea, vomiting, and bradycardia. This complication requires administration of anti-glaucoma medications including beta-blocking agents such as timolol, topical or systemic carbonic anhydrase inhibitors such as acetazolamide and dorzolamide, prostaglandin analogue such as latanoprost, and alpha-2 adrenergics such as brimonidine. All these medications can cause adverse reactions. While the adverse reactions of topical medications are often restricted to the eye surface, causing ocular pruritus, allergy, or foreign body sensation and dryness, now and then there are secondary reactions that affect other organs. Topical beta-blockers may produce headache, bronchospasm, heart block, and exacerbation of congestive heart failure; carbonic anhydrase inhibitors may cause paresthesias, headache, polyuria, and dyspepsia; prostaglandin analogs may result in a rash; and alpha-2 adrenergics may produce somnolence, dry mouth, and hypertension.

FURTHER READING

Cionni, R. J., Snyder, M. E., & Osher, R. H. Cataract surgery. In Tasman, W. & Jaeger, E. A., eds. *Duane's Clinical Ophthalmology*, vol 6. Philadelphia, PA: Lippincott, Williams and Wilkins, 2002.

Krachmer, Mannis, Holland. Cornea: *Surgery of the Cornea and Conjunctiva*, Vol III. Mosby-Year Book, Inc., 1997.

Meredith, T. A. *Atlas of Retinal and Vitreous Surgery*. St. Louis: Mosby, 1999.

Mills, M. R. & Fricker, S. J. Surgical management of strabismus. In Albert, D. M. & Jakobiec, F. A., eds. *Principles and Practice of Ophthalmology*, 2nd edn. Philadelphia, PA: W. B. Saunders, 2000: 4379–4393.

101

Cataract surgery

G. Baker Hubbard, III, Enrique Garcia-Valenzuela, and Thomas M. Aaberg, Sr.

Emory University School of Medicine, Atlanta, GA

Cataracts are characterized by opacity of the crystalline lens of the eye and are the primary cause of preventable blindness in the world. They may be congenital or age related; secondary to exposure to drugs, toxins, or radiation; or the product of various metabolic diseases. Visually significant cataracts are a major public health issue and are found in 50% of persons 65 to 74 years of age and 70% of persons 75 years of age or older.

Modern cataract extraction with placement of an intraocular lens (IOL) is a highly effective and efficient operation to restore visual acuity and contrast sensitivity in patients with severe cataracts. Presently, the operation has evolved to the point where it involves constructing a small (2.5–3.5 mm) wound at the edge of the cornea. The incision is carefully shelved to minimize leakage through the wound, viscoelastic material is injected into the anterior chamber to protect the cornea, and the anterior capsule of the lens is removed. An ultrasound probe (phacoemulsification tip) is then inserted into the anterior chamber and used to fragment and remove the cataractous lens, though the capsule of the lens is left intact except for a small opening in the anterior portion through which the phaco tip had been inserted. An IOL with appropriate focusing power to neutralize any refractive error is chosen based on the size and corneal curvature of the patient's eye. It is folded and inserted through the incision into the "bag" formed by the residual native lens capsule, after which it unfolds and comes to rest in the location of the original native lens and is supported by the native capsule. After the instruments are removed, the wound is usually self-sealing and watertight. Some ophthalmologists place one or more sutures in the wound, though most do not. Despite the fact that cataract surgery requires a significant degree of skill and is a technically challenging procedure, experienced surgeons can perform the operation in 30 minutes or less.

As the procedure has progressed, outcomes have steadily improved and the rate of complications has diminished. In the absence of other ocular disease, postoperative visual acuity is routinely 20/20 or better, often within 1 week of surgery and without glasses. As the risks of the surgery have been reduced and outcomes have improved, the indications for the operation have changed. For patients without coexisting ocular disorders, primary current indications are a symptomatic reduction in visual acuity to worse than 20/40 or complaints of reduction in visual function due to glare (difficulty driving at night) in the setting of cataractous lens changes visible to the examiner. Cataract extraction may also be performed to improve visualization and management of posterior segment disorders.

Cataract extraction is usually performed under local anesthesia with intravenous sedation. The most recent trend is more towards topical anesthesia with drops than retrobulbar block. Stress to the patient is minimal and cataract extraction may be possible and beneficial even in the sickest and most debilitated of patients.

Usual postoperative course

Expected postoperative hospital stay

The vast majority of cataract extractions are performed on an outpatient basis. The patient must be examined on the first postoperative day by his or her ophthalmologist, usually in an office setting.

Operative mortality

Extremely rare.

Special monitoring required

None necessary.

Medical Management of the Surgical Patient: A Textbook of Perioperative Medicine, ed. M. F. Lubin, R. B. Smith, T. F. Dobson, N. Spell, H. K. Walker. 4th edn. Published by Cambridge University Press. © Cambridge University 2006.

Patient activity and positioning

Routine daily activities may be resumed almost immediately, though patients must wear protective glasses or a protective shield over the operated eye during the early postoperative period. Eye rubbing is to be avoided. After several days, face and hair washing may be performed with eyes closed. Excessively strenuous exercise or heavy lifting should be avoided for approximately 1 week.

Alimentation

Regular preoperative diet may be resumed when sedation has worn off.

Antibiotic coverage

Topical corticosteroid and antibiotic drops are used. The antibiotic drop is typically discontinued after 1 week and the steroid drop is tapered off over several weeks.

Postoperative complications

In the hospital

Corneal or macular edema

Some swelling of these structures during the postoperative period is expected. The edema is usually mild and self-limited. Severe or prolonged edema requires treatment to prevent permanent visual disability.

Wound dehiscence or wound leak

Leaks must be identified and treated promptly to prevent microorganisms from gaining access to the inside of the eye.

Dislocation of the intraocular lens

This usually results from a defect in the capsule from the native lens that was left in place to support the implant. Treatment requires reoperation with an alternative form of IOL fixation.

Residual lens fragments

Fragments of lens left behind after cataract surgery can be highly inflammatory and often must be removed with a second operation.

Elevated intraocular pressure

Mild pressure elevations are common after cataract extraction and usually respond well to topical pressure lowering medications. More severe elevations may cause pain, nausea, and vomiting. Even so, response to topical medication is usually good and the duration is usually limited.

After discharge

Retinal detachment

This is a late complication of cataract extraction that can occur months or years after the operation. The standard treatment is to perform a scleral buckle and/or vitrectomy to reattach the retina.

Infection

Endophthalmitis is a rare but devastating complication of cataract extraction. Treatment involves injection of intraocular antibiotics as well as topical and intravenous antibiotics. When visual acuity is light perception or worse, vitrectomy is indicated.

FURTHER READING

Cionni, R. J., Snyder, M. E., & Osher, R. H. Cataract surgery. In Tasman, W. & Jaeger, E. A., eds. *Duane's Clinical Ophthalmology*, vol 6. Philadelphia, PA: Lippincott, Williams, & Wilkins, 2002.

Datiles, M. B. III, Clinical evaluation of cataracts. In Tasman, W. & Jaeger, E. A., eds. *Duane's Clinical Ophthalmology*, vol 1. Philadelphia, PA: Lippincott, Williams, & Wilkins, 2002.

102

Corneal transplantation

C. Diane Song, Enrique Garcia-Valenzuela, G. Baker Hubbard, III, and Thomas M. Aaberg, Sr.

Emory University School of Medicine, Atlanta, GA

Corneal transplant, also known as penetrating keratoplasty, has a 90% success rate as defined by clear grafts in 1 year. The primary indication for the procedure is a hazy or opaque cornea causing decrease in vision. The etiologies of corneal opacities include congenital defects, hereditary dystrophies, infection, and trauma. Occasionally, corneal transplants are performed simultaneously with cataract surgery, intraocular lens exchange, or with posterior segment surgery, depending on other conditions affecting vision. The procedure is not as common as lamellar keratoplasty, in which only the anterior surface of the cornea is grafted, leaving the posterior surface intact.

For most patients, the operation is performed on an outpatient basis under local anesthesia with monitored anesthesia care. Under special circumstances, a patient may require general anesthesia and overnight stay in the hospital. Depending on whether or not other intraocular surgeries are performed at the same time, the operation lasts between one half to two hours and involves removing the patient's hazy cornea and replacing it with a clear donor cornea that is sewn in place with nylon sutures. It is performed under an operating microscope and requires the patient to lie still. When the operation is complete, the patient is given topical medications and the eye should be patched overnight. Blood loss is minimal to none during the procedure.

Usual postoperative course

Expected postoperative hospital stay
Most patients go home on the day of surgery.

Operative mortality
Extremely low and generally associated with the anesthetic used.

Special monitoring required
The eye is usually patched and a shield may be placed over the patch to minimize trauma to the eye. Although the patch is removed the next day, the shield should be worn during the first 2–3 weeks of healing period.

Patient activity and positioning
Minimal physical restrictions are required after surgery and most patients can resume their usual activities. The patient must avoid direct blows to the eye. Other activities to avoid during the first few weeks are heavy lifting, bending the head below the waist, any straining action that requires holding one's breath, and – to minimize risk of infection – swimming.

Alimentation
Dietary restrictions are unnecessary. Regular preoperative diet is usually resumed when the patient recovers from anesthesia.

Antibiotic coverage
Topical antibiotics and steroids are used during the early postoperative period. Antibiotics are prescribed for approximately 1 week, though steroids may be continued indefinitely to decrease the risk of rejection.

Postoperative follow-up
There will be frequent follow-up visits during the first few months, beginning with the day after surgery, then 1–2 weeks later, then monthly for the first few months. There is little discomfort during the healing process. Visual recovery is slow and stabilization occurs over months. Once vision is stable, glasses or contact lenses are prescribed to maximize vision. As desired, sutures may be removed at any time.

Medical Management of the Surgical Patient: A Textbook of Perioperative Medicine, ed. M. F. Lubin, R. B. Smith, T. F. Dobson, N. Spell, H. K. Walker. 4th edn. Published by Cambridge University Press. © Cambridge University 2006.

Postoperative complications

In the hospital

Aqueous leaks

In the early postoperative period, wound leaks may occur. If the leak is small, it can be managed with patching or by a bandage contact lens and is usually self-limited. If the leak is large, additional sutures are necessary.

Infection

This is a serious complication that can occur at any time. Topical antibiotics are used to minimize this risk; however, if an infection develops, local injections of antibiotics may be used. A serious infection could lead to total vision loss.

After discharge

Cataract, glaucoma, and retinal detachment

Eyes that have undergone any intraocular surgery, including corneal transplants, are at increased risk of developing cataract, glaucoma, and retinal detachment because of the unavoidable surgical stress on the eye. If unintended injury occurs to intraocular structures, these risks become significantly higher.

Graft rejection

While risk of this complication is highest during the first year after operation, it remains a lifelong possibility. The four major signs of rejection are increased redness of the eye, sensitivity to light, decreased vision, and pain. Since early treatment can reverse the process, the patient should report any of these signs immediately. If rejection cannot be reversed, repeat corneal transplant can be performed.

FURTHER READING

Krachmer, J. H., Mannis, M. J., & Holland, E. J. (eds.) *Cornea: Surgery of the Cornea and Conjunctiva.* Vol III. St. Louis, MO: Mosby-Year Book, Inc. 1997.

103

Vitreoretinal surgery

G. Baker Hubbard, III, Enrique Garcia-Valenzuela, and Thomas M. Aaberg, Sr.

Emory University School of Medicine, Atlanta, GA

Vitreoretinal surgical techniques are used to address disorders of the posterior segment of the eye. Great strides have been made in the ability to safely and effectively operate in the posterior segment over the last 20 years. With the evolution of advanced micro-surgical instruments, computerized infusion and aspiration systems, endolaser probes, perfluorocarbon heavy liquid for manipulation of detached retinal tissue, implantable slow-release pharmacological devices, wide angle optical viewing systems, and long-acting gases and silicone oil for intraocular tamponade, the spectrum of disorders which are amenable to operative intervention has broadened significantly. The treatment of intraocular tumors with radioactive episcleral plaques has also become well established in recent years. However, in many cases of primary retinal detachment, the most appropriate treatment remains the standard scleral buckling operation that has been performed for over 60 years.

The scleral buckling operation consists of placing a strip of silicone around the outside of the globe to cause a slight indentation or buckle of the eye wall. The buckle achieves its purpose because the indentation helps close the causative retinal tear inside the eye. A combination of support from the buckle and chorioretinal scarring induced by treating the tear with cryotherapy maintain closure of the retinal tear. Complex retinal detachments with very large or posteriorly located retinal tears, significant retinal scarring, vitreous hemorrhage, or severe cataract formation are usually approached with a combination of scleral buckle and the more advanced intraocular vitrectomy techniques listed above.

In addition to retinal detachment, the list of disorders that may be appropriate for vitreoretinal surgical intervention includes macular hole, macular pucker, subretinal neovascularization due to macular degeneration and other disorders, proliferative diabetic retinopathy, vitreous hemorrhage, choroidal melanoma and other intraocular tumors, CMV retinitis and other retinal infections, retained lens fragments after cataract surgery, dislocated intraocular lens implants, intraocular foreign bodies, and endophthalmitis.

Vitreoretinal surgery is most often performed under local anesthesia with retrobulbar block and intravenous sedation. However, in the setting of reoperation after scleral buckle, general anesthesia is preferred as adequate local anesthesia is often difficult to accomplish. In addition, the duration of some operations makes local anesthesia undesirable. Lower back pain exacerbated by lying flat, claustrophobia, and an inability to remain still are relative indications for general anesthesia.

Usual postoperative course

Expected postoperative hospital stay

The trend of performing vitreoretinal procedures on an outpatient basis is growing. However, many patients with disorders of the posterior segment of the eye also have significant medical problems. Given the stringent positioning requirements after many vitreoretinal operations, admission to the hospital for at least one night is often mandatory for monitoring and to insure compliance with positioning and medical regimens.

Operative mortality

Very low and generally associated with anesthesia.

Special monitoring required

Based on the underlying disease.

Medical Management of the Surgical Patient: A Textbook of Perioperative Medicine, ed. M. F. Lubin, R. B. Smith, T. F. Dobson, N. Spell, H. K. Walker. 4th edn. Published by Cambridge University Press. © Cambridge University 2006.

Patient activity and positioning

Strict requirements for head position are common after vitreoretinal operations. After the operation, eyes are frequently left with gas or silicone oil filling the posterior segment to provide tamponade; the tamponade is generally used to help close a retinal tear. Due to the buoyancy of the gas or oil, strict head position is necessary to maintain the tamponade in the correct location inside the eye. The duration of positioning requirements range from 1 to 14 days or more. Aside from these requirements, patients can usually resume normal daily activities within several days. Eye protection in the form of a shield or protective glasses should be worn for at least several weeks postoperatively.

Alimentation

Regular preoperative diet is usually resumed when the patient recovers from anesthesia.

Antibiotic coverage

Usual postoperative regimens include a topical corticosteroid, a topical antibiotic, and a topical muscarinic antagonist (atropine or scopolamine) to reduce the pain associated with spasm of the ciliary muscle. The latter two are stopped after one week and the corticosteroid is tapered over several weeks.

Postoperative complications

In the hospital

Elevated intraocular pressure

Mild pressure elevations are common after vitreoretinal operations and usually respond well to topical pressure lowering medications. More severe elevations may cause pain, nausea, and vomiting. Even so, response to topical medication is usually good and the duration is usually limited.

Vitreous hemorrhage

Some bleeding into the posterior segment after vitrectomy is fairly common, particularly in the setting of proliferative diabetic retinopathy. Most postoperative hemorrhages clear spontaneously but some require reoperation.

Retinal detachment

The rate of postoperative retinal detachment depends on the underlying disease but is generally 1%–5%. This is the most common cause for reoperation.

Infection

While rare, endophthalmitis and infections of scleral buckle elements are devastating complications that usually result in severe visual loss. Treatment involves removal of infected buckle elements, injection of intraocular antibiotics, and administration of topical, oral, and intravenous antibiotics.

After discharge

Cataract

Some degree of cataract formation is inevitable after vitrectomy in all but young adults and children. The time to onset of visually significant cataract may be months to years after the vitrectomy.

Intraocular gas related complications

As noted above, intraocular gas is frequently used after vitreoretinal surgery to provide retinal tamponade. These gas bubbles last between 1 and 8 weeks before complete reabsorption. If a patient undergoes another operation using nitrous oxide anesthesia during this period, the gas will expand and may cause extreme elevations of intraocular pressure resulting in permanent severe visual loss. Patients with intraocular gas therefore must not be given nitrous oxide. Air travel likewise causes expansion of intraocular gas and must be avoided until the gas bubble resolves.

FURTHER READING

Hart, R. H., Vote, B. J., Borthwick, J. H., McGeorge, A. J., & Worsley, D. R. Loss of vision caused by expansion of intraocular perfluoropropane (C(3)F(8)) gas during nitrous oxide anesthesia. *Am. J. Ophthalmol.* 2002; **134**: 761–763.

Meredith, T. A. *Atlas of Retinal and Vitreous Surgery*. St. Louis, MO: Mosby, 1999.

104

Glaucoma surgery

Anastasios P. Costarides, G. Baker Hubbard, III, Enrique Garcia-Valenzuela, and Thomas M. Aaberg, Sr.

Emory University School of Medicine, Atlanta, GA

Multiple ocular conditions can lead to the development of glaucoma, which is the most common optic neuropathy. All therapeutic interventions are directed towards lowering the condition's greatest risk factor, intraocular pressure.

Typically, therapy is instituted in an ascending fashion, with topical medical therapy being the first and simplest option. Medications include topical beta adrenergic blockers, prostaglandin analogs, carbonic anhydrase inhibitors, alpha adrenergic agonists, and miotics; these agents, used alone or in combination, are often sufficient for control of intraocular pressure. In cases of open angle glaucoma requiring greater management of intraocular pressure, laser trabeculoplasty, an outpatient procedure, is used in conjunction with medications. For angle closure glaucoma, outpatient laser iridotomy is applied to relieve the pupillary block mechanism.

Incisional intraocular surgery is the most frequent choice when medical and outpatient laser procedures fail to diminish intraocular pressure, with trabeculectomy and aqueous tube shunt placement being the most commonly used procedures. Both approaches lower intraocular pressure by allowing aqueous humor to leave the anterior chamber and collect in the subconjunctival space. When other interventions have either failed or are unfeasible, such cyclodestructive procedures as laser ablation or cryoablation of the ciliary processes may be done. Incisional surgery is done in an operating room, usually on an outpatient basis; cyclodestructive operations are performed in a clinic setting; and local anesthesia is standard for both methods.

Usual postoperative course

Expected postoperative hospital stay

Glaucoma surgery usually does not require hospitalization, though monocular patients undergoing incisional surgery may be hospitalized.

Operative mortality

Very rare and related to anesthesia.

Special monitoring required

None required.

Patient activity and positioning

Activity restrictions are limited only to patients who have undergone incisional intraocular surgery. An eye pad and shield is usually placed over the affected eye for the first postoperative night, after which the patient wears an eye shield while sleeping for the first 3 postoperative weeks. Patients are instructed to avoid lifting weights greater than 20 pounds for the first postoperative week or as long as the eye is hypotonous. Any strenuous exercise is off-limits for at least the first postoperative week.

Alimentation

Dietary restrictions are unnecessary.

Antibiotic coverage

After incisional surgery, topical corticosteroids and antibiotics are administered. Antibiotics are typically stopped during the first postoperative week, and topical corticosteroids are slowly tapered over several weeks. Topical cycloplegics may also be utilized. These agents are used most frequently when the eye is hypotonous and the anterior chamber has shallowed or flattened.

Medical Management of the Surgical Patient: A Textbook of Perioperative Medicine, ed. M. F. Lubin, R. B. Smith, T. F. Dobson, N. Spell, H. K. Walker. 4th edn. Published by Cambridge University Press. © Cambridge University 2006.

Postoperative complications

In the hospital

Hypotony

Excessive filtration of aqueous humor from the anterior chamber following trabeculectomy or aqueous tube placement can markedly reduce intraocular pressure to a nonphysiologic level. Postoperative hypotony is usually transient, but may have long term pathologic consequences. The complication may be accompanied by a shallow or flat anterior chamber, a choroidal effusion or hemorrhage, optic disc edema, and hypotony maculopathy. Surgical intervention may be crucial to reverse the manifestations of hypotony and to preserve vision.

After discharge

Infectious endophthalmitis

Characterized by a red, painful eye accompanied by visual loss. Blindness is a distinct risk, thus requiring rapid and aggressive intervention. Intravitreal administration of antibiotics or pars plana vitrectomy is necessary for management. It should be emphasized that infectious endophthalmitis can occur years following a trabeculectomy due to breakdown of the surgical filtration site with subsequent bacterial invasion.

FURTHER READING

Katz, L. J., Costa, V. P., & Spaeth, G. L. Filtration surgery. In Ritch, R., Shields, M. B., & Krupin, T., eds. *The Glaucomas*, 2nd edn. St. Louis, MO: Mosby-Year Book, 1996.

105

Refractive surgery

C. Diane Song, Enrique Garcia-Valenzuela, G. Baker Hubbard, III, and Thomas M. Aaberg, Sr.

Emory University School of Medicine, Atlanta, GA

Done to reduce dependence on glasses or contact lenses, refractive surgery involves reshaping the cornea with incisions, heat, or laser to decrease myopia, astigmatism, or hyperopia. Presently, the most frequently performed refractive surgical procedure is laser-assisted in situ keratomileusis (LASIK).

LASIK can correct refractive error within a wide range. To deduce whether LASIK is a good option for a patient, a thorough preoperative eye exam is necessary. Indications may include intolerance to contact lenses, improved conditions for job-related or hobby-related activities, or a desire to lessen reliance on glasses and contact lenses.

Performed in an outpatient setting with topical anesthesia, the operation usually lasts about 15 minutes with the patient experiencing minimal discomfort. Both eyes may be operated on the same day. After it is cut, the thin corneal flap is lifted and reflected to allow the laser to reshape the cornea. The laser is programmed with the patient's refractive error; once that refractive error is corrected, the corneal flap is realigned into place.

Usual postoperative course

Expected postoperative hospital stay

Most surgeries are performed in a surgicenter on an outpatient basis.

Special monitoring required

The patient's eyes are generally not patched, though sunglasses may be necessary if there is sensitivity to light. Discomfort is minimal postoperatively.

Patient activity and positioning

Most patients will be able to see well enough on the first postoperative day to return to regular activity, though they require reading glasses for near vision if they are in the presbyopic age range. Care must be taken not to rub the eye during the first few days. Swimming should also be avoided during the first few weeks to minimize risk of infection.

Alimentation

Dietary restrictions are unnecessary.

Antibiotic coverage

The patient instills topical antibiotics and steroids for the first week or two. Steroids may need to be continued longer to modulate the healing response. The eyes may feel dry during the first few months, and patients may use artificial tears as needed.

Postoperative follow-up

Follow-up is conducted on the first day after surgery, then usually 1–2 weeks later. Additional follow-up visits are generally at 3 months, 6 months, and 1 year. There may be small fluctuations in vision up to 2–3 months after surgery. Some patients may require more than one session if they are under- or overcorrected.

Postoperative complications

Failure to identify preexisting corneal conditions

LASIK can accelerate corneal ectasia in eyes with keratoconus; therefore, the procedure is contraindicated for such patients. A thorough preoperative screening examination is necessary to evaluate for conditions that may increase risk of complications.

Medical Management of the Surgical Patient: A Textbook of Perioperative Medicine, ed. M. F. Lubin, R. B. Smith, T. F. Dobson, N. Spell, H. K. Walker. 4th edn. Published by Cambridge University Press. © Cambridge University 2006.

Halos and glare

Complications with LASIK are rare. Some patients may experience halos and glare at night depending on factors such as pupil size and the amount of refractive error.

Infection

Topical antibiotics are used to minimize the risk of this serious complication, which can occur anytime and could lead to loss of vision.

Decentered laser ablation, irregular corneal surface

While there is a small risk of complications that will lead to an aberrant corneal refractive surface, they may occasionally be improved with more laser ablation.

FURTHER READING

Buratto, L. & Brint, S. *LASIK; Surgical Techniques and Complications.* Thorofare, NJ: Slack Inc., 2000.

106

Eye muscle surgery

Amy K. Hutchinson, G. Baker Hubbard, III, Enrique Garcia-Valenzuela, and Thomas A. Aaberg, Sr.

Eye muscle surgery is performed to correct strabismus, which is any horizontal, vertical, or torsional misalignment of the eyes that affects both children and adults. The disease can be congenital, acquired, restrictive, or paralytic. The purpose of surgery is to restore the eyes to their normal, anatomical position; to maximize the potential for binocularity; and, in some cases, to eliminate diplopia. Either one or multiple muscles may be involved in the operation and bilateral procedures are common. In cooperative children and adults, a postoperative adjustment of the muscle position may be performed once the effects of anesthesia have dissipated.

Strabismus surgery is most often performed under general anesthesia, though local anesthesia and even topical anesthesia can be used in adults.

Usual postoperative course

Expected postoperative hospital stay

Most strabismus surgery is performed on an outpatient basis. Hospitalization is unusual.

Operative mortality

Related to anesthesia. The incidence of malignant hyperthermia may be slightly higher in strabismus patients than in the general population.

Special monitoring required

None necessary.

Patient activity and positioning

For 2 weeks, patients are advised to avoid swimming and other activities that may introduce contaminated material into their eyes. Young children should be properly supervised and discouraged from rubbing their eyes. Dressings are usually unnecessary.

Alimentation

Oral intake should be resumed gradually, since nausea and vomiting are common after strabismus surgery, especially in children.

Antibiotic coverage

Topical antibiotic or antibiotic/steroid combination drops may be used optionally.

Postoperative complications

In the hospital

Slipped or lost muscle

A slipped muscle occurs when there is retraction of the muscle within its capsule; a lost muscle occurs when a muscle becomes completely detached from the sclera. Patients present with an obvious change in their ocular alignment and limited or absent duction of the muscle. Surgical exploration is indicated.

Diplopia

While transient diplopia is a common occurrence after strabismus surgery, persisting diplopia is unusual. When it is encountered, the patients are primarily adults. Additional surgery, prism glasses, or occlusion may be needed in such cases.

Anterior segment ischemia

An uncommon complication that results from insufficient blood flow to the anterior segment of the eye as a result of transection of the ciliary vessels during surgery. It generally occurs in older patients who have compromised

Medical Management of the Surgical Patient: A Textbook of Perioperative Medicine, ed. M. F. Lubin, R. B. Smith, T. F. Dobson, N. Spell, H. K. Walker. 4th edn. Published by Cambridge University Press. © Cambridge University 2006.

circulation or when surgery is performed on three or more muscles in one eye. Patients present with decreased vision, ocular pain, and anterior chamber inflammation. Treatment is with steroids. Most cases resolve, but hypotony and phthisis bulbi can ensue.

After discharge

Infections

Periocular infections are uncommon but can occur, especially in children with poor hygiene or those who rub their eyes. Onset is usually 1–5 days following operation. Patients present with pain, edema, and erythema of the eyelids. Mild cases can be treated with oral antibiotics but may require hospitalization for intravenous antibiotic administration if the infection is severe. Endophthalmitis is very rare following strabismus surgery but can occur even without scleral perforation.

Unsatisfactory postoperative alignment

Multiple operations may be necessary to achieve the desired alignment and candidates should be appropriately counseled preoperatively. Patients should be observed for 4 to 6 weeks or until alignment is stable before reoperation is undertaken.

FURTHER READING

Mills, M. R. & Fricker, S. J. (2000). Surgical management of strabismus. In Albert, D. M. & Jakobiec, F. A., eds. *Principles and Practice of Ophthalmology*, 2nd edn. Philadelphia, PA: W. B. Saunders, vol., 2000: 4379–4393.

107

Enucleation, evisceration and exenteration

Enrique Garcia-Valenzuela, G. Baker Hubbard, III, and Thomas M. Aaberg, Sr.

Emory University School of Medicine, Atlanta, GA

Ophthalmic surgeons may want to remove ocular structures when they are affected by neoplasia, when they are distressed by a severe infectious process, or when an end-stage ocular disease is causing pain. There are three types of ophthalmic intervention:

Enucleation

Removal of the entire eyeball, including sclera and cornea, leaving a stump of the optic nerve and the extraocular muscles. An intraorbital prosthesis is usually implanted.

Evisceration

Removal of all intraocular structures, leaving only sclera and sometimes cornea. An ocular prosthesis is usually implanted.

Exenteration

Removal of the eyeball and the orbital contents which may include removal of orbital bone.

Enucleation is the most frequently performed surgical approach for elimination of intraocular structures. When ocular disease has rendered an eye completely blind (incapable of perceiving the brightest light), any possibility of visual recovery is minimal. Frequently, such severity of pathology makes an eye painful and cosmetically unacceptable in spite of medical treatment. Although there are several procedural choices, the most widely accepted surgery is removal of the eye or enucleation because of its long-term outcome and safety. A frequent scenario where enucleation is recommended is after severe ocular trauma. A blind eye should be enucleated within 2 weeks after trauma to prevent sympathetic ophthalmia, a rare complication where the exposed uveal tissue leads to autoimmune attack of the contralateral healthy eye. Other indications for enucleation include infectious endophthalmitis, end-stage glaucoma, and malignant intraocular tumors.

Evisceration has been regarded as an alternative to enucleation due to the belief that it leads to improved prosthesis motility and because of the hypothesis that the operation has a reduced risk of contaminating orbital tissue in cases of infectious endophthalmitis. Nevertheless, it is seldom employed, with most ophthalmologists preferring enucleation.

Exenteration is rarely performed and typically reserved for unusual cases where a malignant orbital neoplasm (such as cancer of the lacrimal gland) or a severe infectious process within the orbit (such as mucormycosis in a diabetic patient) poses the threat of spreading intracranially.

For medical and psychological reasons, given the negative implications these three procedures have in the minds of most patients, they are usually performed under general anesthesia.

Usual postoperative course

Expected postoperative hospital stay

Although overnight hospital stays may be unnecessary after these operations, it is not unusual to admit patients for 1 to 3 days, particularly after exenteration.

Operative mortality

Very low and generally associated with anesthesia. In the case of exenteration, postoperative mortality can occur if the ophthalmic disease progresses to involve other cranial structures.

Special monitoring required

Observation may be necessary for underlying systemic diseases. Typically, no special monitoring is required other than an ophthalmologic examination 1 day after and in subsequent weeks. The surgical area is typically

Medical Management of the Surgical Patient: A Textbook of Perioperative Medicine, ed. M. F. Lubin, R. B. Smith, T. F. Dobson, N. Spell, H. K. Walker. 4th edn. Published by Cambridge University Press. © Cambridge University 2006.

left under the protection of a pressure dressing. In cases of enucleation and evisceration, many surgeons leave a plastic conformer in the conjunctival cul-de-sac to prevent shortening due to soft tissue scarring.

Patient activity and positioning

Minimal physical restrictions are required after surgery and most patients can resume their usual activities as soon as postoperative discomfort improves.

Alimentation

No dietary restrictions are necessary. Regular preoperative diet is usually resumed when the patient recovers from anesthesia.

Antibiotic coverage

Postoperative medications are often limited to topical antibiotics. When the indication for surgery was infectious, systemic antibiotics are frequently used.

Psychological support

Most patients find removal of an eye to be much more disturbing than complete blindness in one eye. At times, patients may be devastated and require emotional support. The treating physician should always be aware of the potential grief caused by the procedure.

Fitting of an external prosthesis

After several weeks of uncomplicated course, patients are referred to a professional ocularist for crafting of an external prosthesis, such as an ocular shell. For cosmetic reasons, the prosthesis is designed to match the contralateral side of the patient's face. Patients are then trained in the care of their external prostheses: how to remove them, clean them regularly, and place them in position.

Medical follow-up

Depending on the indication for removal of an eye, the internist may be more or less involved during the postoperative course of the patient. If the case was characterized by infectious endophthalmitis of unknown endogenous etiology, an urgent systemic work-up for a source of infection is needed. If the indication was a malignant neoplasm, the patient requires serial metastatic work-ups over the course of years, typically performed by their oncologist.

Postoperative complications

In the hospital

Orbital and periorbital edema

Complications rarely occur after these procedures. Patients commonly complain of edema of the remaining periocular tissue and some postoperative hemorrhage may occur. Neither edema nor minimal bleeding is of great concern, and both tend to resolve spontaneously. The customary pressure patch is meant to minimize these problems.

Sympathetic ophthalmia

A feared but extremely rare complication of evisceration is sympathetic ophthalmia. Of the three operations, only evisceration is capable of causing an autoimmune reaction to the contralateral eye because of possible remnants of uveal tissue attached to the sclera inside the ocular cavity. Systemic steroids are indicated if this complication occurs.

Death

Exenteration is one of the few ophthalmic operations that has significant postoperative mortality given the usual seriousness of the underlying disease process.

After discharge

Extrusion of the implant

An infrequent complication, the implanted spherical prosthesis extruding through the periocular soft tissues requires additional surgery to replace the implant.

FURTHER READING

Dortzbach, R. K. & Woog, J. J. Choice of procedure: enucleation, evisceration, or prosthetic fitting over globes. *Ophthalmology* 1985; **92**: 1249.

Nerad, J. A., Kersten, R., Neuhans, R. *et al.* Orbit, eyelids and lacrimal system. *Am. Acad. Ophthalmol. BCSC*, Section 7, 1996: 116–117.

Nunery, W. R. & Hetzler, K. Enucleation. In Hornblass, A., ed. *Oculoplastic, Orbital, and Reconstructive Surgery*, Vol 2. Baltimore, MD: Williams & Wilkins, 1990: 1200–1220.

Raflo, T. G. Enucleation and evisceration. In Tasman, W. & Jaeger, E. A., eds. *Duane's Ophthalmology*. Vol. 5, Chap. 82. Philadelphia, PA: Lippincott, Williams & Wilkins, 2000.

Orthopedic surgery

108

Arthroscopic knee surgery

Alonzo T. Sexton, II and John W. Xerogeanes

Emory University School of Medicine, Atlanta, GA

Advances in surgical technique and technology have led to increasing indications for arthroscopy. The advantages of arthroscopic surgery include small incisions with lowered risks for operative complications such as infection and excessive blood loss. Video capture systems and the ability to take still photographs provide illustrations of specific points during the operation for the medical record. The benefits also carry over to the postoperative period in the form of lower requirements for analgesia, shortened hospital stays, and earlier initiation of rehabilitation protocols. Arthroscopic surgery is the most common type of orthopedic surgery, with the knee being the most frequent site of surgical treatment.

While the utility of arthroscopy has primarily been observed in its ability for administering therapeutic maneuvers, the arthroscope is also a powerful diagnostic tool for knee pathology. Therefore, the diagnostic portion of the case is the most important step in any arthroscopic procedure, as it allows for the identification of any pathology present and for development of a treatment plan. Surgeries that are performed most regularly include partial meniscectomy, meniscal repair, and ACL reconstruction. The arthroscope is also utilized for complex ligament reconstructions (ACL, MCL, PCL), meniscal transplantation, articular cartilage transplantation, and septic joint irrigation and debridement.

Indications for arthroscopy include the various injuries to the ligamentous and cartilaginous structures about the knee. Patients with meniscal pathology will often report a specific injury to their knee, describing a sharp pain on the medial or lateral side of the knee or occasionally in the back of the knee. Mechanical symptoms such as catching, clicking, or locking are highly suggestive of a flap of meniscal cartilage that is physically impairing knee motion. Patients will likely have tenderness to palpation along the joint line, a positive McMurray's test, or pain with hyperflexion or hyperextension of the knee. Physical findings

may be confirmed by an MRI study. The decision whether to perform a meniscal repair or partial meniscectomy is made at the time of operation.

Patients with injuries to the anterior cruciate ligament (ACL) usually have a twisting injury to the knee and report immediate swelling and pain. Subsequently, they may have a sensation of "looseness" or instability in their knee that manifests when attempting to turn on the knee. Upon examination, the patient may have an effusion and positive Lachman test (most sensitive), anterior drawer or pivot shift test. MRI is also highly sensitive and specific for visualizing ACL rupture. An ACL tear in and of itself is not an indication for reconstruction. The decision for operation should be individualized, as low demand patients do not require an ACL for functions of daily living, and lifestyle modification to avoid certain sports will allow for reasonable outcomes in a majority of patients. For more active patients that are uninterested in lifestyle modification and will commit to vigorous rehabilitation postoperatively, ACL reconstruction is a reasonable option.

Articular cartilage injuries pose a particular difficulty to the treating orthopedic surgeon due to the limitation of healing potential in this tissue type. Newer techniques of cartilage transplantation and stimulation of the healing process through microfracture techniques have provided tools for dealing with this challenging problem. Patients with such injuries may have symptoms and physical findings that are difficult to explain, but cartilaginous or osteochondral lesions may be appreciated on imaging modalities (X-ray, MRI). Failure of conservative therapy may lead to surgical intervention.

Meniscus

Knowledge regarding the importance of the meniscal cartilage in its shock absorbing and joint stabilizing properties has gone through significant evolution. Once thought

Medical Management of the Surgical Patient: A Textbook of Perioperative Medicine, ed. M. F. Lubin, R. B. Smith, T. F. Dobson, N. Spell, H. K. Walker. 4th edn. Published by Cambridge University Press. © Cambridge University 2006.

to be vestigial tissue, menisci were routinely excised when injured. During diagnostic arthroscopy, a characterization of the meniscal tear can be made. Various patterns of tears occur, but an important distinction that affects treatment is the location of the tear within the meniscal substance. Due to the local vascular supply of the menisci, only the peripheral 1/3 receives a blood supply adequate enough to support a repair attempt. After identifying the tear, the portion of the meniscus that is torn may be removed using a mechanical shaver under direct visualization through the arthroscope. Surgery for an isolated meniscal tear can be performed in between 30 and 45 minutes and the blood loss is minimal, making blood transfusion unlikely. If a meniscal repair is possible, it may be done completely arthroscopically or by making a small incision to pass needles through the meniscus and place sutures. Extreme caution must be taken, particularly when repairing posterior horn tears as the popliteal vessels are nearby. As with most arthroscopic procedures, these are performed on an ambulatory basis.

Anterior cruciate ligament

The poor performance of primary repair of ACL tears has led to the development of techniques for arthroscopically assisted ACL reconstruction. The three most popular choices include autograft bone–patellar tendon–bone, autograft hamstring, or allograft. While there is some dependence on surgeon preference, the pros and cons can be described as follows. Allograft tissue lowers the morbidity and pain associated with the surgery by avoiding donor site complications. The major concern with allograft lies in how difficult it is to sterilize soft tissue grafts and the subsequent infection risks. Despite the number of these grafts done each year, there are but a handful of reports of infections with the graft identified as the source. Bone–patellar tendon–bone grafts harvest a portion of the inferior pole of the patella, the central third of the patella tendon, and a wedge of bone from the tibial tubercle. These grafts are extremely stout and are easily secured because the graft has bone on either side, but there are risks of fracturing the patella postoperatively, of tendon rupture, and of anterior knee pain. Hamstring autografts are relatively simple to harvest using a small incision over the insertion on the medial tibia, allowing for less postoperative pain, better cosmesis, and shorter operative time. While there was early concern about its durability, newer techniques have made hamstring fixation reliable.

Once the graft is selected, the arthroscope is used to determine where the graft will be placed. Any remnant of the torn ACL is removed and then bone tunnels are drilled through the tibia and the femur in the anatomic direction of the ACL. The graft is then threaded through the tunnel and secured on both ends. The operation is somewhat more involved than meniscal surgery, requiring between 45 minutes and 2 hours of operative time on average, use of a pneumatic tourniquet, more postoperative analgesia, and a significantly longer rehabilitation. The procedure may be performed under general or spinal anesthesia. Blood loss remains minimal, as a majority of the procedure is performed arthroscopically, and patients are discharged immediately.

Cartilage

A discrete cartilage defect can be the source of pain and lead to increased contact pressures in the knee and development of post-traumatic arthritis. Newer techniques have begun to show some success in the treatment of these lesions. A microfracture procedure perforates the subchondral region in order to introduce bleeding into the local environment to stimulate a healing response. This is a relatively easy procedure, but requires the patient to be non-weight-bearing status for nearly 6 weeks to allow for healing. Additional procedures have been developed, including osteochondral autograft transplantation (OATS), which harvests osteochondral plugs from non-weight-bearing portions of the femoral condyle and transfers them to the area of the osteochondral lesion.

Osteoarthritis

The effectiveness of arthroscopy for degenerative disease is less clear. Mosely *et al.* reported on arthroscopic debridement and lavage for osteoarthritis of the knee and found it to be no more effective than placebo in terms of function or pain control. The result of these procedures is unpredictable at best. However, it is believed that there is a subset of patients with degenerative disease that arthroscopy may benefit, namely those with mechanical symptoms of locking, catching, or clicking that is the result of a meniscal or articular cartilage flap.

Usual postoperative course

Expected postoperative hospital stay
Many procedures are done on an ambulatory basis.

Operative mortality
Rare fatalities are related to anesthetic complications or thromboembolism.

Special monitoring required
None.

Patient activity and positioning

After surgery, patients are given crutches to assist with ambulation; they may be discarded when the patient is able to walk without a limp. This is typically not an issue with partial meniscectomies, but for ACL reconstructions and meniscal repairs patients are usually on crutches for 1 week. Again, patients undergoing cartilage procedures are non-weight-bearing for 6 weeks.

Alimentation

As tolerated.

Antibiotic coverage

Preoperative broad spectrum prophylaxis.

Pain management

During surgery, it is customary to inject local anesthetic into the portal sites and incisions to cause pre-emptive desensitization of nociceptors. Many surgeons also inject morphine and local anesthetic into the knee joint prior to and after the procedure, which has been shown to affect peripheral opioid receptors. Postoperative pain ranges from minimal after arthroscopic menisectomy to moderate after ACL reconstruction. Narcotic analgesics may be required for several days.

Rehabilitation

Protocols vary, depending on the surgery and the surgeon, but some basic principles are followed in all patients. All patients need to understand that the rehabilitation after ACL reconstruction is strenuous and time consuming. For active patients, it will be 9–12 months before they can play sports after ACL surgery. In the early healing period, the basic principle of the rehabilitation process is that motion is key. Immediately after operation, patients work on regaining a normal range of motion and on mild strengthening exercises. More aggressive strengthening may begin when the repair has been afforded time to heal. This is slowly combined with functional activities and then sports specific activities, finally ending with return to competition on a gradual basis. Patients undergoing meniscal surgery do not require extensive rehabilitation and are able to return to full activity when strength and range of motion are optimized.

Postoperative complications

In the hospital

A number of retrospective studies have shown a complication rate between 0.56% and 1.8%. The most common complications are hemarthrosis (60.1%), infection (12.1%), thromboembolic disease (6.9%), anesthesia complications (6.4%), instrument failure (2.9%), complex regional pain syndrome (2.3%), ligament injury (1.2%), and fracture or neurological injury (0.6% each).

Hemarthrosis

May occur in approximately 1% of cases and is more common after release of the lateral patellofemoral retinaculum due to the disruption of the superior lateral geniculate artery.

Thromboembolic disease

Has been described in between 0.1% and 0.17% of arthroscopies in published reports. Several factors have been associated with greater risk for patients, such as being over 40 years of age, undergoing prolonged operating or tourniquet time, and having a history of prior thrombosis or embolus.

Infections

While a rare occurrence, infections are a horrendous complication. They often require arthroscopic lavage and debridement, followed by 4 to 6 weeks of intravenous antibiotics.

Neurological injury

Such injuries may be due to direct damage, compartment syndrome, or external compression due to positioning of the patient or tourniquet compression. Most direct injuries are seen with meniscal repairs.

Compartment syndrome

Caused by fluid extravasation into the thigh or calf via rupture in the suprapatellar pouch or the semimembranosus bursa, respectively.

After discharge

Delayed problems generally relate to persistent or recurrent pain or instability and may require additional treatment.

FURTHER READING

Allum, R. Complications of arthroscopy of the knee. *J. Bone Joint Surg.* 2002; **84B**: 937–945.

Arnoczky, S. P. & Warren, R. F. Microvasculature of the human meniscus. *Am. J. Sports Med.* 1982; **10**: 90–95.

Engebretsen, L., Benum, P., Fasting, O., Molster, A., & Strand, T. A prospective, randomized study of three surgical techniques for treatment of acute ruptures of the anterior cruciate ligament. *Am. J. Sports Med.* 1990; **18**: 585–590.

Fairbanks, T. J. Knee joint changes after meniscectomy. *J. Bone Joint Surg.* 1948; **30B**: 664–670.

Grontvedt, T., Engebretsen, L., Benum, P. *et al.* A prospective, randomized study of three operations for acute rupture of the anterior cruciate ligament: five year follow-up of one hundred and thirty-one patients. *J. Bone Joint Surg.* 1996; **78A**: 159–168.

Jackson, R. W. Current concepts review. Arthroscopic surgery. *J. Bone Joint Surg.* 1983; **65A**: 416–420.

Moseley, J. B., O'Malley, K., Petersen, N. J. *et al.* A controlled trial of arthroscopic surgery for osteoarthritis of the knee. *N. Engl. J. Med.* 2002; **347**(2): 81–88.

Rodeo, S. A., Forster, R. A., & Weiland, A. J. Current concepts review. Neurological complications due to arthroscopy. *J. Bone Joint Surg.* 1993; **75A**: 917–926.

Small, N. C. Complications in arthroscopic surgery performed by experienced arthroscopists. *Arthroscopy* 1988; **4**: 215–221.

Total knee replacement

Mark Hanna and James Roberson

Emory University School of Medicine, Atlanta, GA

The primary indication for total knee replacement is pain and dysfunction due to degenerative or inflammatory arthritis. The artificial knee consists of a resilient, highly polished metal alloy which is designed to cap the femur and articulate with a high-density cross-linked polyethylene tibial component. The polyethylene is often held in place on top of the tibia with a metal tray. Resurfacing the patella with a rounded piece of polyethylene is commonly performed. Most total knee devices use bone cement for fixation; however, some designs have porous metal surfaces which allow for bony ingrowth.

The procedure is commonly performed through a midline skin incision over the anterior aspect of the knee. An incision is then made along the medial border of the patella and the patella is everted laterally, providing full exposure of the ends of the tibia and femur so that they can be prepared by making several cuts using special guides. Careful attention is given to the alignment of the components and the balancing of the knee ligaments. The operation usually takes less than 2 hours, though complicated total knee replacements can take longer. General, spinal, and epidural anesthesia are routinely used. The surgery is usually performed with a tourniquet on the upper thigh to limit intraoperative blood loss. Postoperative bleeding will occasionally require a transfusion, though this complication is more common in total hip arthroplasty. Based on the likelihood of the need for transfusion, which is usually low for primary total knee arthroplasty, autologous blood donation is recommended.

Despite the fact that this has been done for over 20 years, unicompartmental knee replacement is becoming more popular and involves replacement of either the medial or lateral compartment only. Its performance is usually similar to that described above, though it can be done through a much smaller incision without everting the patella, creating less soft tissue damage and allowing for much faster recovery.

Usual postoperative course

Expected postoperative hospital stay
3–5 days.

Operative mortality
Less than 1%.

Special monitoring required
Neurovascular checking of the extremity should be performed during the early postoperative period to rule out neural or vascular injury, which are rare. Monitoring for clinical signs of deep vein thrombosis should be conducted during the remainder of the hospital stay.

Patient activity and positioning
Early mobilization is encouraged following total knee replacement. Patients are made weight bearing as tolerated and asked to walk on the first postoperative day. Before becoming completely independent, they will need to use either a walker or crutches for a month followed by a cane for another month. Physical therapy is consulted to encourage ambulation as well as range of motion exercises. Some surgeons use constant passive motion machines or knee immobilizers to assist with motion. Patients should be able to get out of bed, walk in the hall, and maneuver a few stairs prior to going home. If individuals are slow to achieve these goals, then a short stay in a rehabilitation hospital is recommended.

Alimentation
Diet is advanced as tolerated. Postoperative ileus is rare. Oral pain medicines are usually started on the second postoperative day.

Medical Management of the Surgical Patient: A Textbook of Perioperative Medicine, ed. M. F. Lubin, R. B. Smith, T. F. Dobson, N. Spell, H. K. Walker. 4th edn. Published by Cambridge University Press. © Cambridge University 2006.

Antibiotic coverage

A first-generation cephalosporin is administered just before the incision is made and then continued 24 hours postoperatively. Vancomycin is given to patients who have a significant penicillin allergy.

Postoperative complications

In the hospital

Fever

Similar to that of total hip replacement and many other orthopedic surgeries, postoperative fever is ubiquitous with total knee replacement. Low grade temperatures of up 101.5 °F for 2 to 4 days are probably related to marrow emboli created during preparation of the femur and tibia. Investigation of postoperative fever in these patients is usually negative unless other clinical findings are apparent.

Thromboembolism

Without prophylaxis, deep vein thrombosis occurs in 50% to 80% of patients following total knee replacement. Prophylactic measures such as early mobilization, sequential compression devices, epidural anesthesia and aspirin, low molecular weight heparin, or warfarin reduce the incidence to 30%–40%. Symptomatic pulmonary embolism occurs in 2%–7% of patients and fatal pulmonary embolism has been reported in 0.2%–0.7% of patients. Use of pharmacologic prophylaxis must be weighed against the possibility of bleeding complications.

Bleeding

Postoperative bleeding and hematoma can be very serious problems following total knee replacement. Meticulous hemostasis after deflating the tourniquet and the use of drains postoperatively help prevent hematoma formation. Bleeding may be due to a pre-existing condition or medications used for prophylaxis. As mentioned in the total hip replacement chapter, full anticoagulation without proof of a suspected pulmonary embolus or deep vein thrombosis in the early postoperative period may lead to an unnecessary hematoma and associated morbidity. Hematomas often result in postoperative stiffness and can lead to prolonged serous drainage; the latter condition should be treated aggressively. If the wound continues to drain more than 5 to 7 days despite immobilization and local wound care, operative debridement is recommended. Infection is imminent in such situations.

Neurovascular injury

While rare, injury to nerves and blood vessels should be detected in the immediate postoperative period with neurovascular examination. Peroneal nerve palsy is usually associated with preoperative valgus deformity or flexion contracture. If the patient demonstrates a peroneal nerve palsy, the bandage should be immediately loosened and the knee flexed.

After discharge

Patellofemoral problems

Resurfacing of the patella can lead to many problems, such as patellar fracture, patellofemoral instability, and loosening of the patellar component. If the patella is not resurfaced, 50% of patients will have anterior knee pain. Other potential problems are rupture of quadriceps tendon or the patellar ligament.

Infection

This is a dreaded complication because it usually requires removal of the prosthesis and a prolonged antibiotic course. Persistent infections despite aggressive therapy can lead to amputation. Hematogenous seeding of the prosthetic joint is an unlikely, but permanent, possibility. However, routine prophylaxis following total knee replacement prior to dental procedures, cystoscopy, colonoscopy, etc., is no longer endorsed. Antibiotic prophylaxis is recommended for patients with predisposing conditions (immunosuppression, rheumatoid arthritis, hemophilia, etc.) or active acute/chronic infection near the area of the proposed procedure. Cephalexin or clindamycin is recommended if prophylaxis is indicated.

Stiffness

Expected and usually related to pain and swelling; it often resolves in 6–8 weeks. Manipulation and further work-up should be considered at 3 months. Skillful surgical technique and patient education regarding expectations and goals following surgery can usually prevent problems with stiffness.

Polyethylene wear and loosening

As the metal femoral component articulates with the polyethylene tibial component, microscopic wear particles are released into the joint. In a process known as osteolysis, the most common cause of loosening in total knee replacement, these particles stimulate an inflammatory response which can break down bone. Surgical technique in total knee replacement is critical because a malpositioned component will lead to abnormal stresses, increased wear, and early failure. Affected patients develop a limp and pain with weight bearing. Reoperation is often necessary; revision surgery has less predictable outcomes and more complications.

FURTHER READING

Ayers, D. C., Dennis, D. A., Johanson, N. A., & Pelligrini, V. D. Common complications of total knee arthroplasty. *J. Bone Joint Surg. Am.* 1997; **79**: 278–311.

Deacon, J. M., Pagliaro, A. J., Zelicof, S. B., & Horowitz, H. W. Current concepts review: prophylactic use of antibiotics for procedures after total joint replacement. *J. Bone Joint Surg. Am.* 1996; **78**: 1755–1770.

Geerts, W. H., Heit, J. A., Clagett, G. P. *et al.* Prevention of Venous Thromboembolism, Sixth ACCP Consensus Conference on Antithrombotic Therapy. *Chest* 2001; **119**(1S): 132S–175S.

Hatzidakis, A. M., Mendlick, R. M., McKillip, T., Reddy, R. L., & Garvin, K. L. Preoperative autologous donation for total joint arthroplasty. *J. Bone Joint Surg. Am.* 2000; **82**: 89–100.

Westrich, G. H., Haas, S. B., Mosca, P., & Peterson, M. Meta-analysis of thomboembolic prophylaxis after total knee arthroplasty. *J. Bone Joint Surg. Br.* 2000; **82**: 795–800.

Total hip replacement

Mark Hanna and James Roberson

Emory University School of Medicine, Atlanta, GA

Pain and limitation of function due to hip arthritis are the primary indications for total hip arthroplasty. The artificial hip is most commonly a metal-on-polyethylene design. The femoral component is a high strength metal alloy fashioned into a spherical head, which articulates with the acetabular component, a high-density cross-linked polyethylene shaped like a socket. Metal-on-metal and ceramic-on-ceramic hips are also used. The femoral component is placed within the medullary canal after preparation of the femur and the acetabular component is fixed to the pelvis. Both mechanisms are inserted using bone cement or in a "press–fit" fashion. The "press–fit" components have a porous-coated surface which allows for bone growth into the prosthesis and, therefore, permanent biologic fixation.

Total hip replacement usually takes 2 hours or less, though such complicated cases as revision of a failed replacement require much more time. Depending on surgeon and patient preference, general, spinal, or epidural anesthesia can be used. The average blood loss is 500 ml and postoperative blood transfusion is often required. Patients are asked to donate blood preoperatively based on their age and the type of surgery planned.

Usual postoperative course

Expected postoperative hospital stay
3–5 days.

Operative mortality
Less than 1%.

Special monitoring required
Neurovascular examination of the extremity should be performed in the early postoperative period. Monitoring for clinical signs of deep vein thrombosis must continue during the subsequent hospital stay.

Patient activity and positioning
The patient is mobilized and encouraged to walk on the first postoperative day. Generally, patients are allowed to weight bear as tolerated unless otherwise specified by the surgeon. Patients should be able to get out of bed, walk in the hall, and maneuver a few stairs prior to leaving the hospital. If the patient is having difficulty achieving these goals in a timely manner, a short stay at a rehabilitation hospital is encouraged. Either a walker or crutches are required for a month, followed by a cane for the second month. Patients are instructed to avoid extremes of hip motion for 3 months to minimize the possibility of dislocation. The hip should not be flexed more than 90 degrees or hyperextended. Hip adduction must also be avoided.

Alimentation
Patients are allowed clear liquids on the day of operation and diet is advanced as tolerated. Occasionally, postoperative ileus occurs, delaying oral intake.

Antibiotic coverage
Prophylactic antibiotics have been shown to decrease the infection rate following total hip arthroplasty. A first-generation cephalosporin is given in the operating room prior to the skin incision and then continued for 24 hours after surgery. Vancomycin is used in patients who are allergic to cephalosporins.

Postoperative complications

In the hospital

Fever
Although commonly observed following surgery, fever is ubiquitous after hip replacement. Because of the extensive

Medical Management of the Surgical Patient: A Textbook of Perioperative Medicine, ed. M. F. Lubin, R. B. Smith, T. F. Dobson, N. Spell, H. K. Walker. 4th edn. Published by Cambridge University Press. © Cambridge University 2006.

work done within the marrow of the femur and pelvis, virtually all patients have fevers as high as 101.5 °F for 2 to 4 days. This may be related to bone marrow fat being filtered in the lungs on a subclinical level without causing changes in the chest radiograph. Embarking on an investigation for infection during this period is expensive and invariably negative if no other clinical findings are apparent.

Thromboembolism
As many as 50% of patients undergoing total hip arthroplasty have been found to have deep venous thrombosis on routine venograms. This incidence can be reduced by prophylactic measures such as low molecular weight heparin, aspirin, or warfarin; sequential compression stockings; and early mobility. Despite these measures, deep vein thrombosis still occurs in 15% to 30% of patients. Most of these are asymptomatic and are at, or below, the popliteal vein. Symptomatic pulmonary embolus transpires in about 1% of patients and fatal pulmonary embolus takes place in 0.1% to 0.2% of cases. The type of prophylaxis used depends on the surgeon's training and previous experience and must be weighed against the risk of bleeding.

Bleeding
Postoperative bleeding and hematoma are usually prevented by meticulous hemostasis prior to wound closure. As mentioned before, blood transfusion for postoperative anemia is not uncommon. The medications used for prophylaxis of deep vein thrombosis and pulmonary embolism increase the risk of bleeding. In addition, when a pulmonary embolus is suspected in the early postoperative period, proof of the embolus with a spiral chest CT or VQ scan is highly recommended prior to full anticoagulation. Pulmonary embolus is less likely to occur in the first few days following the procedure and full anticoagulation within 48 to 72 hours following total hip replacement greatly increases the risk of hematoma and its subsequent morbidity. Hematomas are usually observed but occasionally require operative decompression and debridement.

Nerve damage and leg length discrepancy
These complications are rare and are more likely to occur following difficult revision surgery.

After discharge

Dislocation
Occurring when the hip is placed in extremes of flexion or extension, this complication is noted in about 2% of prosthetic hips in the first year and increases to 7% by 25 years. Patient education of their limitations in the early postoperative period is critical to helping to prevent this problem. Closed reduction under conscious sedation or general anesthesia is usually successful, but recurrent dislocations may require reoperation and revision of the components.

Infection
This dreaded complication usually requires removal of the prosthesis and a prolonged course of antibiotics prior to reimplantation. Acute postoperative infections are possible but rare. Later hematogenous seeding of the prosthetic joint is an unlikely, but permanent, possibility. However, routine prophylaxis following total hip replacement prior to dental procedures, cystoscopy, colonoscopy, etc., is no longer recommended. Antibiotic prophylaxis is recommended for patients with predisposing conditions (immunosuppression, rheumatoid arthritis, hemophilia, etc.) or active acute/chronic infection near the area of the proposed procedure. Cephalexin or clindamycin is recommended if prophylaxis is indicated.

Prosthetic wear and loosening
Deterioration in the total hip prosthesis occurs with each step. As the metal femoral head contacts the polyethylene acetabulum, small microscopic particles are deposited in the soft tissues and throughout the joint. In the process known as osteolysis, which is the most common cause of late prosthetic loosening, these small particles stimulate an inflammatory response that can absorb bone. Firm fixation of the components is required for painless function and, if loosening occurs, the patient may develop thigh pain and a limp. Radiographs often show lucent lines around the prosthesis. For various reasons, about 1% of hip replacements require revision operations each year; the procedures are technically difficult and associated with increased operative time, blood loss, and complications.

FURTHER READING

Deacon, J. M., Pagliaro, A. J., Zelicof, S. B., & Horowitz, H. W. Current concepts review: prophylactic use of antibiotics for procedures after total joint replacement. *J. Bone Joint Surg. Am.* 1996; **78**: 1755–1770.

Freedman, K. B., Brookenthal, K. R., Fitzgerald, R. H., Williams, S., & Lonner, J. H. A metaanalysis of thromboembolic prophylaxis following elective total hip arthroplasty. *J. Bone Joint Surg. Am.* 2000; **82**: 929–938.

Hatzidakis, A. M., Mendlick, R. M., McKillip, T., Reddy, R. L., & Garvin, K. L. Preoperative autologous donation for total joint arthroplasty. *J. Bone Joint Surg. Am.* 2000; **82**: 89–100.

Roberson, J. & Nasser, S., eds. Complications of total hip arthroplasty. *Orthop. Clin. North Am.* 1992; **23**.

Salvati, E. A., Pelegrini, V. O., Sharrock, N. E. *et al.* Recent advances in venous thromboembolic prophylaxis during and after total hip replacement. *J. Bone Joint Surg. Am.* 2000; **82**: 252–270.

111

Fractures of the femoral shaft

Lisa K. Cannada and Robert M. Harris

Emory University School of Medicine, Atlanta, GA

The femur is the largest and strongest bone in the body and has a significant soft tissue envelope protecting it. The femoral shaft is defined as the diaphyseal portion of the bone, from below the lesser trochanter to above the metaphyseal portion of the distal femur. Most femoral shaft fractures occur after high-energy trauma such as motor vehicle collisions, vehicles striking pedestrians, falls, gunshots, and sports injuries. Such injuries warrant a complete evaluation according to guidelines established by the American College of Surgeons in the Advanced Trauma Life Support courses. High-energy femoral shaft fractures may be associated with significant damage, including head, thoracic, abdominal, or other extremity injuries. Once the trauma evaluation is complete, one may concentrate on the femoral shaft fracture, which can be associated with significant blood loss in the soft tissue envelope of anywhere from 500–1500 ml or more. The patient must be resuscitated and monitored closely.

The gold standard in the treatment of femoral shaft fracture remains the antegrade locked intramedullary nail. Advances in design and technique offer additional options for nailing: retrograde nailing and reconstruction nailing through a greater trochanter starting point. Additional options include open reduction with a plate and screws and external fixation as a temporizing measure or definitive treatment. The patient's additional injuries, body size, and pre-existing comorbid conditions combined with the personality of the fracture assist the surgeon in determining a treatment plan. The non-operative treatment of femoral shaft fractures in the adult patient is only of historical interest. Open femur fractures require emergent debridement and fixation. The patient may be placed in skeletal traction as a temporizing measure before operative fixation.

The timing of surgery is important. In patients with isolated femoral shaft fractures and those with multiple injuries, any delay in definitive stabilization of more than 24 hours can be detrimental, potentially resulting in an increased incidence of lung problems, such as adult respiratory distress syndrome (ARDS), fat embolization, and pneumonia; a longer intensive care unit (ICU) and hospital stay; and an increased cost of hospitalization. The goals of surgical treatment include rigid fixation to allow for early patient mobilization and joint motion.

Usual postoperative course

Expected postoperative hospital stay

Dependent on the presence of associated injuries. A patient with an isolated femoral shaft fracture usually remains hospitalized for 2–4 days.

Operative mortality

The mortality after femoral shaft fractures is low; however, the risk of death is highly dependent on associated injuries. In patients with bilateral femoral shaft fractures, the mortality rate is increased to as high as 25%. Mortality in these patients is more closely related to associated injuries and physiologic parameters than to their bilateral femur fractures.

Special monitoring required

Following operation, the patient's neurovascular status should be assessed and the limb followed closely for compartment syndrome. In addition, the patient's ongoing resuscitation should be evaluated through postoperative laboratory values (including hematocrit) and urinary output. The victim's mental status and oxygenation levels should also be addressed to assess the possibility of fat emboli syndrome, ARDS, and risk of pulmonary embolism.

Medical Management of the Surgical Patient: A Textbook of Perioperative Medicine, ed. M. F. Lubin, R. B. Smith, T. F. Dobson, N. Spell, H. K. Walker. 4th edn. Published by Cambridge University Press. © Cambridge University 2006.

Patient activity and positioning

With rigid fracture fixation, early mobilization and weight bearing are the goals. Once a femoral shaft fracture is stabilized, the patient is expected to be mobilized on the day following surgery. The nature of their injury, type of implant, and surgeon preference dictate the exact postoperative therapy orders. Early active motion of the hip and knee joint is encouraged.

Alimentation

Clear liquids are permitted with advancement to a regular diet as the bowel sounds return. In the multiply injured trauma patient, metabolic requirements are significantly increased. Early alimentation is initiated through tube feedings or intravenous hyperalimentation, with advancement as the patient's condition improves.

Antibiotic coverage

A first-generation cephalosporin administered preoperatively and then for 24 hours postoperatively is an accepted standard for isolated, closed femoral shaft fractures. For open fractures, a first generation cephalosporin is used for Grade I and II open fractures. For Grade IIIA open fractures, an aminoglycoside is added. For grossly contaminated fractures, Grade IIIB and IIIC injuries, a penicillin is administered. In addition, patients with open fractures should have appropriate tetanus prophylaxis.

Clinical and radiographic evaluation

Patients should return for their first clinical visit 10–14 days after operation for wound check and suture/staple removal. Radiographs are recommended on a monthly basis until fracture union is noted, then at 6 and 12 months after injury. Clinical evaluation should also include monitoring of progress in range of motion, motor strength, and return to functional activities.

Postoperative complications

In the hospital

Fat embolism syndrome

Usually occurs 24–72 hours after trauma in 3%–4% of patients with long bone fractures; can be fatal in 10%–15% of cases. The classic symptoms include tachypnea, tachycardia, hypoxemia, mental status changes, and petechiae. Treatment includes mechanical ventilation with high levels of PEEP. More importantly, prevention includes early skeletal stabilization of long bone fractures.

Thromboembolism

Deep venous thrombosis is common in patients with lower extremity fractures and multiple trauma victims. It may lead to a fatal pulmonary embolism (PE). PE should be suspected in patients with acute onset tachypnea, tachycardia, mental status changes, and pleuritic pain. Evaluation should include EKG (to look for a right bundle branch block), chest X-ray, and arterial blood gas. A duplex ultrasound may be used to diagnose deep venous thrombosis in the limb. In the case of a PE, a spiral CT scan, ventilation–perfusion scan or pulmonary angiography (gold standard) may be used for the diagnosis. Preventive measures include mechanical with the use of sequential compression devices and chemical with subcutaneous heparin, warfarin (rarely in trauma patients), or low molecular weight heparin (LMWH). Early surgical stabilization and subsequent mobilization are important, controllable measures.

Adult respiratory distress syndrome (ARDS)

ARDS is acute respiratory failure with pulmonary edema. It can be due to multiple etiologies and is known to occur after trauma and shock. The patient may be difficult to ventilate secondary to decreased lung compliance. Other signs/symptoms include tachypnea, tachycardia, and hypoxemia. Treatment is with high PEEP. The mortality can be up to 50%. From an orthopedic surgeon's perspective, early stabilization of long bone fractures helps to decrease the incidence of ARDS.

Compartment syndrome

This complication is characterized by elevated pressures within a soft tissue envelope of an extremity and can occur when there has been significant trauma. The increased pressures within a contained space (the muscle compartment) can lead to ischemia and irreversible damage to the nerve and muscle within the compartment. Compartment syndrome after femur fractures is rare; however it can occur in any of the compartments of the upper and lower extremity after trauma. The classic findings include a tense compartment, pain out of proportion to injury, paresthesias, and possibly pulselessness. An emergent fasciotomy is necessary when the diagnosis of compartment syndrome is confirmed.

Nerve paresis

Femur fractures may be fixed on the fracture table and result in a pudendal nerve palsy. This is thought to be due to excessive traction while the patient is on the fracture table and/or improper positioning against the perineal post. It results in a loss of sensation in the genital region. A peroneal nerve neuropraxia with resulting foot drop may also occur if excessive traction is used.

After discharge

Non-union, delayed union, malunion

The rate of non-unions after treatment of femoral shaft fractures with a locked, intramedullary nail is low. The diagnosis is based on the clinical symptoms and radiographic appearance. Treatment is exchange nailing with a slightly larger intramedullary nail. An infected non-union requires more significant surgical treatment and the use of long-term antibiotics, but fortunately is rare after femur fractures. Delayed unions are slightly more common and may be more likely to occur in the multiple trauma patient. Removal of the interlocking screw may allow compression across the fracture site and permit union to occur. The occurrence of malunion after femur fractures is not as well documented in the literature. There may be multiple etiologies and the choice of treatment depends on the cause of the malunion. It has been reported that up to 20% of patients may have rotational deformities but most patients are asymptomatic.

Hardware failure and recurrent fracture

With reamed, statically locked nailing of femur fractures the occurrence of hardware failure is low. The closer a fracture is to the interlocking screw placement the greater the stresses placed on the hardware. If a patient has removal of a femoral plate or intramedullary nail, they must remain non-weight bearing for an extended period of time to minimize the risk of refracture.

Heterotopic ossification

The insertion site for an antegrade nail involves soft tissue dissection. As a result, some patients may develop heterotopic ossification about the hip. In some studies, it has been reported to occur in up to 26% of patients. The clinical significance of this problem is usually minimal, but in severe cases of heterotopic ossification there may be limitation in motion about the hip. This problem does not occur after retrograde intramedullary nailing.

FURTHER READING

Bone, L. B., Johnson, K. D., Weigelt, J., & Scheinberg, R. Early versus delayed stabilization of femoral fractures. *J. Bone Joint Surg. Am.* 1989; **71**: 336–340.

Brumback, R. J., Ellison, P. S., Poka, A., Lakatos, R., Bathon, G. H., & Burgess, A. R. Intramedullary nailing of open fractures of the femoral shaft. *J. Bone Joint Surg. Am.* 1989; **71**: 1324–1330.

Brumback, R. J., Wells, D., Lakatos, R., Poka, A., Bathon, G. H., & Burgess, A. R. Heterotopic ossification about the hip after intramedullary nailing for fractures of the femur. *J. Bone Joint Surg. Am.* 1990; **72**: 1067–1073.

Copeland, C. E., Mitchell, K. A., Brumback, R. J., Gens, D. R., & Burgess, A. R. Mortality in patients with bilateral femur fractures. *J. Orthop. Trauma* 1998; **12**: 315–319.

Patterson, B. M., Routt, M. L. C., Benirschke, S. K., & Hansen, S. V. Retrograde nailing of femoral shaft fractures. *J. Trauma* 1995; **38**: 38–43.

Riska, E. B. & Myllynen, P. Fat embolism in patients with multiple injuries. *J. Trauma* 1982; **22**: 891–894.

Winquist, R. A., Hansen, S. T., & Clawson, D. K. Closed intramedullary nailing of femoral fractures: a report of five hundred and twenty cases. *J. Bone Joint Surg. Am.* 1984; **66**: 529–539.

112

Surgery for hip fractures

Brett S. Sanders and Lisa K. Cannada

Emory University School of Medicine, Atlanta, GA

The term hip fracture is used collectively to refer to fractures of the femoral neck and trochanteric region (i.e., intertrochanteric and subtrochanteric) that occur in two demographic populations: the young and the elderly. Hip fractures in the young result from high velocity trauma to normal bone, while fracture mechanism in the elderly is low velocity and usually involves underlying bone pathology (osteoporosis). Currently, there are 350 000 hip fractures per year in the USA, and this figure is expected to double by 2050. Healthcare cost of treatment of this injury is estimated at 10–15 billion dollars per year, defining it as an enormous burden to society.

Hip fractures may be managed operatively or non-operatively. Non-operative management consisting of early mobilization and adaptive training may be instituted in patients who are non-ambulatory or of unacceptable medical risk. The majority of patients, however, will require operative management to optimize the chance of meaningful functional recovery to premorbid status. Minimally displaced femoral neck fractures in the elderly and many non-displaced femoral neck fractures in the young are treated with percutaneous screw fixation. Displaced femoral neck fractures in the elderly (greater than 65 years of age) often have high complication rates with internal fixation and are best treated with prosthetic replacement. Peritrochanteric fractures are treated with rigid internal fixation according to fracture type and surgeon preference.

The operation that will be least stressful to the patient but allow early mobility and the best chance of recovery is chosen depending on the clinical situation. General endotracheal anesthesia is utilized unless medical comorbidities dictate the use of a regional block and a limited (percutaneous) treatment. Percutaneous screw fixation requires a small incision, minimal operative time, and results in blood loss of 100–300 ml. Prosthetic replacement and open reduction with internal fixation require more extensive exposure and engender a blood loss that may exceed 500 ml. Operative time may take 2 or more hours and the patient is exposed to increased risk of postoperative anemia requiring transfusion.

Usual postoperative course

Expected postoperative hospital stay

May range from 3–7 days, depending on the nature and severity of premorbid medical problems and postoperative complications. Many patients require a short course of rehabilitation. Psychiatric illnesses such as dementia, delirium, and depression may delay recovery of mobility and prolong hospital stay. Absence of social support may also impede discharge.

Operative mortality

Anesthetic mortality rate approaches 1%, depending on ASA classification status; however, 1 year mortality rates are clearly higher in patients with hip fractures compared to age matched controls (14% vs. 9%, respectively). More than 4% of patients die during their hospitalization and 1 year mortality rates range from 10%–35% in some series. Operative mortality is reduced by half in previously ambulatory relatively healthy patients (ASA I or II) if the operation is performed within 2 calendar days of admission. However, patients with severe medical disease may require operative delay for medical optimization. Factors related to increased mortality rates include male sex, preexisting psychiatric illness, and three or more comorbidities.

Special monitoring required

As determined by the patient's physical status. Preoperative anticoagulation should be discontinued and

Medical Management of the Surgical Patient: A Textbook of Perioperative Medicine, ed. M. F. Lubin, R. B. Smith, T. F. Dobson, N. Spell, H. K. Walker. 4th edn. Published by Cambridge University Press. © Cambridge University 2006.

coagulation values normalized. The hematocrit level should be followed daily for the first 3 days to assess continuing blood loss and postoperative hemodilution. Anticoagulants and preoperative medications may need specialized monitoring. Routine serial physical examination is used to assess mental function and neurovascular status of the affected limb. Bone radiographs are an important part of the postoperative clinical follow-up.

Patient activity and positioning

The majority of patients should be mobilized to a chair postoperative on day 1. Weight-bearing status is determined by fracture stability and surgeon preference. Most patients will self-modulate actual weight-bearing secondary to pain. Physical therapy is consulted to assess the patient's need for assistive devices, to instruct regarding hip precautions, and to help with mobilization. If possible, wheelchair use is avoided because it discourages mobility and slows rehabilitation.

Alimentation

After recovery from anesthesia, clear liquids are permitted and diet is advanced as tolerated. As many as half of elderly patients exhibit findings of malnutrition on admission. Because protein-calorie malnutrition may influence infection rates and healing potential, postoperative dietary supplementation and nutritional evaluation may be necessary. Narcotic pain medication, diminished physical activity, and advanced age may lead to constipation and/ or ileus.

Antibiotic coverage

Administration of an intravenous first generation cephalosporin for the first 24 to 48 hours provides adequate prophylactic coverage for skin flora. Some surgeons may continue coverage until the surgical drains are removed. Supplemental use of an aminoglycoside may be necessary in the presence of a nosocomial infection or chronic indwelling foley catheter.

Postoperative complications

In the hospital

Hypotension

May result from blood loss or dehydration. An adequate preoperative assessment is essential for prevention of the latter. Crystalloid and blood products are administered as needed. The patient's cardiac function must be considered in balancing input and monitoring output.

Thromboembolism

Hip fracture patients who do not receive prophylactic anticoagulation experience deep venous thrombosis (DVT) rates of 40% to 50%. Even with current prophylactic modalities, venous thrombosis occurs in 20% of all hip surgeries and fatal pulmonary thromboembolism is reported at 2%–10%, making it the single most prevalent cause of postoperative mortality. To reduce the incidence of DVT, the measures that should be instituted in all hip fracture patients both pre- and postoperatively include sequential compression devices and various anticoagulants such as warfarin, subcutaneous heparin, and low molecular weight heparin (LMWH). LMWH is touted to have improved safety and efficacy without the need for monitoring due to a predictable pharmacokinetic profile. Patients who are elderly with decreased mobility and patients who have undergone hemiarthroplasty should be anticoagulated for 4 to 6 weeks postsurgically on some form of chemoprophylaxis.

Decubitus ulcers

By the fifth hospital day, as many as 20%–70% of patients with hip fractures may develop decubitus ulcers affecting the sacrum and heels. The incidence of these ulcers correlates with age, paralysis, sensory impairment, malnutrition, and incontinence. Preventive measures such as foam padding, frequent turning, excellent nursing care, and rapid mobilization should be rigorously enforced as the hospital mortality rate in these patients is reported to be 27%.

Urinary retention and urinary tract infection

The incidence of these complications is 30%–50% and 10%–20%, respectively. Narcotic analgesics, anesthetics, and prostatic hypertrophy in males are contributors to urinary retention, while infection is usually related to an indwelling catheter. Prophylactic use of an indwelling catheter with discontinuation within 24 hours of operation can decrease the occurrence of retention without increasing the risk of infection.

Altered mentation

Occurs in 30%–50% of elderly patients in the postoperative setting. There is a well known relationship between mental status change and poor functional outcome with prolonged hospital course. Etiologies of delirium include medications, infection, cardiovascular dysfunction, hypoxemia, thromboembolism, electrolyte and glucose abnormalities, and aspiration. Delirium usually abates within one week with appropriate management. A preoperative geriatric consultation may be helpful in reducing the incidence of this complication.

After discharge

Recovery time and functional outcome

A hip fracture often heralds a functional decline. Many patients lose the ability to live independently and over half do not regain their prefracture level of mobility. Although bone healing occurs in 4 to 6 weeks, it may take months of rehabilitation before the patient meets functional goals, if at all. Preoperative health status and mobility are the most valuable predictors of postoperative outcome. Preoperative dementia, severe medical problems, impaired ambulatory status, and residence in a nursing home have a negative impact on mortality, but only recently have outcome data become available. When activities of daily living are used as the measure, only 41% of patients regain prefracture function. Positive postoperative functional outcome correlates with age less than 85 years, premorbid independent living, and a fracture of the femoral neck. Recovery time is generally longer for intertrochanteric and subtrochanteric fractures than for fractures of the femoral neck.

Prevention of subsequent hip fracture

Falls and fractures are symptoms of underlying medical and social issues which require evaluation. Since many hip fracture patients never regain function, and 20% to 25% of patients will fracture the contralateral hip within five years, prevention is paramount. Preventive measures include treatment of underlying osteoporosis and education regarding prevention of falls at home with appropriate use of assistive devices. The use of hip protectors has proven efficacy for patients at risk for further falls.

Prosthetic dislocation and loosening

Prosthetic dislocation occurs in 0.3% to 11% of patients and usually happens in the early postoperative period. Loosening is the most common late complication of prosthetic replacement.

Non-union, malunion, and failure of fixation

These complications are related to vascular insufficiency, location of fracture, fracture stability, implant options, bone quality, and presence or absence of infection. These may occur as frequently as 10% in fractures about the hip. The need for reparation depends on etiology, physical status, and symptoms of the patient.

FURTHER READING

Bray, T. J., Smith-Hoefer, E., Hooper, A., & Timmerman, L. The displaced femoral neck fracture: internal fixation versus bipolar endoprosthesis: results of a prospective randomized comparison. *Clin. Orthop.* 1988; **230**: 127–140.

Holmes, J. Psychiatric illness predicts poor outcome after surgery for hip fracture: a prospective cohort study. *Psychol. Med.* 2000; **30**(4): 921–929.

Kenzora, J., McCarthy, R., Lowell, D., & Sledge, C. Hip fracture mortality: relation to age, treatment, time of surgery, and complications. *Clin. Orthop.* 1984; **186**; 45–55.

Koval, K. Clinical pathways for hip fractures in the elderly: the hospital for joint disease experience. AAOS 70th annual meeting: symposium C. Presented Feb 5, 2003.

Koval, K. J., Friend, K. D., Aharonoff, G. B., & Zukerman, J. D. Weight bearing after hip fracture: a prospective series of 596 geriatric hip fracture patients. *J. Orthop. Trauma* 1996; **10**: 526–530.

Marcantonio, E. R., Flacker, J. M., Michaels, M., & Resnick, N. M. Delirium is independently associated with poor functional recovery after hip fracture. *J. Am. Geriatr. Soc.* 2000; **48**(6): 618–624.

Morris, A. & Zuckermann, J. National Consensus Conference on improving the continuum of care for patients with hip fracture. *J. Bone Joint Surg. Am.* 2002; **4**: 640.

Smith, T. K. Prevention of complications in orthopedic surgery secondary to nutritional depletion. *Clin. Orthop.* 1987; **222**: 91–97.

Zimlich, R. H., Fulbright, B. M., & Friedman, R. J. Current status of anticoagulation therapy after total hip and total knee arthroplasty. *J. Am. Acad. Orthop. Surg.* 1996; **4**: 54–62.

Zuckerman, J. D., Skovron, M. L., Koval, K. J., Aharonoff, G., & Frankel, V. H. Postoperative complications and mortality associated with operative delay in older patients who have a fracture of the hip. *J. Bone Joint Surg. Am.* 1995; **77**: 1551–1555.

113

Lumbar spine surgery

Andrew E. Park and John G. Heller

Emory University School of Medicine, Atlanta, GA

Lumbar surgery in adults can be divided into three general levels of complexity and associated morbidity. The simplest and most common disorder is the herniated lumbar disk. Lumbar stenosis can affect multiple motion segments that will require decompression via a laminectomy. A lumbar diagnosis requiring fusion with or without decompression represents an incremental technical and physiologic event. With the recent advances in spinal instrumentation and biotechnology of bone graft substitutes, an anterior lumbar fusion procedure may be a viable substitute for some posterior fusion operations with less blood loss and faster recovery.

Patients with a lumbar disk herniation present with radiculopathy in a dermatomal pattern and may exhibit motor weakness or reflex changes which correspond to the anatomic level of neural compression. The host is typically a young adult in good health. Axial back pain is not a predominant symptom of this condition and is generally unimproved with a diskectomy. If the symptoms produced by lumbar disk herniation fail to respond to appropriate non-operative therapy, laminotomy and diskectomy are indicated. Patients are placed either prone or in the knee–chest position on a specially designed operating table; the latter position affords decompression of the abdominal cavity and the epidural veins. The procedure is performed with either loupe magnification or the surgical microscope through a posterior midline incision measuring 2.5 to 5 centimeters. The operative level is confirmed radiographically to prevent harming an otherwise normal intervertebral disk. Blood loss is minimal and the total anesthetic time is usually 1 to 2 hours.

Operative treatment of lumbar spinal stenosis requires a laminectomy with or without foraminotomies. The typical patient with spinal stenosis is older than the herniated disk patient and complains of leg pain, heaviness, numbness and/or tingling in one or both lower extremities. The symptoms are claudicating in character, as they increase with weight-bearing activity and are relieved by sitting or supine rest. While axial back pain is not a primary feature of spinal stenosis, a fusion may be added to the laminectomy in selected cases when it is clinically significant. Fusion is also indicated in conjunction with a laminectomy when instability is present on the preoperative radiographs, such as with a degenerative spondylolisthesis or degenerative scoliosis. The term laminectomy refers to the removal of one or more spinous processes and their associated laminae, traditionally for the purpose of decompressing the cauda eguina or lumbar nerve roots. Such exposure of the spinal canal allows the removal of facet joint osteophytes and thickened ligamentum flavum (foraminotomy), which may contribute to neural compression. Compared with laminotomy and diskectomy, laminectomy takes longer to perform, requires a larger incision, and engenders more blood loss (usually less than 500 ml). As stenosis patients are usually older, they often have more coexisting medical conditions and operative risk factors than diskectomy patients. Their preoperative medical clearance and perioperative medical care must account for these incremental risks.

Under certain circumstances, fusion of a lumbar motion segment may be required, which can be done by itself or in concert with either of the decompressive procedures described earlier. If lumbar instability exists before operation or is created during a laminotomy or laminectomy, fusion is performed. Posterolateral (intertransverse) fusion requires a far more extensive posterior muscle dissection. Bleeding from the branches of the lumbar segmental vessels can be copious, with blood loss increasing with each additional level fused. Significant blood loss also occurs from the posterior iliac crest during the harvest of autologous bone graft. Therefore, patients in suitable

Medical Management of the Surgical Patient: A Textbook of Perioperative Medicine, ed. M. F. Lubin, R. B. Smith, T. F. Dobson, N. Spell, H. K. Walker. 4th edn. Published by Cambridge University Press. © Cambridge University 2006.

health may wish to donate two to four units of autologous blood preoperatively or employ erythropoietin to stimulate marrow function, thus reducing the probability of their exposure to banked blood products. Intraoperative red blood cell salvage is another common adjunct to reduce transfusion exposure. Laminectomy and fusion procedures generally require 3½ to 5 hours. If segmental pedical screw fixation is used as an adjunct to the fusion procedure, operative times may increase by one to two more hours. While the use of such instrumentation increases the risk of certain technical complications and the volume of blood loss, it also improves the likelihood of achieving a successful fusion.

Fusion of lumbar motion segments can also be performed via an anterior procedure, which can be either transabdominal or through a retroperitoneal approach. The operation may be performed with autologous iliac crest bone, allograft bone, or a bone graft substitute such as the recently released bone morphogenic protein-2 (InFuse™, Medtronic Sofamor Danek, Inc., Memphis, TN). Any of the available techniques can be performed in conjunction with various forms of spinal instrumentation systems. A single level fusion can generally be completed in 1½ to 3 hours. The advantages of this approach are easier recoveries, generally less postoperative pain, and avoidance of lumbar muscle disturbance. The foraminotomy is accomplished indirectly with this technique by restoring height to the intervertebral space and the neural foramen. A disadvantage is that decompression of spinal stenosis from facet osteophytes and ligamentum flavum cannot be addressed with this technique. There are additional considerations unique to transabdominal or retroperitoneal surgery. They include inadvertent visceral injury, prolonged ileus, intraabdominal adhesions, vascular injury, deep venous thrombosis, and retrograde ejaculation.

Usual postoperative course

Expected postoperative hospital stay
Though some lumbar diskectomies are performed on an outpatient basis, it is common to expect one postoperative hospital day. The inpatient stay will then increase in proportion to the magnitude of the surgical dissection: 2 to 4 days for a laminectomy and 4 to 6 days for a posterior fusion procedure. Unless prolonged by an ileus, anterior lumbar interbody fusion techniques generally allow shorter hospital stays on the order of 2 to 4 days. Medical comorbidities may impact the duration of hospitalization and may also necessitate acute inpatient rehabilitation.

Operative mortality
Generally under 1%, though it increases in proportion to the magnitude of the procedure and the preoperative medical status of the patient.

Special monitoring required
Frequent neurologic evaluation should be performed during the first 24–48 hours after the operation. Any significant change should be reported at once, with appropriate and prompt investigation to be pursued in the event of objective change. Bleeding into the paraspinal tissues continues for two to three days, especially after posterior fusion procedures. The hematocrit decreases after surgery in proportion to the magnitude of the procedure, generally reaching its nadir by postoperative day 3. Platelet counts and coagulation studies should be monitored after large volumes of blood have been lost. For anterior lumbar procedures, pedal pulses should be checked pre and postoperatively since manipulation of the aorta, vena cava, and iliac vessels is occasionally needed for surgical exposure. Additionally, postoperative ileus may be more common for anterior procedures; consideration should be given to the use of nasogastric suction and the withholding of oral intake until the ileus resolves. Fevers below 38.5 °C are the rule more than the exception following fusion procedures; however, persistent or higher temperatures should be investigated thoroughly.

Patient activity and positioning
Ambulation begins on the first postoperative day after laminotomy and laminectomy and on the second postoperative day after fusion procedures. Patients should receive preoperative instruction regarding isometric trunk and lower extremity exercises, body mechanics, and bending and lifting restrictions. A lumbar support may be worn for comfort after laminotomy and laminectomy but is not required. The need for rigid bracing after fusion varies according to the specifics of the procedure and the preference of the surgeon. Unrestricted activity can be expected within 6 to 12 weeks after laminotomy and laminectomy and within 4 to 6 months after a fusion procedure.

Alimentation
Identifiable nutritional deficiencies should be corrected prior to operation, especially in patients undergoing fusion. After the procedure, food intake is advanced as tolerated. Patients undergoing fusion may have a significant adynamic ileus. If oral feeding is delayed more than 3 days, parenteral support should be contemplated.

Antibiotic coverage

Prophylaxis with a first-generation cephalosporin is the standard of care for spinal surgery. Additional doses are given during surgery (based on the duration of the procedure and the magnitude of blood loss) and for 24 hours afterwards. Antibiotics with a broader spectrum of activity may be used in patients who are compromised hosts, who have colonized urinary tracts, or who have required prolonged preoperative hospitalization.

Deep venous thrombosis

Prophylaxis to guard against this condition is recommended. Thigh-high elastic hose should be used in combination with sequential pneumatic compression stockings throughout the operative procedure up to when the patient has achieved independence with ambulation. Pharmacologic treatment with low dose warfarin or low-molecular weight heparin is generally not required. The use of low molecular weight heparin can result in an increased risk of bleeding complications and should be applied with caution. If a patient is at particularly high risk, a vena cava filter should be placed prior to surgery. Circumstances which warrant consideration of a filter include a history of deep venous thrombosis or pulmonary emboli, hypercoagulable states (e.g., protein S deficiency), morbid obesity, anticipation of prolonged immobility or bed rest, paraplegia or quadriplegia, and combined anterior/posterior spinal procedures.

Blood transfusion

Autologous blood donation is encouraged before fusion procedures and complex or revision laminectomies. Intraoperative red cell salvage and reinfusion is practiced during posterior fusion procedures. Bone marrow stimulation with erythropoietin may also be considered. The need for transfusion must be weighed against the patient's general medical condition, degree of anemia symptoms, and their wishes regarding blood product use.

Cigarette smoking

Tobacco interferes with bone graft and wound healing. Fusion potential may be maximized by preoperative cessation of all tobacco and nicotine products. Nicotine patches and analogous products are contraindicated when fusion is included in the procedure.

Medications

Medications that impair platelet function should be discontinued 2 to 4 weeks before operation to minimize intraoperative bleeding, especially when a fusion is planned. Oral narcotics may be appropriate as an alternative analgesic during the preoperative period. Non-steroidal anti-inflammatory drugs should not be used for at least three months after fusion procedures as they have been shown to inhibit the fusion process.

Postoperative complications

In the hospital

Hematoma

Subcutaneous hematomas or seromas are most common when the iliac crest is exposed through the same midline incision. Such collections are best prevented through careful wound closure and drainage of the wound as determined by the operating surgeon at the time of closure. Surgical evacuation is seldom required. Epidural hematomas usually present within 2 to 4 days as a cause of severe back or leg pain with progressive neurologic deficit. Emergent surgical exploration and decompression is required.

Infection

This complication's incidence varies from 0.5% to 5%, depending on the complexity of the case. Diagnosis can be delayed since the appearance of the wound is often deceptively normal. Treatment is by surgical debridement, closure over drains, and administration of parenteral antibiotics. Half-hearted attempts at treatment with antibiotics alone or in combination with local wound care are strongly discouraged, especially in the presence of bone grafts and/or spinal instrumentation.

Cerebrospinal fluid leakage

A dural tear should be surgically repaired when it is identified. If primary repair or patching of the dura is not possible, a closed subarachnoid drain should be used to divert the cerebrospinal fluid. Strict supine bed rest may be necessary for up to 48 hours after a dural repair. The wound dressing should be inspected for cerebrospinal fluid and patients observed for signs of meningitis. Prophylactic antibiotic coverage may be extended during the period that a subarachnoid drain is in place, but the agent chosen should have good blood–brain barrier penetration.

Persistent or recurrent radicular pain or neurologic deficit

Such complications may result from operation at the wrong level, incomplete removal of the herniated material or recurrence at the same level, unrecognized or inadequately decompressed foraminal stenosis, or just inflamed neural elements despite appropriate decompression. Malposition of hooks or pedicle screws may also cause such symptoms after an instrumented fusion. If sufficient symptoms or signs persist, myelography with computed tomography or magnetic resonance scanning is recommended to clarify such issues in the immediate postoperative period. Generally speaking, it is both wiser and easier to address identifiable problems early in the postoperative course rather than later after a period of wishful thinking has passed.

Bowel or bladder dysfunction

Injury to the sacral nerve roots resulting in neurogenic bowel or bladder dysfunction is rare. More often, especially in the elderly, an underlying degree of dysfunction caused by high-grade stenosis and bladder or prostate problems is unmasked under the influence of bed rest, bladder catheterization, and various medications. An intermittent catheterization program should be instituted as soon as possible to minimize the risk of urinary tract infection. Urologic consultation is advised if the symptoms do not resolve rapidly once patients are ambulatory. Retrograde ejaculation, which occurs in at least 5% of males undergoing anterior interbody fusions, should be discussed with the patient preoperatively, especially in regards to family planning. If the dysfunction persists, urologic consultation may be beneficial.

After discharge

Recurrent radicular pain

If this recurs after hospital discharge, each of the causes mentioned earlier should be reconsidered. In addition, postlaminectomy instability or fatigue fracture of the pars interarticularis can cause similar symptoms.

Back pain

The quantity and duration of local wound pain is proportional to the magnitude of the procedure performed. Incisional pain should be managed with analgesics as needed for a reasonable period. Debilitating postdiskectomy back pain may occur in 15% of patients and can be treated by lumbar fusion if warranted. Intervertebral diskitis or deep wound infection should also be considered, especially if the pain persists at night and is associated with diaphoresis and/or low grade temperatures. The external appearance of an infected wound may be deceptively normal, but the sedimentation rate and C-reactive protein levels are consistently elevated and should therefore be checked. Recurrent or new back pain may also be related to postlaminectomy instability or failed fusion.

Pseudarthrosis

The incidence of failed fusion varies with the number and location of segments, use of instrumentation, and the type of bone graft used. Pain is usually activity related. The diagnosis is made with appropriate radiographic studies, bearing in mind that plain radiographs are commonly misleading.

Instrumentation failure

Broken or loose implants are a hallmark of pseudarthrosis. Surgical repair of the non-union is recommended if the symptoms are sufficiently severe.

Wound infection

This complication is mentioned again because the diagnosis of a postoperative spinal wound infection is frequently delayed. Increasing back pain in association with malaise, sweats, chills, and an elevated erythrocyte sedimentation rate and c-reactive protein strongly suggests this diagnosis. Treatment is surgical, followed by administration of parenteral antibiotics.

Psychosocial dysfunction

For many patients who have undergone back surgery, reentry into the workplace requires a coordinated effort by patient, doctor, therapists, employer, and others. Patients must be strongly motivated to help themselves resume a normal lifestyle.

FURTHER READING

Garner, J. S. (1985) Guideline for prevention of surgical wound infections. Hospital Infections Program Centers for Infectious Diseases, Centers for Disease Control.

Herkowitz, H. N. & Sidhu, K. S. Lumbar spine fusion in the treatment of degenerative conditions: current indications and recommendations. *J. Am. Acad. Orthop. Surg.* 1995; **3**: 123–135.

Kjellby-Wendt, G. & Styf, J. Early active training after lumbar discectomy: a prospective randomized and controlled study. *Spine* 1998; **23**: 2345–2351.

Spivak, J. M. Degenerative lumbar spinal stenosis. *J. Bone Joint Surg. A.* 1998; **80**: 1053–1066.

Velmahos, G. C., Kern, J., Chan, L. S., Oder, D., Murray, J. A., & Shekelle, P. Prevention of venous thromboembolism after injury: an evidence based report. Part I: Analysis of factors and evaluation of the role of vena caval filters. *J. Trauma* 2000; **21**(9), 132–139.

Wood, K. B., Kos, P. B., Abnet, J. K., & Ista, C. Prevention of deep-vein thrombosis after major spinal surgery: a comparison study of external devices. *J. Spinal Disord.* 1997; **10**: 209–214.

Surgery for scoliosis or kyphosis in adults

William C. Horton and John M. Rhee

Emory University School of Medicine, Atlanta, GA

The most common indication for surgery in adults with scoliosis or kyphosis is debilitating pain from the deformity or associated spinal stenosis with neurological symptoms. Other indications include documented progression of the deformity or instability that hinders erect posture. Disease that threatens cardiopulmonary function is rare, but significant restrictive lung disease or cor pulmonale may be seen in patients with scoliosis greater than 90–100 degrees, thoracic lordosis, or disorders that affect chest mechanics (muscular dystrophy, ankylosing spondylitis, etc.). When indicated, pulmonary function tests should be correlated to arm span rather than height in the deformity patient. If significant cardiac failure is present preoperatively, the prognosis for life is usually not improved by correcting the deformity and surgery may be ill-advised. If the deformity is progressive and severe enough (more than 45–50 degrees), it is often preferable to perform surgery during adolescence because in adults the complications are more frequent, rehabilitation more extensive, and the operative risk greater. However, in adult patients, debility from chronic severe pain may force consideration of surgical intervention even with significant comorbidity. Depending on the exact nature of the surgery, the physiologic insult sustained by the adult deformity patient may be on par with or exceed that of a liver transplant. As a result, careful preoperative screening, risk stratification, and medical optimization in consultation with medical specialists is paramount to successful outcomes.

Either a posterior, anterior, or combined operative approach may be used. The principal goals of surgery are decompression of symptomatic neural structures, correction of major spinal imbalance, and stabilization of the deformity with fusion. Reconstruction usually requires autologous bone grafting and the use of metal internal fixation devices. Regardless of the operative approach used, the procedure constitutes a severe surgical stress.

Operations last 4 to 14 hours and blood loss may range from 500 to 5000 ml, involving multiple transfusions and significant fluid shifts. If the procedure is expected to last longer than 12 hours, it may be divided into anterior or posterior stages performed on different days. General endotracheal anesthesia is used, as is somatosensory or motor evoked spinal cord monitoring in most cases.

Usual postoperative course

Expected postoperative hospital stay

Approximately 1 to 2 weeks; most patients are fully independent at the time of discharge. If the anterior and posterior portions need to be staged and separated by several days, then the hospital course will be longer. Depending on the magnitude of surgery, postoperative stays in the intensive care unit are often necessary. Common ICU issues include postoperative intubation until airway edema subsides and monitoring for coagulopathy and neurologic changes. Spinal deformity patients occasionally need inpatient rehabilitation prior to their ultimate discharge.

Operative mortality

Ranges from under 1% in average cases to 6%–8% in patients with severe comorbidities.

Special monitoring required

In most cases, central venous access is necessary to manage volume resuscitation both intra- and postoperatively. Because spinal deformity surgery can place major metabolic and nutritional demands on the patient, dedicated central venous access is useful for postoperative hyperalimentation in patients who have staged surgery or are likely to have a prolonged ileus. An arterial line is also used

Medical Management of the Surgical Patient: A Textbook of Perioperative Medicine, ed. M. F. Lubin, R. B. Smith, T. F. Dobson, N. Spell, H. K. Walker. 4th edn. Published by Cambridge University Press. © Cambridge University 2006.

intraoperatively for hemodynamic monitoring (especially since hypotensive anesthesia may be employed to minimize blood loss) and observation of arterial blood gases.

Postoperative intubation is common in the spinal deformity patient because of prolonged surgery with large volume shifts, facial and airway edema from prone positioning, or the need for a transthoracic approach with surgical trauma to the lung and chest. However, patients are rapidly weaned as conditions permit, and tracheostomy is rarely required.

Patient activity and positioning

In order to prevent thromboembolic, pulmonary, and decubitus complications, early mobilization is desirable in the recovery of the deformity patient. Initially, patients are logrolled frequently (every 2–3 hours) while in bed and encouraged to spend time in the lateral position to prevent pressure sores to the extremities and any posterior incision. The head of the bed may be raised 30–45 degrees. Aggressive pulmonary toilet includes deep breathing, coughing, and incentive spirometry in every patient, but may initially be limited due to pain. Primarily for mobilization and gait training, physical therapy is prescribed in the hospital starting on postoperation day 1 or 2.

Spinal stability is a multifactorial situation, but patients with instrumentation are usually stable for mobilization. Patients having severe osteoporosis, a staged initial procedure without fixation, or corrective osteotomies may have a relatively unstable spine; mobilization in these cases should be decided on an individualized basis. In rare circumstances, early mobilization may be contraindicated. Most patients are encouraged to get out of bed and ambulate 2 to 4 days after surgery. If the patient sustained an intraoperative spinal fluid leak, they may need to lie with the head of the bed flat for 24–72 hours to allow the dural repair to seal without excessive hydrostatic pressure. While bracing may be necessary, it is being used much less because of improvements in spinal fixation implants.

Alimentation

Postoperative ileus is common for 1–4 days, especially in patients undergoing anterior lumbar spine surgery. Postoperative narcotics and slow mobilization contribute to the problem. Oral feedings should be delayed until the ileus resolves and the patient passes flatus, but judicious consumption of ice chips is generally well tolerated. Because of the severe metabolic demands placed on the postsurgical deformity patient, nutritional supplementation is mandatory. Proper nutrition is critical to healing and avoidance of wound and infectious complications. Although oral nutrition is instituted as soon as possible, intravenous hyperalimentation should be used if the period of ileus is expected to be prolonged. In patients undergoing staged deformity surgery, studies have demonstrated a clear benefit to hyperalimentation unless specific contraindications exist.

Antibiotic coverage

Intravenous cephalosporin or vancomycin is administered for 24 to 48 hours and may be used longer if a chest tube remains in place.

Pain management

Severe pain is common for 1 to 5 days following surgery. The patient controlled analgesia pump (PCA) is commonly used with transition to oral medications as ileus resolves. Non-steroidal anti-inflammatory drugs (NSAIDS) are avoided due to deleterious effects on platelets and on fusion formation. Epidural catheters may be used, but close neurologic monitoring is mandatory.

Blood loss

This is common postoperatively and results from the raw cancellous bone surface exposed by the fusion procedure. Even with aggressive intraoperative resuscitation with blood products, postoperative coagulopathies can develop from transfusions, hypocalcemia, and factor/platelet consumption. The INR, PT, PTT, and platelet count are followed for 2–3 days after operation. Postoperative bleeding is monitored by suction drain output and serial hematocrits and usually decreases to less than 30 ml per shift within 72 hours. Coagulation defects are aggressively corrected while active bleeding occurs. Postoperative anemia should be anticipated and addressed as medically necessary.

Thromboembolism prophylaxis

Some form of prophylaxis for thromboembolism is necessary, but early anticoagulation is risky because of the expected ongoing bleeding from decorticated cancellous bone in the fusion area and the potential for epidural hematoma. Therefore, elastic stockings, pneumatic compression boots, frequent turning, early leg motion, and mobilization as conditions allow are prescribed instead.

Postoperative complications

In the hospital

Spinal cord and nerve root injury

Spinal cord and nerve root injury is a serious potential problem in all patients undergoing this surgery. Spinal cord evoked potential monitoring is useful during the operation and may occasionally be used in the postoperative phase. Late neurologic changes can arise 1 to 3 days postoperatively. Therefore, detailed and well-documented serial neurologic examinations (motor, sensory, reflexes, and rectal) are the keystone of postoperative monitoring. Any new complaints of postoperative numbness, weakness, clonus, perianal anesthesia, or incontinence should be quickly evaluated. Signs of acute spinal cord dysfunction should prompt consideration of high dose steroids (methylprednisolone), aggressive correction of any significant anemia, hypoxia, or hypotension, and an urgent diagnostic work-up of the spine.

Wound infection

Progressive and increasing incisional pain suggest possible infection. Fever, drainage, and an elevated white blood cell count may or may not be present. A rising C-reactive protein (CRP) or increasing pain are highly suggestive. If infection is suspected, aspiration of the hematoma using meticulous sterile technique may be helpful. Surgical incision and drainage should proceed promptly if infection is seriously considered.

Pulmonary insufficiency

The prophylactic use of incentive spirometry and pulmonary therapy is important. Poor ventilation and splinting from pain are especially common after thoracotomy, thoracoplasty, or anterior approach to the spine. If a patient has pre-existing pulmonary compromise or if the procedure is associated with surgical trauma to the chest cavity, supplemental chest physical therapy or intermittent positive pressure breathing (IPPB) treatments given with a bronchodilator (e.g., albuterol nebulizer) every 4–6 hours may be very helpful. Pneumonia, pulmonary embolus, and pulmonary edema may be causes of postoperative pulmonary insufficiency, but the possibility of pneumothorax must also be entertained in patients who underwent a transthoracic approach or had a central line placed. Appropriate physical examinations, serial chest radiographs, pulse oximetry, and arterial blood gas determinations may be indicated.

Myocardial infarction

Patients are at risk of coronary complications from major spinal deformity surgery as they would be from any operation of similar magnitude. Prolonged prone surgical positioning with pads pressing on the sternum and ribs may cause local chest pain or costochondritis that can be confused with a cardiac etiology. If a patient

sustains a myocardial infarction, the standard treatment measures should be considered. However, decision making regarding the use of thrombolytics and anticoagulants must be tempered by the potential for severe surgical site bleeding and the risk of paralysis from epidural hematoma.

Pulmonary embolism

If embolism occurs, standard therapy is necessary, but anticoagulants should be avoided for at least 48–72 hours following operation because of extensive bone bleeding and the risk of epidural hematoma when a decompression or osteotomy has been done. If the risk of thrombosis is unusually high, a caval filter should be considered or anticoagulants given with great caution.

Bladder atony

Postoperative bladder atony is common from narcotics and immobilization. In general, Foley catheters should be removed 2–4 days postoperatively when the patient is mobile and can more comfortably void. Removing the catheter too soon risks reinsertion if the patient develops urinary retention; prolonged catheterization risks infection. Intermittent sterile catheterization can be performed as needed, but the residual volumes should be kept low in order to prevent a cycle of bladder stretching and atony.

Ileus

Postoperative pain in this patient population can be severe for 1 to 4 days. The PCA pump is commonly used, with the high doses of narcotics frequently required for pain control prolonging the ileus induced from surgery, anesthesia, and immobilization. Oral intake is restricted until peristalsis is established. A nasogastric tube may occasionally be necessary for persistent ileus.

Anemia secondary to blood loss

Postoperative hematocrit levels are used to monitor for anemia related to blood loss, and replacement should be given as necessary with close attention to orthostatic symptoms and signs.

After discharge

Bone graft pain

Donor site pain from the harvest of autologous bone is common but gradually dissipates over 1 to 3 months. Increasing pain at the graft site should raise the suspicion of infection.

Skin ulceration under a brace or cast from pressure and friction

Patients must be closely monitored, especially if very thin or when severely deformed where there may be a poorly fitting brace or cast. Cast revision or brace modification should be done immediately if skin irritation occurs.

Wound infection

Many wound infections manifest at 2–4 weeks postoperatively. Progressive and increasing (rather than decreasing) incisional pain suggests possible infection. Fever, chills, and drainage may not be present, but must all be aggressively evaluated. An elevated white blood count may or may not be present. The sedimentation rate and C-reactive protein should be checked in those with suspected infection, but may be artificially high due to the postoperative state. In general, the sedimentation rate may take up to 7 weeks to normalize postoperatively, whereas the C-reactive protein usually normalizes as early as 2–3 weeks postoperatively. Surgical management is recommended for the majority of postoperative infections except the most benign superficial infections.

Implant failure

Internal fixation devices occasionally loosen or break. This may occur as an early postoperative problem if bone stock is poor (1–3 months) or a later problem if the fusion fails to heal (6–12 months). There may be associated new pain or possible deformity, but radiographic examination is necessary for diagnosis. Revision is usually required but is done as much for the failed fusion as for the implant.

Pseudoarthrosis

Failure of the fusion to solidly heal can occur for any number of reasons related to the mechanical environment (poor bone quality, inadequate fixation of the spine, technical surgical factors), patient noncompliance (smoking or the use of non-steroidal anti-inflammatory drugs in the early postoperative period), or the biological milieu (malnourishment, immunocompromise, inadequate bone graft, or multiple prior operations with scar). Smoking, in particular, has negative effects on the healing of fusions and many spinal surgeons will not perform elective fusions on smokers. Pseudarthrosis usually manifests as increasing pain at the site of nonunion. Implant breakage and/or loosening is a commonly associated finding and progression of deformity may also be seen. The diagnosis is not always evident on plain radiographs alone; thin-cut computed tomography and bone scans may be necessary. Revision surgery is usually required and may necessitate anterior, posterior, or combined approaches.

Acknowledgment

The authors wish to thank Vicki Prevatte for administrative assistance and Dr. Thomas E. Whitesides, Jr., for input to this chapter.

FURTHER READING

An, H. S. & Glover, J. M. Complications and revision surgery in adult spinal deformity. In Bridwell, K. H. & Dewald, R. L. *The Textbook of Spinal Surgery*. 2nd edn. Philadelphia, PA: J. B. Lippincott-Raven, 1997.

Bradford, D. S. Adult scoliosis: current concepts of treatment. *Clin. Orthop.* 1988; **229**: 70–87.

Dickson, J. H., Mirkovic, S., Noble, P. C., Nalty, T., & Erwin, W. D. Results of operative treatment of idiopathic scoliosis in adults. *J. Bone Joint Surg.* 1995; **77A**: 513–523.

Nickel, V. L., Perry, J., Affeldt, J. E., & Dail, C. W. Elective surgery on patients with respiratory paralysis. *J. Bone Joint Surg.* 1957; **39A**: 989–1001.

Polly, D. W. & Kuklo, T. R. Perioperative blood and blood product management for spinal deformity surgery. In Dewald, R. L., ed. *Spinal Deformities*. 1st edn. New York, NY: Thieme, 2003.

115

Surgery of the foot and ankle

Sameh A. Labib

Emory University School of Medicine, Atlanta, GA

The foot is a highly specialized organ that connects us to the ground, providing support and balance, shock absorption, and finally, push-off power and direction. Through its complex bony, ligamentous, and musculo-tendinous units, the foot is able to adapt from a flexible structure that conforms to uneven surfaces to a fairly rigid and solid platform that can provide push-off and spring during various activities. Throughout ambulation, the foot may have to support repetitive loads equal to eight times body weight. In order to resume normal function after foot surgery, it is important to allow enough time for bony and soft tissue healing.

The following is a discussion of common foot surgical procedures:

Surgery of the diabetic foot

Diabetic foot ulcers and infection are a common cause of hospital admissions. Patients usually present with non-healing ulcers and superficial or deep infections and will require immediate antibiotic treatment. Management and prognosis depends on the extent of the infection, vascular and sensory status of the extremity, and foot deformity. Interdisciplinary collaboration between medical subspecialists, nurses, physical therapists, and social workers is needed to provide effective treatment.

Surgical debridement is indicated for patients with bony infection such as osteomyelitis. Amputations may be necessary if the infection cannot be controlled with conservative treatment or if the foot remaining after adequate debridment is judged to be inadequate for ambulation.

Hospital course and postoperative rehabilitation

The duration of hospital stay is dictated by the severity of the infection and the associated medical problems. Broad spectrum antibiotics should be started after appropriate deep tissue cultures are obtained. In the presence of osteomyelitis, surgical debridement is followed by 6 weeks of appropriate antibiotics.

Postoperative activity

Rest and non-weight bearing splint or cast are important adjuncts to medical and surgical treatment. Once infection is brought under control, a well-padded total contact cast is applied to relieve local pressure on healing tissues; this has been shown to be the most successful method to heal chronic foot ulcers.

Discharge plan

Dressing and cast changes are done weekly to follow healing and ensure complete resolution of infection and closure of the ulcer.

Recurrence

Diabetic patients are at high risk for recurrence of ulceration or infection. Diabetic foot care must be done daily and patients should be prescribed appropriate shoes and inserts to prevent recurrent ulceration.

Foot fusion

Degenerative and inflammatory arthritis are common causes of foot pain and deformity. Often, well prescribed medications, orthoses, and shoe modification can provide relief for these disabling conditions. Elective surgical procedures are offered to those patients who fail conservative treatment. Fusion of various foot joints has been the mainstay of treatment for correcting advanced arthritis.

Hospital course and postoperative rehabilitation

Patients are admitted on the day of operation. Fusion surgery is usually done through a longitudinal incision

Medical Management of the Surgical Patient: A Textbook of Perioperative Medicine, ed. M. F. Lubin, R. B. Smith, T. F. Dobson, N. Spell, H. K. Walker. 4th edn. Published by Cambridge University Press. © Cambridge University 2006.

made directly over the involved joint. Transverse and plantar incisions are generally avoided in the foot. Internal fixation and supplemental autologous or allograft bone are routinely used to improve fusion rate. After surgery, the patient is placed in a below the knee non-walking cast or splint. Drains may be used and are usually removed within 48 hours. Prophylactic antibiotics are given for 24 hours or until drains are discontinued.

Discharge plan
The patient is discharged in a below the knee cast and should remain non-weight bearing with crutches or a walker for six weeks. Dressing changes and suture removal are done at 10–14 days following operation.

Foot trauma and fracture treatment

Recent studies have documented an increase in motor vehicle accident related lower extremity trauma. During an accident, airbag deployment may afford protection to the upper torso but leave the lower extremities vulnerable to injury. Moreover, foot trauma is commonly missed, resulting in delayed diagnosis in the multiply injured patient. Failure to diagnose the foot injury in a timely way may lead to long term foot pain and deformity that could be avoided. Therefore, it is imperative for the treating physician to be vigilant and to help manage foot trauma if it is discovered.

Hospital course and postoperative rehabilitation
Most patients will require cast treatment and non-weight bearing following surgery. Acute foot compartment syndrome can present in the perioperative period and should be treated surgically.

Discharge plans
Continue non-weight bearing for 6 weeks. Foot elevation, ice packs, and rest are necessary for recovery.

Usual postoperative course

Expected postoperative hospital stay
Majority of patients are managed without hospital admission.

Operative mortality
Related to associated major injuries.

Special monitoring required
Neurovascular monitoring is required in the immediate postoperative period. Tight casts or bandages should be recognized and corrected.

Patient activity and positioning
Foot rest and elevation is encouraged to minimize postoperative pain and swelling. Ice packs may be applied. Patients are usually non-weight-bearing on the operated foot. Crutches or walker are provided and patients are encouraged to ambulate early.

Alimentation
No change in diet is needed following foot surgery except for postanesthetic nausea or vomiting.

Antibiotic coverage
First generation cephalosporins are routinely given before tourniquet use and for 24 hours postoperatively. Appropriate substitutes are given to patients with known allergic reactions.

Venous thrombosis
Only indicated in high-risk patients during hospital stay and discontinued with resumed ambulation.

FURTHER READING

Coughlin, M. & Mann, R., eds. *Surgery of the Foot and Ankle.* St. Louis, MO: Mosby, 1999.

Koval, K. J., ed. Orthopedic Knowledge Update 7: A home syllabus. *Am. Ann. Orthop. Surg.* 2002.

116

Lower extremity amputations

Alonzo T. Sexton and Lamar L. Fleming

Emory University School of Medicine, Atlanta, GA

Lower extremity amputations are performed for tumors, trauma, peripheral vascular disease, infection, or congenital deformity. The goal of treatment is to return the patient to a functional level allowing pain-free ambulation, which is best achieved through a multi-disciplinary approach involving physician, physical therapist, and prosthetic team. Due to the psychological aspects of care it is important to involve the patient in the decision-making process in order to help the patient understand and concur with the medical staff regarding the importance and necessity of performing the amputation.

The vast majority of amputations are performed for vascular disease and infection resulting from diabetic neuropathy; the most common level is a below knee amputation (BKA). The more proximal the amputation, the greater the metabolic cost of walking. Studies have shown that walking speed is decreased and oxygen consumption is increased with more proximal amputations.

The preoperative consideration of several important factors will directly affect the patient's ability to successfully heal from the amputation. The goal of surgery is to leave enough viable tissue that will heal and allow for fitting with a prosthesis. A serum albumin level below 3.5 g/dl indicates a malnourished patient and an absolute lymphocyte count below 1500/mm^3 is a sign of immune deficiency; these values should be corrected prior to any elective amputation case. Some advocate the optimization of serum glucose levels in diabetics, but this is not entirely clear. Assessing the vascular status of the lower extremity and thus the healing potential of an amputation is an essential step in the preoperative plan. Standard Doppler ultrasound measurements of arterial pressure may be falsely elevated in patients with diabetes and peripheral vascular disease; measurements of toe pressures are more accurate. The gold standard is to determine the transcutaneous partial pressure of oxygen which reflects the oxygen delivering capacity of the vascular system: values greater than 40 mm Hg correlate with acceptable wound healing rates and values less than 20 mm Hg suggest poor healing potential.

Lower extremity amputations are performed under general anesthesia or regional (spinal or epidural) block. The duration of operation ranges from 45 minutes for a transmetatarsal amputation, 1 hour for a below-knee amputation, and as long as 2 hours or more for a hip disarticulation. The magnitude of the surgical stress is directly related to the level of amputation. When a tourniquet is used, blood loss is usually minimal; in more proximal amputations, 2 to 4 units of packed red blood cells may be required.

Usual postoperative course

Expected postoperative hospital stay
Usually 3–5 days after BKA if course is uncomplicated.

Operative mortality
Depends on the level of amputation, age, and general medical condition of the patient and indication for amputation. Mortality rates range from 0.5% for young patients undergoing amputation for trauma to 20% for elderly patients undergoing above knee amputation for vascular insufficiency.

Special monitoring required
A well-padded splint or cast should be used postoperatively to facilitate wound healing, prevent flexion contractures, and reduce stump edema. Postoperatively, care should be taken immediately in the placement of casts as swelling may lead to severe patient discomfort due to impingement on the cast, which may require splitting.

Medical Management of the Surgical Patient: A Textbook of Perioperative Medicine, ed. M. F. Lubin, R. B. Smith, T. F. Dobson, N. Spell, H. K. Walker. 4th edn. Published by Cambridge University Press. © Cambridge University 2006.

Drains are often used to prevent postoperative hematoma and may be removed once the drain output measures less than approximately 30 ml per 8 hour shift.

Patient activity and positioning

Patients are mobilized out of bed on the first postoperative day and physical therapy – including quadriceps, abductor, and hip extension strengthening exercises – is begun on the second day. The cast or rigid dressing is changed 5–7 days after operation, both to allow inspection of the wound and to ensure proper cast fitting after the early postoperative edema has subsided. Skin sutures are removed at about 2 weeks and the cast is changed again at 3–4 weeks. A temporary prosthesis is fitted to the limb when the incision has healed. Touch down weight bearing with the use of crutches or a walker is then increased over the next month to weight bearing as tolerated. When the stump size has not changed in 6 weeks, a permanent prosthesis may be fitted. Young patients with well-vascularized stumps may be candidates for early fitting of their prosthesis and immediate weight bearing.

Alimentation

Because trauma or infection increases energy requirements 30%–50% above basal values, patients should undergo at least baseline nutritional assessments, including serum albumin and total lymphocyte counts. Nutritional supplementation should be provided as necessary.

Antibiotic coverage

Prophylactic antibiotics (usually first-generation cephalosporin) are administered at the initiation of the surgical procedure and continued for 24 hours postoperatively. In infected cases, cultures should be obtained and broad spectrum antibiotics should be initiated until the cultures and sensitivities return. Antibiotics should then be tailored to cover the identified organisms.

Postoperative complications

In the hospital

Wound necrosis

Insufficient arterial circulation, excessive local pressure, hematoma formation, or skin closure under tension account for most cases of wound necrosis. Small areas of necrosis often heal by secondary intention with local wound care and dressing changes. Flap revision or more proximal amputation may become necessary for the treatment of larger areas of necrosis, especially in patients with poor vascularity.

Joint contracture

Best prevented with early physical therapy, proper positioning, and extension splinting or casting. Knee flexion contractures greater than 15 degrees and hip flexion contractures greater than 25 degrees make conventional prosthetic fitting difficult.

Wound infection

The risk of infection increases in patients with vascular insufficiency, diabetes, or previous distal infection. Wound debridement, irrigation, and appropriate antibiotic coverage are the standard treatment, although revision of the amputation to a more proximal level is sometimes necessary.

Pulmonary embolism

Deep vein thrombosis and thromboembolism are potential threats to elderly, partially immobilized patients undergoing lower extremity surgery. Prophylaxis with subcutaneous heparin or Lovenox may be appropriate.

After discharge

Stump edema

Postoperative edema may impede wound healing and make prosthetic fitting difficult. The edema should be treated with compressive dressings. Edema developing after stump maturation is typically due to a poorly fitted prosthesis.

Phantom sensation

Non-painful awareness of the amputated limb. This sensation lasts a variable amount of time and may be permanent in some patients. It is a normal phenomenon and treatment is unnecessary.

Phantom pain

A burning, painful sensation in the amputated part. It occurs in 2%–10% of adults and is most frequently observed in patients with pain in the limb prior to surgery. Organic causes such as neuroma, compartment syndrome, and infection should be ruled out. It may be diminished by prosthetic use, physical therapy, compression, and transcutaneous nerve stimulation. There is controversy over the effectiveness of other treatments, such as epidural injections, Beta blockers, gabapentin, or regional neural blockade.

Residual limb pain

This pain in the stump most often resolves with the healing of the incision in 2–3 weeks.

Skin problems

Abrasion of the skin from excessive local pressure or blisters from friction between the skin and the prosthesis may be managed by providing local skin care and temporarily discontinuing use of the prosthesis. Areas of local pressure should be treated by redistributing the pressure over a larger area of the skin through modification of the prosthetic socket liner.

Psychosocial issues

These should be considered preoperatively as well as after discharge. Studies have shown that young children adapt well to amputations, while adolescents are particularly sensitive to peer acceptance or rejection and may require more assistance. The elderly may be at greater risk than other groups in regards to development of psychiatric disturbances such as depression. A proper support staff is needed for amputation patients to address issues with limb loss.

FURTHER READING

Bodily, K. C. & Burgess, E. M. Contralateral limb and patient survival after leg amputation. *Am. J. Surg.* 1983; **146**: 280–282.

Chapman, M. W. & Madison, M. *Operative Orthopaedics*, vol 1. Philadelphia, PA: J. B. Lippincott, 1988: 603–615.

Crenshaw, A. H. *Campbell's Operative Orthopaedics*. 8th edn., vol 2. St Louis, MO: C. V. Mosby, 1992, 689–710.

Eneroth, M. & Persson, B. M. Risk factors for failed healing in amputation for vascular disease: a prospective, consecutive study of 177 cases. *Acta Orthop. Scand.* 1993; **62**: 369–372.

Evarts, C. M. *Surgery of The Musculoskeletal System*. 2nd edn., vol 5. New York, NY: Churchill Livingstone, 1990: 5121–5161.

Knetsche, R. P., Leopold, S. S., & Brage, M. E. Inpatient management of lower extremity amputations. *Foot Ankle Clin.* 2001; **6**: 229–241.

Volpicelli, L. J., Chambers, R. B., & Wagner, F. W. Jr. Ambulation levels of bilateral lower extremity amputees: analysis of one hundred and three cases. *J. Bone Joint Surg. Am.* 1983; **65**: 559–605.

117

Surgical procedures for rheumatoid arthritis

Gary R. McGillivary

Emory University School of Medicine, Atlanta, GA

Despite markedly improved and more aggressive medical management, rheumatoid arthritis continues to be, for many, a progressive disease that ultimately leads to significant joint destruction. The primary indication for almost all surgical procedures remains pain relief, with functional improvement and prevention of deformity being lesser goals.

Common operative procedures include the following.

Arthroplasty

Primarily joint replacement, such as total hip, knee, shoulder, elbow, wrist and metacarpophalangeal joints, but occasionally other anomalies such as interpositional arthroplasty.

Arthrodesis

Joint fusion remains an excellent procedure in some areas, such as the wrist, interphalangeal joints, ankle, spine, and selected others in certain clinical situations.

Soft tissue procedures

Synovectomy, tenosynovectomy, carpal tunnel release, tendon transfers, and tendon repair all have roles in certain patients. These occasionally are prophylactic and may help alter the course of the disease.

In general, the surgical stress involved is related to the magnitude of the specific procedure. On occasion, multiple procedures may be carried out at one time if they aren't too substantial. For more significant interventions, such as revision arthroplasty, isolated procedures tend to be the standard approach. Most primary procedures, alone or in combination, do not require more than two to three hours of anesthesia. Complicated operations, of course, may demand more.

Procedures on the distal portions of the extremities (below the shoulder and hip) are generally done with tourniquet control, with blood loss being minimal. Although shoulder surgery is done without tourniquet control, the amount of bleeding is usually not excessive and transfusion is fairly uncommon. In the knee, despite the use of a tourniquet, postoperative losses through drains and into the joint tend to be greater and may require eventual replacement. Most often, two units are enough; with preoperative planning and coordination, autologous blood may be used. Stimulants of the hematopoietic system are also being utilized more commonly in such patients.

Many rheumatoid arthritis patients have significant disease of their cervical spines. In addition to a routine history and physical examination, cervical spine films and even preoperative consultation with a spine surgeon and anesthesiologist may be necessary to prevent a serious untoward outcome.

The staging and timing of surgical procedures is primarily dependent upon patient needs and wants, which basically means that the most symptomatic joints are usually treated first. However, if there is no clear indication from the patient, lower extremity procedures are probably best done before upper extremity corrections, thus avoiding the problem of crutch weight bearing down on reconstructed upper extremity joints. In the lower extremity, foot and ankle problems are preferentially done ahead of more proximal joints to provide a stable weight bearing base. In such instances, treatment doesn't always have to be surgical it may be achieved with braces and/or orthotics. The sequencing of hip and knee arthroplasty can vary depending on the degree of joint contracture involved at

Medical Management of the Surgical Patient: A Textbook of Perioperative Medicine, ed. M. F. Lubin, R. B. Smith, T. F. Dobson, N. Spell, H. K. Walker. 4th edn. Published by Cambridge University Press. © Cambridge University 2006.

each level. If there is a choice, the hip should be done before the knee as it is easier to rehabilitate a hip with a bad knee than vice versa. Currently, simultaneous bilateral hip or knee arthroplasties are done more frequently. However, the patients must be chosen carefully, and if problems arise at the end of the first procedure one should not hesitate to stop there.

The goals of upper extremity surgery are simply to allow the patient to position a functional hand in space. Due to the fact that wrist deformity aggravates deformity at the metacarpophalangeal joints, wrist surgery should either proceed or be done in conjunction with metacarpophalangeal procedures. Again, shoulders and elbows usually have the sequence determined by the patient, but shoulder contracture may make positioning for elbow surgery difficult if it is severe.

Usual postoperative course

Expected postoperative hospital stay
Even in patients with rheumatoid arthritis, the hospital stay can be as brief as overnight. Following major lower extremity surgery, patients may stay longer than usual due to increased difficulties with physical therapy. In this situation, 7–10 day stays would not be uncommon.

Operative mortality
Should be less than 0.3%.

Special monitoring required
Occasionally spine surgery will require somatosensory evoked potentials intraoperatively. Beyond that, monitoring is dictated by the general condition of the patient.

Patient activity and positioning
This will vary a great deal based on the previous level of function, general health and conditioning, the specific surgical procedure, and the intra-operative problems encountered such as poor bone quality. Most patients will need physical or occupational therapy. It seems that hips and elbows require less intensive therapy than other joints. Patients undergoing hip arthroplasty very often need to use abduction pillows in bed for several months and may require other aids such as an elevated toilet seat. The use of continuous passive motion machines for knees, elbows, and shoulders has been advocated by some but remains unproven and controversial. Following hand surgery, prolonged use of special splinting techniques may be necessary.

Alimentation
No special dietary requirements are recommended.

Antibiotic coverage
Antibiotic prophylaxis is recommended in all patients that have implants placed, the standard being the use of a first-generation cephalosporin. The initial dose is given preoperatively in the operating room, followed by three doses postoperatively.

Corticosteroid therapy
Patients that have been on long-term steroids will need stress doses of intravenous corticosteroid perioperatively due to suppression of their adrenocortical axis. Typically, 100 mg of hydrocortisone is given in the operating room and then tapered over a few days.

Postoperative complications

In the hospital

Infection
Wound infection typically does not present until approximately 5 days after surgery. In this patient population there is a greater risk of infection due to immunosuppression, both from their disease and many of the medications they take. Most post surgical infections require surgical debridement and antibiotics are supplemental.

Acute adrenal insufficiency
Despite perioperative corticosteroid supplementation, this may still occur and needs to be considered in the gravely ill patient with hypotension, nausea, vomiting, weakness, and hyperthermia. The associated hyponatremia, hyperkalemia, and low hematocrit mandate aggressive and urgent treatment with glucocorticoid replacement.

Delayed wound healing
The rheumatoid condition and many of its medical treatments lead to an impaired ability to heal wounds. Skin, soft tissues, and bone are all affected. Skin sutures may be left in place for prolonged periods.

After discharge

Postoperative fractures
Osteoporosis is such a severe problem in patients with rheumatoid arthritis that postoperative fractures are not uncommon.

Late infection

Occasionally, an artificial joint may become infected well after the immediate postoperative period. This is often due to seeding from another source as these patients are at increased risk due to chronic immunosuppression.

Loosening of prosthesis

All total joint arthroplasties may fail over time, with the most frequent cause being loosening or loss of fixation. This tends to occur at roughly the same rate for all artificial joints, about 1% to 2% per year. The patient usually complains that the joint has once again become painful.

Disease progression

Since nothing that is done either medically or surgically will cure this disease, its progression may ultimately affect the long-term outcome of any surgical procedure.

FURTHER READING

Green, D. P., ed. *Operative Hand Surgery*, 2nd edn. New York, NY: Churchill Livingstone, 1988, Vol. 3, 44: 1655–1784.

Hollander, J. L., ed. *Arthritis and Allied Conditions*, 8th edn. Philadelphia, PA: Lea & Febiger, 1972.

Millender, L. H. & Sledge, C. B. Symposium on rheumatoid arthritis. (Foreword) *Orthop. Clin. North Am.* 1975; **6**: 601–602.

Otolaryngologic surgery

118

Otologic surgery

Douglas E. Mattox

Emory University School of Medicine, Atlanta, GA

Otologic surgery encompasses a wide variety of surgical procedures involving the ear with the goal of eliminating infection and/or restoring hearing. Chronic drainage from the ear suggests a tympanic membrane perforation or cholesteatoma (benign squamous keratocyst) of the middle ear or mastoid. Tympanoplasty (repair of tympanic membrane perforation) usually uses autologous temporalis fascia or perichondrium and may be combined with mastoidectomy, of which there are two types, when inflammatory disease or cholesteatoma extends into the mastoid. In canal-wall-up mastoidectomy, the external auditory canal is kept intact and the mastoid cavity drains through the middle ear as is normally the case. Canal-wall-down mastoidectomy is used for more severe disease and exteriorizes the mastoid cavity through an enlarged external meatus.

Reconstructive surgery for hearing – ossicular reconstruction and stapedotomy – is used when trauma, infection, or otosclerosis (stapedotomy) has damaged the middle ear sound conductive mechanism.

Otologic procedures may be performed under general anesthesia or local anesthesia with sedation. Muscle relaxants are avoided if cranial nerve monitoring is needed intraoperatively. Most otologic procedures are accomplished in one to four hours. Significant blood loss and/or transfusion are not expected.

Usual postoperative course

Expected postoperative hospital stay

Most otologic surgery is performed as an outpatient or ambulatory inpatient procedure with 23-hour observation.

Operative mortality

Equals the anesthetic risk.

Special monitoring required

Since the surgical field is in close proximity to the facial nerve, muscle relaxants are avoided so that facial activity may be monitored intraoperatively. Epinephrine is used as a vasoconstrictor agent; therefore, cardiac monitoring is required.

Patient activity and positioning

The patient may resume normal daily activity within a few days of surgery. Heavy physical exercise, lifting, air travel, and nose blowing are avoided for four weeks until the graft is fully healed.

Alimentation

Regular diet as tolerated.

Antibiotic coverage

A single dose of preoperative antibiotics is used in all cases. Postoperative oral antibiotics may be continued if a prosthesis is left in the middle ear space. Antibiotic eardrops are used to soften the ear canal packing and make its removal easier.

Wound care

The ear canal is packed with dissolvable sponge material for one to two weeks after operation. This packing must be kept dry except for the application of antibiotic eardrops.

Postoperative complications

In the hospital

Nausea and vertigo

Excessive nausea, vomiting, vertigo and/or hearing loss suggest irritation of the labyrinth (inner ear) during the

Medical Management of the Surgical Patient: A Textbook of Perioperative Medicine, ed. M. F. Lubin, R. B. Smith, T. F. Dobson, N. Spell, H. K. Walker. 4th edn. Published by Cambridge University Press. © Cambridge University 2006.

procedure. The surgical procedure should be carefully reviewed and the ear possibly re-explored if these symptoms are persistent. The administration of intravenous fluids and antiemetic drugs may be needed.

Cerebrospinal fluid leak

The roof of the mastoid is a party wall with the floor of the middle cranial fossa. Removal of excessive bone can lead to a temporal lobe encephalocele and penetration of the dura produces an intraoperative cerebrospinal fluid leak. A CSF leak should be repaired immediately when recognized. Lumbar drainage is not routinely used for small leaks, but it may be helpful in large defects or vigorous leaks.

Facial paralysis

The facial nerve traverses both the middle ear and the mastoid. The bony covering over the nerve may be naturally dehiscent or eroded by disease exposing the nerve to intraoperative injury. Any surgical procedure with an unexpected facial paralysis should be re-explored, decompressed, repaired or grafted according to the extent of the injury.

After discharge

Postoperative otorrhea

A small amount of blood tinged or brownish drainage is expected as the ear canal packing dissolves. Purulent or mucoid drainage suggests persistent or postoperative infection. Oral or intravenous antibiotics, cleaning of the canal or mastoid bowl, or debridement of the wound may be required.

Recurrent disease

Poor Eustachian tube function is the root cause of chronic ear disease. The ear may develop recurrent perforation, retraction, or cholesteatoma in cases where antibiotics, decreased inflammation, and surgical correction are unsuccessful in restoring Eustachian tube function. Continued monitoring is critical to detect recurrent disease at an early stage.

Dizziness

Dizziness may be persistent after discharge if the labyrinth has been opened either intentionally or unintentionally. Vestibular suppressive drugs are helpful in the early acute phase, but should be avoided long term because they may impede the vestibular habituation needed for full recovery. Vestibular rehabilitation exercises can be extremely helpful in promoting full recovery.

Canal stenosis

Stenosis of the external canal is an infrequent complication that may need reoperation if the canal or mastoid cavity cannot be examined and cleaned.

Cavity care

A canal-wall-down mastoidectomy leaves the ear canal and the mastoid as one continuous skin-lined space. Ideally, the cavity will be self-cleaning; however, cleaning with suction and operating microscope may be needed at 6- to 12-month intervals.

FURTHER READING

Glasscock, M. E., Gulya, A. J., Shambaugh, G. eds. *Surgery of the Ear*. 5th edn. Hamilton, Ontario, Canada: B. C. Decker Inc., 2002.

119

Myringotomy and tubes

Douglas E. Mattox

Emory University School of Medicine, Atlanta, GA

The placement of myringotomy or pressure equalization (PE) tubes is the most common pediatric procedure and is also frequently required in the geriatric population. The Eustachian tube normally opens during swallowing and yawning, replacing the air absorbed through the middle ear mucous membrane while the tube is closed. Failure of this mechanism from immaturity of the tube in children or atrophy of the peritubal muscles in the elderly causes retraction of the tympanic membrane, fluid effusion resulting in hearing loss, and recurrent acute infections.

Myringotomy tubes are placed through a small incision in the tympanic membrane with either topical anesthesia in the office or, for children, a quick general anesthetic.

Usual postoperative course

Expected postoperative hospital stay
Outpatient procedure.

Operative mortality
Negligible and essentially related to anesthesia risk.

Special monitoring required
None.

Patient activity and positioning
Normal activity may be resumed immediately after the procedure.

Alimentation
No limitation.

Antibiotic coverage
As indicated to treat existing otitis.

Expected postoperative course
Tube placement is typically done in the office or as an outpatient procedure. Otorrhea for 2 to 3 days while the effusion clears from the middle ear and mastoid is not unusual. Topical quinolone otic drops are customarily prescribed during this period.

Water precautions
Since water in the ear canal can enter the middle ear space through the tube and initiate an acute infection, the ear should be kept free of water and shampoo. Ear plugs and custom swim molds are helpful in preventing such contamination, but nothing is consistently waterproof. Exposure to non-chlorinated swimming water should be strictly avoided.

Postoperative complications

In the hospital

Hearing loss
Hearing should immediately and dramatically improve after placement of myringotomy tubes. An incorrect diagnosis or the occasional impingement of the tube on the ossicular chain is indicated if this doesn't occur.

Otorrhea
Usually, results intermittently from water contamination or an upper respiratory infection. Such infections usually respond promptly to a combination of oral antibiotics (amoxicillin/clavulanic acid) and topical otic drops (quinolone). In the event of persistent and prolonged otorrhea unresponsive to antibiotics, culture-directed intravenous antibiotics should be administered. Occasionally in such

Medical Management of the Surgical Patient: A Textbook of Perioperative Medicine, ed. M. F. Lubin, R. B. Smith, T. F. Dobson, N. Spell, H. K. Walker. 4th edn. Published by Cambridge University Press. © Cambridge University 2006.

instances, the tube must be removed as a presumed nidus of persistent infection.

After discharge

Flying

Since the patient should be completely free of any symptoms of decompression/recompression since the air pressure is equalized through the tube, there is no contraindication to flying immediately after tube placement. For individuals who fly frequently, consistent otalgia from pressure changes during commercial airline flights is a rare but legitimate indication for myringotomy tubes.

Extrusion

Extrusion of standard collar button style tubes is expected 6 months after insertion, though the range of duration is from a few weeks to permanent retention. Fortunately, tubes rarely migrate into the middle ear space but are always extruded into the extraauditory canal. Persistent tubes may have to be removed if they are no longer useful.

Reinsertion

Myringotomy tubes are merely a convenient substitute for the natural function of the Eustachian tube. If the underlying pathophysiology of the Eustachian tube has resolved, usually by growth and development, the patient will have normal middle ear function after extrusion of the tube. If Eustachian tube function remains poor, tubes may need to be reinserted. Reinsertion of tubes in children is often combined with adenoidectomy in an attempt to improve Eustachian tube function. In refractory cases, semipermanent "T" tubes may be used for long-term ventilation.

Nasopharyngeal carcinoma

A rare but serious cause of middle ear effusion in adults is an occult malignancy in the nasopharynx. Middle ear effusion in middle-aged adults, especially if it is unilateral, should prompt a thorough endoscopic investigation of the nasopharynx.

Monitoring

The ear should be examined at 2- to 4-month intervals to monitor for infection and extrusion of the tube. Most importantly, the ear must be observed after tube extrusion for recurrence of the primary Eustachian tube problems.

Perforation

Approximately 2% of myringotomies will have a persistent perforation after extrusion or removal. In many cases this is fortunate, as it obviates the necessity of reinsertion of a new tube. In other cases it is presumed that Eustachian tube function has improved and it is desirable to close the perforation (tympanoplasty).

Cholesteatoma

This is a benign squamous keratocyst in the middle ear or mastoid that develops in ears with chronically poor Eustachian tube function. Occasionally, cholesteatoma is directly related to skin growing into the middle ear space adjacent to a myringotomy tube. More commonly, cholesteatoma is a result of severe Eustachian tube dysfunction that does not respond to tube placement. In either event, surgical removal of the cholesteatoma is required.

FURTHER READING

Glasscock, M. E., Gulya, A. J., & Shambaugh, G. E. *Glasscock–Shambaugh Surgery of the Ear*. 5th edn. Philadelphia, PA: B. C. Decker, 2002.

120

Tonsillectomy and adenoidectomy

John M. DelGaudio

Emory University School of Medicine, Atlanta, GA

In the past, tonsillectomy and adenoidectomy (T & A) was one of the most frequent surgical procedures performed on children, the most common indication being recurrent sore throat, though these procedures are performed much less often today. Currently, the most common indication for tonsillectomy in children is tonsillar hypertrophy with upper airway obstruction that results in snoring and sleep apnea. Other indications include recurrent tonsillitis and chronic tonsillitis. In adults, the most common indications are sleep apnea (as part of a uvulopalatopharyngoplasty), chronic tonsillitis, and concern for malignancy.

The adenoids are lymphoid tissue located in the nasopharynx. Adenoid hypertrophy results in nasal airway obstruction, mouth breathing, rhinorrhea, and sleep apnea. Due to the natural atrophy that occurs by puberty, adenoidectomy is usually only performed in children. It is frequently, but not always, done in conjunction with a tonsillectomy. The presence of significant adenoid tissue in an adult raises the concern for neoplasm or HIV infection.

T & A is performed under general anesthetic, usually in the outpatient setting. A careful preoperative history is necessary to rule out coagulation disorders. Bleeding is usually mild but can be considerable. Procedures are done using a combination of electrocautery and cold dissection; the use of electrocautery can reduce bleeding but may increase postoperative pain.

Usual postoperative course

Expected postoperative hospital stay

Patients are usually discharged on the day of surgery following a couple of hours of postoperative observation to assure that they can drink and hold down liquids. Overnight stays are sometimes necessary in patients undergoing T & A for obstructive sleep apnea.

Operative mortality

Extremely rare and usually related to anesthetic complications or excessive bleeding.

Special monitoring required

Unnecessary in most cases. In children with significant obstructive sleep apnea from adenotonsillar hypertrophy, postoperative pulse oximetry is recommended if the patient is admitted to the hospital.

Patient activity and positioning

Activities are reinitiated as early as tolerated by the patient. Light activities are recommended for approximately 2 weeks.

Alimentation

Patients are encouraged to begin oral intake as early as possible. In order to prevent dehydration, which can worsen pharyngeal pain, they are instructed to drink plenty of liquids. Foods that are crunchy and may abrade the pharynx, such as pretzels and chips, should be avoided. Otherwise, the diet can be advanced as tolerated, though patients usually prefer a soft diet.

Antibiotic coverage

Antibiotics have been found to reduce pain, fever, and mouth odor related to tonsillectomy. Preoperatively intravenous ampicillin or cefazolin are used, and patients are placed on 7 days of amoxicillin postoperatively.

Analgesia

Narcotic pain medication, usually acetaminophen with codeine, is given in liquid form and is administered every 4 hours while patients are awake during the first several days. Taking the pain medication 20 or 30 minutes before

Medical Management of the Surgical Patient: A Textbook of Perioperative Medicine, ed. M. F. Lubin, R. B. Smith, T. F. Dobson, N. Spell, H. K. Walker. 4th edn. Published by Cambridge University Press. © Cambridge University 2006.

attempting to eat will allow better oral intake. Adults usually require stronger narcotics such as oxycodone.

Postoperative complications

In the hospital

Hemorrhage
Early (first 24 hours) and delayed (7–10 days) bleeding are the most common adverse events, and are estimated to occur in less than 5% of patients. Bleeding can manifest as frank blood in the mouth or as hematemesis of swallowed blood. Postoperative bleeding should be treated aggressively rather than expectantly, with return to the operating room for blood vessel electrocautery or ligation.

Dehydration
Patients are encouraged to maintain oral intake of fluids to avoid dehydration. Dysphagia in the immediate postoperative period can prevent adequate oral intake. Intravenous hydration may be required.

Severe pain
Throat pain is expected after tonsillectomy and is generally better tolerated by children than adults. Pain can also be referred to the ear. Adequate analgesia is required.

After discharge

Hemorrhage
Bleeding is most common in the first 24 hours after operation, and then approximately 7–10 days postoperatively.

Patients should be seen by their physician if any bleeding occurs. Occasionally minimal bleeding can be controlled with cautery in the office.

Dehydration
Prolonged sore throat can result in inadequate oral intake and dehydration. Intravenous hydration is indicated in these patients, along with adequate analgesia.

Nasopharyngeal stenosis
Excessive scarring of the nasopharynx after adenoidectomy can result in nasopharyngeal stenosis and nasal obstruction.

Velopharyngeal insufficiency
Hypernasal voice and nasopharyngeal regurgitation may result after an adenoidectomy performed on a child with an unrecognized submucous cleft palate.

FURTHER READING

Darrow, D. H. & Siemens, C. Indications for tonsillectomy and adenoidectomy. *Laryngoscope* 2002; **112**: 6–10.

Johnson, L. B., Elluru, R. G., & Myer, C. M. 3rd. Complications of adenotonsillectomy. *Laryngoscope* 2002; **112**: 35–36.

Postma, D. S. & Folsom, F. The case for an outpatient "approach" for all pediatric tonsillectomies and/or adenoidectomies: a 4-year review of 1419 cases at a community hospital. *Otolaryngol. Head Neck Surg.* 2002; **127**(1): 101–108.

Telian, S. A., Handler, S. D., Fleisher, G. R. *et al.* The effect of antibiotic therapy on recovery after tonsillectomy in children. *Arch. Otolaryngol. Head Neck Surg.* 1986; **112**: 610–615.

121

Uvulopalatopharyngoplasty

John M. DelGaudio

Emory University School of Medicine, Atlanta, GA

Uvulopalatopharyngoplasty (UPPP) is a procedure performed on adults for the treatment of obstructive sleep apnea (OSA). UPPP involves removing the posterior aspect of the soft palate including the uvula and lateral pharyngeal mucosa (or tonsils if present) to reduce redundant tissue, thereby enlarging the oropharyngeal and nasopharyngeal airway.

OSA is a condition affecting 4% of the adult population and manifests by repeated episodes of apnea or hypopnea during sleep. During deeper levels of sleep, especially that characterized by rapid eye movement (REM), there is loss of the normal tone of the pharyngeal and tongue muscles that keep the pharynx open, resulting in collapse of the oropharyngeal and nasopharyngeal airway and varying degrees of airway obstruction. Narrowing of the airway causes increased velocity of inspiratory airflow in the pharynx, causing decreased intraluminal pressure, further tissue collapse, and increased airway obstruction (Bernoulli's principle). In instances of complete airway obstruction, the patient will experience apnea, a cessation of breathing for at least 10 seconds. Incomplete obstruction may result in hypopnea, a reduction in airflow with associated oxygen desaturation, which is more common. Each apnea or hypopnea episode continues until the patient awakens to a more shallow level of sleep, which results in a recovery of pharyngeal muscle tone and recovery of airway integrity. The more frequent the apnea and hypopnea the more fragmented the sleep, resulting in greater sleep deprivation due to the lack of adequate REM activity.

Surgical treatment for sleep apnea is directed at the specific site of obstruction, such as the palate, tongue, or nasal cavity. Frequently multiple levels are involved and each must be addressed. In patients with multilevel obstruction, only treating the palate surgically will not adequately improve the OSA. UPPP attempts to decrease the pharyngeal mucosal redundancy, thereby relieving or improving the oropharyngeal airway during deeper levels of sleep.

UPPP is indicated in patients who have sleep apnea with retropalatal obstruction. Patients should have failed or be unable to tolerate nasal continuous positive airway pressure (CPAP) treatment. When used as the only treatment, UPPP is less than 50% effective in significantly improving sleep apnea. Therefore, UPPP should be combined with other site-directed surgery and weight loss for better results.

Usual postoperative course

Expected postoperative hospital stay

Typically, patients usually stay overnight and are discharged the next day after demonstrating the ability to take fluids orally.

Operative mortality

Operative mortality is rare.

Special monitoring required

Intensive care unit observation may be prudent for patients with severe OSA postoperative pulse oximetry. Patients with mild to moderate severity OSA do not require postoperative monitoring.

Patient activity and positioning

Postoperatively, the head of the patient's bed should be elevated approximately 30 to 45 degrees to help with edema. Ambulation should be initiated as early as possible. Strenuous activities should be avoided for 2 weeks.

Alimentation

Patients receive a liquid diet the day of operation and are advanced to a soft diet on the first postoperative day.

Medical Management of the Surgical Patient: A Textbook of Perioperative Medicine, ed. M. F. Lubin, R. B. Smith, T. F. Dobson, N. Spell, H. K. Walker. 4th edn. Published by Cambridge University Press. © Cambridge University 2006.

Severe throat pain is common after UPPP and requires strong analgesia to make oral intake tolerable.

Antibiotic coverage

Intravenous ampicillin or cefazolin is administered preoperatively and for 24 hours postoperatively. Patients are continued on oral antibiotics in liquid form for 7 days.

Analgesia

Postoperative pain is usually severe and can severely compromise the patient's oral intake. Oral narcotics, usually oxycodone in liquid form, are necessary for up to 2 weeks postoperatively.

Postoperative complications

In the hospital

Bleeding

Postoperative bleeding can occur in the immediate postoperative period. Minor mucosal bleeding can be observed, since this will usually resolve spontaneously. More significant bleeding requires return to the operating room for control.

Velopharyngeal insufficiency

Due to involuntary splinting of the palate in an attempt to reduce pain, nasopharyngeal reflux of liquids and a hypernasal voice are common in the immediate postoperative period. As pain diminishes, so will the condition.

After discharge

Velopharyngeal insufficiency (VPI)

Permanent VPI is rare but can occur if excessive resection of the soft palate is performed. This is a difficult problem to remedy.

Nasopharyngeal stenosis

During healing, nasopharyngeal stenosis can occur with posterior contraction of the palate and tonsillar fold, resulting in nasal obstruction, a hyponasal voice, and resumption of sleep apnea symptoms. Conservative resection of the posterior tonsillar pillars and avoiding injury to the posterior pharyngeal wall reduces the likelihood of this complication.

FURTHER READING

Fujita, S., Conway, W., Zorick, F., & Roth, T. Surgical correction of anatomic abnormalities in obstructive sleep apnea syndrome: uvulopalatopharyngoplasty. *Otolaryngol. Head Neck Surg.* 1981; **89**: 923–934.

Mickelson, S. A. & Hakim, I. Is postoperative intensive care monitoring necessary after uvulopalatopharyngoplasty? *Otolaryngol. Head Neck Surg.* 1998; **119**: 352–356.

Riley, R. W., Powell, N. B., Guilleminault, C., Pelayo, R., Troell, R. J., & Li, K. K. Obstructive sleep apnea surgery: risk management and complications. *Otolaryngol. Head Neck Surg.* 1997; **117**: 648–652.

Sher, A. E., Schectman, K. B., & Piccirillo, J. F. The efficacy of surgical modifications of the upper airway in adults with obstructive sleep apnea syndrome. *Sleep* 1996; **19**: 156–177.

122

Endoscopic sinus surgery

Giri Venkatraman

Emory University School of Medicine, Atlanta, GA

Chronic sinusitis is a frequently seen and debilitating disease, affecting about 30 million patients in the USA, and approximately 6 billion dollars is spent annually on treating the condition. Sinusitis is defined as inflammation of the mucosa of the paranasal sinuses and the nasal cavity. Etiologies of sinusitis can be classified into three broad categories: environmental (pollution/allergies, viral URIs), systemic (diabetes, HIV), and host issues (autoimmune diseases, cystic fibrosis). Regardless of the inciting event(s), the mucosal inflammation leads to obstruction of the sinus ostia, stasis of secretions, and often a bacterial infection. Sinusitis is usually diagnosed by a symptom complex that includes congestion, facial pressure (not headache), purulent or discolored rhinorrhea, postnasal discharge, and occasionally anosmia. Fever, if it does occur, is usually low grade. The causative organisms in the acute setting are usually *Streptococcus pneumoniae*, *Hemophilus influenzae*, and *Moraxella cattharalis*. Accurate diagnosis is often quite difficult since viral URIs and allergic rhinitis can often present with the same symptoms, leading to inappropriate use of antibiotics.

Sinusitis is a medical disease and initially should be treated as such. Treatment involves antibiotics, mucolytic agents/decongestants, and steroids for a minimum of 2 weeks. Adjuvant therapies such as hot steam or nasal saline irrigations provide symptomatic relief but have not been shown to expedite bacterial clearance. While most cases of acute sinusitis resolve completely, the inflammation persists in certain subsets of patients, leading to chronic symptoms (CRS), recurrent episodes of acute sinusitis, or the occasional development of inflammatory polyps. Endoscopic sinus surgery is usually reserved for such patients.

Endoscopic sinus surgery (ESS) is currently the procedure of choice for surgical management of CRS. Other indications for ESS include excision of benign tumors of the nose and sinus cavities (papillomas in particular, nasal angiofibromas), repair of CSF leaks and encephaloceles (spontaneous or iatrogenic), correction of exophthalmos related to Graves' disease, and to drain intraorbital abscesses due to complications of sinusitis.

Studies have shown that mucociliary clearance in the paranasal sinuses is always directed toward the natural ostium of the respective sinus. A major advantage of ESS over open sinus procedures is the ability to visually identify diseased mucosa or polyps, then to remove them and accurately identify the various sinus ostia. The ostia are then widened, thus maintaining and augmenting the native mucociliary flow patterns. The anatomy and pneumatization patterns of the ethmoid sinuses are probably the most variable in the human body. Proper visualization and accurate identification of the more invariable portions of the intranasal anatomy such as the maxillary sinus ostium and the skull base are keys to successful ESS.

Usual postoperative course

Expected postoperative hospital stay

Usually ESS is an outpatient procedure. Exceptions are patients with severe reactive lower airway disease or children. The major postoperative issues include postoperative nausea or vomiting (mostly from blood in the pharynx which may be swallowed).

Operative mortality

Currently, almost non-existent after ESS.

Special monitoring required

None is required, except in cases where patients have CRS in association with severe asthma where the respiratory status needs monitoring.

Medical Management of the Surgical Patient: A Textbook of Perioperative Medicine, ed. M. F. Lubin, R. B. Smith, T. F. Dobson, N. Spell, H. K. Walker. 4th edn. Published by Cambridge University Press. © Cambridge University 2006.

Patient activity and positioning

Patients are advised not to lift items above 10 lb to reduce the likelihood of nasal bleeding from the raised intra-abdominal/intrathoracic pressure. This is especially important after endoscopic repairs of CSF leaks or encephaloceles. In such cases, a mild laxative is also prescribed to avoid straining.

Alimentation

There are no dietary restrictions after ESS.

Antibiotic coverage

Patients are usually placed on antibiotics for a week or two prior to their ESS; this is usually continued postoperatively. A broad-spectrum antibiotic is used but may be tailored in the postoperative period based on the intraoperative culture data.

Analgesia

Postoperative pain is fairly mild and easily controlled with mild narcotic analgesics.

Late postoperative course

Postoperative management after ESS is probably as important as the surgery itself. Patients are discharged with antibiotics, steroid taper, analgesics, and nasal saline irrigations. A regimen of aggressive nasal saline irrigations is started to minimize the blood clots and collection of mucus and crusts. These are also debrided in the office as part of the postoperative care to expedite mucosal healing and, more importantly, to minimize synechia formation. Aberrant scarring leading to obstruction of the sinus ostia is probably the most important reason for revision surgery.

Postoperative complications

Major complications of ESS are ophthalmologic and intracranial. Minor complications include bleeding and synechia formation.

In the hospital

Cerebrospinal fluid leak

This usually occurs in the region of the sphenoid and at or near the cribriform area when the skull base is very thin. Management involves early recognition (somewhat difficult since blood-tinged CSF is difficult to differentiate from blood-tinged mucus in the acute setting), and

immediate patching of the leak with a mucosal graft. Postoperatively, these patients are admitted and observed for at least 24 hours to rule out meningitis and/or pneumocephalus. Very rarely, more significant violations of the skull base occur, with injuries to the subfrontal or olfactory areas. The skull base defects may also be repaired endoscopically, but require free bone grafts from the calvarium or temporal bone to seal the defect. In such cases, neurosurgical input is generally requested.

Bleeding

Usually minimal and controlled with topical oxymetazoline with or without topical cocaine. More major bleeding may require postoperative nasal packing. Occasionally, major arterial supplies to the nose such as the sphenopalatine or anterior ethmoid arteries are injured, which may necessitate open approaches for proximal control. These complications, fortunately, are quite rare since the vessels course through bony canals.

Ophthalmic complications

Includes the possibility of blindness. Most problems occur when the lamina papyracea is violated and there is bleeding into the orbit, leading to increased intraorbital pressure and optic nerve damage. Immediate recognition is paramount, followed by steps to reduce intraorbital pressure – steroids, mannitol, and a lateral canthotomy, which also helps to drain the blood and clots. Occasionally, the optic nerve itself is injured, especially in the setting of sphenoid sinusitis.

After discharge

Synechia formation

Probably the most common complication, requiring diligent, aggressive postoperative surveillance and lysis of the adhesions in the office.

FURTHER READING

Glicklich, R. & Metson, R. The health impact of chronic sinusitis in patients seeking otolaryngologic care. *Otolaryngol. Head Neck Surg.* 1995; **113**: 104–109.

May, M., Levine, H., Mester, S., & Schaitkin, B. Complications of endoscopic sinus surgery: analysis of 2108 patients – incidence and prevention. *Laryngoscope* 1994; **104**: 1080–1083.

Ray, N., Baraniuk, J., & Thamer, M. Healthcare expenditures for sinusitis in 1996: contributions of asthma, rhinitis and other airway disorders. *J. Allergy Clin. Immunol.* 1999; **103**: 408–414.

123

Cleft palate surgery

Charles E. Moore

Emory University School of Medicine, Atlanta, GA

Congenital deformities of the head and neck and cleft palate surgery in particular can present surgical and long-term management challenges. Not only can cleft palate involve both the primary and secondary palate, the clefting itself may also vary in width and length. Given this range in palatal defects, the goal of surgical intervention is to provide both functional and esthetic correction of the deformity. The most immediate concern with a palatal defect involves feeding difficulties and the potential for airway compromise. Obstruction of the airway may especially occur with isolated clefts of the secondary palate. Most cases of airway compromise are mild and can be managed effectively by positioning the child in the prone position. In more severe cases, a tongue–lip adhesion may have to be performed while exceptional cases will require a tracheostomy.

Advances in surgical techniques for repair of cleft palate have greatly enhanced the functional aspect, allowing improved speech development and swallowing function, though the effects on facial growth remain controversial. Timing and technique are the two most influential factors in determining the outcome of cleft-palate repair. While the timing of repair continues to be controversial as well, it is generally not attempted before the child is 10 months of age, has 10 g of hemoglobin, and weighs at least 10 lb.

All palatal repairs are done under general anesthesia. Operative time varies according to the severity of the cleft and the surgical approach chosen. Generally, it ranges from 30 minutes to 2 hours. The anatomical needs should dictate the surgical technique used. For example, the Veau–Wardill–Kilner V–Y push back procedure allows for palatal lengthening, though it has the disadvantage of possibly leading to large denuded areas of palatal bone that must heal by secondary intention. Consequently, the procedure may contribute to maxillary growth restriction. Other techniques, such as bipedicled mucoperiosteal flaps as described by Langenbeck or a two-flap technique as described by Bardach, may provide an advantage over V–Y pushback techniques by decreasing the amount of denuded bone. Furlow describes an increasingly popular technique that entails a double-opposing Z-plasty for velar repair that allows for velar lengthening and prevents longitudinal scar contracture. Improved speech has been reported by Furlow's technique as compared to others.

Usual postoperative course

Expected postoperative hospital stay
Generally 2 days.

Operative mortality
1% or less.

Special monitoring required
Continuous pulse oximetry is performed for 24 hours.

Patient activity and positioning
Patients are observed in an intensive care unit or intermediate care setting that allows for continuous monitoring of respiratory status.

Alimentation
Subjects are maintained by intravenous hydration for 24 hours. A liquid diet is started on the second postoperative day and continued until the first postoperative visit in approximately 1 week.

Antibiotic coverage
Cleft palate repair is performed in a contaminated field and therefore requires perioperative broad-spectrum

Medical Management of the Surgical Patient: A Textbook of Perioperative Medicine, ed. M. F. Lubin, R. B. Smith, T. F. Dobson, N. Spell, H. K. Walker. 4th edn. Published by Cambridge University Press. © Cambridge University 2006.

antibiotics. Antibiotics are administered intraoperatively and continued for 2 days. The antibiotic chosen should cover gram-positive, aerobic and anaerobic bacteria; gram negative coverage may also be added to the antibiotic regimen.

Humidity

Face tent humidification in conjunction with continuous pulse oximetry is maintained for 24 hours.

Analgesia

Pain is preferably controlled with meperidine for the first 24 hours. Morphine can be used, but the potential for respiratory depression must be appreciated and monitored. Tylenol with codeine elixir will usually provide adequate pain relief in subsequent days.

Postoperative complications

In the hospital

Respiratory compromise

Palatal edema may lead to decreased oronasal competence. Continuous monitoring by pulse oximetry and staff experienced in the signs and treatment of respiratory compromise are imperative.

Poor oral alimentation

Oral intake may be limited if there is significant palatal edema. Steroid therapy will facilitate resolution of this problem. Intravenous fluids are continued until oral nutritional intake is adequate. In rare situations, it is necessary to initiate intravenous hyperalimentation.

After discharge

Oroantral fistula

In about 5% to 10% of patients wound dehiscence may develop into an oroantral fistula. This usually results from a tight surgical closure or from vascular compromise of the palatal flaps.

Velopharyngeal dysfunction

Hypernasal resonance and nasal air escape indicating velopharyngeal dysfunction may be a transient or long-term complication of cleft palate repair. If it persists, it is treated by speech therapy or a revision palatal procedure to limit the nasal air escape.

Speech difficulty

Persistent speech difficulty can be associated with development of compensatory errors in articulation and further impair speech intelligibility. Speech therapy can usually rectify this problem.

Maxillary growth retardation

Delayed or retarded maxillary growth as well as impaired dental development may result from the surgical manipulation and scarring of the maxilla during repair of a cleft palate. Patients with significant maxillary retrusion may be candidates for a LeFort I osteotomy or maxillary distraction. Dental consultations should be initiated early in this process.

FURTHER READING

Anastassov, G. E., Joos, U., & Zollner, B. Evaluation of the results of delayed rhinoplasty in cleft lip and palate patients. Functional and aesthetic implications and factors that affect successful nasal repair. *Br. J. Oral Maxillofac. Surg.* 1998; **36**(6): 416–424.

Andrews-Casal, M., Johnston, D., Fletcher, J., Mulliken, J. B., Stal, S., & Hecht, J. T. Cleft lip with or without cleft palate: effect of family history on reproductive planning, surgical timing, and parental stress. *Cleft Palate Craniofac. J.* 1998; **35**(1): 52–57.

Kaufman, F. L. Managing the cleft lip and palate patient. *Pediatr. Clin. North Am.* 1991; **38**(5): 1127–1147.

Murray, J. C., Daack-Hirsch, S., Buetow, K. H. *et al.* Clinical and epidemiologic studies of cleft lip and palate in the Philippines. *Cleft Palate Craniofac. J.* 1997; **34**(1): 7–10.

Pensler, J. M. & Bauer, B. S. Levator repositioning and palatal lengthening for submucous clefts. *Plast. Reconstr. Surg.* 1988; **82**(5): 765–769.

Ruiz-Razura, A., Cronin, E. D., & Navarro, C. E. Creating long-term benefits in cleft lip and palate volunteer missions. *Plast. Reconstr. Surg.* 2000; **105**(1): 195–201.

Wallace, A. F. A history of the repair of cleft lip and palate in Britain before World War II. *Ann. Plast. Surg.* 1987; **19**(3): 266–275.

124

Facial surgery

Seth A. Yellin

Emory University School of Medicine, Atlanta, GA

Facial plastic surgery is conceptually divided into aesthetic and reconstructive disciplines. Indications for aesthetic plastic surgery include the sequelae of facial aging: rhytidosis, facial and cervical skin laxity and redundancy, brow ptosis, dermatochalasis and generalized periorbital aging, soft tissue atrophy, and cervical fat excess. Additional indications include the desire for nasal refinement and correction of malformed ears, a weak or prominent chin, and cheekbone or lip enhancement. Reconstructive procedures are indicated for correction of nasal airway obstruction and reconstruction following facial trauma, cancer therapy, and birth defects. The operations vary in complexity and duration based on the indications and goals of the surgical procedure. Regardless of the indication, facial plastic surgery is most often an elective procedure done to improve the patient's quality of life. Blood loss from aesthetic and reconstructive procedures is usually minimal with cases requiring transfusions the rare exception. Medications with antiplatelet activity such as salicylates and non-steroidal anti-inflammatory agents as well as vitamin E and herbal products known to increase bleeding such as ginkgo, ginseng, and supplements of ginger and garlic must be avoided in the perioperative setting. Facial surgery should reinforce the need to make sun protection a lifelong habit.

The choice of anesthetic techniques for these procedures is evenly divided between general anesthesia and a combination of local anesthesia with intravenous sedation. Patient's preference, surgical expertise, and expected duration of the procedure are all considerations in anesthetic decisions.

Usual postoperative course

Expected postoperative hospital stay

Most patients undergo operations on an outpatient basis. The remainder of patients can usually be discharged from the hospital after overnight observation.

Operative mortality

Under 1%. Most of these procedures are performed in an elective setting on patients with few coexisting medical conditions. In cases of complex reconstructive procedures on patients with multiple medical problems, the mortality rates rise proportionally.

Special monitoring required

None necessary.

Patient activity and positioning

Patients are permitted to ambulate on the evening of their procedure. They are advised to avoid straining, bending over, heavy lifting, or – in cases involving nasal procedures – vigorous nose blowing. When in bed, patients are advised to have their head elevated 30° and ice placed on the affected areas. Ice should be maintained for 48 hours intermittently while awake to reduce postoperative ecchymosis and edema.

Alimentation

A regular diet is permitted as tolerated.

Antibiotic coverage

Perioperative prophylactic antibiotics are routinely used. The antibiotics selected should have good gram positive coverage for most routine facial plastic surgery procedures as well as anaerobic coverage when operating inside the

Medical Management of the Surgical Patient: A Textbook of Perioperative Medicine, ed. M. F. Lubin, R. B. Smith, T. F. Dobson, N. Spell, H. K. Walker. 4th edn. Published by Cambridge University Press. © Cambridge University 2006.

mouth. Selection is further determined by the patient's allergy profile.

Postoperative complications

In the hospital and after discharge

Nasal surgery

Nasal discharge and bleeding may persist for several days. Most bleeding is mucosal in origin and self-limited. Profuse arterial bleeding can arise from the anterior or posterior ethmoid or sphenopalatine arteries. Significant bleeding usually responds to nasal packing with expandable Merocel sponges or topical hemostatic agents. Occasionally, surgical intervention is indicated. Infection is a rare occurrence with a reported incidence of 0.8% to 1.6%. Following osteotomies, some facial and periorbital ecchymosis is expected. Periostitis with its associated tenderness can persist along the bone incision sites; however, this problem should resolve without therapy. Injury to the lacrimal duct can also occur but is rare. Excessive scar tissue resulting in contour deformities can often be addressed with the judicious use of subcutaneous steroid injections. Undesirable cosmetic results requiring surgical correction occur with an incidence of 5%–10% depending on whether the nasal surgery is a primary or secondary procedure. If concomitant septoplasty is performed, septal hematoma and perforation are complications that must be identified and addressed. Finally, nasal airway obstruction and an altered sense of smell is an expected short-term consequence of any nasal procedure. However, long-term problems may persist. Permanent changes in airflow, particularly following significant dorsal hump reduction, must be corrected surgically.

Eyelid surgery

Of particular importance is the risk of bleeding following periorbital fat removal. If the patient complains of deep eye pain, visual changes, or acute swelling and bruising of one eye relative to the other, expeditious action is critical. Should bleeding occur in the soft tissues surrounding the globe followed by hematoma development, its extent and time of presentation will guide management. Large hematomas that present early and continue to expand with evidence of symptomatic retrobulbar extension (decrease in visual acuity, proptosis, ocular pain, ophthalmoplegia, progressive chemosis), demand immediate exploration and hemostatic control. Urgent ophthalmologic consultation and orbital decompression are the mainstays of treatment. Untreated, retrobulbar hemorrhage can lead to blindness, the most feared potential complication of blepharoplasty. This occurs with an incidence of approximately 0.04%, typically presenting within the first 24 hours after surgery and often associated with orbital fat removal. Infection can occur but is rare. Lid malposition, asymmetries and contour irregularities may develop and can be treated by a secondary procedure. Lagophthalmos, or difficulty fully closing the upper lid, is often transitory and responds to massage. Temporary treatment with artificial tears and lacrilube often suffices. Long-term difficulty due to overzealous upper lid skin excision can lead to persistent dry eye problems including epiphora, requiring correction. Apparent ptosis is often due to upper lid edema, which is self-limiting; true ptosis from injury to the levator apparatus can occur and demands surgical correction. Ocular injury, including corneal abrasion, globe puncture, and extraocular muscle imbalance, can occur and should be evaluated by an ophthalmologist. Wound dehiscence, suture line milia, and hypertrophic scarring can complicate normal wound healing. Vertical contracture forces of the lateral lid may lead to scleral show and ectropian of the lower lid as well as lateral hooding of the upper lid. Proper treatment should be directed at reorienting the contracting vectors.

Facial flap surgery

Given the robust blood supply to this area, bleeding is a potential complication after any surgical procedure involving the face. In the male face, the rich vascular supply associated with facial hair growth makes hematoma formation more common, with a reported incidence of 7% vs. 0.7% in women following rhytidectomy. Monitoring for hematoma formation should be routine following any operation that involves flap elevation. Rising unilateral facial pain following bilateral procedures or rising pain of any unilateral flap that is associated with increasing swelling, ecchymosis, drainage, and a feeling of pressure should be evaluated. If a dressing is in place, it should be removed and facial proportions and the incision site evaluated. Depending on severity, the hematoma may be treated with local drainage or may require a return to the operating room. Untreated, hematomas can lead to devitalization of skin and cartilage. Skin necrosis and sloughing can also occur secondary to excess tension at the closure site and a compromised flap vascular supply. Infection is uncommon but can manifest on the third or fourth postoperative day and is identified as a dissecting, often fluctuant pocket with overlying skin erythema and tenderness. Treatment should include opening the flap, draining and culturing the wound, and treating with the appropriate antibiotics. Injury to either motor or sensory nerves can occur and may improve with time. Surgical correction, if required, is often less than satisfactory in reconstituting the preinjury state. Following any flap procedure, facial asymmetries and contour irregularities may result but can often be corrected with additional surgery. When implants are used, malposition, asymmetry, and either under- or overcorrection are possible and may necessitate a corrective procedure. Flaps that involve hair-bearing tissues can result in transient alopecia. Finally, hypertrophic or keloid scarring can occur. Treatment includes serial steroid injection and scar revision.

Skin resurfacing

Regardless of the technique used, laser, dermabrasion, and chemical peeling can all result in similar complications. Expected sequelae are skin erythema and sun sensitivity often lasting several months following the procedure. Bacterial infection and herpes simplex outbreaks can occur within several days following resurfacing and should be aggressively treated with standard antibiotics and antiviral medications. Undesirable hyperpigmentation can be reduced with skin lighteners, steroid creams, and sun avoidance. Permanent hypopigmentation may require micropigmentation for correction. Hypertrophic scarring is a disastrous sequela but should not occur with properly performed resurfacing; its occurrence indicates too great a depth of injury. Telangectasias may persist and can be treated with a variety of techniques. Of particular note are the cardiotoxic complications of phenol chemical peeling, which are further exacerbated by liver or kidney dysfunction. Skin resurfacing should not be performed routinely on darker skinned individuals. The significantly higher incidence of dyschromia precludes predictable recovery.

FURTHER READING

Nauman, H. H., Tardy, M. E., & Kastenbauer, E. R. *Head and Neck Surgery*. Vol. 1. New York, NY: Thieme, 1995: 124–167.

Papel, I. D., ed. *Facial Plastic and Reconstructive Surgery*. 2nd edn. New York, NY: Thieme; 2002: 153–246, 276–297, 452–460.

Papel, I. D. & Nachlas, N. E., eds. *Facial Plastic and Reconstructive Surgery*. St. Louis, MO: Mosby Year Book, 1992: 129–183, 256–349.

Resnick, S. S. & Resnick, B. I. Complications of chemical peeling. *Clin. Plast. Surg.* 2001: **28**: 231–234.

125

Tracheotomy

William J. Grist

Emory University School of Medicine, Atlanta, GA

Tracheotomy is performed to establish an airway in patients with existing or impending airway obstruction, such as those with neoplasia of the upper aerodigestive tract and those with trauma to the face, oral cavity, or neck in whom edema, bleeding, and loss of function produces airway compromise. The procedure also provides access to the trachea for suctioning and clearance of secretions. In an emergency situation, mask ventilation or endotracheal intubation is done to gain control of the airway, followed by tracheotomy under more controlled circumstances.

For patients who cannot be ventilated or intubated, cricothyroidotomy is preferable since tracheotomy is a poor emergency procedure. Performed between the larynx and the cricoid cartilage, cricothyroidotomy involves a higher anatomic level than that of tracheotomy. The highly vascular thyroid gland is avoided and airway access can be established in seconds. Immediately following emergency cricothyroidotomy, tracheotomy is done to reposition the tube in a more suitable location in the trachea so that injury to the cricoid cartilage can be avoided and subglottic stenosis will not develop.

Tracheotomy is also performed to prevent complications from prolonged endotracheal intubation. Although low-pressure cuffs on endotracheal tubes have decreased the frequency of such complications, long-term intubation requires careful management. Improper position and excessive pressure in the cuff as well as relative movement between the tube and the patient can produce severe injury to the trachea. There is no exact juncture when an intubated patient should be converted to a tracheotomy, though the procedure should be considered for any patient that has been intubated for 7–10 days and should be done even sooner if an extended duration of intubation can be foreseen early in the patient's course.

Another indication for tracheotomy is severe obstructive sleep apnea which remains unaffected following the performance of more conservative measures. In such cases, patients can be fitted following maturation of the tracheotomy site with a self-retaining airway appliance or button that is relatively inconspicuous and can be occluded during the day. Before retiring for sleep, the device is opened to produce a patent airway that eliminates the sleep apnea.

Tracheotomy can be performed either in the operating room under local or general anesthesia or at the bedside with local and topical anesthesia, the choice depending on various factors such as the stability of the patient, the patient's neck anatomy, and the availability of equipment, support personnel, and the operating room. The goal is to perform a safe, efficient, and cost-effective procedure that is comfortable for the patient, and the surgeon's skill, experience, and judgment should determine the most effectual way to accomplish this objective. Percutaneous tracheotomies involving a needle passed through the anterior midline of the neck into the trachea are performed regularly at hospital bedsides with safety and efficacy. Using the Seldinger technique, a wire passed through the needle guides increasingly larger dilators through the skin, soft tissue, and the anterior trachea into the tracheal lumen.

Usually, fiberoptic bronchoscopy is performed simultaneously through the existing endotracheal tube to ensure proper placement of the dilators and the tube. Regardless of the technique, the end result should be the same: a dependable, stable airway in the lower neck. Tracheotomy in children should always be performed in the operating room, where anesthesia, monitoring, adequate light, suction, and assistance are available. In most cases patients are initially fitted with a cuffed tracheotomy tube. The balloon cuff helps to keep blood out of the trachea and can usually be deflated 24 hours after the procedure unless the patient is being mechanically ventilated. Following the placement of a tracheotomy,

Medical Management of the Surgical Patient: A Textbook of Perioperative Medicine, ed. M. F. Lubin, R. B. Smith, T. F. Dobson, N. Spell, H. K. Walker. 4th edn. Published by Cambridge University Press. © Cambridge University 2006.

adequate measures must be taken to ensure that accidental displacement doesn't occur. Until a tract has formed, a displaced tracheotomy tube can be very difficult to replace. Traction sutures should be placed in the trachea and the tracheotomy tube should be sewn to the skin of the patient. In addition, a security strap should be placed around the patient's neck. The retaining sutures are usually removed 3–5 days after the procedure.

Usual postoperative course

Expected postoperative hospital stay
Usually depends on the underlying reason for the tracheotomy.

Operative mortality
The operative mortality rate is <1% for elective procedures and 10%–50% for emergency procedures.

Special monitoring required
If possible, all patients with a new tracheotomy should be monitored closely in the intensive care unit for bleeding from the tracheotomy site and for security of the tube to avoid displacement from the trachea. Tracheal suctioning should be performed as needed and continuous pulse oximetry is required. A chest radiograph is not routine except in children, but should be considered for patients whose hemoglobin–oxygen saturations are low.

Patient activity and positioning
Patients should have their head elevated, and a high-humidity collar is essential for the first few days. Ambulation is dependent on the patient's overall status and on the underlying condition responsible for the tracheotomy. If the patient is being ventilated, the cuff pressure should be kept just above the pressure at which air leak occurs during inspiration. Mucosal capillary perfusion pressure is approximately 25 cm of water; cuff pressures above this level can potentially damage the tracheal mucosa. If the cuff or the cuff valve begins leaking, the tube will need to be replaced. Otherwise, there is no need to automatically change a tracheotomy tube as long as it is functioning properly.

If a patient is alert and does not require mechanical ventilation, the original cuffed tracheotomy tube can be changed to a non-cuffed tube on the third day after allowing time for a tract to form around it. Following placement, the patient may be able to phonate by occluding the tube. In some cases, the tube can be fitted with a one-way valve that allows the patient to speak without digital occlusion.

When a tracheotomy is no longer needed, it can be removed and the tract is allowed to close. While most tracts close spontaneously, there are occasions where a persistent tracheocutaneous fistula requires surgical closure.

Alimentation
Oral intake may be resumed after operation if the oral cavity and gastrointestinal tract are normal and if the patient's mental status permits. However, due to tethering of the trachea by the tube, the larynx fails to rise normally during swallowing and aspiration is common. Similarly, if gastroesophageal reflux above the upper esophageal sphincter occurs, the patient may aspirate even if they are not allowed oral intake.

Antibiotic coverage
Patients are often on antibiotics for other reasons when undergoing tracheotomy; if not, perioperative antibiotics should be given using a first generation cephalosporin or, if the patient is penicillin allergic, clindamycin.

Postoperative complications

In the hospital

Displacement of the tube
Coughing is often vigorous during the first few hours and can displace the tube unless it is well secured.

Bleeding
The most common site is from the thyroid gland and can usually be controlled with surgical gauze or oxidized cellulose packed around the tube.

Infection
Wound infection is uncommon but aspiration may cause tracheal secretions to increase and to become more purulent.

Obstruction
Thick, tenacious secretions can be difficult to clear. Irrigation with 3–5 ml of sterile saline solution, and use of humidified air or oxygen delivered by tracheotomy collar are helpful. Suctioning should be performed as needed.

Pulmonary edema
Acute relief of airway obstruction can cause post-obstructive pulmonary edema, which is recognized by frothy abundant secretions and hemoglobin-oxygen

desaturation. Positive pressure ventilation is often necessary and diuretics may be helpful.

Pneumothorax

Occurs in 25% of infant tracheotomies because of the high reflection of the pleura into the root of the neck. Chest auscultation and postoperative chest radiographs should identify the condition.

Cervical or mediastinal emphysema

Pneumothorax should be considered. No treatment is necessary unless pneumothorax is present.

After discharge

For successful applications, patient education in care and maintenance of the tracheotomy is crucial. Patients should be instructed on cleaning the tube and the tracheotomy site, and instructions detailing what to do if the tube becomes obstructed or displaced should be given.

Home health services can provide home nursing or respiratory therapy care, providing continued reinforcement of tracheotomy care principles while also relieving much patient anxiety.

A home humidifier can help keep secretions moist. A suction machine can also be useful but requires additional patient and caregiver instruction. Deep suctioning of the trachea is uncomfortable and unnecessary if the patient has a good cough.

If the conditions responsible for tracheotomy are no longer present or the patient has improved, the tracheotomy can be removed. Decannulation should be performed only after careful consideration of the patient's pulmonary mechanics and airway patency.

FURTHER READING

Heffner, J. E. & Hess, D. Tracheotomy management in the chronically ventilated patient. *Clin. Chest Med.* 2001; **22**(1): 55–69.

Pryor, J. P., Reilly, P. M., & Shapiro, M. B. Surgical airway management in the intensive care unit. *Crit. Care Clin.* 2000; **16**(3): 473–488.

Stock, M. C., Woodard, C. G., Shapiro, B. A. *et al.* Perioperative complications of elective tracheotomy in critically ill patients. *Crit. Care Med.* 1986; **14**: 861–863.

Weissler, M. C. Tracheotomy and intubation. In Bailey, B. J., ed. *Head and Neck Surgery – Otolaryngology*. Philadelphia, PA: Lippincott, Williams, & Wilkins, 2001; 677–688.

Weymuller, Ernest, A. Jr. Acute airway management. In Cummings, C. W., ed. *Otolaryngology: Head and Neck Surgery, 3rd edn.* St. Louis, MO: Mosby Year Book, Inc., 1998; 2368–2381.

126

Surgical management of head and neck cancer

Amy Y. Chen

Emory University School of Medicine, Atlanta, GA

Head and neck cancer or cancer of the upper aerodigestive tract is an unusual malignancy comprising only 3% of all newly diagnosed cancers in the USA. However, in many parts of the world, particularly in India and France, head and neck cancer is a major cause of death. Four sites encompass the upper aerodigestive tract: the oral cavity, oropharynx, hypopharynx, and the larynx. The oral cavity includes the lips, oral tongue, floor of the mouth, alveolar ridge, and buccal mucosa; the oropharynx comprises the base of the tongue, the lateral pharyngeal wall, and the tonsil; the hypopharynx consists of the pyriform sinus, the posterior pharyngeal wall, and the postcricoid region; and the larynx includes the epiglottis, the endolarynx, and the subglottic region. The most common pathology is that of squamous cell carcinoma encompassing greater than 90% of all tumors in the upper aerodigestive tract. Five-year survival rates have changed little in the past 30 years: Stage III and IV cancer survival rates are 40%–50% and Stage I and II rates are 70%–90%. Treatment includes chemotherapy, radiotherapy, and/or surgery.

Surgery is indicated either as definitive or as salvage treatment. Definitive methods includes glossectomy, composite resection of mandible and part of the oral cavity and/or oropharynx, and laryngectomy. Neck dissections are usually included because of the primary echelon of nodal drainage for these malignancies to be in the neck. Salvage treatment is reserved for residual disease following chemotherapy and/or radiation and may include the same procedures associated with definitive treatment. Surgery as definitive treatment is preferred for oral cavity lesions, whereas chemotherapy and/or radiation are preferred for oropharynx lesions. Laryngeal preservation protocols (chemotherapy and/or radiation) are currently in favor unless there is extensive thyroid or cricoid cartilage invasion, paretic vocal cord, or incompetent airway. Salvage neck dissections are often performed for residual cervical adenopathy after chemotherapy and radiation. Again, total laryngectomy is indicated for persistent tumor after chemotherapy and radiation.

Glossectomy can be performed transorally or by splitting the mandible. A tracheotomy is often performed in order to protect the airway and to ensure that is adequate. Laryngectomy is often performed in conjunction with a neck dissection. The resulting stoma is the distal trachea sutured to the skin to establish the airway. The rest of the nasopharyngeal airway is not patent in a patient who has had a laryngectomy. Neck dissections are performed routinely for these lesions.

Usual postoperative course

Expected postoperative hospital stay
Generally, two nights for neck dissections and 7 to 10 days for composite resections and total laryngectomies. Surgeries that require extensive reconstruction by plastic surgeons usually require a longer length of stay.

Operative mortality
<1% but extremely dependent on the patient's comorbidities.

Special monitoring required
None.

Patient activity and positioning
Patients who receive a tracheotomy as part of their surgical procedure are usually observed overnight in the surgical intensive care unit (ICU). In addition, patients who require reconstruction by plastic surgery remain in the ICU until the reconstruction is deemed stable, usually 3 days. The head of the bed is customarily elevated to no

Medical Management of the Surgical Patient: A Textbook of Perioperative Medicine, ed. M. F. Lubin, R. B. Smith, T. F. Dobson, N. Spell, H. K. Walker. 4th edn. Published by Cambridge University Press. © Cambridge University 2006.

more than 30 degrees. In addition, the patient's head should be in the midline position because of tenuous arterial and venous anastomoses. Closed suction drains are placed in the operative field and removed when output diminishes to less than 30 ml in a 24-hour period.

Alimentation

Most commonly, patients are not able to take nutrition by mouth, with the exception of simple neck dissections and some surgeries in the oral cavity that do not violate the pharynx. For patients who are rendered NPO, a thin flexible feeding tube is placed through the nares into the stomach. On occasions where prolonged tube feedings are anticipated, a percutaneous gastrostomy tube is placed at the time of surgical extirpation of the tumor. Tube feedings are begun once there is adequate bowel function, manifested by return of bowel sounds. Pharyngeal closures usually require a period of 5–10 days n.p.o. before a trial of clear liquids is begun. Reconstruction of the pharynx utilizing free tissue transfer necessitates a barium swallow prior to initiating oral intake to ensure adequacy of closure and absence of fistula. Nutritionists can provide excellent advice regarding adequacy of nutritional support and need for parenteral nutrition.

Antibiotic coverage

With the exception of neck dissections, head and neck surgery is performed in a clean, contaminated field. Antibiotic coverage to include gram-positive, gram-negative, and anaerobic organisms is important during and for at least 72 hours after operation.

Management of the tracheotomy/tracheostoma

Humidity is important throughout the postoperative period for patients with a fresh tracheotomy or tracheostoma to prevent bleeding and scabbing.

Analgesia

Patients who receive extensive reconstruction consisting of free tissue transfer usually require sedation and ventilator assistance for 24 hours after operation. Other patients do not require such management unless there are significant pulmonary comorbidities. Intravenous narcotics are usually necessary for 24–48 hours after surgery. Oral analgesics such as hydroxycodone and codeine derivatives are sufficient after the immediate postoperative period.

Speech therapy/physical therapy/occupational therapy

After extirpation of head and neck tumors, patients can have significant speech and swallowing problems. It is optimal to obtain a speech/swallowing consult prior to

surgery and to implement it in the immediate postoperative period to assist in the rehabilitation of swallowing and speech. In addition, after neck dissections, the spinal accessory nerve can be affected and result in decreased shoulder mobility, pain, and stiffness. Intervention by a physical therapist can help facilitate rehabilitation and prevent long-term dysfunction.

Management of comorbidities

Consultations are often obtained from the critical care team or hospitalist service to assist with patients who have complex medical issues. Representatives from these services can be instrumental in decreasing length of stay and recommending effective medical interventions.

Postoperative complications

In the hospital

Bleeding

Such major vessels as the internal jugular vein and carotid artery are encountered routinely during surgery of the head and neck. In addition, for advanced tumors of the neck that produce erosion into the great vessels of the neck, there is a high propensity for carotid artery "blowout."

Infection

Fortunately, this is relatively uncommon given the amount of clean contamination that takes place during such cases. Gram-negative and anaerobic coverage in addition to gram-positive coverage must be considered.

Fistula

A communication between the oropharynx or oral cavity and the neck can occur after surgery, especially if extensive loss of native tissue occurs. As a part of the laryngectomy, a pharyngotomy is created. Occasionally, the repair of the pharyngotomy is unsuccessful and the patient develops a fistula. Close observation and meticulous wound care are usually sufficient for treating this complication.

Speech and swallowing impairment

At times this is inevitable. However, impairment is aggravated by cranial neuropathies, particularly of the hypoglossal, glossopharyngeal, and vagus nerves.

Shoulder pain/weakness

As part of a routine neck dissection, the spinal accessory nerve is dissected and traced in order to unwrap the facial envelope of nodes away from the nerve. In this triangle, cervical lymphadenopathy often resides and, therefore, it is extremely important to be meticulous in this area. As a result of the dissection, the cranial nerve can suffer neuropathy. Usually, physical therapy can assist with this.

Esophageal perforation

This uncommon complication carries with it great morbidity and mortality. Perforations and/or tears in the distal esophagus can particularly lead to mediastinitis and lung abscesses that can be fatal. To successfully manage this complication, prompt identification of the symptoms (e.g., severe chest pain, pneumomediastinum) and consultation with a thoracic surgeon are essential.

Airway obstruction

An emergent awake tracheotomy may be necessary if there is sufficient edema post surgery to obstruct the airway. This may be prevented by performing an elective tracheotomy at the time of surgical resection of the tumor.

Chylous fistula

An infrequent complication that usually occurs after a left neck dissection because of the location of the thoracic duct. Management usually consists of close observation.

After discharge

Tumor recurrence

Careful postoperative surveillance is necessary to identify and treat local or distant tumor persistence or recurrence.

FURTHER READING

Brazilian Head and Neck Cancer Study Group. Results of a prospective trial on elective modified radical classical vs. supraomohyoid neck dissection in the management of oral squamous carcinoma. *Am. J. Surg.* 1998; **176**: 422–427.

Byers, R. M., Clayman, G. L., McGill, D. *et al.* Selective neck dissections for squamous carcinoma of the upper aerodigestive tract: patterns of regional failure. *Head Neck* 1999; **21**: 499–505.

Johnson, J. T., Myers, E. N., Bedetti, C. D., Barnes, C. L., Schramm, V. L. Jr., & Thearle, P. B. Cervical lymph node metastases: incidence and implications of extracapsular carcinoma. *Arch. Otolaryngol.* 1985; **111**: 534–537.

Munro, A. J. An overview of randomized controlled trials of adjuvant chemotherapy in head and neck cancer. *Br. J. Cancer* 1995; **71**: 83–91.

O'Brien, C. J., Lahr, C. J., & Soong, S. Surgical treatment of early stage carcinoma of the oral tongue. *Head Neck Surg.* 1986; **8**: 401–408.

Pauloski, B. R., Rademaker, A. W., Logemann, J. A., & Colangelo, L. A. Speech and swallowing in irradiated and nonirradiated postsurgical oral cancer patients. *Otolaryngol. Head Neck Surg.* 1998; **118**: 616–624.

Shumrick, D. A. & Quenelle, D. J. Malignant disease of the tonsillar region, retromolar trigone and buccal mucosa. *Otolaryngol. Clin. Am.* 1979; **12**: 115–120.

Vokes, E. E., Kies, M. S., Haraf, D. J. *et al.* Concomitant chemoradiotherapy as primary therapy for locoregionally advanced head and neck cancer. *J. Clin. Oncol.* 2000; **18**: 1652–1661.

127

Anterior cranial base surgery

Charles E. Moore

Emory University School of Medicine, Atlanta, GA

Anterior cranial base surgery has been greatly enhanced with new advances in diagnostic and surgical techniques that apply a comprehensive, multidisciplinary methodology to the removal of anterior skull-base lesions. Approaching the anterior cranial base from anterior and below has gained increasing popularity because of the minimal amount of frontal lobe retraction. In addition, the technique eliminates the need for facial incisions, therefore avoiding facial scarring. In contradistinction to more traditional techniques that often ensure anosmia, the approach also allows for the preservation of smell depending on the location of the lesion.

Imaging plays an important role in the surgical and reconstructive planning of craniofacial tumors as it allows for assessment of the extent of the disease process and determination of the operability of the lesion. The imaging modalities commonly employed include axial and coronal two-dimensional, three-dimensional, and interactive three-dimensional CT imaging; MR imaging; and angiography.

The use of the subcranial approach in anterior cranial base surgery allows intracranial access extending along the posterior planum sphenoidal, anterior clinoid, and tuberculum sellae. The lateral aspect of the exposure is determined by the type and extent of craniotomy that is performed. Extra-cranial exposure extends to the foramen magnum. After tumor extirpation, closure is routinely accomplished with a pericranial flap. A tracheotomy is rarely necessary if nasal trumpets are placed to divert air away from the skull-base closure.

Anterior cranial base procedures are performed under general anesthesia. Depending on the extent of the disease process, the operative time may range from 3–10 hours. Blood transfusion may be required depending on the tumor pathology. The approach to the brain is sterile via a craniotomy; while the subcranial approach from below is semisterile since the sinuses are exposed.

Usual postoperative course

Expected postoperative hospital stay
Generally expected to be 5 days, though the final determination is decided by neurological status and the ability to tolerate removal of a CSF monitoring device.

Operative mortality
1% or less.

Special monitoring required
A lumbar drain or ventriculostomy is routinely placed intraoperatively to monitor and adjust CSF pressure.

Patient activity and positioning
Each patient is initially observed in the intensive care unit, with the neurological status being closely monitored. The patient may remain intubated for 24 hours, which may be extended based upon neurological status. A lumbar drain or ventriculostomy along with nasal trumpets are in place for approximately 5 days.

Alimentation
Patients are not allowed to have any oral intake if they have ventilatory support. Otherwise, a liquid diet is initiated and progressed to a regular diet based on the patient's tolerance.

Antibiotic coverage
Antibiotics are administered intraoperatively and continued until the lumbar drain or ventriculostomy is removed.

Medical Management of the Surgical Patient: A Textbook of Perioperative Medicine, ed. M. F. Lubin, R. B. Smith, T. F. Dobson, N. Spell, H. K. Walker. 4th edn. Published by Cambridge University Press. © Cambridge University 2006.

The chosen antibiotic should have good central nervous system penetration.

Humidity

Irrigation of the nasal trumpets is performed while they are in place in order to prevent their occlusion.

Analgesia

Pain is routinely controlled with morphine or meperidine. Prior to their discharge, patients are introduced to an oral pain medication such as Tylenol with codeine to provide pain relief.

Postoperative complications

In the hospital

Excessive pneumocephalus

A certain degree of pneumocephalus is expected as a result of performing a craniotomy. If an air leak continues through the surgical closure, obtundation or herniation may result. The lumbar drain or ventriculostomy combined with the nasal trumpets usually provides adequate time for the surgical closure to seal. In the remote possibility that the closure doesn't seal, a tracheostomy should be performed to divert air from traversing the surgical closure.

Cerebrospinal fluid leak

The chance for a CSF leak increases in direct proportion to the increase in size of the defect and the associated size of the reconstructed surgical site. A lumbar drain or ventriculostomy is rarely inadequate in preventing a CSF leak in the standard period of time. In most cases, continued use of one of these devices in the immediate postoperative period eventually results in resolution of the leak.

Cerebral edema

In addition to being a possible characteristic of the tumor itself, swelling of the brain can be caused by surgical manipulation of the brain. This complication can be monitored by imaging studies and managed by hyperventilation, steroids, mannitol, and furosemide.

Seizures

Tumors that involve the cortex or surgical manipulation of the cortex can lead to seizures. Anticonvulsants are given routinely in an effort to avoid seizure development. The duration of the anticonvulsant therapy is often dependent on the location and pathology of the mass.

Low pressure headache

A protracted headache may occur from the loss or removal of CSF. Most cases will resolve as the CSF pressure equilibrates. A blood patch may prove helpful in low pressure headaches that are prolonged.

After discharge

Delayed cerebrospinal fluid leak

A CSF leak after discharge may present as CSF rhinorrhea. In the later postoperative period, the problem can be treated by elevation of the head of the bed and CSF drainage either by spinal taps or by a continuous device. If persistent, an additional surgical procedure is needed to repair the leak.

Crusting

Severe nasal cavity crusting is common, resulting in nasal obstruction and potential superimposed bacterial infection. This can be avoided by the patient's strict adherence to a nasal irrigation regimen.

Diplopia

Diplopia is a transient complication from mobilization of the orbital contents, particularly the trochlea. In severe cases, an eye patch may be used intermittently until the diplopia resolves.

FURTHER READING

Browne, J. D. & Mims, J. W. Preservation of olfaction in anterior skull base surgery. *Laryngoscope* 2000; **110**(8): 1317–1322.

Darrouzet, V. Subcranial approach to tumors of the anterior cranial base. *Otolaryngol. Head Neck Surg.* 2000; **122**(3): 466–467.

Fliss, D. M., Zucker, G., Cohen, A. *et al.* Early outcome and complications of the extended subcranial approach to the anterior skull base. *Laryngoscope* 1999; **109**(1): 153–160.

Moore, C. E. & Marentette, L. Subcranial approach to tumors of the anterior cranial base. *Otolaryngol. Head Neck Surg.* 2000; **122**(3): 466–467.

Moore, C. E., Ross, D. A., & Marentette, L. J. Subcranial approach to tumors of the anterior cranial base: analysis of current and traditional surgical techniques. *Otolaryngol. Head Neck Surg.* 1999; **120**(3): 387–390.

Raveh, J., Turk, J. B., Ladrach, K. *et al.* Extended anterior subcranial approach for skull base tumors: long-term results. *J. Neurosurg.* 1995; **82**(6): 1002–1010.

128

Surgery for syndromic craniosynostosis

Charles E. Moore

Emory University School of Medicine, Atlanta, GA

Syndromic craniosynostosis encompasses deformity of the cranial vault and facial skeleton, with craniosynostosis specifically defined as premature fusion of one or more of the cranial sutures. Accordingly, syndromic craniosynostosis includes several interacting conditions resulting from diverse causes and factors such as molecular and cellular events, genetic factors, and deformational and mechanical forces in association with a multitude of other clinical entities.

The most common syndromic craniostoses include Apert syndrome, Crouzon syndrome, Pfeiffer syndrome, Carpenter syndrome, and Saethre–Chofzen syndrome. Apert syndrome, known as acrocephalosyndactyly, is autosomal dominant in its inheritance pattern and occurs sporadically. This disease constellation includes craniosynostosis, especially of the coronal sutures, high arched palate, midfacial hypoplasia, symmetric compound syndactyly of the hands and feet, stapes fixation, and patent cochlear aqueduct. Crouzon syndrome, termed craniofacial dysostosis, is autosomal dominant in its inheritance pattern, occurs sporadically, and includes midfacial hypoplasia, craniosynostosis affecting the coronal sutures, exophthalmos, mandibular prognathism and small maxilla, hearing loss, and congenital enlargement of the sphenoid bone. Pfeiffer syndrome is autosomal dominant in its inheritance pattern and includes craniosynostosis, especially of the coronal sutures, broad thumbs and great toes, and occasional partial soft tissue syndactyly of the hands. Carpenter syndrome is autosomal recessive in its inheritance pattern and comprises craniosynostosis of the sagittal and lambdoidal sutures, polysyndactyly of the feet, brachdactyly of the fingers, and dinodactyly. Saethre–Chofzen syndrome is autosomal dominant in its inheritance pattern and usually involves craniosynostosis of the coronal sutures, low-set frontal hairline, upper eyelid ptosis, facial asymmetry, and partial soft tissue syndactyly of the hands.

A craniofacial surgeon and a pediatric neurosurgeon are required to address the surgical needs of these patients. Although a similar approach can be applied to this wide spectrum of conditions, each case should be individualized to respond to particular nuances manifested by each patient. Initially, a functional aesthetic assessment should be taken. Head circumference should be measured which can determine brain growth abnormality. The shape of the head may indicate the pattern of craniosynostosis. Uncompensated craniosynostosis is indicated if the circumference is small. A large circumference may indicate hydrocephalus or compensated growth pattern associated with the craniosynostosis. Evaluation of the periorbital region is paramount in order to determine if hypertelorism and telecanthus, exophthalmos, or hypoplastic orbits exist. In addition, evaluation of the optic discs and fundus can indicate increased intracranial pressure. Growth disturbance of the cranial base results in malar flatness and midfacial retrusion.

Imaging studies and consultations are helpful in the assessment and treatment of patients with syndromic craniosynostosis. A skull series serves to evaluate the cranial sutures and to demonstrate fusion radiographically. A CT scan will assess the structural anatomy of the brain and the bony anatomy including the cranial vault, hydrocephalus, signs of increased ICP, or craniofacial pathology. 3-D imaging may also be useful. MRI can be complimentary in evaluating the brain. A neuroophthalmologic and genetics evaluation will confirm the diagnosis and screen for associated problems. This consultation will assist with establishing the need for further testing and family counseling.

The surgical goal is to reconstruct while creating facial form and symmetry, taking into account growth of the facial skeleton. The timing of release of cranial sutures is controversial. Problems such as increased ICP warrant earlier intervention. The correction of deformities of a child with syndromic craniosynostosis may necessitate a series of operations, the first operation usually being performed at 9–12 months of age and involving a front-orbital advancement. Cranial vault reshaping may be performed in conjunction with this procedure. In less severe cases, no further operations are warranted. In cases involving severe multiple suture synostoses, additional procedures can be combined or staged. The second stage of reconstruction involves a posterior cranial vault expansion combined with a shortening of the height of the cranial vault. The next phase entails midfacial correction by either monobloc advancement or Lefort III advancement and orbital bipartition. Midfacial distraction in the form of osteogenesis may be indicated if conventional surgery is inadequate. The age at which this part of the reconstruction occurs is also controversial. Early intervention considers issues of psychosocial development in comparison to delayed intervention which values stability and decreased number of operations as having more importance.

All reconstructive procedures are performed under general anesthesia. The operative time may range from 3–12 hours depending on the nature and extent of the craniosynostosis and the type of reconstruction needed. A blood transfusion is rarely required during the reconstructive process. Reconstruction of the cranial vault is performed in a sterile environment, while reconstruction of the midface and orbital region is performed in a semisterile environment since the sinuses are exposed.

Usual postoperative course

Expected postoperative hospital stay
Generally expected to be 7 days, though the final determination is decided by neurological status and the ability to tolerate removal of a CSF monitoring device.

Operative mortality
1% or less.

Special monitoring required
A ventriculostomy may be placed intraoperatively to monitor and adjust CSF pressure.

Patient activity and positioning
Each patient is initially monitored in the intensive care unit; the neurological status is closely observed. The patient may remain intubated for 24 hours, though this may be extended based upon the neurological status.

Alimentation
Patients are not allowed to have any oral intake if they have ventilatory support. Otherwise, a liquid diet is initiated and progressed to a regular diet as the patient is able to tolerate oral intake.

Antibiotic coverage
Antibiotics are administered intraoperatively and continued until the ventriculostomy is removed. The chosen antibiotic should have good central nervous system penetration.

Analgesia
Pain is routinely controlled with morphine or meperidine. Patients are introduced to an oral pain medication such as Tylenol with codeine prior to their discharge in order to provide pain relief.

Postoperative complications

In the hospital

Hydrocephalus
An elevated intracranial pressure may develop. Treatment involves placement of a monitor to watch for resolution. A shunt or expansion of the cranial vault or both may be necessary for more expedient resolution.

Airway obstruction
A tracheostomy may be warranted for airway obstruction. If less severe, CPAP or supplemental oxygen with continuous monitoring may be utilized.

Severe exposure of globes
If corneal desiccation occurs, it should be treated with patching, topical ophthalmic applications, or tarsorrhaphy.

FURTHER READING

Abrahams, J. J. & Eklund, J. A. Diagnostic radiology of the cranial base. *Clin. Plast. Surg.* 1995; **22**(3): 373–405.

Becker, L. E. & Hinton, D. R. Pathogenesis of craniosynostosis. *Pediatr. Neurosurg.* 1995; **22**(2): 104–107.

Hennekam, R. C. & Van den Boogaard, M. J. Autosomal dominant craniosynostosis of the sutura metopica. *Clin. Genet.* 1990; **38**(5): 374–377.

Humphreys, R. P. Apert syndrome. Diagnosis and treatment of craniostenosis and intracranial anomalies. *Clin. Plast. Surg.* 1991; **18**(2): 231–235.

Hoffman, H. J. & Reddy, K. V. Progressive cranial suture stenosis in craniosynostosis. *Neurosurg. Clin. North Am.* 1991; **2**(3): 555–564.

Hoyte, D. A. The cranial base in normal and abnormal skull growth. *Neurosurg. Clin. North Am.* 1991; **2**(3): 515–537.

Mulliken, J. B. & Bruneteau, R. J. Surgical correction of the craniofacial anomalies in Apert syndrome. *Clin. Plast. Surg.* 1991; **18**(2): 277–289.

Ohman, J. C. & Richtsmeier, J. T. Perspectives on craniofacial growth. *Clin. Plast. Surg.* 1994; **21**(4): 489–499.

Persing, J. A. & Jane, J. A. Treatment of syndromic and nonsyndromic bilateral coronal synostosis in infancy and childhood. *Neurosurg. Clin. North Am.* 1991; **2**(3): 655–663.

Posnick, J. C. Craniofacial dysostosis. Staging of reconstruction and management of the midface deformity. *Neurosurg. Clin. North Am.* 1991; **2**(3): 683–702.

Posnick, J. C., Bite, U., Nakano, P., Davis, J., & Armstrong, D. Indirect intracranial volume measurements using CT scans: clinical applications for craniosynostosis. *Plast. Reconstr. Surg.* 1992; **89**(1): 34–45.

Richtsmeier, J. T., Grausz, H. M., Morris, G. R., Marsh, J. L., & Vannier, M. W. Growth of the cranial base in craniosynostosis. *Cleft Palate Craniofac. J.* 1991; **28**(1): 55–67.

Thompson, D. N., Harkness, W., Jones, B., Gonsalez, S., Andar, U., & Hayward, R. Subdural intracranial pressure monitoring in craniosynostosis: its role in surgical management. *Childs Nerv. Syst.* 1995; **11**(5): 269–275.

Urologic surgery

129

Nephrectomy

John G. Pattaras

Emory University School of Medicine, Atlanta, GA

Nephrectomy is a common urologic procedure indicated for malignancy, certain benign conditions of the kidney, and renal transplantation. While simple, radical, partial, donor nephrectomy, and nephroureterectomy all have common surgical steps, they each have unique complications.

Simple nephrectomy is indicated for benign but not trivial conditions. Indications include non-functioning kidneys (causing pain from congenital obstruction or urolithiasis), renovascular disease causing uncontrollable hypertension, benign symptomatic tumors (angiomyolipomas), trauma, or infectious diseases (xanthogranulomatous pyelonephritis, chronic or emphysematous pyelonephritis, and tuberculosis). The kidney is removed within Gerota's fascia along with a small amount of ureter. Patients who undergo nephrectomy for inflammatory conditions can be some of the most difficult to manage due to their medical comorbidities.

Donor nephrectomy is a simple procedure in which a healthy kidney (typically the left kidney because of increased vein length) is removed and transplanted as an allograft in a controlled, scheduled situation. The donor patients are healthy and have had extensive preoperative evaluations. Transplant nephrectomy is a simple nephrectomy in which the renal allograft is removed, usually for rejection complications.

Radical nephrectomy involves the removal of all structures within Gerota's fascia, which includes the ipsilateral, adrenal, kidney, and perirenal tissue. Adrenal sparing radical nephrectomy, especially for lower pole tumors, has become commonplace because of the low incidence of ipsilateral adrenal invasion or metastases. Most renal tumors are found incidentally by advanced radiologic imaging or during hematuria screening. Approximately 95% of enhancing renal masses are malignant; therefore, needle biopsy or pathologic proof before surgery is not routinely performed. Complicated radical nephrectomy includes renal tumor extension via vena cava, tumor thrombus, or large masses invading surrounding organs such as liver, spleen, colon, pancreas, duodenum, or diaphragm. These challenging cases are managed by various approaches, which can even include thoracoabdominal exposure or cardiopulmonary bypass for tumor extension into the right atrium.

Alternatively, upper tract uroepithelial carcinoma differs in surgical and chemotherapeutic management. The entire urothelial lining from the renal pelvis to the urinary bladder should be excised in continuity. Nephroureterectomy involves removing the kidney (sparing the adrenal if not involved) and entire ureter down to and including the ureteral orifice in the bladder.

Nephron-sparing surgery is the goal for today's urologic oncologist. Presently, smaller (less than 4 cm), bilateral tumors or tumors in patients with borderline renal function may be managed by partial nephrectomy with fairly equivalent oncologic results. Depending on tumor location and size, surgical approach may include renal hypothermia, vascular control and temporary occlusion, or renal cortical occlusion. Reconstruction of the renal parenchyma, collecting system, ureter, or major vasculature are additional possibilities. The most recent treatment for small masses is renal tumor ablation therapy with cryosurgery or radiofrequency techniques; however, the modality has limited long-term follow-up and is considered an option only for high-risk surgical candidates. Long term studies investigating the oncologic success of ablation therapy are ongoing, though its efficacy appears to make it a viable option over nephrectomy or partial nephrectomy in certain patients.

Nephrectomy is usually performed under general anesthesia. Incisional placement varies according to

Medical Management of the Surgical Patient: A Textbook of Perioperative Medicine, ed. M. F. Lubin, R. B. Smith, T. F. Dobson, N. Spell, H. K. Walker. 4th edn. Published by Cambridge University Press. © Cambridge University 2006.

surgeon preference/experience, patient body habitus, and surgical goal. If possible, extraperitoneal approaches are favored, though transperitoneal surgery is common for advanced tumors or complex infectious cases. First performed in 1991, laparoscopic nephrectomy is now a standard procedure that can be performed with either the transperitoneal method or the less commonly used retroperitoneal approach. The obvious advantages include less pain, quicker recovery, and better cosmesis. Patients at high anesthetic risk are also candidates for laparoscopy and have been shown to have equivalent surgical outcomes, decreased hospitalization, and decreased convalescence when compared to open nephrectomy. Transfusions for nephrectomy also vary with regard to surgical approach, but generally the overall rate is low. Simple nephrectomy for xanthogranulomatous or emphysematous pyelonephritis can be more difficult than most radical nephrectomies and may require a higher rate of transfusion. Radical nephrectomy with caval tumor thrombus, advanced partial nephrectomy, or extensive dissections all increase the possibility of blood transfusion.

Usual postoperative course

Expected postoperative hospital stay

For simple or uncomplicated radical nephrectomy, 3–5 days is expected. Laparoscopic nephrectomy usually decreases hospital stays to as short as one day for simple retroperitoneal nephrectomies to an average of 3 days for radical cases. Medical comorbidities greatly influence hospital stay; even for laparoscopic cases the duration may extend to 7 days.

Operative mortality

Generally quoted as less than 1% for simple uncomplicated nephrectomy and as high as 5% for advanced, higher risk patients with metastatic disease, extensive dissection, or preexisting medical comorbidities.

Special monitoring required

General anesthesia intraoperative monitoring may include arterial line, central venous pressure, and special attention to urine output. Laparoscopic cases commonly have decreased intraoperative urine output that increases with cessation of pneumoperitoneum. Postoperative urine output and daily chemistries should be closely followed. Transient elevations in creatinine and BUN are common.

Patient activity and positioning

Unless extensive reconstructive or vascular surgery prohibits movement, patients are usually encouraged to ambulate within 24 hours of the procedure.

Alimentation

Open surgery usually is followed by ileus, which can resolve in 24–48 hours or take several days to dissipate. Laparoscopic surgery decreases postoperative ileus. In pure retroperitoneal approaches, patients are fed the same day. High protein diets should be avoided because of potential hyperfiltration injury to the kidney.

Antibiotic coverage

Antibiotics are used for short-term prophylaxis and stopped after 24 hours. Exceptions include simple nephrectomies for complicated pyelonephritis, infected stone surgery, or on opening the gastrointestinal tract. Broad-spectrum antibiotic use should then be continued until clinically stable. Doses should be adjusted according to renal function.

Diaphragmatic/pleural injury

Entry into the pleural cavity is a common and well-known complication of nephrectomy. Intraoperative discovery can be managed by a small chest tube or diaphragmatic closure during deep inspiration. Postoperative chest X-rays should be followed until signs of pneumothorax have resolved.

Drains

While not routinely placed for radical nephrectomies, surgical drains are used for infectious cases, partial nephrectomy with entry into the collecting system, and nephroureterectomy requiring partial cystectomy. Drain fluid can be checked for creatinine levels: creatinines over-exceeding serum levels indicate urinary extravasation.

Laboratory values

After nephrectomy, a transient increase in serum BUN and creatinine is often detected. Pancreatic or hepatic involvement may cause brief rises in amylase and LFTs, respectively. Preoperative anemia may be present in large tumors, paraneoplastic syndromes, or renal insufficiency.

Analgesia

Pain control varies in relation to surgical approach. Thoracoabdominal or flank approaches may require epidural placement. Laparoscopic approaches necessitate minimal parenteral analgesia, quickly switched to oral medication. Non-steroidal anti-inflammatory medication should be avoided in the immediate postoperative period and should be limited lifelong to avoid nephrotoxic effects.

Postoperative complications

In the hospital

Ileus

Short-term ileus may occur from any surgical approach and should resolve promptly. Nasogastric decompression and bowel rest are usually curative. A prolonged ileus should be evaluated by CT with oral contrast to rule out herniation or volvulus.

Wound infection

An uncommon complication even in patients with renal infections. Obesity and malnutrition are predisposing factors. Local wound care and drainage may be necessary.

Pneumothorax

A postoperative chest X-ray in the recovery room may reveal this complication, which can be managed conservatively by observation for a small, asymptomatic pneumothorax. For larger or symptomatic collections, chest tube placement, oxygen supplementation, and positive pressure inspiration aid in resolution.

Deep venous thrombosis and pulmonary emboli

These are serious complications that often result from extensive dissection of the vena cava or iliac veins. Prevention starts with placement of sequential compression stockings in the operating room prior to anesthesia induction. In addition, prophylactic subcutaneous heparin (5000u b.i.d or t.i.d) can be administered to hemodynamically stable patients.

Bowel injury

Somewhat unique to laparoscopy, bowel injury is a rare and potentially life threatening complication that can occur from an unrecognized thermal injury. The classic peritoneal symptoms are frequently absent. Nausea/vomiting, trocar site pain, fever, and leukocytosis are indications that should be immediately investigated by CT. Exploration or CT drainage with conservative management are emergently necessary.

After discharge

Flank/abdominal hernia or weakness

Abdominal wall herniation or weakness in the flank is more common in obese, elderly, or malnourished patients. Hernia occurs from a disruption of the fascial closure. Herniations may occur at larger trocar sites even when fascial closure is performed. Surgical intervention is necessary for incarceration or symptomatic hernias. Flank weakness results from a denervation of the musculature secondary to injury of the intercostal and subcostal nerve branches. Weakness may not be correctable, but vigorous physical therapy sometimes helps.

Renal insufficiency/failure

After nephrectomy, the occurrence of this complication can be transient, stable, or progressive. If possible, the contralateral kidney should be evaluated preoperatively to aid the decision of whether to perform total nephrectomy or nephron-sparing surgery.

FURTHER READING

Baldwin, D. D., Dunbar, J. A., Parekh, D. J. *et al.* Single-center comparison of purely laparoscopic, hand-assisted laparoscopic, and open radical nephrectomy in patients at high anesthetic risk. *J. Endourol.* 2003; **17**(3): 161–167.

Bishoff, J. T., Allaf, M. E., Kirkels, W. *et al.* Laparoscopic bowel injury: incidence and clinical presentation. *J. Urol.* 1999; **161**: 887–890.

Desai, M. M. & Gill, I. S. Current status of cryoablation and radio-frequency ablation in the management of renal tumors. *Curr. Opin. Urol.* 2002; **12**(5): 387–393.

Kerbl, K., Clayman, R. V., McDougall, E. M. *et al.* Transperitoneal nephrectomy for benign disease of the kidney: a comparison of laparoscopic and open surgical techniques. *Urology* 1994; **43**: 607–613.

130

Cystectomy and urinary diversion

Peter T. Nieh

Emory University School of Medicine, Atlanta, GA

Cystectomy is most often performed for aggressive bladder cancer that has invaded into the muscular layer of the bladder. In males, the procedure usually includes removal of the prostate; in such cases, the operation is known as cystoprostatectomy. A nerve-sparing technique originally described for radical prostatectomy to preserve the neurovascular bundle for erectile function may be used in cystoprostatectomy in younger patients. In women, the traditional radical cystectomy includes hysterectomy, oophrectomy, and removal of the anterior vaginal wall, which is also referred to as anterior pelvic exenteration. More recently, there has been a trend towards preservation of the anterior vaginal wall.

When dealing with bladder cancer, pelvic lymphadenectomy is usually performed to complete the surgical staging, though more recent reports have also demonstrated a therapeutic role for lymphadenectomy in patients with node-positive disease showing improved survival when the lymph nodes are removed. Thus, a more extensive dissection to include the common iliac nodal tissue has become routine. With such extended dissections in the pelvis/retroperitoneum, there is more risk for lymph leak, bleeding, and third spacing in the early postoperative period.

Other indications for cystectomy include neurogenic bladder, pyocystis from defunctionalized bladder, salvage cystoprostatectomy for radiation therapy failure for prostate cancer, radiation cystitis, and refractory interstitial cystitis.

Once the bladder has been removed, reconstruction of the urinary tract is performed. The ideal bladder replacement would fill and empty without leakage, would protect the kidneys from reflux or obstruction, would have no metabolic or nutritional consequences, would not require an appliance or instrumentation, and would have low risk of infection or stones. Numerous types of urinary diversions have been described, each with advantages and disadvantages, but none have attained the ideal. Currently, there are several options for permanent urinary diversion.

The ileal loop or conduit, popularized by Bricker in 1950, uses a short 15–20 cm segment of the distal ileum to continuously transport urine to the skin surface through a stoma where an external appliance collects the effluent. The ureters are anastomosed separately to the proximal end of the ileal segment in a refluxing fashion. Factors that contributed to the widespread use of this technique were the generous length of small bowel available, even after pelvic radiation; the reliable vascular arcades of the small bowel mesentery; ease of construction; fewer metabolic complications compared with ureterosigmoidostomy; and the improved urinary drainage with use of silicone stents.

Continent reservoirs permit urine to collect in a bowel reservoir and are drained by intermittent catheterization through a small, often recessed, skin stoma. This type of diversion is necessary when the urethra has been removed for disease beyond the bladder neck or involving the urethra, or unsuitable for orthotopic neobladder, such as following radiation therapy. Continent reservoirs are created using lengthy (50–75 cm) segments of small bowel only, combinations of small and large bowel (ileocecal, ileocolonic), and occasionally a wedge of stomach, which are then detubularized to diminish intrareservoir pressures and reshaped into spherical reservoirs. The ureters are anastomosed to the reservoir, relying on either an isoperistaltic ileal segment or "chimney," intussuscepted nipple, or tunneled reimplant into the tenia of the large bowel to prevent reflux. The catheterizable stoma may be created from appendix or tubularized small bowel using a tunneled implant into the reservoir. These reservoirs take several months to expand to a volume permitting catheterization at 6-hour intervals. Younger patients who wish

Medical Management of the Surgical Patient: A Textbook of Perioperative Medicine, ed. M. F. Lubin, R. B. Smith, T. F. Dobson, N. Spell, H. K. Walker. 4th edn. Published by Cambridge University Press. © Cambridge University 2006.

to avoid an external appliance are the best candidates for this approach. Selected patients for this technique must be highly motivated and well informed of the more rigorous rehabilitation than that of ileal loop diversion.

Continent orthotopic neobladder, avoiding an external appliance and any type of stoma, is feasible when the urethra has been preserved. In this form of diversion, the detubularized bowel reservoir is placed in the pelvis and attached to the native urethra, making the external sphincter responsible for continence. Similar to postradical retropubic prostatectomy vesicourethral anastomosis, this procedure was originally used only in males, though the indications have now been extended to females, where preservation of the distal two-thirds of the urethra maintain excellent continence. Patients void by abdominal straining, have a less forceful stream, and may sometimes need self-catheterization to empty completely. The rehabilitation period – during which the reservoir gradually increases in capacity – is more prolonged than ileal loop, taking up to several months before achieving 6-hour intervals between voids. While daytime continence is excellent, most patients will also need to awaken at night to empty or risk nocturnal incontinence. This occurs because the small bowel mucosa permits free water to equilibrate with the more concentrated urine excreted by the kidneys at night, increasing urine volume despite dehydration. An important caveat about continent reservoirs, whether orthotopic or catheterizable, is to avoid them in patients with impaired renal function ($C_r > 2.0$) for they are more likely to have significant metabolic problems from the large absorptive surface.

The combination of cystectomy, pelvic lymphadenectomy, and urinary diversion is an extensive surgical procedure, taking 5–8 hours to perform depending on the type of diversion. Patients require a full mechanical bowel preparation starting the day before operation and receive standard perioperative parenteral antibiotics. Most patients perform the bowel preparation at home and are admitted the day of surgery. However, those more debilitated patients with bowel dysfunction, including fragile diabetics or those with a neurogenic bladder such as myelomeningocele patients, require inpatient bowel preparation with cleansing enemas and may need intravenous fluids to prevent volume contraction due to the preparation. Venous thrombosis prophylaxis with lower extremity venous compression devices and minidose heparin is employed. Arterial and central venous monitoring is routine, since significant fluid shifts from the extensive pelvic dissection require aggressive crystalloid resuscitation. Even with use of the cell saver, blood replacement may be necessary.

Usual postoperative course

Expected postoperative hospital stay
6–10 days.

Operative mortality
Approximately 4%.

Special monitoring required
As many bladder cancer patients have a smoking history with compromised pulmonary function, monitoring of blood gases during weaning from assisted ventilation is necessary. Since many also have coronary disease, the hematocrit must be maintained above 30. Urine output should exceed 50–60 ml/h. Patients have significant third spacing, which will mobilize around the third postoperative day.

Patient activity and positioning
Early mobilization from bed on postoperative day 1 and ambulation on postoperative day 2 are recommended for prevention of deep venous thrombosis.

Alimentation
Use of postoperative nasogastric tube drainage is according to the surgeon's preference. This author prefers to remove the tube in the recovery room, as many patients perform air-swallowing from the tube-induced posterior pharyngeal discomfort, with resultant increase in gaseous distention and more prolonged ileus. Patients are permitted to moisten their lips and oral cavity with swabs, but are not allowed oral intake until bowel activity returns. Stimulation of lower gut function with Dulcolax suppositories begins on the second day. Bowel function usually returns around the third or fourth postoperative day, when clear liquid diet is started. The diet is then advanced to regular as tolerated.

Antibiotic coverage
Pre-existing urinary infections are treated beginning a few days before surgery. Perioperative broad spectrum antibiotic coverage for prophylaxis is routine, beginning just before the procedure and continued for two days afterwards. To minimize problems with *C. difficile* colitis, prolonged courses of broad spectrum antibiotics should be avoided. A low-dose uroselective antibacterial such as nitrofurantoin may be used until catheters are removed.

Postoperative complications

In the hospital

Ileus

In any procedure where the bowel is manipulated, there is risk for delayed return of bowel activity. Prolonged ileus occurs in 2.4% of cases. In such patients with abdominal distension, nausea, and vomiting, placement of a nasogastric tube may be necessary for relief. Persistent ileus may prompt evaluation with CT scan to ascertain contributing causes for the ileus, such as urinary leak, small or large bowel leak, obstructed ureteral stent, or infected lymphocele.

Stomal ischemia

The distal end of the bowel used for creating the stoma may have its blood supply compromised when the mesentery is released to deliver adequate length of bowel through the fascia to create a protruding stoma. The mucosa may appear edematous and dusky for the first 48 hours, but still result in a healthy stoma. If it becomes darker, however, there may be compromised perfusion of the entire bowel segment requiring surgical intervention. One can avoid this problem in obese patients by using a loop–end Turnbull stoma, where the terminal segment of the stoma is brought to the skin surface with the mesentery intact, and the stoma is created by everting the bowel through a transverse opening in the bowel.

Infarcted urinary diversion

This catastrophic complication may be recognized at surgery when the vascular pedicle to the bowel segment is damaged by excessive traction, compression, or surgical injury. The entire bowel segment becomes dark, the pulse cannot be palpated in the mesenteric pedicle, and intraoperative Doppler interrogation confirms lack of perfusion. Delayed infarction may occur following hemorrhage into the mesenteric pedicle. Surgical resection and revision is required.

Urinary leak

The use of ureteral stents and drainage catheters has minimized urinary leaks. Whenever there is persistent drainage from a suction or Penrose drain, analysis of the fluid for creatinine should quickly determine whether the leak is urine or lymph. Irrigation of catheters or stents to eliminate mucous occlusion might be required. Most urine leaks resolve with conservative management.

Oliguria or anuria

Inadequate fluid resuscitation accounts for most low urinary output situations, but mucous or blood clot obstruction must be evaluated to prevent overdistension of the reservoir in the early postoperative period. Careful and regular irrigation of catheters should be performed. Edema of the ileal loop stoma may obstruct drainage; insertion of a small catheter into the loop should relieve this blockage.

Bleeding

Most oozing stops once the abdominal cavity is closed and coagulation abnormalities are corrected. Ongoing bleeding through drains or from the vaginal wound may require re-exploration if no medically correctable bleeding problems exist and the patient demonstrates ongoing transfusion requirement.

Deep venous thrombosis and pulmonary embolus

In major pelvic surgery, particularly with extended pelvic lymphadenectomy where there is dissection around the iliac veins, and surgery that addresses malignancy, there is an increased risk of deep venous thrombosis. If clinical signs of deep venous thrombosis or pulmonary embolism occur, either full anticoagulation or inferior vena caval filter placement should be considered depending on bleeding risk in the postoperative period.

Obturator nerve injury

While rare, the obturator nerve may be damaged during the pelvic lymphadenectomy or by excessive traction from a deep retractor blade. If possible, the injury should be repaired when recognized at operation. Patients with this complication may have difficulty with leg adduction, ambulation, and possibly driving.

Urosepsis

Perioperative antibiotics should cover most urinary tract organisms, but repeat colonization may lead to active infection during prolonged hospital stays. Judicious antibiotic use, central venous pressure monitoring, and volume resuscitation are required. In addition, a CT scan or ultrasound should be performed to identify upper tract obstruction from poorly positioned or obstructed stent or to locate any fluid collection in the abdomen or pelvis (possible infected lymphocele, urinoma, mucous collection, or hematoma) which would require percutaneous drainage.

Mucus production

In the early postoperative period with continent reservoirs, mucus may occlude the catheters or stents. Regular and rigorous irrigation with 50 ml volumes of saline or bicarbonate solution will prevent such mucus plugs from causing leakage. As the reservoir expands, the increased urinary volume tends to diminish this problem.

After discharge

Incontinence

In the early months after a continent reservoir, urinary incontinence is common as the reservoir has relatively high intraluminal pressures from high wall tension with small reservoir diameters (LaPlace's Law). The wall tension and intraluminal pressure drops as the pouch gradually distends, permitting improved continence.

Difficult catheterization

In the older reservoirs, the cutaneous stoma was created with a wide lumen with redundancy of the suprafascial portion of the stoma, resulting in buckling of the catheter. Use of the appendix or tailoring of the stoma over a smaller catheter improves this problem.

Stomal stenosis

Typically caused by chronic scarring and occasionally accelerated by urine-induced skin irritation, stomal narrowing occurs in about 20% of ileal loop patients. When urinary infection or hydronephrosis occurs, surgical correction is needed.

Nocturnal incontinence

While most patients achieve daytime continence, nocturnal control is more difficult. Contributing factors are surgical injury to distal sphincter complex; pelvic nerve damage affecting reflex recruitment from bladder distension that normally increases to maintain sphincter tone; increased intrapouch pressures at capacity despite detubularization; and the absence of the usual diurnal variation in urine volume, with more free water being drawn passively into the pouch lumen through the reservoir wall to equilibrate the osmolarity as the urine becomes more concentrated. Ileum is slower to achieve osmotic equilibrium than jejunum but more rapid than colon or stomach. Patients may need to awaken to catheterize or void to prevent overdistension and incontinence.

Metabolic or nutritional disorders

Each bowel segment used in the urinary tract has different metabolic consequences. Stomach may cause a hyponatremic, hypochloremic metabolic alkalosis, which may be useful in patients with pre-existing metabolic acidosis; jejunum can produce a hyponatremic, hypochloremic, hyperkalemic metabolic acidosis; and ileum and colon are associated with hyperchloremic metabolic acidosis, as chloride is exchanged for bicarbonate. These metabolic abnormalities are related to amount of bowel used and rarely occur in patients with normal renal function. Concerns that chronic acidosis from ileal diversion would result in bone loss have not been substantiated.

The use of lengthy segments of ileum (up to 75 cm) for continent reservoirs is rarely (<1%) associated with intractable diarrhea or malabsorption. However, loss of more than 50 cm of terminal ileum may result in vitamin B_{12} malabsorption, increasing the risk of megaloblastic anemia or irreversible neurologic symptoms. As the liver stores of vitamin B_{12} last approximately 3 years, it is recommended that vitamin B_{12} levels be monitored beginning from 1 to 5 years after an operation that utilizes more than 50 cm of terminal ileum. Replacement therapy for vitamin B_{12} is 100 µg intramuscularly every month.

Urinary tract infection

With the freely refluxing ileal loop, bacteria introduced into the stoma can ascend into the upper tracts. Thus, any stomal stenosis or appliance difficulties might predispose to pyelonephritis. Chronic infections may result in renal deterioration, and prompt stomal revision or conversion to a non-refluxing system.

Bacteriuria is common in intermittently catheterized continent reservoirs because of bacterial adherence on the extensive mucosal surface provided by the villi. While urine cultures are often positive, most patients are asymptomatic. When these patients develop symptomatic infection ("pouchitis"), they tend to experience more local discomfort, having the sense of pouch fullness despite recent catheterization, sudden onset of urinary incontinence from the stoma or the urethra, fever, abdominal pain in the region of the stoma, low back pain, nausea, and increased mucous drainage with cloudy, strong-odored urine. While the initial picture may resemble pyelonephritis, these patients respond more rapidly. By maintaining self-catheterization to drain the reservoir regularly and proper antibiotic selection, excellent tissue and urinary antibiotic levels are achieved that are enhanced by the active reabsorption of antibiotic through the permeable pouch wall.

Calculus formation

Stone formation occurs in association with exposed staples, hair or other foreign bodies introduced with self-catheterization, mucus, and chronic urinary infection. Most stones will be detected incidentally, but the remainder may present with symptomatic urinary tract infections or new onset urinary incontinence. Most of these stones are struvite and can become quite sizable, causing obstruction and upper tract infections. The smaller stones may be fragmented by extracorporeal shock wave lithotripsy or endoscopic lithotripsy and removed via standard endoscopic instruments through the older wide-caliber stomas or by the percutaneous route for patients with the tailored or tunneled stomas, where repeated instrumentation would endanger the continence mechanism. Generous irrigation to remove all fragments, particularly the primary nidus (staple or foreign body) of the stone, is necessary. However, the larger calculi may require open surgical removal.

Metabolic factors also contribute to stones in continent reservoirs. Such patients tend to have increased urinary calcium, phosphate, and magnesium excretion. Many will also have metabolic acidosis, which further promotes hypercalciuria and hypocitraturia. Thus, a complete metabolic evaluation with 24-hour urine collections is recommended for recurrent stone formers. Treatment with oral citrates may be necessary.

Pouch distension

An overdistended pouch may occur with any type of continent urinary reservoir if the regular catheterizations are not performed on schedule. Rupture of a continent reservoir is extremely rare, but augmented bladders in children for neurogenic bladder are more susceptible to spontaneous rupture. Patients experience severe cramping abdominal pain with nausea and vomiting from the distended small bowel of the reservoir, which produces a tense lower abdomen around the stoma. The entry into the reservoir may become acutely angulated with distension, making passage of the relatively flimsy smaller catheters difficult. When the pouch is distended to this degree, catheters, scopes, and most guidewires usually fail to negotiate the angulation. Using ultrasound guidance, draining a small volume of urine from the pouch under local anesthesia with a spinal needle will decrease the pouch pressure sufficiently to straighten out the catheterizable stoma so that regular catheterization may be resumed.

Parastoma hernia

This may occur where the mesenteric portion of the stoma is most difficult to secure to the abdominal wall fascia and thus vulnerable to herniation. Most herniations are asymptomatic bulges, but some may affect adherence of the appliance or become symptomatic. Either of these last situations requires parastomal hernia repair. With tapered or tailored catheterizable stomas, the risk of fascial defect and parastomal hernia is significantly reduced.

Hydronephrosis

Hydronephrosis may occur from reflux, obstruction from stenotic stoma or afferent nipple, stricture at the ureterointestinal anastomosis, or recurrent cancer. Most patients are asymptomatic, while the remainder present with urinary tract infections. Urine cytology should be ordered; if recurrent disease is present, surgical resection is necessary. For benign obstruction, endoscopic dilation or incision and stenting of the obstruction has limited success, as ischemia is often the underlying problem. Surgical revision is required for durable relief.

Cancer at ureterointestinal anastomosis

Cancer of the bowel has been reported in patients 15–20 years following ureterosigmoidostomy diversions. Periodic endoscopic monitoring of the reservoir is recommended, particularly if gross hematuria is present.

FURTHER READING

Bricker, E. M. Symposiums on clinical surgery: bladder substitution after pelvicevisceration. *Surg. Clin. North Am.* 1950: **30**: 1151–1521.

McDougal, W. S. Metabolic complications of urinary intestinal diversion. *J. Urol.* 1992; **147**: 1199–1208.

Nieh, P. T. The Kock pouch urinary reservoir. *Urol. Clin. North Am.* 1997; **24**: 755–772.

Stein, J. P., Cai, J., Groshen, S., & Skinner, D. G. Risk factors for patients with pelvic lymph node metastases following radical cystectomy with en bloc pelvic lymphadenectomy: concept of lymph node density. *J. Urol.* 2003; **170**(1): 35–41.

131

Radical prostatectomy

Fray F. Marshall

Emory University School of Medicine, Atlanta, GA

Radical prostatectomy is indicated for localized prostate cancer, involves total removal of the prostate and surrounding tissue including the seminal vesicles and ampullae of the vas deferens, and is classically associated with a bilateral pelvic lymph node dissection. The operation is performed using a perineal or retropubic approach. The earlier perineal approach initially produced less morbidity and lower blood loss; however, the retropubic approach allows for a bilateral pelvic lymphadenectomy and a nerve sparing operation that can also provide for improved potency compared to the perineal method. In addition, rectal or anal problems are rare during or after a retropubic approach but may be more likely with a perineal operation. Therefore, the radical retropubic prostatectomy (RRP) has been performed with higher frequency in recent years. Using a small incision (8 cm), a mini-laparotomy (mini-lap) radical retropubic prostatectomy can provide the advantages of minimally invasive surgery with the nerve sparing component as well. In addition, the minilap radical retropubic prostatectomy compares favorably with laparoscopic radical prostatectomy, which is usually performed via an intra-abdominal approach under general anesthesia and requires an excess of 4 hours of surgery. The mini-lap retropubic prostatectomy can be performed in half the time under regional anesthesia with similar hospitalization and morbidity. In addition, the nerve-sparing component for potency with the laparoscopic approach remains more certain.

Typically, indications for radical prostatectomy are patients with organ-confined disease (stage T_1 and T_2 disease) that are under 70 years of age and are in good medical condition. The most common group of patients (stage T_{1c}) are diagnosed by an elevated prostatic specific antigen (PSA). The operation is performed through a vertical incision made above the pubic symphysis, after which the rectus fascia is divided in the midline (no rectus muscle is divided), and an initial bilateral pelvic lymphadenectomy is performed. The radical prostatectomy is performed with careful dissection at the apex of the prostate preserving the urethral external sphincter and its fascial support for continence as well as the neurovascular bundles for maintenance of potency. The bladder neck is divided and the anastomosis is carefully completed joining the bladder neck to the urethra. Typically, an 18 F catheter is left in place for 2 weeks. The operation is performed with one surgical assistant and the Omni-Tract Retractor (Minnesota Scientific Inc.), a specifically designed retractor system that allows performance of the operation through this small incision. Complications have been infrequent. The need for allogeneic blood transfusion has been reduced to 3.5% and there have been no operative deaths in more than 1000 patients. The operation usually takes 2–2.5 hours and can be performed under either regional or general anesthesia.

Usual postoperative course

Expected postoperative hospital stay
Patient is in the hospital 2–3 days and is sent home for an additional 12–14 days of recuperation before catheter removal.

Operative mortality
No hospital deaths in more than 1000 operations performed by author.

Special monitoring required
Observation for postoperative hematuria.

Patient activity and positioning
Quiet in bed for 1 day; ambulatory the next.

Medical Management of the Surgical Patient: A Textbook of Perioperative Medicine, ed. M. F. Lubin, R. B. Smith, T. F. Dobson, N. Spell, H. K. Walker. 4th edn. Published by Cambridge University Press. © Cambridge University 2006.

Alimentation

As tolerated.

Antibiotic coverage

Perioperative administration only.

Pain control

Patients take few, if any, pain medications after discharge and appear to tolerate well the small lower abdominal incision. The indwelling catheter often causes the patient more discomfort than the incision.

Postoperative complications

In the hospital

In-hospital complications have been relatively rare, as patients are assessed medically prior to the operation.

After discharge

Incontinence

Mini-lap radical retropubic prostatectomy patients have excellent continence levels. After 9 months in the last several hundred patients, 95% are wearing either a small pad or no pad. It is common to have good levels of continence in the first 4–8 weeks. Some reports from elsewhere are not as favorable. Older patients, especially those over 70 years of age, may have a higher incidence of incontinence.

Impotence

Potency depends on many factors including age and comorbid features such as diabetes and hypertension. As many as two-thirds of patients will maintain potency, though it often takes more than 9–12 months for full return. There is significant variability in potency results from different series. Younger patients do considerably better than older patients, particularly those over the age of 65. In the past, perineal prostatectomy appeared to have a better continence rate than radical retropubic prostatectomy, but these differences have partially disappeared with improved surgical techniques using the retropubic approach. Potency with perineal prostatectomy has had poorer results with relatively few reports overall.

Bladder neck contracture

Can occur 2–3 months following the operation and develops in 2%–8% of prostatectomies. It can usually be managed with urethral dilation or an endoscopic incision, if necessary.

FURTHER READING

Abbou, C. C., Salomon, L., Hoznek, A. *et al.* Laparoscopic radical prostatectomy: preliminary results. *Urology* 2000; **55**(5): 630–634.

Marshall, F. F. Mini-laparotomy staging pelvic lymphadenectomy (mini-lap). Point/Counterpoint Series. *Contemp. Urol.* 1997; **9**: 39–48.

Walsh, P. C., Lepor, H., & Egleston, J. C. Radical retropubic prostatectomy with preservation of sexual function. *Prostate* 1983; **4**: 473–485.

Young, H. H. Cure of cancer of prostate by radical perineal prostatectomy (prostate-seminal vesiculectomy): history, literature, and statistics of Young's operation. *J. Urol.* 1945; **53**: 188–252.

132

Transurethral resection of the prostate (TURP)

Muta M. Issa and Dwayne Thwaites

Emory University School of Medicine, Atlanta, GA

Transurethral resection of the prostate (TURP) is considered the gold standard surgical treatment for benign prostatic hyperplasia (BPH) throughout the world. In the 1986 National Health Survey, 96% of patients undergoing prostate surgery for BPH had TURP. It was estimated that 350 000 Medicare patients had a TURP that year. During the last 5 years, the number of these procedures performed has decreased to less than 150 000 per year (Medicare data) because of the increasing number of patients managed by watchful waiting, medical therapy, and minimally invasive thermal therapy.

TURP is the treatment of choice in patients with moderate to severe BPH symptoms and significant compromise to their quality of life who fail or are unable to tolerate other forms of management, are in urinary retention thought to be secondary to BPH, have recurrent urinary infection secondary to BPH, have bladder stones secondary to BPH, have renal failure secondary to BPH, or have recurrent bleeding (gross hematuria) secondary to BPH.

Spinal or general anesthesia can be used for the procedure, though the former is the preferred method since it permits closer intraoperative monitoring of the patient and allows for easier postoperative recovery. The patient is placed in dorso-lithotomy position. The urologist uses a specially designed cystoscopic instrument (resectoscope) to perform the procedure under direct vision. The resectoscope has an energy-active (radiofrequency) metal loop that is used to resect the obstructing prostatic tissue into small chips (1/2 to 1 gram). The tissue fragments are then evacuated out of the bladder and hemostasis is secured by coagulating all bleeding vessels on the resected surface of the prostate. A three-way Foley catheter is then inserted into the bladder and placed on traction by taping it stretched onto the patient's thigh, the traction allowing the Foley balloon to tamponade the vessels at the resected surface. Continuous bladder irrigation (CBI) is instituted by running normal saline through the Foley to circulate inside the bladder before draining out, which prevents clot formation during the initial postoperative period. Once the urine clears, the Foley traction and the CBI are discontinued. Prior to discharge, the Foley is removed and the patient is given a voiding trial. Most patients (>90%) will void spontaneously. However, some patients may require a prolonged period of Foley catheterization. All prostatic chips resected during TURP are sent for pathological examination. The pathologist will confirm the diagnosis of BPH. There is often an inconsequential degree of inflammatory changes in the specimen (prostatitis). In approximately 10% of patients, prostate cancer is incidentally found in the specimen. The patient is then referred to as having either stage T1a or T1b prostate cancer depending on the percentage of tissue affected by cancer and its histological grade (Gleason grade).

Usual postoperative course

Expected postoperative hospital stay
Hospitalization ranges from one to three days depending on the size of the prostate, extent of the resection, and overall health status of the patient.

Operative mortality
Over the past 50 years, there has been a gradual reduction in operative mortality due to improvement in instrumentation and technique of TURP as well as anesthesia; the rate has dropped from 5% (1930s) to 0.2% (1980s). In 1995, The Veterans Affairs Study Group reported similar mortality rate between TURP and watchful waiting.

Special monitoring required
Urinary output and degree of hematuria should be observed as long as the catheter remains in place.

Medical Management of the Surgical Patient: A Textbook of Perioperative Medicine, ed. M. F. Lubin, R. B. Smith, T. F. Dobson, N. Spell, H. K. Walker. 4th edn. Published by Cambridge University Press. © Cambridge University 2006.

Patient activity and positioning

The resected "raw" prostatic fossa usually takes 4–8 weeks to heal completely. During this period, patients are requested to refrain from excessive physical activities, straining, heavy lifting, and sports since such activities may precipitate delayed bleeding. For the same reason, it is not unusual for patients to experience gross hematuria after a bowel movement or physical activity such as walking. A clot or "scab" may also pass in the urine during this recovery period and patients should be warned about this. It is unusual for the patient's voiding symptoms to resolve immediately after TURP. Improvement in voiding will take a few weeks and occasionally several months.

Alimentation

To avoid constipation, patients should be placed on oral hydration, a fiber rich diet, and stool softeners.

Antibiotic coverage

Broad spectrum prophylactic antibiotics are given perioperatively.

Bladder function

Many years of urinary obstruction cause the bladder muscle to hypertrophy in order to push the urine out through a narrowed channel. Following TURP and relief of the obstruction, the bladder continues to function abnormally for a few weeks until readjustment. During this period, patients are warned of continued symptoms of frequency, urgency, and nocturia.

Postoperative complications

In the hospital

Bleeding

Generally, an average of 10 ml of blood is lost for every gram of prostate tissue resected. However, this may be variable, with less bleeding emanating from those prostates referred to as "dry glands" (2–5 ml per resected gram of tissue), and more bleeding from those prostates referred to as "wet glands" (15 ml per resected gram of tissue). The frequency of blood transfusion is low, estimated at 4–5%.

Prostatic capsular perforation

Occurs in approximately 2% of cases and may be associated with urine extravasation outside the prostate into the pelvis. In the majority of cases, this can be managed conservatively by Foley catheter drainage for an extended period. Occasionally, extensive extravasation may necessitate placement of a suprapubic drain for a few days.

TUR syndrome

The hypotonic irrigation fluid used during TURP may be absorbed through the opened blood vessels of the prostate, resulting in some degree of fluid overload and hyponatremia. In a small percentage of patients (2%), the amount of fluid absorption is excessive and causes the patient to develop "TUR syndrome," characterized by mental confusion, nausea, vomiting, hypertension, slow heart rate, and visual disturbances (related to the glycine content of the irrigation fluid). The risk is increased when the prostate gland is larger than 35 grams and resection time exceeds 90 minutes. Early recognition of the syndrome is important, after which the procedure should be terminated and a diuretic given. Occasionally, hypertonic saline is infused to counteract the blood dilution. In the majority of cases, patients recover without sequelae.

Urinary retention

The Foley catheter may be blocked by a residual prostate chip or a blood clot that develops in the bladder, causing urinary retention. This is treated by evacuating the obstruction.

Urinary infection

Prior to the TURP, every effort should be made to ensure that the patient has sterile urine and that any active infection is treated adequately. Prophylactic antibiotics are recommended to reduce the possibility of dissemination of an unrecognized urinary infection, but patients may develop signs of infection despite these precautions. This is usually treated successfully with antibiotics.

After discharge

Urinary incontinence

True urinary stress incontinence – which occurs in less than 1% of patients – results from damage to the external urinary sphincter during the procedure, rendering it weak and incapable of retaining urine. The risk increases in patients with previous TURPs, significant prostate cancer, or severely damaged bladders. True permanent "stress-type" urinary incontinence should be distinguished from the more common transient "urge-type" urinary incontinence, which is self-limiting and resolves when the healing is complete.

Erectile dysfunction (impotence)

Since the nerves for erection are situated between the prostate and the rectum, there is a risk of nerve damage during the procedure that probably results from the heat generated by the resecting loop. Although the risk is small (approximately 10%), it is more likely to occur in patients with some pre-existing erectile dysfunction.

Retrograde ejaculation (RGE)

Retrograde ejaculation is a backward flow of the ejaculatory fluid (semen) into the bladder instead of the normal forward propulsion through the urethra. It is a direct result of the anatomical debulking of the prostate with associated bladder neck incompetency and is seen commonly after TURP (70%–90%). While most patients are unconcerned by this complication, in some, especially the young, it may be considered undesirable. In these individuals, a more conservative resection should be performed to minimize the risk of developing RGE.

Bladder neck contracture

Obstruction from scar formation at the bladder neck may occur in 7%. After confirming the diagnosis on cystoscopy, the contracture is treated by transurethral incision of the bladder neck (TUIBN).

Urethral strictures

Instrumentation during TURP causes a certain amount of trauma to the urethra. In the majority of cases the urethra heals without sequelae. However, in a small percentage of patients (<10%), scar formation develops and causes the lumen to stricture. This complication is treated by dilation or transurethral incision to re-establish patency.

Regrowth BPH

Since the peripheral rim of the prostate is left in place after TURP, there is a potential risk for the residual tissue to grow in the years following the operation. The risk for this growth to become symptomatic is 20% during the initial 10 years after operation. A number of patients may require a second TURP after 15–20 years.

New modified TURP procedures

Over the past decade, various modifications of the standard TURP procedure have become available. One such modification is transurethral electrovaporization of the prostate (TUEVP), in which the obstructing prostate is vaporized with a specially designed roller-ball device. Significantly higher radiofrequency energy is utilized during TUEVP to produce very high temperatures required for evaporation. Another modification is transurethral vaporesection of the prostate (TUVRP), which modifies the configuration of the standard TURP loop component

to allow a combination of resection and vaporization of tissue. The theoretical objective of all of these modified procedures is to provide less blood loss and fluid absorption during the procedure.

In our experience, the best new TURP device is the bipolar system that allows for hemostatic tissue resection in a normal saline medium. With the use of this new instrument in our practice, the perioperative and short-term complication rate has become negligible.

Transurethral incision of the prostate (TUIP)

Transurethral incision of the prostate is an efficacious surgical therapy for BPH. TUIP consists of establishing incisions (usually two) along the obstructing prostate to release the obstruction. It only works on relatively small BPH glands (<20 grams), but is a simpler and safer technique and carries less risk of urinary incontinence, impotence, and retrograde ejaculation.

New minimally invasive thermal therapies

The last 10 years have seen the emergence of various forms of minimally invasive thermal therapies as well, including interstitial laser thermal therapy (ILTT) (see Chapter 133), transurethral needle ablation (TUNA), transurethral microwave thermotherapy (TUMT), and high intensity focus ultrasound (HIFU) thermal therapy. These modalities utilize various forms of energy to achieve the desired effect, including laser, radiofrequency (RF), microwave, and ultrasound. Irrespective of the type of energy used, the final common objective is to achieve sufficient therapeutic intra-prostatic temperatures, usually in the range of 80–110 °C.

The advantages these minimally invasive thermal therapies offer include the option of performance as an outpatient procedure in a clinic setting or cystoscopy suite; local anesthesia with sedation can be used rather than spinal or general anesthesia; complications such as bleeding, impotence, retrograde ejaculation, and urinary incontinence tend to be lower; efficacy in the treatment of BPH, though not as much as with standard surgical therapy; more safety than conventional surgical therapy; and patients can resume work and regular daily activities within a few days. While the adoption of these methods by the urological community continues to face challenges due to high cost, inconsistent reimbursement, limited patient selection, lower treatment efficacy, and unknown long term durability, we believe that this type of therapy has an important place in the armamentarium of BPH surgical treatment.

FURTHER READING

Issa, M. M. & Marshall, F. F. *Contemporary Diagnosis and Management of Diseases of the Prostate*. Handbooks in Healthcare Co., 1999: 153–161.

McConnell, J. D., Barry, M. J., Bruskewitz, R. C. *et al.* Benign prostatic hyperplasia diagnosis and treatment. *Clinical Practice Guideline, Agency of Health Care Policy and Research (AHCPR) Publication.* 2003.

Roger, S. K. & McConnell, J. D., eds. *Benign Prostatic Hyperplasia.* 4th edn. Health Press Publishers, 2002: 47–54.

Wasson, J. H., Reda, D. J., Bruskewitz, R. C. *et al.* A comparison of transurethral surgery with watchful waiting for moderate symptoms of benign prostatic hyperplasia. The Veterans Affairs Cooperation Study Group of Transurethral Resection of the Prostate. *N. Engl. J. Med.* 1995; **332**: 75–79.

133

Interstitial laser thermal therapy for benign prostatic hyperplasia

Muta M. Issa and Rafael Bouet-Blasini

Emory University School of Medicine, Atlanta, GA

Although TURP is a very efficacious treatment for BPH, its risks, morbidity profile, inconveniences, and recovery time concerns patients and urologists. The wide gap that existed for years between simple medical therapy and TURP coupled with the need for simpler, less morbid alternatives to TURP, led to the development of minimally invasive thermal therapies such as interstitial laser thermal therapy (ILTT), which achieves its therapeutic effect through thermal ablation of the prostatic tissue (110 °C). Various other nomenclatures have been used in the literature for this procedure, including interstitial laser coagulation (ILC), interstitial thermal therapy (ITT), interstitial laser therapy (ILT), laser-induced thermal therapy (LITT), and laser delivered interstitial therapy (LDIT).

These are numerous advantages over conventional surgical therapy offered by ILTT, including the fact that it can be performed on an outpatient basis rather than in the operating room; it requires local anesthesia rather than spinal or general anesthesia; it is safe and has negligible morbidity profile with regard to bleeding, impotence, retrograde ejaculation, and urinary incontinence when compared to TURP; it is efficacious in the treatment of BPH; patients can often resume work and normal daily activities within a few days after the procedure; and it can be performed safely on high surgical risk patients, the elderly, and those on anticoagulation therapy.

Currently, the most widely used technology for the procedure in the USA is the Indigo Optima Laser System (Ethicon Endo-Surgery Inc., Johnson & Johnson, Cincinnati, Ohio, USA), which consists of a diode laser generator that utilizes a diode pump source and gallium–aluminum–aresenide as a lasing medium to generate 830 nm wavelength laser with a power range of 2–20 watts. The generator has a fully automated energy delivery program that continuously adjusts the power wattage to achieve an efficient and smooth rise in the intraprostatic

temperature to 110 °C. During treatment, the sensor system at the tip of the laser fiber monitors intraprostatic temperatures and provides continuous feedback information. The Indigo Diffuser-Tip laser fiber is an optical laser fiber with an outer diameter of 1.5 mm and a distal end designed to emit laser energy in a radial (360 degree angle) fashion along a 1 cm segment located near the tip.

ILTT is performed in an outpatient clinic setting without the need for hospitalization. The patient is placed in the lithotomy position with his legs up in stirrups. Local anesthesia is achieved by transperineal prostatic block and topical intra-urethral lidocaine. Using a standard 19 F cystoscope, the laser fiber is inserted into the prostate gland and laser energy is then delivered according to the system treatment protocol. The intraprostatic temperature reaches the target therapeutic temperature of 110 °C within 30 seconds and is thereafter maintained at that level for the 1½ minute treatment session. The duration of the procedure is dependent on the number of treatment sites required. Laboratory and human studies have demonstrated each ILTT lesion to be 5–7 ml in volume.

Proper technique regarding positioning of the laser fiber tip within the prostate is very important, as improper positioning too close to the prostatic urethra may cause thermal injury to the urethra with subsequent increased likelihood for prolonged catheterization, exacerbation of irritative voiding symptoms, tissue sloughing, and the potential for retrograde ejaculation. At Emory, our experience with a new technique of intraprostatic laser fiber insertion designed to minimize such urethral thermal injury has resulted in more consistent urethral preservation and significantly lower postoperative complications.

Several studies have shown ILTT to be an efficacious treatment for symptomatic BPH as judged by the improvement in both subjective and objective parameters. A recent review of the world literature on ILTT included a

Medical Management of the Surgical Patient: A Textbook of Perioperative Medicine, ed. M. F. Lubin, R. B. Smith, T. F. Dobson, N. Spell, H. K. Walker. 4th edn. Published by Cambridge University Press. © Cambridge University 2006.

total of 785 patients (14 series, 1994–1996) with a follow-up of 2–12 months. Overall improvement in voiding symptoms and urinary flow averaged 70% and 98%, respectively. The re-treatment rate is <10%. Similarly in a recent multi center randomized US study, ILTT compared favorably with TURP.

Postoperative complications

In the hospital

Urinary tract infection

The most common adverse event seen following ILTT is reported in 27%–35% of patients during the early postoperative period. This high incidence is attributed to the inconsistent use of antibiotics and to the prolonged duration of the bladder catheters in the initial postoperative period. With the use of prophylactic antibiotics, the incidence decreased to 16.5%. In our institution, urinary infection is prevented by the use of prophylactic fluoroquinolone antibiotics which is continued for 5 days through the postoperative period.

Irritative voiding symptoms with tissue sloughing

Seen in only 11%–12% of patients, which is significantly less than with the old laser procedures.

Postoperative bleeding

Rare (<2%), as is the need for blood transfusion (0.4%).

Transient stress urinary incontinence

In one series of 239 subjects, this condition was reported in a single patient (0.4%). The potential risk for true urinary incontinence is extremely small.

After discharge

Urethral strictures and bladder neck contractures

At <5% at 1-year follow-up. Postoperative erectile sexual dysfunction has not been reported.

Retrograde ejaculation

Ranges between 3% and 11.9%.

It is to be emphasized that ongoing improvements in this technology as well as increasing experience will continue to reduce the morbidity profile of this procedure. For example, the initial 10–14 day requirement of bladder catheterization has been decreased significantly following recent modifications in the surgical technique that allowed for protection of the prostatic urothelium from thermal injury. Using this technique, the duration of postoperative Foley catheterization has decreased from 13.3 to 0.5 days.

FURTHER READING

Issa, M. M., Ritenour, C., Greenberger, M., Hollabaugh, R. & Steiner, M. The prostate block for outpatient prostate surgery. *World J. Urol.* 1998; **16**(6): 378–383.

Issa, M. M., Townsend, M., Jiminez, V. K., Miller, L. E. & Anastasia, K. A new technique of intra-prostatic fiber placement to minimize thermal injury to prostatic urothelium during indigo interstitial laser thermal therapy. *Urology* 1998; **51**: 105–110.

Kiursh, E. D., Conception, R., Chan, S. *et al.* Interstitial laser coagulation versus transurethral resection for treating benign prostatic obstruction: a randomized trial with 2-year follow-up. *Urology* 2003; **61**(3): 573–578.

Muschter, R. Interstitial laser therapy of benign prostatic hyperplasia. In Graham, S. D. Jr. & Glenn, J. F., eds. *Glenn's Urological Surgery*. 5th edn. Philadelphia, PA: Lippincott-Raven, 1998: 1111–1117.

134

Management of upper urinary tract calculi

John G. Pattaras

Emory University School of Medicine, Atlanta, GA

The term "endourology" was adopted for the minimally invasive endoscopic surgery of upper urinary calculus disease. Since the introduction of shock wave lithotripsy, this modality has become the most common form of stone therapy as it allows virtual hands-off treatment for radio opaque calculi. Owing to the technological advances of endourologic procedures such as ureteroscopy and percutaneous nephrolithotomy, the incidence of open kidney stone surgery is almost non-existent. Despite the evolution of surgical intervention for nephrolithiasis, it is important to note that the medical management and prevention of complicated urolithiasis remains difficult.

Nephrolithiasis affects as much as 12% of the population in industrialized nations. Urolithiasis patients will agree that the sensation of stone passage is perhaps the most painful and intense experience of their lives. Urolithiasis may present as hematuria (ranging from asymptomatic microscopic hematuria to painful gross hematuria), abdominal/flank/back pain, urinary tract infection, renal failure, or an incidental radiologic finding. Decompression of the acutely obstructed system with either cystoscopic stenting or percutaneous nephrostomy drainage is emergently mandatory for patients with a solitary kidney, infected obstruction, immunocompromised state (diabetes, AIDS, transplant), history of renal insufficiency, and worsening renal function.

The absolute minimum work-up of the potential nephrolithiasis patient should include: general history, determination of any prior history or family history of nephrolithiasis, physical examination, urine analysis (and culture for any hematuria, pyuria, fevers, or elevated WBC count), and radiologic examination if clinically warranted. The gold standard radiologic examination of stone disease had been the intravenous urogram (IVU), but this has generally been replaced by non-contrast helical computerized tomography (CT) of the abdomen/pelvis. The distinct advantages of being able to visualize other abdominal pathology and lack of intravenous contrast make the CT an attractive alternative to IVU.

While it is still practiced in contemporary urology, open surgical management of renal and ureteral calculi is limited to less than 1% of stone therapy. American Urological Association practice guidelines were established for ureteral and staghorn renal calculi and should be referred to for procedural options regarding stone size, location, and clinical status. The most common treatment for renal calculi is shock wave lithotripsy (SWL), a non-invasive management technique that relies on focused sound energy to fragment calculi. Absolute contraindications to SWL include pregnancy, active complicated urinary tract infection, uncontrollable hypertension, and irreversible coagulopathy. Ureteroscopy can be performed using semirigid scopes for lower ureteral calculi (below iliac vessels). For upper ureteral or renal stones, flexible ureteroscopes as small as 7 F (2.5 mm) can be introduced for basket extraction or laser lithotripsy. While it is more invasive than SWL, the direct visual lithotripsy of ureteroscopy lends a higher success rate. The technique is indicated for almost any calculus under 1.5 cm, calculi which have failed SWL, or high-risk patients that present with coagulopathy, arrhythmias, or pregnancy. Percutaneous nephrolithotomy (PCNL) is indicated for stone burden greater than 1.5–2 cm, lower pole stones that have failed SWL, and infectious or staghorn calculi. PCNL involves creating a percutaneous nephrostomy tract(s), dilating the tract (24–30 F), and using a rigid or flexible scope for lithotripsy. "Second look procedures" are performed through an established tract when excessive stone burden or complicated staghorn calculi can't be managed in a single setting. Laparoscopic ureterolithotomy or pyelolithotomy have been described but are more invasive than endoscopy and, therefore, performed less

Medical Management of the Surgical Patient: A Textbook of Perioperative Medicine, ed. M. F. Lubin, R. B. Smith, T. F. Dobson, N. Spell, H. K. Walker. 4th edn. Published by Cambridge University Press. © Cambridge University 2006.

frequently. Ultrasonography or non-contrast CT in a patient with suspected complications can generally delineate the problem. Interventional or surgical correction of the obstruction, especially in medically frail or infected patients, should be accomplished in a timely fashion.

Usual postoperative course

Expected postoperative hospital stay

Ureteroscopy and SWL are routinely performed as outpatient procedures. Medical comorbidities can require admission for observation or postoperative care. Percutaneous nephrolithotomy and laparoscopic procedures usually require 2 to 4 days of hospitalization.

Operative mortality

The overall operative mortality for stone procedures is 0.01% to 1% for more invasive procedures such as PCNL.

Special monitoring required

General anesthesia monitoring for ureteroscopy and PCNL is standard. While SWL can be performed under i.v. sedation, it still requires continuous electrocardiography observation due to the possibility of shock-induced arrhythmias. PCNL procedures require diligent electrolyte monitoring to assess the absorption of intraoperative irrigating fluids. Postoperative chest X-ray is necessary for nephrostomy placement above the tenth rib or if a pneumo- or hydrothorax is suspected.

Patient activity and positioning

Intraoperative patient positioning differs by procedure. SWL is usually performed supine for most stones and prone for mid-ureteral calculi, ureteroscopy is performed in dorsal lithotomy but can also be accomplished in split-leg prone, PCNL is commonly accomplished in the prone position, and second look procedures are done in lateral decubitus position. Immediate ambulation is normal for outpatient procedures.

Alimentation

In most cases, oral food intake is immediate in the absence of ileus, nausea, or vomiting.

Antibiotic coverage

Patients undergoing SWL should have a negative urine culture; therefore, they rarely require antibiotics. Since irrigation fluid and drains increase chances of complicated urinary infection, all patients undergoing ureteroscopy and PCNL procedures should receive preoperative intravenous antibiotics at least 1 hour prior to the procedure. Medically complicated and infectious stone patients should be admitted 24 to 48 hours prior to surgery for intravenous antibiotics, with the coverage continued orally for 7 days postprocedure. Fevers are common after PCNL operations and are not always infectious in source.

Drains

An internal double-J ureteral stent should be placed for SWL procedures performed for stones greater than 1.5 cm or solitary kidneys. Stents are commonly placed for ureteroscopy procedures and are the surgeon's preference for PCNLs. For uncomplicated procedures stents are left indwelling for 3–7 days, though complications such as ureteral perforation or stricture disease will increase the duration of placement. Ureteral stents can either be removed by the urologist as a simple outpatient procedure or by the patient by means of a string that exits the urethra. PCNLs require an established nephrostomy tract for infectious stones at least 24 hours prior to definitive procedure. Otherwise, nephrostomy tubes can be placed intraoperatively. Postoperatively, the tubes are left to straight drainage for 24–48 hours, capped if the patient experiences no obstructive symptoms, and removed if significant hematuria has resolved and all stone burden has been relieved.

Postoperative complications

In the hospital

Fever

Fever is common after percutaneous surgery, especially with infected stones. Patients should be kept on appropriate antibiotics until afebrile. Fevers may occur from release of bacteria from lithotripsy, renal trauma, or pulmonary atelectasis. Clinical assessment is mandatory for prolonged fever.

Gross hematuria

Commonly seen during and after SWL, though it should dissipate within 24 hours after the procedure. Because of the more invasive nature of PCNL, gross hematuria may last for several days and eventually resolve, though it may recur as late as 2 weeks postsurgery. In routine cases, ureteroscopy usually produces the least amount of hematuria because of the absence of an incision and the focal nature of stone basketing or intracorporeal lithotripsy. In patients with undiagnosed coagulopathies, undisclosed blood thinners (ASA), and uncontrolled hypertension, hemorrhage and hematomas may occur.

Renal/ureteral obstruction

Stone fragments or ureteral edema may cause transient yet substantial obstruction, resulting in pain, nausea, and infection in the unstented patient. *Steinstrasse* is ureteral obstruction from a lead fragment followed by smaller fragments of stone passing quickly through the ureter after SWL. Stenting, nephrostomy placement, or ureteroscopy with lead fragment lithotripsy are treatment options for steinstrasse.

Pain

A multitude of sources could be responsible for postprocedural discomfort. Therefore, potent analgesia medications may be required for several days.

After discharge

Urinoma

Instrumentation can perforate the collecting system or ureter. Nephrostoureterogram is usually performed at the end of PCNLs but may not identify a small tear with urinary extravasation. Complicated ureteroscopy with laser perforation or difficult stone extraction may also produce a ureteral tear. CT scan or ultrasound may identify free fluid in the retroperitoneum.

Subcapsular hematoma

Subcapsular renal hematomas are seen in 0.1–0.3% of SWLs and are usually a self-limiting, pain-causing complication. Close follow-up with radiographic imaging and blood pressure monitoring should be performed. A resultant Page kidney from capsular distension may occur and necessitate nephrectomy.

Organ damage

There are minimal reports about surrounding organ damage from the shockwave path during SWL. Colonic perforation may occur during percutaneous tube placement, especially in patients with previous colonic or gastric surgery.

Late-onset hypertension

While yet to be substantiated, delayed hypertension after SWL has been reported.

FURTHER READING

Collado, S. A., Huget, P. J., Monreal, G. F. *et al.* Renal hematoma as a complication of extracorporeal shockwave lithotripsy. *Scand. J. Urol. Nephrol.* 1999; **33**(3): 171–175.

Menon, M., Parulkar, B., & Drach, G. Urinary lithiasis: etiology, diagnosis and medical management. In Walsh, P., Retik, A., Vaughn, E. D. *et al.*, eds. *Campbell's Urology*, 7th edn. Philadelphia, PA: W. B. Saunders, 1998: 2659–2733.

Segura, J. W., Preminger, G. H., Assimos, D. G., *et al.* The American Urological Association. Ureteral Stones Clinical Guidelines Panel summary report on the management of ureteral calculi. *J. Urol.* 1997; **158**(5): 1915–1921.

Segura, J. W., Preminger, G. H., Assimos, D. G. *et al.* The American Urological Association Nephrolithiasis Clinical Guidelines Panel. Nephrolithiasis Clinical Guidelines Panel summary report on the management of staghorn calculi. *J. Urol.* 1994; **151**(6): 1648–1651.

135

Female urinary incontinence surgery

Niall T. M. Galloway

Emory University School of Medicine, Atlanta, GA

More than 20 million Americans are estimated to have moderate or severe urinary incontinence. Despite the severe symptoms this common problem causes, many patients fail to seek medical help due to the social stigma associated with the condition; a typical patient will suffer symptoms for more than seven years before seeking help. For the elderly, problems of incontinence often lead to institutional care. It is estimated that more than 200 000 surgical procedures are done each year for the treatment of urinary incontinence.

There are many causes for stress urinary incontinence, and surgery is not always needed to resolve it. For some patients, the symptoms of stress incontinence will resolve with simple non-surgical measures. Current practice guidelines clearly mandate that reversible factors should be identified and treated first. Behavioral treatments are often effective: fluid restriction, diet and bowel management, and pelvic floor exercises. Operative treatment should be reserved for those who have failed these methods, especially pelvic floor muscle strengthening, and who have demonstrable anatomical abnormalities that can only be corrected by surgical procedures.

The current vogue is to construct a compensatory abnormality at surgery – injection of bulking agents, placement of slings, or fixation of tissues to aberrant locations – in an effort to correct incontinence. Surgeons have been swept along by these trends because such procedures are simple and quick to perform in an outpatient setting. The marketing of new surgical products and techniques has been aggressive and directed to both patients and the medical community, resulting in a stampede for surgical care. The short-term claims for these treatments and the brief procedure and recovery times are attractive, but adverse outcomes and complications must be considered.

There is a wide spectrum of individual variations in pelvic floor structure and function. Individuals with the best structures have the best quality of function, while those with incompetent structures have a greater tendency to develop bladder and pelvic floor problems including pelvic organ prolapse and bowel dysfunction. There is a tendency for bladder and bowel and pelvic floor problems to "run in the family." A variety of acquired diseases may have a part to play in urinary incontinence, such as diabetes, lumbar, or cervical disc disease, spinal canal stenosis, and pelvic floor insults such as vaginal delivery. Surgical procedures in the pelvis or retroperitoneum may also disturb function, as can radiation therapy in the field of the neurospinal axis and peripheral neuropathy.

Surgery for stress urinary incontinence is elective. There is rarely any immediate need to treat or to accept a patient for surgery in less than optimal condition. Initial evaluation should include clinical history, physical examination, post void residual, urinalysis, and review of the patient's bladder diary. Assessment of gait, the lumbosacral spine, lower extremities, and the feet should be included. The innervation of the feet, S2 and 3, are immediately adjacent to the innervation of the pelvic floor and sphincters, S3, 4 and 5. The feet are like a mirror that will help to reflect the integrity of the nerves in the most distal segments of the spinal cord. On abdominal examination, one looks for evidence of abdominal distention; surgical scars and hernias should be noted. Two-point discrimination should be tested in the perianal and postanal dermatomes, and muscle tone and grip of the circumvaginal and anal sphincter muscles noted on the right and left. Examination of the perineum should be done when the bladder is full and with the patient in the standing as well as supine position. One should use both a bivalve (Graves') speculum to examine the vaginal vault and a Sim's speculum to examine the anterior and posterior vaginal walls.

All patients should be asked to keep a bladder diary of every voided volume and the time of the void; a standard

Medical Management of the Surgical Patient: A Textbook of Perioperative Medicine, ed. M. F. Lubin, R. B. Smith, T. F. Dobson, N. Spell, H. K. Walker. 4th edn. Published by Cambridge University Press. © Cambridge University 2006.

graduated measuring "hat" that fits in the commode will assist in making these recordings. Patients are instructed to maintain their usual practices during the recording period so that the fluid intake will reflect their usual pattern. The resulting chart provides critical information about the largest voided volume (functional bladder capacity), the pattern of voiding throughout the day and night, and the total output in 24 hours. Total 24-h urine volume should be on the order of 1.5 to 2 liters for the average adult, but it is not unusual to find that patients with urinary frequency and incontinence may have daily voided volumes in excess of 6 to 8 liters a day. If there is no organic cause, moderation of fluid intake can readily improve or eliminate their troublesome urinary symptoms. Non-surgical treatments are offered to almost every patient in this instance. The treatment plan must be tailored to the needs of the individual patient and every effort made to initially address the most troublesome symptom. Preliminary strategies might include fluid restriction, bowel management, and review of prescription and non-prescription medications; timed or prompted voiding might also be considered. It is often effective to team the patient with a continence nurse for coaching and personal support.

If the symptoms are moderate or severe and the patient has persisting anatomical defects that could be corrected, one should proceed with urodynamic evaluation. Patients who need urodynamics have demonstrable moderate or severe incontinence, have failed conservative management, desire further treatment, and are usually candidates for surgical correction. One should evaluate the pelvic support anatomy and plan surgical repair of all significant anatomical support defects. In the female pelvis, responsibility for care is divided between different specialists: urologists, gynecologists, and colorectal surgeons. In the prevailing surgical climate, it is common to treat only one part of the problem and to ignore other correctable anatomical support defects. Lack of an integrated care plan promotes incomplete treatment and imperfect outcomes that will often demand further surgical revisions.

Surgical procedures for stress incontinence should change the patient's anatomy. If the cause of incontinence is one or more anatomical defects, correction of those defects is likely to resolve the continence problem. If there are other causes, incontinence is likely to persist in spite of surgery. Since there is no standard operation to treat stress urinary incontinence, many approaches are used, all of which have their own risks and benefits. These include traditional open suprapubic procedures (MMK and Burch) that have been applied for more than 40 years and have been well studied. Gynecologists tend to favor vaginal repairs for cystocele, including Kelly plication and anterior colporrhaphy. Needle suspensions (Peyrera and Raz) were the first generation of minimally invasive procedures but have generally failed to provide sustained benefit. Recently developed minimally invasive techniques are now popular, including tension free vaginal tape and tension free obturator tape. These procedures are appealing because they can be done under local anesthesia in an outpatient setting, but there is limited information regarding their long-term efficacy.

Preparation of the patient should include a general medical assessment and consideration of comorbidities and risk factors. Such patients may be taking hormone replacement therapy, which should be withheld 1 week prior to surgery to reduce the risk of deep venous thrombosis and pulmonary embolism.

Usual postoperative course

Expected postoperative hospital stay

1–3 days.

Operative mortality

Not greater than 0.1%.

Special monitoring required

A urinary catheter may be used in the first 24 hours to maintain bladder drainage and to monitor urinary output.

Patient activity and positioning

The patient is positioned in a modified dorsal lithotomy position for surgery. Serial compression is applied to the legs as prophylaxis against deep venous thrombosis.

Alimentation

Fluid diet is prescribed for 2 days prior to operation, and use of laxatives or bowel preparation with an enema the day before and the morning of surgery are recommended. Food intake is permitted as tolerated following surgery with the first passage of flatus.

Antibiotic coverage

A preoperative antibiotic (single dose fluoroquinolone 1 hour before operation) is appropriate. A urinalysis should be done 1 week preoperatively and a urine culture is appropriate if the urinalysis suggests possible infection. Urinary tract infection should be resolved or thoroughly treated before elective surgery.

Instrumentation

Cystoscopy is appropriate for all patients.

Urodynamic studies

Urodynamics involve measurement of intravesical volume and pressure during bladder filling and provocative maneuvers to provoke leakage and mimic patient symptoms. Primary surgical correction may be done without urodynamics if the clinical features and findings are clear; however, for secondary procedures and when features are not typical, pressure studies are recommended to confirm the clinical diagnosis and to guide the surgical plan.

Postoperative complications

In the hospital

Bleeding

Typically, intraoperative blood loss is minimal, but bleeding disorders or inappropriate medications might provoke a risk. Patients should avoid aspirin and non-steroidal anti-inflammatory medications for 5 days prior to operation. Wound hematoma and vaginal bleeding are uncommon.

Abdominal distention

This is generally due to inertia of the large bowel rather than paralytic ileus. Minimal use of opiates, anticholinergic medications, and epidural analgesia may limit the bowel problems.

Early voiding difficulty and incomplete bladder emptying

These are to be expected for most patients when the catheter is removed on the first postoperative day. Pain and local swelling might impair voiding function at first. Some surgeons leave a suprapubic catheter in place for a few days and remove it after a successful voiding trial; others prefer to teach clean intermittent catheterization to empty the bladder after voiding efforts in order to measure the residual volumes. Bladder function is usually better when bowel function has resumed. Catheterization is usually continued until the bladder is emptying well (residuals consistently less than 100 ml).

After discharge

Wound problems

Uncommon, but late hematoma or wound infection may occur. Worsening pain at the operative site together with feeling of malaise and fever suggest infection. Local signs of swelling, heat, redness, tenderness, and discharge confirm the clinical suspicion. It may be necessary to open the wound to allow for optimal drainage and to encourage healing by secondary intention. Antibiotics are indicated.

Urinary tract infection

Problems with increased frequency and bladder pain might suggest urinary infection. It is appropriate to use a daily antimicrobial such as nitrofurantoin as a prophylactic against infection for the patient who is learning to manage clean catheterization.

Urinary frequency, urgency, and nocturia

These symptoms suggest incomplete emptying or a small bladder capacity. Pelvic hematoma can form a capsule around the urinary bladder, reducing the space that is necessary to permit effective bladder filling and causing a tendency to frequency and urgency until the hematoma resolves. At times, a similar pattern of urinary symptoms can be provoked by constipation and bowel inertia.

Deep venous thrombosis

Special measures should be used to minimize the possibility in high-risk patients. Early ambulation in the hospital and sustained daily walking exercise after discharge are to be encouraged.

Postoperative anemia

Since signs of anemia are sought and treated effectively before surgery and the operative blood loss is typically small, this is a rare difficulty. At times, postoperative treatment with iron supplements may be indicated.

FURTHER READING

Blaivas, J. G., Appell, R. A., Fantl, J. A. *et al.* Definition and classification of urinary incontinence: recommendations of the Urodynamics Society. *Neurourol. Urodyn.* 1997a; **16**: 149–151.

Blaivas, J. G., Appell, R. A., Fantl, J. A. *et al.* Standards of efficacy for evaluation of treatment outcomes in urinary incontinence: recommendations of the Urodynamics Society. *Neurourol. Urodyn.* 1997b; **16**: 145–147.

Burch, J. C. Urethrovaginal fixation to Cooper's ligament in the treatment of cystocele and stress incontinence. *Prog. Gynecol.* 1963; **4**: 591–600.

Fantl, J. A., Newman, D. D. K., Colling, J. *et al.* Urinary incontinence in adults: acute and chronic management. *Clinical Practice Guideline No. 2, 1996 Update* (AHCPR Publication No. 96–0682). Rockville, MD, US Department of Health and Human Services, Public Health Service, Agency for Health Care Policy and Research, March 1996.

Leach, G. E., Dmochowski, R. R., Appell, R. A. *et al.* Female stress urinary incontinence clinical guidelines panel summary report on surgical management of female stress urinary incontinence. *J. Urol.* 1997; **158**: 875–880.

Index